Medical Effects of Ionizing Radiation

Medical Effects of Ionizing Radiation

THIRD EDITION

Fred A. Mettler, Jr., MD, MPH

Chief, Radiology and Nuclear Medicine
New Mexico V.A. Health Care System
Clinical Professor
Department of Radiology, University of New Mexico School of Medicine
Albuquerque, New Mexico

Arthur C. Upton, MD

Clinical Professor
Department of Environmental and Community Medicine
Robert Wood Johnson Medical School
University of Medicine and Dentistry of New Jersey
Piscataway, New Jersey

SAUNDERS

ELSEVIER

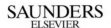

1600 John F. Kennedy Blvd.
Ste 1800
Philadelphia, PA 19103-2899

MEDICAL EFFECTS OF IONIZING RADIATION   ISBN: 978-0-7216-0200-4
THIRD EDITION

Notice

Knowledge and best practice in this field are constantly changing. As new research and experience broaden our knowledge, changes in practice, treatment and drug therapy may become necessary or appropriate. Readers are advised to check the most current information provided (i) on procedures featured or (ii) by the manufacturer of each product to be administered, to verify the recommended dose or formula, the method and duration of administration, and contraindications. It is the responsibility of the practitioner, relying on their own experience and knowledge of the patient, to make diagnoses, to determine dosages and the best treatment for each individual patient, and to take all appropriate safety precautions. To the fullest extent of the law, neither the Publisher nor the Editors assume any liability for any injury and/or damage to persons or property arising out or related to any use of the material contained in this book.

Library of Congress Cataloging-in-Publication Data
Mettler, Fred A.
Medical effects of ionizing radiation / Fred A. Mettler, Jr., Arthur C. Upton.—3rd ed.
  p. ; cm.
 Includes bibliographical references and index.
 ISBN 978-0-7216-0200-4
1. Ionizing radiation—Toxicology. 2. Ionizing radiation–Dose-response relationship. 3. Radiation carcinogenesis. 4. Radiation injuries. I. Upton, Arthur C. II. Title.
  [DNLM: 1. Radiation Effects. 2. Dose-Response Relationship, Radiation. 3. Radiation, Ionizing. WN 620 M595m 2008]

RA1231.R2M474 2008
616.9'897—dc22   2007019407

Acquisitions Editor: Rebecca Gaertner
Design Direction: Steven Stave

Printed in the United States of America.

Last digit is the print number: 9 8 7 6 5 4 3 2 1

This book is dedicated to our wives, Gloria and Elizabeth, who have been infinitely understanding and who have provided encouragement to us in our professional pursuits; and to those of our colleagues who devote their time and effort, through service on the committees of many professional societies and organizations, for the purpose of bringing pertinent medical and scientific knowledge to bear on radiation-related issues.

There are, in fact, two things, science and opinion; the former begets knowledge, the latter, ignorance.

Hippocrates

Preface to First Edition

This book was written as a source book for professionals interested in effects of ionizing radiation on humans. Its intended audiences are those with a background in the health field, including physicians, nurses, health physicists, allied health professionals, and lawyers with a medicolegal background.

This text generally does not include animal data. The reason for this is that although interspecies comparison is sometimes useful for experimental studies, it is rarely directly applicable to humans without some major assumptions. In addition, inclusion of the large amount of available animal data would create a multivolume work, and extensive reviews are already available in the publications of the United Nations Scientific Committee on the Effects of Atomic Radiation (UNSCEAR) and the National Academy of Sciences Committee on the Biological Effects of Ionizing Radiation (BEIR). Most of the data concerning radiation effects in human beings comes from three sources: radiation therapy, accidental or occupational exposures, and the atomic bomb survivors.

Radiation therapy involves treatment of localized body volumes with doses higher than can be tolerated by the entire body. Such exposures provide information concerning the tolerance of and long-term effects on specific organs and tissues. This information is valuable because the radiation doses are well measured in the treated tissue. A major drawback in use of radiotherapy information is that the radiation is usually given in fractionated doses over several weeks, and, thus, application of these data to accident situations involving single acute or chronic exposures is limited. Radiation therapy exposure has been included not only as a source of human experience, but also because it is widely practiced and, therefore, has the potential for a large number of adverse reactions.

Accidental exposures have provided a limited amount of information concerning acute single doses absorbed across the body.

The greatest source of data concerning generalized whole body exposure comes from the atomic bomb survivors at Hiroshima and Nagasaki. These persons have been extensively followed by the Atomic Bomb Casualty Commission (ABCC) and its successor, the Radiation Effects Research Foundation (RERF). Their exposures consisted of a mixture of gamma and neutron radiation. At the time of this writing, the exact quantity of neutron exposure, particularly at Hiroshima, is in doubt. While reevaluation of the dosimetry will have some impact on the knowledge of the risks of neutron exposure in humans, it is not expected to cause large changes in the gamma radiation risk estimates.

This book discusses the effects of high-level as well as low-level exposures. The reason for this is that although there is interest in human exposures at low levels, there is such a limited quantity of relevant human data that estimates of low-level effects can be made only by extrapolation from high-dose data. Because of their importance both the method and rationale for these extrapolations have been included.

The sources of exposure to ionizing radiation as well as the dose–effect relationships and their statistical implications are systematically treated in the text. Direct effects, carcinogenic effects, and genetic effects of ionizing radiation are examined in detail. Radiation exposure in utero is considered as a special case. Perception and acceptance of risk are considered, as well as some specific analysis of probability of causation. An extensive glossary and a collection of useful tables are appended.

Preface to Second Edition

This second edition follows the first edition by 9 years. In the interim, there have been a number of important developments in the understanding of the medical effects of ionizing radiation. These developments include new concepts in radiation protection, better understanding of the molecular and genetic basis of radiation carcinogenesis, publication of a large body of observations concerning late effects of radiotherapy, a greater understanding of direct effects on humans as a result of the Chernobyl accident, and an embryologic basis for in utero effects of ionizing radiation on the brain. There are, of course, other areas in which the book has been updated, and an effort has been made to expand the epidemiologic data relative to carcinogenesis. The overall purpose of the book remains the same as does the intended readership. It is hoped that both professional researchers and the public at large will benefit from this work.

Preface to Third Edition

The third edition follows the first edition by 22 years and the second edition by 13 years. Primary changes in the interval have included the increased magnitude of radiation exposure to the population from medical exposure, molecular and cellular insights into the potential mechanisms of effects at low doses, and additional information from the epidemiologic literature on site-specific cancer risks. There have also been many additional scientific publications on the deterministic effects of radiation.

Chapter 9 has been expanded to include information on radium. Chapter 10 has been significantly rewritten to include a broader perspective on the attribution of radiation effects. Chapter 11 has been expanded to include more information on psychological aspects. Appendix 6 on normal tissue toxicity grading has been added as well. There have also been recent comprehensive reports by the BEIR VII and UNSCEAR 2006 committees; we have tried to include this information where applicable.

Acknowledgment

We would like to acknowledge RuthAnne Bump and James Janis for their help with the illustrations and Ingrid Hendrix for her help with the references.

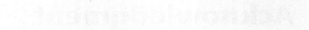

Contents

1 Basic Radiation Physics, Chemistry, and Biology 1

2 Sources of Radiation Exposure 27

3 Effects on Genetic Material 47

4 Cancer Induction and Dose-Response Models 71

5 Carcinogenesis of Specific Sites 117

6 Deterministic Effects of Radiation 285

7 Effects of Radiation in Combination with Other Agents 389

8 Radiation Exposure in Utero 401

9 Uranium, Plutonium, and Radium 423

10 Attribution of Radiation Effects and Probability of Causation in a Specific Individual 437

11 Perception of Radiation and Psychological Effects 459

12 Hormesis 473

Appendix 1 Glossary 477

Appendix 2 Radiation Source Term Table 491

Appendix 3 Conversion Tables 495

Appendix 4 Absorbed Dose Estimates from Radionuclides 497

Appendix 5 Specific Gamma Ray Constants 503

Appendix 6 SOMA Normal Tissue Radiotoxicity Tables 505

Index 531

Basic Radiation Physics, Chemistry, and Biology

Understanding the basic concepts and mechanisms in radiation physics, chemistry, and biology is important not only for a coherent approach to radiation-induced abnormalities but also for derivation of radiation protection principles. Much of the basic understanding of mechanisms has come from animal research and from study of more primitive biologic systems, as well as from human cells that have been maintained in tissue culture. In considering radiobiologic effects, any number of parameters may be examined, ranging from the gross changes of cell death to smaller changes such as loss of certain functional capabilities or even more subtle biochemical and genetic changes. Several excellent reviews of radiation physics, chemistry, and biology have been published, and the reader is referred to these for more in-depth treatment than is presented here.[1–6]

PHYSICAL FACTORS

The first step in evaluating either radiochemical or radiobiologic effects is to define the physical parameters of the ionizing radiation exposure. These parameters include (1) type of radiation (e.g., x-ray, gamma, neutron, alpha, or beta); (2) dose rate (e.g., gray and rad/minute); (3) temporal period of exposure (single-dose, fractionated dose, or chronic exposure); (4) energy of the radiation; and (5) exposure mode (i.e., whether the exposure is external, internal, homogeneous, or inhomogeneous).

Atomic Structure

Matter is composed of atoms. Each atom has a central nucleus that contains protons and neutrons. The protons are positively charged, and the neutrons have no electrical charge. Neutrons appear to be necessary to help bind protons together. A cloud of electrons surrounds the nucleus. Electrons are negatively charged and travel in orbits that have discrete energy levels. The electrons closer to the nucleus are more tightly bound than the outer electrons because of the attraction between the positive charge of the protons and the negative charge of the electrons. The mass of the proton and that of the neutron are each approximately equal to 1 atomic mass unit (AMU): one twelfth of a carbon 12 atom. If this mass is converted into energy, 931 million electron volts (MeV) are released. The electron is much lighter than a neutron or a proton and has a mass that is only 0.00055 AMU. If the mass of an electron were converted into energy, 0.51 MeV of energy would be liberated. The stability of an atom is the result of a balance of the forces of the various nuclear components. An atom that is unstable will attempt to reach stability by releasing energy in various ways, often resulting in the emission of ionizing radiation. Ionizing radiation represents only a small part of the electromagnetic spectrum. This spectrum includes radio waves, radar, microwaves, ultraviolet radiation, and even electric power (Fig. 1-1).

Ionization

The transfer of energy to a medium by either electromagnetic or particulate radiation may be sufficient to overcome the binding energy of an electron, and the electron may be ejected from the atom. This process is called *ionization*. Each ionization event causes approximately 33 electron volts (eV) of energy to be deposited into the absorbing medium. Compared with other types of radiation that may be absorbed, ionizing radiation deposits a relatively large amount of energy into a small area. In fact, the 33 eV from one ionization is more than enough energy to disrupt the chemical bond between two carbon atoms. The method by which incident radiation interacts with the medium to cause ionization may be direct or indirect. Electromagnetic radiations (x-rays and gamma photons) are *indirectly ionizing*, that is, they give up their energy in various interactions, and the energy is then used to produce a fast-moving charged particle such as an electron. It is the electron that then secondarily may react with a target molecule. Charged particles, in contrast, strike the tissue or medium and directly react with target molecules such as oxygen and water. These particulate radiations are *directly ionizing* radiation. Examples of directly ionizing particles include alpha and beta particles. Indirectly ionizing radiations include x-rays, gamma rays,

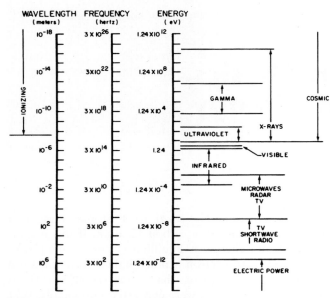

THE ELECTROMAGNETIC SPECTRUM

Figure 1-1 • Comparison of the wavelength, frequency, and energy of the electromagnetic spectrum. Ionizing radiation represents that portion of the spectrum in which the energy exceeds approximately 10 eV.

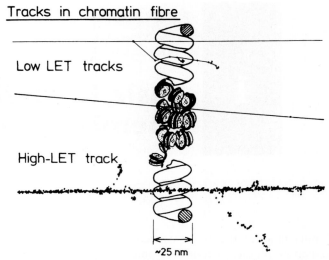

Tracks in chromatin fibre

~25 nm

Figure 1-2 • Diagram of high- and low-LET tracks passing through a section of chromatin (a mixture of DNA and protein). Low-LET radiation causes relatively sparse ionization along the track of the radiation, whereas high-LET radiation causes very dense ionization along the radiation path with a cluster of radiation at the end of the path (the Bragg peak). (From International Commission on Radiological Protection (ICRP): 1990 Recommendations of the International Commission on Radiological Protection. ICRP Pub. No. 60, Annals of the ICRP, Oxford, Pergamon Press, 1991.)

and neutrons and are almost always more penetrating than directly ionizing particulate radiations.

Mass, charge, and velocity of a particle all affect the rate at which ionization occurs. The higher the charge of the particle and the lower the velocity, the greater is the propensity to cause ionization. Heavy, highly charged particles (such as alpha particles) lose energy rapidly with distance and, therefore, do not penetrate deeply. When a particle causes ionization, it loses energy and slows down. A particle may give off most of its energy just prior to stopping. This effect causes more energy to be given off just as the maximum range of the particle is reached and is referred to as the *Bragg peak*.

The amount of energy deposited into tissue can be measured as a function of distance along the track of the radiation. Various types of ionizing radiation are divided into high-LET and low-LET radiation; LET refers to linear energy transfer, or the amount of energy deposited in a unit of track length (Fig. 1-2). LET is normally expressed in units of kiloelectron volts/micron (keV/μ). LET increases with the square of the charge on the incident particle. Some specific LET values can be found in Table 1-1.

The biologic effects of radiation depend upon the energy transferred to the tissue, and these effects are, therefore, a function of the LET. Scientifically it would be preferable to specify the LET of each radiation used in experiments. Unfortunately, because many radiation qualities are used in experimentation, overall comparison of experiments is extremely difficult. A more general term, the *relative biologic effectiveness* (RBE), is normally reported.

In using RBE, one determines the effectiveness of a given type of experimental radiation and then compares it to 250 kilovolt (peak) x-rays. In general, most x-rays and gamma rays have an RBE of approximately 1, whereas fast neutrons and alpha particles have RBEs that are substantially larger than 1.0. Not all low-LET radiations have the same effectiveness and, in specific experimental radiobiology systems, 200 kV x-rays have been shown to be twice as effective at low doses compared to high-energy gamma rays. To a large extent, the RBE is related to the LET (Fig. 1-3). Table 1-2 gives ranges, because the RBE may be slightly different from tissue to tissue and may also be different if early and late radiation effects are compared.[7]

Table 1-1 • Relative Energy and Linear Energy Transfer Values for Various Types of Radiation of Different Energies		
Radiation	**Energy**	**LET (keV/μ)**
X-ray	250 keV	3.0
Cobalt 60	1.17, 1.33 MeV	0.3
X-ray	3 MeV	0.3
Beta minus	10 keV	2.3
Beta minus	1 MeV	0.25
Neutron	2.5 MeV	20
Neutron	19 MeV	7
Proton	2 MeV	16
Alpha	5 MeV	100
Fission fragments	High	5000

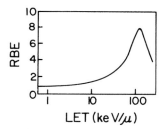

Figure 1-3 ● The relationship of RBE to LET. Up to 100 keV/μ, RBE increases with increasing LET.

The biologic effectiveness of ionizing radiation is usually due to the rather localized deposition of energy, which may affect critical structures such as the genetic material (e.g., DNA). The total amount of energy delivered in a lethal dose of radiation is, in fact, extremely small but is effectively used. A total body dose of 7 Gray (Gy) represents absorption of only 1 calorie (cal) in a 70-kg man. In terms of a temperature rise, this would represent an increase of less than 0.002°C.

Electromagnetic Radiations

Both gamma rays and x-rays originate from energy given off by an unstable atom. Both sometimes display wave phenomena and sometimes act as a stream of packets of energy. The wavelength (λ) is inversely proportional to energy and frequency. A simple formula for determining the energy of a particular wavelength x- or gamma ray is given as follows:

$$\lambda = \frac{12.4}{E}$$

In this formula, lambda (λ) refers to wavelength in angstroms, and E refers to energy in keV. Thus, the energy of a gamma ray with a wavelength of $^1/_{100}$ of an angstrom (0.01Å) is 1240 keV. The short electromagnetic wavelengths that characterize x-rays and gamma photons contain enough energy to cause ionization in a target material.

There are three major ways in which x-rays and gamma rays may be absorbed and indirectly result in ionization. These processes are the photoelectric process, Compton effect, and pair production. At low energies,

the *photoelectric process* predominates; this occurs when an incident photon (gamma or x-ray) interacts with an orbital electron (usually in the K, L, or M orbit of the absorbing material). If the energy of the photon is greater than that of the binding energy of the electron, the electron is released from the orbit with a kinetic energy equal to that of the incident photon minus the binding energy. If the process results in ejection of an electron in an orbit relatively close to the nucleus (the K orbit is the closest), then this orbit is filled by another electron "falling in" from an outer orbit. As the loosely bound electron in the outer orbit moves to an inner, more tightly bound status, it loses potential energy, which is given off as additional electromagnetic radiation. Because there are discrete energy levels for each orbit, the amount of energy given off for a transition from one orbit to another is constant for a particular transition and is called *characteristic radiation*.

Photoelectric absorption varies as a function of the atomic number (Z) (specifically it is proportional to Z^3). When the incident photon (gamma or x-ray) has somewhat higher energy, the *Compton effect* occurs. At energy levels normally encountered in diagnostic radiology, both the photoelectric process and Compton effect are important in absorption of the radiation. In the Compton effect phenomenon, the incident photon interacts in sort of a "billiard ball" fashion with an electron in a very peripheral orbit or shell. This peripheral orbital electron in an atom of absorbing medium may be referred to as a *free electron*, because the binding energy is very small. Part of the incident photon energy is given to the free electron as kinetic energy, and the residual amount of energy continues on as a less energetic deflected photon. Most of the patient dose and biologic damage in diagnostic radiology are due to energy absorbed from Compton effect recoil electrons and to a lesser extent from photoelectrons. At energy levels above 1.02 MeV, the incident photons may be absorbed through a process known as *pair production*. As a result of this process, a positron and an electron are produced in the absorbing material. A positron has essentially the same mass as an electron but has a positive charge. The positron travels only a very short distance in the absorbing medium before it interacts with an electron. When this happens, there is annihilation of both the positron and electron. In this annihilation process, the entire mass of both the electron and positron is converted to energy, and emission of two photons in exactly opposite directions results. The energy conversion is such that each of the photons has an energy of 0.51 MeV.

It is often important to know how much radiation reaches a certain depth in tissue. For gamma radiation and x-rays, one can determine the half-value layer (HVL) from tables and use this to determine dose at depth in a given medium.[8] The *half-value layer* is that depth of target medium that absorbs half of the incident radiation.

Table 1-2 ● **Approximate Relative Biologic Effectiveness (RBE) of Ionizing Radiations**		
Type of Radiation	**LET (keV/μ)**	**RBE**
Gamma and x-rays	0.3–10	1.0
Beta radiation	0.5–15	1–2
Neutrons	20–50	2–5
Alpha radiation	80–250	3–20

Table 1-3 • Half-Value Layer (HVL) for Photons

Photon Energy (MeV)	Water (cm)	Concrete (cm)	Lead (cm)
0.1	4.2	1.7	0.015
0.2	5.0	2.3	0.065
0.4	6.5	3.0	0.27
0.6	7.8	3.6	0.5
0.8	8.8	4.0	0.7
1.0	9.6	5.0	0.9
2.0	14.0	7.0	1.3
5.0	23.0	11.0	1.5

Table 1-5 • Maximum Penetration of Beta Radiation (cm)

Beta Energy (MeV)*	Air	Water†	Lead
0.1	15	0.015	0.001
0.2	40	0.05	0.004
0.3	65	0.08	0.006
0.4	94	0.12	0.009
0.5	130	0.16	0.013
0.7	200	0.24	0.021
1.0	315	0.40	0.034
2.0	790	0.96	0.081
3.0	1360	1.70	0.144
4.0	2020	2.30	0.210

*Beta-emitting radionuclides emit a spectrum of energies. Average energy is about one third of the maximum energy.
†A useful rule of thumb is that the range in centimeters in water or tissue is equal to the energy in MeV divided by 2.

Although radiations may be characterized by HVL in aluminum, copper, or even lead, for biologic purposes, the HVL in water is more important because it is very close to that of soft tissue (Table 1-3). As an example, suppose that for a 100-kVp beam of x-rays, the HVL in water is 6 cm, and we want to know what percentage of the surface dose is present 12 cm deep in the tissue. At 6 cm, there would only be half of the surface dose (or 50%). After another 6 cm, the dose would be half of 50% (25%) of the surface dose. Often for diagnostic radiology calculations, a tissue dose-to-air exposure ratio can be used.

Particulate Radiation

In addition to indirectly ionizing electromagnetic radiation (x-rays and gamma rays), directly ionizing particulate radiations also are important. Examples of these include protons, electrons, alpha particles, neutrons, negative pi mesons, and other charged ions (Table 1-4). Protons are positively charged particles normally residing in the nucleus of an atom. The mass is approximately 2000 times greater than that of an electron. Electrons (negatrons or beta minus particles) can be emitted as particulate radiations from either an accelerator or a radionuclide. Beta (minus) particles can penetrate up to several centimeters into the body (Table 1-5). A beta particle of at least 70 keV is required to penetrate the protective layer of skin (0.07 mm). A general rule for calculating the dose rate from a beta source is that the dose rate at 1 foot from a beta source (of strength in Curies [Ci]) is equal to about 3 Gy × Ci/hour.

Any subatomic particles that have an associated electrical charge can be accelerated in various electrical devices. Linear accelerators, cyclotrons, and betatrons can accelerate electrically charged particles to produce a beam of particulate radiation. Because neutrons have no charge and, therefore, cannot be electrically accelerated, they are produced either by a reaction of a charged particle with a target or by fission. Energetic neutrons may be obtained by accelerating a beam of *deuterons* (a nucleus of deuterium consists of a proton and a neutron) into a tritium target. When this happens, a neutron is emitted at 14 MeV. Another common method of neutron production is cyclotron acceleration of deuterons (which have an electrical charge) into a beryllium target. The beryllium is converted to boron with ejection of a high-energy neutron. Fission neutrons are produced inside a nuclear reactor through fissioning of uranium 235. Fission neutrons have a wide range of energies, which center about 1 MeV but may extend as high as 6 MeV. Some rare radionuclides undergo spontaneous fission and may give off a mixture of neutrons and gamma rays. An example of a neutron-producing radionuclide is californium 252. Because neutrons are uncharged, they do not easily interact with the target medium and, therefore, are

Table 1-4 • Particulate Radiation

Particle	Charge	Mass (AMU)	Comments
Proton	+1	1.008	—
Neutron	0	1.009	—
Electron	−1	0.0005	Also called *negatron* or *beta minus*
Positron	+1	0.00054	Also called *beta plus*
Deuteron	+2	2.015	Also called *heavy hydrogen*; consists of a proton and a neutron
Alpha	+2	4.034	Consists of two protons and two neutrons

much more penetrating than a proton of the same energy. Neutrons are indirectly ionizing and are absorbed by interaction with the nuclei of the atoms of the absorbing material. When this happens, there is production of fast-recoil protons, alpha particles, and other heavy nuclear fragments. At energies between 100 keV and 20 MeV, if an incident neutron collides with the nucleus of an atom, part of its energy is transferred to the nucleus, and part is retained by a deflected neutron. This process is called *elastic scattering*. Most of the elastic scattering process in tissue is the result of interaction between incident neutrons and hydrogen nuclei. The best shielding of neutrons is provided by paraffin because of its high hydrogen content. The HVL in water for 8 MeV neutrons is 9.25 cm. At incident neutron energies above 16 MeV, inelastic scattering begins with the production of alpha particles. Alpha particles do not penetrate tissues well because they are heavy, travel relatively slowly, and carry a substantial electrical charge. The range of alpha particles is shown in Table 1-6.

Heavy ions, such as the nuclei of carbon and oxygen, can be accelerated in special linear accelerators. These high-LET, directly ionizing particles have a path with a large number of ionizations along it. As the particle slows down near the end of its range, it has more time to interact with the surrounding medium. As mentioned earlier, there are increased ionizations and energy depositions near the terminal depth of the ion (the Bragg peak).

Radioactivity and Radionuclides

The atom may be thought of as a collection of protons, neutrons, and electrons. A formal set of symbols is used to express their numerical relationship. The number of neutrons in an atom is usually abbreviated by N, and the number of protons is represented by Z (also called the *atomic number*). The atomic mass number or the total number of nuclear particles is represented by A and is simply the sum of N and Z.

The symbolism used to designate atoms of a certain element having the chemical symbol X is given by $^A_Z X_N$.

The symbol $^{131}_{53} I_{78}$ refers to one isotope of iodine. In this instance, 131 refers to the total number of protons and neutrons in the nucleus. By definition, all isotopes of a given element have the same number of protons and differ only in the number of neutrons. Thus, all isotopes of iodine have 53 protons. Many isotopes are stable; it is a common misconception that an isotope is necessarily radioactive. There may be many isotopes of a given element, with some having configurations of protons and neutrons that are unstable. Such unstable isotopes will seek greater stability by decay or disintegration of the nucleus to a more stable form. Of the known nuclides, most have even numbers of neutrons and protons. When nuclides have an odd number of neutrons and protons, they are usually unstable. Nuclear instability may result from either neutron or proton excess. Nuclear decay may involve a release of energy from the nucleus or may actually change the number of protons or neutrons within the nucleus. Isotopes attempting to reach stability by emitting radiation are *radionuclides*.

Radioactive Decay Mechanisms

Radionuclides may have more than one mechanism of decay to achieve stability (Fig. 1-4).

Alpha Emission

In alpha emission, an alpha particle (α) consisting of two protons and two neutrons is released, with a resulting decrease in the atomic mass number (A) by 4 and

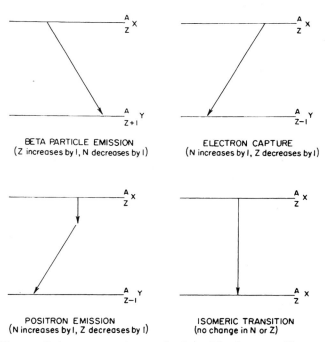

Figure 1-4 ● Decay schemes of radionuclides from unstable states (*top line*) to more stable states (*lower line*). If the number of protons (Z, or the atomic number) increases, the arrow points down and to the right. If Z decreases, the arrow points to the left.

Table 1-6 ● Range of Alpha Particles*

Energy (MeV)	Mean Range in Air (cm)	Range in Water (μ)
0.5	0.25	—
1.0	0.5	7.2
2.0	1.0	—
3.0	1.5	—
4.0	2.5	—
5.0	3.5	45
6.0	4.6	—
7.0	6.0	60
8.0	7.4	80

*An alpha particle requires at least 7.5 MeV to penetrate the protective layer of skin (0.07 mm, or 70 μ).

reduction of both Z and N by 2. The mass and charge of alpha particles are so great that they travel only a few centimeters in air and are unable to penetrate paper. These properties cause alpha emitters to be hazardous only if there is internal contamination (i.e., if the radionuclide gets ingested, inhaled, or otherwise absorbed).

Beta Negative Decay

Beta particle (β^-) emission is another process used to achieve stability, usually by nuclides that have a neutron excess. In this case, one of the neutrons may be thought of as being transformed into a proton, which subsequently remains in the nucleus. In beta negative decay an electron is emitted, accompanied by an antineutrino. Beta particle emission decreases the number of neutrons (N) by 1 and increases the number of protons (Z) by 1, while A remains unchanged. In this case when Z is increased, the arrow in the decay scheme points toward the right; when it points down it indicates a more stable state (see Fig. 1-4). The energy spectrum of radionuclide beta particle emission ranges from a certain maximum down to 0, with the mean energy of the spectrum being about one third of the maximum. Beta minus emitting radionuclides can cause injury to the skin and superficial body tissues but mostly present an internal contamination hazard.

Positron Emission

In cases in which there are too many protons in the nucleus (*neutron-deficient nuclide*), *positron emission* may occur. In this case a proton may be thought of as being converted into a neutron, and a positron (β^+) is emitted, accompanied by a neutrino. This increases N by 1, decreases Z by 1, and again leaves A unchanged. A schematic representation of this process is indicated in Figure 1-4. The arrow points down, indicating a more stable state; it points to the left to indicate that Z is decreased. Positron emission from a radionuclide cannot occur unless at least 1.02 MeV of energy is available.

Electron Capture

Electron capture occurs in a neutron-deficient nuclide when one of the orbital electrons is captured by a proton in the nucleus, forming a neutron and a neutrino. This can occur when there is not enough energy available for positron emission. Because the proton is essentially changed to a neutron, N increases by 1, Z decreases by 1, and A remains unchanged. This also can be seen in Figure 1-4.

Isomeric Transition

If, in the previously mentioned attempts at stabilization, the nucleus still has excess energy, this may be emitted with Z and N remaining the same (see Fig. 1-4). Any process in which energy is given off and the numbers of protons and neutrons are not changed is called *isomeric transition*. Isomeric transition includes gamma ray (photon) emission as well as internal conversion. In *internal conversion*, the excess energy of the nucleus is transmitted to one of the orbital electrons, and the electron may be ejected from the atom. This process usually competes with gamma ray emission. Internal conversion can occur only if the amount of energy given to the orbital electron exceeds its binding energy. The ratio of internal conversion electrons to photons is designated by the symbol α. (This should not be confused with the same symbol, alpha, which is also used to indicate an alpha particle.)

In many instances a gamma ray photon is emitted almost instantaneously after beta decay. If the emission of the gamma ray photon is isomeric, and the product remains in the excited state with a half-life of longer than 10^{-9} seconds, the isotope is referred to as "metastable." The most well-known metastable isotope is technetium 99m (Tc 99$_m$), in which the m indicates the metastable state.

Production of Radionuclides

Most radioactive materials can be produced by bombardment or by fission, although many exist "naturally." Both production methods alter neutron-proton ratios to produce an unstable isotope. In the case of bombardment, the equations are usually written so that the target and bombardment particles are listed on the left-hand side of the equation, with an arrow pointing to the right indicating the product and other particles that are produced, for example:

$$_Z^Y A + n \rightarrow {}_Z^{Y+1} A + \gamma$$

This is referred to as an (n,γ) reaction, and an example is ^{98}Mo $+ n \rightarrow {}^{99}$Mo $+ \gamma$. It will be noted that this makes a stable isotope radioactive by adding a neutron. A nuclide being made radioactive by bombardment with neutrons in a reactor will reach half the theoretical maximum in one half-life of the produced nuclide and 75% of the theoretical maximum in two half-lives. It should be obvious that not all ^{98}Mo will be changed to ^{99}Mo; thus, it is not possible to produce carrier-free isotopes in this way. A *carrier-free isotope* is one that has none of the stable element accompanying it. The neutrons present because of fissioning of uranium in a reactor can also cause the materials of the reactor and impurities in the water to become radioactive. These are referred to as *activation products*. Activation products in a reactor usually have atomic mass numbers of less than 80 (e.g., cobalt 60). A second method of radionuclide production is by *fission*, or splitting of atoms (usually uranium 235). When uranium is split in the fission process, a multitude of radioactive materials, which usually have atomic mass numbers in the range of approximately half that of uranium, are produced. Typical fission products include strontium 90 and iodine 131. Unlike (n,γ) products, fission products are normally carrier-free (i.e., free of stable isotope).

Radioactive Decay

The amount of radioactivity present, or the number of disintegrations each second, is referred to as *activity*. In the past, the unit of radioactivity has been the curie (3.7×10^{10} disintegrations each second). Thus, 1 millicurie (mCi) is 3.7×10^7 disintegrations each second. Because this is a somewhat inconvenient unit, it has been replaced by an international unit called a *becquerel* (Bq), which is essentially one disintegration each second. *Specific activity* is the activity in a unit mass of material (e.g., Bq/g). For an isotope with no stable atoms of the element present (carrier-free), the longer the half-life of the isotope, the lower will be the specific activity. Radionuclides decay exponentially, and the term *half-life* is often used casually to characterize radionuclides. This term usually refers to the physical half-life, or the amount of time necessary for a radionuclide to be reduced to half of some given activity. The physical half-life ($T_{1/2}$) is equal to $0.693/\lambda$, where λ is the decay constant. Half-lives range from fractions of a second to millions of years. The physical half-life is unique to each radionuclide and is unchangeable. A useful formula to be familiar with and to be able to use is

$$A = A_0 e^{-\frac{0.693}{T_{1/2}}t}$$

This formula can be used to find the activity (A) present at a given time (t) when one began with a certain activity (A_0) at time $t = 0$. For example: If you had 5 mCi of iodine 131 at 9:00 AM today, how much would remain at 9:00 AM tomorrow? In this case, $T_{1/2}$ of iodine 131 is 193 hours, and t is 24 hours. Thus, the formula is

$$A = A_0 e^{-\frac{0.693}{T_{1/2}}t}$$

$$A = A_0 e^{-\frac{0.693}{193h}t}$$

$$A = 5 \text{ mCi}(e^{-\frac{0.693}{193h}24\text{hr}})$$

$$A = 5 \text{ mCi}(e^{-0.0036 \times 24})$$

$$A = 5 \text{ mCi}(e^{-0.086})$$

$$A = 5 \text{ mCi}(e^{\frac{1}{0.086}})$$

$$A = 5 \text{ mCi}(0.917)$$

$$A = 4.59 \text{ mCi}$$

Thus, after 24 hours, the amount of iodine 131 remaining is 4.59 mCi. The activity of any radionuclide is reduced to less than 1% of the original activity after seven half-lives have elapsed. It should be mentioned that in addition to the physical half-life, or the physical decay, of the radionuclide, two other concepts are commonly used: biologic half-life and effective half-life. The *biologic half-life* is the time an organism takes to eliminate a compound or chemical on a strictly biologic basis. Thus, if a stable chemical compound were given to an individual

and half of it were eliminated by the body (perhaps in urine) within 3 hours, the biologic half-life would be 3 hours. The *effective half-life* incorporates both the physical and biologic half-lives. Thus, in speaking of the effective half-life of a radionuclide in the human, one needs to know the physical half-life as well as the biologic half-life. If these are known, the following formula can be used to calculate the effective half-life:

$$\frac{1}{\text{effective half-life}} = \frac{1}{\text{biologic half-life}} + \frac{1}{\text{physical half-life}}$$

For example, if the biologic half-life is 3 hours and the physical half-life is 6 hours, the effective half-life is 2 hours. Note that the effective half-life is always shorter than either the physical or biologic half-life. In no instance can the effective half-life be equal to or greater than the physical or biologic half-life.

RADIATION UNITS AND QUANTITIES

Prior to 1928, there were no units to measure radiation "dose," and usually only exposure factors (such as time, voltage, and current) were given. This was quite unsatisfactory because the x-ray tubes were not well calibrated and measurement of voltage and other factors was still primitive. As an alternative, the *skin erythema dose* was often used. This was the dose of radiation required to produce erythema of the skin of the patient or, too frequently, of the operator of the machine. Again, this method was unsatisfactory because the skin erythema dose varies among individuals and in different portions of the body.

Roentgen

In 1928, the International Commission on Radiologic Units (ICRU) proposed as the exposure unit the roentgen (R), which was defined slightly differently in 1938. The roentgen is the amount of x- or gamma rays that produces a given amount of ionization in each unit of air—0.000258 coulomb in each kilogram (coul/kg) or 1.0 electrostatic unit (ESU) in 0.000123 g. This is a unit of "exposure" in air and not "absorbed dose" in tissue; in addition, it is not applicable to high-energy x-rays (greater than 2 MeV) or to particulate radiations. For many situations (e.g., a single diagnostic x-ray exposure), the roentgen is too large a unit, and therefore such exposure is usually measured in milliroentgens. A milliroentgen (mR) equals 0.001 R. In the International System (SI), the unit of exposure is coul/kg or air; 1 R equals 2.58×10^{-4} (coul/kg). For most biologic purposes, a temporal reference is needed (e.g., R/minute).

Gray (Rad)

The rad was proposed in 1953 to avoid some of the problems cited. It measures absorbed energy or dose. The *rad* is defined as 100 ergs/g of tissue (or other absorbing material). The rad has been replaced by the international unit, the *gray* (Gy); 1 Gy (1 joule of energy absorbed in each kilogram of absorbing material) is 100 rad, and 1 rad equals 10 mGy. This unit is not restricted to air and can be measured in other absorbing media. For low-LET radiations such as x- and gamma rays, exposure to 1 R causes energy deposition of 93 ergs/g, or almost 1 rad, and, thus, in these circumstances roentgens and rads are almost interchangeable. As with the roentgen, for biologic purposes, a time frame is usually provided for use with the rad and gray (e.g., Gy/hour).

Kerma

For very-high-energy radiation and for particulate radiation, another type of unit is sometimes used: the *kerma* (an acronym for kinetic energy released in matter). This quantity is used because it includes not only the energy deposited in a local area but also the additional energy deposited as a result of *bremsstrahlung*, or "braking radiation." Bremsstrahlung is produced when an electron is deflected and slowed by the nucleus of an atom with the differential energy being given off as a photon. For most work, the rad and kerma are interchangeable. The major exception in this text is in the calculation of doses for the atomic bomb survivors where the ratio of organ dose to kerma dose ranges from 0.4 to 0.7 for gamma radiation and 0.12 to 0.55 for neutron radiation.[9]

Sievert (Rem)

The radiation units mentioned so far concern only physical parameters. A unit that reflects the biologic response and that could be used to compare effects of different radiations would be extremely useful; toward this end, a unit of "dose equivalence" was derived, the *rem* (acronym of roentgen equivalent man). An international unit called the *sievert* (Sv) has since replaced the rem; 1 Sv equals 100 rem, and 1 rem equals 10 mSv.

Specific Quantities

Exposure and doses from radiographic studies are reported in different ways. The easiest measurement is *exposure at the entrance skin surface*; however, such a measurement cannot be exactly related to absorbed dose. Another quantity given is *entrance skin dose*, which is calculated from skin exposure and includes scattered radiation. This dose is usually the highest of any point in the body. To calculate the absorbed dose at a given depth in tissue, the beam quality must be known. Occasionally, the *midline tissue dose* (MTD) is reported, although this is more commonly used for radiation therapy or whole-body exposure situations. Doses to specific radiosensitive organs (such as the gonads or eye) are usually reported separately. The bone marrow dose can be calculated at a particular spot in the patient;

however, it is usually weighted with respect to the amount of active marrow in the body and in the past has been reported as *mean bone marrow dose*.

Becquerel (Curie)

The unit for measurement of radioactivity is the International Unit, the becquerel. The becquerel (Bq) is a recipricol second and thus effectively equals 1 disintegration every second; 1 curie (Ci), therefore, equals 3.7×10^{10} Bq.

CHEMICAL FACTORS

Free-Radical Formation

The physical absorption of radiation in a human cell that results in ionization or, less likely, excitation, causes a chemical reaction known as free-radical formation. A free radical is an atom or molecule that has a single unpaired electron in one orbit (as compared with most electron orbits that have pairs of electrons). Following ionization, the two substances most likely to be involved in free-radical formation are oxygen and water. When a photon interacts with water and ejects an electron, the following takes place:

$$H_2O + \text{ionizing radiation} \rightarrow H_2O^+ + e^-$$

$$H_2O^+ + H_2O \rightarrow OH\cdot + H_3O^+$$

Water may also be excited (H_2O^*) causing hydrogen and hydroxyl free-radical production as follows:

$$H_2O + \text{ionizing radiation} \rightarrow H_2O^* \rightarrow H\cdot + OH\cdot$$

The hydroxyl radical (OH·) is the major *oxidizing* species resulting from radiation interaction with water. Water is of particular interest because it is the major component of the human body. Although free radicals are an extremely reactive chemical species, in cells most free radicals in these reactions recombine to form oxygen and water in a matter of about 10^{-9} seconds without causing any "injury" or biologic effects. Biologic effects may occur when there is free-radical interaction with DNA creating a DNA radical or they react with other chemical compounds in a number of ways, with the exact reaction depending on the chemical environment in which the free radical finds itself. Free radicals may act as either oxidizing or reducing agents and may form peroxides when they react with water. They may inactivate cellular mechanisms directly, or they may interact with the genetic material (DNA or ribonucleic acid [RNA]). It is thought that free radicals can diffuse a short distance to reach a critical target (e.g., to reach DNA from within a cylinder with a diameter about twice that of the DNA helix). It has been suggested that about two thirds of x-ray damage to mammalian cells is mediated by the hydroxyl radical.[4]

Modifiers

Although radiochemical events may not immediately appear to have much clinical relevance, they form the basis of many principles in radiation protection and radiation therapy. Because their presence causes cells or organisms to be sensitive to radiation, oxygen and water are termed *modifiers* of radiation effects. Lack of oxygen (anoxia) is particularly important in radiation therapy. Radiation oncologists learned many years ago that normal cells and well-oxygenated tumor cells in the periphery of a tumor are moderately sensitive to radiation, whereas the cells located centrally in a necrotic tumor are anoxic or hypoxic, are much more resistant to radiation, and thus can survive higher absorbed radiation doses. The ability of oxygen to enhance radiation damage is known as the *oxygen effect*. Experimental situations are often examined with and without the presence of oxygen, and an *oxygen enhancement ratio* (OER) can be determined. In general, the OER is greatest for low-LET radiation (Fig. 1-5).

The induction of free radicals as an initial step in production of radiation damage has implications for development and use of radioprotective and radiosensitizing agents. For the most part, radioprotective agents are free-radical scavengers, preventing the free radicals from interacting with other cellular compounds and thus averting radiation injury. Some compounds also affect DNA repair, selected gene modulation, cell cycle checkpoints, or cytokine induction. As might be expected, these agents must be present in the cell at the time of radiation to be effective. Examples of these compounds are sulfhydryl amines such as cysteine and cysteamine and S- (2-aminoethyl) isothiuronium (AET). Because of their side effects, these compounds have not been used clinically as radioprotective agents with the exception of the aminothiol Amifostine (WR-2721).[10]

In addition to radioprotective agents, multiple agents are radiosensitizers. As previously discussed, oxygen is probably the most important chemical radiosensitizer. In clinical experience, dose-modifying factors for fully oxygenated tissues compared to anoxic tissues yield modifying factors of 2.5–3.0 for low-LET radiation. For high-LET radiation, the dose-modifying factor or OER is much smaller. It is important to note that for a sensitizing effect, oxygen must be present at the time the radiation is administered. The introduction of oxygen, even fractions of a second after radiation exposure, will not have a significant effect. This relation of the OER to RBE has led to the investigation of high-LET radiations for radiotherapy (particularly for anoxic tumors). It is hoped that use of such high-LET radiations will cause a situation in which the anoxic cells in the central portion of the tumor will not be much more resistant than the peripheral, better-oxygenated tissues. Some radiosensitizers are oxygen-mimetic and electron affinic, such as metronidazole, misonidazole, SR 2509, and other nitroimidazoles. DNA analogs such as halogenated pyrimidines also are known to increase cellular sensitivity, as will chemotherapeutic agents including actinomycin D, doxorubicin, methotrexate, and 5-flourouracil. The sensitizing action of the halogenated pyrimidines is only seen if the compounds are available to the cells for several generations and have time to become incorporated into the genetic material. As will be discussed in later chapters, some cancer chemotherapeutic agents can increase complication rates as well as affect the incidence of second malignancies. Even caffeine has been shown to cause reduced survival in cells exposed to x-ray. Some physical factors, such as hyperthermia, also can enhance the cell-killing effects of radiation. Modifiers of radiation effects are more fully discussed in the discussion of combined effects (see Chapter 7).

BIOLOGIC FACTORS

Target

In evaluating the interaction of radiation within the subcellular system, a number of theories that may apply to specific situations have been proposed. These include the *single-target model*, in which the sensitive site needed to express a desired effect is a single site and may be inactivated with a single hit. In addition to this model, there exist *single-hit multitarget*, *multihit single-target*, and *multihit multitarget models*. The *hit* usually is an ionization, and the *target* is usually DNA. At typical environmental dose rates of about 1 mGy per year, each cell nucleus (assumed to be about 8 μm in diameter) receives about one ionizing track per year. At dose rates of 1 Gy, about 1000 tracks through the cell nucleus result in an average spacing between ionizations of about 160 nanometer (nm). This is quite large compared with the diameter of DNA (about 2 nm) or the likely diffusion distances of the radiolysis products of water (about 5 nm).

The number of DNA breaks induced by ionizing radiation varies based on radiation type, dose rate,

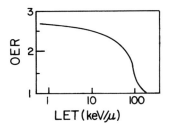

Figure 1-5 • The relationship of OER to LET. Overall, the OER is much more pronounced for low-LET radiation than for high-LET radiation.

and other factors. However, for mammalian cells, the number of lesions per cell immediately after 1–2 Gy of x-ray is about 1000 single-strand breaks (SSBs), 40 double-strand breaks (DSBs), and over 1000 areas of base damage. Chromosomal DNA is the principal target for cellular effects. Ionizing radiation produces several kinds of DNA damage including single-strand breaks, double-strand breaks, DNA-DNA covalent crosslinks, DNA-protein crosslinks, and oxidative changes in bases.

The molecular lesion generally agreed to be responsible for cell death after irradiation is a double-stranded DNA break, whereas single-stranded breaks may cause mutations or be repaired. About 65% of DNA strand breaks are due to the OH· radical. This radical is also responsible for causing damage to DNA bases. Although such theories may be suitable for the subcellular level, the more complex clinical effects in humans are not suitable for study with such simplified direct action models.

As mentioned earlier, the energy from an ionizing radiation is deposited along the track of the particle. The energy deposited from secondary electrons may occur in "packets" and can produce clusters of OH· radicals. The deposition is not uniform but occurs in many event sizes.[11] Recently, the various size events have been termed "spurs" (about 3 ion pairs, up to 100 eV and diameter of 4 nm), "blobs" (about 12 ions pairs, 100–500 eV and diameter of 7 nm) and "short tracks." In the case of photons, 95% of the energy is deposited as spurs whereas for neutrons or alpha particles more blobs tend to occur.

Since both blobs and spurs have diameters similar to the DNA helix (2 nm), if the events overlap, multiple complex free-radical-induced lesions may occur in a sort segment of DNA. These are referred to as *locally multiply damaged sites* (LMDS) and the damage may include DSB, SSB, and base damage. The yield and type of complex damage varies significantly based upon the type and LET of the incident radiation as well as the DNA microenvironment. LMDS production increases with LET. The production of LMDS is independent of dose rate since it results from the passage of a single particle track. Complex damage may represent 60% of total DNA damage after low-LET radiation and as much as 90% after high-LET radiation.

DNA in the cell is basically unstable, with thousands of spontaneously occurring depurination and deamination reactions per day. While the chemistry may be similar, clustered damage due to radiation is different from the randomly spaced damage occurring spontaneously as a result of oxidative free-radical formation. Another difference in the mechanisms is relatively increased production of peroxyl radicals by ionizing radiation that do not cause DNA strand breaks but can cause oxidized base damage.

Cellular changes that may follow radiation exposure are schematically shown in Figure 1-6.

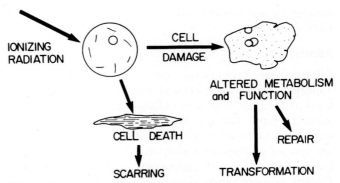

Figure 1-6 • Possible cellular changes following exposure to ionizing radiation. If radiation exposure is high enough, cell death and ultimately tissue scarring may result if the organism survives. If the cell recovers on an acute basis, there remains a possibility of altered metabolism and function, which may be repaired, or there may be transformation to a carcinogenic cell.

Epigenetic Responses

In the last one to two decades there has been a growing body of evidence identifying genomic or cellular effects without the requirement for directly induced DNA damage.[4,12] Such effects are termed epigenetic and are often divided into two classes: (1) genomic instability and (2) bystander effects.

RADIATION INDUCED GENOMIC INSTABILITY

Conventional DNA damage from radiation is usually expressed within one to two cell cycle divisions. In contrast, genomic instability refers to an initial chromosomal aberration that results in an increase in chromosomal aberrations, gene mutations, or apoptosis (cell death) occurring many generations later. Additional mechanisms have also been proposed, including persistence of reactive oxygen species over several generations, telomere loss, alterations in signal transduction pathways, and alterations in nucleotide pools.[13–18]

Reduction in cell cloning efficiency several generations post irradiation may be due to genomic instability. An increase in de novo mutations (with a similar spectrum to spontaneous mutations) also may be due to genomic instability. Genomic instability has been found in established lines and cell culture, although it may be that only a certain fraction of cells or those in a certain part of the cell cycle are susceptible. Searches for this phenomenon in humans and mice have been largely negative or inconclusive, and the biological basis and potential relationship to radiation-induced cancer remain poorly understood.

POSTIRRADIATION BYSTANDER SIGNALING (BYSTANDER EFFECT)

The bystander effect refers to various deleterious (and occasionally beneficial) effects that an irradiated cell has on nearby nonirradiated cells.[19–28] This may involve induction of mutations, micronuclei formation, cell-killing, changes in signal transduction, genomic instability, malignant transformation, and, in at least one experiment, increased survival. The bystander effect may be a response to a "signal" from the irradiated cell (possible molecules transmitted through gap junctions in the cell membrane or diffusion of a substance through the cell culture media). These may be related to stress reactions or release of clastogenic (chromosome damaging) factors. There is also another complexity in that some experiments have shown that a radiation-induced adaptive response could partially cancel a bystander effect.

The majority of bystander effects have been reported after microbeam experiments with high-LET radiations, but there are some positive studies on low-LET bystander effects as well.[20,29–32] It should be pointed out here that this research into basic mechanisms has no effect on epidemiologically derived cancer risk estimates presented later in this book, since the risk coefficients would have included all underlying mechanisms. At very low doses it has been speculated that existence of a bystander effect could result in a convex, downward-curving dose response relationship and that extrapolation from high to low doses could lead to an underestimate of the risk at low doses. To date, however most studies have not shown the bystander effect at doses of less than 50 mGy. The BEIR VII report concluded that until reproducible effects are demonstrated in an intact organism and are reproducibly observed for low-LET radiation in the range of 1–5 mGy, a bystander effect of low-dose, low-LET radiation resulting in a dose response curving either upwards or downwards should not be assumed.[4]

Adaptive Responses

Adaptive responses have been found in some experimental systems. The term refers to a reduced response to a second dose of radiation when the cells have been "primed" with an initial radiation dose.[33–39] The reduced response may be in the form of DNA repair, transformation frequency, or cell lethality. This phenomenon is not found in all cells either in vivo or in vitro and there is considerable variability among individuals of the same species. The response appears to require initial priming doses above several tens of milligray and challenge doses on the order of 1–2 Gy. To date, no consistent reduction in tumor yield or immune effects has been identified in humans or animals attributable to an adaptive response. The BEIR VII report indicates that on the basis of current information, the assumption is unwarranted that any stimulatory effects of low doses of ionizing radiation substantially reduce long-term deleterious radiation effects in humans.[4] The broader concept of hormesis is discussed in detail later in the text (see Chapter 12).

Cell Cycle

The typical cell undergoes a generation cycle that can be characterized by periods of DNA replication and division. The time between divisions of the cell is referred to as *interphase*. Interphase includes a G_1 *period*, which is the time between the end of cell division and the beginning of DNA synthesis (Fig. 1-7). The G_1 phase has the most variable length of the phases, however. Some cells lose proliferative ability (e.g., some neural cells) and are in a subpopulation referred to as G_0. Following the G_1 phase is an *S phase*, or synthetic phase, which is the time required for replication of the DNA. During the S phase, the cell reproduces DNA so that it has enough genetic material to provide each daughter cell with a complete complement following division. A G_2 *phase* is then encountered; in it, DNA synthesis has stopped and the proteins and RNA required for division are synthesized. Last is an *M (mitosis) phase*, during which division actually occurs.

The cellular sensitivity to radiation is markedly different in different phases of the DNA synthetic cycle and varies with cells that have a long or a short G_1 period. Cells having a short G_1 period are most sensitive in G_2 and mitosis, less sensitive in G_1, and most resistant during the end of S. Those cells having a long G_1 period are different, in that the G_1 period is relatively resistant until the very end of G_1. The differences in sensitivity during various portions of the cell cycle can account for radiosensitivity differences in the same cell line by factors of as much as 2 or 3. Generally, the majority of cells are considered to be most radiosensitive during mitosis and most resistant in late S phase. Although radiation may affect many cellular structures, cellular radiosensitivity is usually measured in terms of *reproductive death*: after irradiation, a cell may lose the ability to undergo mitosis either immediately or after one or more generations. Reproductive death is the cell's loss of unlimited ability to divide; its mechanism is not well understood.

Cell cycle checkpoint genes exist and these will not allow initiation of a later phase in the cell cycle if the preceding phase is incomplete. With radiation exposure there is a halt of the cell in G_2, during which there is

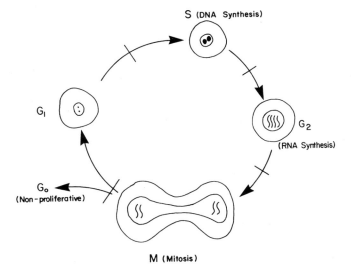

Figure 1-7 • Phases of the cell cycle based upon DNA replication.

evaluation of chromosome damage, DNA damage, and opportunities for repair before the cell proceeds into mitosis. If the biochemical balance is unfavorable, apoptosis (programmed cell death) may occur. This is an alternative mechanism to DNA repair for elimination of potentially harmful effects.

Cell Survival Curves

Most information concerning the basic subcellular and cellular mechanisms involved in radiation effects has come from experiments on cultured mammalian cells. In these tissue culture systems, mammalian cells have been removed from the body and maintained in tissue culture with adequate nutrients and environment. Such cells will generally reproduce for an indefinite period of time during which they may be studied. They are put in solution, plated on culture media, and examined for colony-forming ability. A colony usually arises from a single cell and is taken as evidence of reproductive survival. The first mammalian cell radiation survival curve was developed by Puck and Marcus in 1956.[40] Most mammalian cell cultures exposed to low-LET radiation demonstrate a dose-response curve such as is seen in Figure 1-8. Survival curves are usually expressed by using semilog plots. An irradiated cell population is cultured, and the colony-forming ability of cells for different doses is plotted along a linear scale of the dose. The reciprocal of the slope of the linear portion of the curve is a constant (D_0) and is also called the D_{37}. This is the dose required to reduce the number of cells to 37% of their former value. In general, the steeper the slope of the curve, the more sensitive are the cells or the more effective is the radiation.

The *shoulder*, or initial curvilinear portion of the curve, indicates that there is some process in which the

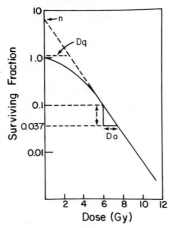

Figure 1-8 • Schematic survival dose-response curve for mammalian cells in tissue culture exposure to low-LET radiation. The extrapolation number (n) is derived by extension of the linear portion of the curve back to 0 dose. The quasithreshold dose (D_q) is the dose measured at 100% survival; the reciprocal of the slope of the linear portion of the curve (D_0), also called the D_{37}, expresses the radiation sensitivity of the cells. The steeper the linear portion of the curve, the more sensitive the cells are to radiation.

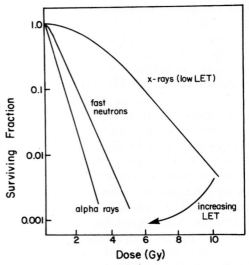

Figure 1-9 • The effect of increasing LET upon the cell survival curve. The higher the LET, the steeper is the curve. Most cells in tissue culture exposed to low-LET radiation demonstrate an initial shoulder on the curve, indicating ability to repair radiation damage. With exposure to high-LET radiations, there is little or no ability to repair damage.

radiation at low doses is less effective than at higher doses. The extrapolation number, n, is derived by extension of the linear portion of the curve back to 0 dose. This is a measure of the width of the shoulder. Another measure of the shoulder width is D_q (the quasithreshold dose), measured at 1.0 surviving fraction (100% survival). This shoulder may be due to a cellular process of accumulating damage or a repair mechanism that is operational within the cell itself. Cells irradiated with low-LET radiation may show a pronounced shoulder, although the same cells irradiated with high-RBE fast neutrons may have a linear plot only (Fig. 1-9). The differential sensitivity of cells in various phases of the cell cycle and with different degrees of oxygenation can also be shown by using cell survival curves (Figs. 1-10 and 1-11). The full potentiating

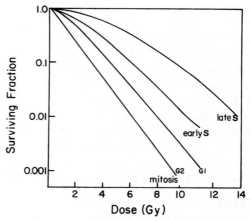

Figure 1-10 • Cellular radiosensitivity as a function of stage in the cell cycle. Overall, the most resistant portion is during late S phase, and the most radiosensitive portion is during mitosis.

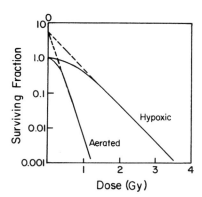

Figure 1-11 • Relationship of the oxygenation of cells to their radiosensitivity. Well-oxygenated cells demonstrate a relatively narrow initial shoulder and steep linear portion of the survival curve, indicating a greater radiosensitivity.

effect of oxygen is found when the partial pressure of arterial blood will not cause additional radiosensitivity.

Repair of sublethal radiation damage is extremely rapid and can be shown by these survival curves. If a cell population is irradiated to a certain dose level and immediately exposed to more radiation, no additional shoulder is identified on the curve, but cell killing continues. If, on the other hand, the cells are irradiated and then allowed to incubate for several hours, they again demonstrate the shoulder on the curve or the capacity to repair additional sublethal damage (Fig. 1-12). The ability of the cells to regain the capacity to repair sublethal damage is one important aspect in the reduced radiation damage or effects noted when low-LET radiation is administered in either chronic or fractionated scheme. Human tissue culture experiments have, in fact, demonstrated that there is repair of sublethal radiation damage to the DNA.

Subcellular Repair of Radiation Damage

At low doses of radiation, the critical cellular component injured is DNA. Radiosensitivity of a cell, in terms of producing reproductive death, is proportional to its DNA content. When there is relatively sparse radiation damage, single-stranded DNA breaks may be produced. This low-dose, low-LET radiation may cause damage that can be repaired at a relatively rapid rate. This probably happens at single acute doses up to 100 mGy. One of the reasons that single-stranded DNA repair may be so rapid is that the remaining intact DNA strand probably serves as a guide to repair. The effect of dose rate upon repair of sublethal damage is schematically represented in Figure 1-13. Thus, as a given absorbed dose is spread out over time, it is much less effective in producing damage, particularly with low-LET radiation. As a dose becomes very protracted, there is even less effect, because not only is there repair of sublethal damage, there is also cellular repopulation due to continued cellular mitosis.

It has been recently recognized that there exist a number of DNA damage response genes (ATM, NBS, and DNA PK$_{cs}$ proteins). These pathways suggest that error-prone repair of complex DNA lesions is responsible for the majority of effects including chromosome aberrations, gene mutations, and cell killing. The potential for error-free DSB repair is small and mostly occurs in later phases of the cell cycle. Additional information on DNA repair mechanisms is presented in Chapter 3.

Cellular Death

With doses of low-LET radiation in the range of 0.5–5 Gy, cellular reproductive death appears to be due to death occurring after one or more divisions of an irradiated parent cell. This usually occurs in the first generation, although it may happen generations later. In contrast to single-strand DNA breaks, which can be

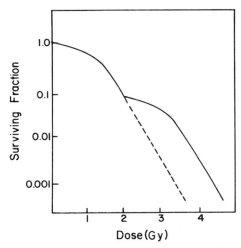

Figure 1-12 • The effect of fractionation upon the cell survival curve. If an initial dose of 2 Gy is given, cells are reduced to the linear portion of the curve, and if they are then allowed to rest several hours before a second dose, they are able to recover their ability to repair sublethal damage. This is indicated by a second shoulder seen on the cell survival curve.

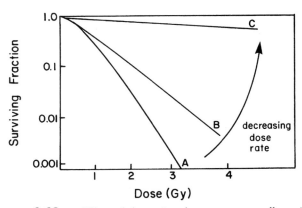

Figure 1-13 • Effect of decreasing dose rate upon cell survival curves. As the dose rate decreases from a relatively high rate (A) to a moderate rate (B), the cells are able to repair radiation damage; therefore, fewer cells are killed. Markedly decreased dose rate has little effect upon cell survival (C) because cells can repair radiation damage and repopulate.

repaired, higher-radiation doses probably cause double-strand DNA breaks. These are considered to be irreparable in most cases and probably to lead to cell death. Finally, extremely large doses (usually greater than 5 Gy) of radiation may cause direct cell death before division (*interphase death*). As will be noted in other chapters, small lymphocytes are intensely sensitive to this interphase death compared with other cells. Interphase death probably results from direct interaction of the free radicals upon essential cellular mechanisms, such as enzymes, required for continuation of the cell.

Radiation Effects on Cell and Organ Systems

Morphologic Cell Changes

With radiation, morphologic changes in the cell itself can be appreciated. At low-dose levels, changes occur predominantly in the nucleus with the clumping of the nuclear chromatin and swelling of the nucleus. With higher doses, the nucleus often becomes dense and disfigured; there may be swelling and loss of the nuclear membrane. Outside the nucleus, the cytoplasm may demonstrate swelling, with distortion of the mitochondria and degeneration of the endoplasmic reticulum. These changes are probably not primary, but rather the result of some other internal process within the cell.

Cellular Radiosensitivity

The sensitivity, in terms of cellular death, of various cell lines can differ markedly, and a given organ in the human body necessarily has different cell lines, for example, structural, functional, and vascular (Table 1-7). In 1906, Bergonié and Tribondeau examined cells that were radiosensitive.[41] The *Bergonié-Tribondeau law* states that (1) actively proliferating cells are the most sensitive to radiation, (2) the degree of differentiation of cells is inversely related to their radiosensitivity, and (3) radiosensitivity of cells is proportional to the duration of mitotic and developmental activity that they must pass through. In other words, rapidly dividing cells that are poorly differentiated and that have a long mitotic period are very radiosensitive. The major exception to these principles is the small circulating lymphocyte which is very sensitive to radiation and rarely, if ever, divides.

The clinical radiation effect observed following radiation damage depends not only on the sensitivity of the various cell lines, but also upon the nature of the function performed by them. Rubin and Casarett[42] have devised a system for classifying cells according to radiosensitivity into four groups. This system is much more useful on a clinical basis than the cell cycle radiosensitivity classification; cells are categorized according to type, function, and mitotic activity. The classes of cells, listed in increasing order of sensitivity, are shown in Figure 1-14.

Table 1-7 • Radiosensitivity of Normal Cells

Radiosensitivity*	Cell Types
Very high	Lymphocytes
	Immature hematopoietic cells
	Intestinal epithelium
	Spermatogonia
	Ovarian follicular cells
High	Urinary bladder epithelium
	Esophageal epithelium
	Gastric mucosa
	Mucous membranes
	Epidermal epithelium
	Epithelium of optic lens
Intermediate	Endothelium
	Growing bone and cartilage
	Fibroblasts
	Glial cells
	Glandular epithelium of breast
	Pulmonary epithelium
	Renal epithelium
	Hepatic epithelium
	Pancreatic epithelium
	Thyroid epithelium
	Adrenal epithelium
Low	Mature red cells
	Muscle cells
	Mature connective tissues
	Mature bone and cartilage
	Ganglion cells

*Refers to cell death not neoplastic transformation.

The category of *vegetative intermitotic cells* (group I) includes the most radiosensitive cells. These cells divide very regularly and include most primitive stem cells of the bone marrow and the gastrointestinal tract, as well as spermatogonia, granulosa cells of the ovary, and basilar germinal cells of the dermoid tissues. Another category, *differentiating intermitotic cell* (group II), is somewhat less radiosensitive, and the cells are also usually short-lived.

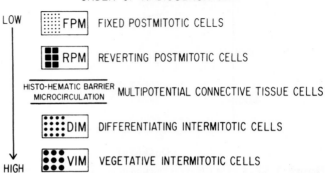

Figure 1-14 • Cellular radiosensitivity as a function of cell type. Cells that do not divide (*fixed postmitotic cells*) have low radiosensitivity; as cells become less differentiated and divide more quickly, radiosensitivity increases. (From Rubin P, Casarett GW: Clinical Radiation Pathology. Philadelphia, Saunders, 1968.)

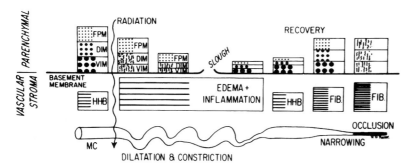

Figure 1-15 • The events following radiation exposure in a rapid renewal system such as the intestinal mucosa. After radiation exposure, destruction of the *vegetative intermitotic cells* and *differentiating intermitotic cells* at the base of the crypts occurs. This is accompanied by edema and inflammation below the basement membrane in the histohematic barrier (HHB) and some dilatation and constriction of the microcirculation (MC). Following sloughing of the mucosa, there may be recovery of the parenchymal mucosal cells; however, this is accompanied by increasing HHB fibrosis and MC occlusion, which ultimately, if severe enough, causes mucosal death. (From Rubin P, Casarett GW: Clinical Radiation Pathology. Philadelphia, WB Saunders, 1968.)

Division and some degree of differentiation may occur. Included are the more differentiated spermatogonia and spermatocytes, as well as the dividing, differentiating cells of the bone marrow. *Multipotential connective tissue cells* include the cells of the microcirculation (particularly endothelial cells), fibroblasts, and mesenchymal cells and are intermediate in sensitivity between groups II and III. *Reverting postmitotic cells* (group III) are generally relatively resistant to radiation and have relatively long lives, undergoing division only under unusual circumstances. Included in this class are epithelial parenchymal cells, and the duct cells of the liver, kidney, pancreas, salivary glands, and endocrine glands. Other examples in this category include reticulum cells in the bone marrow, smooth muscle, and interstitial tissue of the lung. Finally, the most radioresistant category of cells consists of *fixed postmitotic cells* (group IV), which have lost the ability to divide. The class includes long-lived neural tissue and striated muscle, erythrocytes, and polymorphonuclear granulocytes.

Organ Radiosensitivity

Clearly, the pathologic changes identified after irradiation of a given organ depend not only upon the physical parameters of the exposure, but also upon the radiosensitivity of the various organ components. In cases in which the functional or parenchymal cells of the organ are either vegetative intermitotic or differentiating intermitotic cells, loss of function of these cells will be the initial critical factor (Fig. 1-15), although later vascular compromise may become important. After substantial radiation exposure, failure of the organ system may result relatively

quickly. An example of an organ system with very sensitive parenchymal cells is the gastrointestinal system. Marked abnormalities can be seen within several days after a moderate dose of radiation.

When the organ irradiated has parenchymal cells that are part of a slow renewal system, that is, reverting postmitotic cells or fixed mitotic cells, the controlling factor is the more sensitive multipotential connective tissue cells (i.e., the microcirculation supplying blood to the parenchymal cells; Figs. 1-16 and 1-17). An example of such an organ is the brain.

Rubin and Casarett have also divided clinical manifestations of radiation injury into periods of arbitrary length. The *acute clinical period* is the first 6 months; *subacute*, 6 to 12 months; *chronic clinical period*, 12 months through 5 years; with *late clinical period* being greater than 5 years following radiation. The *acute clinical period* includes the initial destructive processes and various repair processes of the organ system. Whether the organ actually survives depends on the total dose, volume of the organ irradiated, radiosensitivity, and physical and chemical parameters discussed earlier. If the radiation dose is high enough, the tolerance of the organ parenchyma will be exceeded, and failure of that system during the acute period will result. With moderate exposures, there may be some parenchymal damage, and the organ may recover either full or partial function (Fig. 1-18). If the parenchymal cells of the organ are relatively radioresistant, no changes may be noted during the acute period. However, this should not be construed as indicating that no clinical radiation damage will result. Vascular changes

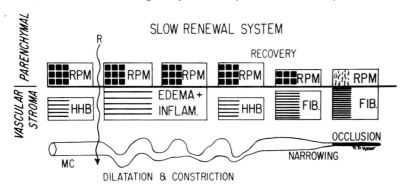

Figure 1-16 • Events following radiation (R) of the slow renewal system such as mature cartilage or pulmonary epithelium. In this renewal system, radiation has relatively little effect upon the *reverting postmitotic cells* (RPM); ultimate parenchymal atrophy over several months results from HHB fibrosis and MC occlusion. (From Rubin P, Casarett GW: Clinical Radiation Pathology. Philadelphia, WB Saunders, 1968.

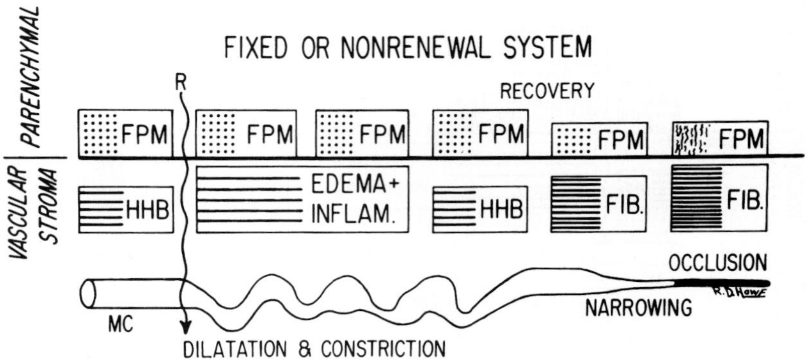

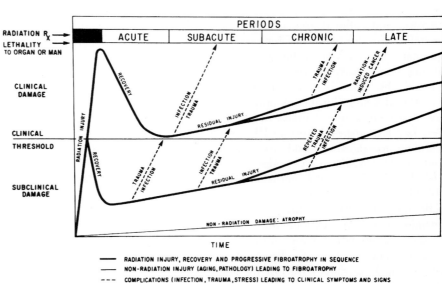

Figure 1-17 • Mechanism of injury in fixed or non-renewal cellular system following radiation exposure (R). An example of such a system is neural or muscle tissue. The mechanism of injury is very similar to that seen in the slow renewal system with initial edema and inflammation in the HHB followed by MC occlusion and fibrosis that causes death *of the fixed postmitotic cells.* (From Rubin P, Casarett GW: Clinical Radiation Pathology. Philadelphia, WB Saunders, 1968.)

Figure 1-18 • Clinicopathologic course. This figure represents a general scheme of radiation injury over time. Injury may cause only subclinical damage, and recovery of this damage may occur, as in the lower set of curves. Over time, with changes in the MC, damage may be apparent in the chronic and late stages or earlier if there is associated trauma or infection. Alternatively, the damage may initially be extensive enough to be recognized clinically. If the individual does not die in the early stages, recovery usually results, however, residual injury remains, and infection or trauma that otherwise may have been minor may lead to substantially greater complications, including death. (From Rubin P, Casarett GW: Clinical Radiation Pathology. Philadelphia, WB Saunders, 1968.)

as a result of arteriolar narrowing may occur later with associated complications. Vascular changes are often responsible for the limiting dose that may be given to an otherwise radioresistant organ.

In the *subacute period* (6 to 12 months after exposure), underlying radiation damage in parenchymal cells may become manifest in terms of clinically significant problems. These may also be complicated by vascular deterioration due to fibrosis, myointimal proliferation, and hyaline sclerosis of the subintimal and medial regions of small arteries and arterioles. During the *chronic clinical period* (12 months to 5 years), an organ system may demonstrate further deterioration of vascularity and secondary degeneration of the parenchyma that can lead to decreased resistance to various sorts of stress. In the *late clinical period*, there is a slow progression of residual radiation damage and formation of dense fibrous tissue due to hypoperfusion. A major problem identified in this late period is radiation carcinogenesis.

FRACTIONATION OF RADIATION EXPOSURE

In general, as previously discussed in the section on cellular repair of sublethal damage, dividing a low-LET

radiation dose and giving it in two fractions separated by several hours will allow the system to repair some of the radiation injury. Thus, *fractionation of radiation exposure*, or protraction of the dose over a period of time, almost always reduces the effect of the dose. There are a few exceptions to this rule; for example, irradiation of the male gonads at specifically selected time periods can cause a much greater effect than if the dose were given all at once because of selective radiosensitivity of certain cells at different stages in the cell cycle. The radiation dose will selectively kill those cells in sensitive phases of the cycle, essentially synchronizing the remainder of the cell population. If the second fraction of radiation is then given during a period of peak radiosensitivity in the cell cycle, the effect is maximized. These exceptions notwithstanding, it is generally true that as a given absorbed dose of radiation is extended over a longer time period, the effects manifested are lessened.

DOSE AND DOSE RATE EFFECTIVENESS FACTOR (DDREF)

The reduced effectiveness of low-LET radiation at low doses or low-dose rates can be expressed by a dose and dose rate effectiveness factor (DDREF). This may be done for cancer or noncancer end points. Choice of a DDREF involves subjective judgments on the choice of data sets, dose range, and statistical uncertainty. The United Nations Scientific Committee on Effects of Atomic Radiation (UNSCEAR) 2000[2] and the International Council on Radiation Protection (ICRP) 1991[6] and 2006[43] have used a DDREF for cancer end points. The BEIR VII committee reviewed human and animal cancer data and selected a factor of 1.5 although 2 was also compatible with the data.[4] For animal experiments involving low-LET radiations and induced cancers, the DDREF ranges from values of 1 to 10. Similar values may be seen for reduction in cell killing with fractionation.

INVERSE DOSE RATE EFFECT

The inverse dose rate effect refers to a situation in which the cells become more radiosensitive as the dose rate is reduced. This phenomenon has been reported for some cells of human origin. While the mechanism is not well understood in human tissue, the cause has been found in yeast to be mutation of a G_2 molecular checkpoint gene. This results in accumulation of cells in G_2, which is a radiosensitive portion of the cell cycle. With higher chronic or fractionated doses, on the other hand, the cell is frozen in the stage of the cell cycle that they are in at the beginning of irradiation.

FRACTIONATION IN RADIOTHERAPY

There are many reasons why radiation oncologists may choose to fractionate the dose, including reducing the release of toxic products, increasing oxygen available to the remaining tumor cells, and taking advantage of a differential recovery rate between normal and neoplastic tissue. Fractionation of radiation treatment is extremely important in management of malignant tumors. The "four R's" of radiobiology are also often quoted as being particularly important for the treatment of tumors with radiation; these are repair, repopulation, reassortment, and reoxygenation. *Repair* is correction of sublethal damage. *Repopulation* is an increase in cell numbers by means of cellular division following a treatment. Fractionation in a radiation therapy regime allows the normal cells to repair and repopulate more than the tumor cells. *Reassortment* is redistribution in the cell cycle of the cells that have been somewhat synchronized by selective killing by an initial radiation dose. *Reoxygenation* refers to the phenomenon that most tumors have hypoxic cells; after a radiation dose they become oxygenated and therefore more radiosensitive. Thus, in contrast to normal tissues, tumor cells usually experience more damage from fractionated radiotherapy regimes than from single doses (primarily because of reoxygenation between treatments).

Nominal Standard Dose (NSD)

To compare various fractionated radiation exposure regimens, radiation oncologists have used the concept of the *nominal standard dose* (NSD). The NSD is a single absorbed dose of radiation that causes the same biologic effect that the fractionated treatment does. Thus, the NSD would always be less than the cumulative radiation exposure given in a fractionated course of therapy. Although the NSD in its original form is rarely used in current practice, it has provided an instructive concept in comparing the radiosensitivities of different tissues and a rough estimation of effects of fractionated exposures. The following formula for NSD was suggested by Ellis[44,45]:

$$NSD = dose \times F^{-0.24} \times t^{-0.11}$$

In this formula, *dose is the total absorbed dose in rad; F* is the total number of fractions, and *t* is the total number of elapsed days.

Biologically Effective Dose (BED)

A linear-quadratic concept can be used to compare the acute and late deterministic biological effects of various radiation dose and fractionation schemes on different tissues. For a single acute dose (*D*), the biologic effect (*E*) is given by

$$E = \alpha D + \beta D^2$$

The α symbol represents the linear portion of the cell survival curve and is the $\log_e$ of the cells killed per Gy. The β symbol represents the quadratic portion of the curve and is the $\log_e$ of cells killed per Gy^2.

To compare radiation effects from different fraction schemes the biologically effective dose can be calculated.

The general formula is:

$$BED = (total\ dose) \times (relative\ effectiveness)$$

The total dose is the product of the number of separate fractions (*n*) and the dose (*d*) per fraction. The relative effectiveness is the quantity

$$1 + \left(\frac{d}{\alpha/\beta}\right)$$

The specific formula for BED then is

$$E/\alpha = (nd) \times \left(1 + \frac{d}{\alpha/\beta}\right)$$

The BED has units of dose and is usually expressed in Gy. Alpha/beta ratios are also expressed in Gy and differ depending on the specific tissue and whether it is an early or late responding tissue. In general, the α/β ratio is about

10 Gy for early-responding tissues and about 3 for late-responding tissues.

Hall and Giaccia[1] have provided examples of how this methodology can be used to compare expected early and late effects from two different radiotherapy protocols.

In the first, a patient receives 30 fractions of 2 Gy given at one fraction per day 5 days per week (i.e., 30F × 2Gy/6 weeks).

For early effects:

$$E/\alpha = (nd) \times \left(1 + \frac{d}{\alpha/\beta}\right)$$

$$= 60\left(1 + \frac{2}{10}\right)$$

$$= 72 \text{ Gy}_{10}$$

For late effects:

$$E/\alpha = (nd) \times \left(1 + \frac{d}{\alpha/\beta}\right)$$

$$= 60\left(1 + \frac{2}{3}\right)$$

$$= 100 \text{ Gy}_3$$

This can then be compare to potential effects of a protocol in which the patient received 70 fractions of 1.15 Gy given twice daily, 6 hours apart, 5 days per week, for an overall treatment time of 7 weeks (i.e., 70F × 1.15 Gy twice daily/7 weeks).

For early effects:

$$E/\alpha = (nd) \times \left(1 + \frac{d}{\alpha/\beta}\right)$$

$$= 80.5\left(1 + \frac{1.15}{10}\right)$$

$$= 89.8 \text{ Gy}_{10}$$

For late effects:

$$E/\alpha = (nd) \times \left(1 + \frac{d}{\alpha/\beta}\right)$$

$$= 80.5\left(1 + \frac{1.15}{3}\right)$$

$$= 111.4 \text{ Gy}_3$$

The higher values for early and late effects of the latter protocol indicate that there will be a higher expected adverse reaction rate for both early and late effects.

Tolerance Dose (TD)

A tolerance dose (TD) is usually expressed in Gy. Examination of radiation tolerance doses is useful in ascertaining the probability of various side effects. A tolerance dose with 5% severe complication rate within 5 years is referred to as $TD_{5/5}$, and the tolerance dose with 50% severe complications within 5 years is expressed as $TD_{50/5}$. Tolerance doses are shown in Table 1-8.

Although the tolerance doses generally express various authors' experience, they are included here as an indication of the wide range of doses that may be tolerated by a given tissue.[42,46] Tolerance doses also demonstrate the relative radiosensitivity of different organs under a radiation therapy treatment scheme. As pointed out earlier, particular fractionation schemes may cause significantly different results. Therefore, in a given circumstance, all of the parameters must be assessed as carefully as possible before the expected result of radiation exposure in a given individual may be predicted with even moderate accuracy. Orton and Ellis[47–49] have developed useful tables that include time, dose, and fractionation (TDF) factors for comparing different radiotherapy regimens. In addition, they have developed a decay factor table to be used in instances in which the radiation regimen is interrupted by a given time, or "rest" period.

There has been some continued refinement, predominantly as a result of empirical experience gained by radiotherapists over the last several decades. The TDF method is the simplest to apply and least prone to mathematical error; however, it has been criticized for the reason that the equations are purely empirical rather than derived radiobiologically, and that the parameters do not change from tissue to tissue, which appears to be necessary. In the last decade, several modifications have occurred. One of these has been to relate TDF to NSD by using the following formula:

$$\text{TDF} = \text{NSD}^{1.538} \times 10^{-3}$$

The 10^{-3} factor was included to make a TDF of 100 approximately represent skin tolerance. In addition, tissue specific scaling factors (K) and volume factors have also been incorporated.[50]

Some radiotherapists use a second methodology, proposed by Barendsen,[51] termed the *extrapolated dose response* (ERD) model, that includes modifications of a linear quadratic model. The ERD is a bioeffect dose unit, and the model divides radiation into high- and low-LET components. The model also includes potential solutions for tumor as well as both early and late reacting tissue. At the present time, there is no uniform agreement among radiotherapists about which methodology to use, and some radiotherapists use the NSD model for one tissue and the ERD model for other tissues. The best that can be said is that while the models provide some guidance, they are certainly not absolute laws of radiobiology and should not override clinical experience.

Table 1-8 • **Radiation Tolerance Doses (in Gy)**

Organ	Injury at 5 Years	1–5% (TD$_{5/5}$)	25–50% (TD$_{50/5}$)	Volume or Length
Skin	Ulcer, severe fibrosis	55	65	100 cm^3
Oral Mucosa	Ulcer, severe fibrosis	60	75	50 cm^3
Esophagus	Ulcer, stricture	50	68	Whole
		60	72	1/3
Stomach	Ulcer, perforation	50	65	Whole
	Hemorrhage	60	70	1/3
Intestine	Ulcer, perforation	40	55	whole
	Obstruction, fistula	50	65	1/3 or 1/2
Colon	Ulcer, stricture	45	65	No effect
Rectum	Ulcer, stricture, fistula	60	80	100 cm^3
Salivary	Xerostomia	32	46	1/3 or 1/2
Liver	Hepatitis	30	40	Whole
		50	55	1/3
Kidney	Nephrosclerosis	23	28	Whole
		50	—	1/3
		—	40	2/3
Bladder	Ulcer, contracture	65	80	2/3
		80	85	1/3
Ureters	Stricture, obstruction	70	100	5–10 cm
Testes	Permanent sterilization	1	2	Whole
Ovary	Permanent sterilization	2–3	6–12	Whole
Uterus	Necrosis, perforation	>100	>200	Whole
Vagina	Ulcer, fistula	90	>100	Whole
Breast (child)	No development	10	15	Whole
Breast (adult)	Atrophy and necrosis	>50	>100	Whole
Lung	Pneumonitis, fibrosis	17.5	24.5	Whole
		45	65	1/3
Capillaries	Telangiectasia, sclerosis	50–60	70–100	—
Large arteries, veins	Sclerosis	80	100	10 cm
Heart	Pericarditis, pancarditis	40	50	Whole
		60	70	1/3
Bone (child)	Arrested growth	20	30	Whole
Bone (adult)	Necrosis, fracture	60	100	10 cm^3
Cartilage (child)	Arrested growth	10	30	Whole
Cartilage (adult)	Necrosis	60	100	Whole
Brain	Necrosis, infarction	45	60	Whole
		60	75	1/3
Spinal cord	Necrosis, transection	47	—	20 cm
		50	70	5–10 cm
Peripheral nerve	Neuritis	60	100	
Eye	Panophthalmitis, hemorrhage	55	100	Whole
Cornea	Keratitis	50	>60	Whole
Lens	Obvious cataract	5	18	Whole
Retina	Blindness	45	65	Whole
Ear (inner)	Deafness	>60	—	Whole
Ear (vestibular)	Meniere's syndrome	60	100	Whole
Thyroid	Hypothyroidism	45	150	Whole
Adrenal	Hypoadrenalism	>60	—	Whole
Pituitary	Hypopituitarism	45	200	Whole
Muscle (child)	No development	20	40	Whole
Muscle (adult)	Fibrosis	60	80	Whole
Bone marrow		2.5	4.5	Whole
		30	40	Localized
Lymph nodes	Atrophy	50	70	—
Lymphatics	Sclerosis	50	80	—
Fetus	Death	2	4	Whole

Note: There are no dose data available for the pancreas, gallbladder, or aorta.
Modified from Hall E, Giaccia A: Radiobiology for the Radiologist. Philadelphia, Lippincott Williams & Wilkins, 2006.

CONCEPTS AND QUANTITIES IN RADIATION PROTECTION

Many concepts have been derived specifically for use in radiation protection (i.e., at low doses and low-dose rates). Often these concepts have been misused and mistakenly applied to high-dose situations. Radiation protection is concerned with protection of groups of individuals, their progeny, and the human race as a whole. It is with this aim in mind that dose limits for the population, occupational dose limits, and maximum permissible dose levels have been derived. Radiation protection prior to the 1950s was mostly directed at protecting those individuals who received occupational exposure; however, in the mid-1950s the concern was widened to include the population at large.

Absorbed Dose

Absorbed dose is usually defined as the average absorbed dose over an organ or tissue. Of course, this represents a simplification of the actual situation. Normally when an organ or individual is irradiated, the dose is not uniform throughout the volume of the organ but is rather inhomogeneous. A simplification used is the assumption that the detriment will be the same whether the organ is uniformly or nonuniformly irradiated. In extreme circumstances, this is obviously not the case; however, if the nonuniformity is less than 50% or so across the organ or individual of interest, the mean organ dose probably can be used effectively.

Equivalent Dose

Knowledge of absorbed dose alone is not very useful in predicting the severity of the effects unless other factors are taken into account. Two major factors are the quality of the radiation and the product of all other modifying factors. Historically, the *dose equivalent, H,* was given by the equation $H = DQN$, where D was the absorbed dose, Q was related to the quality of the radiation, and N was undefined but related to modifying factors. In 1990, the ICRP introduced equivalent dose using radiation weighting factors that are closely related to the previously used quality factor (Q) and are also related to LET and RBE. For radiation protection purposes, the RBE for tumor induction is generally used. The radiation weighting factors (w_R) given by the ICRP in their 1990 and 2006 draft recommendations are shown in Table 1-9.

The absorbed dose in an organ multiplied by a weighting factor for that particular type of radiation (w_R) allows for differences in energy distribution. This is called the equivalent dose in tissue (H_T), and it is expressed in joules per kilogram and measured in sieverts (Sv). The formula for equivalent dose is as follows:

$$H_T = \sum_R D_{TR}$$

Where D_{TR} refers to dose in a particular tissue or organ for a given type of radiation, w_R refers to the radiation weighting factor for that radiation. When the product of these is summed over all radiations, it equals the equivalent dose for that tissue (H_T). It is the equivalent dose that is used for evaluating radiation risk to an organ.

Effective Dose Equivalent and Effective Dose

In an attempt to compare detriment from absorbed dose of a limited portion of the body with the detriment from total body dose, in 1977 the ICRP derived a concept of *effective dose equivalent* (H_E). In 1990, the ICRP modified its definitions and weighting factors. The tissue weighting factor (w_T) was developed based on differing sensitivities of

Table 1-9 • Radiation Weighting Factors*

Type and Energy Range	RADIATION WEIGHTING FACTOR (w_R)	
	ICRP 1990	ICRP 2006
Photons, all energies	1	1
Electrons and muons, all energies[†]	1	1
Neutrons, energy <10 keV	5	2.5
10 keV to 100 keV	10	2.5–7.5[‡]
>100 keV to 2 MeV	20	7.5–20[‡]
>2 MeV to 20 MeV	10	20–7.0[‡]
>20 MeV	5	7.0–2.5[‡]
Protons and charged pions	5	2
Alpha particles, fission fragments, heavy nuclei	20	20

*All values relate to the radiation incident on the body or, for internal sources, emitted from the source.
[†]Excluding Auger electrons emitted from nuclei bound to DNA.
[‡]A continuous (bell-shaped) function rather than a step function is now recommended.
Adapted from ICRP: The 1990 Recommendations of the International Commission on Radiological Protection. ICRP Pub. No. 60, Annals of the ICRP, Oxford, Pergamon Press, 1991 and 2006 Draft ICRP Recommendations. Accessed August 1, 2006 at www.icrp.org.

Table 1-10 • ICRP Tissue Weighting (w_T) Factors

Tissue	Effective Dose Equivalent (1997)	Effective Dose (1990)	Effective Dose (2006)
Breast	0.15	0.05	0.12
Red bone marrow	0.12	0.12	0.12
Lung	0.12	0.12	0.12
Colon	—	0.12	0.12
Stomach	—	0.12	0.12
Remainder	0.30	0.05	0.12*
Gonads	0.25	0.20	0.08
Thyroid	0.03	0.05	0.04
Bladder	—	0.05	0.04
Liver	—	0.05	0.04
Esophagus	—	0.05	0.04
Skin	—	0.01	0.01
Bone surface	0.03	0.01	0.01
Brain	—	—	0.01
Salivary glands	—	—	0.01
Total	1.00	1.00	1.00

*Remainder organs include adrenals, extrathoracic region, gallbladder, heart, kidneys, lymphatic nodes, muscle, oral mucosa, pancreas, prostate, small intestine, spleen, thymus, uterus/cervix.

From International Commission on Radiological Protection (ICRP): 1977 Recommendations of the International Commission on Radiological Protection. ICRP Report No. 26, Oxford, Pergamon Press, 1977; ICRP: 1990 recommendations of the International Commission on Radiological Protection, ICRP Pub. No. 60, Oxford, Pergamon Press, 1991; ICRP: 2006 draft recommendations of the International Commission on Radiological Protection. Accessed August 1, 2006 at www.ICRP.org.

various tissues to tumor induction. The ICRP weighting factors for the different tissues are shown in Table 1-10. With development of the weighting factor for tissue radio-sensitivity (w_T), it is now possible to improve upon the equivalent dose that was discussed earlier. The product of the equivalent dose in tissue (H_T) and the tissue weighting factor (w_T) summed over all tissues leads to the effective dose (E). The effective dose is expressed in sieverts. The definition of the concept of effective dose allows comparison of risks to a person exposed to different sources of radiation and to different portions of the body. For example, average effective dose from natural background radiation is 2.5 mSv per year, the effective dose from a chest x-ray is about 0.1 mSv, and this can be compared to the annual dose from living in a highly contaminated settlement near Chernobyl that yields approximately 6 mSv per year.

The effective dose E is calculated as $\sum w_T H_T$ where w_T is the weighting factor for a tissue and H_T is the equivalent dose in that organ. As an example of use of the system, suppose one wanted to compare the risk from 4 mSv equivalent dose to the lung with a similar dose to whole body. This would be calculated as 4 mSv gonadal dose × 0.12 = 0.48 mSv effective dose; in other words, the "detriment" from a lung dose of 4 mSv should be about the same as what one could expect from a whole-body dose of 0.48 mSv. Quantities and units are summarized in Table 1-11. It should be pointed out that effective dose cannot be used to evaluate risk to a given organ. Under the proper circumstances it can be used to compare detriment from various sources of radiation.

Collective Equivalent or Effective Dose

For low doses of radiation delivered to a population, one may choose to express detriment in terms of a *collective equivalent or effective dose* (S_T) that relates to a specified tissue or organ. In a given population, this is defined as $S_T = \sum E_i N_i$. In this equation, E_i is the mean effective dose, and N_i represents the members of an exposed subgroup. In simplified terms, if 100 people were each exposed to 1 mSv, then the collective dose would be 0.1 man Sv. This essentially equates the effects that one

Table 1-11 • Quantities and Units of Radiation Dose Quantity

Symbol	SI Unit	Nonstandard Unit	Relationship Among Quantities	Relationship Between Units
Absorbed dose D	gray (Gy)	rad	1 Gy = 1.0 J/kg 1 rad = 0.01 J/kg	1 mGy = 100 mrad 1 Gy = 100 rad
Equivalent dose H	sievert (Sv)	rem	H (Sv) = w_R × D (Gy) H (rem) = w_R × D (rad)	1 mSv = 100 mrem 1 Sv = 100 rem
Effective dose H_E	sievert (Sv)	rem	H_E (Sv) = $\sum w_T H_T$ (Sv) H_E (rem) = $\sum w_T H_T$ (rem)	Same as for equivalent dose

would expect in 100 people, each receiving 1 mSv with the detriment that one person could suffer from receiving 100 mSv. As with the concept of dose uniformity, the concept of collective dose has the limitation that it necessarily implies linearity between radiation dose and detrimental effect and that there is no threshold. The reliability of this assumption is difficult to prove; however, most human experience indicates that such linear approximations are not unreasonable.

The other major limitation of the collective dose equivalent is that it cannot be applied to high doses. For example, giving 10,000 individuals 10 mSv clearly will not have the same effect as giving one person 100 Sv. In such an extreme example, the one individual would clearly die within hours, whereas the group of 10,000 individuals would have only a minimal increase in cancer risk. If the equivalent dose to the individuals is in the low-dose range, then many radiation protection groups have used the collective equivalent dose as a basis for radiation protection limits. It has also been used for comparison between different practices involving radiation exposure. Groups that have used this approach include the UNSCEAR and the National Council on Radiation Protection and Measurements (NCRP). The concept was originally derived and set forth by the ICRP. Several theoretical problems with use of the collective equivalent dose include the following: (1) because of the dose level restrictions, the concept cannot be applied to radiation therapy as a source of exposure to the population; and (2) the concept requires a uniform population of all ages and an individual of intermediate sex. Thus, calculations and comparisons in situations in which the population distribution is substantially skewed (such as in mammography exposure) may be limited. At present, however, these concepts have been used to examine the possible detriment from natural background radiation and to compare it to the potential detriment from other radiation sources.

When the radiation source is one that will result in exposure delivered over time (such as fallout), it is occasionally necessary to invoke another concept, the *collective equivalent or effective dose commitment*. This concept is also used in certain, very restrictive circumstances involving a single intake of radioactive material into the body. Under such a situation, the quantity of *committed equivalent or effective dose* (H_{50}) to a given organ may be expressed; this quantity is the equivalent dose that would be accumulated over 50 years for adults and 70 years for children from that single particular intake of radionuclide. Usually no reductions in the detriment due to exposure over time as compared to an instantaneous exposure are included in the calculations.

Maximum Permissible Doses and Dose Limits

Using the concepts previously outlined, both the ICRP and the NCRP have proposed maximum permissible doses and dose limits. The *maximum permissible dose* (MPD) is "the dose of ionizing radiation that, in the light of present knowledge, is not expected to cause appreciable bodily injury to a person at any time during his lifetime."[10] *Appreciable bodily injury* is any bodily injury or effect that the average person would regard as being objectionable or that competent health authorities would regard as being deleterious to the health and well-being of the individual. Historically, radiation dose limits have been consistently lowered. In the late 1920s and early 1930s, the first value of a *daily tolerance dose* was derived. It was suggested that this be one tenth of a skin erythema dose in a year, calculated to be 0.24 R per day. This number was rounded down to 0.1 R per day or 0.7 R per week. In 1949, the NCRP recommended lowering the permissible dose for radiation workers to half of this value, or approximately 0.3 rem per week, even though there had not been a single observation of injury at the earlier dose levels. The reason for this recommendation was the expectation of widespread expansion of industrial and medical applications of radiation. Although the expansion was not so great as anticipated, the recommendations of the NCRP quickly became embedded in regulatory guides and limitations.[11]

In 1956 and 1957, the NCRP recommended again lowering the permissible dose limit, this time to 5 rem per year. This was actually directed at a gonadal dose, again without any evidence of genetic injury at the previous dose levels. At that time, a formula was introduced for radiation workers for the cumulative permissible dose, which was expressed by the relationship $5(N - 18)$ rem, where N is the person's age and N is greater than 18. This formula was intended to permit a degree of averaging to offset minor administrative overruns of exposure, and it was not intended to be an exposure limit for the population as a whole. The 2004 U.S. Nuclear Regulatory Commission (NRC) occupational radiation dose limits are as shown in Table 1-12; 1990 NCRP recommended dose limits are shown in Table 1-13; and 2006 ICRP recommended dose limits are shown in Table 1-14. The limits do not include contributions from background radiation or from medical procedures. Several philosophies for radiation protection have been proposed over the last several decades. Both the NCRP and the ICRP had recommended that radiation doses be kept *ALAP*, or "as low as practicable." The ICRP subsequently changed to another philosophy, which was adopted in 1977 by the NRC. It was recommended that even though radiation dose limits do exist, radiation exposure should be kept "as low as reasonably achievable" (ALARA).[14] In this circumstance, *ALARA* has been defined by the NRC as "as low as reasonably achievable taking into account the state of technology and economics of improvement in relationship to benefits to the public health and safety as well as inclusion of other societal and socioeconomic considerations." Clearly, this definition represents a subjective philosophy rather than a numerical limiting system.

Table 1-12 • U.S. Nuclear Regulatory Commission Dose Limits (2004)

A. Occupational exposures (annual)
  1. Whichever is more limiting:
    a. Total effective dose equivalent   50 mSv
      or
    b. Sum of deep dose equivalent and committed dose equivalent to any organ/tissue except lens of the eye (nonstochastic)   500 mSv
  2. Eye dose equivalent   150 mSv
  3. Shallow dose equivalent to skin/ extremity   500 mSv
  4. Minors (occupational under the age of 18) 10% of above

B. Public exposures
  1. Total effective dose equivalent (annual)   1 mSv
  2. Dose in unrestricted area (in any one hour)   0.02 mSv/hr

C. Embryo-fetus exposures
  1. Total dose (after pregnancy declared)   5 mSv

D. Planned special occupational exposure
  1. In any year   As in A, above
  2. In individual's lifetime   5 × A, above

E. Required notification of NRC*
  1. Immediate
    a. Total effective dose equivalent   0.25 Sv
    b. Eye dose equivalent   0.75 Sv
    c. Shallow dose equivalent   2.5 Gy
  2. Within 24 hours
    a. Total effective dose equivalent   0.05 Sv
    b. Eye dose   0.15 Sv
    c. Shallow dose equivalent   0.5 Sv
  3. 30 days
    Any doses in excess of occupational, public or embryo/fetus limits

*If licensee is in a U.S. Nuclear Regulatory Commission state. If licensee is in agreement state reporting to the state may vary but is usually very similar.

Table 1-13 • National Council on Radiation Protection and Measurements Recommended Dose Limits (1990)*

A. Occupational exposures
  1. Effective dose limits
    Annual   50 mSv
    Cumulative   10 mSv × age
  2. Equivalent dose annual limits for
    Lens of eye   150 mSv
    Skin, hands, and feet   500 mSv

B. Public exposures (annual)
  1. Effective dose limit
    Continuous or frequent exposure   1 mSv
    Infrequent exposure   5 mSv
  2. Equivalent dose limits for
    Lens of eye   15 mSv
    Skin, hands, and feet   50 mSv
    Embryo/fetus
    Monthly equivalent dose limit   0.5 mSv

C. Negligible individual dose (annual)   0.01 mSv

*Sum of external and internal exposures but excluding natural and personal medical doses.
From National Council on Radiation Protection and Measurements: Limitation of Exposure to Ionizing Radiation. Report No. 116, Bethesda, MD, 1993.

It should be noted that there are other limits that are imposed in special situations. Included in these is the occupational exposure of women during pregnancy. The current recommendations in the United States are that the dose to the fetus not be allowed to exceed 5.0 mSv during the nine months of gestation. Thus, the fetus is treated as a member of the general public that finds itself in a radiation environment without its consent. In accidental and emergent exposure situations, dose limits have also been suggested. Unfortunately, these vary among organizations. In 1990 the ICRP recommended that in immediate and urgent situations, effective

Table 1-14 • International Commission on Radiological Protection Recommended Dose Limits (2006)*

	DOSE LIMIT	
Application	**Occupational**	**Public**
Effective dose	20 mSv per year, averaged over defined periods of 5 years[†]	1 mSv in a year[‡]
Annual equivalent dose in		
The lens of the eye	150 mSv	15 mSv
The skin[§]	500 mSv	50 mSv
The hands and feet	500 mSv	—

*The limits apply to the sum of the relevant doses from external exposure in the specified period and the 50-year committed dose (to age 70 years for children) from intakes in the same period.
[†]With the further provision that the effective dose should not exceed 50 mSv in any single year. Additional restrictions apply to the occupational exposure of pregnant women.
[‡]In special circumstances, a higher value of effective dose could be allowed in a single year, provided that the average over 5 years does not exceed 1 mSv/yr.
[§]The limitation on the effective dose provides sufficient protection for the skin against stochastic effects. An additional limit is needed for localized exposures to prevent deterministic effects.
From International Commission on Radiological Protection (ICRP): 2006 Draft Recommendations of the International Commission on Radiological Protection. Accessed August 1, 2006 at www.icrp.org.

doses should not exceed 0.5 Sv except for life-saving actions. The equivalent dose to the skin should not be allowed to exceed about 5.0 Sv, again except for life-saving actions. In application of radiation protection principles, it often is not possible to use equivalent dose, and under such circumstances, limits may be used for environmental circumstances that would be expected to lead to a certain absorbed equivalent dose. Such limits are known as *derived limits* and may relate to contamination levels in air or limits on surface contamination. In some institutions or plants, working limits below the derived limits may be used; these are commonly known as *authorized limits*.

Application of dose limits is much more complicated in attempts to derive limits for intake of radionuclides. In such circumstances, the dose distribution throughout the body is markedly inhomogeneous, and the dose may be absorbed over quite a long period of time. Under such conditions, limits for the activity of radionuclide, known as the *maximum permissible body burden* (MPBB), have been derived. In general, an MPBB is of very little medical significance in contrast to the importance that its name appears to carry. It is a level, which if maintained, is expected to cause very little risk to the individual compared with everyday accepted risks.

REFERENCES

1. Hall, E. and A. Giaccia, Radiobiology for the Radiologist. 2006, Philadelphia: Lippincott Williams & Wilkins.
2. United Nations, Scientific Committee on the Effects of Atomic Radiation (UNSCEAR), Sources and effects of ionizing radiation: UNSCEAR 2000 report to the General Assembly, with scientific annexes. 2 vols. 2000, New York: United Nations.
3. Wagner, L.K., Radiation Bioeffects and Management: Test and Syllabus. 1991, Reston, Va: American College of Radiology.
4. National Research Council (NRC), Committee on the Biological Effects of Ionizing Radiations (BEIR), Health risks from exposure to low levels of ionizing radiation. BEIR VII, Phase 2. 2006, Washington, DC: NRC Press.
5. International Commission on Radiological Protection (ICRP), Nonstochastic effects of ionizing radiation. Ann ICRP, 1984. 14(3):1–33.
6. International Commission on Radiological Protection (ICRP), 1990 Recommendations of the ICRP. Ann ICRP, 1991. 21(1–3):1–201.
7. International Commission on Radiological Protection (ICRP), RBE for deterministic effects: A report of a Task Group of Committee I of the ICRP. Ann ICRP, 1989. 20(4):1–57.
8. Shleien, B., The Health Physics and Radiological Health Handbook. 1992, Silver Spring, Md: Scinta Press.
9. Kerr, G.D., Organ dose estimates for the Japanese atomic-bomb survivors. Health Phys, 1979. 37(4):487–508.
10. Seed, T.M., Radiation protectants: Current status and future prospects. Health Phys, 2005. 89(5):531–545.
11. Hall, E.J., Radiobiology for the Radiologist. 5th ed. 2001, New York: Harper and Row.
12. United Nations Scientific Committee on the Effects of Atomic Radiation (UNSCEAR), UNSCEAR 2000 report. Health Phys, 2001. 80(3):291.
13. Barber, R.C. and Y.E. Dubrova, The offspring of irradiated parents, are they stable? Mutat Res, 2006.
14. Preston, R.J., Radiation biology: Concepts for radiation protection. Health Phys, 2005. 88(6):545–556.
15. Lorimore, S.A., P.J. Coates, and E.G. Wright, Radiation-induced genomic instability and bystander effects: Inter-related nontargeted effects of exposure to ionizing radiation. Oncogene, 2003. 22(45):7058–7069.
16. Little, J.B., Genomic instability and radiation. J Radiol Prot, 2003. 23(2):173–181.
17. Smith, L.E., et al., Radiation-induced genomic instability: Radiation quality and dose response. Health Phys, 2003. 85(1):23–29.
18. Mothersill, C. and C. Seymour, Radiation-induced bystander effects, carcinogenesis and models. Oncogene, 2003. 22(45):7028–7033.
19. Azzam, E.I., et al., Intercellular communication is involved in the bystander regulation of gene expression in human cells exposed to very low fluences of alpha particles. Radiat Res, 1998. 150(5):497–504.
20. Brenner, D.J., J.B. Little, and R.K. Sachs, The bystander effect in radiation oncogenesis: II. A quantitative model. Radiat Res, 2001. 155(3):402–408.
21. Djordjevic, B., Bystander effects: A concept in need of clarification. Bioessays, 2000. 22(3):286–290.
22. Mothersill, C. and C. Seymour, Radiation-induced bystander effects: Are they good, bad or both? Med Confl Surviv, 2005. 21(2):101–110.
23. Mothersill, C. and C. Seymour, Genomic instability, bystander effects and radiation risks: Implications for development of protection strategies for man and the environment. Radiat Biol Radioecol, 2000. 40(5):615–620.
24. Mothersill, C. and C.B. Seymour, Radiation-induced bystander effects—implications for cancer. Nat Rev Cancer, 2004. 4(2):158–164.
25. Prise, K.M., M. Folkard, and B.D. Michael, Bystander responses induced by low LET radiation. Oncogene, 2003. 22(45):7043–7049.
26. Seymour, C. and C. Mothersill, Cell communication and the "bystander effect." Radiat Res, 1999. 151(4):505–506.
27. Seymour, C.B. and C. Mothersill, Relative contribution of bystander and targeted cell killing to the low-dose region of the radiation dose-response curve. Radiat Res, 2000. 153:508–511.
28. Zhou, H., et al., Radiation-induced bystander effect and adaptive response in mammalian cells. Adv Space Res, 2004. 34(6):1368–1372.
29. Brenner, D.J., Is it time to retire the CTDI for CT quality assurance and dose optimization. Med Phys, 2005. 32(10):3225–3226.
30. Ponnaiya, B., et al., Biological responses in known bystander cells relative to known microbeam-irradiated cells. Radiat Res, 2004. 162(4):426–432.
31. Sawant, S.G., et al., The bystander effect in radiation oncogenesis: I. Transformation in C3H 10T½ cells in vitro can be initiated in the unirradiated neighbors of irradiated cells. Radiat Res, 2001. 155(3):397–401.
32. Randers-Pehrson, G., et al., The Columbia University single-ion microbeam. Radiat Res, 2001. 156(2):210–214.
33. Mothersill, C. and C.B. Seymour, Radiation-induced bystander effects and the DNA paradigm: An "out of field" perspective. Mutat Res, 2006. 597(1–2):5–10.
34. Mothersill, C. and C. Seymour, Radiation-induced bystander effects and adaptive responses—The Yin and Yang of low dose radiobiology. Mutat Res, 2004. 568(1):121–128.

35. Preston, R.J., The LNT model is the best we can do—today. J Radiol Prot, 2003. 23(3):263–268.
36. Calabrese, E.J. and L.A. Baldwin, Defining hormesis. Hum Exp Toxicol, 2002. 21(2):91–97.
37. Upton, A.C., Carcinogenic effects of low-level ionizing radiation: Problems and prospects. In Vivo, 2002. 16(6):527–533.
38. Upton, A.C., Radiation hormesis: Data and interpretations. Crit Rev Toxicol, 2001. 31(4):681–695.
39. Sinclair, W.K., The linear no-threshold response: Why not linearity? Med Phys, 1998. 25(3):285–290; discussion 300.
40. Puck, T. and P. Marcus, Action of x-rays on mammalian cells. J Exper Med, 1956. 103:653–666.
41. Bergonie, J. and L. Tribondeau, Interpretation de quelques resultants de la radiotherapie et essai de fixation d'une technique rationnelle. Comptes Rendus Hebdomed des Seances de Acad Sci (Paris), 1906. 143:983.
42. Rubin, P. and G. Casarett, Clinical radiation pathology. 1966, Philadelphia: Saunders.
43. International Commission on Radiological Protection (ICRP), 2006 Draft Recommendations of the International Commission on Radiological Protection. Accessed August 1, 2006 at www.icrp.org.
44. Ellis, F.T., Nominal standard dose and the ret. Brit J Radiol, 1971. 44:101–108.
45. Ellis, F.T., Dose time and fractionation: A clinical hypothesis. Clin Radiol, 1969. 20:1–7.
46. Emami, B., et al., Tolerance of normal tissue to therapeutic irradiation. Int J Radiat Oncol Biol Phys, 1991. 21(1):109–122.
47. Beal, K., et al., Radiation pneumonitis in breast cancer patients treated with taxanes: Does sequential radiation therapy lower the risk. Breast J, 2005. 11(5):317–320.
48. Orton, C.G. and L. Cohen, A unified approach to dose-effect relationships in radiotherapy. I. Modified TDF and linear quadratic equations. Int J Radiat Oncol Biol Phys, 1988. 14(3):549–556.
49. Orton, C.G. and F. Ellis, A simplification in the use of the NSD concept in practical radiotherapy. Br J Radiol, 1973. 46(547):529–537.
50. Orton, C.G. and E. Ellis, A simplification in the use of the NSD concept in practical radiotherapy. Brit J Radiol, 1973. 46:529–537.
51. Barendsen, G.W., Dose fractionation, dose rate and iso-effect relationships for normal tissue responses. Int J Radiat Oncol Biol Phys, 1982. 8(11):1981–1987.

2 Sources of Radiation Exposure

Exposure to ionizing radiation comes from two major sources: natural (background) radiation and technologically induced radiation. The latter category is often referred to as "man-made" radiation, although many of the technologically modified sources simply represent a rearrangement or concentration of naturally occurring radiation sources. In many countries natural sources of radiation constitute the major source of exposure to the population, with the next largest source being medical applications of ionizing radiation. The relative contribution of medical exposure varies substantially, depending on the technologic state of the country involved (for an extensive review of the sources of ionizing radiation, see the 2006 United Nations Scientific Committee of the Effects of Atomic Radiation [UNSCEAR] report).[1] In 2006 in the United States, medical exposure exceeded natural background as a source, with annual effective doses from various sources estimated as shown in Table 2-1 and Figure 2-1.

NATURAL RADIATION SOURCES

Natural radiation is of particular importance because this source is the largest contributor to the collective dose of the world's population.[1,2] Distinctive characteristics of natural irradiation are that it is incurred at a relatively constant rate and that humans have always been exposed to it. Absorbed doses from various natural sources are shown in Figure 2-2.

Cosmic Sources

Cosmic Rays

There are three main sources of cosmic radiation: galactic, solar, and radiation from the earth's (van Allen) radiation belts. All but the highest energy cosmic rays originate within our own galaxy. Galactic cosmic ray fluence varies with solar activity and it lowers when solar flare activity is higher. Outside the earth's atmosphere the equivalent dose during solar minimum is slightly above 1 Sv per hour. Solar cosmic radiation originates from solar flares and can produce high dose rates at high altitudes but only the most energetic protons contribute to doses at ground level. There are two van Allen radiation belts, one at about 3000 km above the earth's surface and

another at about 22,000 km. The protons and electrons in these belts can result in doses in excess of tens of Sv per day. Normally, this is not an issue except that manned orbital flights need to avoid the South Atlantic anomaly where the inner belt comes much closer to the earth's surface. Cosmic rays originate predominantly from galactic sources; only a small fraction are normally solar in origin, but the solar component becomes significant after solar flares associated with cyclic sun spot activity.[4,5]

Cosmic rays are 85% protons, 14% alpha particles, and about 1% nuclei of atomic number between $Z = 4$ and $Z = 26$. These particles are highly penetrating and have a mean energy of 10^{10} eV and maximum energies up to 10^{19} eV. The higher-energy primary particles interact with atmospheric nuclei and undergo nuclear reactions (*spallation*), producing neutrons, protons, pions, and kaons, as well as a variety of reaction products (*cosmogenic nuclides*). The high-energy spallation particles thus formed react (*cascade*) to form secondary particles. The pions decay into muons or photons, initiating other cascades. At sea level mesons (*muons*) account for about 80% of cosmic radiation and electrons for about 20%. Less than 0.05% of the primary cosmic protons penetrate to sea level. The typical sea-level effective dose rate is about 34 nSv per hour.

The reaction of the cosmic rays with the atmosphere causes attenuation of the cosmic rays; in other words, the atmosphere provides us with shielding equivalent to a layer 10 m thick of water. As a result, the higher one is above sea level, the greater cosmic ray exposure becomes (Table 2-2), doubling every 1500 m above the earth's surface. In addition to variations in cosmic ray dose with altitude, there are variations with latitude. Primary cosmic rays are substantially affected by the earth's magnetic field, which deflects the lower-energy radiation back into space. As a result of this process, the flux of cosmic rays is greater at the north and south poles than it is at the equator (Table 2-3). The cosmic ray flux at the poles is high enough that their atmospheric interactions are visualized as the aurora borealis.

A typical absorbed dose rate in air at sea level from the ionizing component of cosmic radiation is 32 nGy per hour. Because the quality factor is 1.0, this is also the effective dose rate. For the neutron portion the estimate of effective dose is 3.6 nSv per hour. The annual effective dose

Table 2-1 • Estimated Annual Effective Dose in the U.S. Population 2006

Source	Number of People Exposed	Average Annual H_E* in the Exposed Population (mSv)	Annual Collective Effective Dose Equivalent (person-Sv)	Average Annual H_E in the U.S. Population (mSv)
Natural sources				
Radon	300,000	1.9	570,000	1.9
Other	300,000	1.1	330,000	1.1
Occupational	930	2.3	2,000	0.009
Nuclear fuel cycle[†]	—	—	136	0.0005
Consumer products	—	—	30	0.1
Tobacco[‡]	50,000	—	—	—
Other	120,000	0.05–0.3	12,000–29,000	0.05–0.13
Miscellaneous environmental sources	~25,000	0.006	160	0.0006
Medical				
Diagnostic x-rays	—[§]	—	720,000	2.4
Nuclear medicine	—[§]	—	230,000	0.8
Rounded total	300,000	—	~1,900,000	~6.2

*H_E is the effective dose equivalent.
[†]Collective doses were calculated to the regional population within 80 km (50 miles) of each facility.
[‡]Effective dose difficult to determine; dose to a segment of bronchial epithelium estimated to be 0.16 Sv/yr.
[§]Number of persons exposed is not known.

from cosmic rays at sea level is 260 μSv. This can be compared with a high-altitude city such as Denver, where the dose is 570 μSv. Cosmic ray dose in some other cities is shown in Table 2-4.

There is some attenuation by buildings, and an average reduction of cosmic rays by 20% is usually assumed indoors. If one takes into account variations in altitude and buildings, the average annual effective dose from cosmic rays is approximately 380 μSv. The directly and indirectly ionizing components contribute 300 and 80 μSv, respectively. The worldwide collective effective dose is approximately 1.9×10^6 man Sv. About 90% of this occurs in the northern hemisphere due to the population distribution. Because altitude is an important factor, about one half of the collective dose is received by about one third of the population that lives below 0.5 km in altitude. One-fiftieth of the population lives above 3 km and receives one tenth of the collective dose. With increases in altitude, neutrons become a more important component. In general, the range of individual annual effective dose from cosmic rays is 260 to 2000 μSv.

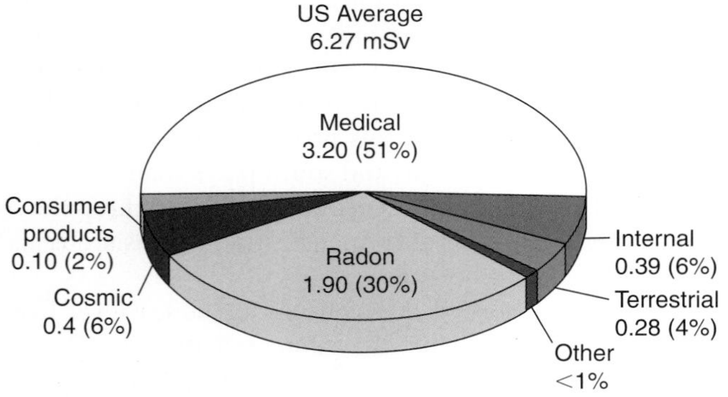

Cosmogenic Radionuclides

Most cosmogenic radionuclides contribute little to natural background radiation exposure. Of the many nuclides produced by cosmic radiation (Table 2-5), only tritium (^{3}H),

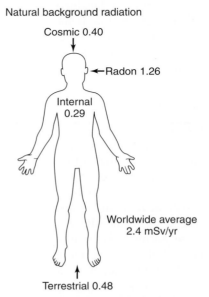

Figure 2-2 • Contribution of various natural sources of radiation to the annual per caput effective dose worldwide.

US Average
6.27 mSv

Medical
3.20 (51%)

Consumer products
0.10 (2%)

Cosmic
0.4 (6%)

Radon
1.90 (30%)

Internal
0.39 (6%)

Terrestrial
0.28 (4%)

Other
<1%

Figure 2-1 • Contribution of various sources of radiation to the annual effective dose in the United States in 2006.

Table 2-2 • Incremental Increase in Cosmic Dose Rates with Altitude

Elevation (ft)	Cosmic Ray Dose Rate (mSv/yr EDE)
Sea level	0.26
Up to 1000	Add 0.02/yr
1000–2000	Add 0.05/yr
2000–3000	Add 0.09/yr
3000–4000	Add 0.15/yr
4000–5000	Add 0.21/yr
5000–6000	Add 0.29/yr
6000–7000	Add 0.40/yr
7000–8000	Add 0.53/yr
Above 8000	Add 0.70/yr

Table 2-4 • Average Annual Effective Dose from Cosmic Rays in Different Locations

	Population (millions)	Altitude (m)	Effective Dose (μSv/yr)
La Paz, Bolivia	1.0	3900	2.02
Lhasa, China	0.3	3600	1.71
Quito, Ecuador	11.0	2840	0.57
Mexico City, Mexico	17.3	2240	0.82
Denver, United States	1.61	1610	0.57
Teheran, Iran	7.5	1180	0.44
Sea level			0.26
World average			0.38

with a half-life of 12.3 years, beryllium (^{7}Be), with a half-life of 53.6 days, carbon 14 (^{14}C), with a half-life of 5730 years, and sodium 22 (^{22}Na), with a half-life of 2.6 years, contribute appreciably; the major contributor is carbon 14.[3]

The major source of natural tritium is the interaction of cosmic ray neutrons with nitrogen and oxygen in the atmosphere. It is then converted to tritiated water and participates in the normal water cycle. The average concentration of natural tritium in continental surface waters is 400 Bq/m^3; for ocean waters the average natural tritium is 100 Bq/m^3. Annual individual intake is about 500 Bq, and, if one assumes that the specific activities of ^{3}H in body tissues are the same as those in the continental surface waters before nuclear explosions began, the annual absorbed doses from natural tritium are of the order of 10^{-8} Gy, in all tissues. The annual effective dose for tritium is about 0.01 μSv.

The concentration of ^{7}Be is approximately 30 mBq/m^3 in air and 700 Bq/m^3 in rainwater. The main pathway to humans for ^{7}Be is through the ingestion of leafy vegetables, resulting in an annual intake of about 1000 Bq. The absorbed doses in tissue are approximately 12 μGy in the walls of the

lower large intestine and somewhat lower in other tissues. The annual effective dose is about 0.03 μSv.

Carbon 14 is produced in the upper atmosphere by the interaction of slow cosmic neutrons with nitrogen 14. Carbon 14 is usually metabolized as carbon dioxide and appears in the photosynthetic cycle in plants. This cosmogenic radionuclide is the basis for carbon 14 dating. Plant materials that have undergone recent photosynthesis have a higher activity of carbon 14 than do plants that participated in the photosynthetic cycle hundreds or millions of years ago. The specific activity of carbon 14 in air has decreased because of the diluting effect of releases into the atmosphere of carbon dioxide from the burning of fossil fuels. If one assumes the natural specific activity of carbon 14 to be 227 Bq/kg of carbon with an annual intake

Table 2-3 • Variation with Latitude in Cosmic Ray Dose Rates Outdoors at Sea Level*

Latitude (Degrees)	Directly Ionizing Component	Neutron Component	Total
80–90	32	11	43
70–80	32	11	43
60–70	32	10.9	42.9
50–60	32	10	42
40–50	32	7.8	39.8
30–40	32	5.3	37.3
20–30	30	4	34
10–20	30	3.7	33.7
0–10	30	3.6	33.6

*Effective dose rate (nSv/hr).

Table 2-5 • Cosmogenic Radionuclides (Produced by Cosmic Rays Interacting with Earth's Atmosphere)

Radionuclide	TROPHOSPHERIC CONCENTRATION	
	(Bq/kg air)	(pCi/kg air)
^{3}H	1.8×10^{-3}	3.2×10^{-22}
^{7}Be	1.0×10^{-2}	0.28
^{10}Be	1.3×10^{-9}	3.2×10^{-8}
^{14}C	1.3×10^{-1}	3.4
^{22}Na	1.1×10^{-6}	3.0×10^{-5}
^{24}Na	(15-yr half-life)	
^{32}Si	2.0×10^{-8}	5.4×10^{-7}
^{32}P	2.3×10^{-4}	6.3×10^{-3}
^{33}P	1.3×10^{-4}	3.4×10^{-3}
^{35}S	1.3×10^{-4}	3.5×10^{-3}
^{36}Cl	2.5×10^{-10}	6.8×10^{-9}
^{38}S	(2.87-hr half-life)	
^{38}Cl	(27.3-min half-life)	
^{39}Cl	(55.5-min half-life)	

of 20 kBq, the annual absorbed doses in tissue range from 5 to 24 µGy; the annual effective dose is therefore 12 µSv.

The annual intake of ^{22}Na by ingestion is 50 Bq. The annual absorbed dose in tissue ranges from 0.1 to 0.3 µGy, corresponding to an annual effective dose of about 0.15 µSv. Despite the very small production rate and concentration of ^{22}Na, the annual absorbed doses are higher than for tritium because of the metabolic behavior of sodium and of the decay properties of ^{22}Na.

Terrestrial Sources

Primordial Radionuclides

In addition to cosmogenic radionuclides, there is another main category of radionuclides that have existed on the earth's crust since its formation; referred to as *primordial radionuclides*, they are the source of terrestrial radiation. The relative abundance of isotopes now present on earth is derived from the isotopic ratios produced when the earth was formed. Despite the surprising uniformity of the ratios of the elements (not only in this galaxy, but even in extragalactic nebulas), minor shifts in isotope ratios do occur gradually in nature as a result of mass-sensitive physiochemical and geologic processes. The primordial radionuclides that now remain in the earth's crust are those with half-lives comparable to the age of the universe. Those with half-lives of less than approximately 10^8 years have become undetectable in the 30 or so half-lives since their creation. Radionuclides having half-lives of greater than 10^{10} years have decayed very little up to the present time. It is estimated that 95% of the world's population lives in areas of "normal" background, and receive an outdoor absorbed dose rate from primordial radionuclides of 56 nGy per hour. This corresponds to a yearly effective dose in the United States of 0.28 mSv. Primordial radionuclides produce secondary radionuclides by radioactive decay. Table 2-6 lists the primordial radionuclides and their half-lives.

There are three distinct chains of primordial radioactive elements: (1) the uranium series, which originates with ^{238}U; (2) the thorium series, which originates with ^{232}Th; and (3) the actinium series, which originates with ^{235}U. All are found in the earth's crust and account for much of the exposure to terrestrial radioactivity (Tables 2-7 to 2-9).[4,5] The natural content of some primordial radionuclides in soil and human tissues is shown in Tables 2-10 and 2-11.

The uranium normally found in nature consists of three isotopes having mass numbers of 234, 235, and 238. ^{238}U, the parent of the uranium series, is present in the amount of 99.28% and is in equilibrium with ^{234}U, which is present in the amount of 0.0058%. ^{235}U, present in the amount of 0.71%, is the parent isotope of the actinium series and is the principal nuclide used in the fission process. Uranium is found in various quantities in most rocks and soils. Because the uranium isotopes are alpha emitters, they do not contribute to the gamma ray

Table 2-6 • Primordial Radionuclides

Radionuclide	Physical Half-life (yr)
^{40}K	1.26×10^9
^{50}V	6×10^{15}
^{87}Rb	4.8×10^{10}
^{115}In	6×10^{14}
^{123}Te	1.2×10^{13}
^{138}La	1.12×10^{11}
^{142}Ce	$>5 \times 10^{16}$
^{144}Nd	2.4×10^{15}
^{147}Sm	1.05×10^{11}
^{148}Sm	$>2 \times 10^{14}$
^{146}Sm	$>1 \times 10^{15}$
^{152}Gd	1.1×10^{14}
^{156}Dy	$>1 \times 10^{18}$
^{174}Hf	2×10^{15}
^{176}Lu	2.22×10^{10}
^{180}Ta	1×10^{12}
^{187}Re	4.3×10^{10}
^{190}Pt	6.9×10^{11}
^{232}Th	1.4×10^{10}
^{235}U	7.04×10^8
^{238}U	4.47×10^9

background. They are present in too low a concentration to contribute significantly to the internal alpha dose delivered to humans; however, as would be expected from the presence of uranium in soils and in fertilizers, it is possible to demonstrate the presence of uranium in food and human tissues.[6,7] The uranium content of the "standard" adult male has been estimated to be 100 to 125 µg, in equilibrium with a daily intake of 1 to 1.4 µg of uranium.

From the point of view of potential ionizing radiation exposure from naturally occurring radioactive substances, the isotope ^{226}Ra (radium—originating in the uranium series) and its daughter products are of special importance. ^{226}Ra is an alpha emitter that is present in varying amounts in all rocks, soils, and water. Radium 226, with a half-life of 1622 years, decays to ^{222}Rn (radon). Radon is a noble gas radionuclide with a half-life of 3.8 days that emits *alpha* particles but also adds to the *gamma* activity of the environment through its gamma-emitting descendants. Radium, chemically similar to calcium, is absorbed from the soil by plants and passes through the food chain to humans.[8] In the body, 70% to 90% of radium is contained in bone. The radium content of foods varies in relation to the considerable variability in the radium content of soils and in its rate of absorption by plants, which is, in turn, related to the amount of exchangeable calcium in the soil. The ^{226}Ra content of total diets ranges from 1.9×10^{-2} Bq/kg to 2.7×10^{-2} Bq/kg. The average person has 850 mBq of ^{226}Ra (for each) kilogram of calcium, and a total of 850 mBq in the skeleton. This corresponds to an annual effective dose equivalent of 7µSv from ^{226}Ra intake. Because of the tendency of the Brazil nut trees to concentrate barium, a chemical very similar to radium, the radium content of Brazil nuts varies from

Table 2-7 • Uranium Series

Nuclide	Historical Name	Half-life	MAJOR RADIATION ENERGIES (MeV) AND INTENSITIES					
			α		β		γ	
$^{238}_{92}$U	Uranium I	4.47×10^9 yr	4.15 4.20	(23%) (77%)	—		0.0496	(0.07%)
$^{234}_{90}$Th	Uranium X$_1$	24.1 d	—		0.096 0.189	(19%) (73%)	0.0633 0.0924	(3.8%) (2.7%)
$^{234}_{91}$Pa^m	Uranium X$_a$	1.17 m	—		2.28	(99%)	0.766 1.001	(0.21%) (0.59%)
99.87% ⎸ 0.13%								
$^{234}_{91}$Pa	Uranium Z	6.75 h	—		0.53 1.13	(66%) (13%)	0.132 0.570 0.926–0.946	(20%) (11%) (23%)
$^{234}_{92}$U	Uranium II	2.47×10^5 yr	4.72 4.77	(27%) (72%)	—		0.053 0.121	(0.12%) (0.04%)
$^{230}_{90}$Th	Ionium	7.7×10^4 yr	4.62 4.68	(23%) (76%)	—		0.068 0.142	(0.4%) (0.07%)
$^{226}_{88}$Ra	Radium	1602 yr	4.60 4.78	(6%) (94%)	—		0.186	(3%)
$^{222}_{86}$Rn	Emanation Radon (Rn)	3.823 d	5.49	(99.9%)	—		0.510	(0.08%)
$^{218}_{84}$Po	Radium A	3.05 m	6.00	(~100%)	0.33	(~0.019%)	—	
99.98% ⎸ 0.02%								
$^{214}_{82}$Pb	Radium B	26.8 m	—		0.67 0.73 1.03	(48%) (43%) (6%)	0.295 0.352	(19%) (37%)
$^{218}_{85}$At	Astatine	~2 s	6.66 6.70	(6%) (90%)	—		—	
$^{214}_{83}$Bi	Radium C	19.9 m	5.45 5.51	(0.012%) (0.008%)	1.42 1.51 3.27	(8%) (36%) (18%)	0.609 1.120 1.765	(46%) (15%) (16%)
99.98% ⎸ 0.02%								
$^{214}_{84}$Pb	Radium C′	164 μs	7.69	(100%)	—		0.799	(0.010%)
$^{210}_{81}$Ti	Radium C″	1.3 m	—		1.3 1.9 2.3	(25%) (56%) (19%)	0.292 0.800 1.31	(80%) (99%) (21%)
$^{210}_{82}$Pb	Radium D	22.3 yr	3.72	(0.000002%)	0.016 0.063	(80%) (20%)	0.047	(4%)
$^{210}_{83}$Bi	Radium E	5.01 d	4.65 4.69	(0.00007%) (0.00005%)	1.161	(~100%)	—	
~100% ⎸ 0.00013%								
$^{210}_{84}$Po	Radium F	138.4 d	5.305	(100%)	—		0.803	(0.0011%)
$^{206}_{81}$Tl	Radium E″	4.20 m	—		1.571	(100%)	—	
$^{206}_{82}$Pb	Radium G	Stable	—		—		—	

Adapted from Shleien B: The Health Physics Radiological Health Handbook. Silver Spring, MD, Scinta, Inc., 1992.

10.1 to 262.7 Bq/kg, approximately 1000 times greater than the radium concentration in the average diet.[9]

The average annual effective dose from terrestrial radionuclide gamma rays in various countries is shown in Table 2-12. There are regions in the world where the terrestrial radiation substantially exceeds the normal range of variation for most of the earth's surface. Monazite sand areas in Kerala, India, as well as selected areas in Brazil, have been best investigated dosimetrically. In addition, high-background regions are known to exist in Italy (provinces of Latio and Campania, 200 nGy/hour), southwest France (10 to 10,000 nGy/hour), Ramsar, Iran (70 to

Table 2-8 • Thorium Series

Nuclide	Historical Name	Half-life	MAJOR RADIATION ENERGIES (MeV) AND INTENSITIES					
			α		β		γ	
$^{232}_{90}$Th	Thorium	1.41×10^{10} yr	3.95 4.01	(24%) (76%)	—		0.059 0.126	(0.19%) (0.04%)
$^{228}_{88}$Ra	Mesothorium I	6.7 yr	—		0.0389	(100%)	—	
$^{228}_{89}$Ac	Mesothorium II	6.13 hr	—		1.17 1.74 2.08	(32%) (12%) (8%)	0.338 0.911 0.969	(11%) (27%) (17%)
$^{228}_{90}$Th	Radiothorium	1.910 yr	5.34 5.43	(28%) (71%)	—		0.084 0.214	(1.6%) (0.3%)
$^{224}_{88}$Ra	Thorium X	3.64 d	5.45 5.68	(6%) (94%)	—		0.241	(3.7%)
$^{220}_{86}$Rn	Emanation Thoron (Tn)	55 s	6.29	(100%)	—		0.55	(0.07%)
$^{216}_{84}$Po	Thorium A	0.15 s	6.78	(100%)	—		0.128	(0.002%)
$^{212}_{82}$Pb	Thorium B	10.64 hr	—		1.334 0.586	(85%) (14%)	0.239 0.300	(45%) (3.4%)
$^{212}_{83}$Bi	Thorium C	60.6 m	6.05 6.09	(25%) (10%)	1.58 2.25	(5%) (48%)	0.040 0.727 1.620	(1%) (11.8%) (2.8%)
$^{214}_{84}$Pb	Thorium C′	304 ns	8.78	(100%)	—		—	
$^{208}_{81}$Tl	Thorium C″	3.10 m	—		1.28 1.52 1.80	(25%) (21%) (50%)	0.511 0.583 0.860 2.614	(21%) (86%) (12%) (100%)
$^{208}_{82}$Pb	Thorium D	Stable	—		—		—	

(branching: 64.0% / 36.0%)

Adapted from Shleien B: The Health Physics Radiological Health Handbook. Silver Spring, MD, Scinta, Inc., 1992.

17,000 nGy/hour), Madagascar, China, and Nigeria. Although quantitative information on outdoor absorbed dose rates in air in such unusual areas is limited, rates from 4×10^{-7} to 5×10^{-5} Gy per hour have been reported. In Kerala, India, the thorium concentration in the monazite sand is the highest known in the world. The absorbed dose rate for a few people in this area may be as high as 5000 nGy per hour, and the average absorbed dose rate for the 70,000 persons residing in this area is about 1500 nGy per hour. There are several high-background areas in Brazil, a monazite sand region along the Atlantic coast comprising the towns of Guarapari, Meaipe, and Cumuruxatiba. Absorbed dose ranges in the air in these towns are as high as 5400 nGy per hour, or 175 mGy per year in selected spots on the beach. In addition to these areas, there are several volcanic regions in the state of Minas Gerais. Absorbed dose rates in air of up to 3×10^{-6} Gy per hour have been reported; however, this particular area is uninhabited and quite small. Other high-background areas have also been identified. On the Egyptian and Ganges Delta, dose rates are estimated to be in the range of 4×10^{-7} Gy per hour. In areas where there is a lot of

uranium, such as in Ramsar, Iran, on the Caspian Sea, dose rates up to 3×10^{-5} Gy per hour have been reported. Extremely high levels have also been found in localized areas in Sweden, which range up to 1×10^{-4} Gy per hour. The highest levels in the United States are in Denver and the Reading Prong section in New Jersey, which are both about 180 nGy per hour absorbed dose rate in air.

Both cosmogenic and primordial radionuclides produce internal radiation doses when they are inhaled or ingested. The average body burden of such radionuclides in a 70-kg man are as follows:

1. Potassium 40: 4.4×10^3 Bq
2. Rubium 87: 455 Bq
3. Carbon 14: 330 Bq
4. Hydrogen 3 (tritium): 40 Bq
5. Radium 226: 4 Bq
6. Thorium 232: <4 Bq

Although they are not considered in discussions of internal body burden, the short-lived decay products of radon 222 are the most important, accounting for more

Table 2-9 • Actinum Series

Nuclide	Historical Name	Half-life	α		β		γ	
			MAJOR RADIATION ENERGIES (MeV) AND INTENSITIES					
$^{235}_{92}$U	Actinoranium	7.04 × 10^8 yr	4.37 4.40 4.5–4.6	(18%) (56%) (11%)	—		0.144 0.186 0.205	(11%) (54%) (5%)
$^{231}_{90}$Th	Uranium Y	25.5 hr	—		0.205 0.287 0.304	(15%) (49%) (35%)	0.026 0.0842	(14.8%) (6.5%)
$^{231}_{91}$Pa	Protoactinium	3.28 × 10^4 yr	4.95 5.01	(23%) (26%)	—		0.027 0.303	(9.6%) (4.6%)
$^{227}_{89}$Ac 98.6% | 1.4%	Actinium	21.8 yr	4.95 4.95	(0.53%) (0.66%)	0.043	(~99%)	0.070 0.10	(0.02%) (0.32%)
$^{227}_{90}$Th	Radioactinium	18.7 d	5.76 5.98 6.04	(20%) (23%) (24%)	—		0.050 0.236 0.30–0.33	(8%) (11%) (5.8%)
$^{223}_{87}$Fr	Actinium K	22 m	5.44	(~0.005%)	1.15	(~100%)	0.050 0.080 0.235	(34%) (9%) (3%)
$^{223}_{88}$Ra	Actinium X	11.43 d	5.61 5.71 5.75	(24%) (52%) (9%)	—		0.154 0.270 0.32–0.34	(6%) (13%) (6%)
$^{219}_{86}$Rn	Emanation Actinon (An)	3.96 s	6.42 6.55 6.81	(7%) (12%) (81%)	—		0.271	(10%)
$^{216}_{84}$Po ~100% | 0.00023%	Actinium A	1.78 ms	7.38	(~100%)	0.74	(~0.00023%)	0.439	(0.04%)
$^{211}_{82}$Pb	Actinium B	36.1 m			0.26 0.97 1.37	(4.8%) (1.4%) (93%)	0.405 0.427 0.832	(3%) (1.4%) (2.8%)
$^{215}_{85}$At	Astatine	~0.1 ms	8.03	(~100%)	—		—	
$^{211}_{83}$Bi 0.28% | 99.7%	Actinium C	2.14 m	6.28 6.62	(16%) (84%)	0.58	(0.27%)	0.351	(13%)
$^{211}_{84}$Po	Actinium C′	0.52 s	7.42	(99%)			0.570 0.90	(0.5%) (0.5%)
$^{207}_{81}$Tl	Actinium C″	4.77 m	—		1.42	(99.8%)	0.897	(0.24%)
$^{207}_{82}$Pb	Actinium D	Stable	—		—		—	

Adapted from Shleien B: The Health Physics Radiological Health Handbook. Silver Spring, MD, Scinta, Inc., 1992.

Table 2-10 • Natural Radionuclide Content in Soil in the United States (Bq/kg)

Radionuclide	Mean	Range
^{40}K	370	100–700
^{238}U	35	4–140
^{226}Ra	40	8–160
^{232}Th	35	4–130

From United Nations Scientific Committee on the Effects of Atomic Radiation (UNSCEAR): Sources and effects of ionizing radiation: UNSCEAR 1993 report to the General Assembly, with scientific annexes. New York, United Nations, 1993.

than 70% of the effective dose from internal emitters. In decreasing order of importance for internal irradiation are potassium 40 (13%), decay products of radon 220 (13%), and lead and polonium 210 (8%). There are other natural radionuclides such as tritium, but they are of less importance. Uranium 238 decays into 15 major nuclides, including uranium 234, thorium 230, radium 226, radon 222, polonium 214, lead 210, and polonium 210. For uranium, thorium, and radium, a small amount is inhaled; however, much more enters the body via ingestion. In contrast, radon 222 mainly exposes humans via the

Table 2-11 • Reference Values for Radionuclides of the Uranium and Thorium Series in Human Tissues*

Nuclide	Lung	Liver	Kidney	Muscle and Other Tissues	Bone
^{238}U	20	3	30	5	100
^{230}Th	20	9	5	1	20–70
^{226}Ra	4	4	4	4	260
^{210}Pb	200	600	600	100	2400
^{210}Po	200	600	600	100	2400
^{232}Th	20	3	3	1	6–24
^{228}Ra	20	3	2	2	100

*Concentration in mBq/kg.
From United Nations Scientific Committee on the Effects of Atomic Radiation (UNSCEAR): Sources and effects of ionizing radiation: UNSCEAR 1993 report to the General Assembly, with scientific annexes. New York, United Nations, 1993.

inhalation route. Values of radon concentration in outdoor air range between 0.1 and 10 Bq/m^3. In some countries, the dose to humans caused by inhaled radon daughter radionuclides constitutes more than 60% of the radiation dose from natural sources. Radon 222 (^{222}Rn) is produced by the decay of radium 226, and decays by alpha emission with a half-life of 3.8 days to polonium 218 (radon A), then to lead 214 (radon B), bismuth 214 (radon C), polonium 214 (radon C^1), and, finally, to stable lead 206. These daughter products have a half-life of only about 30 minutes. The major alpha dose to the tracheobronchial region is from the polonium 218, rather than from the radon 222 itself. Thoron (^{220}Rn) is produced by decay of radium 224 in the

Table 2-12 • National Estimates of the Average Annual Effective Dose from Terrestrial Gamma Rays

Country	μSv
Bulgaria	450
Canada	230
China	550
Denmark	360
Finland	490
Germany	410
Japan	300
Norway	480
Spain	400
Sweden	650
United Kingdom	350
United States	280

The conversion coefficient of 0.7 Sv/Gy is used to convert absorbed dose in air to effective dose.
From United Nations Scientific Committee on the Effects of Atomic Radiation (UNSCEAR): Sources and effects of ionizing radiation: UNSCEAR 1993 report to the General Assembly, with scientific annexes. New York, United Nations, 1993.

thorium series and decays by alpha emission to polonium 216 and subsequently to stable lead 208.

Radon and its breakdown products are in the decay chain from uranium 238. Uranium 238 decays to radium 226, which has a half-life of 1600 years.[10] Radon is a noble gas that is colorless, odorless, and chemically nonreactive. Radon 222 is produced by alpha decay of radium 226. Because radon is a gas, it diffuses from the point of origin. The amount depends on factors such as soil porosity, local concentrations of radium 226, temperature, and atmospheric pressure. Concentration in the open air is low due to rapid mixing, although radon can build up in enclosed spaces. Radon moves by diffusion and pressure flow into basements and buildings. Radon itself poses little biologic threat. Like other inert gases it is breathed in and out of the lungs without significant interaction with body tissues. Alpha particles generated by radon outside the body do not penetrate the skin. The biologic danger arises from the radon daughters. A fraction of these aerosols can be deposited in the tracheobronchial tree. Both polonium isotopes, 218 and 214, emit alpha particles.

Radon activity is measured either in curies (Ci) or becquerels (Bq). The typical concentrations in air are expressed as picocuries per liter or becquerels per cubic meter. Measurement of radon daughter activity, however, is historically derived from monitoring done in uranium mines. One working level (WL) is defined as any combination of radon daughters in 1 liter of air that results in the release of 1.3×10^5 MeV of alpha energy. This is approximately the amount of alpha energy imparted by the radon daughters in equilibrium with a radon concentration of 3700 Bq per cubic meter (100 pCi/L). Exposure entails time, as well as activity, and, therefore, literature usually expresses exposure in terms of working level months (WLM). One month is defined as 170 hours (a figure based on a 40-hour work week). Continuous exposure from the environment at an average of 1 WL for 168 hours per week, therefore, will produce a cumulative exposure of over 4.3 WLM per month. WL, or WLM, are a measure of exposure and not of dose. Relationship of exposure to dose is complex for radon and its daughter products. Typically, radon concentration is easier to measure than radon daughters, but the conversion of radon concentration to WL is close only if the gas is in equilibrium with its daughter products. Another uncertainty is what proportion of the radon daughters attaches to aerosols. Most of them do, but a small proportion does not. All of the unattached fraction deposits in the bronchial tree and, therefore, has a greater biological impact.

Measurement of radon is much cheaper and easier than measuring radon daughters. It can be done with a number of devices. For long-term measurements an etched track detector is widely used. Other measurements are determined by using small canisters that contain activated charcoal. Typical outdoor levels of radon (^{222}Rn) are about 7 Bq/m^3 (0.2 pCi/L). Typical indoor concentrations of radon are about 45 Bq/m^3 (1.2 pCi/L). Outdoors, there are both diurnal and seasonal variations of radon. Radon concentration is highest at midnight and at a minimum at approximately noon. The variation (of radon) during the day is a function of mixing of the air, although radon concentration usually decreases with altitude. The seasonal variations include a minimum concentration of radon in the spring and summer caused by mixing of the air. It is estimated that about 9.25×10^{20} Bq/m^3 (2.5×10^8 Ci) is released predominantly from the soil on a global annual basis. This leads to an average outdoor air concentration over land masses of 7.4×10^4 Bq (200 pCi/m^3); concentrations of radon in air over oceans and arctic areas are one or two orders of magnitude lower.

Radon concentration is much higher indoors than outdoors (discussed further in the section Technologically Modified Sources). With respect to the thorium 232 decay series, there are strong similarities with the uranium 238 decay series, and there are some isotopes of the same elements, including radium, radon, lead, and polonium. Of this series, radon 220 is probably the most important, with inhalation again being the major exposure route. The outdoor concentration of radon 220 is estimated to be approximately 0.2 Bq/m^3 (0.007 pCi/L). Of the primordial radionuclides other than the uranium, thorium, and actinium series, only ^{40}K and ^{87}Rb are significant internal sources of radiation. Potassium is an essential element with an average concentration of about 2 g of potassium in each kilogram of body weight. The isotopic ratio of ^{40}K is 1.18×10^{-4}, and the average activity concentration of ^{40}K in the body is about 60 Bq/kg. Potassium 40 is quite abundant in muscle tissue and can be used to give estimates of the lean body mass. The highest annual absorbed dose of 270 μGy is received by the red bone marrow. The annual effective dose from ^{40}K is approximately 165 μSv for adults and 185 μSv for children. The average activity concentration of ^{87}Rb in the body is 8.5 Bq/kg; bone-lining cells receive the highest annual dose of any body tissues, approximately 14 μGy. The annual effective dose from ^{87}Rb is estimated to be about 6 μSv. The worldwide average, annual effective dose from external exposure to terrestrial radionuclides is 0.46 mSv and the committed dose from annual intakes is 0.25 mSv.

Summary

In summary, natural sources of radiation include cosmic rays, cosmogenic radionuclides, and primordial radionuclides, which result in both external and internal radiation exposure. The annual absorbed dose resulting from radionuclides in the soil, as well as the cosmic ray component due to altitude, varies substantially throughout the country and world (Fig. 2-3 and Table 2-13). The average outdoor absorbed dose rate in air from terrestrial sources is 6×10^{-8} Gy per hour. The relative contributions of

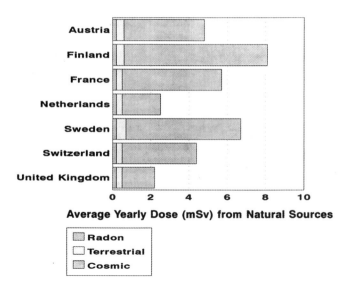

Figure 2-3 • Variation in effective dose from natural radiation sources in countries located near each other. The largest contributor is radon.

^{40}K, ^{238}U, and ^{232}Th are about 35%, 25%, and 40%, respectively. Decay products of the uranium 238 decay series (particularly radon 222) account for more than half of the effective dose. Worldwide averages for effective doses from natural background are shown in Table 2-14.

TECHNOLOGICALLY MODIFIED SOURCES

Radiation exposure may be enhanced in several ways by technologic processes, through modification of natural sources of radiation (e.g., enhanced exposure to cosmic rays from air travel), or by technologic modifications and production of radiation sources (such as occupational exposure or nuclear weapons fallout).

Modification of Natural Radiation Sources

Technology may modify natural sources so that the radiation exposure to the population is decreased rather than increased. However, in terms of radiation effects, only activities that increase radiation exposure to the population will be considered here.

Fossil Fuel

Although fossil fuel contains a small amount of cosmogenic radionuclides, the major source of radiation exposure following the burning of fossil fuel results from dispersion of primordial radionuclides and potassium 40. Coal contains more radionuclides than the other types of fossil fuels, and burning coal produces a large amount of particulate emissions. The major pathway for population radiation exposure around coal-fired power plants is through inhalation. Fly ash from such plants has substantially more radioactivity than the coal itself. Coal has the

Table 2-13 • Total Average Annual Doses (mSv/yr) Effective Dose Equivalent in Various States

State	Cosmic	Terrestrial	Radon	Total
Alabama	0.271	0.225	1.70	2.196
Alaska	0.266	0.292	0.97	1.529
Arizona	0.315	0.292	2.50	3.107
Arkansas	0.275	0.191	1.42	1.886
California	0.268	0.232	1.26	1.76
Colorado	0.475	0.426	6.10	7.001
Connecticut	0.264	0.327	1.80	2.391
Delaware	0.263	0.201	1.12	1.584
District of Columbia	0.264	0.227	No data	Not enough data
Florida	0.262	0.143	0.091	1.315
Georgia	0.276	0.257	2.73	3.263
Hawaii	0.263	0.292	No data	Not enough data
Idaho	0.368	0.292	3.42	4.08
Illinois	0.274	0.266	3.43	3.97
Indiana	0.276	0.287	4.01	4.573
Iowa	0.283	0.292	7.27	7.845
Kansas	0.292	0.292	4.74	5.324
Kentucky	0.277	0.278	4.70	5.255
Louisiana	0.266	0.146	No data	Not enough data
Maine	0.268	0.292	2.86	3.42
Maryland	0.264	0.207	4.76	5.231
Massachusetts	0.264	0.29	2.28	2.834
Michigan	0.276	0.292	2.26	2.828
Minnesota	0.285	0.251	3.83	4.366
Mississippi	0.266	0.146	1.60	2.012
Missouri	0.276	0.287	3.50	4.063
Montana	0.363	0.292	No data	Not enough data
Nebraska	0.293	0.292	3.61	4.195
Nevada	0.366	0.212	1.64	2.218
New Hampshire	0.273	0.292	3.78	4.345
New Jersey	0.262	0.28	0.98	1.522
New Mexico	0.457	0.337	2.69	3.484
New York	0.265	0.288	2.23	2.783
North Carolina	0.278	0.244	2.68	3.202
North Dakota	0.299	0.292	7.30	7.891
Ohio	0.277	0.28	4.17	4.727
Oklahoma	0.29	0.288	2.47	3.048
Oregon	0.274	0.292	0.99	1.556
Pennsylvania	0.272	0.232	2.93	3.434
Rhode Island	0.263	0.274	No data	Not enough data
South Carolina	0.259	0.234	No data	Not enough data
South Dakota	0.307	0.292	9.03	9.629
Tennessee	0.276	0.251	5.11	5.637
Texas	0.281	0.182	1.65	2.113
Utah	0.418	0.292	1.96	2.67
Vermont	0.273	0.292	No data	Not enough data
Virginia	0.272	0.214	2.60	3.086
Washington	0.269	0.292	0.79	1.351
West Virginia	0.289	0.299	1.97	2.558
Wisconsin	0.278	0.292	2.93	3.50
Wyoming	0.504	0.292	2.60	3.396
National average*	0.295	0.266	3.03	3.59

*Values differ from Table 2-1 due to different dosimetry methodology.
From Mauro, J: Assessment in Variations in Radiation Exposure in the United States, Report for the U.S. Environmental Protection Agency (EPA), Contract No. EP-D-05-002. Washington, DC, EPA, July 2005.

following concentrations of radionuclides: ^{40}K 50 to 100 Bq/kg, ^{238}U series 16 to 17 Bq/kg, and ^{232}Th series 8 to 27 Bq/kg. For fly ash the values are 250 to 700, 200 to 900, and 50 to 150, respectively; UNSCEAR has estimated the collective effective dose commitment resulting from atmospheric releases from coal-fired power plants on the basis of unit of energy generated.[1] The best estimate is 2 man sieverts for each gigawatt of energy generated. Worldwide effective dose commitment is estimated to be 10^5 man sieverts.

Table 2-14 • Average Annual Contribution to Effective Dose (mSv) from Various Sources of Natural Background Radiation in the World

Element of Exposure	In Areas of Normal Background	In Areas of Elevated Exposures
Cosmic rays	0.39*	2.0
Terrestrial gamma rays	0.48	4.3
Internal irradiation	0.25	0.6
Radon and its decay products		
Inhalation of radon 222	1.15	10
Inhalation of radon 220	0.1	0.1
Ingestion of radon 222	0.005	0.1
Total	~2.4	†

*Includes 10 mSv from cosmogenic radionuclides.
†A total value is not given, because elevated doses from all elements of exposure would not be expected to coincide at a single location.
From United Nations Scientific Committee on the Effects of Atomic Radiation (UNSCEAR): Sources and effects of ionizing radiation: UNSCEAR 1993 report to the General Assembly, with scientific annexes. New York, United Nations, 1993.

Phosphate Fertilizers

Phosphate rock is mined and used primarily as fertilizer, but some of the by-products are used in the building industry. Radiation exposure due to phosphate usage comes predominantly from the uranium 238 decay series of primordial radionuclides. The predominant by-product use is that of gypsum as a building material in homes. Although only 10% of by-product gypsum is so used, this is by far the most important contributor to the total dose from uses of phosphate rock. The worldwide collective effective dose commitment for 1977 production was estimated to be 3×10^5 man sieverts, of which only 6×10^3 man sieverts was due to commitments from portions of the phosphate cycle other than gypsum use.

Buildings

Many kinds of building materials such as stone and brick (as well as gypsum) lead to higher-than-average external absorbed doses. As mentioned earlier, the dose rate outdoors from terrestrial gamma rays is about 56 nGy per hour. The overall effect of building material surrounding persons indoors is to increase the dose rate by 40% to 50%. Thus, the average for indoor measurements is about 80 nGy per hour. This, obviously, varies substantially, depending on the building construction. In granite houses in the United Kingdom dose rates are approximately 100 nGy per hour. In houses made with mud blocks in Jamaica, the rates are 200 nGy per hour. Measurements in Czechoslovakia, where some houses are made with outside walls containing uraniferous coal slag, indicate dose rates approaching 1000 nGy per hour. In addition to the actual construction materials, radon is captured within the building and may reach significant concentrations. Thoron 220 also can enter a building; however, the annual effective dose from thoron and its decay products is essentially insignificant when compared to radon 222. Ventilation can reduce any indoor radon concentration effectively to outdoor concentrations, but this requires about 4 air changes each hour. Such ventilation rates are rarely attained in buildings, and thus indoor concentrations of radon are usually substantially higher than outdoor levels.[11] Radon exposure in dwellings is caused primarily by radium in the soil itself, although radon in water may be a source of radon in the air in some dwellings. Natural gas may contain radon, although when natural gas is used, it is normally vented. Radon and thoron may also be released by the walls, floor, or ceilings if they are constructed of rock or soil. The radium concentration in soil and rocks can vary substantially, even in different regions of the same country. Of course, there is significant variation of indoor radon concentrations around the world. As is obvious from examination of the means and the maximum values, the national mean values mask marked regional variations within a country. Very high radon concentrations are generally found adjacent to areas of uranium mining. The soil in unpaved crawl spaces is a major radon source in some houses in the United States. Typically, remedial action in homes is suggested when the radon concentration exceeds 400 Bq/m^3 (11 pCi/L).

The relative significance of different radon sources in a reference house is shown in Table 2-15. NCRP Report 78[10] indicates that the annual absorbed doses to basal cells in the bronchial epithelium from the "average" indoor and outdoor activities of the population are as

Table 2-15 • Variation in Radon Concentration and Resulting Lung Doses with Type of Structure

		MEAN AIR CONCENTRATION (pCi/m³)		
	Working Level (WL)	Mean	Range	Mean Lung Dose (mSv/yr)
Outdoors	0.0016	180	(100–300)	1.2
First Floor	0.0041	830	(150–3000)	5.7
Cellars	0.0081	1700	(340–4000)	10.2

1 WL = 100 pCi/L = 3700 Bq/m^3.
From National Council on Radiation Protection and Measurements (NCRP): Radiation exposure of the U.S. population from consumer products and miscellaneous sources. NCRP report no. 95. Bethesda, MD, NCRP, 1987.

follows: male, 1.9 mGy; female, 1.7 mGy; 10-year-old child, 3 mGy; 1-year-old infant, 1.7 mGy. The average lifetime exposure is about 17 WLM. The average dose over 50 years of adult life is about 0.01 Gy for a male and 0.09 Gy for a female. In the United States, this yields a collective annual absorbed dose of about 2.2×10^5 Gy per year to the bronchial epithelial basal cells, or a collective effective dose of about 1.7×10^4 Sv per year. As with the outside air concentrations of radon, inside concentrations also vary diurnally and seasonally. Radon activity in houses is lowest at noontime and highest early in the morning and is approximately twice as high in the winter as in the summer. These variations are a function of the use of cooling units and attempts to keep windows and doors closed during the winter.

Recently, many programs have been developed to conserve energy, including switching off ventilation systems, operating at reduced levels, and sealing of windows and doors. These procedures effectively reduce admission of outside air to the building. Ventilation rate substantially changes the dose rate of the absorbed dose from radon daughters. As the ventilation in the building is reduced from 2 air changes an hour to 1, the dose rate rises approximately fourfold, and if this figure is reduced to 1 air change every 2 hours, it increases approximately eightfold.[11] In general, the indoor environment, because of radon inhalation, produces exposures approximately 20% higher than the outside environment does. For concrete buildings a value of 50% higher is used. Inhalation of radon predominantly results in exposure to the lungs from the inhaled radon daughters. Radon daughters have two basic target tissues: the tracheobronchial basal layer and the pulmonary epithelium. The dose to the lung depends substantially on the size distribution of the aerosol dust to which the daughter products of radon and thoron are attached. On the average, the bronchial basal layer receives a dose five to eight times higher than that to the pulmonary region.

Conversion coefficients relating annual average concentrations to effective dose equivalent have been the subject of a number of publications. As mentioned earlier, the conversion depends substantially on the estimated fraction that is attached to aerosol as well as the dosimetry model used. The conversion of radon gas concentration to effective dose equivalent is typically between 25 and 50 μSv per year per Bq/m^3. For mines and workplaces, the conversion coefficient for effective dose is about 10 mSv per WLM. The effective dose from 1 Bq per hour per m^3 is estimated by UNSCEAR 1993 to be 9 nSv.[12] The average annual effective dose from inhalation of radon progeny outdoors is estimated to be 0.13 mSv and for radon indoors it is estimated to be 1.0 mSv. This assumes 80% of the time is spent indoors and 20% outdoors. The annual dose from inhaled radon that becomes dissolved in tissues is 0.05 mSv. Thus the total average annual effective dose is 1.2 mSv from radon and 0.07 mSv from thoron.

These numbers vary slightly based on assumptions regarding equilibrium coefficients, attached fraction, and residency times.

Exposure to Cosmic Rays

Air travel significantly affects cosmic ray doses. The actual dose received depends on altitude, flight pattern, and duration (Table 2-16). Typical commercial aircrafts operate at altitudes of 7 to 13 km. In 1989 there were 1.8×10^{12} passenger km flown, which translates into 3×10^9 passenger hours. The collective dose from this in terms of global air travel is about 10,000 man Sv. The annual average individual dose in North America is about 10 μSv.

Aircraft crew members, professional couriers, and frequent fliers all receive more than this annual dose. Aircraft crew members receive 1800 μSv, professional couriers receive about 3600 μSv, and a frequent flier receives an annual effective dose of approximately 90 μSv. Supersonic planes, such as the Concord, typically operated at altitudes of 15 km. The average dose was approximately 12 μSv per hour, but it can reach a maximum of 40 μSv per hour. This can be contrasted with the typical dose rate for regular commercial airliners of 4 to 8 μSv per hour at altitudes of 9 to 12 km and a latitude of 50 degrees. Dose rates at lower latitudes are generally lower and a dose rate of 4 μSv per hour is generally the average for long haul (transatlantic) flights. For short haul flights the altitude is lower and the dose rate is about 3 μSv per hour. For the supersonic planes, annual doses to the air crew are about 2.5 mSv, but maximums of 17 mSv have been recorded.

Space travel also increases the cosmic ray component.[13] The effective doses vary substantially depending on orbit, shielding, solar activity, and other factors. Space flight in low earth orbits, measured on U.S. shuttle missions and Russian space missions, range from 100 to 700 μSv per day.

Consumer Products

Many consumer products contain various radionuclides.[14] In general, these are deliberately incorporated to use the radioactive decay. Items included in these categories are

Table 2-16 • Cosmic Ray Doses to a Person Flying in Aircraft (Dose/Roundtrip)*

	Subsonic Flight (μGy)	Supersonic Flight (μGy)
Los Angeles to Paris	48	37
Chicago to Paris	36	26
New York to Paris	31	24
New York to London	29	22
Los Angeles to New York	19	13

*Under normal circumstances without solar flares.
Adapted from Wallace, R: Measurements of the cosmic radiation dose in subsonic commercial aircraft compared to the city–pair dose calculation. Lawrence Berkeley Laboratory Report No. 1505, 1975.

radioluminous timepieces (such as watches), electronic and electrical devices (such as television sets), antistatic devices, smoke detectors (0.07 mSv/year), and miscellaneous items such as the older Coleman lantern mantles (which contained 1.3 kBq of thorium 232). Radium 226, promethium 147, and hydrogen 3 (tritium) are used to make the luminous numbers on watches and clocks. For old wristwatches containing radium 226, the annual gonadal dose is almost always less than 40 µGy. Most watches, however, use tritium rather than radium, and the external dose to the individual wearer from tritium is essentially negligible. This is because tritium emits only very low-energy beta-minus particles. The annual dose to the wearer of such a watch is approximately 0.3 µGy. Liquid crystal watch displays often use gaseous tritium light sources. For these applications, the tritium content is higher than in a painted watch. There is some absorption of the beta particles in the glass tube in the face of the watch, and, therefore, the dose to the wearer is essentially the same as that from a tritium-painted watch. UNSCEAR estimated the per capita annual effective dose from such radioluminous timepieces to be in the range of 5×10^{-7} Sv.[12]

Electronic equipment, particularly television sets with cathode ray tubes, may emit a small amount of x-radiation, and high-pressure mercury lamps, ignition devices for fluorescent lamps, and some other electronic components may contain radioactive substances. From a public viewpoint, most concern appears to emphasize possible radiation emissions from cathode ray tubes and video display terminals. The video display terminal is quite similar in basic mechanism to a standard television set and is commonplace for airline scheduling, word processing, and computer entry terminals. Many reports have indicated that video display terminals emit little, if any, ionizing radiation under normal operating conditions.[15–17] Performance standards limit x-ray emissions from television receivers to 1.3×10^{-7} C/kg per hour at 5 cm from the surface of the set. Emissions for television sets have been reviewed in a publication from the U.S. Department of Health and Human Services.[18] For the most part, on the older, tube-type sets, once the radiation emissions exceeded allowable standards, the picture quality deteriorated to the point that the set was no longer useful. The newer solid-state televisions emit a negligible amount of radiation and then only when the picture is visible. The primary source of ionizing radiation in the video display terminal is the cathode ray tube. Most of this radiation does not escape from the image tube because of the attenuation provided by the high-lead-content glass envelope. Testing of tube-type video display terminals has indicated that likely emission is in the range of 0.26 $\times 10^{-7}$ C/kg per hour or less. If one assumes viewing of 6 hours per day, 5 days a week, and 50 weeks per year, the annual radiation dose to the individual 2 inches in front of the surface of the screen emitting 0.26×10^{-7} C/kg per hour would be 1.5 mSv. Essentially nobody views the terminal from a distance as close as 2 inches, and the radiation dose decreases substantially with distance. For example, increasing the distance to 2 feet would reduce radiation exposure by a factor over 100.

Nonionizing radiation may also be emitted from video display terminals. These electromagnetic spectrum radiations include ultraviolet, visible light, infrared, microwave, radiofrequency, and radiation in the acoustic spectrum. The biologic effects of these radiations are beyond the scope of the present text; however, measurements of nonionizing radiation from such terminals have been analyzed and reported by the U.S. Department of Health and Human Services.[18] Ultrasound emitted by video display terminals has also been measured. Very high levels of ultrasound have been associated with fatigue, headaches, tinnitus, instability, and nausea. These have been reported at exposures in the range greater than 70 decibels (db). Acoustic measurements of video display terminals by the Bureau of Radiological Health were all below this range. Similarly, measurements of optical radiation and radiation in the near ultraviolet or near infrared region have also been measured and have been found to be substantially lower than existing standards and guidelines. Very high exposure to this type of radiation occasionally results in skin and eye burns and ultimately cataract formation. The Bureau of Radiological Health has suggested that working conditions are the primary cause of video display terminal user complaints rather than any radiation emission because testing of the terminals under normal operating and worst-case conditions all fell within current standards and guidelines for each type of radiation. The health of video display terminal workers has been shown to be affected by items such as fatigue, posture, environment, glare, ambient noise, or duration.

Antistatic devices contain radioactive substances and are widely used. These usually contain 18.5 to 37 MBq polonium 210 sources, which is primarily an alpha emitter. Because the half-life is 138 days, these devices are rarely effective for more than 1 year. UNSCEAR estimated the annual effective dose to be in the range of 10^{-8} Sv.[19] Smoke detectors may be of either the optical type or ionization type. In the ionization smoke detectors, most use americium 241 as the source of the ionization. Smoke detectors in commercial buildings may contain up to 3.7 MBq of ^{241}Am, whereas household units use 185 kBq or less. Other consumer product uses of radionuclides are the inclusion of thorium in incandescent mantles and uranium and thorium in the manufacture of some glass and porcelain. Overall, these substances yield a negligible amount of radiation exposure to individuals unless they are internally ingested. The consumer products that deliver the greatest radiation dose are probably tobacco products (Table 2-17) because of the localized radiation to the bronchial epithelium from radionuclides (such as lead 210 and polonium 210) in tobacco smoke.

Table 2-17 • Radiation Exposure in the United States from Consumer Products and Miscellaneous Sources

Source	Average Annual Effective Dose Equivalent to an Exposed Person (μSv)	Annual Collective Effective Dose Equivalent in U.S. (person Sv)
Televisions (tube type)	<10	<2300
Video display terminals	<10	<500
Airport luggage x-ray	0.021	0.6
Tritium watches and clocks	1	12
Smoke detectors	0.08	8
Road materials	40	200
Building materials	70	8400
Domestic water (radon)	10–60	2300–14,000
Fertilizers	5–50	<2000
Combustible fuels		
Coal	0.3–3.0	80–700
Natural gas	22	790
Propane	1.3	23
Tobacco products	160,000*	—

*Bronchial epithelium dose equivalent.
Note: At the time this table was compiled, standard measurement of dose was "effective dose equivalent." Since that time the measurement has been changed to "effective dose." The two measurements vary slightly. The data in this table are calculated according to "effective dose equivalent."
Data from National Council on Radiation Protection and Measurements (NCRP): Radiation exposure of the U.S. population from consumer products and miscellaneous sources. Report no. 95. Bethesda, MD, NCRP, 1987.

Security Screening Devices

Inspection of hand-carried baggage in airports and other forms of cargo screening has also been a subject of interest. It has been estimated that the average exposure to the traveler in each trip from the inspection of such luggage is less than 4×10^{-10} coul/kg of luggage. This corresponds to an effective dose of 7×10^{-9} Sv, or about 1% of the radiation incurred during a transcontinental flight. Scanners for screening of individuals themselves are either backscatter or transmission systems.[20] For current x-ray backscatter systems the effective dose for an anterior scan is 0.03 μSv and 0.01 to 0.02 μSv for a posterior scan. The dose to the operator or to a nearby person (outside the primary beam) is indistinguishable from background. The current transmission x-ray system gives an effective dose of 3 to 6 μSv per scan. Cargo container scanners usually use ^{137}Cs or ^{60}Co sources or machine-generated x-rays or neutrons. Depending on the system, doses to an individual hiding in a container could range from 0.1 to approximately 100 μSv per scan.[20]

Summary

Technologic enhancement of natural sources occurs under many circumstances. The largest technologically enhanced source of radiation dose to the population is a result of energy conservation and exposure to radon in buildings. Of the various other activities, the highest calculated effective dose equivalent probably results from tobacco products and to a much smaller extent the wearing of radioluminous watches. Items that have received extensive public attention (including video display terminals) are essentially negligible in terms of exposure to the individual.

TECHNOLOGIC PRODUCTION OF RADIATION

Fallout

Atmospheric nuclear testing began in 1945. Very large weapons test programs were conducted between 1954 and 1962 and have continued. There have been 502 atmospheric and 1876 underground nuclear explosions as of 2000. A well-contained underground nuclear explosion delivers an extremely low-dose commitment, if any, to any group of people, although there is occasional "venting" of such tests. The estimated yields of all the underground tests are approximately 90 megatons (MT). The estimated yields of atmospheric nuclear explosions between 1943 and 2000 by country are as follows: United States, 197 MT; USSR, 219 MT; United Kingdom, 21 MT; France, 45 MT; China, 22 MT; for a total of 504 MT. Current estimates are that the world inventory of nuclear arsenals is more than 40,000 weapons with a total yield of over 13,000 MT. Each weapon on the average contains 4 kg of plutonium. Radionuclides released in atmospheric explosions may enter the body or may be deposited on the earth's surface. Deposited radionuclides result in either external radiation or internal radiation through ingestion. Most estimates of fallout exposure to the world's population do not include tropospheric (local) fallout but are rather concerned with atmospheric (particularly stratospheric) fallout. Particles carried into the stratosphere give rise to worldwide fallout, accounting for most of the worldwide contamination of long-lived fission products. Fallout and weapons testing result in internal irradiation of individuals by tritium (hydrogen 3), carbon 14, manganese 54, iodine 131, iron 55, strontium 89 and 90, ruthenium

106, cesium 136 and 137, barium 140, cerium 144, and plutonium and transplutonic elements. Estimates of the collective effective dose commitment to the world's population from the various radionuclides involved in weapons explosions are shown in Table 2-18.

The radionuclide that contributes the highest percentage (70%) of the total effective dose commitment from weapon testing is carbon 14. This commitment, however, will be delivered over thousands of years to the population and not to any one generation. Cesium 137 accounts for 14% of the commitment; zirconium 95, 5.3%; strontium 90, 3.2%; ruthenium 106, 2.2%; cerium 144, 1.4%; tritium, 1.2%; and all the rest, less than 1%. In considering fallout radionuclides, the contribution from ingestion is about four times higher than that of external irradiation, and external irradiation is five times greater than doses from inhalation of those radionuclides. UNSCEAR indicates that the collective effective dose commitment to the world population over 10,000 years for nuclear explosions carried out to the end of 1980 is 22.3×10^6 man Sv.[24] This corresponds to exposing a member of the population to an additional 3 years of natural background radiation over his or her lifetime. The commitment is slightly higher in the northern hemisphere than in the southern hemisphere. The annual per capita absorbed dose from fallout radionuclides is approximately 45 µSv. The average effective dose from global fallout received by the world's population from all pathways before 2000 was 994 µSv, projected doses from 2000–2100 are 253 µSv, and doses beyond the year 2100 are estimated to be 2240 µSv.

Nuclear Power Production

Exposures from nuclear power production include those occupational exposures incurred during mining, uranium fuel fabrication, reactor operation, and waste storage and disposal.[21] An additional source is environmental dispersion of radionuclides, particularly krypton 85, tritium, carbon 14, and iodine 129. Accidents occurring in reactors also contribute a small portion of the exposure to the population. The overall impact of nuclear power generation on total population exposure is very small. The collective effective dose is two orders of magnitude less than that from atmospheric weapons testing. Worldwide annual collective effective dose is 4×10^5 man Sv, which is a per capita effective dose of about 0.1 µSv. This represents only 0.005% of the average exposure to natural sources of radiation. The majority of the collective effective dose comes from the atmospheric releases of radionuclides, particularly carbon 14 (25%) and radon 222 (75%). The former is released from reactors, and the latter is from mine tailings. As discussed earlier in the section on fossil fuel, atmospheric releases of radionuclides from fossil fuel plants (particularly coal plants without scrubber systems) may be substantially greater than environmental releases of radionuclides from nuclear plants. The relative

Table 2-18 • Collective Effective Dose Commitment to the World's Population from Various Radionuclides in Fallout

Radionuclide	Stratospheric Input	Collective Effective Dose Equivalent Commitment
Tritium (hydrogen 3)	186 EBq*	1.9×10^5 man Sv‡
Carbon 14	213 PBq†	2.6×10^7 man Sv
Manganese 54	3.9 EBq	130 man Sv
Iron 55	1.5 EBq	3.10^4 man Sv
Krypton 85	160 PBq	20 man Sv
Strontium 89	117 EBq	3.2×10^3 man Sv (ingestion)
		5.8×10^3 man Sv (inhalation)
Strontium 90	0.6 EBq	2.8×10^4 man Sv
Ruthenium 103	247 EBq	
Ruthenium 106	12 EBq	9.6×10^4 man Sv
Iodine 131	675 EBq	1.1×10^5 man Sv
Cesium 137	0.95 EBq	1.2×103 man Sv (inhalation)
		6.9×10^5 man Sv (ingestion)
Barium 140	759 EBq	670 man Sv
Cerium 144	31 EBq	1.2×10^5 man Sv
Plutonium 238	0.33 PBq	0.3×10^4 man Sv
Plutonium 239	6.5 PBq	10×10^4 man Sv
Plutonium 240	4.4 PBq	6×10^4 man Sv
Plutonium 241	142 PBq	3×10^4 man Sv
Americium 241	Unknown	2×10^4 man Sv

*EBq = exa or 10^{18} becquerel = 2.7×10^7 Ci.
†PBq = peta or 10^{15} becquerel = 2.7×10^4 Ci.
‡man Sv = man sievert.
Data from United Nations Scientific Committee on the Effects of Atomic Radiation (UNSCEAR): Ionizing radiation: Sources and effects. UNSCEAR report to the General Assembly, in annex K: Radiation = induced life shortening. New York, United Nations, 1982.

Table 2-19 • Local and Regional Individual Doses (µSv) to the Public from Nuclear Power Production

Mining and milling	6.7
Fuel fabrication	<0.1
Reactor operation	6
Fuel reprocessing	1.9
Transportation	2.2
Total	~17

Data from United Nations Scientific Committee on the Effects of Atomic Radiation (UNSCEAR): Sources and effects of ionizing radiation: UNSCEAR 1993 report to the General Assembly, with scientific annexes. New York, United Nations, 1993.

contribution of each portion of the nuclear fuel cycle is shown in Table 2-19.

The dose to the population is a function of distance from the nuclear power plant; however, under normal operating conditions, U.S. regulations limit the annual absorbed dose to the population at the site boundary to less than 50 µSv. This is the maximal dose that can be incurred by an individual who spends 365 days a year at the site boundary and who participates in the ecologic cycle of plants and animals at the site boundary.

In addition to normal operation, nuclear accidents both at civilian nuclear reactors and military installations have contributed to radiation exposure to the world's population. The Three Mile Island accident near Harrisburg, Pennsylvania, had relatively small environmental releases. Most releases were from xenon 133 and iodine 131. Individual doses within 80 km of the plant averaged 15 µGy, and the collective whole-body dose within 80 km of the plant was 20 man Sv. The releases from Chernobyl were much higher. The major radionuclides of interest are iodine 131 and cesium 134 and 137. The collective effective dose from the accident was estimated to be about 600,000 man Sv, of which 40% was received in the former Soviet Union, 57% in the remainder of Europe, and 3% in the other countries of the northern hemisphere. An accident occurred at a graphite reactor in Windscale in the United Kingdom in 1957. The major release was of iodine 131, and to a lesser extent, cesium 137 and xenon 133. A small amount of polonium 210 was also released. The collective effective dose from this accident in the United Kingdom and Europe was estimated to have been 2000 man Sv. Another accident occurred in the early 1950s at a plutonium production center near Kyshtym in Russia. Exposure was due to strontium 90, and the collective effective dose was between 1000 and 3000 man Sv. A number of other accidents have occurred, which generally have resulted in less collective effective dose. These include accidents involving transported nuclear weapons, satellite reentry, and accidents involving medical or industrial radioactive materials.

Occupational Exposure

Occupational exposures occur in management of the nuclear fuel cycle, medical uses of radiation, research, industry, and in miscellaneous sources activities, such as aviation, nonuranium mining, and use of phosphate fertilizers.[22] In the United States there are about 1.1 million persons who are potentially exposed on an occupational basis. About one half of these receive a measurable dose. The mean yearly dose equivalent for all workers is about 1.1 mSv, and the total annual collective effective occupational dose in the United States is about 2000 man Sv. The annual collective effective dose worldwide in 1985 to 1989 was estimated to be 4400 man Sv. The components of this are 1900 man Sv from the nuclear fuel cycle, 1200 man Sv from industrial uses, 240 man Sv from defense activities, and 110 man Sv from medical uses. UNSCEAR 2000 has estimated that worldwide occupational collective dose annually from 1990 to 1994 for 11.1 million monitored workers was 14,000 man Sv with an average annual effective dose to monitored workers of 0.1 mSv. The majority of this (11,700 man Sv) came from natural radiation sources such as radon. As might be expected, most is received by workers who are between 20 and 39 years of age, with the mean age being 33 to 34 years. The number of occupationally exposed persons has increased rapidly in the United States from 0.3 million in 1960 to 0.8 million in 1970 and 1.3 million in 1980. However, during the 1960 to 1981 period, the mean annual dose equivalent decreased from 1.8 mSv to 1.1 mSv. About 80% of workers received an annual dose equivalent of less than 1 mSv, 95% received less than 10 mSv, and 99.9% received less than the allowable limit of 50 mSv. The individual occupational annual dose equivalent for workers at nuclear power plants varies with the reactor type: 2.1 mSv for pressurized water reactors, and 2.3 mSv for boiling water reactors. Exposures in both uranium and nonuranium mines contribute significantly to occupational exposure. In the United States it is estimated that about 51,000 coal miners and 15,000 others are engaged in mining—a total of 66,000 persons. Exposure to radon and decay products in coal mines is approximately 0.1 WLM per year. At the present time there are very few operational uranium mines in the United States. Radon levels in uranium mines vary significantly as a function of concentration of uranium, ventilation, and other factors. The mean cumulative exposure for miners in the uranium mines in New Mexico from 1950 to 1985 was 111 WLM. In the Colorado mines, the mean cumulative exposure from 1951 to 1982 was 882 WLM. The number of people potentially exposed to radiation by occupation in the United States in the period 1985 to 1989, and the relative contributions of some types of occupational exposures, are shown in Table 2-20.

Overall, Table 2-20 indicates that occupational exposure is approximately equal for workers in power reactor

Table 2-20 • Occupational Exposure of Monitored Workers in the United States (1990–1994)

Occupation	Annual Number of Workers (thousands)	Average Annual Effective Dose (mSv)	Annual Collective Effective Dose (man Sv)
Well logging*	7.6	1.4	10
Industrial radiography	5.6	3.3	18
Accelerators*	4	0.5	2
Isotope production	4	1.6	7
Uranium mining	0.3	—	1
Uranium enrichment	3	0.12	0.4
Fuel fabrication	9	0.6	5
Fuel cycle research*	32	1.6	19
Fuel reprocessing	5	0.3	1.6
Nuclear reactors			
Pressurized water	114	1.3	154
Boiling water	40	1.7	131
Defense activities	73	0.6	69
Education and research*	17	0.4	6
Medical*	734	0.4	280
Airline crews*	97	1.7	165

*Refers to the period 1985–1989.
Data from United Nations Scientific Committee of the Effects of Atomic Radiation (UNSCEAR): Sources and effects of ionizing radiation: UNSCEAR 2000 report to the General Assembly, with scientific annexes. 2 vols. New York, United Nations, 2000.

operation, medical care, and flying in airplanes. Airline crews generally receive absorbed doses of radiation greater than those of diagnostic x-ray technologists.

MEDICAL EXPOSURE

Medical irradiation is normally divided into three categories: (1) diagnostic x-ray examinations, (2) use of radiopharmaceuticals in nuclear medicine, and (3) therapeutic applications of radiation. In many countries, medical exposure is the largest contributor of technologically induced radiation exposure to the population. In well-developed countries with a high degree of medical technology, the exposure from medical sources has approached the contribution from natural sources and has been increasing on an annual basis. Medical exposure as a source is different from most of the other sources discussed previously. Probably the most significant difference is that the person receiving the exposure is the direct recipient of a presumed benefit. Another difference is that medical radiation is almost always delivered to a portion of the body rather than to the whole body and at a high dose rate. To compare this source to the other sources, it is necessary to use the ICRP weighting system and the concept of effective dose discussed in Chapter 1.[23] Use of the concept of effective dose is not completely satisfactory for comparison with other sources because the concept was derived for low-level radiation and radiation protection purposes. The concept involves the implicit assumption that there is a similar age and sex distribution of the exposed populations. This does not occur in most medically irradiated populations. In the United States well over half of x-ray procedures and nuclear medicine

examinations are performed in the over-45-year-old age groups, and over one fourth of this exposure occurs in the over-64-year-old age group.

The frequency and absorbed dose from most diagnostic radiologic procedures in the United States was analyzed in 1964, 1970, and 1980[24–26] and is currently being reanalyzed. The effective doses for various x-ray and nuclear medicine procedures are shown in Table 2-21.

The frequency of diagnostic x-ray examinations performed in the United States has increased dramatically over the last four decades but particularly so in the last decade. The most marked growth has been in computed tomography (CT). CT scans increased from 3 million in 1980, 21 million in 1995, to 67 million in 2006. They are a relatively high-dose procedure with effective doses of about 10 mSv per examination. Increasing use of interventional techniques (particularly coronary angiography with angioplasty and stent placement) have also raised doses in medicine. Other changes in dose from medical procedures have occurred as radiology departments have switched from film to digital receptors. Outpatient x-ray examinations account for about two thirds of the total number of diagnostic x-ray examinations. The estimated total number of medical x-ray examinations in the United States in all settings in 2006 is shown in Table 2-22 and the ratio of examinations to population is shown in Table 2-23. Dental x-rays are probably the most commonly performed diagnostic x-ray examination. The effective dose per intraoral examination is about 5 μSv. The per caput annual dose in the United States in 2006 is about 0.6 mSv from typical radiography and an additional 1.2 mSv from CT scanning.

The UNSCEAR 2000 report estimated that in developed countries from 1991 to 1996 there was a total

Table 2-21 • Effective Doses from Medical Examinations

Examination	Effective Dose per Examination (mSv)
Diagnostic Radiology	
Skull	0.1
Cervical spine	0.20
Thoracic Spine	1.0
Lumbar Spine	1.5
Chest (2 views)	0.1
Abdomen	0.7
Pelvis	0.6
Hip	0.7
Extremity	0.001
Mammography	0.4
Upper Gastrointestinal	6.0
Barium Enema	8.0
Intravenous Pyelogram	3.0
CT scan head	2.0
CT scan chest	7.0
CT scan abdomen and pelvis	14.0
Dental intraoral	0.005
Nuclear Medicine	
Brain	6.9
Hepatobiliary	3.1
Liver/Spleen	2.1
Bone	6.3
Lung Ventilation/Perfusion	2.5
Thyroid	1.9 (with iodine 123)
Infection (WBC)	7.0
Tumor (PET with fluorodeoxyglucose)	14.0
Tumor (non-PET)	13.0
Cardiac (perfusion) (stress test)	9.5
Cardiac blood pool	7.8
Urinary	2.0
PET/CT scan	37.0

Table 2-22 • Estimated Numbers of Selected X-ray Examinations (×1000) Performed in the United States Hospitals

	2006
Skull	330
Head and face	2400
Chest (radiographic)	126,000
Abdomen	15,000
Lumbar spine	
Total spine	17,600
Upper gastrointestinal	4000
Barium enema	700
Pyelograms	1100
Pelvis/hip	20,000
Extremities	57,000
Computed tomography	67,000
Mammography	34,000
Total	345,000

population of 1.3 billion persons and about 1.4 billion medical x-ray examinations were performed annually. This resulted in an annual per caput dose of about 1.2 mSv from medical radiography and 0.01 mSv from dental examinations. The total annual collective effective dose in developed countries was estimated to be 2×10^6 man Sv. The worldwide annual collective effective dose from medical radiography and 1.9 billion examinations was estimated to be between 2.5×10^6 man Sv and the annual per caput dose estimated to be about 0.4 mSv.[27]

Nuclear Medicine

The diagnostic use of radiopharmaceuticals has also increased rapidly in the United States from 3.3 million in 1972, 6.4 million in 1980, to about 20 million examinations annually in 2006 (Table 2-24). Much of the growth has occurred from the relatively high dose stress-rest myocardial perfusion examination. The effective dose from this examination is about 10 mSv. Additional growth and increasing doses are now occurring with the widespread

use of positron emission (PET) and CT scans. These studies have an effective dose of about 37 mSv. Absorbed doses to the whole body, gonads, and critical organs from various radiopharmaceuticals are listed in Appendix 2. At the present time, over 85% of radiopharmaceuticals are labeled with technetium 99m. The administered activity usually is in the range of 100 to 1100 MBq. The effective dose for the most common examinations is in the range of 1 to 10 mSv for each examination. The major exception to use of technetium-99m-labeled radiopharmaceuticals is the increasing used of fluorine 18 fluoro-deoxyglucose and the application of iodine 123 for thyroid uptakes and scans. The per caput effective dose equivalent from nuclear medicine procedures in the United States in 2006 was about 0.8 mSv, and the collective effective dose was about, 230,000 man Sv.

UNSCEAR 2000 estimated that for diagnostic nuclear medicine examinations during the period 1991–1996 in developed countries, there were 29 million examinations annually resulting in an annual per caput dose of 0.08 mSv; the annual collective effective dose was 1.2×10^5 man Sv.[27] For all the countries in the world,

Table 2-23 • Estimated Medical X-Ray Procedures in the United States

	Examinations (Millions)	Population (Millions)	Ratio of Examinations to Population
1964	105	190	0.55
1970	130	203	0.64
1980	180	227	0.79
1990	250–315	250	1.00–1.26
2006	345	300	1.15

Table 2-24 • Estimated Number of Nuclear Medicine Examinations (×1000) in the United States

	1972	1975	1980	1990	2005
Brain	1250	2100	870	—	<100
Hepatobiliary	25	—	50	—	—
Liver	450	680	1150	—	Total GI 1210
Bone	80	220	1300	—	3450
Lung	330	600	900	—	740
Thyroid	450	630	650	—	<100
Tumor	10	20	130	—	340
Cardiovascular	25	50	600	—	9800
Urinary	110	150	200	—	470
Miscellaneous (including infection)	500	350	200	—	380
Total	3230	4800	5850	7500	19,000
U.S. population (millions)	209	215	227	250	300

UNSCEAR 2000 estimated there were 32 million nuclear medicine examinations and that the annual collective effective dose from nuclear medicine was estimated to be between 1.5×10^5 man Sv with a per caput dose of 0.03 mSv.

Radiation Therapy

Radiation therapy has been used predominantly to treat malignant neoplasms, although it does have some limited applications for benign conditions. The therapeutic use of radiation falls into three general categories: (1) external beam therapy, (2) brachytherapy, and (3) radiopharmaceutical therapy. Benign disease conditions often receive doses between 10 and 20 Gy, whereas most malignant conditions require absorbed doses in the range of 50 to 70 Gy, which are usually fractionated over 5 to 6 weeks. These high doses lead to direct, or *nonstochastic*, effects, such as cell killing, arteriolar narrowing, and so on. Some of the normal tissues that lie within or nearby the treatment volume may receive high doses of radiation as well, and thus incur some risk of late effects. Many patients receiving treatment for malignancies have limited life expectancies and are often beyond the childbearing age group; thus, one cannot easily calculate a reasonable effective dose, collective effective dose, or genetically significant dose. In addition, the ICRP weighting factors were designed for radiation protection purposes at low doses and are, therefore, not applicable.

Recently, attention has been directed toward curative therapeutic regimes in young patients, particularly those having the possibility of long-term survival (e.g., children with leukemia, adolescents with Hodgkin's disease). If these individuals survive the malignancy, they are at long-term risk for radiation carcinogenesis; it is important to assess the number of such individuals at risk. Unfortunately, data are not easily available. Annualy there are about 1 million patients in the United States receiving radiotherapy. The chief therapeutic application of radionuclides is the use of sodium iodide 131. Occasionally, phosphorus 32 is used for treatment of polycythemia and strontium 89 is used to treat metastases from prostate cancer. Doses to the gonads and target organs from these radionuclides are indicated in Appendix 2. UNSCEAR estimated that for therapeutic radiation in developed countries, there were approximately 2.9 million procedures and 5.5 million worldwide.[27]

SUMMARY

The major sources of radiation exposure to the population are natural background and medical exposure. Radon is an important and often overlooked portion of natural background exposure. Marked increases in relatively high dose medical examinations in the United States have resulted in the annual per caput dose from medical uses increasing from 0.54 mSv in 1980 to 3.2 mSv in 2006 and exceeding that from natural background radiation (2.3 mSv). The estimated collective doses to the U.S. population from various sources are shown in Table 2-25.

Table 2-25 • Annual Estimate of U.S. Population Collective Dose 2006

	Man Sievert	Percent
Natural background	900,000	48
Medical radiation	960,000	51
Consumer products, building materials	20,000	1
Nuclear energy	136	<1
Occupational	2000	<1
Total (approximate)	1,860,000	100

REFERENCES

1. United Nations Scientific Committee of the Effects of Atomic Radiation (UNSCEAR), Sources and effects of ionizing radiation: 2006 report to the General Assembly with annexes. 2006, New York: United Nations.

2. National Council on Radiation Protection and Measurements (NCRP), Exposure of the population in the United States and Canada from natural background radiation: Recommendations of the NCRP report, no. 94. 1987, Bethesda, Md: NCRP.

3. Perkins, R.W. and J.M. Nielsen, Cosmic-ray produced radionuclides in the environment. Health Phys, 1965. 11(12):1297–1304.

4. Eisenbud, M., Environmental Radioactivity. 2nd ed. 1973, New York: Academic Press.

5. Bureau of Radiological Health, Radiological Health Handbook, PHS Pub. no. 2016. 1970, Washington, DC: U.S. Department of Health, Education, and Welfare.

6. Welford, G.A. and R. Baird, Uranium levels in human diet and biological materials. Health Phys, 1967. 13(12):1321–1324.

7. Hamilton, E.I., The concentration of uranium in man and his diet. Health Phys, 1972. 22(2):149–153.

8. Shleien, B., Evaluation of 226-Ra in total diet samples, 1964 to June 1967. In Radiological Health Reports. 1969, Washington, DC: Bureau of Radiological Health, U.S. Food and Drug Administration.

9. Penna-Franca, E., et al., Radioactivity of Brazil nuts. Health Phys, 1968. 14:95–99.

10. National Council on Radiation Protection and Measurements (NCRP), Evaluation of occupational and environmental exposures to radon and radon daughters in the United States: Recommendations of the NCRP. Report no. 78. 1984, Bethesda, Md: NCRP.

11. Phillips, C., S. Windham, and J. Broadway, Radon and radon daughters in buildings. A survey of past experience. In Radon in Buildings. 1980, Washington, DC: National Bureau of Standards.

12. United Nations Scientific Committee on the Effects of Atomic Radiation (UNSCEAR), Sources and effects of ionizing radiation: UNSCEAR 1993 report to the General Assembly, with scientific annexes. 1993, New York: United Nations.

13. Langham, W., Radiobiological Factors in Manned Space Flight. 1967, Washington, DC: National Academy of Sciences.

14. National Council on Radiation Protection and Measurements (NCRP), Radiation exposure of the U.S. population from consumer products and miscellaneous sources. NCRP report no. 95. 1987, Bethesda, Md: NCRP.

15. Center for Disease Control (CDC), A report on electromagnetic radiation surveys of video display terminals. 1977, Washington, DC: U.S. Dept. of Health, Education and Welfare.

16. Wolbarsht, M., et al., Electromagnetic emissions for visual display units: A non-hazard. SPIE, Society of Photo-optical Instrumentation Engineers, 1980. 229:187.

17. Peterson, R., et al., Non-ionizing electromagnetic radiation associated with video display terminals. SPIE, Society of Photo-optical Instrumentation Engineers, 1980. 229:179.

18. U.S. Food and Drug Administration (FDA), An evaluation of radiation emission from video display terminals. 1981, Washington, DC: U.S. Dept. of Health and Human Services.

19. United Nations Scientific Committee on the Effects of Atomic Radiation (UNSCEAR), Ionizing radiation: Sources and effects. UNSCEAR report to the General Assembly, in annex K: Radiation-induced life shortening. 1982, New York: United Nations.

20. National Council on Radiation Protection and Measurements (NCRP), Screening of humans for security purposes using ionizing radiation systems. 2003, Bethesda, Md: NCRP.

21. National Council on Radiation Protection and Measurements (NCRP), Public radiation exposure from nuclear power generation in the United States: Recommendations of the NCRP. Report no. 92. 1987, Bethesda, Md: NCRP.

22. National Council on Radiation Protection and Measurements (NCRP), Exposure of the U.S. population from occupational radiation: Recommendations of the NCRP. Report no. 101. 1989, Bethesda, Md: NCRP.

23. International Commission on Radiological Protection (ICRP), 1990 Recommendations of the ICRP. Ann ICRP, 1991. 21(1–3):1–201.

24. Center for Devices and Radiological Health, Radiation Experience Data 1980: A survey of hospital practice. 1984, Washington, DC: Center for Devices and Radiological Health, U.S. Food and Drug Administration.

25. Center for Devices and Radiological Health, Population exposure to x-rays, United States 1964. 1966, Washington, DC: Center for Devices and Radiological Health, U.S. Food and Drug Administration.

26. Center for Devices and Radiological Health, Population exposure to x-rays, United States 1970. 1973, Washington, DC: Center for Devices and Radiological Health, U.S. Food and Drug Administration.

27. United Nations Scientific Committee on the Effects of Atomic Radiation (UNSCEAR), Sources and effects of ionizing radiation: UNSCEAR 2000 report to the General Assembly, with scientific annexes. 2 vols. 2000, New York: United Nations.

3 Effects on Genetic Material

With the discovery by H.J. Muller in 1927 that x-rays caused mutations in *Drosophila* (fruit flies), attention turned toward examination of the genetic effects of radiation and the risks that they might pose to future generations. Mutations of DNA may occur in any cell, either spontaneously or through the action of physical, biologic, or chemical agents. Mutations in "germ" cells have potential consequences for future generations, whereas mutations in "somatic" cells are not passed on to progeny and affect only those who are exposed. Maintaining the integrity of the genetic material (DNA) is crucial; very small changes may have significant consequences. In general, radiation-induced mutations are recessive rather than dominant and, therefore, may not be detected for a number of generations. The long generation time in humans, lack of dosimetric data, and the few populations known to be exposed to significant amounts of radiation have all added to the difficulty of detecting and assessing the impact of heritable effects of radiation in humans. Although animal data have been indispensable, there is enough variation among species so that extrapolation of risk estimates to humans is of limited value. Advances in human genetics have shown hereditary function to be much more complicated than previously thought. Nevertheless, the data from long-term studies on children and grandchildren of atomic bomb survivors can be used to set upper limits on radiation risk estimates, and they indicate that the heritable effects of acute exposure on a large human population are minimal and pose less risk than the carcinogenic effects on the same population. This chapter will deal with heritable genetic effects and with genetic effects on somatic cells. Although the mechanisms of radiation-induced cancers probably have their basis in genetic changes, the nature of such changes and the extent to which susceptibility to their induction may vary among different members of the population, are discussed separately in Chapter 4.

BACKGROUND

Before discussing radiation-induced genetic changes, it will be helpful to review some of the basic concepts of genetics. A *gene* is a DNA segment with a linear sequence of nucleotide pairs that contain the genetic code. The four bases used to make such pairs are: adenine (A), thymine (T), guanine (G), and cytosine (C). In the specific pairing of the bases A is joined with T and G with C. The genetic material in the DNA has multiple triplet frames (called codons), each of which contains three nucleotides. Because these nucleotides code for an amino acid in a protein, any change in the nucleotide sequence causes that triplet to code for a different amino acid (*point mutation*). A string of codons, which is the basic unit of genetic information (gene), can determine the structure and function of a protein. Three specific codons act as "stop" signals in the reading of the genetic sequence. Because genetic material is read in a sequential fashion, any change in the sequence can result in a change of the DNA code. Addition or deletion of a nucleotide from DNA will shift the triplet-frame-reading sequence of the code; thus, the information and ultimate protein production will be modified. When such a mutation occurs in a *germ* cell, it may cause phenotypic changes in a subsequently conceived offspring, a consequence that is more likely if an entire chromosome is involved. In contrast, a major genetic change in one of an individual's *somatic* cells may cause the death or neoplastic transformation of that cell but will have no effect on the individual's offspring. Genes are arranged in a linear order to form *chromosomes* (Fig. 3-1). In metaphase, each chromosome has a constricted central portion and four "arms." In the human, there are 46 chromosomes (23 pairs). Chromosomes in a given individual are normally paired, with one chromosome of each pair originating from the mother and one from the father. One of the pairs determines the sex of the individual (*sex chromosomes*); the chromosomes of the other pairs are called *autosomes*. The chromosome pairs are usually numbered from 1 to 23 with the last pair (23) being the sex chromosomes.

The human genome (the complete set of human chromosomes) is estimated to contain about $3–7 \times 10^9$ base pairs of DNA.[1] In general, however, few of the nucleotides in a given gene comprise coding (exon) sequences; the great majority appear to comprise intervening, noncoding (intron) sequences, the function of which remains to be determined. Furthermore, only a small proportion of

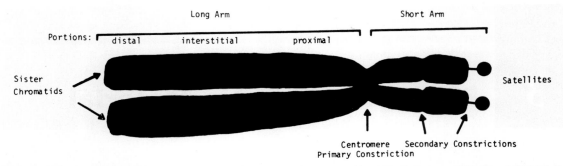

Figure 3-1 • Morphology of a metaphase chromosome. (From Dalrymple GV, Gaulden ME, Kollmargen GM, Vogel HH: Medical Radiation Biology. Philadelphia, WB Saunders, 1973.)

the genes are expressed in any one tissue. Alternative forms of a gene that may be present at a given locus on a chromosome are called *alleles*. Although there may be many alleles in the human population, normally only two of them may occur in a single individual. An individual is *homozygous* for a given gene if both of the homologous alleles derived from the two parents are alike, and he or she is *heterozygous* if the homologous alleles differ. Different alleles arise by genetic mutation.

From a simplified standpoint, genes may be classified as dominant or recessive. A *dominant* gene will express itself in the presence of a recessive allele (heterozygosity). On the average, a dominant trait in one parent will be passed on to 50% of his or her offspring. Affected individuals will usually have an affected parent. Not all dominant traits are expressed to the same extent. Some persons in a family may be severely affected and others only mildly affected. In an extreme case of low expressivity, a parent may carry the dominant gene and appear phenotypically normal. Recessive traits or disorders are those that are usually expressed only when both alleles at a given genetic locus are abnormal (homozygosity). Recessive traits are also expressed, however, when one abnormal allele, but no normal allele, is present (hemizygosity). Hemizygosity occurs normally in males for the X chromosome because males have an X chromosome from their mother and a Y chromosome from their father. Damage or loss of genes on the X chromosome can be expressed in the male in the form of X-linked traits. Consanguinous marriages are a cause of the expression of rare recessive alleles. In evaluation of the incidence of genetic abnormalities in populations, it is important to assess the rate of this type of marriage. Occasionally, both parents pass on two different but abnormal alleles. In this circumstance, the offspring could have a combination disorder that is different from that seen with either allele alone, or each gene could compensate for the other's defects and produce an individual who is phenotypically normal. Several types of nontraditional inheritance have recently been described, making evaluation of radiation risks more complex. The mechanisms that have been recognized include mosaicism, genomic imprinting, uniparental disomy,

cytoplasmic inheritance, genetic expansion, and gene amplification.

Mosaicism refers to a mix of cells that differ genetically within the same individual. This can result from the occurrence of a mutation or chromosome anomaly within a somatic cell at some time during development, in which case not all of the cells in the individual carry the defect. Mosaicism can also exist in germ-line cells. If this happens, disorders may develop that essentially skip a generation, because the germ cells of the carrier parent are formed during embryogenesis of the grandparent.

Genomic imprinting is a phenomenon in which an abnormal gene is expressed differently depending on whether it was received from the mother or father. The "imprinted" gene is inactivated. Examples of this are the Prader-Willi and Angelman syndromes. Both occur as a result of deletions in the same region of the long arm of chromosome 15 (15q11–13 region). The syndromes are very different clinically, and it appears that the former is only paternally derived, and the latter is always maternally derived. Similar differences have been observed for paternally transmitted retinoblastoma and maternally transmitted sarcomas resulting from mutations of the rb gene on chromosome 13.

Uniparental disomy occurs when a cell has a normal number of chromosomes, but both are derived from one parent instead of one set being maternal and the other paternal. Under these circumstances a child can be homozygous and, therefore, express a recessive gene from one parent. The nucleus of a cell is not the only cellular organelle that carries genetic information.

Genetic inheritance also occurs through the cytoplasm. For example, mitochondrial DNA is derived strictly from the mother. Disorders such as Leber optic atrophy, myoclonic epilepsy, and progressive external ophthalmoplegia have been shown to be the result of mitochondrial DNA mutations. Mitochondrial genes have also been shown to have a significantly higher rate of spontaneous mutations than nuclear genes.

Genetic expansion is a phenomenon that results in a disorder becoming progressively more severe with each subsequent generation. With myotonic muscular dystrophy, the children are usually much more severely affected than the parent with the gene. A similar phenomenon has been observed as a result of allelic expansion, in which the gene size is increased. In these circumstances a repetition of a defective gene sequence can result in a more severe form of the disease. This has been noted in the fragile-X syndrome as well as in X-linked spinal bulbar atrophy. Gene amplification is a result of a gene or large portions of a gene being duplicated. This can cause more of a certain product of the gene to be manufactured. In turn, this may lead to either a protective benefit or a disease.

MUTATIONS

Most mutants are heterozygous, and the major impact on health and fitness is from heterozygous rather than homozygous mutations. Gene and genetic point mutations are sometimes classified as nonlethal, sublethal, or lethal. A *dominant lethal gene* is one that causes death before the individual reaches reproductive age. Because many human characteristics are the result of expression of multiple genes of different expressiveness at different foci, only severe dominant genetic mutations are generally discernible and quantifiable within the first several generations. In general, such mutations would have a great impact initially but would be eliminated from the population because of reduction in survival and fertility. Less severe mutations would have less initial impact but would take longer to be eliminated. Up to 10% of spontaneous point mutations may be attributable to background radiation, although the actual percentage may be lower if all known mutagens (such as those present in food) are accounted for. If repair of genetic material is considered in the low-dose range below 0.5 Sv, the production of point mutagens probably follows a linear quadratic relationship. Although it is a moot point, some authors believe that the frequency of point mutagens in germ cells is a function of the interval between radiation exposure and mating. Genes differ in their mutation rates, and even specific portions of individual genes have varying mutation rates. The susceptible spots on the genome for point mutations appear to depend on the sequence organization. CpG dinucleotide sequences are "hot spots" for transition-type mutations involving A to G, G to A, C to T, and T to C transitions.

While most spontaneous mutations tend to be small point mutations, the majority of radiation-induced mutations involve larger DNA deletions.[2-6] This has important consequences in limiting risk estimations made for radiation exposures on the basis of such concepts as the "doubling dose," which will be discussed later. Spontaneous mutation rates appear to be in the range of 5 to 6×10^{-6} per locus per generation, 2×10^{-8} per codon, and 6×10^{-9} per base. In addition to permanent point mutational changes in a gene, there may be larger changes of the amount of DNA in chromosomes that will cause a "frameshift" and change the reading sequence. This is the result of addition or deletion of DNA base nucleotides. Specific events may cause a change in the structure and/or number of whole chromosomes; these changes are referred to as *chromosome aberrations* or *chromosome mutations*, in contrast to the gene, point, or frameshift mutations. Human chromosomes from peripheral lymphocytes may be studied during metaphase by placing the lymphocytes in a culture medium and stimulating division by addition of phytohemagglutinin (PHA). Once the lymphocytes have begun to divide, colchicine is added to arrest cells in division. The cells are then placed on a slide and stained, so that the metaphase chromosomes are visible. A *karyotype* is made by taking a photograph of the chromosomes, cutting out the chromosomes, and arranging them in order of decreasing size (Fig. 3-2). In addition to numbering the chromosomes of each pair from 1 to 23, they are also divided into alphabetical or letter groups as follows: 1–3 (A), 4–5 (B), 6–12 (C), 13–15 (D), 16–18 (E), 19–20 (F), 21–22 (G), and 23 (sex chromosomes).

By examining the karyotype, various chromosomal aberrations or mutations can be identified. The easiest identification is that of changes in the numbers of whole chromosomes. The number of chromosomes found in a human gamete (sperm or egg) is 23, referred to as the *haploid number*. In the normal zygote or somatic cell, 46 chromosomes are present (*diploid number*). *Polyploidy* denotes the presence of more than two sets of chromosomes in a cell, most commonly three (*triploidy*) or four

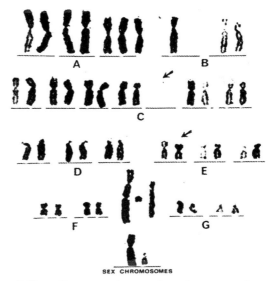

Figure 3-2 • Karyotype of a metaphase chromosome from a lymphocyte of an early diagnostic radiologist. The third chromosome in A is trisomic and the first group in B is monosomic. The fifth pair in group C has no chromosomes (nullisomic, *upper arrow*). The first chromosome pair of E (chromosome 16) is mismatched (*lower arrow*), and between F and G groups are a dicentric chromosome and two acentric fragments. (From Dalrymple GV, Gaulden ME, Kollmargen GM, Vogel HH: Medical Radiation Biology. Philadelphia, WB Saunders, 1973.)

(*tetraploidy*) sets. Entire extra sets of chromosomes may occur in some body cells but are rarely found in all cells in a given person. *Aneuploidy* is the change in number of chromosomes of one or more given sets. Examples of this condition are individuals with Down syndrome ("mongolism"), who have three chromosomes of set 21 (*trisomy* 21) rather than two chromosomes. If both chromosomes of a given set are absent, this is *nullisomy*, and if only one chromosome of the set is present, it is *monosomy*. Other chromosome mutations that occur result from chromosome breaks. Many chromosome breaks rejoin normally with no lesion resulting. In the case of a single break in only one chromosome, the two pieces may not rejoin; in this case a *terminal deletion* occurs. The centric fragment containing the centromere of the chromosome will remain, but the acentric fragment is usually resorbed. Two breaks in a chromosome can result in a variety of mutational events (Fig. 3-3). The segment between the two breaks may be lost: when the segment is long, this is an *interstitial deletion;* when the segment is very short, it is referred to as a *dot deletion*. An inversion occurs when the segment between the two breaks is inverted and the pieces rejoined. A ring can result when both ends of the segment of the chromosome lying between the two breaks are joined together.

When a single break occurs in each of two chromosomes, there may be an exchange of fragments between the chromosomes (*translocation*). An example of a translocation associated with a neoplasm is the *Philadelphia chromosome*, found in 90% of patients with chronic myelogenous leukemia. If no detectable effects are observed, the translocation is balanced. When a fragment containing a centromere (*centric* fragment) is transferred to another centric fragment, a *dicentric* results. Dicentrics are an important biologic dosimeter. The radiation dose-response curve for single chromosome breaks is, as expected, linear, whereas two-hit break aberrations, as might be expected, follow a linear-quadratic curve with low-LET radiation, relatively few double-hit breaks in a chromosome being produced at low doses. In a manner similar to that for "hot spots" on the gene, "hot spots" for radiation-induced breaks have been identified on the chromosomes of peripheral blood lymphocytes. These susceptible spots are in the T bands, which contain many GC and Alu sequences. T bands represent only 15% of all bands but contain 42% of all radiation-induced breaks.[4]

In addition to single-gene and chromosome disorders, a third category of multifactorial or polygenic disorders has been described. These comprise a vast number of diverse disorders that do not follow standard Mendelian hereditary patterns. They are thought to be the result of expression of a number of genes and also due to exposure to environmental factors. An example of such a disorder is neural tube defect, a group of anomalies of the developing

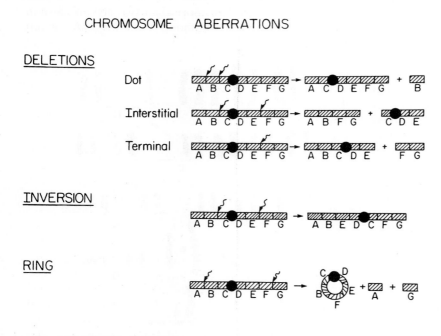

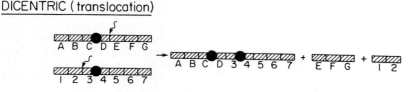

Figure 3-3 • Varieties of chromosome aberrations. Single-hit damage may result in a terminal deletion; if two chromosomes are involved in single breaks, a dicentric may result. Two-hit, or two chromosome breaks are necessary for dot and interstitial deletions, as well as inversions and ring chromosomes.

brain and spinal cord. Neural tube defects have a higher incidence in females and lower socioeconomic groups. They are seen with high incidence in persons with Celtic or East Indian heritage. Some families have a high incidence, as well. Recently, supplementing the diet with folic acid has been shown to reduce the risk of recurrence in subsequent offspring. Other disorders that are thought to be multifactorial include cardiovascular disease and cancer. Obviously, the risk of both of these is somewhat familial but is also influenced by diet and environmental factors like smoking. The common occurrence of diseases that may have at least a partial genetic basis has led many authors to try to formulate mathematical models for the distribution and recurrence of risk. Unfortunately, it is clear that each disorder requires a separate model, and, often, recurrence rates are very different from one family to another. The effect that radiation may have on the severity and incidence of such disorders is undoubtedly small, as will be evident later in this chapter in the discussion of the atomic bomb survivors.

Normal Incidence of Genetic Defects and Malformations

To assess the impact of radiation-induced genetic changes in humans, it is necessary to assess the prevalence of naturally occurring genetic defects in the human population. In a survey in British Columbia, 9.4% of diseases were inferred to be of genetic origin.[7] The data were obtained from several registries and surveillance systems between 1952 and 1972. In another survey, performed in Northern Ireland, the total frequency of genetic disease was estimated to be similar (10.5%).[8,9] One percent of genetic diseases were found to be dominant and X-linked, 0.1% recessive, 0.4% chromosomal, 4.3% congenital malformations, and 4.7% multifactorial or irregularly inherited diseases. Surveys include those by Czeizel covering a seven-year period in Hungary, 1970 through 1976.[10,11] The frequency of malformed babies averaged 3.1%, which is not significantly different from the British Columbia estimate of 3.6%.[7] A study performed in the United States by Myrianthopoulos and Chung examined over 53,000 single deliveries.[12] In a different approach, the study examined children not only at birth but up to 1 year of age. There were 1004 fetal deaths (2%), and 15.6% of the children were born with known malformations, with 13% of these having only a single malformation. The higher incidence of malformations reported in this study is probably due to the one-year follow-up. One third of the congenital abnormalities were recognized at birth and, notably, males had significantly more malformations than females. This study also indicated that among whites in the United States, 2051 of 24,153 (8.5%) deliveries resulted in children with one or more major congenital abnormalities. Carter[13] and Leck[14] have examined the transmissibility of common malformations and found

that the prevalence at birth in siblings of patients with malformations was between 2% and 7% and ranged between 2% and 13% in the offspring of these patients. Thus, it is clear that the rates are much lower than would be expected if the malformations were each due to a single gene and that most common malformations were probably due to a number of causes or genes. Leck has attempted to identify lethal or handicapping malformations and estimates these to number 24.4 cases in 1000 total births, or 2.4%.[14] The relation of genetic mutations to health has been discussed at considerable length by Neel.[15–17] It is an important topic since many diseases with previously obscure etiologies are now known to be due to absence of (1) enzyme activity, (2) an enzyme, or (3) a receptive protein.[18] Many such changes are probably due to continuing mutations. Such mutations are often termed *null mutations* and may occur spontaneously in humans, with a frequency of 2×10^{-5} per locus in a generation. Because there are at least 5000 vulnerable proteins in humans, it is possible that a *zygote* (fertilized egg) could be homozygous for one of these 9% to 10% of the time. It is not known how many of these homozygotes would survive to term during pregnancy. Carter has indicated that if recessive null mutations do occur with the frequency suggested, the frequency in the population must be kept low by selection processes.[19] In addition to gene mutations at a single locus in the chromosome, larger chromosome abnormalities may occur, as described earlier. To assess the significance of chromosome aberrations, one faces the task of determining the normal incidence of chromosome aberrations in the populations at large. This is normally done through cytogenetic metaphase analysis of the chromosomes in circulating lymphocytes. The 1977 United Nations Scientific Committee on Effects of Atomic Radiation (UNSCEAR) report, in reviewing the literature, indicated that cytogenetic analysis in 55,679 live-born infants demonstrated abnormal chromosomes in 1.05%.[20] The 1982 UNSCEAR[21] report included some new data[22,23] but excluded the data of Lin et al.[24] and Bochkov et al.[25] The reason some of the earlier data were excluded was the use of banding techniques and possible selection in the studies. To determine an index of harm, one must examine not only the incidence but also the clinical significance of chromosome abnormalities. A study by Hook and Hamerton indicated that approximately one half of all chromosomal abnormalities detected in newborns were clinically significant by their definition.[26] In their analysis, balanced structural abnormalities and sex chromosomal mosaics were excluded. UNSCEAR 1982[21] suggested that this may be an underestimate of the true clinical significance for several reasons, one of which is the need for long-term studies.[27]

Apparently, balanced, or *euploid*, structural rearrangements have been found in a higher proportion of mentally retarded individuals.[28–30] In addition, chromosome abnormalities have been reported to occur more frequently than normal in those infants dying during the perinatal period.[31-36] The incidence of chromosomal abnormalities in spontaneous abortions was extensively reviewed in the 1977 UNSCEAR report[20] and additional data have been reviewed in the more recent UNSCEAR[21,36-39] and Biological Effects of Ionizing Radiations (BEIR) reports.[6,40] These reviews have indicated that the overall frequency of chromosomal abnormalities in spontaneous abortions may be as high as 50%. In this group, trisomies accounted for 50% of all chromosomal abnormalities; monosomy X, 18%; triploidy, 17%; tetraploidy, 6%; and others, 9%. With increasing maternal age, trisomies increase substantially. Hook has also estimated that 15.5% of all conceptuses recognized at the fifth week of gestation do not survive to live birth, and that the proportion of recognizable conceptions with a chromosomal anomaly is 5%.[26]

The mutation rate for chromosomal anomalies in live-born children was estimated by UNSCEAR 1993[36] to be about 8.3×10^{-4} per gamete per generation for autosomal errors, corresponding to a total of 1.51×10^{-4} per gamete per generation. However, additional anomalies may soon be recognized. Advances in fusion of human spermatozoa with zona pellucida eggs of the golden hamster has allowed direct study of the chromosome constitution in a given population.[41] In addition, the application of banding techniques[42,43] to chromosomes has demonstrated partial monosomies and trisomies, as well as the heritability of at least 17 fragile sites.[44,45] About 20% of mentally retarded persons have a chromosomal abnormality (with about 75% of these being Down syndrome). An update of the data from the British Columbia Registry and from a study in Massachusetts[46,47] confirms a 2% to 3% incidence of severe congenital anomalies in live-borns in all populations which significantly and adversely affect the life of the individual in the absence of medical intervention. Another 2% to 3% incidence of serious congenital anomalies will be found by 5 years of age. In an additional 5% to 13% of the population minor anomalies will be detected. Baird et al. also found that before the age of 25 years more than 53 per 1000 live-born individuals will have diseases that have an important genetic component (Table 3-1).[48] If all congenital anomalies are considered, the incidence rate is about 80 per 1000 live-born individuals. If one includes congenital anomalies that are not felt to have a genetic component, like congenital inguinal hernia, the incidence is approximately doubled.

With an increasing number of malformation registries around the world, it is clear that some regional and ethnic differences do exist. For example, in Western Australia aboriginal newborns have a higher incidence of nervous system and cardiovascular defects than nonaboriginals, but the former have a lower incidence of urogenital abnormalities and pyloric stenosis. Such comparisons are useful particularly if the data are from one registry. When trying to compare data across registries, one needs to ascertain that the same methodology was used to obtain the data. Items of interest in this regard are the inclusion of stillborns, the effect of elective abortion, how individuals with multiple anomalies were reported, and the population size of the registry. The background incidence of congenital anomalies and especially multifactorial diseases has been a matter of debate. The UNSCEAR 1996 report used a figure of 60,000 per million for congenital anomalies and 600,000 per million (or 60% of the population) for multifactorial diseases.[49] More recently, the BEIR VII report[6] likewise estimated congenital anomalies to number 60,000 per million, and other disorders of complex etiology, such as heart disease, cancer, and other diseases to number 650,000 per million. The problem in interpreting such estimates is that a major causal component of the diseases in question is the result of voluntary and avoidable behavior such as smoking.

Table 3-1 • Incidence of Spontaneously Occurring Genetic or Partially Genetic Diseases Having Serious Health Consequences Before Age 25

Type	Rate per Million Live-born	Percent of Total Births
Known Genetic Etiology		
Dominant	1395	0.14
Recessive	1655	0.17
X-linked	532	0.05
Chromosomal	1845	0.18
Multifactorial	46,583	4.64
Other	1164	0.12
Total known genetic	55,175	5.32
Serious Congenital Anomalies		
Nongenetic	26,224	2.62
Known genetic included above	26,584	2.66
Total genetic and other serious congenital anomalies	79,399	7.94

From Baird PA, Anderson TW, Newcombe HB, et al: Genetic disorders in children and young adults: A population study. Am J Hum Genet 1998:42:677–693.

Radiation Risk Estimates

Until about 1956, estimates of radiation-induced genetic risks were obtained predominantly from *Drosophila*, and mouse data were only beginning to become available. In spite of this fact, the potential for genetic harm dominated radiation protection philosophy. Only in recent decades have somatic effects been weighted more heavily. Until 1956, guiding genetic principles included the concepts that (1) mutations were usually harmful, (2) irradiation of reproductive cells entailed some genetic risk, (3) the number of mutations was proportional to the dose, and (4) the effect was independent of the dose rate. There was little awareness of sex and tissue differences or genetic repair mechanisms. The concept of *doubling dose*, defined as the dose or amount of radiation required to produce a mutation rate equal to that which occurs spontaneously, was introduced to aid in genetic risk assessment. In the 1950s, the doubling dose for humans was thought to lie between 50 mGy and 1.5 Gy, with 400 mGy taken to be a reasonable "average" value. Subsequently, the doubling dose of chronic low-LET radiation for the induction of heritable mutations at seven specific loci in the mouse was found to be 4.7 Sv, implying that earlier estimates for humans might have been too low. Major changes in approach also occurred as a result of an increased appreciation of somatic risks in the derivation of radiation protection guidelines and new knowledge about genetics. During this time, the number of recognized genetic diseases in the human population increased significantly, and there were advances in understanding of the chemical structure of the gene and increased realization that chromosome aberrations may cause substantial genetic damage.

In the last three decades, evaluation of data from mice and from the children of atomic bomb survivors (discussed later in the chapter) has suggested that earlier estimates of genetic risk were too high. Irradiation of male mice at a low dose rate has been found to produce considerably fewer genetic effects than the same dose delivered at a high dose rate, and the descendants of irradiated mice have shown substantially fewer harmful effects than were expected. Concomitantly, extensive studies of the children of A-bomb survivors have failed to detect significant evidence of radiation-induced genetic effects in this population.[50,51] The net effect of the mutation process is still thought to be harmful,[6] even though it may have been useful in an evolutionary sense.[52,53]

Although few significant data on the heritable effects of radiation in humans have become available as yet, estimates of such effects have been important for radiation protection purposes. To meet the need, therefore, animal data have been used as a basis for estimating such effects in humans. The two most commonly used approaches have been the direct and indirect methods, both of which extrapolate from data on the rate of radiation-induced mutations in mice to obtain quantitative estimates of the corresponding rates for humans. In the direct method the estimate of damage in the first generation is based directly on the frequency of phenotypic damage observed in that generation. The indirect method is based on an extrapolation back to the first generation from a prediction at genetic equilibrium. The indirect method is also called the doubling-dose method. Both methods have advantages and disadvantages. The direct method usually involves applying a multiplication factor (commonly 10) to the frequencies of dominant skeletal malformations and cataracts that are produced in mice by a given dose to estimate the total number of mutations that would be produced by the same dose in humans. The method is probably simplistic, however, in view of the complexity and varying sensitivity of the human genome. It must be remembered that both dominant skeletal mutations and cataracts in mice arise from connective tissue; it is not known if other tissues respond similarly to DNA damage. Nevertheless, the direct method uses observed, rather than estimated, numbers of malformations in the first generation. The indirect (doubling-dose) method suffers from the inherent assumption that radiation will cause the same relative frequencies and types of mutations as occur spontaneously, in spite of the large body of scientific evidence indicating that doubling doses in mice differ appreciably, depending on the end point chosen for examination. In this connection, it is noteworthy that scanning of the offspring of irradiated male mice on a genome-wide basis has shown the average rate of induced mutations in such animals to be several times lower than that based on the seven specific locus test.[54] The limitations of the direct and indirect methods notwithstanding, both methods have been used to estimate genetic risks in humans. Fortunately, some human evidence can now be used to place bounds on estimates made from the animal data.

Although risk estimates have commonly been based on the rates of spontaneous and induced mutations in mice, on the assumption that the rates of both types of mutations are similar in the two species, the rates of spontaneous mutations are likely to differ between the species, for various reasons.[5,6,55,56] The latest risk estimates for Mendelian and chronic multifactorial diseases have therefore used human data on spontaneous mutation rates and have used mouse data only on induced mutation rates.[6] Based in part on such animal data and the absence of significant evidence of heritable genetic effects of radiation in the children of atomic bomb survivors, discussed later in this chapter, the doubling dose for genetic effects in humans exposed chronically to low-LET radiation is now estimated to approximately 1 Sv,[6] a value that is currently used in radiation protection.[57-59] In estimating the risks of radiation-induced genetic diseases the doubling dose is of central importance, but it is only one of the factors to be considered in the process. Other factors include: (1) the relative increase in the prevalence of a given disease that can be expected to be produced per unit relative increase in the mutation rate (the so-called *mutation component* [MC] of the disease), (2) the proportion of human genes in which a mutation can be expected to be expressed in live-born offspring (the so-called *potential recoverability correction factor* [PRCF] for the mutation), and (3) the concept that the adverse effects of radiation-induced genetic damage are likely to be expressed predominantly in the form of multisystem developmental abnormalities in the offspring of irradiated individuals.[6]

The use of the MC is based on the rationale that the relationship between mutation and disease varies among different classes of genetic disorders, being simple for autosomal dominant and X-linked diseases, slightly complex for autosomal recessive diseases, and highly complex for multifactorial diseases.[60] Therefore, in the most recent BEIR risk estimates, the MC has been inferred to vary accordingly, being assigned a value of 0.3 for autosomal dominant diseases in the first post-irradiation generation, 0.51 for autosomal dominant diseases in the second postirradiation generation, 0 for autosomal recessive diseases, 0.02 for multifactorial diseases in the first and second postirradiation generations, and no value for congenital abnormalities, since the estimates for these disorders were based on mouse data for developmental abnormalities and did not use the doubling dose.[6]

The need for inclusion of the PRCF in the risk estimation process derives from the differences between spontaneous disease-causing mutations in humans and radiation-induced disease-causing mutations in mice. The former comprise a wide variety of molecular alterations, from simple base changes to multigene deletions, but most depend on the DNA sequence of the affected genes and their genomic context. Radiation-induced mutations, in contrast, are often multigene deletions that cause loss of function through haplo-insufficiency, and their recoverability in live-born young seems to depend on whether they are compatible with viability in heterozygotes. The values assigned to the PRCF in the BEIR VII report[6] ranged from 0.15 to 0.3 for autosomal dominant and X-linked diseases, and from about 0.02 to 0.09 for multifactorial diseases; no PRCF was given for autosomal recessive diseases, since such diseases do not result from autosomal recessive mutations within the first few generations.

The equation incorporating these factors for risk estimation is, therefore:

$$\text{Risk per unit dose} = P \times (1/DD) \times MC \times PRCF$$

Where P is the baseline frequency of the disease class under consideration, $1/DD$ is the relative risk of mutations per unit dose, MC is the disease class–specific mutation component, and $PRCF$ is the disease class–specific potential recoverability factor.[6] The risk estimates derived with the use of this formula are shown in Table 3-2.

Genetic Studies on Exposed Populations

There have been continuing studies to identify possible radiation-induced mutations affecting protein structure in the population of both Hiroshima and Nagasaki.[61,62]

Table 3-2 • Estimated Risks of Genetic Diseases in Humans Resulting from Exposure to 0.01 Gy (1 rad) of Chronic Low-LET Radiation

Disease Class	Normal Incidence per Million Live Births	RISK PER MILLION PER 0.01 Gy*	
		First Generation	Second Generation[†]
Mendelian			
Autosomal dominant and sex-linked	16,500	7.5–15	13–25
Autosomal recessive	7,500	0	0
Chromosomal	4,000	‡	‡
Multifactorial			
Chronic multifactorial	650,000[§]	0.03–0.1	2.5–12
Congenital abnormalities	60,000	20[‖]	24–30
Total	738,000	30–47	40–67
Total risk as a percentage of the normal, baseline risk		0.004–0.006	0.005–0.009

*Values rounded.
[†]Assuming conditions of continuous radiation exposure in every generation.
‡Assumed to be subsumed in part under the risks of autosomal dominant and X-linked diseases and in part under the risks of congenital abnormalities.
[§]Frequency in the population.
[‖]Calculated from the mouse data on developmental abnormalities, without use of the doubling-dose method.
Data from National Research Council (NRC), Committee on the Biological Effects of Ionizing Radiations (BEIR): Health risks from exposure to low levels of ionizing radiation. BEIR VII. Washington, DC, NRCUSNA Press, 2005.

These Japanese populations are of particular interest because the data obtained come from a large, relatively homogeneous and initially healthy population. Although the dosimetry, particularly in Hiroshima, continues to be reexamined, this does not appear to be of major significance. In these studies, the survivors are usually divided into groups of parents exposed within 2000 m of the bomb hypocenter and those more than 2500 m from the hypocenter, who received essentially no radiation. The total number of children examined has been approximately 27,000 in each of the two groups. The current studies indicate that there was only one "possible" mutation in the proximally exposed group. The mutation rates per locus per generation were estimated to be 6×10^{-6} (95% CI: $2-15 \times 10^{-6}$) for the exposed group and 6.4×10^{-6} (95% CI: $1-19 \times 10^{-6}$) for the nonexposed group. The number of loci screened was 6.67×10^4 in both the exposed group (those who had parents within 2 km of the hypocenter) and in the control group. The studied cohort of children from exposed parents was 31,150. The control group consisted of an age- and sex-matched group of 41,066 children. The average combined gonadal dose from both parents of the exposed group was 0.4 Sv.[27,63,64]

The atomic bomb survivor data have been used to estimate the doubling doses for various outcomes.[65–68] The doubling-dose 95% confidence limits for various outcomes are as follows: untoward pregnancy, which includes stillbirth, neonatal death, and major congenital abnormalities (0.18 to 0.29 Sv), F_1 mortality (0.68 to 1.1 Sv), F_1 cancer (0.05 to 0.11 Sv), sex chromosome aneuploids (1.6 Sv), and loci encoding proteins (2.27 Sv). In summing all outcomes, the best estimate of doubling dose in humans is between 1.7 and 2.2 Sv. Because the atomic bombs represent an acute, high-dose-rate exposure situation, the minimal estimate of a doubling dose in humans for chronic exposure is about 4 Sv. These studies also suggest that humans are not as sensitive to the genetic effects of radiation as projected from the mouse paradigm.[65,69]

A 1988 report confirmed that there was no statistically significant increase in the frequency of chromosome abnormalities in the offspring of the atomic bomb survivors.[70] However, perplexing and as yet unexplained differences in the chromosome aberration rates between Hiroshima and Nagasaki remain. At 0 dose the chromosome aberration rate in Nagasaki is 10% higher than in Hiroshima.[70]

At least two studies have been done to assess the effect of the Chernobyl accident on the background incidence of genetic diseases and anomalies. Czeizel et al. have reported that in Hungary no increase in mutation rates was detected.[71] The International Chernobyl Project reviewed pre- and post-Chernobyl data from affected republics and concluded that no statistically significant increase in malformations could be attributed to the accident as of 1990.[72]

The 2006 Chernobyl Forum concluded that there was no evidence of radiation effects on infant mortality, although a quite a high rate of infant mortality compared to other countries was noted in both contaminated and noncontaminated regions.[73] There were excellent data from Belarus on well-defined congenital malformations. This data registry was in place long before the Chernobyl accident and the data show a relatively constant rise in reported congenital malformations over the period 1983–1999 (Fig. 3-4).[74] Actually, the rise was similar but slightly higher in the less contaminated areas. Evaluation of the incidence of Down syndrome in Belarus is unremarkable, with the exception of a spike in January of 1987 and another in May of 1990 (Fig. 3-5). Sever et al. have reported on congenital malformations and occupational exposure at the Hanford site.[75] Of 12 specific malformation types, two (hip dislocation and tracheoesophageal fistula) show an association with employment but not with radiation dose. There is also data, which is largely negative, regarding potential heritable effects after medical exposures. Diagnostic x-rays for scoliosis[76] and radiotherapy for hemangiomas in childhood[77] have not been linked to congenital malformations nor has low-dose radiotherapy used ostensibly to treat infertility.[78] Maconochie et al. have examined the sex ratio in over 46,000 children born to U.K. nuclear industry workers and found no evidence of a radiation exposure effect.[79]

Analysis of the offspring of 2286 survivors of childhood cancer who had been treated either with radiation to the abdomen or gonads or with alkylating agents showed no evidence of an increase in either congenital abnormalities or change in sex ratio.[80]

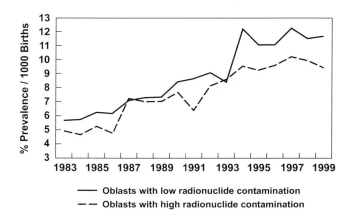

Figure 3-4 ● Incidence of nine easily recognized and clearly defined congenital malformations by year, before and after the Chernobyl accident in areas of high and low contamination in Belarus. Note that the incidence of malformations in both areas rises with time (probably due to increased reporting) and the incidence is higher in the areas with less radiation. (From Lazjuk G, Verger P, Gagniere B, et al: The congenital anomalies registry in Belarus: A tool for assessing the public health impact of the Chernobyl accident. Reprod Toxicol 2003;17:659–666.)

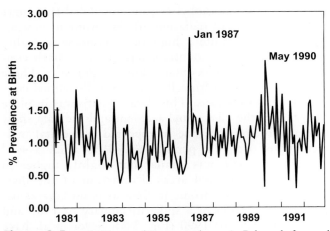

Figure 3-5 ● Incidence of Down syndrome in Belarus before and after the Chernobyl accident. The spike occurring about nine months after the accident is unexplained and may be due to statistical noise as another almost identical spike is seen later unrelated to the accident. (From Lazjuk G, Verger P, Gagniere B, et al: The congenital anomalies registry in Belarus: A tool for assessing the public health impact of the Chernobyl accident. Reprod Toxicol 2003;17:659–666.)

A somewhat smaller but similar study after leukemia treatment was reported by Nygaard et al., with the same conclusions.[81] Similar conclusions have been reached by a number of additional authors.[80,82–86] Boice et al. have reported a U.S. series of 4214 children born to cancer survivors.[87] In this group there were 3.7% with genetic diseases compared to 4.1% among the controls. In a parallel but smaller Danish study the rate of birth defects in children of cancer survivors was 6.1% compared to 5.0% among controls.

Also of particular interest are a number of reports that have examined the possibility of germ-cell mutations in parents causing increased cancer in the offspring. Hawkins et al. examined the cancer risk in 382 offspring of survivors of childhood leukemia and lymphomas and did not find any cancer for a median period of almost 6 years.[83]

Andersson et al. have studied the offspring of patients given injections of Thorotrast and found no association either in terms of cancer incidence or mortality from all causes.[88] To date, no statistically significant differences have been found in a cohort of 31,150 offspring of atomic bomb survivors compared to 41,066 persons in a control group.[89–94]

A case-control study by Gardner et al. of leukemia and lymphoma occurring in young people near the Sellafield nuclear plant in the United Kingdom raised a question about paternal gonadal chronic exposure as a contributing cause to leukemia in children.[95–97] The study involved 52 cases of leukemia and 22 cases of non-Hodgkin's lymphoma. Increased risk was found for fathers who worked at the plant and who had gonadal doses equal to or above 10 mSv. The authors admitted that their results conflicted with the data from the atomic bomb survivors. It should

be noted that the gonadal exposures of the atomic bomb survivors were much higher than those of the fathers of leukemic children at Sellafield. In addition, the elevated risks were derived almost entirely from four children. Most of the other leukemic children had fathers in other industries. Gardner's results at Sellafield not only conflict with the atomic bomb survivor data but are problematical on a biologic basis.[98,99] Most childhood leukemias result from mutations that are so severe that germ-cell viability is doubtful, which means that inheritance of such a mutation would be very unlikely.[100] Another study of leukemia near the Dounreay nuclear plant (also in the United Kingdom) failed to reveal an increase in leukemia related to paternal radiation exposure,[101] as did a comparable study of the offspring of Canadian radiation workers.[102] Other studies of fathers who worked at British, French, and Canadian nuclear installations also have failed to reveal a correlation between paternal dose and leukemia in offspring.[103] Draper et al.[104] and Roman et al.[105] conducted studies of over 35,000 children in the United Kingdom who were diagnosed with cancer to see if their fathers were radiation workers. No relationship was found. Similar conclusions were reached by Sorahan regarding the Oxford Survey of Childhood Cancers.[106,107] A retrospective study by Wakeford et al. of areas in the United Kingdom (besides Sellafield) that had excesses of childhood leukemia and non-Hodgkin's lymphoma failed to find a relationship with paternal radiation exposure.[108] A final point suggesting that Gardner's observation may not be related to radiation is that the cases of leukemia in the children of fathers who had received over 100 mSv only occurred if the children lived in the village of Sellafield. No leukemia was found in children of fathers with the same dose who had raised their children outside the village itself. This argues more for an environmental rather than a genetic causal effect.[102,103,109,110]

The most recent risk estimates for hereditary risks from radiation have been presented in the BEIR VII report.[6] The results are shown in Table 3-2. The International Commission on Radiological Protection (ICRP) has estimated the risk of multifactorial diseases to be about 0.5×10^{-2} per Sv, and the total risk of severe hereditary effects for all generations to be about 1×10^{-2} per Sv.[58]

Down Syndrome

Because Down syndrome accounts for the largest group of recognized chromosomal abnormalities, it will be discussed here in some detail. It is the best known autosomal aneuploid. Over 95% of the cases are due to trisomy 21; 2% to 5% are due to translocation, usually with chromosome 14; and 1% to 2% of patients with Down syndrome are mosaics. The most common condition (trisomy 21) appears to arise by nondisjunction during gametogenesis, most often in the mother, appearing to be maternal in 66% of the cases and paternal in 34%.[111] A slightly higher maternal incidence (81%) has been reported by Mikkelson and coworkers.[112] The risk of recurrence after having one child with Down syndrome appears to be slightly elevated above the incidence in the general population and is about 1% to 2%.[113]

The effect of maternal age on the incidence of Down syndrome relates only to the primary trisomy for chromosome 21. Translocation Down syndrome and mosaics do not exhibit any maternal age dependency.[114–116] The risk of a standard trisomy 21 in a mother less than 20 years of age is 1 in 2500. The risk increases rapidly after the age of 30, and a mother 45 years old has a 1 in 50 chance of having a child with Down syndrome. Multiple studies have been performed to examine the possible increased risk of Down syndrome caused by preconception parental irradiation. The only studies showing a positive effect of radiation are those of Alberman et al.[117,118] and Uchida and Curtis.[119,120] Most studies have shown no significant effect of radiation exposure.[121–128]

The incidence of Down syndrome was examined as a part of the study of populations in China that were living in areas of high and low natural background radiation.[129,130] While congenital abnormalities or cancer mortality in the high background area were not unusually high, there was a significant excess of Down syndrome. Some unusual factors must be taken into consideration before one accepts these findings as evidence of a radiation effect. The rate of Down syndrome in the control area was 1.8 per 10,000 newborns and was 8.7 per 10,000 in the area of high background. Both of these figures are much lower than commonly reported for other countries in the world (13 to 14 per 10,000). The most likely explanation for them is underreporting of the syndrome in both groups. Also 12% of mothers in the high background area were over 35 years of age compared with 4.4% in the low background area.

In Hungary, after the Chernobyl accident, the incidence of Down syndrome did not increase.[71] Sperling et al. reported a cluster of 12 cases in West Berlin (compared to 2 to 3 expected) nine months after the Chernobyl accident.[131,132] Burkart et al. also reported an increase in Down syndrome in northern Bavaria.[133] In both of these instances the radiological exposure was very low and Burkart indicated that biological considerations argued against Chernobyl fallout as a cause. De Wals et al. reported on chromosomal abnormalities, including Down syndrome in Europe and found no increase after the Chernobyl accident in May 1986.[134,135] There is a single report of an increase in Down syndrome in children conceived during the period of highest radiation exposure in Belarus (May 1986) and born in January 1987.[136] No overall trend was identified and a similiar high spike was seen in May of 1990 but not at other times. These spikes may simply be due to statistical noise. No increase in Down syndrome was found in the offspring of the atomic bomb survivors; only one case of Down syndrome was reported; a male was born in 1966 to a father exposed in Hiroshima.[70]

A very small study looking for trisomy 21 in the offspring of mothers who had undergone preconceptual medical radiography also failed to find an association.[137]

Chromosomal Studies in Atomic Bomb Survivors

A 1981 study by Schull et al. reappraising the genetic effects of the atomic bomb is very important because it included integrated estimates based on children born over a 21-year period following irradiation of a heterogeneous human population.[138] The findings indicated no identifiable significant trend of increasing untoward outcomes of pregnancy with increasing maternal or paternal exposure, and the total parental gonadal dose appeared to have no significant effect. Overall, the risk of untoward pregnancy outcome accompanying exposure from the atomic bomb appeared to be substantially lower than that associated with inbreeding. When the survival of live-born infants was examined, there was no evidence of increasing mortality with increasing parental gonadal dose. The study also examined chromosomal abnormalities. Unfortunately, in the F_1 generation mortality study, blood samples were not obtained until the children were 13 years old. Therefore, most children with autosomal aneuploidy would have died, with the possible exception of those with trisomy 21. The findings, therefore, are only valid when one considers balanced translocations and sex chromosome aneuploids. Through 1979, 12 individuals with sex chromosome abnormalities and 5 individuals with balanced autosomal structural rearrangements in 5058 children of parents with no significant exposure were identified. There were 16 chromosome abnormalities and 10 balanced rearrangements identified in the 5762 children of parents one or both of whom were proximally exposed. The mean joint gonadal exposure for parents in the proximally exposed group whose children were examined was 820 mSv, based on a neutron RBE of 5. These frequencies indicate a slight increase in the exposed group, but the increase is not of statistical significance. This information has implications for estimation of the genetic doubling dose of radiation in humans. There is little doubt that radiation has some initial genetic effect because chromosomal changes in peripheral lymphocytes were identified in the survivors for extended periods. The doubling dose for untoward pregnancy outcomes, including major congenital defects, stillbirth, or death during the first week of life, has been estimated to be 690 mSv. An estimate of any dose below 180 mSv would be excluded at the 5% probability level. The doubling dose for deaths during infancy and childhood was estimated to be 1.47 Sv per gamete with 290 mSv being the lower limit at the 5% confidence level. The doubling dose for sex chromosome aneuploids is estimated to be 2.52 Sv.[139]

The doubling dose for mutations of protein phenotypes is more difficult to estimate. The revised Japanese data, as well as those from other population studies, have failed to demonstrate an increase in electrophoretically detectable mutations. One might, therefore, arbitrarily set the human mutation rate at 0.2×10^{-5} per locus for each generation, a figure emerging from the investigations on *Drosophila*. The "average" doubling dose when all three categories are considered is 1.56 Sv. In summary, in the atomic bomb survivors, no statistically significant genetic effects of parental exposure have been observed. This does not mean that radiation has no genetic effects in humans. Low-LET acute radiation delivered to the mouse indicates a doubling dose of 300 to 400 mSv but it now appears that the doubling dose in humans is significantly higher (i.e., the human is significantly more resistant to radiation-induced genetic defects).

GENETIC MARKERS USED FOR BIOLOGIC DOSIMETRY

Somatic Mutations

A number of studies have examined induction of hypoxanthine guanine phosphoribosyltransferase (*HPRT*) gene mutations in peripheral T-lymphocytes. These have been seen in atomic bomb survivors[140,141] (Fig. 3-6) and after radioimmunological therapy.[142] Of interest is that significant elevations of this mutation have been reported following chemotherapy[143] and may also be associated with environmental radon levels.[144] The number of mutations declines with time. The assay requires about two weeks to perform and uses a large amount of blood.

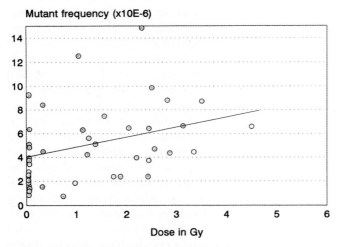

Mutant frequency (x10E-6)

HPRT mutant frequency (A-bomb DS86 RERF TR 18-87)

Figure 3-6 • Relationship between DS86 dose and *HPRT* mutant frequency in atomic bomb survivors. Note the marked individual scatter for a given dose level. (From Hakpda H, Akiyama M, Kyoizumi S, et al: Increased somatic cell mutant frequency in atomic bomb survivors. RERF Technical Report 18-87, Hiroshima, Japan, Radiation Effects Research Foundation, 1987.)

Another problem is that in vivo the dose-response relationship is quite shallow. All of these factors limit the use of this technique for dosimetry estimation. The T-cell receptor (TCR) is expressed in almost all mature T-lymphocytes and is associated with antigen recognition and cell inactivation. The mutant frequency increases significantly with age and the relevant gene is quite mutable. TCR gene analysis is another method that has been investigated for use as a genetic biological dosimeter. Mutant cells are defective in expression of this gene. One advantage of the TCR method is that only 1 to 2 mL of blood are required, whereas larger volumes (20 to 50 mL) are needed for the dicentric and *HPRT* analyses. The method also uses a commercially available antigen. The glycophorin A (GPA) assay also uses only 1 to 2 mL of blood but can be used only on persons who are MN heterozygous. An analysis of atomic bomb survivors showed more TCR mutations in males than females but no radiation dose effect. In six patients who had received Thorotrast exposure, and in some radioiodine therapy patients, there was reported to be a dose-related increase in mutation frequency; there was a large increase in one Chernobyl survivor estimated to have received 3 to 4 Gy.[145,146] A later study of 18 Thorotrast patients by the same group reported again that TCR gene mutations were elevated but not erythrocyte glycophorin mutations.[147,148] In contrast, in atomic bomb survivors the opposite was found; that is, exposure could be detected by GPA assay but not by TCR. The exact reason for this remains unclear, but this finding limits the use of either method for general biological dosimetry.[147,149–151] As a part of the International Chernobyl Project, TCR analysis was conducted on populations living in clean and in contaminated areas around the Chernobyl plant for 5 years. There was no evidence of an effect of the contamination on mutation frequency.[72]

The GPA assay is conducted on erythrocytes, and elevated levels of mutations at the chromosome location 4q have been found in atomic bomb survivors 40 years after exposure.[149] The method uses a pair of monoclonal antibodies conjugated with different fluorescent dyes to detect erythrocytes that lack expression of the M or N allele of the GPA gene. The method uses a small amount of blood, and blood samples can be stored or shipped long distances before analysis. While there is some relationship with dose when groups of people are examined, there is so much variation among individual persons that the method is unlikely to be useful for clinical purposes or individual dose estimation (Fig. 3-7). GPA analysis was done during the International Chernobyl Project comparing persons living in clean and in highly contaminated villages around the Chernobyl plant. The mutation frequency was higher in the contaminated villages but the difference was not statistically significant. This study was limited in size but examined chromosome aberrations as well as somatic mutations.

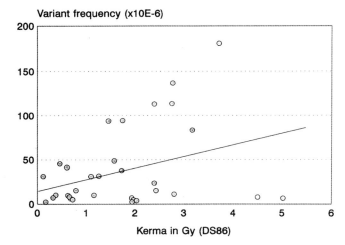

MM mutant dose response (A-bomb)

Figure 3-7 • Relationship between dose and MM mutant frequency in atomic bomb survivors. (From Kyoizumi S, Nakamura N, Hakoda M, et al: Detection of somatic mutation at the glycophorin—A locus in erythrocytes of atomic bomb survivors using a single beam flow sorter. RERF Technical Report 9-88, Hiroshima, Japan, Radiation Effects Research Foundation, 1988.)

The chromosome dicentric frequency was higher than expected; however, there was no difference between clean and contaminated village populations. There was no statistically detectable increase in either GPA or TCR gene mutation frequencies. The dose levels to which these persons were exposed were less than 0.1 Sv and the exposure was chronic. Based on risk factors generated by other studies, increases in mutations were not expected to be detected.[72]

In patients treated with iodine 131 for thyroid cancer, the frequency of N/O GPA variant erythrocytes has been observed to increase with the dose to the bone marrow, at a rate of roughly 10.9×10^{-6} per cell per Sv, which is about one half of that produced by rapid, whole-body external irradiation.[152]

Chromosome Aberrations in Peripheral Lymphocytes

Over the last two decades, evaluation of chromosome aberrations in peripheral lymphocytes has been used as a biologic dosimeter, particularly in radiation accidents in which the exposure is uniform.[153,154] It is of more limited value in the assessment of partial-body, or nonuniform, exposures and in cases of internal contamination. Evaluation of chromosome aberrations is the most sensitive biologic dosimeter for whole-body radiation. Radiation-induced aberrations that may be observed are of chromosome type and chromatid type. *Chromatid type aberrations* are produced only after the chromosome has split into the two chromatids (late G_2 stage or subsequently). When the cell is irradiated during G_1 stage, only chromosome aberrations are observed,

although they may also be seen after chromosome replication. Several unique factors make the evaluation of peripheral lymphocytes particularly useful. They circulate throughout the body and for all practical purposes are all in the postmitotic pre-DNA synthetic G_0 state. Lymphocytes that circulate are classified either as T-lymphocytes or B-lymphocytes. *T-lymphocytes* are dependent on the thymus and are the lymphocytes of interest. They are relatively long-lived, with a half-life of several years, allowing analysis of stable aberrations to be used for dosimetric estimates for a long period after an accident or exposure. Scheid et al. have examined the time course of disappearance of chromosomal aberrations in the peripheral lymphocytes of a person who was involved in a radiation accident.[155] They concluded that there was a sevenfold decline in identified aberrations in the 4 years after the accident. Even though there is a decline with time, stable chromosome aberrations are still detectable in atomic bomb survivors 40 years later. Even persons who have received partial-body radiotherapy or a large dose from medical fluoroscopy have statistically significant elevations decades later. In these persons there does not appear to be any evidence that the yield of aberrations varies with age at exposure.[156] It should be noted that chromosome breaks can be caused by other noxious agents also, including chemotherapeutic agents (specifically alkylating agents). There is no agreement on an exact disappearance half-time, but 3 years appears to be a reasonable value. Although the half-life of the T-lymphocytes in the biologic circulation is long, there is significant individual variation, depending on the health of the person affected.

In evaluation of a blood sample, the T-lymphocytes are cultured and stimulated by PHA, causing the lymphocytes to resume mitotic activity and allowing a karyotype to be performed. The culture time is extremely important since one wishes to evaluate only the incidence of dicentric chromosomes at first metaphase. Addition of bromodeoxyuridine (BrdU) allows positive identification of first metaphase division. In general, most medically significant full-body exposures can be identified by evaluating 200 to 500 lymphocytes. Cytogenetic analysis of such numbers of cells is time-consuming and involves at least two days of two-person microscope work, a major limitation of the technique. The practical lower limit of detection for whole-body radiation exposure is approximately 0.25 Gy. Even if as many as 600 cells are scored, wide confidence intervals in the dose estimates remain. This can be seen easily from Figure 3-8. To ascertain an exposure of 50 mGy with a 95% certainty, 5000 to 10,000 cells must be examined. This would take a trained technologist nearly a year to accomplish. Finally, the analysis requires about 20 mL of blood and lymphocytes that are relatively sensitive, making sample transport and storage a problem. It is possible that some new techniques such as premature chromosome condensation (PCC) or computer image

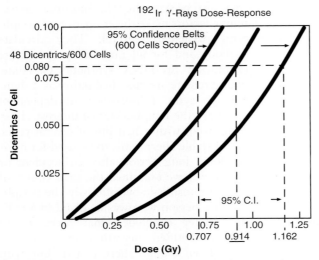

Figure 3-8 • In vitro dose-response curve for dicentric induction in human lymphocytes exposed to gamma rays from iridium 192. Also shown are the methods for point and interval estimation of an accident victim who demonstrated 48 dicentrics in 600 lymphocyte metaphases. Uncertainties shown on the data points are standard errors based on the assumption of a Poisson distribution. (From Littlefield LG, Joiner EE, Dufrain RJ, et al: Cytogenetic dose estimates from in-vivo samples from persons involved in real or suspected radiation exposures. In Hubner KF, Fry SA [eds]: The Medical Basis of Radiation Accident Preparedness. New York, Elsevier/North Holland, 1980.)

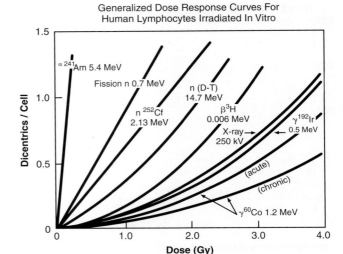

Figure 3-9 • Dose-response curves for dicentric chromosome induction in human lymphocytes irradiated in vitro. (From Dufrain RJ, Littlefield LG, Joiner EE, et al: In vitro human cytogenetic dose-response systems. In Hubner KF, Fry SA [eds]: The Medical Basis of Radiation Accident Preparedness. New York, Elsevier/North Holland, 1980.)

analysis may reduce the time required to perform the analysis.

Lymphocyte chromosome aberrations may be classified as stable or unstable. The *unstable aberrations* include pericentric inversions and translocations. Their instability prevents them from being particularly useful for dosimetric purposes. The *stable aberrations* include dicentrics, centric rings, and acentrics. Many environmental mutagens are known, including caffeine, chemicals, and some drugs. In addition, viruses may act as mutagens. Most of these agents cause chromatid damage. Thus, exposure to viral or chemotherapeutic agents does not cause background aberrations that could interfere with the dicentrics or centric ring aberrations that one expects from radiation exposure. The reported background frequencies for dicentrics and acentric aberrations are $(1.2–1.3) \pm 0.25 \times 10^{-3}$ and $3.3 \pm 0.4 \times 10^{-3}$, respectively.

In general, dosimetric estimates are made from extrapolation coefficients derived from in vitro irradiation of human blood.[157] Many researchers have reported the usefulness of these methods.[153,158–165] Exposure to radiation causes varying dose-response curves for the dicentrics, with the shape of the curve depending on the type of radiation involved as well as the dose rate. With high-LET radiation (such as alpha particles and neutrons), the slope is steep and the curve is rather linear, whereas with low-LET radiation (such as beta or gamma rays), a linear-quadratic curve is found (Fig. 3-9). The high-LET linear curve may be expressed as $Y = \alpha D$, where Y is the frequency

of dicentrics found in each cell, and α represents the slope coefficient with D given in rad. For neutron exposure, as the energy of the neutron increases, the LET decreases, and a linear-quadratic equation of the form $Y = \alpha D + \beta D^2$ becomes appropriate. This linear-quadratic formula is also usual for describing the response to acute doses of low-LET radiation. The alpha and beta coefficients for generalized dose for different types of radiation are reported in Table 3-3. The dose rate of low-LET radiation affects the yield of dicentrics in each cell, as shown in Figure 3-10.

It is important to realize that the induction of chromosome aberrations in human lymphocytes is a random process in circumstances involving low-LET radiation and, therefore, may be described by a Poisson distribution. This indicates that the number of cells that have two lesions would be relatively low. Overrepresentation of cells with two- and three-chromosome aberrations with respect to the cells having only a single aberration should raise the suspicion of either nonuniform external exposure or internal contamination with alpha emitters. The observed dispersion for varying doses of both gamma rays and alpha particles is presented in Table 3-4. This table is used as illustrated by the following example: If dicentrics were identified in 10% of cells in a given patient, and the affected cells had only a single dicentric aberration in each, an acute whole-body gamma dose of 1 Gy would be assumed. But if the distribution consisted of 1 cell with 3 dicentrics, 6 cells with 2 dicentrics, and 23 cells with 1 dicentric, the overdistribution of cells with multiple dicentrics should suggest the possibility of a nonuniform, or partial-body, exposure. Very few of the studies used to

Table 3-3 • Reported Coefficients of Dose-Response Relationships for Human Lymphocytes Irradiated In Vitro

Type of Radiation	$\alpha \times 10^{-4}$	$\beta \times 10^{-4}$
^{60}Co γ 1.2 and 1.3 MeV	1.6	5.0
^{60}Co γ 1.2 and 1.3 MeV (chronic)	1.8	2.9
^{60}Co γ 1.2 and 1.3 MeV	3.9	8.2
^{60}Co γ 1.2 and 1.3 MeV	0.9	6.8
^{60}Co γ 1.2 and 1.3 MeV	2.7	4.8
^{60}Co γ 1.2 and 1.3 MeV (chronic)	2.7	3.0
^{60}Co γ 1.2 and 1.3 MeV	5.7	3.2
^{137}Cs γ 0.67 MeV	6.8	1.7
^{192}Ir γ 0.59, 0.47 MeV	3.2	6.1
^{3}H β 0.006 MeV	3.1	12.0
e$^-$ 15 MeV (microseconds)	0.9	6.1
e$^-$ 15 MeV	0.6	5.7
e$^-$ 3 MeV	2.6	3.5
X-ray 30 kV	11.1	8.7
X-ray 150 kV	-0.2	7.4
X-ray 180 kV	4.0	2.6
X-ray 180 kV	9.1	6.3
X-ray 200 kV	7.5	7.1
X-ray 220 kV	7.8	4.2
X-ray 220 kV	7.9	5.4
X-ray 250 kV	5.6	5.5
X-ray 250 kV	3.6	6.7
X-ray 250 kV	4.8	6.2
X-ray 250 kV	6.3	6.5
X-ray 1.9 MeV	0.9	4.3
$-\Pi$ Ions (plateau)	13.4	2.8
$-\Pi$ Ions (peak)	23.4	4.8
D-T neutrons 15.0 MeV	14.1	3.8
D-T neutrons 14.7 MeV	26.2	8.8
D-T neutrons 14.1 MeV	25.0	3.7
D-Be neutrons 7.6 MeV	47.8	6.4
D-Be neutrons 6.2 MeV	33.8	—
^{252}Cf neutrons 2.13 MeV	60.0	—
D-Be neutrons 2.0 MeV	74.5	—
Fission neutrons 1.5 MeV	64.8	—
Fission neutrons (Nereide)	87.4	—
Fission neutrons (Crac)	90.1	—
Fission neutrons (IRT-200)	26.6	—
Fission neutrons 0.7 MeV	84.9	—
Fission neutrons 0.90 MeV	72.8	—
Fission neutrons 0.85 MeV	78.4	—
Fission neutrons 0.70 MeV	83.5	—
^{241}Am α 5.5 MeV	489.8	—

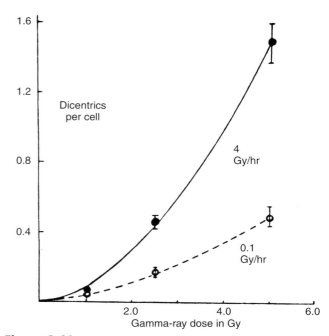

Figure 3-10 • Frequency of dicentrics in human lymphocyte cultures at different gamma radiation dose rates. (From Webster EW: On the question of cancer induction by small x-ray doses. AJR, 1981.137:647–666.)

derive the dicentric dose-response curves in humans have employed a total-body homogeneous exposure. Silberstein et al. have cautioned that individual variation in cytogenetic response to therapeutic radiation may be substantial.[166]

Nonetheless, chromosomal aberration analysis has been used for over a decade with fairly good agreement between biologic cytogenetic data and physical methods of dose estimation.

Radiation-induced dicentrics and other chromosome aberrations can be relatively easily studied in the peripheral lymphocytes. The frequency of dicentrics for each lymphocyte has been shown to correlate well with varying types of irradiation. The main use of the technique to date has been in the evaluation of suspected radiation accidents rather than in evaluation of medically significant exposures, although it certainly could be helpful in such cases (Lloyd et al.).[167,168–170]

One of the minor problems with the dicentric aberration technique is that the dicentrics are unstable and disappear over years. There has been a search for a method that will allow identification of the stable chromosome aberrations. Conventional and banding analyses were developed, but were too time-consuming for routine analysis. Recently the development of a fluorescence in situ hybridization technique (FISH) or "chromosome painting" has proved to be useful.[171] In this technique, the DNA is thermally denatured to provide single strands of DNA. These targeted strands are incubated with nontarget DNA probes that bind to the DNA sequences that are homologous. The target DNA is stained, and the nontarget DNA is counterstained. Under a fluorescence microscope the target DNA appears yellow, and the nontarget DNA appears red. In the case of a translocation, the affected DNA strand will appear to be partially red and partially yellow. This method detects only a fraction of the translocations, so that it is necessary to apply a multiplication factor to estimate total translocation frequency. This method has been tested in atomic bomb survivors and yields a general dose-response

Table 3-4 • Distributional Analysis of Induced Dicentric Chromosomes by Gamma Rays and Alpha Particles

Dose	Dicentrics	Cells	Mean/ Cell	Observed Frequency of Cells with Number of Dicentrics Indicated						
				0	1	2	3	4	5	6
Gamma Irradiation										
0.5 Gy	7	300	0.023	293	7	0	0	0	0	—
1.0 Gy	20	200	0.10	180	20	0	0	0	0	—
2.0 Gy	33	100	0.33	74	20	5	0	0	0	—
4.0 Gy	218	200	1.09	59	80	46	14	1	0	—
Alpha Irradiation										
8.5 mGy	19	400	0.475	386	10	3	1	0	0	0
17 mGy	15	200	0.75	187	11	2	0	0	0	0
34 mGy	33	200	0.165	178	14	5	3	1	0	0
68 mGy	67	200	0.335	160	23	12	2	2	0	1

Adapted from DuFrain RJ, Littlefield LG, Joiner EE, et al: In-vitro human cytogenetic dose-response systems. In Hubner KF, Fry SA (eds): The Medical Basis for Radiation Accident Preparedness. New York, Elsevier/North Holland, 1980.

relationship, although, like the GPA assay, it is subject to a lot of individual variation for a given radiation dose level (Fig. 3-11).[172]

In addition to the FISH technique, other chromosomal methods have been developed. Because chromosome fragments that occur as a result of radiation exposure can fail to be incorporated into the daughter nuclei during cell division, they can remain in the cytoplasm as micronuclei. The relationship between micronuclei in human lymphyoctyes and radiation exposure appears to be linear up to 4 Gy.[173] Micronuclei are scored by microscopic analysis, and they are lighter than, or the same color as, the nucleus, while being one third or less in diameter than the main nuclei. The response to gamma irradiation is linear quadratic but linear with neutron dose. High dose rates of gamma irradiation are about 1.5 times more effective in micronuclei production than low dose rates[174]; however, a dose-dependent increase has been observed in patients treated with iodine 131 for thyroid cancer.[175] Micronucleus frequencies, spontaneous and induced, appear to increase with donor age.[176,177] Reciprocal translocations are another promising biomarker in that their frequency in individuals exposed to whole-body radiation is dose-dependent, easily measured, and relatively stable with time.[178] Other biosimetric techniques deserving of further investigation include the use of the polymerase chain reaction to identify mutant genes in irradiated cells,[165,179] the selective painting of PCCs,[165,180,181] and assays for radiation-induced expression of proto-oncogenes.[182]

CLINICAL PERIPHERAL CHROMOSOME STUDIES

The evidence from a number of populations indicates an increase in spontaneous frequency of chromosome aberrations with the age of individuals. Thus, a positive correlation with radiation dose in any study must be examined and corrected for age bias. It should be emphasized that although lymphocytes provide a biologic dosimeter at relatively high radiation exposure levels, the clinical significance of chromosomal changes in lymphocytes is apparently negligible. Because the ratio of chromosomal aberrations between lymphocytes and germ cells varies among species, it is not possible at present to extrapolate from chromosomal changes in circulating lymphocytes to genetic hazard in progeny. Many studies have examined the incidence of chromosome aberrations in peripheral lymphocytes in various exposed populations. Overall,

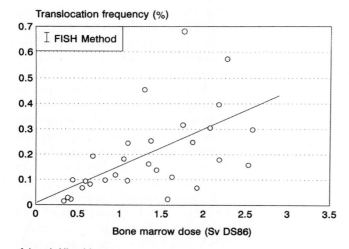

A-bomb Hiroshima

Figure 3-11 • Relationship between dose and translocation frequency in 36 Hiroshima atomic bomb survivors. (From Kodama Y, Nakano M, Ohtaki K, et al: Biotechnology contributes to biological dosimetry. RERF Update Winter, Hiroshima, Japan, Radiation Effects Research Foundation, 1992.)

because of radiation doses often less than 0.2 Gy, research has provided few statistically significant findings related to radiation exposure, and such data often have been contradictory in their conclusions. Studies are usually complicated by lack of adequate control populations and confounding effects of other environmental mutagens.

Areas of High Natural Background

The radon thermal springs in the area of Badgastein, Austria, contribute significantly to high natural radiation, particularly in the spas. Pohl-Ruling and Fischer have classified the individuals working and living in the area into groups estimated to have "blood burdens" of 100 to 340 mR per year from gamma ray exposure and 1 to 1600 mR per year of alpha exposure.[183] One hundred and eighty blood samples were examined from 122 persons. Even at these very low-dose levels, a dose-effect relationship appeared for chromosome fragments, dicentrics, and interstitial deletions. From 1972 to 1975, over 73,000 inhabitants of the Guangdong Province in China were studied because the monazite in the region causes natural background radiation levels to be three times higher than in neighboring areas.[184] Cytogenetic study revealed almost identical frequencies of chromatid and chromosome aberrations in the high-radiation area and the control population. The frequency of hereditary diseases and congenital abnormalities was actually lower in the high-background region. Only the incidence of Down syndrome was higher in the high-background region, but this was not at a statistically significant level. Exposure differed for individuals in the high-background and control regions, at 25 mR per month and 9 mR per month, respectively. These levels are so low that given current risk estimates, larger populations must be studied to find statistically significant effects. In addition to population groups that have been exposed to high levels of background radiation, persons either occupationally or accidentally exposed have been the subjects of chromosomal studies. Thus, residents of the vicinity of the Semipalatinsk nuclear explosion site have been observed to show an elevated frequency of micronuclei in their peripheral blood lymphocytes,[185] as have the residents of radioactively contaminated buildings in Taiwan, in whom the elevations gradually decreased after leaving the contaminated areas.[186]

Occupational Exposure

During one 10-year period, Evans et al. studied 197 workers who had been exposed to neutron and gamma radiation while refueling submarine nuclear reactors in England.[187] The study is particularly interesting because it employed a control blood sample obtained from the workers before exposure to serve as a personal control, with subsequent samples taken as dose was accumulated. Film badges were used to estimate the dose. Almost all exposures were below the 0.05 Sv annual limit. The findings indicated a positive dose-effect relationship for dicentrics, acentric fragments, and unstable aberrations but not for symmetrical rearrangements. The rate of dicentric aberrations produced was about 1.4×10^{-4} dicentrics per cell for each 0.01 Sv. The dicentric yield was 1 in 700 cells prior to exposure, rising to about 1 in 200 after accumulated doses of 0.2 to 0.3 Sv. A similar study performed in the Federal Republic of Germany involved 57 male workers at nuclear power plants receiving gamma- and x-ray exposure.[188] Eleven healthy males were used as controls. Although the radiation workers all received less than the allowable annual limits of 0.05 Sv, the frequency of dicentrics and acentrics was significantly higher than in the controls. This increase in chromosome abnormalities was not dependent on either the total accumulated absorbed dose or age of the worker. The difference in findings from the English study may be the result of a smaller sample and lack of individual data before exposure.

Eighty uranium miners and 10 controls have been examined by Brandom et al. in the United States.[189] The exposure estimates were based on working time and measurements of radon levels in the mines. The group receiving exposures of up to 3000 working level months (WLM) showed a statistically nonsignificant but threefold increase in chromosome aberrations other than dicentrics and rings. The group of miners receiving the highest exposure (greater than 3000 WLM) actually showed a decrease in dicentrics and rings compared to the other groups. Brandom et al. have also examined plutonium workers.[190] Plutonium burdens and dose estimates of 343 workers were obtained by urine bioassay and lung counting. External dose was estimated by film badge readings. Workers were subdivided on the basis of organ and systemic plutonium burden. Those workers with systemic plutonium burdens of 37 to 370 Bq were unremarkable, but those workers who had both systemic and lung burdens of 37 Bq to 1.48 kBq had significant increases in the frequency of dicentrics, rings, inversions, and translocations. The rate for complex deletions was 0.5 per 100 cells in controls and about 3.5 per 100 cells in the exposed group. Total aberrations went from 1 per 100 in controls up to 5 per 100 in the exposed group. The analysis indicated that age, external irradiation, and lung burden were all statistically significant variables. Stable chromosome aberrations also have been observed to increase with the accumulated dose in the lymphocytes of workers at the Sellafield nuclear facility; the rate of increase—0.79 ± 0.22 aberrations per 100 cells per Sv—being several times lower than that observed in atomic bomb survivors, suggesting a dose-rate effectiveness factor of about 6 for chronic exposure.[191] In the same study population, the frequency of GPA variant erythrocytes showed no correlation with dose. The frequency of micronuclei in peripheral blood lymphocytes has been found to increase systematically with age but to correlate only weakly with accumulated dose in other groups of radiation workers exposed within the permissible dose range.[192]

Atomic Bomb Survivors

Some of the genetic effects on the atomic bomb survivors have been discussed previously in this chapter in the context of heritable effects. Many studies of somatic chromosomes in this population have also been performed. These demonstrate that the chromosome aberrations induced in circulating lymphocytes are proportional to dose and may persist for up to three decades.[57,193,194] Sofuni et al.[195] and Stram et al.[196] analyzed 23 survivors who received 1 to 8.5 Gy of gamma and neutron irradiation. This study is of interest because it demonstrated that a trypsin-Giemsa banding stain showed slightly higher frequencies of aberrant lymphocyte chromosomes than the conventional orcein stain. Use of the ordinary stain revealed 23% aberrant cells in the 1.0 to 1.9 Gy group versus 26% with the G-banding method. In the 4 to 4.9 Gy group, the frequencies were 29% and 34%, respectively. Other studies consist of analysis of cultured lymphocytes from blood samples obtained from 1245 atomic bomb survivors between 1968 and 1980. Structural chromosome abnormalities were related to dose, but the percentage of cells with at least one aberration increased less rapidly with dose in Nagasaki than in Hiroshima. The magnitude of the intercity difference is less with the dosimetry estimates from 1986 (DS86) than with the tentative 1965 (T65D) dose estimates (Fig. 3-12). However, the differences still remain statistically significant. This is one of several intercity differences in radiation effects that have been difficult

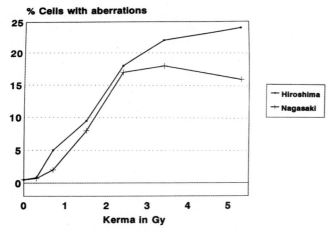

% Cells with aberrations

— Hiroshima
+ Nagasaki

Kerma in Gy

A-bomb DS86

Figure 3-12 • Percent of lymphocytes with aberrations in atomic bomb survivors from Hiroshima and Nagasaki (DS86 dosimetry). (From Preston D, McConney M, Awa A, et al: Comparison of the dose-response relationships for chromosome aberration frequencies between the TD65 and the DS86 dosimetries. RERF Technical Report 7-88, Hiroshima, Japan, Radiation Effects Research Foundation 1988.)

to explain but may in part be due to variations in the neutron doses. The frequency of erythrocytes mutant at the GPA locus has also been observed to increase significantly with dose, age, and number of cigarettes smoked, with a doubling dose similar to that for the incidence of solid cancer, and with no significant intercity or sex differences.[197]

Accidents

Analysis of chromosomal aberrations has been useful for analysis of patients at a number of radiation accidents, including those at Chernobyl and Goiania, Brazil. Even this technique can yield a wide variety of dose estimates for a given individual based on the laboratory. If uniform methodology and training of the technicians are used, agreement can be acceptable between laboratories.[198]

In the Chernobyl accident, in firemen and others who suffered from acute radiation syndrome, lymphocyte analysis revealed a high incidence of chromosome aberrations, which was one method that was used to estimate patient doses. Other methods included the hematologic response and initial patient symptomatology. There have been a number of lymphocyte chromosomal analyses in persons living in areas of Chernobyl fallout. While some authors in southern Germany reported elevated aberration rates after Chernobyl, these results have not been duplicated by other groups who have pre-Chernobyl data.[199,200] The International Chernobyl Project, conducted in 1990, also examined about 100 persons living in clean as well as highly contaminated villages around the plant. Although the study was limited, no differences in chromosome dicentrics or somatic mutations were identified.[72] These results are not surprising, because absorbed doses even in the highly contaminated villages were less than 0.1 Gy, and lymphocyte chromosome analysis is not accurate at radiation levels this low. Populations residing in less heavily contaminated regions of Norway have, likewise, shown no increase in the frequency of chromosome aberrations, with the possible exception of dicentrics (0.3% per cell).[201] More recently, however, germ-line mutations at eight minisatellite loci have been observed to be increased in frequency in men residing in areas heavily contaminated by radionuclides from the Chernobyl accident.[202] Also, follow-up FISH analysis has revealed the frequency of symmetrical translocations in the peripheral blood lymphocytes of 12 of the highly irradiated accident victims to be elevated persistently over the period of observation from 1991 to 1994.[203] The frequencies of *HPRT* mutant T lymphocytes[204] and of lymphocytes with chromosome aberrations were, likewise, found to be elevated at the outset in people exposed to cesium 137 gamma radiation in the Goiania accident; on follow-up, however, both types of abnormality gradually declined, the half-life for the *HPRT* mutant lymphocytes approximating 2.1 years.[204]

SUMMARY

The ultimate aim of the examination of available data is to arrive at estimates of genetic risk from radiation and to quantify the impact. If this can be done, then it is possible to evaluate radiation risk in relation to other risks. It must be borne in mind that the radiation risk estimates used for humans derive some of their strength from animal data, which are used for testing qualitative hypotheses, particularly at low-dose ranges where large numbers of subjects are required for statistical significance. An extensive review of the animal data may be found in the UNSCEAR 2001 report.[39] The human data that were presented previously in this text provide confirmatory evidence that the scientific principles are reasonably similar. A number of new concepts and hereditary mechanisms have been identified and described during the last decade that indicate that human genetics is much more complicated and the biology more resilient than previously thought. Radiation does cause genetic changes, but they are much less common and somewhat different from the spectrum of spontaneously occurring mutations. A large number of animal studies have been done that have helped in understanding the genetic effects of radiation. Unfortunately, all of these have some limitations and require major assumptions to have application to human risk estimates. Fortunately, we do not have to rely solely on animal data, because there are a number of human studies. As UNSCEAR 1993 states,[36]

While people who have been exposed to radiation have been shown to suffer direct effects from exposure, such as increased cancer rates, the data on the survivors of the atomic bombings of Hiroshima and Nagasaki indicate that acute irradiation at moderate doses results in a negligible adverse effect on health of the subsequent generation. Any minor effects that might be produced are so small that they are submerged in the background noise of naturally occurring mutational effects. They cannot be demonstrated even by the refined epidemiological methods that have been employed over the last 5 decades.

Other studies support this view as well. There are nonheritable radiation effects on the genetic material of somatic cells. These effects are only reliably demonstrated at acute doses that exceed 0.1 Gy. They have been seen both in red blood cells and peripheral lymphocytes. These changes cause no apparent clinical harm and many serve as a useful basis for biologic dosimetry in radiation accidents. Radiation carcinogenesis in an irradiated individual occurs as a result of genetic changes in somatic cells that are very complex and difficult to identify. These issues are discussed in Chapter 4.

REFERENCES

1. McKusick, VA. Mendelian inheritance in man. Accessed September 24, 2007 at www.ncbi.nlm.nih.gov/sites/entrez?db=OMIM.
2. Sankaranarayanan, K., Genetic effects of ionising radiation in man. Ann ICRP, 1991. 22(1):75–94.
3. Sankaranarayanan, K., Ionizing radiation and genetic risks. I. Epidemiological, population genetic, biochemical and molecular aspects of Mendelian diseases. Mutat Res, 1991. 258(1):3–49.
4. Sankaranarayanan, K., Ionizing radiation, genetic risk estimation and molecular biology: Impact and inferences. Trends Genet, 1993. 9(3):79–84.
5. Sankaranarayanan, K., Ionizing radiation and genetic risks. III. Nature of spontaneous and radiation-induced mutations in mammalian in vitro systems and mechanisms of induction of mutations by radiation. Mutat Res, 1991. 258(1):75–97.
6. National Research Council (NRC), Committee on the Biological Effects of Ionizing Radiations (BEIR), Health risks from exposure to low levels of ionizing radiation. BEIR VII. 2005, Washington, DC: NRCUSNA Press.
7. Trimble, B. and M. Smith, The incidence of genetic disease and the impact on man of an altered mutation rate. Can J Genet Cytol, 1977. 19:375–385.
8. Stevenson, A., The load of hereditary defects in human populations. Radiat Res, 1959. 1(Suppl): S306–S325.
9. Vogel, F.S. and R. Rathenburg, Spontaneous Mutations in Man: Advances in Human Genetics, vol. 5, H. Harris and K. Hirchhorn, eds. 1975, New York: Plenum Press.
10. Czeizel, A., The Hungarian congenital malformation monitoring system. Acta Paediatr Acad Sci Hung, 1978. 19(3):225–238.
11. Czeizel, A., The baseline data of the Hungarian Congenital Malformation Register, 1970–1976. Acta Paediatr Acad Sci Hung, 1978. 19(2):149–156.
12. Myrianthopoulos, N.C. and C.S. Chung, Congenital malformations in singletons: Epidemiologic survey. Report from the Collaborative Perinatal project. Birth Defects Orig Artic Ser, 1974. 10(11):1–58.
13. Carter, C.O., Genetics of common single malformations. Br Med Bull, 1976. 32(1):21–26.
14. Leck, I., Congenital malformations and childhood neoplasms. J Med Genet, 1977. 14(5):321–326.
15. Neel, J.V., Some considerations pertinent to monitoring human populations for changing mutation rates. In 14th International Congress of Genetics. 1978: Moscow.
16. Neel, J.V., Mutation and disease in man. Can J Genet Cytol, 1978. 20:295–306.
17. Neel, J.V., Mutation and diseases in humans. In Banbury Report I: Assessing Chemical Mutagens: The Risk to Humans, V. McElheny and S. Abrahamson, eds. 1979, Cold Spring Harbor, NY: Cold Spring Harbor Laboratory.
18. Miwa, S., Hereditary haemolytic anaemia due to erythrocyte enzyme deficiency. Acta Haematol Japan, 1973. 36:573–615.
19. Carter, C., Contribution of gene mutations to genetic disease in humans. In Progress in Mutation Research, vol. 1. 1981, Amsterdam: Elsevier/North-Holland Biomedical Press.
20. United Nations Scientific Committee on the Effects of Atomic Radiation (UNSCEAR), Sources and effects of ionizing radiation. Report to the General Assembly with annexes. 1977, New York: United Nations.
21. United Nations Scientific Committee on the Effects of Atomic Radiation (UNSCEAR), Ionizing radiation: Sources and effects. UNSCEAR report to the General Assembly, in annex K: Radiation-induced life shortening. 1982, New York: United Nations.

22. Buckton, K.E., et al., A G-band study of chromosomes in liveborn infants. Ann Hum Genet, 1980. 43(3):227–239.

23. Maeda, T., et al., A cytogenetic survey of consecutive liveborn infants: Incidence and type of chromosome abnormalities. Jap J Hum Genet, 1978. 23:217–224.

24. Lin, C.C., et al., Chromosome analysis on 930 consecutive newborn children using quinacrine fluorescent banding technique. Hum Genet, 1976. 31(3):315–328.

25. Bochkov, N.P., et al., Population cytogenetic investigation of newborns in Moscow. Humangenetik, 1974. 22(2):139–152.

26. Hook, E. and J. Hamerton, The frequency of chromosome abnormalities detected in consecutive newborns studies—differences between studies—results by sex and by severity of phenotypic involvement. In Population Cytogenetics: Studies in Humans, E. Hook and I. Porter, eds. 1977, New York: Academic Press.

27. Neel, J.V., et al., Search for mutations altering protein charge and/or function in children of atomic bomb survivors: Final report. 1987, Hiroshima, Japan: Radiation Effects Research Foundation.

28. Jacobs, P., Correlation between euploid structural chromosome rearrangements and mental subnormality in humans. Nature, 1974. 147(6):164–165.

29. Tharapel, A.T., et al., Apparently balanced de novo translocations in patients with abnormal phenotypes: Report of 6 cases. Clin Genet, 1977. 11(4):255–269.

30. Funderburk, S.J., M.A. Spence, and R.S. Sparkes, Mental retardation associated with "balanced" chromosome rearrangements. Am J Hum Genet, 1977. 29(2):136–141.

31. Alberman, E.D. and M.R. Creasy, Frequency of chromosomal abnormalities in miscarriages and perinatal deaths. J Med Genet, 1977. 14(5):313–315.

32. Bochkov, N.P. Monitoring of human populations in connection with the environmental pollution by the evaluation of chromosome anomalies. In Environmental Mutagens: 4th Annual Meeting of the European Environmental Mutagen Society. 1977, Berlin: Akademie-Verlag.

33. Kuleshov, N., Chromosome anomalies of infants dying during the perinatal period. Hum Genet, 1976. 23:151–160.

34. Machin, G.A. and J.A. Crolla, Chromosome constitution of 500 infants dying during the perinatal period: With an appendix concerning other genetic disorders among these infants. Humangenetik, 1974. 23(3):183–198.

35. Sutherland, G., R. Bauld, and A. Bain, Chromosome abnormality in perinatal death. Lancet, 1974. 1:752.

36. United Nations Scientific Committee on the Effects of Atomic Radiation (UNSCEAR), Sources and effects of ionizing radiation: UNSCEAR 1993 report to the General Assembly, with scientific annexes. 1993, New York: United Nations.

37. Walsh, L., W. Ruhm, and A.M. Kellerer, Cancer risk estimates for gamma-rays with regard to organ-specific doses. Part I: All solid cancers combined. Radiat Environ Biophys, 2004. 43(3):145–151.

38. United Nations Scientific Committee on the Effects of Atomic Radiation (UNSCEAR), Sources and effects of ionizing radiation: UNSCEAR 2000 report to the General Assembly, with scientific annexes. 2000, New York: United Nations.

39. United Nations Scientific Committee on the Effects of Atomic Radiation (UNSCEAR), Hereditary effects of radiation: UNSCEAR 2001 report to the General Assembly, with scientific annex. 2001, New York: United Nations.

40. National Research Council (NRC), Committee on the Biological Effects of Ionizing Radiations (BEIR), Health effects of exposure to low-levels of ionizing radiation. BEIR V. 1990, Washington, DC: N.A. Press.

41. Rudak, E., P. Jacobs, and R. Yamagimachi, Direct analysis of the chromosome constitution of human spermatozoa. Nature, 1978. 174:911–913.

42. Dutrillaux, B. and J. LeJeune, New techniques in the study of human chromosomes: Methods and applications. In Advances in Human Genetics, vol. 5, H. Harris and K. Hirschhorn, eds. 1975, New York: Plenum Press.

43. Dutrillaux, B., New chromosome techniques. In Molecular Structure of Human Chromosomes, J. Yunis, ed. 1977, New York: Academic Press.

44. Dekaban, A.S., Persisting clone of cells with an abnormmal chromosome in a woman previously irradiated. J Nucl Med, 1965. 6:740–746.

45. LeJeune, J., et al., Endore-duplication selective du bras long du chromosome 2 chez une femme et sa fille. Comptes Rendus Hebdomed des Seances de Acad Sci (Paris), 1968. 266:24–26.

46. Baird, P.A., Measuring birth defects and handicapping disorders in the population: The British Columbia Health Surveillance Registry. CMAJ, 1987. 136(2):109–111.

47. Nelson, K. and L.B. Holmes, Malformations due to presumed spontaneous mutations in newborn infants. N Engl J Med, 1989. 320(1):19–23.

48. Baird, P.A., T.W. Anderson, and H.B. Newcombe, et al., Genetic disorders in children and young adults: A population study. Am J Hum Genet, 1988. 42(5):677–693.

49. United Nations Scientific Committee on the Effects of Atomic Radiation (UNSCEAR), Sources and effects of ionizing radiation: UNSCEAR 1996 report to the General Assembly, with scientific annex. 1996, New York: United Nations.

50. Otake, M., W.J. Schull, and J.V. Neel, Congenital malformations, stillbirths, and early mortality among the children of atomic bomb survivors: A reanalysis. Radiat Res, 1990. 122(1):1–11.

51. Neel, J.V., et al., The children of parents exposed to atomic bombs: Estimates of the genetic doubling dose of radiation for humans. Am J Hum Genet, 1990. 46(6):1053–1072.

52. Crow, J.F., A century of mammalian genetics and cancer: Where are we at midpassage? Prog Clin Biol Res, 1981. 45:309–323.

53. Crow, J.F. and C. Denniston, The mutation component of genetic damage. Science, 1981. 212(4497):888–893.

54. Asakawa, J., et al., A genome scanning approach to assess the genetic effects of radiation in mice and humans. Radiat Res, 2004. 161(4):380–390.

55. Baverstock, K.F. and K. Sankaranarayanan, Alpha-particles and leukaemia. Nature, 1992. 357(6377):370.

56. Sankaranarayanan, K., R. Chakraborty, and E.A. Boerwinkle, Ionizing radiation and genetic risks. VI. Chronic multifactorial diseases: A review of epidemiological and genetical aspects of coronary heart disease, essential hypertension and diabetes mellitus. Mutat Res, 1999. 436(1):21–57.

57. International Commission on Radiological Protection (ICRP), Risk estimation for multifactorial diseases: A report of the ICRP. Ann ICRP, 1999. 29(3–4):1–144.

58. International Commission on Radiological Protection (ICRP), 1990 Recommendations of the ICRP. Ann ICRP, 1991. 21(1–3): 1–201.

59. National Council on Radiation Protection and Measurements (NCRP), Risk estimates for radiation protection; Limitation of exposure to ionizing radiation; Research needs for radiation protection; Radiation protection in the mineral extraction industry. NCRP Report nos. 115–118. 1993, Bethesda, Md: The Council.

60. Denniston, C., R. Chakraborty, and K. Sankaranarayanan, Ionizing radiation and genetic risks. VIII. The concept of mutation component and its use in risk estimation for multifactorial diseases. Mutat Res, 1998. 405(1):57–79.

61. Neel, J.V., et al., Search for mutations affecting protein structure in children of atomic bomb survivors: Preliminary report. Proc Natl Acad Sci U S A, 1980. 77(7):4221–4225.

62. Neel, J.V., H.W. Mohrenweiser, and M. Meisler, Rate of spontaneous mutation at human loci encoding protein structure. Proc Natl Acad Sci U S A, 1980. 77:6037.

63. Neel, J.V. and S.E. Lewis, The comparative radiation genetics of humans and mice. Annu Rev Genet, 1990. 24:327–362.

64. Neel, J.V. and W.J. Schull, The Children of the Atomic Bomb Survivors, Neel, J.V. and W.J. Schull, eds. 1991, Washington, DC: National Academy Press.

65. Schull, W.J. and J.V. Neel, Radiation and the sex ratio in man. Science, 1958. 128(3320):343–348.

66. Neel, J.V., et al., Implications of the Hiroshima-Nagasaki genetic studies for the estimation of the human "doubling dose" of radiation. In 16th International Congress of Genetics. 1988: Toronto, Canada.

67. Neel, J.V., et al., Implications of the Hiroshima-Nagasaki genetic studies for the estimation of the human "doubling dose" of radiation. Genome, 1989. 31(2):853–859.

68. Otake, M., W.J. Schull, and J.V. Neel, Congenital malformations, stillbirths, and early mortality among the children of atomic bomb surviviors: A reanalysis. 1989, Hiroshima, Japan: Radiation Effects Research Foundation.

69. Neel, J.V., The past and the future in the study of radiation-induced mutation in the germ-line of mice and humans. Environ Mol Mutagen, 1989. 14(1):55–60.

70. Awa, A., et al., Cytogenetic study of the offspring of atomic bomb survivors, Hiroshima and Nagasaki. 1988, Hiroshima, Japan: Radiation Effects Research Foundation.

71. Czeizel, A.E., C. Elek, and E. Susanszky, The evaluation of the germinal mutagenic impact of Chernobyl radiological contamination in Hungary. Mutagenesis, 1991. 6(4):285–288.

72. International Atomic Energy Agency (IAEA), The International Chernobyl Project: Report of an International Committee. 1991, Vienna: IAEA.

73. Chernobyl Forum and World Health Organization (WHO), Health effects of the Chernobyl accident and special health care programmes. 2005, Geneva: WHO.

74. Lazjuk, G., et al., The congenital anomalies registry in Belarus: A tool for assessing the public health impact of the Chernobyl accident. Reprod Toxicol, 2003. 17(6):659–666.

75. Sever, L.E., et al., A case-control study of congenital malformations and occupational exposure to low-level ionizing radiation. Am J Epidemiol, 1988. 127(2):226–242.

76. Goldberg, M.S., et al., Adverse reproductive outcomes among women exposed to low levels of ionizing radiation from diagnostic radiography for adolescent idiopathic scoliosis. Epidemiology, 1998. 9(3):271–278.

77. Kallen, B., et al., Outcome of reproduction in women irradiated for skin hemangioma in infancy. Radiat Res, 1998. 149(2):202–208.

78. Kaplan, I., Genetic effects in children and grandchildren of women treated for infertility and sterility by roentgen therapy: A report of the study of 33 years. Radiology, 1959. 72:518–521.

79. Maconochie, N., et al., Sex ratio of nuclear industry employees' children. Lancet, 2001. 357(9268):1589–1591.

80. Hawkins, M.M., Is there evidence of a therapy-related increase in germ cell mutation among childhood cancer survivors? J Natl Cancer Inst, 1991. 83(22):1643–1650.

81. Nygaard, R., et al., Reproduction following treatment for childhood leukemia: A population based prospective cohort study of fertility and offspring. Med Pediatr Oncol, 1991. 19:459–466.

82. Hawkins, M.M., Pregnancy outcome and offspring after childhood cancer. BMJ, 1994. 309(6961):1034.

83. Hawkins, M.M., G.J. Draper, and D.L. Winter, Cancer in the offspring of survivors of childhood leukaemia and non-Hodgkin lymphomas. Br J Cancer, 1995. 71(6):1335–1339.

84. Byrne, J., et al., Genetic disease in offspring of long-term survivors of childhood and adolescent cancer. Am J Hum Genet, 1998. 62(1):45–52.

85. Blatt, J., Pregnancy outcome in long-term survivors of childhood cancer. Med Pediatr Oncol, 1999. 33(1):29–33.

86. Chiarelli, A.M., L.D. Marrett, and G.A. Darlington, Pregnancy outcomes in females after treatment for childhood cancer. Epidemiology, 2000. 11(2):161–166.

87. Boice J.D., Jr., et al., Genetic effects of radiotherapy for childhood cancer. Health Phys, 2003. 85(1):65–80.

88. Andersson, M., et al., Effects of preconceptional irradiation on mortality and cancer incidence in the offspring of patients given injections of Thorotrast. J Natl Cancer Inst, 1994. 86(24):1866–1867.

89. Yoshimoto, Y., et al., Mortality among the offsprings (F₁) of the atomic bomb survivors, 1946–85. 1991, Hiroshima, Japan: Radiation Effects Research Foundation.

90. Yoshimoto, Y., et al., Malignant tumors during the first two decades of life in the offspring of atomic bomb survivors. Am J Hum Genet, 1990. 46(6):1041–1052.

91. Yoshimoto, Y., et al., Frequency of malignant tumors during the first two decades of life in the offspring (F₁) of atomic bomb survivors. 1990, Hiroshima, Japan: Radiation Effects Research Foundation.

92. Yoshimoto, Y., H. Kato, and W.J. Schull, Risk of cancer among children exposed in utero to A-bomb radiations, 1950–84. Lancet, 1988. 2(8612):665–669.

93. Yoshimoto, Y., et al., Mortality among the offspring (F₁) of atomic bomb survivors, 1946–85. J Radiat Res (Tokyo), 1991. 32(4):327–351.

94. Kato, H., Y. Yoshimoto, and W.J. Schull, Risk of cancer among children exposed to atomic bomb radiation in utero: A review. IARC Sci Publ, 1989(96): 365–374.

95. Taylor, G.N., et al., Comparative toxicity of ^{226}Ra, ^{239}Pu, ^{241}Am, ^{249}Cf, and ^{252}Cf in C57BL/Do black and albino mice. Radiat Res, 1983. 95(3):584–601.

96. Gardner, M.J., et al., Results of case-control study of leukaemia and lymphoma among young people near Sellafield nuclear plant in West Cumbria. BMJ, 1990. 300(6722):423–429.

97. Gardner, M.J., et al., Methods and basic data of case-control study of leukaemia and lymphoma among young people near Sellafield nuclear plant in West Cumbria. BMJ, 1990. 300(6722):429–434.

98. Wakeford, R., et al., The Seascale childhood leukemia cases—The mutation rates implied by paternal preconceptional radiation doses. J Radiat Prot, 1994. 14(1):17–24.

99. Little, M.P., A comparison of the risk of stillbirth associated with paternal pre-conception irradiation in the Sellafield workforce with that of stillbirth and untoward pregnancy outcome among Japanese atomic bomb survivors. J Radiol Prot, 1999. 19(4):361–373.

100. Evans, H.J., Gardner report. Leukaemia and radiation. Nature, 1990. 345(6270):16–17.

101. Black, R.J., et al., Incidence of leukaemia and other cancers in birth and schools cohorts in the Dounreay area. BMJ, 1992. 304(6839):1401–1405.

102. McLaughlin, J.R., et al., Paternal radiation exposure and leukaemia in offspring: The Ontario case-control study. BMJ, 1993. 307(6910):959–966.

103. Doll, R., H.J. Evans, and S.C. Darby, Paternal exposure not to blame. Nature, 1994. 367(6465):678–680.

104. Draper, G.J., et al., Cancer in the offspring of radiation workers: A record linkage study. BMJ, 1997. 315(7117):1181–1188.

105. Roman, E., et al., Cancer in children of nuclear industry employees: Report on children aged under 25 years from nuclear industry family study. BMJ, 1999. 318(7196):1443–1450.

106. Sorahan, T., et al., Cancer in the offspring of radiation workers: An investigation of employment timing and a reanalysis using updated dose information. Br J Cancer, 2003. 89(7):1215–1220.

107. Sorahan, T., et al., Childhood cancer and paternal exposure to ionizing radiation: A second report from the Oxford Survey of Childhood Cancers. Am J Ind Med, 1995. 28(1):71–78.

108. Wakeford, R. and L. Parker, Leukaemia and non-Hodgkin's lymphoma in young persons resident in small areas of West Cumbria in relation to paternal preconceptional irradiation. Br J Cancer, 1996. 73(5):672–679.

109. Gardner, M., Leukemia in children and paternal radiation exposure at the Sellafield nuclear site. Monogr Natl Cancer Inst, 1992. 12:133–135.

110. Gardner, M.J., Paternal occupations of children with leukemia. BMJ, 1992. 305(6855):715.

111. Vrema, R., H. Dosik, and L. Ha, Interrelationship between parental age and source of non-disjunction during first and second meiotic division of extra chromosome 21 in Down syndrome: A report of six cases with review. Mammalian Chromosome Newsletter, 1978. 19(1,2)56.

112. Mikkelsen, M., et al., Non-disjunction in trisomy 21: Study of chromosomal heteromorphisms in 110 families. Ann Hum Genet, 1980. 44(Pt 1):17–28.

113. Carter, C. and K. Evans, Risk of parents who have had one child with Down syndrome (mongolism) having another child similarly affected. Lancet, 1961. 2:785.

114. Penrose, L. and G. Smith, Down Anomaly. 1966, London: Churchill.

115. Richards, B., Mosaic mongolism. J Ment Defic Res, 1969. 13:66–83.

116. Gorlin, R., Classical chromosome disorders. In New Chromosomal Syndromes, vol. 8, J. Yunis, ed. 1977, New York: Plenum Press.

117. Alberman, E., et al., Parental exposure to x-irradiation and Down's syndrome. Ann Hum Genet, 1972. 36(2):195–208.

118. Sigler, A., et al., Radiation exposure in parents of children with mongolism (Down syndrome). Bull Johns Hopkins Hosp, 1965. 117:374–399.

119. Uchida, I. and E. Curtis, A possible association between maternal radiation and mongolism. Lancet, 1961. 2:848–850.

120. Uchida, I., R. Holunga, and C. Lawler, Maternal radiation chromosome aberrations. Lancet, 1968. 2:1045–1949.

121. Sankaranarayanan, K., The role of non-disjunction in aneuploidy in man: An overview. Mutat Res, 1979. 61(1):1–28.

122. Cohen, B.L., A. Lilienfeld, and S. Kramer, Parental factors in Down syndrome: Results of the second Baltimore case-control study. In Population Cytogenetics: Studies in Humans, E. Hook and I.H. Porter, eds. 1977, New York: Academic Press.

123. Villumsen, A., Environmental factors in congenital malformations. In A Perspective Study of 9006 Human Pregnancies. 1970, Copenhagen: FADL Forlag.

124. Schull, W.J. and J.V. Neel, Maternal radiation and mongolism. Lancet, 1962. 1:537–538.

125. Lunn, J.E., A survey of mongol children in Glasgow. Scott Med J, 1959. 4:368–372.

126. Carter, C., K. Evans, and A. Stewart, Maternal radiation and Down syndrome (mongolism). Lancet, 1961. 2:1042.

127. Stevenson, A., R. Mason, and K. Edwards, Maternal diagnostic x-irradiation before conception and the frequency of mongolism in children subsequently born. Lancet, 1970. 2:1335–1337.

128. Stevenson, A. and V. Matousek, Medical x-ray exposure history of the parents of children with Down syndrome (mongolism). 1961, Oxford: Medical Research Council, Population Genetics Research Unit.

129. Deng, S., Birth survey in background radiation area. Chin J Radiol Med Prot, 1982. 2:60.

130. Cui, Y., Hereditary diseases and congenital malformation survey in high background area. Chin J Radiol Med Prot, 1982. 2:55–57.

131. Sperling, K., et al., Fallout from Chernobyl: Authors stand by study that Chernobyl increased trisomy 21 in Berlin. BMJ, 1994. 309(6964):1299.

132. Sperling, K., et al., Significant increase in trisomy 21 in Berlin nine months after the Chernobyl reactor accident: Temporal correlation or causal relation? BMJ, 1994. 309(6948):158–162.

133. Burkart, W., B. Grosche, and A. Schoetzau, Down syndrome clusters in Germany after the Chernobyl accident. Radiat Res, 1997. 147(3):321–328.

134. de Wals, P., et al., Chromosomal anomalies and Chernobyl. Int J Epidemiol, 1988. 17(1):230–231.

135. De Wals, P., et al., Epidemiologic surveillance of congenital abnormalities using the EUROCAT Register. Rev Epidemiol Sante Publique, 1988. 36(4–5): 273–282.

136. Zatsepin, I., et al., Cluster of Down syndrome cases registered in January 1987 in the Republic of Belarus as a possible consequence of the Chernobyl accident. Int J Radiat Med (in press).

137. Francis, J. and M. Snee, A case control study of trisomy 21 and maternal pre-conceptual radiography. Clin Radiol, 1991. 43(5):343–346.

138. Schull, W.J., M. Otake, and J.V. Neel, Genetic effects of the atomic bombs: A reappraisal. Science, 1981. 213(4513):1220–1227.

139. Schull, W.J., M. Otake, and J.V. Neel, Hiroshima and Nagasaki: A reassessment of the mutagenic effect of exposure to ionizing radiation. In Population and Biological Aspects of Human Mutation. 1981, New York: Academic Press.

140. Hakoda, M., et al., Increased somatic cell mutant frequency in atomic bomb survivors. 1987, Hiroshima, Japan: Radiation Effects Research Foundation.

141. Hakoda, M., et al., Increased somatic cell mutant frequency in atomic bomb survivors. Mutat Res, 1988. 201(1):39–48.

142. Nicklas, J.A., et al., In vivo ionizing irradiations produce deletions in the hprt gene of human T-lymphocytes. Mutat Res, 1991. 250(1–2):383–396.

143. Branda, R., J. O'Neill and L. Sullivan, Factors influencing mutation at the hprt locus in T-lymphocytes: Women treated for breast cancer. Cancer Res, 1991. 511:6603–6607.

144. Bridges, B.A., et al., Possible association between mutant frequency in peripheral lymphocytes and domestic radon concentrations. Lancet, 1991. 337(8751):1187–1189.

145. Kyoizumi, S., et al., Frequency of mutant T-lymphocytes defective in the expression of the T-cell antigen receptor gene among radiation exposed people. 1990, Hiroshima, Japan: Radiation Effects Research Foundation.

146. Kyoizumi, S., et al., Frequency of mutant T lymphocytes defective in the expression of the T-cell antigen receptor gene among radiation-exposed people. Mutat Res, 1992. 265(2):173–180.

147. Umeki, S., et al., Flow cytometric measurements of somatic cell mutations in Thorotrast patients. Jpn J Cancer Res, 1991. 82(12):1349–1353.

148. Umeki, S., et al., Flow-cytometric measurements of somatic cell mutations in Thorotrast patients. 1991, Hiroshima, Japan: Radiation Effects Research Foundation.

149. Langlois, R.G., W.L. Bigbee, and R.H. Jensen, Measurements of the frequency of human erythrocytes with gene expression loss phenotypes at the glycophorin A locus. Hum Genet, 1986. 74(4):353–362.

150. Langlois, R.G., et al., Evidence for increased somatic cell mutations at the glycophorin A locus in atomic bomb survivors. Science, 1987. 236(4800):445–448.

151. Kyoizumi, S., et al., Detection of somatic mutations at the glycophorin A locus in erythrocytes of atomic bomb survivors using a single beam flow sorter. 1988, Hiroshima, Japan: Radiation Effects Research Foundation.

152. Jensen, R.H., et al., Glycophorin A as a biological dosimeter for radiation dose to the bone marrow from iodine-131. Radiat Res, 1997. 147(6):747–752.

153. Lloyd, D.C., et al., Doses in Radiation Accidents Investigated by Chromosome Aberrations Analysis: IX. A Review of Cases Investigated. 1979, Harwell, UK: National Radiological Protection Board.

154. Dolphin, G.W. and D.C. Lloyd, The significance of radiation-induced chromosome abnormalities in radiological protection. J Med Genet, 1974. 11(2):181–189.

155. Scheid, W., J. Weber, and H. Traut, Chromosome aberrations induced in human lymphocytes by an X-radiation accident: Results of a 4-year postirradiation analysis. Int J Radiat Biol, 1988. 54(3):395–402.

156. Kleinerman, R.A., et al., Chromosome aberrations in relation to radiation dose following partial-body exposures in three populations. Radiat Res, 1990. 123(1):93–101.

157. Bender, M.A., Chromosome aberrations in irradiated human subjects. Ann N Y Acad Sci, 1964. 114:249–251.

158. Dolphin, G., Biological dosimetry with paratular reference to chromosome aberration analysis. In Handling of Radiation Accidents, in Proceedings of a Symposium. 1969, Vienna: International Atomic Energy Agency.

159. Evans, H., Use of chromosome aberration frequencies for biological dosimetry in man. In Advances in Physical and Biological Radiation Detectors, in Proceedings of a Symposium in New Developments in Physical and Biological Radiation Detectors. 1971, Vienna: International Atomic Energy Agency.

160. Abbatt, J., Cytogenetic indicators of radiation (and other) damage calibration—present and future practical applications. In Biochemical Indicators of Radiation Injury in Man. 1971, Vienna: International Atomic Energy Agency.

161. Bender, M.A., Status of Human Chromosome as a Biological Radiation Dosimeter in the Nuclear Industry. 1978, Upton, NY: Brookhaven National Laboratory (BNL).

162. Dufrain, R., et al., In-vitro human cytogenetic dose-response system. 1979, Oak Ridge, Tenn: Oak Ridge Associated Universities.

163. Edwards, A.A., D.C. Lloyd, and R.J. Purrott, Radiation induced chromosome aberrations and the Poisson distribution. Radiat Environ Biophys, 1979. 16(2):89–100.

164. WF, B., et al., Radiation exposure assessment using cytological and molecular biomarkers. Rad Prot Dosimetry, 2001. 97(1):17–23.

165. Blakely, W.F., et al., Radiation exposure assessment using cytological and molecular biomarkers. Radiat Prot Dosimetry, 2001. 97(1):17–23.

166. Silberstein, E.B., et al., The human lymphocyte as a radiobiological dosimeter after total body irradiation. Radiat Res, 1974. 59(3):658–664.

167. Lloyd, D.C., et al., Doses in Radiation Accident Investigated by Chromosome Aberration Analysis. 1982, Oxford: National Radiological Protection Board.

168. Schneider, G., B. Chone, and T. Bloonigen, Chromosomal aberrations in a radiation accident. Radiat Res, 1969. 40:613–617.

169. Littlefield, L., et al., Cytogenetic dose estimates from in-vivo samples from persons involved in real or suspected radiation exposures. In The Medical Basis for Radiation Accident Preparedness, K. Hubner and S.A. Fry, eds. 1980, New York: Elsevier/North-Holland.

170. Edwards, A.A., The use of chromosomal aberrations in human lymphocytes for biological dosimetry. Radiat Res, 1997. 148(Suppl 5):S39–S44.

171. Finnon, P., et al., The ^{60}Co gamma ray dose-response for chromosomal aberrations in human lymphocytes analysed by FISH; Applicability to biological dosimetry. Int J Radiat Biol, 1999. 75(10):1215–1222.

172. Lucas, J.N., et al., Rapid translocation frequency analysis in humans decades after exposure to ionizing radiation. Int J Radiat Biol, 1992. 62(1):53–63.

173. Countryman, P.I. and J.A. Heddle, The production of micronuclei from chromosome aberrations in irradiated cultures of human lymphocytes. Mutat Res, 1976. 41(2–3):321–332.

174. Ban, S., et al., Gamma-ray and fission neutron induced micronuclei in PHA-stimulated and unstimulated human lymphocytes. 1990, Hiroshima, Japan: Radiation Effects Research Foundation (RERF).

175. Catena, C., et al., Micronucleus yield and colorimetric test as indicators of damage in patients' lymphocytes after ^{131}I therapy. J Nucl Med, 2000. 41(9):1522–1524.

176. Ban, S., et al., Radiosensitivity of atomic bomb survivors as determined with a micronucleus assay. 1992, Hiroshima, Japan: Radiation Effects Research Foundation.

177. Ban, S., et al., Radiosensitivity of atomic bomb survivors as determined with a micronucleus assay. Radiat Res, 1993. 134(2):170–178.

178. Lucas, J.N., Dose reconstruction for individuals exposed to ionizing radiation using chromosome painting. Radiat Res, 1997. 148(Suppl 5): S33–S38.

179. Grace, M.B., C.B. McLeland, and W.F. Blakely, Real-time quantitative RT-PCR assay of GADD45 gene expression changes as a biomarker for radiation biodosimetry. Int J Radiat Biol, 2002. 78(11):1011–1021.

180. Durante, M., K. George, and T.C. Yang, Biodosimetry of ionizing radiation by selective painting of prematurely condensed chromosomes in human lymphocytes. Radiat Res, 1997. 148(Supp 5): S45–S50.

181. Prasanna, P.G., et al., Premature chromosome condensation assay for biodosimetry: Studies with fission-neutrons. Health Phys, 1997. 72(4):594–600.

182. Miller, A.C., et al., Proto-oncogene expression: A predictive assay for radiation biodosimetry applications. Radiat Prot Dosimetry, 2002. 99(1–4):295–302.

183. Pohl-Ruling, J. and P.Fischer, The dose effect relationship of chromosome aberrations to alpha and gamma irradiation in a population subjected to an increased burden of natural radioactivity. Radiat Res, 1979. 80:61–81.

184. High Background Radiation Research Group (HBRRG), Health survey in high background radiation areas in China: HBRRG, China. Science, 1980. 209(4459):877–880.

185. Tanaka, K., et al., High incidence of micronuclei in lymphocytes from residents of the area near the Semipalatinsk nuclear explosion test site. J Radiat Res (Tokyo), 2000. 41(1):45–54.

186. Chang, W.P., et al., Follow-up in the micronucleus frequencies and its subsets in human population with chronic low-dose gamma-irradiation exposure. Mutat Res, 1999. 428(1–2):99–105.

187. Evans, H.J., et al., Radiation-induced chromosome aberrations in nuclear-dockyard workers. Nature, 1979. 277(5697):531–534.

188. Bauchinger, M., et al., Chromosome analyses of nuclear-power plant workers. Int J Radiat Biol Relat Stud Phys Chem Med, 1980. 38(5):577–581.

189. Brandom, W.F., et al., Chromosome aberrations as a biological dose-response indicator of radiation exposure in uranium miners. Radiat Res, 1978. 76(1):159–171.

190. Brandom, W.F., B.Archer, and A. Bloom, Chromosome changes in somatic cells of workers with internal depositions of plutonium. In Biological Implications of Radionuclides Released from Nuclear Industries. 1979, Vienna: International Atomic Energy Agency.

191. Tucker, J.D., et al., Biological dosimetry of radiation workers at the Sellafield nuclear facility. Radiat Res, 1997. 148(3):216–226.

192. Thierens, H., A. Vral, and L. De Ridder, A cytogenetic study of radiological workers: Effect of age, smoking and radiation burden on the micronucleus frequency. Mutat Res, 1996. 360(2):75–82.

193. Awa, A.A., Review of thirty years study of Hiroshima and Nagasaki atomic bomb survivors. II. Biological effects. G. Chromosome aberrations in somatic cells. J Radiat Res (Tokyo), 1975. 16(Suppl):S122–S131.

194. Awa, A.A., et al., Chromosome-aberration frequency in cultured blood-cells in relation to radiation dose of A-bomb survivors. Lancet, 1971. 2(7730):903–905.

195. Sofuni, T., et al., A cytogenetic study of Hiroshima atomic bomb survivors. In Mutagen-Induced Chromosome Damage in Man, H.J. Evans and D.C. Lloyd, eds. 1978, Edinburgh: Edinburgh University Press.

196. Stram, D.O., et al., Stable chromosome aberrations among A-bomb survivors: An update. Radiat Res, 1993. 136(1):29–36.

197. Kyoizumi, S., et al., Somatic cell mutations at the glycophorin A locus in erythrocytes of atomic bomb survivors: Implications for radiation carcinogenesis. Radiat Res, 1996. 146(1):43–52.

198. Ramalho, A.T., et al., Frequency of chromosomal aberrations in a subject accidentally exposed to ^{137}Cs in the Goiania (Brazil) radiation accident: Intercomparison among four laboratories. Mutat Res, 1991. 252(2):157–160.

199. Braselmann, H., E. Schmid, and M. Bauchinger, Chromosome analysis in a population living in an area of Germany with the highest fallout deposition from the Chernobyl accident. Mutat Res, 1992. 283(3):221–225.

200. Stephan, G. and U. Oestreicher, Chromosome investigation of individuals living in areas of southern Germany contaminated by fallout from the Chernobyl reactor accident. Mutat Res, 1993. 319(3):189–196.

201. Brogger, A., et al., Chromosome analysis of peripheral lymphocytes from persons exposed to radioactive fallout in Norway from the Chernobyl accident. Mutat Res, 1996. 361(2–3):73–79.

202. Dubrova, Y.E., et al., Elevated minisatellite mutation rate in the post-Chernobyl families from Ukraine. Am J Hum Genet, 2002. 71(4):801–809.

203. Salassidis, K., et al., Chromosome painting in highly irradiated Chernobyl victims: A follow-up study to evaluate the stability of symmetrical translocations and the influence of clonal aberrations for retrospective dose estimation. Int J Radiat Biol, 1995. 68(3):257–262.

204. da Cruz, A.D., et al., Monitoring hprt mutant frequency over time in T-lymphocytes of people accidentally exposed to high doses of ionizing radiation. Environ Mol Mutagen, 1996. 27(3):165–175.

4 Cancer Induction and Dose-Response Models

Cancer induction is the most important somatic effect of radiation at dose levels below 1 Gy. However, almost all of the data used to derive risk estimates for the carcinogenic effects of low-level irradiation have been obtained from situations in which the exposure actually occurred at dose levels above 0.1 Gy. Nevertheless, the bulk of the available experimental and epidemiological data support the assumption that the induction of tumors, whether benign or malignant, is a probabilistic function, or *stochastic effect*, of radiation.[1-3] Hence, as in the case of genetic effects, which also are stochastic, an increase in the dose is assumed to increase the probability of the effect but to have little or no influence on its severity.

Therefore, most scientists assume on philosophical grounds and for radiation protection purposes that there is no threshold for cancer induction and that even a small dose of radiation may, in theory, increase the risk of neoplasia.[2] This assumption can neither be proved nor disproved, as noted below. The cancers induced by radiation are not individually distinguishable, clinically or pathologically, from those due to other causes. Furthermore, although the induced tumors include neoplasms of many types, tissues vary widely in susceptibility to the carcinogenic effects of radiation, and some types of human cancers (e.g., chronic lymphocytic leukemia [CLL]) do not appear to be induced by radiation in significant numbers, if at all (Table 4-1).

MOLECULAR AND CELLULAR ASPECTS

Most, if not all, cancers are clonal growths, each arising from a single cell through a succession of genetic changes.[4-6] The development of cancer is thus typically a multicausal, multistage process, in which the stepwise accumulation of genetic abnormalities in an evolving clone leads to the selection of increasingly autonomous cellular variants. Although the specific changes that are involved vary from one neoplasm to another, the process is commonly subdivided for convenience into the following successive stages: (1) *tumor initiation*, the irreversible change of a normal somatic cell into a cell with preneoplastic proliferative potential; (2) *tumor promotion*, the early clonal expansion of the initiated, preneoplastic cell;

(3) *neoplastic conversion*, the transformation of the preneoplastic cell into an autonomous cellular variant committed to neoplastic proliferation; and (4) *malignant progression*, the accumulation of further changes in the neoplastic cell and its progeny, rendering them capable of invading normal tissue and metastasizing to distant sites, and leading stepwise to progressively more autonomous cellular variants.[2] As implied, these four stages do not all necessarily contain the same number of steps, nor are they all of the same length for different types of tumors.

The *initiating* phase characteristically involves a permanent genetic change, as noted below, and although various epigenetic factors may also be involved in the process,[7] the chemical and physical agents known to be capable of causing tumor initiation are typically genotoxic. *Promoting* agents, in contrast, are not genotoxic themselves, although some are able to induce free radical formation and damage DNA indirectly. Typically, promoting agents have low oncogenic potential when acting alone, but they can greatly increase the probability of neoplasia when acting on initiated cells. Usually repeated or chronic exposure to a given promoting agent is necessary, and its effects may be reversible, in contrast to those of an initiating agent, which are characteristically irreversible.[8,9] Promoting agents comprise a large number of chemicals, including bioacid, phenobarbital, phorbol esters, growth factor hormones, and various dietary components; in animal systems, tissue wounding and stress also may act as promoting agents. In general, promoting agents disturb cellular homeostasis, stimulate hyperplasia, and may also induce inflammation. Ionizing radiation, through its ability to damage tissue and cause regenerative hyperplasia, can act as a promoting agent, but its promoting effects are likely to be significant only at doses that are large enough to cause substantial cell inactivation. Since the process of tumor promotion is essentially a supernormal proliferative response, which may result in part from the loss of intercellular communication, substances such as retinoids that increase intercellular communication may act as antipromoters. Virus infections also have been associated with the development of certain human neoplasms; for example, Kaposi's

Table 4-1 • Comparative Susceptibility (Based on % Increases in Background Incidence/Unit Dose) of Different Tissues to Radiation-induced Cancer	
High	Kidney
Bone marrow (leukemia other than CLL)	Larynx
	Nasal sinuses
Breast (female)	
Salivary glands	**Very low or absent**
Thyroid (more common in females)	Cervix
	Chronic lymphatic leukemia
Moderate	Oral cavity
Bladder	Esophagus
Colon	Melanoma
Stomach	Prostate
Liver	Uterus
Lung	Pancreas
Ovary	Rectum
Skin	Gallbladder
	Hodgkin's disease
Low	Lymphatic system and myeloma
Bone	Testes
Brain	Muscle
Connective tissue	

sarcoma, T-cell leukemia, lymphoma, nasopharyngeal carcinoma, and cancers of the liver, cervix, anus, larynx, and skin.[10–12]

Malignant progression denotes the accumulation of further genetic changes in association with genomic instability. The principle characteristic of the process is the progressive dedifferentiation of the neoplastic cells, exemplified by their acquisition of the ability to invade normal tissues, penetrate blood vessels and/or lymphatic systems, and metastasize to distant sites. Steps involved in this process include the action of various digestive enzymes to allow the neoplastic cells to penetrate normal tissues, as well as changes in cell surface receptors to allow reattachment of the cells at distant sites. Also, for the cells to form a tumor at a distant site, a blood supply (angiogenesis) must be recruited for the purpose, a process mediated by growth factors.

The specific types of genetic abnormalities that are involved in the various stages of radiation carcinogenesis, their modes of action, and the mechanisms by which they may be produced are questions at the forefront of a fast-moving and complex research field. (For in-depth and excellent reviews of the topic, see the recent United Nations Scientific Committee on the Effects of Atomic Radiation (UNSCEAR)[13,14] and Committee on the Biological Effects of Ionizing Radiation (BEIR)[2] reports and articles by Cox[15,16] and Little.[17]

In brief, the process of carcinogenesis has been observed to involve changes in several classes of regulatory genes, including *tumor-suppressor* genes of the so-called

gatekeeper type, tumor genes of the so-called caretaker type, and tumor genes of the *oncogene* type.[2,6] The cells of a given cancer often contain changes in several such genes, and there is evidence of complementary interactions between different tumor genes. The requirement for multiple, interacting genes to be involved may account in part for the age-distribution of most cancers in the general population and for the long latent period that typically occurs between irradiation and the clinical appearance of a tumor.

The specific genetic determinants of the process of *tumor initiation* are incompletely known. For a growing number of solid tumors, however, the data point to the involvement of tumor-suppressor genes of the so-called gatekeeper type, loss or inactivation of which allows the affected cell to escape from normal regulation and embark on a phase of abnormal clonal expansion.[2,6,14,18] Examples include the *RBI* gene in retinoblastoma and osteosarcoma, the *RET* gene in thyroid carcinoma, the *VHL* gene in kidney carcinoma, the *APC* gene in colorectal cancer, and the *PTCH* (*Patched*) gene in basal cell carcinoma.[2,14,19] Suppressor genes have also been described for tumors of the endometrium, breast, cervix, lung, bladder, meninges, central nervous system (astrocytoma, acoustic neuroma, neuroblastoma, neurofibromatosis of type 1 and type 2), skin (melanoma), kidney (Wilms' tumor), adrenal (pheochromocytoma), and multiple endocrine gland neoplasia type 2.[20] The loss of function of such genes can occur through point mutation, intragenic deletion, gross chromosomal change, or epigenetic silencing.[18,21] For example, specific chromosome deletion at 13q occurs in retinoblastoma and at the gene site 11p in Wilms' tumor. Additionally, segment 21 on chromosome 5 (5q21) is associated with human familial adenomatous polyposis and colorectal carcinoma.

From the foregoing, it is evident that the loss or inactivation of gatekeeper genes has been observed primarily in solid tumors. In the pathogenesis of leukemias and lymphomas, a different genetic mechanism appears to be involved; namely, the activation of tissue-specific proto-oncogenes, through juxtaposition of DNA sequences by specific chromosomal rearrangements.[22,23]

Another broad and overlapping class of genes implicated in various stages of carcinogenesis includes the so-called caretaker genes, which are involved in the maintenance of genomic integrity. The loss or inactivation of such genes can lead to deficiencies in DNA repair, chromosomal segregation, cell cycle control, and/or apoptotic response,[18] resulting in a genomic instability that has been postulated to be an important factor in radiation carcinogenesis.[17] Examples of human tumor genes of the caretaker type and their associated neoplasms include the *BRCA1,2* genes (cancers of the breast and ovary), the *ATM* gene (lymphocytic leukemia), the *TP53* gene (many types of cancer), the *MSH2, MLH1, PMS* genes (cancers of the colon and endometrium), and the *XPA-G* gene

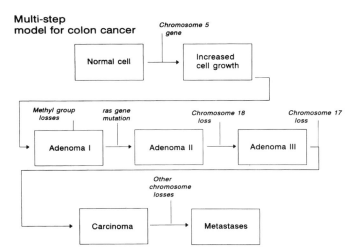

Figure 4-1 • Possible multistep model for induction of colon cancer. (From Fearon E, Logelstein B: A genetic model for colorectal tumourigenesis. Cell 1990;61:759–767.)

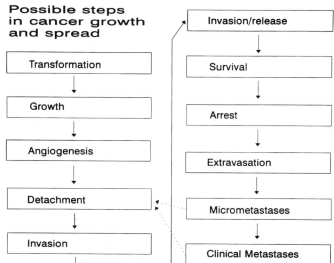

Figure 4-2 • Possible steps involved in the induction and spread of cancer. (From Hart I, Saini A: Biology of tumour mestastasis. Lancet 1992;339:1453–1457.)

(squamous and basal cell carcinomas and melanomas of the skin).[2]

As noted above, multiple genetic interactions are commonly required for tumor induction. In the development of human colorectal cancer, for example, the sequential loss and/or activation of one, two, or three genes are required for benign changes, whereas at least four or five genes must be mutated before full malignant conversion occurs (Fig. 4-1).[5,24]

Overall, it appears that tumors may be induced by a combination of events, including positive signals from activated oncogenes and loss of negative signals from tumor-suppressor genes, which may be followed by a number of nonmutational events such as DNA methylation and modifications of the activities of two classes of proteins, particularly kinases and cyclines. Because chromosomal rearrangements occur in various tumors, there has been interest as to whether all sites on the chromosome have the same strength or resistance to breakage or deletion. Sites of chromosomal instability, also called fragile sites, are known to exist. These have been demonstrated by induction with different types of chemical treatment, and it is not yet clear whether these same sites are preferentially damaged or broken by ionizing radiation. Furthermore, although damage to certain portions of the DNA can cause major changes in cellular properties if it remains unrepaired or is misrepaired, damage in other, noncoding areas may have little or no consequence. By the same token, although all cells in a given individual contain the same genes, the genes are not equally active in every cell; differences in gene activation are critical to the normal development, structure, and function of the different organs, and the differences are subject to mediation through secondary processes, including the action of hormones and other compounds. Not surprisingly, therefore, a given radiation-induced change

in DNA cannot be expected to cause the same biological effect in all types of cells. A generalized scheme for multistage oncogenesis is shown in Figure 4-2.

PREDISPOSITION TO RADIATION-INDUCED MALIGNANCY

Because the phases of oncogenesis depend heavily on genetic changes and characteristics, it is not surprising that a family history of early-onset cancer is associated with an increased risk of a second malignant neoplasm,[25] and that certain inherited disorders are associated with increased risks of specific neoplasms. Familial traits are associated with DNA sequence loss for retinoblastoma, Wilms' tumor, and multiple endocrine neoplasia. The breast cancer susceptibility gene *BRCA1* has been localized to a region on chromosome 17q and the *BRCA2* gene to a region on 13q12-q13. There are also the rare but relatively well-documented genetic disorders of *xeroderma pigmentosum* (XP) and ataxia-telangiectasia (A-T). Cells from A-T patients clearly are more radiosensitive in terms of cell inactivation than normal or than the cells from patients who have other DNA repair deficiencies. Likewise, there is evidence suggesting that deficiencies in DNA repair may be related to the development of thyroid tumors after radiotherapy to the head and neck in childhood.[26]

In all, some 641 spontaneous cancer-prone genetic disorders have been identified, but the incidence of any one of them is quite low.[27] Most are in the range of 1-in-5000 to 1-in-100,000 live births[2,3] (Table 4-2). Overall, based on the frequency of known, highly penetrating mutations, experts have generally concluded that genetic susceptibility to cancer is not a major factor to be considered in formulating radiation risk estimates for the

Table 4-2 • Estimates of the Frequency of Some Cancer-prone Human Mutations

Mutation	Principal Neoplasms	Phenotypic Manifestations	Chromosomal Location	Frequency per Live Births
Ataxia-telangiectasia (homozygotes)	Leukemias, lymphomas	Recessive	11/a/	~1 per 100,000
Ataxia-telangiectasia (heterozygotes)	Mammary carcinoma	Recessive	11/a/	1 per 100*
Retinoblastoma	Retinoblastoma, osteosacrcoma	Dominant	13q	~1 per 20,000
Wilms'-aniridia	Nephroblastoma	Dominant	11p	~1 per 30,000
Basal cell nevus syndrome	Skin carcinoma, medulloblastoma	Dominant	9q	< 1 per 50,000
Neurofibromatosis	Neurofibromas, CNS tumors	Dominant	17q	~ 1 per 5,000
Familial adenomatous polyposis	Colorectal carcinomas	Dominant	5q	~ 1 per 10,000
Nonpolyposis colorectal cancer	Colorectal carcinomas	Dominant	2p	†
Familial breast cancer	Mammary and ovarian carcinomas	Dominant	17q	? 1 in 200
Li-Fraumeni syndrome	Wide range of malignancies	Dominant	17p	< 1 per 50,000

*The number and location of ataxia-telangiectasia genes has yet to be conclusively determined; the number of genetic complementation groups in ataxia-telangiectasia is a major determinant of heterozygote frequency.
†Accounts for 14% of colorectal cancers in the population.
Data from United Nations Scientific Committee on the Effects of Atomic Radiation (UNSCEAR): Sources and effects of ionizing radiation: UNSCEAR 1993 report to the General Assembly, with scientific annexes. New York, United Nations, 1993.

general population.[2,13] Systemic factors that are known to be associated more commonly with the risk of cancer include hormonal status, particularly for tumors of the breast, ovaries, testes, and prostate, for which hormones may act as tumor promoters or cocarcinogens.[28] The influence of endocrine factors on radiation-induced tumors is relatively well documented in the appearance of radiation-induced breast cancer. That irradiated female children usually do not express an increased incidence of such tumors until after having reached the age of sexual maturity, when breast cancer is seen in the general population, indicates that hormonal status is a major determinant in the development of breast cancer, and that the initiated cell from which each tumor arises may remain dormant for long periods.[2] That the latent period may be influenced by other factors as well is indicated by the fact that in female atomic bomb survivors who were irradiated before the age of 20 the relative risk of the disease was 13 times higher in those developing breast cancer before age 35 than in those diagnosed at older ages, suggesting that the former represented a genetically susceptible subgroup.[29–31]

Dietary factors, particularly fat intake, appear to influence the risks of many neoplasms. Some such factors may act predominantly as promoting agents, but whether they have any other specific interactive effects with radiation-initiated cells is uncertain. Likewise, some immunodeficiency diseases of genetic origin can increase susceptibility to specific neoplasms, possibly through the involvement of oncogenic DNA viruses in some instances[11]; in general, however, immune responses mediated by T- and B-cells are thought not to play a major role in moderating the oncogenic effects of radiation.[2,13] Also, in contrast to radiation, some chemicals appear to produce neoplasms in only one or a few specific organs; examples of the latter include vinyl chloride–induced hepatic angiosarcomas and asbestos-induced mesotheliomas. The relatively high organ specificity in such cases may reflect chemical-specific interactions with DNA in the particular organs affected, and contrasts sharply with the effects of ionizing radiation, which is capable of producing a wide variety of neoplasms in many different organs. That some neoplasms, however, such as CLL, do not appear to be induced by radiation for reasons yet to be determined, suggests that the major molecular and genetic mechanisms for radiation-induced neoplasia may differ from those for spontaneous neoplasia.

In this connection, whereas spontaneous mutations are predominantly point mutations, rather than deletions, ionizing radiation exerts its mutagenic action principally through the induction of DNA deletions.[2,32–34] It must be recognized, however, that the radiation-induced mutations that have been analyzed thus far have been produced by irradiation at relatively high doses and high-dose rates. Whether they would remain the same under other conditions remains a matter of research.

The realization that certain genetic mutations are associated with either specific tumors (e.g., the defective *RB* tumor suppressor gene causing retinoblastoma and the defective *WT* gene in Wilms' tumors) or with general tumor gene activation has spurred research to examine patients who are suspected of having radiation-induced tumors, in the hope of becoming able to identify retrospectively radiation-induced tumors from spontaneously occurring tumors. A number of authors have reported abnormalities in the thyroid after irradiation.[35] While mutations of the RAS gene appear to have the same prevalence in spontaneously occurring and radiation-associated thyroid cancers, *K-RAS* mutations appear to occur more often in radiation-associated thyroid cancers.[36] The codon 61 of the *c-Ha-RAS* gene is mutated more often in iodine-deficiency thyroid cancers. When present, the RAS mutations do not appear to have been a primary event in the induction of the tumors caused by radiation, as opposed to chemicals.[37] Instead, it appears that they are downstream from the initiating event, in which case they probably cannot be used as a radiation signature. Collart et al. have reported finding alteration of a *c-fms* gene in a patient with leukemia who had previously received Thorotrast, but they were unable to find an alteration in the *c-mos* locus even though abnormalities in this region have been reported in a number of individuals exposed to radium.[38]

Studies of leukemia in atomic bomb survivors, as compared with unirradiated controls, have detected no significant differences between the two groups in terms of mutations or sites of base substitution in the *N-RAS* or *K-RAS* oncogene sequences.[39-41] On the basis of present knowledge, it is not feasible to determine with certainty whether a particular tumor has been induced by radiation or some other cause.[2,3]

The majority of chemical carcinogens appear to act principally by causing point mutations. Chemical agents that have established carcinogenic activity in humans have been reviewed elsewhere and are discussed later in Chapters 10 and 11.[42] One of the questions of interest in relation to risk assessment concerns the number of ionizations that it would take on average to cause a malignancy, or the converse, that is, the probability that a single-track intersection in a target cell would give rise to a cancer. The International Commission on Radiological Protection (ICRP) has estimated that the chance of a 1 mGy dose of gamma rays depositing energy in a 2 nm segment of DNA is less than 10^{-9}, or less than one chance in a billion.[1] By using a number of rough assumptions, this probability of a malignant transformation has been calculated to approximate 10^{-15}. Obviously, such a calculation depends on a number of biological assumptions relating to the number of stem cells at risk, the rates of gene inactivation and gene loss mutations, and the inherent cellular metabolism, as well as the dose rate. Noteworthy in this connection is the hypothesis that acute lymphatic leukemia is induced by radiation mainly through mutagenic effects on stem cells that already carry a preleukemic translocation prior to their exposure.[43] According to this hypothesis, the risk of radiation-induced ALL in the general population is attributable almost entirely to its occurrence in a small subgroup (< 4%) of predisposed carriers of spontaneously acquired clones of preleukemic cells.[43]

Cancer genes of low penetrance do not appear to play a major role in cancer etiology and there is little evidence to support the concept of general inheritance of cancer susceptibility. A very large Danish study by Olsen et al.[44] has shown that the cancer rate of the parents of children with cancer was not different from the general population. Similar results have been obtained by others.[45-49]

ICRP has estimated that the overall incidence of high penetrance cancer-predisposing mutations in Western populations is likely to be less than 1% and that they probably account for about 5% of total lifetime cancer.[50] This is somewhat age dependant with more occurring in children

and young to middle-aged adults and it is more likely with solid tumors than with lympho-hematopoietic neoplasms. The largest genetic component appears to be in cancers of the breast, colon, and prostate, and since these are relatively common cancers they make up the greatest overall genetic impact. Quantification of the degree that familial cancers have toward tumors arising from radiation has uncertainties but ICRP has judged that the increase based on human data is less than about 10-fold. This is approximately the same factor that occurs in the absence of radiation exposure (e.g., in breast cancer–prone families). ICRP also has indicated that based on the above assessments there is not likely a need to change existing radiation risk factors and that the available data provide no evidence of a major familial component of radiation risk. It is also clear that any genetically prone persons with an increase in radiation sensitivity are already included in epidemiological studies.

ICRP has provided an illustrative example of this point using one of the most radiosensitive organs in the body.[50] A theoretical disorder is postulated in which the lifetime risk of breast cancer is 40% and that the radiation risk is increased 10-fold over the normal value. Using a normal radiation risk estimate of 0.2% per Sv for breast cancer in the total population of all ages, the risk in females would be 0.4% per Sv. In a female with the postulated disorder, the radiation risk would be 10-fold greater or 4% per Sv for fatal breast cancer and another 4% for nonfatal breast cancer. In spite of a 10-fold greater absolute risk, following a protracted dose of 100 mSv the risk of fatal breast cancer would rise from 40% to 40.4% and for total cancer from 80% to 80.8%. Finally, in assessment of assigned share or probability of causation of a tumor arising in a particular individual, the estimated value is not likely to be significantly affected, since the ratio of increased risk on a genetic basis alone and that due to radiation exposure are likely to be about the same.

SPECIFIC SYNDROMES

In addition to the familial cancer syndromes discussed above, there are individuals in whom sensitivity to various types of ionizing or nonionizing radiation is increased by genetic and chromosomal defects. These include persons with (1) xeroderma pigmentosum, (2) ataxia-telangiectasia, (3) Fanconi anemia, (4) Bloom's syndrome, and (5) Cockayne's syndrome. The major findings for each of these are listed in Table 4-3. Other traits in which increased radiosensitivity has been observed include the Nijmegen breakage syndrome.[51]

Xeroderma Pigmentosum

In patients with XP, the basis for neoplastic predisposition is an abnormality in the repair of DNA damage and, possibly, depressed immune function in the skin itself. The increase in the incidence of cancer appears to be small.

Table 4-3 • Genetic Disorders Associated with Increased Sensitivity to Radiation

Disorder	Clinical Features
Xeroderma pigmentosum	Marked sensitivity of the skin to sunlight, sunburn, freckling, hyperpigmentation, skin carcinomas, and melanomas; usually death occurs before age 30
Ataxia-telangiectasia	Progressive cerebellar ataxia, conjunctival and cutaneous telangiectasia, frequent infections, predisposition to carcinoma, usually lymphoreticular; death usually occurs before age 20 from infection or malignancy
Fanconi anemia	Progressive marrow failure, anemia, leukopenia and thrombocytopenia, growth retardation, hypoplasia or aplasia of the radius and thumb, brownish pigmentation of the skin; other associated anomalies of the heart and kidney
Bloom's syndrome	Severe growth retardation, telangiectatic erythema on exposed areas of the skin, and sun sensitivity; multiple infections with impaired immune system; usually half the cancers that develop are nonlymphocytic leukemias
Cockayne's syndrome	Dwarfism, retinal atrophy, deafness, cataracts, photosensitivity, mental retardation, prognathism, and progeria

The frequency of XP in the populations of North America and Europe is approximately 1 in 250,000. The syndrome occurs in homozygotes, although the sensitivity of heterozygotes is not clear. One subgroup of XP (DeSanctis-Cacchione syndrome) is characterized by mental retardation and other neurologic abnormalities.[52-55]

XP cells are highly sensitive to the lethal effects of ultraviolet (UV) radiation and display cross-sensitivity with certain chemical carcinogens. Their sensitivity to UV radiation contrasts with their normal response to damage from ionizing radiation, alkylating agents, and DNA cross-linking agents.[56-60] Although some chromosomes are broken by UV light in XP strains, the chromosomal changes do not appear to be sufficient to be the principal cause of death of the cells. All XP cell lines are defective in one or more DNA repair pathways for UV damage, but their repair of damage from radiation other than UV radiation is essentially normal.

Ataxia-Telangiectasia

Patients with A-T demonstrate increased chromosome breakage in lymphocytes and fibroblasts. Homozygotes for mutations of the *ATM* gene occur approximately once in 100,000 births, and the frequency of heterozygotes may be about 1% in the population. The increase in risk of the heterozygote's dying of cancer is 2 to 10 times greater than that for a normal individual. It has been estimated that approximately 5% of persons dying from any malignancy before the age of 45 may carry the *ATM* gene. Banding studies of the gene have shown specific involvement of chromosomes 7 and 14 in translocation chromosomal rearrangements. The structural rearrangements of chromosome 14 may be to some extent responsible for leukemic transformations.[61] In a study of R-banding of lymphocytes, out of a total of 927 lymphocytes analyzed, 158 chromosomal rearrangements (a frequency of 0.17%) were observed. A similar frequency was identified for fibroblast chromosomal rearrangements, as well. The most common change appeared to be an inversion of chromosome 7 or translocation involving chromosomes 14 and 7.[62]

A number of reports have described patients with A-T who showed unusual radiosensitivity for deterministic effects.[63-65] These include a 10-year-old boy with A-T and a malignant lymphoma, who received a therapeutic dose of 30 Gy to the nasopharynx, and subsequently developed signs of marked cutaneous erythema with associated deep tissue damage. He died, and his autopsy indicated that the radiation was the probable cause of death. In another case, a 9-year-old boy with Hodgkin's disease and A-T who received 28.4 Gy of therapeutic radiation to the mediastinum, subsequently developed severe esophagitis, respiratory damage, and skin damage, and died within four months. The patients also included a 7-year-old boy with A-T and a malignant lymphoma who received 20 Gy to his right lung, after which dysphasia and erythema were noted, and at 30 Gy, treatment was stopped. The patient died subsequently, apparently because of radiation damage.[65] Another report concerns a 44-month-old girl with an immunoglobulin-A deficiency and an A-T-like syndrome who had none of the physical stigmata of A-T. The girl suffered severe radiation damage with "standard" doses of radiotherapy for Hodgkin's disease.[66] A significant percentage of patients with radiation-induced ocular telangiectasia also have been found to be carriers of missense mutations of the *ATM* gene.[67]

Examination of the gamma ray sensitivity of fibroblasts in patients with A-T demonstrates marked radiosensitivity, with a mean D_{37} value of 0.57 Gy plus or minus 0.15 Gy, which is lower by a factor of about 3 than the D_{37} value for normal fibroblasts.[68] The comet assay has been reported to be a useful method for detecting such increases in radiosensitivity.[69,70] The response of A-T cells to chemical carcinogens indicates that they are especially sensitive to those compounds that mimic ionizing radiation. In contrast to their high sensitivity to the induction of chromosome aberrations and cell killing, however, there is some evidence that A-T cells may be relatively resistant to the induction of point mutations by ionizing radiation.[71] The precise biochemical defect responsible for the enhanced radiosensitivity remains unknown.

There have been a number of reports about the incidence of cancer in families affected by A-T. Persons who are homozygous usually have a high risk of leukemia and lymphoma but not of breast cancer. In a study of 161 families, the relative risk of cancer in heterozygotes was found to be 3.8 in males and 3.5 in females when compared with noncarriers.[72] The latter study also indicated a fivefold excess risk of breast cancer in females who had been exposed to diagnostic fluoroscopic examinations, as compared with nonexposed females. At first glance, the differences seem to be significant; however, the study has a number of limitations. The diagnostic radiology involved was almost always of the abdomen, which gives only scatter radiation to the breast at very low doses (less than the annual dose from natural background radiation). This would imply that natural background radiation is responsible for a large number of breast cancers, which is clearly not plausible. Furthermore, the exposed and control groups were of very different ages, and appropriate adjustment for the age differences is not possible.[73] No protein-truncating mutations of the *ATM* gene were found in women without A-T or a family history of the disease who had developed breast cancer after having previously received radiation therapy for Hodgkin's disease.[74]

Fanconi Anemia

Persons with Fanconi anemia demonstrate increased sensitivity to chromosomal breakage and rearrangement, usually of the chromatid type and mainly between nonhomologous sites. The chromatid breaks appear predominantly in chromosomes 1 to 13, between the R- and Q-bands, with the sex chromosomes rarely affected. The incidence of FA at birth is about 1 in 350,000 in North America and possibly as high as 1 in 70,000 in Europe. In the United States, the heterozygote frequency is estimated at 0.33%. In one family the heterozygotes appeared to have an increased incidence of carcinoma, but this finding has not been substantiated in other heterozygote families. The defect in Fanconi anemia cells appears to be defective repair of DNA cross-linking. This is suspected because of the unusually high sensitivity of the cells to DNA cross-linking agents. The repair of x-ray-induced single-strand breaks and sensitivity to gamma irradiation are relatively normal.[50]

Bloom's Syndrome

In patients with Bloom's syndrome, the risk of developing cancer is about 17%, with a large number of the cancers being nonlymphocytic leukemias. It is not known whether heterozygotes are at an increased risk for developing neoplasms. About one half of the reported patients are Ashkenazi Jews from the Ukrainian-Polish border region. The syndrome is one of chromosomal instability with a symmetrical quadriradial figure seen in lymphocytes and fibroblasts. These involve homologous chromosomes and

are so characteristic that their identification should precede a diagnosis of BS.[75] There are also a large number of sister chromatid exchanges present in these cells.[76]

The DNA repair defect in BS cells is unknown. BS fibroblasts are not unusually sensitive to killing by x-rays or UV, nor does exposure to these agents cause an elevated frequency of chromosome aberrations in these cells.

Cockayne's Syndrome

The fibroblasts from persons with Cockayne's syndrome show an increased sensitivity to UV but not to x-rays.[77] This sensitivity may be due to less than the normal amount of DNA polymerase activity.[78]

Retinoblastoma

Children with bilateral retinoblastoma or a family history of the disease have gene mutations that increase the risk of second cancers.[79–81] The cumulative probability of death from such a second neoplasm is about 25% at age 40 years,[82] but the risk is greatly reduced in patients who are more than one year old at the time of irradiation.[83,84]

RISK ESTIMATION: SYSTEMIC AND POPULATION ASPECTS

A source of uncertainty that arises in assessing the risks from low doses and the risks to specific individuals is the heterogeneity that is characteristic of human populations. A mathematical model designed to address this problem has suggested that if the response of sensitive subgroups had a major influence on the dose-response relationship for cancer induction, the curve would be convex upward in the range below 1 Gy.[85] However, this type of curve has not been supported by the epidemiological data that are available.[2]

Radiation-induced tumors are characterized by the elapse of an appreciable *latent period* between the time of radiation exposure and the clinical appearance of the tumor. The latent period may be conceptualized as comprising at least two portions: the true latent period, or interval from initiation of cells to the beginning of unrestrained growth, and a second portion of tumor growth, or the time to clinical diagnosis or presentation. Although minimum latent periods are 2 to 3 years for leukemia, 3 to 4 years for bone cancer, 4 to 5 years for thyroid cancer, and approximately 10 years for other solid tumors, the mean latent periods are usually substantially longer, approximating 20 to 30 years for most solid tumors. Examples of the mean latent periods for some radiogenic tumors are listed in Table 4-4. If the epidemiological follow-up of individuals is shorter than the minimum latent period, radiation-induced tumors are not observed. Conversely, if tumors are found in a very short interval after radiation exposure, etiologies other than radiogenic induction must be suspected.

It is clear that the latent period depends on the age of the individual at exposure. This has been well documented for breast carcinoma. Most radiation-induced, or *excess*,

Table 4-4 • Estimates of Mean Latent Periods for Various Tumors Following External Irradiation

Tumor Type	Mean Latent Period (yr)
Brain	27
Salivary glands	20
Pharynx, larynx	24
Thyroid	20
Breast	22
Lung	25
Stomach	14
Sarcomas	12
Colon	26
Bone	10–15
Leukemia	7–10
Skin	24

tumors of the female breast are not manifested with a high frequency until the exposed individuals reach the age at which there is a substantial incidence of "spontaneously occurring" breast tumors. Thus, women exposed at age 20 may develop breast cancer within 10 to 20 years; however, girls who were younger than 9 years of age when exposed to atomic bomb radiation in Japan had a much longer latent period and did not begin to demonstrate an excess of breast cancers until they reached 30 to 40 years of age.[86,87] The minimal latent period, therefore, has one component that is invariable with age at exposure, as well as one that is variable and depends on age at exposure. Such variations in latent period as well as actual risk have also been demonstrated for leukemia (Fig. 4-3).

Risk estimates derived from the observation of excess cancer rates can be underestimated if the follow-up of the exposed group is too short. A population that is exposed at a very young age must therefore be followed throughout life if the carcinogenic effects on the population are to be fully manifested and recorded. Likewise, a low-risk estimate may be obtained if a very elderly group is exposed to radiation, since the latent period in this case may exceed

the average lifespan of the exposed individuals. Risk estimates derived in such circumstances must not be applied to the general population. In addition to age at exposure, the dose also may appear to affect the length of the latent period in some situations. For leukemia, the data suggest an inverse relationship between absorbed dose and the latent period: the higher the dose, the shorter the latent period.[88] In actuality, however, the higher dose may merely induce more neoplasms with the same mean latent period, but given that the neoplasms follow a Poisson distribution in time, some of them will appear earlier simply on a statistical basis. With most tumors, particularly of the breast and thyroid, there appears to be little relationship between the dose and the latent period. Questions about the latent period often arise, particularly when a tumor occurs in a specific individual a short time after exposure. The latent period is that time at which a statistically significant increase is identified as a result of radiation exposure, not when the specific tumor is first observed in the population.[89]

Although a large number of case reports in the literature describe one or several persons who have developed tumors after some radiation exposure, these are not epidemiological studies and make no comparison with an unexposed group to demonstrate a causal association. Even in large epidemiological studies, tumors will appear as a result of natural incidence. Nonscientists often point to these spontaneously occurring tumors and say that the latent period for radiogenic tumors is extremely short because a tumor has appeared in the studied population. As an example, about 1,400,000 persons develop cancer each year in the United States (excluding carcinoma in situ and carcinomas of the skin), and about 570,000 persons each year die from cancer. All of these persons were exposed to radiation from some source in the year prior to diagnosis, such as medical and dental x-rays, natural background, occupational exposure, and even radiation therapy, but these exposures cannot have caused their cancers, for a number of reasons. The simplest reason is tumor "doubling time." Most cancers are at least two cubic centimeters in diameter when they are detected and contain billions of cells. The time required for a tumor to double in size is usually on the order of several months. Working backward to determine a time when the tumor began, it can easily be seen that essentially all tumors must grow for 30 to 35 doublings (at least 5 years) before they become clinically apparent. Several years are also required for the multiple stages and multiple mutations of radiation-induced tumors to be expressed. These have been discussed in earlier paragraphs on the mechanisms of radiation oncogenesis. The only large study to have suggested an increased relative risk of solid tumors within the 5-to-10-year period following exposure is the tumor incidence study of the atomic bomb survivors; in this case, the risk is based on only 10 cases and is not apparent for individual tumor types,

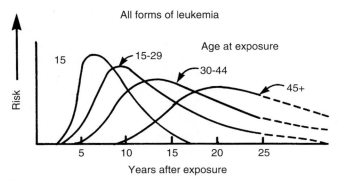

Figure 4-3 • Schematic representation of induction period and risk of leukemia as a function of age at exposure. (From Ishimaru M, Ishimaru T: Leukemia and related disorders. J Radiat Res 1975;16[Suppl]:S89–S96.)

except for cancer of the cervix and uterus, which are not thought to be radiogenic. The risk 5 to 10 years after exposure is apparent only at high doses (1 Gy) and when all tumors are lumped together in a pooled analysis.[90]

In contrast to the incidence data, the mortality data for the same population indicate that the frequency of death from radiation-induced solid tumors did not reach a level of statistical significance until after 1960.[91] Thus, the minimum latent period appears to have been 15 years or longer and may have varied by site of cancer. At the present time, the generally accepted minimum latent period for radiogenic solid tumors other than those of bone and possibly thyroid is 10 years. For non–CLL, the minimum latent period is 2 to 3 years. The ICRP has concluded that "With solid tumors other than those of bone, however, the excess cases do not become evident until 10 or more years after irradiation, following which they tend to increase in numbers with advancing age."[1] UNSCEAR, likewise, has recommended that for risk assessment purposes, most solid tumors should be assumed to have a latent period of at least 10 years, since risks, if any, before that time are extremely small.[92]

DOSE-EFFECT RELATIONSHIP

To estimate the risks of carcinogenic effects from exposures at low doses and low-dose rates, it is necessary to know or to assume the shape of the relevant dose-response curve. In animals, most radiation-induced cancers reach a peak incidence at some intermediate dose, above which the incidence declines at higher doses. The decline in the incidence of tumors at higher doses is thought to reflect severe damage to the DNA or other cellular elements, so that cell death, rather than cancer induction, occurs. At least two human studies demonstrate decreasing risk at high doses. In one of them, an analysis of radiation-induced leukemia in patients treated for cervical cancer with radiation therapy, the risk was found to decrease as the dose exceeded 4 Gy.[93] In the other, a study of women treated for postpartum mastitis, risk of breast cancer peaked at about 3 Gy and decreased at doses over 5 Gy.[94]

The epidemiological data that are available rarely cover a wide dose range and rarely involve a nondiseased, homogeneous population. The only large study group for whom such data exist is the population of atomic bomb survivors. The majority of other studies involve exposures that are usually fractionated over time, focus on selected populations and age groups, and often involve only partial-body exposures. In an attempt to give adequate consideration to all relevant information in formulating risk assessments, heterogeneous assortments of human data are often checked against animal data in an effort to use a coherent, unified risk model. The three mathematical dose-response models most often selected for the purpose are the linear, linear-quadratic, and quadratic models. These are shown schematically in Figure 4-4.

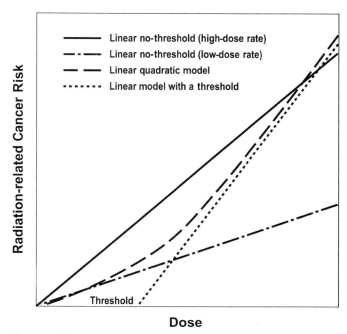

Figure 4-4 • Schematic representation of common mathematical models for induction of radiation-induced tumors. At 0 dose, a measurable effect is due to spontaneous incidence of the effect in the population examined. As radiation dose increases, an increasing effect may be identified. The appropriate mathematical model for any particular situation may depend on many factors, including physical parameters of the radiation, tumor type, and so on. (From National Research Council: Health risks from exposure to low levels of ionizing radiation. BEIR VII. Washington, DC, National Academies Press, 2006.)

Linear Model

The simplest dose-response model is often referred to as the linear-no-threshold (LNT) risk model, which is expressed mathematically as $y = ax$, where y is the incidence of excess cancer, a is a constant, and x is the dose. The LNT model suggests that each time energy is deposited in the susceptible target there is a probability of tumor initiation. If this were true, the effect of each small dose should be additive, and spreading the dose out over a certain time span (or fractionating the dose) should not alter the risk. Most scientific groups have used the LNT model to estimate an upper bound of risk for low–linear energy transfer (LET) radiation.[2,3,95–98] Although it is generally considered to be a conservative approach and has been criticized by opponents as being overly conservative,[99–101] the assumption of linearity may actually lead to an underestimate of the risks of radiation-induced cancers in some instances.[102] For high-LET radiation, the linear dose-response model may be more accurate than for low-LET radiation. From epidemiological analysis of the overall risk of radiation-induced solid tumors, the linear model can neither be excluded nor validated conclusively.[97] The small number of radiogenic cancers that may occur at low doses is swamped by the large number of "spontaneous" cancers, which leads to

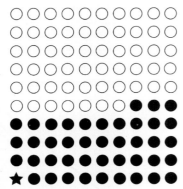

Figure 4-5 • Representation of the risk of "spontaneous" and radiation-induced cancer in a population. In a lifetime, approximately 42 (*solid circles*) of 100 people will be diagnosed with cancer. Calculations of the BEIR VII Committee suggest that approximately 1 cancer (*star*) could result from a single exposure to 0.1 mSv of low-LET radiation above background radiation. (From National Research Council: Health risks from exposure to low levels of ionizing radiation. BEIR VII. Washington, DC, National Academies Press, 2006.)

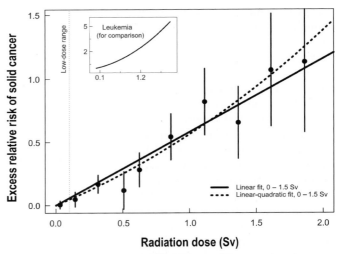

Figure 4-6 • ERR (with 95% CI) of solid cancer for Japanese atomic bomb survivors. Calculations were for a population exposed at age 30 who had attained age 60. Solid and dotted lines represent linear and linear-quadratic models and there is statistically significant difference between the fit of the models. (From National Research Council: Health risks from exposure to low levels of ionizing radiation. BEIR VII. Washington, DC, National Academies Press, 2006.)

large uncertainties in the data points (Fig. 4-5). Even with the large numbers of atomic bomb survivors who have been studied over the last 60 years, it is unlikely that direct empirical risk estimates can be made to remove the necessity for use of mathematical models at low doses.[2,102–104]

Linear-Quadratic Model

The preponderance of animal experiments implies that for low-LET radiation, a linear-quadratic dose-response model is likely to be applicable in most instances. The mathematical form of the linear-quadratic model is $y = ax + bx^2$, where a and b are different constants, and x is the radiation dose. This model gives the best fit for low-LET radiation leukemia risks. It has been pointed out, however, that one or another dose-response curve cannot be assumed to represent or even substantially reflect the pathogenesis of cancer.[2,3,105] Data from the atomic bomb survivors indicate that leukemia and solid tumors clearly have different dose-response curves[17,106,107] (Fig. 4-6). At least one reason for this is the known dose dependence of many of the modifying mechanisms operating at cellular, tissue, and systemic levels. Because each of these factors may change differently with dose, the risk and the shape of the curve in a certain dose region cannot be extrapolated with certainty either up or down, except on the basis of confirmatory epidemiologic data.

The Quadratic Model

The mathematical form of the quadratic dose-response model is $y = ax^2$. In general, the application of the quadratic model to experimental and epidemiological data has not yielded a satisfactory fit. The model predicts that effects at low doses are much less frequent than are

predicted by the other two models. It has, therefore, been used by the BEIR 1980 Committee to obtain a lower set of risk estimates only.[108] In addition, quadratic models predict a very pronounced reduction of the carcinogenic effect from lowering the dose rate or from fractionating the dose. This prediction has not been substantiated by the majority of human epidemiological evidence, particularly in the induction of breast tumors,[2,3,96] as will be discussed in Chapter 5.

The Threshold Model

The threshold model denotes a dose-response relationship in which no effect is produced below a certain level dose. This model predicts that below some level of dose no carcinogenic effect will result from exposure. While the linear dose-response model can be used to place upper bounds on estimates of the risks at low doses, the uncertainties are such that it cannot be distinguished unambiguously from the threshold model. The possibility exists that very low doses may produce no effect. This is not such a far-fetched idea as it may seem, especially at doses of less than 0.01 Gy, given that radiation repair has been shown to exist in many forms. Figures 4-7 and 4-8 show data from the statistically strongest human database (the Japanese atomic bomb survivor study). It is clear from an inspection of these figures that a number of models, from threshold to linear, could fit the data, as has been emphasized elsewhere.[2,3,97,109,110]

As we have seen previously, some of the mortality data from the atomic bomb survivors cannot unequivocally exclude a threshold. Statistical analysis of the data, however, indicates that the linear or linear-quadratic model fit

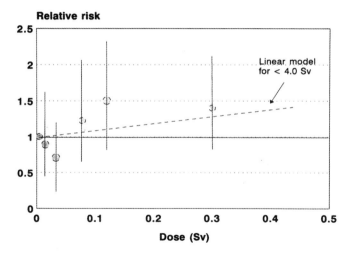

Thyroid cancer incidence (A-bomb LSS)

Figure 4-7 • Thyroid cancer incidence at doses below 0.5 Sv in the atomic bomb survivors. Error bars indicate 95% CIs. (From Shimizu Y, Kato H, Schull W, et al: Dose-response analysis of atomic bomb survivors exposed to low-level radiation. RERF Update, Autumn. Hiroshima, Japan, Radiation Effects Research Foundation, 1992.)

the data better. At small increments of dose above background, the probability of inducing a cancer with radiation is small. Even in a large group of persons the number of radiation-attributable cancers will almost certainly be undetectable, as pointed out earlier. This, however, provides no evidence for a real threshold. Bone tumors constitute the only type of solid tumor for which data seem to support a threshold, as will be discussed more in the appropriate section of Chapter 5. In summary, several mathematical dose-response models have been considered

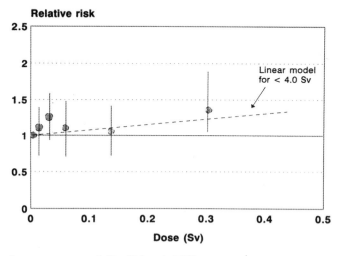

Lung cancer mortality (A-bomb LSS)

Figure 4-8 • Lung cancer mortality at doses below 0.5 Sv in the atomic bomb survivors. Error bars indicate 95% CIs. (From Shimizu Y, Kato H, Schull W, et al: Dose-response analysis of atomic bomb survivors exposed to low-level radiation. RERF Update, Autumn. Hiroshima, Japan, Radiation Effects Research Foundation, 1992.)

for extrapolation of cancer risks from intermediate- to low-dose levels. The generally preferred models are either linear or linear quadratic. The threshold and quadratic models do not provide the best mathematical fit for the bulk of experimental or human data on solid tumors. Although the linear-quadratic model appears to fit the experimental animal data best, the statistical power of most human epidemiological studies does not suffice to exclude the other models, particularly the linear one. Providing examples of applications of these types of models to epidemiological data concerning differing tumor types is difficult because the confidence limits on the data points in most epidemiological studies are wide. At the present time, therefore, most national and international scientific groups recommend a linear dose-response model for those solid tumors known to be induced by radiation.[1–3,96,97]

CARCINOGENIC RISK VERSUS TIME AFTER IRRADIATION

To predict the duration and magnitude of the carcinogenic effect of radiation exposure after the latent period, two risk projection models, the additive (absolute) risk model and the multiplicative (relative) risk model, have been used.[2,96] In the additive (absolute) risk model, the expression of excess risk in an irradiated population begins at some time after exposure, and the excess risk continues at the same rate for some additional period. *Absolute risk* is defined as the excess cancer cases for each unit of population for each unit of time and each unit of absorbed dose. The radiogenic excess of tumors is divided by the number of persons exposed, the average number of years of observation, and the average absorbed dose to which the subjects were exposed. The absolute risk, therefore, may be expressed as an annual absolute risk or a lifetime absolute risk (e.g., *X* number of excess cancer cases in 1 million persons for 1 gray or 0.01 Gy). The age at observation is not critical for determining risk in this model once the latent period has passed. The lifetime absolute risk obviously depends on the age at exposure. Absolute risk is independent of the natural risk of cancer.

In the multiplicative (relative) risk projection model, the excess cancer risk after the latent period is expressed as a fraction or multiple of the natural age-specific cancer risk for that particular population (e.g., a relative risk of 1.5 indicates that a 50% increase over the spontaneous rate may be expected). The estimated magnitude of the excess changes according to the age at observation and varies from one population to another if the populations differ in the "spontaneous," or baseline, incidence of cancer. The relative risk (RR) concept carries the inherent assumption that the risk of a given radiation-induced cancer varies in proportion to the risk of spontaneous cancer development in the organ in question. Whether this is true is uncertain at the present time.

There remains some debate as to whether the multiplicative risk projection model or the additive risk projection model should be used in estimating cancer risk, with both models receiving some support. It is well known that leukemia has a high spontaneous incidence in children and the elderly. Thus, if the multiplicative risk model were correct for all tumors, then young and old people should have a much higher incidence of radiation-induced leukemia. This is clearly not the case in the atomic bomb survivors (see Fig. 4-3). At least for leukemia, therefore, the risk decreases with increasing age at exposure and does not appear to be related to the spontaneous incidence. In addition, there is some difficulty in using the multiplicative risk model when estimates of detriment from carcinogenic effects are to be applied over very different population groups. For example, the RR of radiation-induced stomach cancer in the Japanese may well not be the same as the RR in the U.S. population, because the spontaneous incidence of these tumors is very different between the two populations. Models based on the assumption that cells initiated by acute irradiation are added to the pool of spontaneously initiated cells, and that susceptibility to initiation itself is not age-dependent, have been found to fit the data for the temporal and age distributions of cancers in the atomic bomb survivors.[111–113]

The ICRP, in developing its 1990 recommendations, examined additive and multiplicative models and a U.S. National Institutes of Health (NIH) model.[1] It also averaged cancer rates over five different populations in an attempt to minimize the differences of widely varying cancer rates in different countries. The populations considered were from China, Japan, Puerto Rico, United Kingdom, and the United States. It concluded that each model had certain advantages and disadvantages but that "it is difficult to choose between the multiplicative and the NIH projection models, and it seems not unreasonable to suppose that the truth may lie somewhere in between."[114] The combination of models used by the Commission emphasized the multiplicative model for cancers other than leukemia, with the understanding that "this may overestimate the probability of cancer at older ages."[1] The same combination has since been used in risk assessments by other expert groups, as well.[2,96] The BEIR VII 2005 and International Commission on Radiological Protection (ICRP) 1990 risk estimates are shown in Tables 4-5 and 4-6.[1]

An additional problem in using the multiplicative, or relative, risk projection model is the problem of determining the "natural" cancer risk in a given population, which needs to be known if one is to base an estimate on a multiple of that number. If, for example, one were to select two populations in the United States, only one of which smoked, and were to derive radiation risk factors by the multiplicative method for both of them, the estimated detriment would be substantially different in the two.

Table 4-5 • Lifetime Mortality from Specific Fatal Cancers in a Population of All Ages Attributable to Low-level Irradiation

Type or Site of Cancer	CANCER DEATHS PER 100,000 PER 0.1 SV	
	Males	Females
Lung	140	270
Colon	76	46
Breast	—	73
Leukemia	69	52
Urinary bladder	22	28
Stomach	19	25
Ovary	—	24
Liver	20	11
Prostate*	9	—
Uterus*	—	5
Other	120	132
Total	475	666

*Prostate and uterus are included even though risk estimates are not statistically significant.
Data from National Research Council, Committee on the Biological Effects of Ionizing Radiations (BEIR): Health risks from exposure to low levels of ionizing radiation. BEIR VII. Washington, DC, NRCUSNA Press, 2006, p 491.

Some estimates of the spontaneous cancer incidence and mortality rates in the United States are shown in Table 4-7.

Projection models allow one to estimate lifetime risks from a given exposure. Projections of lifetime risks are based on contemporary cancer rates. One of the problems in doing lifetime estimates with multiplicative models is that cancer risks are changing with time (e.g., due to changes in lifestyle, diet, and smoking habits). The projections of lifetime risk vary somewhat, depending on the methods used by the groups that have calculated them. UNSCEAR 1988 used the term *risk of exposure induced death (REID)*, which was interpreted as the risk that an individual would die from a cancer caused by a given exposure.[115] The BEIR committees[2,116] have used the term *excess lifetime risk (ELR)*, which represents the difference between the proportion of persons dying from a given cause in an exposed population and the proportion dying of this cause in an unexposed population. Overall, the REID will be about 20% larger than the ELR. Another measure that has

Table 4-6 • Nominal Probability Coefficients for Lifetime Cancer Detriment (10^{-2} Sv^{-1})

Exposed Population	Fatal Cancer	Nonfatal Cancer
Adult workers	4.0	0.8
Whole population	5.0	1.0

Data from International Commission on Radiological Protection (ICRP): 1990 Recommendations of the International Commission on Radiological Protection. Pub. no. 60. Ann ICRP 1991;21(1–3):1–201.

Table 4-7 • **Estimated Lifetime Risks of Spontaneously Occurring Cancer in the United States**

Cancer Site or Type	PERCENTAGE DEVELOPING A GIVEN CANCER		PERCENTAGE DYING FROM A GIVEN CANCER	
	Males	Females	Males	Females
Prostate	15.9	—	3.5	—
Breast	—	12.0	—	3.0
Lung	7.7	5.4	7.7	4.6
Colon	4.2	4.2	2.2	2.1
Urinary bladder	3.4	1.1	0.8	0.3
Stomach	1.2	0.7	0.7	0.4
Uterus	—	3.0	—	0.8
Leukemia	0.8	0.6	0.7	0.5
Thyroid	0.2	0.6	0.04	0.0
Other*	12.5	8.8	6.8	5.1
Total	45.9	36.4	21.7	16.8

*Excluding nonmelanomatous skin cancers.
Data from National Research Council, Committee on the Biological Effects of Ionizing Radiations (BEIR): Health risks from exposure to low levels of ionizing radiation. BEIR VII. Washington, DC, NRCUSNA Press, 2006.

been used by both UNSCEAR and ICRP is "loss of life expectancy," usually expressed as the years of life lost per radiation-induced cancer. For the multiplicative risk projection model, the mean life lost per attributable cancer death is estimated to be about 13 to 15 years. The similar figure for the additive risk model is 20 years.

Recognized genetic abnormalities or genetic predispositions to cancer may apply to both natural and radiogenic cancers. If the mechanism of susceptibility to carcinogenesis is a function of constitutional susceptibility, then the multiplicative model is certainly preferable. Multiplicative risk figures by themselves may be a bit misleading initially. For example, a multiplicative risk of 2 with regard to leukemia may appear worse than a multiplicative risk of 1.5 for breast cancer; however, because leukemia is very rare in the population, multiplying the normal incidence by 2 would still result in a very small number of additional cases. On the other hand, the breast cancer population is large, and applying a multiplicative risk factor of 1.5 produces a much larger number of cases than in the case of leukemia.

In general, use of the multiplicative risk projection model leads to higher risk estimates than does use of the additive projection model. This difference in estimated risk may be as much as a factor of 5. Use of the linear and linear-quadratic models usually causes differences in risk estimates on the order of a factor of 1 to 2. Although debate prevails about whether it is better to use the additive or the multiplicative risk model, it is most likely that the truth lies somewhere in between. We know that not all tumors fit either model. Bone cancer and leukemia provide very poor fits to the multiplicative risk model; breast and lung cancers do not correspond well with estimates derived from the additive risk model. It would, of course, be unreasonable to expect that the carcinogenic effects of radiation would be the same in all tissues, because the tissues have different cellular turnover times, hormonal influences, different exposures to environmental

carcinogens, and so on. As analyzed by most models, natural background ionizing radiation is estimated to account for an extremely small proportion (less than 4%) of all "spontaneous" cancers.[2,3]

EPIDEMIOLOGICAL ASPECTS

Although a vast anecdotal literature concerns radiation carcinogenesis, most of the useful information about human radiation carcinogenesis comes from epidemiological studies. Hence it is important to understand the strengths and weaknesses of such studies to analyze their data, conclusions, and validity. Most of the epidemiological data in humans arise from doses in excess of 0.1 Gy and usually in excess of 1 Gy. Although exposures above levels of 1 Gy are relatively rare, there have been sufficient studies to indicate the general magnitude of radiation-induced cancer associated with such exposures. Most of the controversy in the minds of members of the public and patients, and in legal arenas, concerns exposures of less than 0.1 Gy. It is confusing to a lay audience that after 100 years of research and experience with ionizing radiation, scientists are unable to quantify more precisely risks below dose levels of 0.1 Gy. The public does not understand the statistical limitation of trying to observe a very small potential radiation effect superimposed on a large background of spontaneously occurring cancers. Although some publications purport to demonstrate cancer risks at very low levels, there is no proven body of data that establishes an increase in human cancer rates at radiation levels below about 0.1 Gy.[2,97,117]

In the absence of statistically reliable data at these low-dose levels, most organizations that issue radiation protection recommendations assume that there is a LNT dose-effect relationship. With the limited amount of human epidemiologic data at low doses, various statistical procedures are employed to extract as much

Table 4-8 • Sample Size Required for Statistical Precision in Obtaining Dose-Response Data on Carcinogenesis

Dose Level	Sample Size
1 Gy	1,000
0.1 Gy	100,000
0.01 Gy	10,000,000

information from the data as possible. The statistical precision of a risk estimate depends on the expected number of cases, the true excess cases, and the standard deviation. The application of valid statistical methods has been outlined and discussed by Land[118] and others.[2] The sample size needed to find or estimate an increased health risk in a population depends on the size of the risk already present in the population. Thus, to find an excess of an effect that occurs rarely in a population, only a small number of cases may be needed; however, to find a small increase in the incidence of cancer (which occurs spontaneously in 40% of people), a large exposed population group is needed. As the additional risk due to any noxious agent becomes smaller, the sample size must increase as the inverse square of the risk to maintain statistical precision and power. For example, if excess risk is truly proportional to the dose and if a sample of 100,000 persons is necessary to determine the effect of a 0.1-Gy exposure, a sample of approximately 10 million persons will be needed statistically to find the same effect for 0.01 Gy (Table 4-8).

In a more practical context, the annual risk of breast cancer from exposure to 10 mGy is generally assumed to be approximately six cases per 1 million women exposed, after a latent period of 10 years, so that a study to determine the effect of a single high-dose mammographic examination (delivering 1 rad to both breasts) can be calculated to require the follow-up of 50 million women in the exposed group and 50 million women in a nonexposed control group. On the other hand, to examine the radiation risk with respect to leukemia would require a smaller study sample because of the relative rarity of leukemia in the general population. In this case, if 0.01 Gy bone marrow dose were applied, with a follow-up of 15 years, the number of cases required would be one fifteenth that for the breast cancer example.[119,120]

The measures of disease frequency used in epidemiological studies are usually prevalence and incidence. Prevalence is the number of persons with the disease divided by the number of persons in the population at a point in time. Incidence usually means the number of new cases of disease in a given time period divided by the total population at risk. There are a number of types of epidemiological studies. The first are descriptive studies, including correlational studies, case reports, and case series. These studies usually do not have adequate control groups and often cannot test dose-response or temporal relationships. Therefore, they cannot test etiologic hypotheses. To do this requires other types of studies. Many nonexperts incorrectly quote literature containing the former types of studies when attempting to determine or prove causation. Most useful epidemiological studies are of the *cohort* type: an exposed population is identified and followed for the type of malignancy of interest, and similar persons or controls without the radiation exposure are also investigated for the malignancy. The largest cohort study of radiation effects is the study of the Japanese atomic bomb survivors.[121,122] If a suitable control population is available, an estimation of radiation risk is derived by subtracting the observed risk in the control population from the total risk in the exposed population.

The second type of study, which is performed less frequently, is the *case-control* study. In such a study, cancer incidence or cancer deaths are retrospectively reviewed and compared with age- and sex-matched controls. Determining a risk factor by the case-control method is more difficult. In general, what is obtained is an odds ratio (OR), RR, or excess relative risk (ERR) in comparing the control group to the exposed group. A number of factors must be examined critically to determine whether a particular epidemiological study is of value. Because human exposure is not performed on a prospective experimental basis, each epidemiological study will have strengths and weaknesses. Each of these should be examined, and no conclusions should be drawn until this analysis is performed. In addition, any study may have a "statistically significant" result purely on the basis of chance. This would be similar to flipping a coin enough times and relating only the event that occurred when you got six "heads" in a row.

The degree to which chance may account for a given result of a statistical test is given by the *P* value. A *P* value of 0.05 means the probability that the observed result is due to chance is less than 1 in 20 (or 5%). A *P* value of less than 0.05 is considered statistically significant by convention. The *P* value is a reflection of both the magnitude of difference observed and the size of the group. A better value to use is the *confidence interval* (CI). The CI actually shows you the values and range for a given risk estimate. For example, should a study be judged significant if it found an RR of 3 in exposed over unexposed persons? Initially, this looks like a large difference, and if the 90% CI were narrow (perhaps 2.8 to 3.3) and the study population was large, the effect would probably be genuine. On the other hand, a 90% CI of −2.1 to 12.4 would mean that no real effect was shown. The term *statistical significance* is often misinterpreted by authors, readers, and the public. A statistically significant result does not mean that chance cannot have accounted for the finding but only that it is unlikely.

Another often overlooked point is that a statistically significant association does not provide information that two items are causally related or that one causes the other. For example, there is a statistically significant association between the wearing of dresses and being female. This does not mean that being female makes one wear a dress or that wearing a dress makes one a female. They are statistically significantly associated facts but not causally related. Particular epidemiological criteria that should be examined include the following items: study design, sample size, presence and accuracy of information on individual radiation doses, presence and appropriateness of a control (unexposed) group, accuracy of records used (such as hospital records or death certificates), completeness of follow-up, and potential biases related to sex, parity, ethnicity, information recall, concurrent diseases, and other exposures (e.g., chemicals and cigarettes). Even when these items are examined and a "statistically significant" result is obtained, there should be a search for consistency with other similar studies, dose-response relationships, and plausible underlying biological mechanisms. Other items to be examined are strength of association, time sequence, and the presence of a dose-response relationship.[123] When these items have been examined, then, and only then, should one use the data. Another problem that generally goes unrecognized is that of reporting bias.

Often an investigator will not report a study in which no link with radiation was found. This probably occurs even more often with editors of journals who wish to reserve their space for positive findings. Whether this is appropriate is not at issue, but the public is often left with a distorted view of scientific reality, caused by selective reporting of statistical chance associations. A well-designed epidemiological study should examine not only the association between radiation exposure and cancer, but it also should define the temporal pattern and magnitude of the effect. In addition, an attempt should be made to define the effect on those exposed at different ages. The importance of this last factor can be recognized when one is considering leukemia in the atomic bomb survivors. If one ignores the effect of age at exposure, the ERR increases at 3.5% per year, but when correction is made for age at exposure, the ERR actually decreases at 0.9% per year. When ERRs are calculated, they should not be derived by using summary statistics but rather with adjustments for age, sex, and other characteristics of the population. In a recent study of workers at Oak Ridge National Laboratory, misleading results were reported by the authors because they did not control for smoking biases.[124]

In general, when radiation dose and the cancer risk are high in relation to the spontaneous risk, bias factors are not particularly important. However, when the radiation dose is low, and, therefore, the incidence of radiation-induced cancer is low compared to the normal risk, even very small biases can lead to substantial errors. When one examines the risk factor for all types of cancer combined, the numbers of people in a given study must be quite large, because, as mentioned earlier, approximately 40% of the U.S. population will contract cancer sooner or later, and some 20% will die from cancer. A number of terms are used to express strength of association or risk in the various epidemiological studies, and it is often very difficult to compare one study with another because of the different terms and types of analysis used. The most commonly used terms at the moment in cohort studies are RR or ERR. Both are expressions of the risk in the exposed group relative to some nonexposed group. A RR of 1.0 means that the exposed group has the same risk as the control group, which equates to an ERR of 0. If the RR is 2, than the exposed population is twice as likely to develop a condition as the nonexposed control group. This equates to an ERR of 1.0. Obviously, the control group must be of essentially the same age, sex, and so on, as the exposed group for these terms to be legitimately used. Of note in this context, the concept of RR is different from that involved in the multiplicative risk model used for projection. A number of factors should be analyzed when RR estimates for cancer are considered. Data from the atomic bomb survivors indicate that there is a sex difference in ERR. For solid tumors as a group, the ERR for females is larger than for males, but in Japan the natural incidence of cancer in females is about half that of males.[125,126] Therefore, the absolute excess risks are about the same. This pattern is not seen for liver and thyroid cancer, and leukemia. Thus, use of a summary single-risk estimate may mask important tumor-specific differences. These questions will be discussed relative to specific tumors in Chapter 5.

Another factor that should be taken into account when RRs are considered is that an increased RR does not necessarily mean that a given exposure has had an effect. In calculation of RR, two populations are being compared. If the control group has a lower disease or mortality rate than is normally expected, the RR will be above unity (1.0), even though there is not an excess of disease or mortality in the exposed population. For this reason an increased RR or ERR should not be considered until such factors have been clarified. The expression of radiogenic cancer and RR over time is a complex matter complicated in that the pattern is not the same for all tumors. A model in which the ERR for a given age at exposure is constant with passing time provides an adequate fit for mortality for all cancers as a group other than leukemia in the atomic bomb survivors.[125,127,128] This is probably fortuitous, because the RR for breast cancer in women survivors appears to have increased for 15 years and then decreased.[2,116] In Japan, the thyroid cancer RR appears, likewise, to have been highest in those irradiated as children and to decrease with attained age.[129] For carcinoma of the esophagus in the atomic bomb survivors, the ERR has decreased at 19% per year since 1960, while the ERR for urinary tract carcinomas increased at 7% per year.[127] In patients treated with radiation for ankylosing spondylitis, the RR for all cancers other than

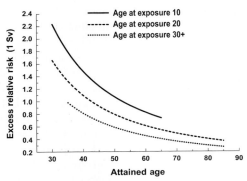
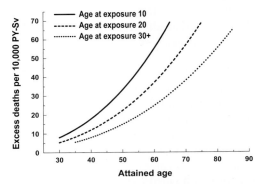

Figure 4-9 • Age-time patterns in radiation-associated risks for solid cancer incidence excluding thyroid and nonmelanoma skin cancer. Curves are sex-averaged estimates of the risk at 1 Sv for people exposed at the ages indicated. (From National Research Council: Health risks from exposure to low levels of ionizing radiation. BEIR VII. Washington, DC, National Academies Press, 2006.)

leukemia or colon cancer has been found to decrease significantly with time.[130]

In persons irradiated in childhood, the radiation-induced ERR appears to decrease with time after exposure.[125,131,132] Use of such a decreasing ERR model for irradiation during childhood decreases RR by 30% to 45%, compared with a constant ERR model. Differences in risk on the basis of ethnic origin also have been found. The rates of excess skin cancer found in children irradiated for ringworm of the scalp (tinea capitis) were very different between whites and blacks; of the irradiated group, 25% were black, but all 41 skin cancer cases were found in whites, suggesting the additive effects of exposure to UV radiation.[133]

Age at exposure is another important factor to be considered in general evaluation of epidemiologic studies. There are fairly profound differences in risk based not only on age at exposure but attained age as well (Figs. 4-9 to 4-11). The variation in risk with age at exposure depends on whether one is considering relative or absolute risks. For many solid tumors, persons exposed early in life have higher-average ERRs and lower-excess absolute risks than those exposed later in life. This effect is quite apparent when the various mortality studies of breast cancer are considered. Standardized mortality ratio (SMR) relates an exposed group to some norm, typically, mortality rates for the country or state. The SMR is often calculated in retrospective cohort-occupational studies. The term *standardized* refers to weighting for person-years of follow-up. If one is considering a group of workers and comparing them with national averages for persons of the same age and sex, the result may not be entirely comparable, because national averages contain persons who are too sick to work. In case-control studies, participants are selected based on having a disease, and, thus, it is not possible to calculate the likelihood of development of that disease based on the presence or absence of exposure. Case-control studies present ORs, which give the odds of having an effect based on exposure. In some instances, the OR can be used as an approximation of RR.

UNCERTAINTIES IN RISK ESTIMATION

Given the problems that are associated with any epidemiological study of radiation carcinogenesis, the question about the level of uncertainty associated with estimation of risks at low doses is often asked.[134–136] Excellent reviews of the topic have been provided by Sinclair,[137]

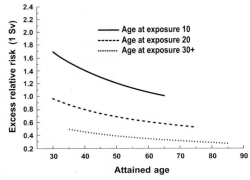
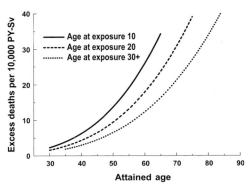

Figure 4-10 • Age-time patterns in radiation-associated risks for all solid cancer mortality. Curves are sex-averaged estimates of the risk at 1 Sv for people exposed at the ages indicated. (From National Research Council: Health risks from exposure to low levels of ionizing radiation. BEIR VII. Washington, DC, National Academies Press, 2006.)

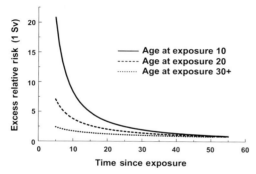
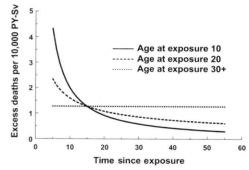

Figure 4-11 ● Age-time patterns in radiation-associated risks for leukemia mortality. Curves are sex-averaged estimates of the risk at 1 Sv for people exposed at the ages indicated. (From National Research Council: Health risks from exposure to low levels of ionizing radiation. BEIR VII. Washington, DC, National Academies Press, 2006.)

Brenner et al.,[102] Wakeford,[138] Land,[139] and the BEIR VII Committee.[2] Because the largest study to date involves the atomic bomb survivors, specific uncertainties relative to this study have been estimated. The first category of uncertainties involves epidemiological issues. These include possible underreporting of cancer, a population that had very few adult males, wartime stresses and rationing, and possible misclassification. The last has been estimated to result in about 15% uncertainty. Another problem is estimation of risk from very few cases of cancer. Between 1950 and 2001, of the 86,500 or so atomic bomb survivors in the study cohort, about 10,300 died of cancer, but the radiation excess is estimated to be only approximately 570 fatal cases.[122] Random or systematic fluctuations about the spontaneous number could decrease or accentuate what appears to be the radiation excess.

Dosimetry considerations represent a second issue. There can be both random and systematic uncertainties,[135,140] which in the risks estimated from atomic bomb survivors are estimated to result in 20% to 40% uncertainty. It has been estimated that such errors can cause risks arrived at by linear extrapolation to be 5% to 10% too low.[134,141] Another problem is the probable effect due to persons being assigned to a dose category higher than the dose actually incurred. At high doses this tends to increase the estimated risks. At dose levels of 0.5 to 4 Gy, this could increase risk estimates for leukemia by 7% and for solid cancers by 11%. A second dosimetry issue is the extent to which neutrons contributed to the total dose at Hiroshima. In the DS86 dosimetry neutrons were assumed to account for about 1% to 2% of organ doses, which has since been criticized as an underestimate.[142]

The third major issue is the model used to project from current experience to lifetime experience. Uncertainty remains because more than half of the atomic bomb survivors are still alive 50 years after the event, and until they reach the end of their lifespan we will not be completely sure of the very late risks of exposure. One of the current models uses a constant RR over lifetime. Some authors think a model based on attained age is more accurate than age at exposure. If this is true, we are currently overestimating risks by a factor of 2.

Another issue is the transfer of risks from a Japanese population to other populations. In the 1990 risk estimates provided by the ICRP, the baseline cancer rates of five populations were merged to minimize application errors. This issue is essential in determining whether to use an absolute (additive) model or a relative (multiplicative) risk model. Breast cancer data would suggest an additive model, but other organs seem to fit better with a multiplicative model. Use of a purely multiplicative model (which is often done) gives higher risk estimates.

The fourth major issue is what adjustment factor to use when extrapolating from high doses and dose rates to low doses or low-dose rates. This factor is called either the dose-rate effectiveness factor (DREF) or dose and dose-rate effectiveness factor (DDREF). Experiments on animals suggest that a factor between 1 and 10 is found with low-LET radiation, depending on the experiment. The average appears to be about 3 to 4. If one examines the yield of lymphocyte chromosome aberrations, a factor of 3 or more is found. Pierce and Vaeth have reported that the low-dose data from the atomic bomb survivors suggests that the low-dose effectiveness factor probably does not exceed 2 or 2.5.[143] Currently, for estimation of human cancer risks, a factor of 2 is used by ICRP, and 1.5 was used by the BEIR VII committee.

As is clear, some of the uncertainties may cause risk estimates to be lowered while others suggest they should be raised. If the uncertainties to estimate the worst-case scenario are considered as a group and in only one direction, the maximum uncertainty is more than a factor of 2 or 3. On the whole, most scientific groups such as BEIR, UNSCEAR, and ICRP consider the current risk estimates to be appropriate and probably conservative.[2]

Many of the inferences about the time and age patterns of excess risk of cancer have been learned from analysis of the combined rates of all cancers (except leukemia) as a group. This is referred to as pooled analysis, which is unsatisfactory in obtaining information about specific tumor types and can mask effects if opposite effects are seen for two tumor types. Even with atomic bomb survivors, detailed analysis of the specific tumor types is limited by the small numbers of cases. A method of joint analysis has been proposed to overcome some of these difficulties, which essentially combines similar types of cancers for analysis.[131]

MAJOR EPIDEMIOLOGIC STUDIES

In general, few studies claim to have found carcinogenic effects of radiation exposure at dose levels below 0.1 Gy. This, of course, is expected in light of the statistical considerations mentioned earlier. These few studies have received a vast amount of public attention, because, if their findings are valid, they suggest that currently used carcinogenic risk estimates may be in error by one or more orders of magnitude. These studies have also been carefully examined for sources of bias; excellent reviews of the subject have been done.[2,3,97,102,117]

Risk estimates have been derived from several major categories of epidemiologic studies. These include: atomic bomb survivors, persons living in areas of higher-than-average natural background radiation levels, persons exposed to radioactive fallout, populations living near nuclear installations, occupational exposures, medical diagnostic exposures (prenatal and adult), and medical therapeutic exposures for benign and malignant diseases.

Each of the categories has strengths and limitations. Usually, these are related to sample size, population composition, certainty of dose, concurrent diseases, and other confounding factors. Each of these factors will be discussed further in the specific studies in the following text.

Atomic Bomb Survivors

In general, most people presume that the major late cause of death at Hiroshima and Nagasaki was radiation-induced cancers. However, as of 2001, radiation-induced cancers actually had accounted for about a 1% increase in the overall death rate. Of 86,572 survivors alive in 1950, 47,685 had died (10,371 from cancer) by 2001 (Fig. 4-12). The excess cancer deaths due to radiation are estimated not to have exceeded 570.[122]

The study of the atomic bomb survivors is the largest, longest, and most comprehensive epidemiological study of radiation carcinogenesis. Its strengths are that it includes a large population of all ages and both sexes who were not selected because of occupation or disease. Other strengths are that it includes a wide range of doses, has included follow-up for over 50 years, and has comprehensive individual dosimetry. Weaknesses of the study are that it began in 1950, 5 years after irradiation, the exposure occurred at a high-dose rate, and the possible contribution of neutrons is somewhat uncertain. That the population is Japanese also raises some question about the transfer of observed risk factors to other populations that may have different baseline cancer rates.

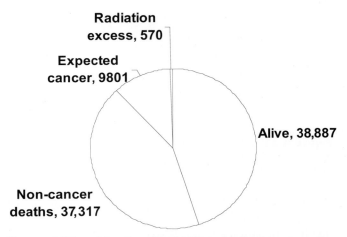

Status of 86,572 A-bomb survivors in 2001

Radiation excess, 570
Expected cancer, 9801
Alive, 38,887
Non-cancer deaths, 37,317

Figure 4-12 • Mortality of the 86,572 atomic bomb survivors alive in 1950 as of 2001. 47,685 had died (10,371 from cancer). The estimated excess cancer deaths due to radiation are 570.

The so-called Life Span Study (LSS) of the survivors began with 120,321 Japanese. Of these, 26,580 were not in the city at the time of the bombings, and for another 7109 persons the dose was unknown. There were 263 persons with doses over 4 Gy and another 6397 who had died or had developed cancer. The latest risk analyses are based on a cohort of 86,611 persons for whom DS02 dose estimates are available.[122] These are compared with 26,000 nonexposed controls. There are two major ongoing studies of cancer rates in the atomic bomb survivors: an incidence study and a mortality study.[126] The incidence study includes 37,270 exposed persons and 42,702 unexposed controls. The group is 55% female and has had a follow-up of 50 years and 3.18 million person-years through 2000.[122] The incidence study has found statistically significant increases in the incidence of leukemia, salivary gland, stomach, colon, liver, gallbladder, lung, female breast, nonmelanoma skin, ovary, and thyroid cancers. It has not found increases in the frequencies of the following cancers: multiple myeloma, oral cavity, esophagus, rectum, pancreas, uterine, prostate, or central nervous system (Fig. 4-13).

The mortality study has 48,104 exposed persons and 38,507 unexposed controls. It is also 55% female and as of 2000 had 50 years of follow-up with 3.18 million person-years of study (Tables 4-9 and 4-10). The LSS mortality study data as of 1997 demonstrated statistically significant increases in the rates of leukemia; cancers of the lung, breast, thyroid, esophagus, stomach, colon, ovary, and urinary bladder; and multiple myeloma. The excess of multiple myeloma has decreased since then and is no longer significant. Cancers of the rectum, gallbladder, pancreas, prostate, uterus, and malignant lymphoma did not increase

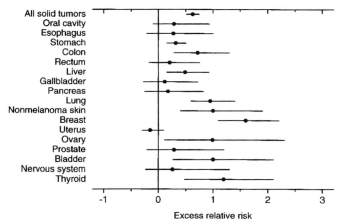

Figure 4-13 • ERR (and 95% CI) at 1 Sv for the incidence of various tumor types in the atomic bomb survivors (1958–1987). (From Thompson DE, et al: Cancer incidence in atomic bomb survivors. Part II: Solid tumors. Radiat Res 1994; 137 (Suppl 2): S17–S67.)

in frequency (Fig. 4-14). Cancer incidence and mortality by dose and cancer site are shown in Table 4-11 and 4-12. In general, the radiation-induced solid tumors appeared after the exposed persons reached the age when spontaneous cancers occur. Sensitivity was about twice as high in children as in adults (see Figs. 4-9 to 4-11).

The dosimetry at Hiroshima and Nagasaki has been evaluated several times. The latest estimate of weapon yield at Hiroshima is 16 kilotons and at Nagasaki 21 kilotons. Originally, the dosimetry system was called T65 (1965 Tentative dosimetry). In 1986 the dosimetry was revised (DS86), and it was revised again in 2002 (DS02). The principal differences include an increase of the

Table 4-9 • Summary of Risk Estimates for Cancer Incidence from Atomic Bomb Survivors

Cancer Site or Type	ERR/Sv*	AR (%)†
Leukemia (excluding CLL)	4.4 (3.2; 5.3)	31
Salivary gland	3.5 (1.5; 7.5)	35
Female breast	1.6 (1.1; 2.2)	32
Thyroid	1.2 (0.48; 2.1)	26
Urinary organs and kidney	1.2 (0.62; 2.1)	22
Nonmelanoma skin	1.0 (0.41; 1.9)	24
Ovary	0.99 (0.12; 2.3)	18
Trachea, bronchus, and lung	0.95 (0.6; 1.4)	19
Colon	0.72 (0.29; 1.3)	14
Liver	0.49 (0.16; 0.92)	11
Pancreas	0.18 (−0.25; 0.82)	3
Stomach	0.32 (0.16; 0.50)	7
Oral cavity and pharynx	0.29 (−0.09; 0.93)	9
Esophagus	0.28 (−0.23; 1.0)	6
Rectum	0.21 (−0.17; 0.75)	4
Prostate	0.29 (−0.21; 1.2)	7
Nervous system	0.26 (−0.23; 1.3)	6
Uterus	−0.15 (−0.29; 0.10)	−3
All solid tumors	0.63 (0.52; 0.74)	12

*90% confidence limits in parentheses.
†In this case attributable risk (AR) denotes the percentage of cases in exposed survivors attributed to their irradiation (values rounded).
Data from National Research Council, Committee on the Biological Effects of Ionizing Radiations (BEIR): Health risks from exposure to low levels of ionizing radiation. BEIR VII. Washington, DC, NRCUSNA Press, 2006.

Hiroshima weapon yield from 12 to 16 kilotons and an increased transmission of gamma rays through tissue (an increase by a factor of 2 to 3 in gamma-ray dose at Hiroshima). In addition, the neutron component at Hiroshima was reduced by a factor of 6 to 10.

Table 4-10 • Actual Numbers of Deaths from Solid Cancer Observed in the Life Span Study (1950–1997)

Cancer Site	MALES Deaths	MALES ERR/Sv*	FEMALES Deaths	FEMALES ERR/Sv*
Lung	716	0.48 (0.23; 0.78)	548	1.1 (0.68; 1.6)
Oral cavity	68	−0.20 (<−0.3; 0.45)	42	−0.20 (<−0.3; 0.75)
Esophagus	224	0.61 (0.15; 1.2)	67	1.7 (0.46; 3.8)
Stomach	1,555	0.20 (0.04; 0.39)	1,312	0.65 (0.40; 0.95)
Colon	206	0.54 (0.13; 1.2)	272	0.49 (0.11; 1.1)
Rectum	172	−0.25 (<−0.3; 0.15)	198	0.75 (0.16; 1.6)
Liver	722	0.39 (0.11; 0.68)	514	0.35 (0.07; 0.72)
Gallbladder	92	0.89 (0.22; 1.9)	236	0.16 (−0.17; 0.67)
Pancreas	163	−0.11 (<−0.3; 0.44)	244	−0.01 (−0.28; 0.45)
Urinary bladder	83	1.1 (0.2; 2.5)	67	1.2 (0.10; 3.11)
Kidney	36	−0.02 (<−0.3; 1.1)	31	0.97 (<−0.3; 3.8)
Brain/CNS	14	5.3 (1.4; 16)	17	0.51 (<−0.3; 3.9)
Female breast	—	—	272	0.79 (0.29; 1.5)
Ovary	—	—	136	0.94 (0.07; 2.0)
Uterus	—	—	518	0.17 (−0.10; 0.52)
Prostate	104	0.21 (<0.3; 0.96)	—	—
All solid cancers	4,451	0.37 (0.26; 0.49)	4,884	0.63 (0.49; 0.79)

*ERR/Sv for age 30 at exposure, computed in an age-constant linear ERR model, 90% confidence limits in parentheses.
Updated from Preston DL, et al: Studies of mortality of atomic bomb survivors. Report 13: Solid cancer and noncancer disease mortality: 1950–1997. Radiat Res 2003;160(4):381–407.

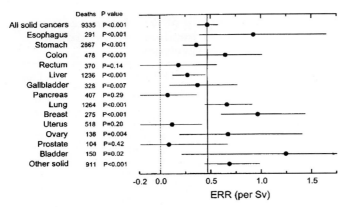

	Deaths	P value
All solid cancers	9335	P<0.001
Esophagus	291	P<0.001
Stomach	2867	P<0.001
Colon	478	P<0.001
Rectum	370	P=0.14
Liver	1236	P<0.001
Gallbladder	328	P=0.007
Pancreas	407	P=0.29
Lung	1264	P<0.001
Breast	275	P<0.001
Uterus	518	P=0.20
Ovary	136	P=0.004
Prostate	104	P=0.42
Bladder	150	P=0.02
Other solid	911	P<0.001

Figure 4-14 • ERR (and 90% CI) at 1 Sv for the mortality of various tumor types in the atomic bomb survivors (1958–1987). (From Preston DL, et al: Studies on mortality of atomic bomb survivors. Report 13: Solid cancer and noncancer disease mortality: 1950–1997. Radiat Res 2003; 160(4):381–407.)

The DS86 changes increased risk estimates for solid cancers by about 30% more than the T65 estimates.[141,144] Under the DS86 and DS02 systems, the neutron doses were very small at both cities. While the differences between the effects at both cities have become smaller, differences that are not well understood still remain. For example, mortality, chromosomal aberrations, epilation, and lens opacities are consistently higher in Hiroshima than in Nagasaki for given doses. At the time of the adoption of the DS86 dosimetry system, physicists were aware of some discrepancies between thermal neutron fluxes based on cobalt-activation measurements or on fast-neutron transport equations. These differences, which were made more apparent by measurements of europium 152 and 154 in soil and of chlorine 35 and 36 in concrete,[142] have since been resolved in the DS02 system.[122] The earlier data from Nagasaki showed reasonably good agreement between estimates of thermal neutrons and estimates made by activation analysis. In the revised DS02 system, however, the neutron doses in both cities have decreased

appreciably compared to those in DS86, while the average gamma-ray doses have increased by about 10% to 12%. Thus, estimates of solid cancer risk per sievert (Sv) based on the DS02 dosimetry are about 5% lower than those based on the DS86 dosimetry.[122] Data on cancer and leukemia mortality at high and lower doses are shown in Figures 4-15 and 4-16.

In spite of the revised dosimetry, differences still exist between the populations of Hiroshima and Nagasaki in addition to those that are attributable to differences in weapon construction and absorbed dose. One example of a confounding variable is the degree of consanguinity. This could certainly have affected the frequency of cancer and mental retardation.

One point of concern raised by Stewart in relation to the LSS was the possible role of immunological and other factors affecting overall resistance as a source of bias.[145,146] It was suggested that reduced immunocompetence and resistance to disease may not only have been a cause of early deaths from infection but also may have played a role in selecting a subpopulation less susceptible to carcinogenesis. An additional possibility is that the surviving population may be inhomogeneous with respect to the control sample. Land reviewed the Japanese data, comparing them with estimates of the carcinogenic effects of radiation in other populations, and found the data overall to be in remarkably close agreement if appropriate age-adjustments of the population are made.[147] Also, the effects on childhood cancer mortality were much less prevalent in prenatally exposed survivors than would have been predicted by Stewart.[148,149] The general argument advanced by Stewart against using the data from the atomic bomb survivors suggests that, in some fashion, depressed immunocompetence and resistance during the cancer latent period is more important for cancers of the immune system than for other cancers and that other diseases or environmental stresses imposed on the population selectively removed persons who ultimately would have developed cancer. It has been pointed out, however, that analysis of the death certificate data from survivors exposed postnatally offers no support for the argument that there is a significant bias in this

Table 4-11 • Number of Incidence Cases of Solid Cancer Excluding Thyroid and Nonmelanoma Skin Cancer and Number of Deaths from Solid Cancer by Sex and Colon Dose in Atomic Bomb Survivors

Colon Dose (Sv)	NUMBER OF INCIDENCE CASES (1958–1998)			NUMBER OF DEATHS (1950–2000)		
	Males	Females	Total	Males	Females	Total
<0.005	2504	2855	5359	2089	2181	4270
0.005–0.1	1900	2295	4195	1603	1784	3387
0.1–0.2	379	547	926	307	425	732
0.2–0.5	473	602	1075	379	436	815
0.5–1.0	294	348	642	241	242	483
1.0–2.0	199	219	418	160	166	326
2.0+	74	89	163	51	63	114
Total	5823	6955	12,778	4830	5297	10,127

Data from National Research Council, Committee on the Biological Effects of Ionizing Radiations (BEIR): Health risks from exposure to low levels of ionizing radiation. BEIR VII. Washington, DC, NRCUSNA Press, 2006.

Table 4-12 • Number of Incidence Cases and Number of Deaths by Cancer Site and Sex in Atomic Bomb Survivors

Cancer Site	NUMBER OF INCIDENCE CASES (1958–1998)			NUMBER OF DEATHS (1950–1997)		
	Males	Females	Total	Males	Females	Total
Stomach	1899	1703	3602	1555	1312	2867
Colon	547	618	1165	206	272	478
Liver	676	470	1146	722	514	1236
Lung	770	574	1344	716	548	1264
Breast	7	847	854	3	272	275
Prostate	281	0	281	104	0	104
Ovary	0	190	190	0	136	136
Uterus	0	875	875	0	518	518
Bladder	227	125	352	83	67	150
Other solid	1416	1553	2969	1036	1175	2211
Total	5823	6955	12,778	4425	4814	9239

Data from National Research Council, Committee on the Biological Effects of Ionizing Radiations (BEIR): Health risks from exposure to low levels of ionizing radiation. BEIR VII. Washington, DC, NRCUSNA Press, 2006.

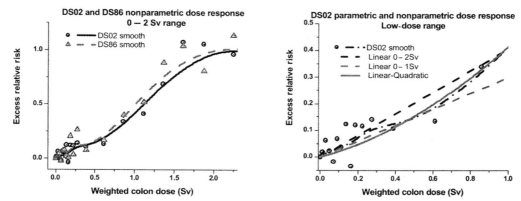

Figure 4-15 • ERR estimates (and 95% CI) of solid tumor incidence in atomic bomb survivors based on DS02 dosimetry and different fits to the data. The right panel shows the data and empirical fits based on the dose range 0–1 Sv. (From Preston, DL, et al: Effect of recent changes in atomic bomb survivor dosimetry on cancer mortality risk estimates. Radiat Res 2004;162[4]:377–389.)

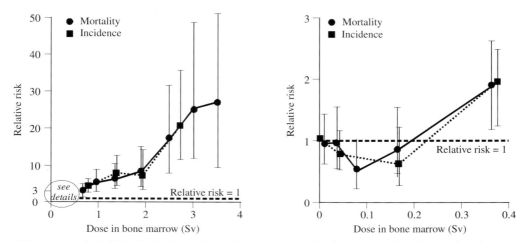

Figure 4-16 • RR estimates (and 95% CI) for leukemia incidence in atomic bomb survivors. Details regarding data in low dose range are presented on the right. (UNSCEAR 2000, Annex I, No. xxviii on p 130. Taken from Little MP, Muirhead, CR: Curative in the cancer mortality dose response in Japanese atomic bomb survivors: Absence of evidence of threshold. Int J Radiat Biol 1998; 74(4):471–480.)

respect.[147] Also, it has been suggested that although some degree of selection cannot be excluded, its effects could be important only in the time period from 1950 to 1958 and appear less likely with the DS86 dosimetry than with the older, T65 estimates of dose.[150] The latter analysis also indicated that even if the alleged selection effect is not an artifact, there is no need to make corrections of risk estimates to the extent suggested by Stewart. A final problem in analyzing data from the atomic bomb survivors lies in determining the "natural," or baseline, cancer rate, since the cancer rate in the surviving population is changing due to differences in diet and smoking habits.

Areas of High Levels of Natural Background Radiation

Relatively few epidemiological studies have been designed to investigate the effects of natural background radiation, owing to the extremely large numbers of people that would be required for the purpose, given that the dose from natural background radiation averages less than 0.01 Gy annually. There are, however, some geographic areas in which the dose rate is higher. These areas are rather limited and are remote from population centers; thus, the number of people available for study in high-natural-background areas has been small. Although most studies of such areas have been negative, they have been useful for setting an upper limit on estimates of the risk of radiation-induced cancer attributable to low doses. Clearly, any risk of cancer mortality that would be postulated to result from natural background radiation cannot exceed the baseline level of cancer mortality that is actually observed. Claims by some "scientists" that linear extrapolation seriously underestimates the risks from low-dose radiation have been refuted on this basis. For example, using this approach to test the validity of the BEIR III Committee's LNT dose-response model for radiation-induced leukemia, Webster found that the rate of leukemia predicted by the model approximated closely the actual mortality rate from the disease in English women aged 20 to 27 during the period 1911 to 1920.[117] Given this concordance, it is clear that a leukemia risk even twice that predicted by the model is not feasible. At least 11 studies of the relationship between leukemia rates and natural background radiation levels have found no significant correlation.[151–161] Two studies, both of which were performed in the United Kingdom, reported to have found an association; however, the first concluded that social and economic factors also needed to be, but were not, considered before a proper interpretation could be made,[162] and the second used statistical methods that were unorthodox and incomprehensible to most scientists.[163]

The question of what proportion of "spontaneously" occurring cancers might be due to natural background radiation has been considered by Darby,[164] who inferred that it is 4% or less, in keeping with the estimates of most other experts.[2,3,116] These calculations are somewhat of a fruitless exercise, however, because given the uncertainties discussed previously, the actual percentage may range between 0% and 4% and will probably never be known with certainty. Even if one uses a linear dose-response hypothesis, the actual number of cancers expected to be induced by background radiation is dwarfed by the statistical noise in the large number of spontaneously occurring cancers as well as those due to other carcinogens that are present in our environment. An increase in background radiation is well known to occur with increasing altitude. Initial attempts to correlate levels of natural background with cancer rates produced negative results.[165] In a study of death rates from leukemia in Colorado, where the contributions from cosmic and terrestrial radiation are almost double those found at sea level, no excess mortality was identified in those counties above 3000 feet, as compared with counties at sea level,[156] in keeping with the results of a later study by Weinberg et al.[157]

A similar type of study in China, which included more than 41,000 people, found no excess of malignancies in an area of high levels (2 mSv/year) of natural background radiation, as compared with an area of low levels (0.7 mSv/year) of natural background radiation.[159] This study was enlarged and updated in 1982 to cover the years 1970–1980.[166] The difference in radiation dose between the high- and low-background areas was 40 to 50 mSv in each generation. The mortality from malignant tumors was lower in the high background area, and the difference was statistically significant. The two populations are quite similar in other respects because they are only approximately 50 miles apart. The results of the study cannot be used to show that living in high-background areas reduces the risk of malignancy; however, they do rule out risk coefficients appreciably higher than those proposed by BEIR and UNSCEAR. Likewise, the suggestion that the rate of mortality from breast cancer is correlated with the concentration of fission products in the diet, based on data from nine census regions in the United States for the years 1984–1988,[167] is severely deficient on methodological and statistical grounds.[168]

There are many studies regarding radon, both with regard to residential exposure and during mining activities. These studies relate almost exclusively to lung cancer and are discussed extensively in that section of Chapter 5. At the present time there is a clear dose-response relationship between lung cancer and residential radon, which has become evident from combined studies in both Europe and North America.[169,170] The relationship with regard to mining and radon is best presented by Lubin et al.[171]

Fallout Studies

There have been a number of studies of populations exposed to radioactive fallout from weapons testing, weapons use, and nuclear plant accidents. Some of these studies involve relatively few persons (as in the Marshall Islands), but most involve thousands or hundreds of thousands of people. One advantage of such studies is that they involve populations of both sexes and all ages. In addition, they may yield information on the effects of chronic exposure. The difficulties in risk assessment arise because the doses are usually quite low and are rarely available on any given individual. Typically, dose estimates are derived from computer modeling of the source term, meteorology, environmental pathways, and assumptions about ingestion pattern and amounts. Often, the dose estimates can be made only collectively. While fallout patterns can be modeled by computers, experience from Chernobyl has shown that individual doses may vary by an order of magnitude from the estimated average.

Weapons fallout studies have been published by the British National Radiological Protection Board and the Nordic countries. No consistent increase in leukemia was observed after the period of high fallout during 1964 to 1965.[172,173] Studies of Swedish Lapps, who breed reindeer and eat their meat, and who might therefore be expected to have higher rates of tumors because of the known concentration of fallout products in the lichen-reindeer food pathway, have found no increased risk of tumors in organs considered to be most sensitive to radiation carcinogenesis.[174]

Among children in Utah exposed to fallout from weapons tests conducted in Nevada from 1951 to 1958, increased mortality from leukemia has been reported in several studies. In one of the early studies,[175] the children were grouped into a "high-exposure" cohort and two "low-exposure" cohorts, and the rate of mortality from leukemia in the high-exposure cohort was found to be approximately twice that in the low-exposure cohorts; however, interpretation of the findings is complicated in that the number of cases of leukemia observed did not differ significantly from the expected number (4.39 vs. 4.23), and cases in the low-exposure cohort were fewer than expected, even in the high-fallout counties. Also, no dosimetric information for the individuals themselves was available, and the "high" and "low" cohort groups differed with respect to the years of exposure that were studied. A subsequent review, using mortality data from the National Center for Health Statistics, found the childhood leukemia rate in southern Utah between 1944 and 1949 to be anomalously low, with no clear relationship between the frequency of the disease and fallout levels.[176] A later study, however, suggested an association between leukemia and fallout in Utah during the period from 1952 to 1958, but found no increase in the frequency of any type of thyroid disease,[177] and a subsequent case-control study, involving 1177 individuals who died of leukemia and 5330 controls, also suggested a weak link between the frequency of leukemia and the estimated bone marrow dose, but the difference was not statistically significant.[178,179] In more recent cohort studies, the

incidence of thyroid cancer has been found to be increased in children of southwestern Utah and Nevada who were exposed to weapons fallout during the 1950s[180,181]; the largest such study, involving the analysis of 4602 deaths from thyroid cancer occurring between 1957 and 1994 and 12,657 incident cases diagnosed between 1973 and 1994 in selected counties of the United States, found the increase to be confined to individuals who were exposed under 1 year of age in the 1950–1959 birth cohort.[181]

An extensive scientific effort has since been made to reconstruct the doses from fallout that were released by weapons testing at the Nevada Test Site. The advantages of this effort include a comprehensive evaluation of the exposures in question, the fact that such exposures were protracted at extremely low dose rates, and the large number of leukemia deaths that may be available for analysis. In spite of the improved dose estimates that have resulted, however, considerable uncertainty in individual doses to the thyroid and bone marrow remains. In addition, the estimated cumulative doses are much lower than those that are received from natural background radiation.

Another type of study has explored the effects of fallout or other environmental releases of radioactivity on personnel participating in atmospheric weapons tests. One early such study involved military personnel who participated in the "Smokey" bomb test in Nevada on August 31, 1957.[182] Of the 3224 men who had been present at the test, approximately 70% were traced, and film badge data for gamma- and beta-ray doses were available; 9 leukemia cases were observed versus 3.5 expected after 20 years of follow-up. Four of the cases were acute myelocytic leukemias, three were chronic myelocytic leukemias, one was an acute lymphocytic leukemia, and one was a hairy-cell leukemia. The mean whole-body dose was 10.6 mGy, with a mean bone marrow dose of 5.3 mGy. Thus, the calculated absolute risk of leukemia amounted to approximately 160 cases per 1 million persons annually for 10 mGy (80 times greater than the BEIR 1980 Committee estimate). As has been pointed out, if the risk factors derived from this study were correct, the equilibrium number of cases of certain types of leukemia caused by background radiation alone would be substantially greater than the numbers actually occurring in the U.S. population.[117] In a follow-up of the same study, the only cancer identified as having a statistically significant increase in incidence and mortality was leukemia[183]; however, there was no increase in the frequency of leukemia with increasing radiation dose, so that the increase reported previously may have been due to chance or factors other than radiation. Subsequently, another study also was interpreted to suggest that lymphomas, melanomas, and cancers of the thyroid, breast, bone, and brain, as well as leukemia, were increased in frequency in the vicinity of the Nevada Test Site,[184] but this suggestion must be questioned in view of the study's methodological limitations. More recently, an increase in the frequency of lymphopoietic cancer deaths in U.S. Navy veterans who participated in Operation Hardtack was reported, the RR amounting to 3.72 (CI 1.28 to 10.83) in those exposed to doses of 50 mSv or more.[185] Men who participated in atmospheric weapons testing in the United Kingdom also have been reported to show suggestive evidence of an increase in mortality from leukemia but no significant excess in the incidence of, or mortality from, any other type of cancer.[186,187]

Studies on the effects of localized fallout from the 1954 BRAVO weapons tests in the Marshall Islands have shown an increase in the frequencies of both thyroid nodules and thyroid cancer in the population of these islands, which numbered less than 8000 persons.[188,189] Advantages of these studies include the facts that the population was unselected, an attempt at individual dosimetry was made, and long-term comprehensive medical follow-up was available; however, the small numbers of persons and tumors remain a problem, as does the uncertainty in dose due to short-lived radioiodines. In addition, surgery and hormonal therapy may have affected the number of subsequent tumors.

Populations exposed to fallout as a result of the Chernobyl accident in 1986 also have been investigated systematically, and they are advantageous for study in that they are large, unselected, and include occupants of highly contaminated villages for which dosimetric measurements are available.[2,3,190,191] The limitations of the studies are their limited length of follow-up to date and the uncertainty of their radioiodine dosimetry. No increase in the frequency or mortality from neoplasms in the exposed population was evident within the first 16 years after the accident (Figs. 4-17 and 4-18).[192] There was, however, a rapidly growing increase in the incidence of childhood thyroid cancer, which became apparent about 4 to 5 years after the accident.[193,194] The increase, which was much earlier and larger than had been reported in any

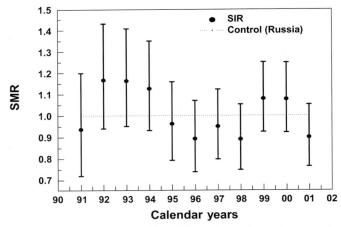

Figure 4-18 • All-solid cancer SIR among residents of 5 contaminated *raions* (counties) of the Bryansk region of Russia compared to the general Russian population (*dotted straight line*) from 1991–2001. (From Ivanov V, et al: Medical Radiological Consequences of the Chernobyl Catastrophe in Russia. St. Petersburg, Russia, Nauka, 2004.)

previous study of thyroid cancer, was quickly followed by case-control and cohort studies to determine whether the increase was a real effect of radiation or merely the result of increased screening or some other cause.[195] Such studies have since multiplied rapidly and now number more than 50 in the published literature. Since they have recently been reviewed elsewhere[2] no attempt is made to cite each of them here. Suffice it to say that the resulting data now establish unequivocally a dose-dependent increase in the incidence of thyroid cancer, the magnitude of which varies inversely with age at exposure,[196] and one study is suggestive of an increase in the incidence of childhood leukemia.[197] A similar increase in the incidence of thyroid cancer is reported to have occurred in the residents of Ozyorsk who were exposed during childhood to radioactive fallout from the Mayak facility.[198]

Studies of the effects of contamination of the Techa River in the eastern part of Russia also have been reported.[199] The strengths of these studies include a wide range of doses, long follow-up, an unselected population, and a large number of persons. In comparison with a population of 394,000 unexposed persons, the exposed population of over 28,000 persons showed a statistically significant increase in the frequency of leukemia, although the ERR per unit dose was about 20% to 50% of that observed in the atomic bomb survivors. The difference may be a result of a dose-rate effect, difficulty in accurately estimating bone marrow doses, or inadequate ascertainment of cases. No excess of solid cancers was observed in members of the study population or in their offspring.[199]

Populations Living Near Nuclear Facilities

Studies of populations living around nuclear power plants have the advantage that they can be well defined if there

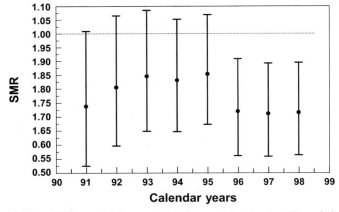

Figure 4-17 • Solid cancer mortality ratio for Russian Chernobyl emergency workers (1991–1998) compared to the general Russian population (*dotted straight line*). (From Ivanov V, et al: Medical Radiological Consequences of the Chernobyl Catastrophe in Russia. St. Petersburg, Russia, Nauka, 2004.)

has been little population mobility. Unfortunately, because mobility is common in the United States, researchers need to ascertain that the cases of cancer detected occurred in persons who were living near the plant before the latent period for cancer induction. The very low doses delivered by emissions from most normally functioning plants make the required sample sizes for statistical significance almost impossible to achieve in circumstances less serious than those at Chernobyl. The reason so many studies of this nature have been done is to respond to reports of "clusters" of leukemia cases or cancers in certain locations. Thus, in recent years, people living in the vicinity of nuclear facilities have become concerned about the possibility that the low doses they receive from such facilities operating under normal conditions might suffice to increase their risks of cancer. On a biological basis, the risk estimates derived by extrapolation from higher-dose epidemiological studies make this possibility seem remote. However, reports of clusters of leukemia around nuclear plants[200–202] have prompted additional, more definitive studies.

One of the first such clusters reported occurred in the U.K. village of Seascale, located 4 miles south of the Sellafield nuclear fuel processing plant. Five deaths from leukemia were reported to have occurred in a little over 1000 children born to mothers living in Seascale in the years 1950–1983, as compared with 0.5 cases expected.[201] However, there were 0 deaths against the 0.8 expected during the same period in 1500 children who had moved into the area after birth, and when the study sample was enlarged to include all cases of leukemia and non-Hodgkin's lymphoma occurring between 1950 to 1988, 11 cases were found to have been diagnosed during this period, and the RRs were computed to be 9.9 for children who were not born in Seascale and 10.2 for those who were born in Seascale.[202] The estimated doses from Seascale in the period before 1960 exceeded those from natural background radiation by only about 20% and after 1960 were even lower. Since such low doses would not be expected to cause a ninefold increase in leukemia rates, some have suggested that the increase could have resulted in part from paternal irradiation prior to conception of the affected children,[203,204] a suggestion that has since been refuted by others,[205,206] as discussed in Chapter 3.

Shortly after the Seascale "cluster" was described, another cluster of leukemia cases was reported around the Dounreay nuclear installation, in which five cases were identified, versus 0.5 expected.[207] On analysis of this report, however, it is clear that the observed case ratio could be obtained only by limiting consideration to the population at the local urban center of Thurso, which was bisected in an arbitrary fashion. If, instead, the perimeter of the study area had been extended to 25 km and the entire exposure period from 1968 up to the time of the publication included in the follow-up, the number of

expected cases would have increased by 2.5, whereas the number of observed cases would have increased by only 1. Furthermore, the incidence of childhood leukemia in the birth cohorts was later found to be increased only nonsignificantly, whereas the incidence in the school cohorts was found to be increased significantly, suggesting that place of birth was not the determining factor.[208–210] Also, the risk in children born to fathers who worked at the Dounreay nuclear facility was later found to bear no relation to the occupational radiation doses that their fathers had received.[211] It is highly unlikely that radiation emitted from the Dounreay plant would cause a significant increase in the incidence of leukemia, since the annual dose from the plant's emissions is estimated to have been smaller than the maximum annual dose delivered by fallout from the atmospheric weapons tests in the early 1960s. It is noteworthy, therefore, that several other clusters of childhood leukemia have been reported near one of three nuclear plant sites in the south of England as well as in the small town of Egremont north of the Sellafield nuclear plant,[212,213] and that follow-up investigations in these areas has indicated that the above-average rates of leukemia are not accounted for by parental employment in the nuclear industry.[205]

The questions raised by the earlier reports, however, have caused a number of larger studies to be undertaken. One such study, examining mortality in the 402 county districts in England and Wales for the period of 1969 to 1978, found no excess in total mortality from cancer in counties containing nuclear installations, but a 15% increase in mortality from leukemia and a 25% increase in mortality from Hodgkin's disease in county districts in which more than 0.1% of the population lived within 16 km of a nuclear installation.[214] The increased frequency of Hodgkin's disease is unlikely to have resulted from irradiation, since no increase in the risk of this disease had been identified in any other irradiated cohort, including the atomic bomb survivors; however, the increased frequency of leukemia prompted the investigators to examine the rates of this disease in populations living near sites of potential or prospective nuclear installations. In the six such sites they subsequently examined, the RRs of mortality from leukemias of all types combined and from Hodgkin's disease were found to be 1.14 and 1.50, respectively, the latter being statistically significant.[215] These findings suggest that the excesses described in the earlier studies were not caused by radiation but probably resulted instead from statistical variation or some other confounding factor or artifact.

This conclusion has since been reinforced by the results of many additional studies of leukemia and other cancers in children living near nuclear power plants in the United States, France, Canada, and Germany.[216–223] In the United States, an extensive study examined the rates of cancer in populations living near all 62 nuclear facilities in the United States that were in service prior to 1982, as well as major Department of Energy facilities for nuclear fuel reprocessing, isotope separation, and other activities involving radioactive material.[220] The study examined cancer deaths occurring from 1950 through 1984 in 107 counties with nuclear facilities and some adjacent counties as well, each county with nuclear facilities being matched for comparison with three similar control counties in the same region. Over 900,000 cancer deaths were found to have occurred in the counties with nuclear facilities and over 1,800,000 cancer deaths in the control areas, and no evidence was found to suggest that the incidence of leukemia or any other form of cancer was higher in study counties than in control counties. For childhood leukemia, the RR in the study counties before plant start-up was 1.08, while after start-up it was 1.03. For leukemia averaged over all ages, the RR was 1.02 before start-up and 0.98 after start-up. The conclusion emerging from the study is that there was no evidence for any cause-effect relationship between particular facilities and cancer rates in nearby populations. In the study's extensive three-volume report, not only are the actual data for each tumor type and each facility presented, an analysis of which results are "statistically significant" is also included. Care needs to be taken in interpreting these data, however, as pointed out in the foregoing discussion on relative risk. For example, the report indicates some RRs that were significantly increased, such as the RR for liver cancer around the Portsmouth gaseous diffusion plant, which is seen on careful analysis to have resulted from a lower-than-expected SMR in the control group. In addition, data for the same plant suggest a "statistically significant" decrease in the RR of breast cancer in the local population, which cannot plausibly be attributed to radiation exposure. In support of the negative results of the studies of childhood cancer rates in areas around nuclear facilities are the similarly negative results of comparable studies of the rates of cancer in the offspring of radiation workers[224] and atomic bomb survivors.[225–230]

Epidemiological studies of populations living near nuclear facilities do not suffice methodologically to exclude an increase in the risk of cancer in such populations or to define the relevant dose-response relationships,[231] but the results of such studies have thus far provided no firm evidence of a radiation-related cancer excess. In fact, the studies in France suggest leukemia rates that are lower than those for the entire nation and control groups. In Germany, likewise, the RRs in regions within a 15-km radius of a nuclear installation have been found to average only 0.97 for all malignancies combined; and the RR for acute leukemia, although 1.06 in children diagnosed before the age of 5 years was actually higher in regions where nuclear power plants had been planned but not yet built.[223] At the present time, therefore, the clusters of childhood leukemia that have been reported around some nuclear installations are generally attributed to chance and/or, possibly, to the spread of infection resulting from the influx of populations from other areas.[138,210,232–234]

Occupational Exposure

Leukemia and other cancers have long been known to have occurred with increased frequency in early radiation workers, whose doses greatly exceeded those encountered in today's workplace.[235,236] The extent to which the risks of such cancers may still be elevated at the much lower doses and dose rates currently encountered has been a subject of continuing interest and debate.[2,96] To address this question, occupational studies constitute a major epidemiological resource, with advantages that include known work records and employment dates, relatively large numbers of persons for study, and quantitative dose measurements; the latter vary in quality, however, from good, for workers in nuclear facilities, to poor for groups such as the early uranium miners.

A large and growing number of occupational studies have been published, many of which have found the rates of cancer mortality in radiation workers to be no different from, or lower than, the average rates in persons of the same age, sex, geographic region, and time period. The interpretation of such studies and assessment of their public health implications are complicated, however, in that the workforce is composed predominantly of young or middle-aged, healthy males, whose risk factors cannot be assumed to be applicable to other populations without allowances for the so-called "healthy-worker" effect, which tends to result in SMRs or standardized incidence ratios (SIRs) that are less than unity. For this reason, the use of internal cohorts is desirable, especially when looking for a dose response. Other confounding factors, such as smoking habits and exposure to chemicals and other agents in the workplace, also can be significant sources of error.

One of the largest occupational groups studied consists of persons who have worked at atomic energy facilities or nuclear installations. A number of early studies of nuclear workers in the United States suggested that the frequencies of multiple myeloma and cancers of the pancreas and other organs were increased in such workers.[237,238] More recently, however, larger and better-designed studies have failed to confirm these findings, as indicated below. Two such studies in the United Kingdom are noteworthy. One of them, an analysis of 3373 deaths among 39,546 atomic energy workers during the period 1946 to 1979, found the SMR in such workers to be 0.74 for all causes and 0.79 for all cancers combined; the death rates for tumors of four types (thyroid, leukemia, testicular, and non-Hodgkin's lymphoma) were reported to be above, but not significantly higher than, the national averages.[239] Another cohort analysis, which included 95,217 workers in the U.K. registry of radiation workers and covered over 1.2 million person-years at risk, found no significant excess in mortality from leukemia or all cancers combined.[240] Likewise, a combined analysis of the mortality from 1946 to 1988 in three U.K. nuclear industry workforces, which included 75,000 employees, found the rates of cancer mortality and all-cause mortality in these workers to be below the national rates, although a positive correlation between mortality from leukemia and external radiation was suggested.[241]

A growing number of occupational studies have been performed in the United States. Some of these have generated a large amount of controversy and merit careful review before their findings can be accepted. Three such reports are commonly quoted without careful analysis. The first of these is a report on the mortality of workers at the Rocky Flats Nuclear Weapons Facility.[242] While this report suggested excesses in mortality from some types of cancer, the excesses have CIs that are usually so wide that no excess risk (unity) is well within the range of estimates. In addition, the analysis assumed latent periods shorter than 10 years for solid tumors, which are biologically implausible; if the usually accepted latent periods of 10 years are used, the reported effects disappear. Similar problems are encountered in the report of another study, in which nonsignificant excesses of cancers of the brain and lung were found if the duration of the latent period for such tumors was assumed to be 0 years, but not otherwise, and no excesses of other cancers or leukemia were found.[243] Also misleading was a subsequent report of mortality in workers from the Oak Ridge National Laboratory, which suggested risk estimates for cancer in this population that were 10 times higher than those based on studies of the atomic bomb survivors.[124] The authors of this report admitted later that they found this result difficult to explain and that confounding factors such as smoking had not been taken into consideration; not unexpectedly, therefore, a later analysis of the data by Gilbert actually found the associations to be largely due to smoking-related cancers.[244] In a study of workers at the Mound facility in Ohio during the period of 1947 to 1979, no significant increase in the overall cancer rate was observed, and the frequency of leukemia was found to be increased only when CLL, which is not known to be related to radiation, was included.[245]

Other publicly prominent and controversial studies involving occupationally exposed workers include an investigation of cancer mortality in employees of the Hanford Laboratory in Richland, Washington, the results of which were reported initially in 1977[237] and again, after reanalysis, in 1978.[238] This study, which compared the mortality of an "exposed" group of workers (average dose 21 mGy) with that of a "nonexposed" group (average dose 16 mGy, reported a 6% increase in mortality from cancer of the pancreas, 7% from cancer of the lung cancer, and 28% from cancers of the bone marrow in the exposed workers.[238] As with the "Smokey" study,[183] however, if these risk estimates were correct, then exposure to medical radiation and natural background radiation should produce more cases of cancer in the U.S. population than are actually observed. The study has been extensively reviewed, and most reviewers have concluded that the only associations of significance were those of multiple myeloma and pancreatic cancer.[246] However, the data from studies of the atomic bomb survivors and other irradiated populations suggest that the few excess cases of multiple myeloma and pancreatic cancer that were observed may represent statistical artifacts or incorrect causes of death rather than radiation effects.[2,96]

Another early and controversial publication was the report of a study of workers in the Portsmouth Naval Shipyard, where nuclear submarines are maintained and serviced, who died of cancer between 1959 and 1977[247] and were divided into "exposed" and "nonexposed" groups, based on telephone interviews with the next of kin, rather than on the actual radiation exposure records kept by the Navy. In the exposed group, there were 6 observed deaths from leukemia, versus 1.1 expected, and 56 from all cancers, versus 31 expected. Because of the wide publicity these data received, the U.S. Congress requested a more complete study of all workers at the shipyard between 1952 and 1977, as well as analysis of the actual radiation exposures. The resulting study revealed no increase in the rates of either leukemia or other cancers among the radiation workers, whose mean radiation dose was estimated to be 27.8 mSv[248]; the absence of any radiation-related increase in such workers has since been borne out by extensive additional analyses.[249]

A combined cohort analysis of workers at Hanford, Rocky Flats, and Oak Ridge National Laboratory has since been performed by Gilbert et al.[250–253] The Hanford cohort included 32,643 workers, with 623,511 person-years at risk; the Rocky Flats cohort included 5952 persons and 81,237 person-years at risk; and the Oak Ridge cohort included 6348 persons and over 138,222 person-years at risk. Each cohort was analyzed for excess risks of leukemia and all other cancers. Whereas an increase in mortality from cancer of the pancreas had been suggested in the previous study of the Hanford cohort, it disappeared with longer follow-up of the cohort, and no statistically significant excess of the disease was found in the combined analysis of the workers at all three facilities. Another, large, combined cohort analysis of nuclear workers in the United States, Canada, and United Kingdom, which included 95,673 subjects and 2,124,526 person-years of follow-up, found the risk of leukemia to be increased in such workers, the increase amounting to an ERR of 2.18 (0.13, 5.7) per Sv.[254] In the past decade other occupational studies have been reported, which are summarized elsewhere.[2,96] The salient estimates of cancer risks resulting from nuclear worker studies are shown in Table 4-13, along with estimates derived from studies of the atomic bomb survivors, which are included for comparison.

Table 4-13 • Estimated Risks of Mortality from All Cancer and Leukemia (Excluding CLL) in Nuclear Workers and Atomic Bomb Survivors

Study Population	All Solid Cancer (ERR/Sv*)	Leukemia (ERR/Sv*)
US nuclear power industry workers (pooled)[†]	0.51 (−2.01; 4.64)	5.67 (−1.84; 24.5)
Canadian nuclear power industry workers (pooled)[‡]	2.80 (−0.038; 7.13)	52.5 (3.97; 225)
UK, US, and Canadian nuclear industry workers (pooled)[§]	−0.07 (−0.39; 0.30)	2.18 (0.13; 5.7)
Atomic bomb survivors (linear model)[‖]	0.43 (0.33; 0.53)	4.55 (2.83; 7.07)

*ERR/Sv, with 90–95% CL in parentheses.
[†]Data from reference 261.
[‡]Data from reference 262.
[§]Data from reference 254.
[‖]Data from reference 122.

In addition to the results of the occupational studies reviewed above, significant information is available on the mortality of workers at the reactor and reprocessing plants at Chelyabinsk (Mayak) in Russia, where relatively large radiation doses were received.[255–260] During the period 1949–1953 most workers received over 0.25 Gy annually, and in a 40-year analysis of 931 workers who received an average accumulated gamma dose of 3.26 Gy, 22.6% died of malignant tumors, and 6.2% died from leukemia. In the reprocessing plant during the period 1949–1953, the average cumulative gamma-ray dose was 2.45 Gy, and in a follow-up of 1812 workers over 62,000 person-years, 197 cancers were observed, versus 153 expected, and 25 leukemias were observed, versus 7 expected. For the 1479 workers of the period 1954–1958, followed over 44,000 person-years, with an average cumulative dose of 7.16 Gy, the results are less dramatic; 55 cancers were observed, versus 61 expected, and 6 leukemias were observed, versus 3.6 expected. Among 2346 workers in the Mayak radiochemical plant, where the exposure was mostly from inhalation, 45 cases of lung cancer were observed, versus 33 expected; there was an increasing trend with dose, but the possible role of chemicals in the etiology of the cancers remains uncertain.[260]

Studies of the mortality of nuclear power industry workers in the United States and Canada have suggested that deaths from leukemia and all cancers combined were increased in frequency in these workers. In the U.S. cohort, which contained 53,698 individuals from 15 nuclear power utilities (52 nuclear plants) who had been employed for some time between 1979 and 1997, the ERRs per Sv for leukemia (excluding CLL) and for all solid cancers combined were calculated to be 5.67 (−2.56, 30.4) and 0.506 (−2.01, 4.64), respectively.[261] In the Canadian cohort, which contained 45,468 workers from the Canadian National Dose Registry, who had been monitored for more than 1 year some time between 1957 and 1994, the ERRs per Sv for leukemia (excluding CLL) and for all solid cancers combined were calculated to be 52.5 (0.205, 291) and 2.80 (0.038, 7.13), respectively.[262] These risk estimates are not inconsistent with those observed in other groups of nuclear workers and in the atomic bomb survivors, but their confidence limits are wide, owing in no small measure to the relatively young ages of the workers in these two cohorts and the comparatively small numbers of them who died during the periods in question.

An international collaborative retrospective study of 407,391 nuclear workers in 15 countries was published by Cardis et al. in 2005.[263,264] The excess risk for cancers other than leukemia was significantly increased at 0.97 per Sv (0.14, 1.97) but the increase was no longer significant when lung and pleural cancers were removed. The excess risk for non–CLL leukemia was not significantly elevated at 1.93 per Sv (<0, 8.47). They concluded that 1% to 2% of deaths from cancer among these workers may be attributable to radiation. An editorial by Wakeford raised a number of issues that caution the interpretation of these findings, including confounding by smoking, most of the positive increase is driven by questionable data from one country (Canada), and the lack of an effect on leukemia and exclusion of certain occupational studies, which are largely negative.[265]

The cancer mortality in British male radiologists who died between 1897 and 1977 also has been examined.[266] Two successive cohorts of radiologists were analyzed, one containing 339 radiologists who entered radiology before 1921, and the other containing about 1000 radiologists who entered afterward; the 1921 date is important because that was when improved radiation protection measures were introduced in Great Britain. Two control populations also were identified in the study. In the pre-1921 cohort, there was a significant excess of cancer deaths (64 versus 37.2 expected), with excesses of cancers of the skin, lung, and pancreas, and leukemia. In the post-1921 cohort, no significant difference between the radiology cohort and all other physicians appeared. Furthermore, in those radiologists entering practice after 1935, fewer cancer deaths were identified than in other physicians (24 versus 30.1 expected).

By the same token, no excess of cancer mortality has been evident in atomic energy workers in India[267] or in U.S. Army technicians trained during World War II.[268] The latter were followed in a study made up of two cohorts of 6000 technologists each, one composed of x-ray technologists and the other a control group of laboratory or pharmacy technologists. The x-ray technologists were originally trained in the Army, and approximately 20% were found to have continued in the field.[268]

The incidence of cancer among medical diagnostic workers in China has been reviewed in a study that compared 27,011 x-ray technologists with 25,782 persons in other medical specialties.[269] The x-ray workers were found to have a 50% higher risk of developing cancer (RR 1.5, 95% CI 1.3 to 1.7), and the risks for leukemia as well as cancers of the breast, thyroid, and skin were increased. Esophageal and liver cancer also showed excesses, but these were not related to dose and were judged to have resulted from other causes. There was no excess in cancers of the lung, oral cavity, bladder, rectum, pancreas, cervix, ovary, brain, lymphoma, or multiple myeloma. The workers often had depressed white blood cell counts, suggesting that their doses were likely to have been on the order or 1 Gy or more, and when this was noted, they were given time off work so that their marrow could recover.[269] Lack of knowledge of individual doses precludes estimation of risk estimates from this study.

Occupationally exposed Danish radiotherapists also have been reported to show an increased RR of cancer, all types combined (RR 1.13), but the RR in this population was much smaller than that in the Chinese study, possibly because the doses in the Danish group were likely to have been smaller.[270] Another important difference is that the major excess risk in the Danish workers that was statistically significant was for prostate cancer (RR 6.25), which was not seen on the Chinese study. This difference, along with prostate cancer generally not being considered to be radiogenic, illustrates the wide variability that can occur between studies. Statistically significant increases are often identified in a single study that are not borne out by the majority of other studies in the literature. It is another example that "statistical significance" alone does not signify that an association denotes a causal relationship.

With the advent of jet airplane travel and the dawn of flights in outer space, the increased levels of ionizing radiation to be encountered at such altitudes have been a subject of potential concern.[271–273] Based on the currently available evidence, however, it has been suggested that the cumulative lifetime occupational dose to the crewmember of a high-flying jet airplane is unlikely to exceed 80 to 180 mSv.[274] If this dose estimate is correct, the resulting cancer risks, if any, are probably too small to be readily detectable epidemiologically.[2]

Finally, there are a large number of other occupational studies that concern the carcinogenic effects of internal emitters, the results of which are not generally applicable to the derivation of numerical risk estimates for many types of cancers. This category includes the large number of studies of uranium miners and other underground miners, and persons exposed in specific industries involving thorium exposure and radium exposure (as in the case of the radium dial painters). These studies will be covered more in Chapter 5, in the sections on lung, liver, and bone cancer, as well as in the section on leukemia.

Medical Diagnostic Exposures

Diagnostic studies have certain advantages, in that the doses and the anatomical fields that are irradiated are reasonably well known, and the exposed populations include people of both sexes and most age groups, many of whom are generally available for long-term follow-up. However, the doses may not be as precise, percentage-wise, as in therapeutic studies, because they are known to be low, and the technical factors are not usually recorded. Furthermore, the doses are generally so low that extremely large sample sizes are required to investigate their effects, and the latter may be confounded as well by preexisting health conditions which prompted the diagnostic examinations in the first place.

Prenatal Irradiation

The risk of carcinogenic effects from prenatal irradiation has been the subject of intense interest, particularly since the studies of the so-called Oxford survey, in which the diagnostic radiation histories of over 7000 children who died of cancer before the age of 10 were compared with those of matched controls.[275–278]

Since the original publication, a number of similar studies have reported RRs of childhood cancer following prenatal irradiation in the range of 1.4, regardless of what the fetal dose appears to have been. A number of doubts as to whether radiation was responsible for this increased risk have been raised, especially because the information on fetal dose is generally poor.[279,280] That case-control studies can be easily biased, and the possibility that an unidentified condition might cause some, and not others, to be x-rayed has been addressed by analysis of twin data within the Oxford study and in two case-control studies of twins in Connecticut, Britain, and Sweden, all of which found an association between prenatal x-irradiation and childhood cancer.[281–283]

There are, however, a number of arguments against a true association between low-dose obstetric x-rays and childhood cancer. The first of these is that in utero exposure during the atomic bombings at Hiroshima and Nagasaki, which involved a mean uterine dose of 0.18 Gy, has not been linked to an increase in childhood cancer. During the first 14 years of life only two cancers and no leukemias were found in the exposed children.[148,284]

A second reason for concern about an association related to prenatal radiation is that most of the previously mentioned studies indicated an RR of leukemia to be 1.4 and the RR for all solid tumors also to be 1.4. Because these two types of neoplasms are known to have very different origins and very different risks after exposure in adult life, the purported similarity in RRs raises questions about the biological plausibility of the assumed effect. Additional questions about biological plausibility arise in view of the fact that Japanese children who were under the age of 10 when exposed to the atomic bomb developed leukemia but no other childhood cancer.[285,286] Hence, the suggestion that in utero exposure leads to both leukemia and childhood cancer at the same rate in some prenatal studies is questionable.

Another puzzling circumstance that needs to be considered relative to the effects of in utero exposure is that ERRs have been found only in the case-control studies, whereas six cohort studies have failed to detect an increase in the frequency of childhood cancer following prenatal irradiation, finding RRs of only about 1.0 or less.[148,287–290] Whether this difference is a result of the small numbers of childhood cases and low statistical power of such studies remains uncertain.

The difference between obstetrical prenatal case-control studies and the data from the atomic bomb survivors who were exposed in utero is different not only in terms of expression and timing but also in terms of the derived risk estimates. If prenatal exposures from obstetrical examinations were in the range of 10 mSv, then the estimated ERR per Sv is 40 for leukemia and 40 for other cancers; however, both pre- and postnatal atomic bomb exposure for persons under the age of 10 yield ERR per Sv of 17 for leukemia and 2 for all other cancers. Most other studies, including cervical cancer series, breast cancer therapy, ankylosing spondylitis, thymic irradiation, peptic ulcer treatment study, and the benign gynecologic disease studies all yield leukemia risk estimates more consistent with the range for the atomic bomb survivors. This will be discussed more in the section on leukemia in Chapter 5. In a study that evaluated adult-onset cancers following prenatal exposure, a significantly increased risk of adult cancer among the 1630 prenatally exposed survivors of the atomic bomb who had been followed through 1984 was observed.[285] In a later follow-up, which continued from 1985 to 1989, no cancers occurred, and, therefore, the risk over the entire period was no longer significantly elevated.[286]

In summary, although the case-control studies have yielded surprisingly consistent and similar risk estimates for leukemia and solid tumors, their results are in marked contrast to the data from cohort studies and studies of the atomic bomb survivors exposed in utero. These differences notwithstanding, the available data are generally inferred to support the view that exposure in utero increases the risk of leukemia and, perhaps, other cancers during childhood and adult life, although the magnitude of the increase is uncertain.[206] Paternal radiation exposure prior to a child's conception, on the other hand, is not thought to increase his or her risk of leukemia or other cancers, as has been discussed in Chapter 3 on hereditary effects.

Postnatal Irradiation

The major studies that involve diagnostic exposure of adults to radiation include studies of the effects of multiple fluoroscopies for pneumothorax therapy in tuberculosis patients, use of Thorotrast as a contrast agent, use of multiple x-rays for scoliosis evaluation, and retrospective studies of diagnostic exposures in general.

Two studies of the effects of fluoroscopy on patients with tuberculosis in the United States[291–293] and one such study on patients in Canada[294] are particularly noteworthy. The strengths of the studies included the fact that nonexposed tuberculosis patients were used as controls, individual dosimetry existed, the exposures were fractionated over a period of years, and a dose-response analysis was possible. Interpretation of their results is complicated, however, by uncertainties concerning the fluoroscopic exposure time and patient orientation in some cases. In addition, tuberculosis may have modified the effects of radiation on the lung, and the use of questionnaires may have resulted in a failure to ascertain some cancers.

Two of the studies used only female patients, because they were concerned specifically about the risk of breast cancer as a secondary tumor; however, the frequency of this disease was found to be increased in all three studies. In the Massachusetts study, which included both males and females, cancer of the esophagus was also significantly increased in frequency, but leukemia and cancer of the lung were not.[291] Thorotrast (which contained thorium) was used as a contrast agent for angiography and to a much lesser extent for sinus studies. This material remains in the body and has been associated with increases in the frequencies of leukemia, and tumors of the liver, gallbladder, bile ducts, and, in cases where the material remained in place, nasal sinuses.[295–300]

In patients receiving diagnostic x-ray examinations for scoliosis, the risk of breast cancer was reported by Hoffman et al. to have been increased[301]; however, this report should be interpreted with caution, because the cancers were found as a result of an intensive screening process, and many of the women were nulliparous, which may have accounted in part for their higher relative risk. Most studies retrospectively examining other plain diagnostic uses of x-rays have been negative, as expected, given the low doses they involved and the large population sample sizes therefore required. In the members of two prepaid health plans in which the number of diagnostic x-rays could be retrospectively assessed by case, the risks of non–CLL were found to be slightly elevated (RR 1.17), but no dose-response relationship was evident when x-ray procedures performed shortly before the time of leukemia diagnosis were excluded.[302] An increase in the frequency of multiple myeloma also was seen in the same study, but, as the authors noted, the increase was not consistent with the results of much larger studies of nuclear workers and atomic bomb survivors, and was, therefore, probably not causally related.

The risks of carcinogenic effects from diagnostic doses of radioiodine administered to perform thyroid scanning also have been a subject of study. One of the largest such studies included 35,074 patients who were matched with the Swedish cancer registry.[303] The strengths of this study are the large number of patients involved, nearly complete ascertainment of cancers, and known amounts of radioiodine administered to each patient. Some of the study's limitations, however, are that some patients were initially being examined for suspicion of thyroid cancer, doses to organs other than the thyroid were very low, and the group was compared with the general population. For all cancers as a group, no excess was detected (SIR of 1.01) nor were excesses of thyroid, breast, kidney, or bladder cancer detected. There were questionable increases in the rates of leukemia and cancers of the central nervous system. With regard to the latter tumors, there is no reason to expect that CNS tumors should have been increased by the doses of radioiodine investigated in this study, because much larger doses were received by organs that are more sensitive to radiogenic tumor induction, and no increases in the frequency of tumors in such organs were seen. Furthermore, no excess of CNS tumors has been seen following higher-dose therapy with radioiodine for hyperthyroidism or thyroid cancer.

Radiotherapy for Benign Diseases

Studies of patients who have received radiation therapy for benign diseases have the advantage of a known exposure field, type of radiation, and usually good dosimetry. The dosimetry can be a problem in some cases where children were irradiated and the organ of interest was near the primary radiation field. In these cases, patient motion could cause substantial uncertainty in actual organ doses of interest. The high doses of radiotherapy allow risk estimates to be derived with relatively small population groups; however, the high doses also introduce the confounding factor of potential cell killing.[304] Other disadvantages typically are patient selection bias, confounding by disease, confounding by other therapies or economic status, and potential loss to follow-up if the disease does not require further treatment. The major follow-up studies of patients treated with radiation for benign diseases include those of patients treated for tinea capitis, suspected thymic hyperplasia, postpartum mastitis, ankylosing spondylitis, peptic ulcer, benign gynecologic diseases, polycythemia, tuberculosis, arthritis, hemangiomas, and hyperthyroidism.

A large investigation of Israeli children treated for tinea capitis, which included 10,834 exposed persons, 16,226 controls, and 686,000 person-years of study, found an increased incidence of thyroid, skin, brain, and salivary gland cancers, but no excess of breast cancer, in the irradiated group.[305,306] The risk factors derived for thyroid cancer in this study are much higher than those observed in other studies, raising the possibility that movement of patients during irradiation caused their actual thyroid doses to be underestimated. Increased risk

in Jewish persons was also felt to be a factor. A similar study of children treated for tinea capitis in New York, which was only about one fifth as large, still demonstrated statistically significant excesses of thyroid and skin cancer, but not of brain cancer, leukemia, or salivary gland cancer.[133] Some scientists are uncertain about the effect that radiation may have had on the pituitary gland in relation to thyroid cancer incidence.

During the early 1950s infants were treated with radiation to the chest in the belief that thymic hypertrophy was the cause of sudden infant death syndrome and that radiotherapy would shrink the gland. A study of such infants in Rochester, which included 2652 exposed persons, 4823 controls, and 221,000 person-years of study, demonstrated increased risks of thyroid and breast cancer in the exposed group.[307,308] The strengths of this study included individual dosimetry, long follow-up, and a sibling control group. The study also was able to evaluate dose fractionation effects and include a dose-response analysis. The weaknesses of the study included varied sizes of the treatment fields, so dosimetry for some sites was uncertain, and the questionnaire follow-up may have caused some underascertainment of cases.

Another practice in the late 1940s and early 1950s was to use radiotherapy for the treatment of benign postpartum mastitis and other conditions. Patients who received this treatment also have shown a subsequent excess of breast cancer.[94,309,310]

For patients with ankylosing spondylitis, a skeletal abnormality resulting in progressive fusion of the sacroiliac joints and the spine, radiotherapy used to be a standard form of treatment and was helpful in relieving pain. The follow-up studies of such patients are statistically strong because large numbers of patients have been included, long-term and complete mortality follow-up has been possible, dosimetry for the leukemia cases is available, and some patients with the disease were not treated with radiation. The series are limited, however, because of the difficulty of applying risk factors from these groups to the general population, some cancers were apparently initially misdiagnosed as spondylitis, and organ doses are uncertain since individual dosimetry is lacking. The practice of treating this disease with radiation has been discontinued, but a follow-up of 14,106 of these patients treated with external beam therapy during 184,000 person-years of study has shown increases in the frequencies of leukemia and of other cancers at anatomical sites (except the colon) in the treatment field.[311] Radium treatment of about 2000 children and adults with this disease in Germany has also been shown to have increased their risks of bone sarcomas, breast cancer, liver cancer, and leukemia.[312–314]

A follow-up study of patients who received radiotherapy for peptic ulcer has shown these individuals, likewise, to be at increased risk of cancer.[315,316] The study involved 1831 exposed patients and 1778 controls, with over 78,000 person-years at risk. Statistically significant increases were identified for cancers of the stomach, pancreas, lung, female breast, non-Hodgkin's lymphoma, and leukemia. There was no excess of cancers of the colon, esophagus, rectum, liver, larynx, bone, connective tissue, bladder, kidney, brain, thyroid, or myeloma.

The strengths of the study include individual dosimetry, 50-year follow-up, and a control group of nonexposed patients with peptic ulcer. Unfortunately, however, a standardized radiotherapy regimen precluded dose-response analysis, and metastatic spread of cancer may have been misclassified as primary liver or pancreatic cancer in some cases.

Studies of patients who have received radiotherapy for benign gynecologic diseases are also useful because they include large numbers of patients, patients who can be followed for long periods and can be compared to women with the same conditions who were not treated with radiotherapy, and patients for whom a dose-response analysis is possible. Difficulties with these studies include uncertainty as to the amount of bone marrow exposed, small numbers of certain secondary cancers, and potential misclassification on death certificates for entities such as pancreatic cancer. A follow-up of patients who received intrauterine radium radiotherapy for benign uterine bleeding, which included 4153 women studied over 110,000 person-years at risk, found excesses of leukemia and cancers of the rectum, pancreas, and genital organs, but no excesses of cancers of the uterus, bladder, colon, pelvic bones, liver, gallbladder, stomach, kidney, or hematopoietic tissues in such women.[317,318] In another report on the same group, an excess of uterine cancer was mentioned.[318] In a third study of similar patients, nonsignificant increases in tumors of the rectum, colon, and nervous system, and a decreased risk of breast cancer were seen.[319]

Polycythemia vera, an overproduction of red blood cells, is treated when severe by phlebotomy, radiation therapy, or chemotherapy. The radiation treatment is usually accomplished by intravenous injection of phosphorus 32 and appears to be associated with the subsequent development of leukemia, but whether the latter is due to the nature of the disease or the radiation treatment has been a matter of debate.[320,321] There is no evidence that polycythemia itself is caused by radiation exposure. The intravenous injection of radium, a procedure formerly used in Europe for the treatment of tuberculosis and found to be ineffective for the purpose, has been observed to increase the risk of bone sarcomas and leukemia.[322,323]

External beam radiotherapy for skin hemangiomas in childhood has been reported to result in increased risks of thyroid and brain cancers but no excess of bone, soft tissue, or breast cancers.[324,325] A number of case reports in the literature relate such radiotherapy to the induction of soft tissue tumors as well, but adequate, supporting epidemiological data are not available. (See section on soft tissue tumors in Chapter 5.)

A large number of patients are treated each year with iodine 131 for hyperthyroidism. In one study of 1762 women who had received such treatment, no increase was found in the SIR when all malignant neoplasms were considered together, and analysis of cancers of the breast, digestive organs, pancreas, brain, or all other sites also failed to show a significant or dose-related increase.[326] Another study of 10,500 patients treated in Sweden found no significant increase in the frequency of leukemia or all tumors considered together, and the increases that were found in cancers of the brain, kidney, and stomach did not vary significantly in relation to iodine dose.[327] The strengths of this study include a large number of patients, nearly complete incidence ascertainment, and known administered activities of radioiodine. Undoubtedly, cell killing due to high doses in the thyroid gland occurred, and comparison was made to the general population rather than to other persons with hyperthyroidism.

In the United States, a Cooperative Thyrotoxicosis Therapy Follow-up Study, which included 19,200 radioiodine-treated patients who were followed for 8 years, found no increase in either leukemia or thyroid cancer in such patients.[328,329] The strengths of the study include the large numbers of patients involved, a comprehensive follow-up effort, and suitable nonexposed comparison groups; its limitations include individual doses that were not calculated, there was no late follow-up, and only leukemia and thyroid tumors were evaluated. Another study, in which 1000 patients treated at the Mayo Clinic were followed for an average of 15 years and compared with surgically treated patients, showed no increase in the risk of leukemia or other cancers, except for cancer of the thyroid; the latter, however, was not attributable to radiation but rather to an unexpectedly low rate of thyroid cancer in the surgically treated patients, from whom considerable amounts of thyroid tissue had been excised previously.[330]

Given that radiotherapy is known to entail some risk of radiation-induced second tumors, however large or small the risk may actually be, it has been recommended that the radiotherapeutic dose be minimized insofar as possible, especially in the treatment of benign conditions and in patients who are young or otherwise unusually susceptible.[331]

Radiotherapy for Malignant Disease

Studies involving patients treated for malignant diseases have among their strengths: well-defined doses, known types of radiation, and localized treatment fields. Their weaknesses, however, include the possibility of concurrent or other therapies that may confound analysis, selection bias due to the disease being treated, the possibility of cell killing rather than cancer induction, and a shortened lifespan for follow-up, due to the high mortality of malignant neoplasms. The studies of persons treated for malignancies that have been followed to determine the incidence of second cancers include women treated for cervical cancer and breast cancer. There are several major cervical cancer follow-up studies, the strengths of which are that they include long-term follow-up, nonexposed comparison patients, individual dosimetry for many organs in some instances, and the possibility of dose-response analyses; however, they are limited in that the large doses they involve cause cell killing, and the partial-body nature of the exposure seriously complicates the dosimetry. In British patients who have developed second primary cancers after previous radiotherapy, for example, the radiation-associated risks of leukemia and cancers of the lung, bone, and ovary have been observed to be significantly lower than those seen in the Japanese atomic bomb survivors, a difference that may be largely attributable to the extent of cell-ster-ilization caused by the larger doses involved in radiotherapy.[332,333]

In a combined study of the incidence of second cancers in women treated for carcinoma of the cervix in Canada, Denmark, Finland, Norway, Sweden, Yugoslavia, the United Kingdom, and the United States, 82,616 exposed women were compared with 99,424 unexposed controls, over 1.28 million person-years at risk, and were found to show excess risks of leukemia and cancers of the esophagus, small intestine, rectum, pancreas, and other genital organs, but no excess risks of cancers of the oral cavity, salivary gland, stomach, colon, liver, lung, breast, uterus, kidney, bladder, bone, skin, myeloma, or lymphoma.[333] In another study, 4188 radiation-treated women who had developed second cancers were compared with 6880 controls and were found to show excess risks of non-Hodgkin's lymphoma, leukemia, and cancers of the bladder, rectum, vagina, cecum, uterus, and stomach.[335] Also as in the previously cited study, cancer of the pancreas was increased in frequency, but the increase was not dose-related, and no excesses of cancers of the breast or myeloma were observed.

In a case-control study of patients treated with radiation for carcinoma of the cervix, the number of subjects was smaller than in the cohort studies mentioned above, but statistically significant excesses of leukemia and cancers of the stomach, rectum, uterus, bladder, and bone were found in such women; no excesses of cancers of the pancreas, small intestine, colon, breast, ovary, vulva, or connective tissues were found.[93] The only second neoplasms found consistently to be in excess in both the case-control and cohort studies were leukemia and cancer of the rectum, both of which originate in tissues that were clearly in the primary radiation field. Breast cancer was not observed to be increased in frequency, in spite of an average estimated dose of 0.3 Gy to the breast. The lack of an excess of breast cancer may have been due to the large number of patients over the age of 35 when treated, since susceptibility to the induction of breast cancer appears to decrease markedly with increasing age at exposure.[336]

A Japanese study of 5725 cervical cancer patients treated with radiotherapy alone and 4161 treated with surgery alone found significant excesses of leukemia and cancers of the rectum and bladder in the radiotherapy group, and an excess of lung cancer in both groups.[337]

There are a number of reports of second tumors after radiotherapy for testicular cancers.[338,339] In a Norwegian study of 876 patients, 65 of whom had developed second cancers, statistically significant excesses of lung cancer and malignant melanoma were found; however, the melanomas were considered not to be radiation-related but rather to have resulted from frequent physical examination and better detection, although chemotherapy also may have played a role.[339] In another study, five malignancies of various types were observed to have developed in 79 men, versus one expected, all but one of the tumors having arisen in the radiation field.[340]

Follow-up studies of women treated with radiation for breast cancer have focused primarily on the risks of cancer in the opposite breast and leukemia.[341-343] Strengths of such studies include individual dosimetry, a wide range of high doses, and large numbers of incident cases; their weaknesses come from the limited numbers of young women who are included and the potential of misclassification of metastases or recurrences. The first of the studies cited above found a statistically significant increase in the frequency of contralateral breast cancer only in women less than 45 years of age at exposure.[341] The other two studies found no effects except for myelodysplastic syndrome.

A number of studies have examined the risks of second tumors after treatment for childhood cancer and have found the risks of secondary carcinomas of the thyroid gland and osteogenic sarcomas to be increased, but not the risk of leukemia.[344-346] Some other studies have suggested that the risks of secondary cancers are increased after therapy for Wilms' tumors also, but the numbers of excess cases in question were small. Such studies have strengths in their individual dosimetry, but cell killing and effects of chemotherapy makes complicate their analysis.

Follow-up studies on patients treated with radioactive iodine for thyroid cancer have been conducted in Sweden,[347,348] the United Kingdom,[348] Denmark,[349] Finland,[350] and the United States.[351] The study in Sweden followed 834 patients, in whom the SIR was above unity for leukemia and all cancers, but none of the increases was statistically significant. The United Kingdom study included 258 patients and showed statistically significant excesses of leukemia and cancers of the urinary bladder, and breast; however, a much larger and more recent study, involving 47,000 Swedish patients who had received radioiodine for thyroid cancer, hyperthyroidism, or diagnostic purposes, failed to show an increased risk of leukemia in that study group.[352]

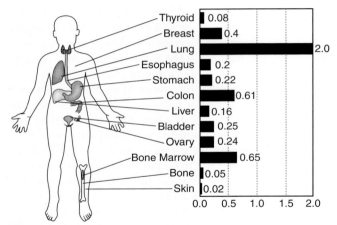

Figure 4-19 • Risk estimates for lifetime mortality from different cancer types as a result of acute radiation exposure. (Data from National Research Council, Committee on the Biological Effects of Ionizing Radiations [BEIR]: Health risks from exposure to low levels of ionizing radiation. BEIR VII. Washington, DC, NRCUSNA Press, 2006.)

Table 4-14 • Probability of Fatal Cancer (100 persons/Sv)

Organ	Updated Value
Thyroid	0.08
Breast	0.4
Lung	2.0
Esophagus	0.2
Stomach	0.22
Colon	0.61
Liver	0.16
Bladder	0.25
Ovary	0.24
Bone marrow	0.65
Bone	0.05
Skin	0.02

Data from National Research Council, Committee on the Biological Effects of Ionizing Radiations (BEIR): Health risks from exposure to low levels of ionizing radiation. BEIR VII. Washington, DC, NRCUSNA Press, 2006.

SUMMARY

In summary, epidemiologic studies of the atomic bomb survivors and other groups have clearly shown a relationship between high-dose radiation exposure and the subsequent risks of many tumors, particularly leukemia, lung, breast, stomach, and thyroid (Fig. 4-19 and Table 4-14). For some tumors, increases in incidence have been difficult to detect even at high doses. This result may be due to inherent cellular, hormonal, or organ system differences. Epidemiologic studies performed to evaluate the possibility of radiation carcinogenesis at doses of less than 0.1 Gy have failed to provide positive evidence that can withstand scrutiny and bias evaluation. Occasionally some authors suggest that the dose-response models commonly used are inadequate and develop their own models to predict future events.[353] Such "personally developed" models have not

been consistent with epidemiologic data and are rarely viewed seriously by scientific groups. As mentioned earlier, if the statistical risk estimates provided by the BEIR Committee, the UNSCEAR Committee, and the ICRP are reasonable, then a sample size of at least 100,000 persons exposed to 0.1 Gy and a similar group of sex-matched controls will be necessary to detect radiogenic cancers at these dose levels. The BEIR VII committee has estimated the lifetime attributable risk for cancer incidence and mortality for cancer site by age at exposure and for acute and chronic exposures (Tables 4-15 to 4-19). Similar data for leukemia is shown in Table 4-20). It must be recognized, however, that the existing negative low-dose data do not rule out the possibility that cancer is induced by doses of radiation less than 0.1 Gy; what such data simply mean is that if a carcinogenic effect is present, it is too small to be detectable by presently available statistical and epidemiological methods.

Table 4-15 • BEIR VII Committee's Preferred Estimates of the Lifetime Attributable Risk of Incidence and Mortality for All Solid Cancers and Leukemia with 95% Subjective Confidence Intervals*

	ALL SOLID CANCERS		LEUKEMIA	
	Males	Females	Males	Females
Excess cases (including nonfatal cases) from exposure to 0.1 Gy	800 (400, 1600)	1300 (690, 2500)	100 (30, 300)	70 (20, 250)
Number of cases in the absence of exposure	45,500	36,900	830	590
Excess deaths from exposure to 0.1 Gy	410 (200, 830)	610 (300, 1200)	70 (20, 220)	50 (10, 190)
Number of deaths in the absence of exposure	22,100	17,500	710	530

*Number cases or deaths/100,000 exposed persons.
Data from National Research Council, Committee on the Biological Effects of Ionizing Radiations (BEIR): Health risks from exposure to low levels of ionizing radiation. BEIR VII. Washington, DC, NRCUSNA Press, 2006.

Table 4-16 • Lifetime Attributable Risk of Site-specific Solid Cancer Incidence*

Cancer Site	AGE AT EXPOSURE (YEARS)										
	0	5	10	15	20	30	40	50	60	70	80
Males											
Stomach	76	65	55	46	40	28	27	25	20	14	7
Colon	336	285	241	204	173	125	122	113	94	65	30
Liver	61	50	43	36	30	22	21	19	14	8	3
Lung	314	261	216	180	149	105	104	101	89	65	34
Prostate[†]	93	80	67	57	48	35	35	33	26	14	5
Bladder	209	177	150	127	108	79	79	76	66	47	23
Other	1123	672	503	394	312	198	172	140	98	57	23
Thyroid	115	76	50	33	21	9	3	1	0.3	0.1	0.0
All solid	2326	1667	1325	1076	881	602	564	507	407	270	126
Leukemia	237	149	120	105	96	84	84	84	82	73	48
All cancers	2563	1816	1445	1182	977	686	648	591	489	343	174
Females											
Stomach	101	85	72	61	52	36	35	32	27	19	11
Colon	220	187	158	134	114	82	79	73	62	45	23
Liver	28	23	20	16	14	10	10	9	7	5	2
Lung	733	608	504	417	346	242	240	230	201	147	77
Breast	1171	914	712	553	429	253	141	70	31	12	4
Uterus[†]	50	42	36	30	26	18	16	13	9	5	2
Ovary	104	87	73	60	50	34	31	25	18	11	5
Bladder	212	180	152	129	109	79	78	74	64	47	24
Other	1339	719	523	409	323	207	181	148	109	68	30
Thyroid	634	419	275	178	113	41	14	4	1	0.3	0.0
All solid	4592	3265	2525	1988	1575	1002	824	678	529	358	177
Leukemia	185	112	86	76	71	63	62	62	57	51	37
All cancers	4777	3377	2611	2064	1646	1065	886	740	586	409	214

*Number of cases/100,000 persons exposed to a single dose of 0.1 Gy. These estimates are obtained as combined estimates based on relative and absolute risk transport and have been adjusted by a dose and dose-rate effectiveness factor (DDREF) of 1.5, except for leukemia, which is based on a linear-quadratic model.
[†]Prostate and uterus are included even though 95% CI for LAR encompassed 0.
Data from National Research Council, Committee on the Biological Effects of Ionizing Radiations (BEIR): Health risks from exposure to low levels of ionizing radiation. BEIR VII. Washington, DC, NRCUSNA Press, 2006.

Table 4-17 • Lifetime Attributable Risk of Site-specific Solid Cancer Mortality*

Cancer Site	AGE AT EXPOSURE (YEARS)										
	0	5	10	15	20	30	40	50	60	70	80
Males											
Stomach	41	34	30	25	21	16	15	13	11	8	4
Colon	163	139	117	99	84	61	60	57	49	36	21
Liver	44	37	31	27	23	16	16	14	12	8	4
Lung	318	264	219	182	151	107	107	104	93	71	42
Prostate[†]	17	15	12	10	9	7	6	7	7	7	5
Bladder	45	38	32	27	23	17	17	17	17	15	10
Other	400	255	200	162	134	94	88	77	58	36	17
All solid	1028	781	641	533	444	317	310	289	246	181	102
Leukemia	71	71	71	70	67	64	67	71	73	69	51
All cancers	1099	852	712	603	511	381	377	360	319	250	153
Females											
Stomach	57	48	41	34	29	21	20	19	16	13	8
Colon	102	86	73	62	53	38	37	35	31	25	15
Liver	24	20	17	14	12	9	8	8	7	5	3
Lung	643	534	442	367	305	213	212	204	183	140	81
Breast	274	214	167	130	101	61	35	19	9	5	2

*Number of deaths/100,000 persons exposed to a single dose of 0.1 Gy at age 10, 30, and 50 years. These estimates are obtained as combined estimates based on relative and absolute risk transport and have been adjusted by a dose and dose-rate effectiveness factor (DDREF) of 1.5, except for leukemia, which is based on a linear-quadratic model.
[†]Prostate and uterus are included even though 95% CI for LAR encompassed 0.

Continued

Table 4-17 • Lifetime Attributable Risk of Site-specific Solid Cancer Mortality*—cont'd

Cancer Site	AGE AT EXPOSURE (YEARS)										
	0	5	10	15	20	30	40	50	60	70	80
Females—cont'd											
Uterus[†]	11	10	8	7	6	4	4	3	3	2	1
Ovary	55	47	39	34	28	20	20	18	15	10	5
Bladder	59	51	43	36	31	23	23	22	22	19	13
Other	491	287	220	179	147	103	97	86	69	47	24
All solid	1717	1295	1051	862	711	491	455	415	354	265	152
Leukemia	53	52	53	52	51	51	52	54	55	52	38
All cancers	1770	1347	1104	914	762	542	507	469	409	317	190

*Number of deaths/100,000 persons exposed to a single dose of 0.1 Gy at age 10, 30, and 50 years. These estimates are obtained as combined estimates based on relative and absolute risk transport and have been adjusted by a dose and dose-rate effectiveness factor (DDREF) of 1.5, except for leukemia, which is based on a linear-quadratic model.
†Prostate and uterus are included even though 95% CI for LAR encompassed 0.
Data from National Research Council, Committee on the Biological Effects of Ionizing Radiations (BEIR): Health risks from exposure to low levels of ionizing radiation. BEIR VII. Washington, DC, NRCUSNA Press, 2006.

Table 4-18 • Lifetime Attributable Risk of Site-specific Solid Cancer Incidence and Mortality*

Cancer Site	INCIDENCE EXPOSURE SCENARIO		MORTALITY EXPOSURE SCENARIO	
	1 mGy/yr Throughout Life	10 mGy/yr from Ages 18 to 65	1 mGy/yr Throughout Life	10 mGy/yr from Ages 18 to 65
Males				
Stomach	24	123	13	66
Colon	107	551	53	273
Liver	18	93	14	72
Lung	96	581	99	492
Prostate[†]	32	164	6.3	32
Bladder	69	358	16	80
Other	194	801	85	395
Thyroid	14	28		
All solid	554	2699	285	1410
Leukemia	67	360	47	290
All cancers	621	3059	332	1700
Females				
Stomach	32	163	19	94
Colon	72	368	34	174
Liver	8.7	44	8	40
Lung	229	1131	204	1002
Breast	223	795	53	193
Uterus[†]	14	19	3.5	18
Ovary	29	140	18	91
Bladder	71	364	21	108
Other	213	861	98	449
Thyroid	75	139		
All solid	968	4025	459	2169
Leukemia	51	270	38	220
All cancers	1019	4295	497	2389

*Number of cases or deaths/100,000 persons exposed to 1 mGy/yr throughout life or to 10 mGy/yr from ages 18–65. These estimates are obtained as combined estimates based on relative and absolute risk transport and have been adjusted by a dose and dose-rate effectiveness factor (DDREF) of 1.5 except for leukemia, which is based on a linear-quadratic model.
†Prostate and uterus are included even though 95% CI for LAR encompassed 0.
Data from National Research Council, Committee on the Biological Effects of Ionizing Radiations (BEIR): Health risks from exposure to low levels of ionizing radiation. BEIR VII. Washington, DC, NRCUSNA Press, 2006.

Table 4-19 • BEIR VII Committee's Preferred Estimates of Lifetime Attributable Risk of Solid Cancer Incidence and Mortality* with 95% Subjective Confidence Intervals[†,‡]

Exposure Scenario	INCIDENCE		MORTALITY	
	Males	Females	Males	Females
0.1 Gy to population of mixed ages	800 (400, 1590)	1310 (690, 2490)	410 (200, 830)	610 (300, 1230)
0.1 Gy at age 10	1330 (660, 2660)	2530 (1290, 4930)	640 (300, 1390)	1050 (470, 2330)
0.1 Gy at age 30	600 (290, 1260)	1000 (500, 2020)	320 (150, 650)	490 (250, 950)
0.1 Gy at age 50	510 (240, 1100)	680 (350, 1320)	290 (140, 600)	420 (210, 810)
1 mGy/yr throughout life	550 (280, 1100)	970 (510, 1840)	290 (140, 580)	460 (230, 920)
10 mGy/yr from ages 18 to 65	2600 (1250, 5410)	4030 (2070, 7840)	1410 (700, 2860)	2170 (1130, 4200)

*These were obtained as the sum of site-specific LAR estimates. The site-specific estimates were obtained as a weighted average (on a logarithmic scale) of estimates based on relative and absolute risk transport. For sites other than lung, breast, and thyroid, relative risk transport was given a weight of 0.7 and absolute risk transport was given a weight of 0.3. These weights were reversed for lung cancer. Models for breast and thyroid cancer were based on data that included Caucasian subjects. The resulting linear estimates were reduced by a dose and dose-rate effectiveness factor (DDREF) of 1.5.
[†]This includes uncertainty from sampling variability, transport, and DDREF. The uncertainty evaluation was based on evaluation of estimates based on analyses of LSS cohort data on all solid cancers analyzed as a single category.
[‡]Number of cases or deaths per 100,000 exposed persons.
Data from National Research Council, Committee on the Biological Effects of Ionizing Radiations (BEIR): Health risks from exposure to low levels of ionizing radiation. BEIR VII. Washington, DC, NRCUSNA Press, 2006.

Table 4-20 • Lifetime Attributable Risk (LAR) of Leukemia Incidence and Mortality*

Exposure Scenario	MALES			FEMALES		
	LAR Based on RR Transport[†]	LAR Based on AR Transport[‡]	Committee's Preferred Estimate[§] (Subjective 95% CI[‖])	LAR Based on RR Transport[†]	LAR Based on AR Transport[‡]	Committee's Preferred Estimate[§] (Subjective 95% CI[‖])
Incidence						
0.1 Gy to population of mixed ages	120	64	100 (33, 300)	94	38	72 (21, 250)
0.1 Gy at age 10	140	85	120 (40, 360)	110	50	86 (25, 300)
0.1 Gy at age 30	87	77	84 (31, 230)	69	49	62 (22, 170)
0.1 Gy at age 59	110	45	84 (24, 290)	84	30	62 (16, 230)
1 mGy/yr throughout life	83	40	67 (19, 230)	68	26	51 (13, 200)
10 mGy/yr from ages 18 to 65	430	240	360 (110, 1140)	340	160	270 (79, 920)
Mortality						
0.1 Gy to population of mixed ages	88	40	69 (22, 220)	71	25	52 (14, 190)
0.1 Gy at age 10	88	42	70 (21, 240)	71	26	53 (13, 210)
0.1 Gy at age 30	70	53	64 (23, 180)	59	36	51 (17, 150)
0.1 Gy at age 59	93	37	71 (20, 250)	74	26	54 (14, 210)
1 mGy/yr throughout life	62	25	47 (13, 180)	53	17	38 (9, 160)
10 mGy/yr from ages 18 to 65	350	170	290 (84, 970)	290	120	220 (61, 820)

*Number of cases or deaths/100,000 exposed persons. All estimates are based on linear-quadratic model.
[†]Based on excessive relative risk model.
[‡]Based on excessive absolute risk model.
[§]Obtained as a weighted mean (on a logarithmic scale) with weights of 0.7 for the relative risk transport estimate and a weight of 0.3 for the absolute risk transport estimate.
[‖]Including uncertainty from sampling variability and transport. Sampling uncertainty includes uncertainty in both linear and quadratic terms of the dose response.
AR, absolute risk; RR, relative risk.
Data from National Research Council, Committee on the Biological Effects of Ionizing Radiations (BEIR): Health risks from exposure to low levels of ionizing radiation. BEIR VII. Washington, DC, NRCUSNA Press, 2006.

REFERENCES

1. International Commission on Radiological Protection (ICRP), 1990 Recommendations of the International Commission on Radiological Protection, Pub. No. 60. Ann ICRP, 1991. 21(1–3):1–201.

2. National Research Council (NRC), Committee on the Biological Effects of Ionizing Radiations (BEIR), Health risks from exposure to low levels of ionizing radiation. BEIR VII. 2006, Washington, DC: NRCUSNA Press.

3. United Nations Scientific Committee on the Effects of Atomic Radiation (UNSCEAR), Sources and effects of ionizing radiation: UNSCEAR 2000 report to the General Assembly, with scientific annexes. 2000, New York: United Nations.

4. Fearon, E.R., S.R. Hamilton, and B. Vogelstein, Clonal analysis of human colorectal tumors. Science, 1987. 238(4824):193–197.

5. Fearon, E.R. and B. Vogelstein, A genetic model for colorectal tumorigenesis. Cell, 1990. 61(5):759–767.

6. Balmain, A., J. Gray, and B. Ponder, The genetics and genomics of cancer. Nat Genet, 2003. 33(Suppl):S238–S244.

7. Kamiya, K., et al., Evidence that carcinogenesis involves an imbalance between epigenetic high-frequency initiation and suppression of promotion. Proc Natl Acad Sci U S A, 1995. 92(5):1332–1336.

8. Streffer, C. and W.U. Muller, Radiation risk from combined exposures to ionizing radiations and chemicals. Adv Radiat Biol, 1984. 11:173–210.

9. Trosko, J.E., C.C. Chang, and B.V. Madhukar, Modulation of intercellular communication during radiation and chemical carcinogenesis. Radiat Res, 1990. 123(3):241–251.

10. Wyke, J., Viruses in cancer. In Introduction to the Cellular and Molecular Biology of Cancer, L. Franks and N. Teich, eds. 1990, Oxford: Oxford University Press.

11. Sharp, G.B., et al., Hepatocellular carcinoma among atomic bomb survivors: Significant interaction of radiation with hepatitis C virus infections. Int J Cancer, 2003. 103(4):531–537.

12. Cologne, J.B., et al., Uncertainty in estimating probability of causation in a cross-sectional study: Joint effects of radiation and hepatitis-C virus on chronic liver disease. J Radiol Prot, 2004. 24(2):131–145.

13. United Nations Scientific Committee on the Effects of Atomic Radiation (UNSCEAR), Sources and effects of ionizing radiation: UNSCEAR 1993 report to the General Assembly, with scientific annexes. 1993, New York: United Nations.

14. United Nations Scientific Committee on the Effects of Atomic Radiation (UNSCEAR) 2000: The United Nations Scientific Committee on the Effects of Atomic Radiation. Health Phys, 2000. 79(3):314.

15. Cox, R., Resolving the molecular mechanisms of radiation tumorigenesis: Past problems and future prospects. Health Phys, 2001. 80(4):344–348.

16. Cox, R., Molecular mechanisms of radiation oncogenesis. Int J Radiat Biol, 1994. 65(1):57–64.

17. Little, J.B., Radiation carcinogenesis. Carcinogenesis, 2000. 21(3):397–404.

18. Vogelstein, B. and K.W. Kinzler, Cancer genes and the pathways they control. Nat Med, 2004. 10(8):789–799.

19. Haber, D. and E. Harlow, Tumour-suppressor genes: Evolving definitions in the genomic age. Nat Genet, 1997. 16(4):320–322.

20. Weinberg, R.A., Tumor suppressor genes. Science, 1991. 254(5035):1138–1146.

21. Mangano, J.J., et al., Elevated childhood cancer incidence proximate to U.S. nuclear power plants. Arch Environ Health, 2003. 58(2):74–82.

22. Rabbitts, T.H., Chromosomal translocations in human cancer. Nature, 1994. 372(6502):143–149.

23. Greaves, M.F. and J. Wiemels, Origins of chromosome translocations in childhood leukaemia. Nat Rev Cancer, 2003. 3(9):639–649.

24. Nishisho, I., et al., Mutations of chromosome 5q21 genes in FAP and colorectal cancer patients. Science, 1991. 253(5020):665–669.

25. Kony, S.J., et al., Radiation and genetic factors in the risk of second malignant neoplasms after a first cancer in childhood. Lancet, 1997. 350(9071):91–95.

26. Leprat, F., et al., Impaired DNA repair as assessed by the "comet" assay in patients with thyroid tumors after a history of radiation therapy: A preliminary study. Int J Radiat Oncol Biol Phys, 1998. 40(5):1019–1026.

27. Doerffer, K. and P. Unrau, Cancer genes and risk assessment. Health Phys, 1998. 74(2):173–180.

28. Moolgavkar, S.H., Hormones and multistage carcinogenesis. Cancer Surv, 1986. 5(3):635–648.

29. Land, C.E., Breast cancer in the RERF Life Span Study. RERF Update. 1993, Hiroshima, Japan: R.E.R. Foundation.

30. Land, C.E., et al., Early-onset breast cancer in A-bomb survivors. Lancet, 1993. 342(8865):237.

31. Chakraborty, R. and K. Sankaranarayanan, Cancer predisposition, radiosensitivity and the risk of radiation-induced cancers. II. A Mendelian single-locus model of cancer predisposition and radiosensitivity for predicting cancer risks in populations. Radiat Res, 1995. 143(3):293–301.

32. Meuth, M., The structure of mutation in mammalian cells. Biochim Biophys Acta, 1990. 1032(1):1–17.

33. Sankaranarayanan, K., Ionizing radiation and genetic risks. III. Nature of spontaneous and radiation-induced mutations in mammalian in vitro systems and mechanisms of induction of mutations by radiation. Mutat Res, 1991. 258(1):75–97.

34. Hollstein, M., et al., p53 gene mutation analysis in tumors of patients exposed to alpha-particles. Carcinogenesis, 1997. 18(3):511–516.

35. Wright, P.A., et al., Radiation-associated and "spontaneous" human thyroid carcinomas show a different pattern of ras oncogene mutation. Oncogene, 1991. 6(3):471–473.

36. van den Berg, E., et al., Cytogenetic study of a nodular hyperplasia of the thyroid after irradiation for Hodgkin's disease. Cancer Genet Cytogenet, 1991. 53(1):15–21.

37. Shi, Y.F., et al., High rates of ras codon 61 mutation in thyroid tumors in an iodide-deficient area. Cancer Res, 1991. 51(10):2690–2693.

38. Collart, F.R., et al., Alteration of the c-fms gene in a blood sample from a Thorotrast individual. Health Phys, 1992. 63(1):27–32.

39. Tanaka, K., M. Takechi, and N. Kamada, Mutation of ras oncogene in atomic bomb radiation-exposed leukemia. J Radiat Res (Tokyo), 1991. 32(4):378–388.

40. Kamada, N., et al., Cytogenetic and molecular changes in leukemia among atomic bomb survivors. J Radiat Res (Tokyo), 1991. 32 (Suppl 2):S257–S265.

41. Kamada, N., Cytogenetic and molecular changes in leukemia found among atomic bomb survivors. J Radiat Res (Tokyo), 1991. 32 (Suppl):S172–S179.

42. Tomatis, L., et al., Evaluation of the carcinogenicity of chemicals: A review of the Monograph Program of the International Agency for Research on Cancer (1971 to 1977). Cancer Res, 1978. 38(4):877–885.

43. Nakamura, N., A hypothesis: Radiation-related leukemia is mainly attributable to the small number of people who carry pre-existing clonally expanded preleukemic cells. Radiat Res, 2005. 163(3):258–265.

44. Olsen, J.H., et al., Cancer in the parents of children with cancer. N Engl J Med, 1995. 333(24):1594–1599.

45. Hrubec, Z. and J.V. Neel, Contribution of familial factors to the occurrence of cancer before old age in twin veterans. Am J Hum Genet, 1982. 34(4):658–671.

46. Sondergaard, J.O., S. Bulow, and E. Lynge, Cancer incidence among parents of patients with colorectal cancer. Int J Cancer, 1991. 47(2):202–206.

47. Pastore, G., et al., Cancer mortality among relatives of children with soft-tissue sarcoma: A national survey in Italy. Cancer Lett, 1987. 37(1):17–24.

48. Burke, E., et al., Cancer in relatives of survivors of childhood sarcoma. Cancer, 1991. 67(5):1467–1469.

49. Moutou, C., et al., The French Wilms' tumour study: No clear evidence for cancer prone families. J Med Genet, 1994. 31(6):429–434.

50. International Commission on Radiological Protection (ICRP), Genetic susceptibility to cancer. ICRP Pub. No. 79. Ann ICRP, 1998. 28(1–2):1–157.

51. Bakhshi, S., et al., Medulloblastoma with adverse reaction to radiation therapy in Nijmegen breakage syndrome. J Pediatr Hematol Oncol, 2003. 25(3):248–251.

52. Robbins, J.H., et al., Xeroderma pigmentosum: An inherited disease with sun sensitivity, multiple cutaneous neoplasms, and abnormal DNA repair. Ann Intern Med, 1974. 80(2):221–248.

53. Swift, M., Malignant neoplasms in heterozygous carriers of genes for certain autosomal recessive syndromes. In Progress in Cancer Research and Therapy, J.J. Mulvihill, et al., eds., vol. 3. 1977, New York: Raven Press.

54. Takebe, H., Genetic aspects of repair deficiency: Concluding remarks in radiation research. In Proceedings of the Sixth International Congress on Radiology Research. 1979, Tokyo, Japan: Japanese Association for Radiology Research.

55. Cleaver, J.E. and D. Bootsma, Xeroderma pigmentosum: Biochemical and genetic characteristics. Annu Rev Genet, 1975. 9:19–38.

56. Takebe, H., et al., High sensitivity of xeroderma pigmentosum cells to the carcinogen 4nitroguinoline-1-oxide. Mutat Res, 1972. 15(1):98–100.

57. Arlett, C., Lethal response to DNA damaging agents in a variety of human fibroblast cell stains. Mutat Res, 1977. 46:106.

58. Fujiwara, Y. and M. Tatsumi, Cross-link repair in human cells and its possible defect in Fanconi's anemia cells. J Mol Biol, 1977. 113(4):635–649.

59. Maher, V. and J. McCormick, Effect of DNA repair on the cytotoxicity and mutagenicity of UV-irradiation and of chemical carcinogens in normal and xeroderma pigmentosum cells. In Biology of Radiation Carcinogenesis, J.M. Yuhas and R. Tannant, eds. 1976, New York: Raven Press.

60. Setlow, R.B., Repair deficient human disorders and cancer. Nature, 1978. 271(5647):713–717.

61. McCaw, B.K., et al., Somatic rearrangement of chromosome 14 in human lymphocytes. Proc Natl Acad Sci U S A, 1975. 72(6):2071–2075.

62. Aurias, A., et al., High frequencies of inversions and translocations of chromosomes 7 and 14 in ataxia telangiectasia. Mutat Res, 1980. 69(2):369–374.

63. Gotoff, S.P., E. Amirmokri, and E.J Liebner, Ataxia telangiectasia: Neoplasia, untoward response to x-irradiation, and tuberous sclerosis. Am J Dis Child, 1967. 114(6):617–625.

64. Morgan, J.L., T.M. Holcomb, and R.W. Morrissey, Radiation reaction in ataxia telangiectasia. Am J Dis Child, 1968. 116(5):557–558.

65. Cunlift, P.N., et al., Radiosensitivity in ataxia-telangiectasia. Br J Radiol, 1975. 48(569):374–376.

66. Pritchard, J., et al., The effects of radiation therapy for Hodgkin's disease in a child with ataxia telangiectasia: A clinical, biological and pathologic study. Cancer, 1982. 50(5):877–886.

67. Mauget-Faysse, M., et al., Idiopathic and radiation-induced ocular telangiectasia: The involvement of the *ATM* gene. Invest Ophthalmol Vis Sci, 2003. 44(8):3257–3262.

68. Paterson, M.C., P.H. Lohman, and M.L. Sluyter, Use of UV endonuclease from *Micrococcus luteus* to monitor the progress of DNA repair in UV-irradiated human cells. Mutat Res, 1973. 19(2):245–256.

69. Alapetite, C., et al., Analysis by alkaline comet assay of cancer patients with severe reactions to radiotherapy: Defective rejoining of radioinduced DNA strand breaks in lymphocytes of breast cancer patients. Int J Cancer, 1999. 83(1):83–90.

70. Oppitz, U., et al., Radiation-induced comet-formation in human skin fibroblasts from radiotherapy patients with different normal tissue reactions. Strahlenther Onkol, 1999. 175(7):341–346.

71. Arlett, C. and A.R. Lehmann, Human disorders showing increased sensitivity to the induction of genetic damage. Ann Rev Genet, 1973. 12:95–115.

72. Swift, M., et al., Incidence of cancer in 161 families affected by ataxia-telangiectasia. N Engl J Med, 1991. 325(26):1831–1836.

73. Boice, J.D., Jr. and R.W. Miller, Risk of breast cancer in ataxia-telangiectasia. N Engl J Med, 1992. 326(20):1357–1358; author reply, 1360–1361.

74. Offit, K., et al., Rare variants of ATM and risk for Hodgkin's disease and radiation-associated breast cancers. Clin Cancer Res, 2002. 8(12):3813–3819.

75. German, J., L. Crippa, and D. Bloom, Bloom syndrome: Analysis of the chromosomal aberration characteristic of this disorder. Chromosoma, 1974. 48:361–366.

76. Schroeder, T.M., Sister chromatid exchanges and chromatid interchanges in Bloom's syndrome. Humangenetik, 1975. 30(4):317–323.

77. Wade, M., E. Chu, and R. Schimickel, Ultraviolet light sensitivity and deficiency in DNA polymerase activity in cultured skin fibroblasts from patients with Cockayne's syndrome. Mutat Res, 1977. 46:162.

78. United Nations Scientific Committee on the Effects of Atomic Radiation (UNSCEAR), Ionizing radiation: Sources and effects. UNSCEAR report to the General Assembly, in annex K: Radiation-induced life shortening. 1982, New York: United Nations.

79. Wong, F.L., et al., Cancer incidence after retinoblastoma: Radiation dose and sarcoma risk. JAMA, 1997. 278(15):1262–1267.

80. Hasegawa, T., et al., Second primary rhabdomyosarcomas in patients with bilateral retinoblastoma: A clinicopathologic and immunohistochemical study. Am J Surg Pathol, 1998. 22(11):1351–1360.

81. Mohney, B.G., et al., Second nonocular tumors in survivors of heritable retinoblastoma and prior radiation therapy. Am J Ophthalmol, 1998. 126(2):269–277.

82. Eng, C., et al., Mortality from second tumors among long-term survivors of retinoblastoma. J Natl Cancer Inst, 1993. 85(14):1121–1128.

83. Abramson, D.H. and C.M. Frank, Second nonocular tumors in survivors of bilateral retinoblastoma: A possible age effect on radiation-related risk. Ophthalmology, 1998. 105(4):573–579; discussion, 579–580.

84. Abramson, D.H., et al., Third (fourth and fifth) nonocular tumors in survivors of retinoblastoma. Ophthalmology, 2001. 108(10):1868–1876.

85. Baum, J.W., Population heterogeneity hypothesis on radiation-induced cancer. Health Phys, 1973. 25(2):97–104.

86. McGregor, H., et al., Breast cancer incidence among atomic bomb survivors, Hiroshima and Nagasaki, 1950–69. J Natl Cancer Inst, 1977. 59(3):799–811.

87. Tokunaga, M., et al., Malignant breast tumors among atomic bomb survivors, Hiroshima and Nagasaki, 1950–74. J Natl Cancer Inst, 1979. 62(6):1347–1359.

88. Land C. and J. Norman, Latent Period for Radiogenic Cancers Occurring among Japanese A-bomb Survivors in Late Biological Effects of Ionizing Radiation, vol. 2. 1978, Vienna: International Atomic Energy Agency (IAEA).

89. Carter, R., R. Sposto, and D. Preston, Estimating the Temporal Distribution of Exposure-related Cancers: Commentary and Review Series. 1992, Hiroshima, Japan: Radiation Effects Research Foundation.

90. Shimizu, Y., et al., Mortality of Life Span Study Sample. 1988, Hiroshima, Japan: Radiation Effects Research Foundation.

91. Shimizu, Y., H. Kato, and W.J. Schull, Cancer mortality in the years 1950–1985 based on the recently revised doses (DS86). 1988, Hiroshima, Japan: Radiation Effects Research Foundation.

92. United Nations Scientific Committee on the Effects of Atomic Radiation (UNSCEAR), Sources and effects of ionizing radiation: UNSCEAR 1994 report to the General Assembly, with scientific annexes. 1994, New York: United Nations.

93. Boice, J.D., Jr., et al., Radiation dose and leukemia risk in patients treated for cancer of the cervix. J Natl Cancer Inst, 1987. 79(6):1295–1311.

94. Shore, R.E., et al., Breast cancer among women given x-ray therapy for acute postpartum mastitis. J Natl Cancer Inst, 1986. 77(3):689–696.

95. Sinclair, W.K., The linear no-threshold response: Why not linearity? Med Phys, 1998. 25(3):285-290; discussion, 300.

96. United Nations Scientific Committee on the Effects of Atomic Radiation (UNSCEAR), Sources and effects of ionizing radiation: UNSCEAR 2006 report to the General Assembly with annexes. 2006, New York: United Nations.

97. National Council on Radiation Protection and Measurements (NCRP), Evaluation of the linear-nonthreshold dose-response model for ionizing radiation: Recommendations of the NCRP report no. 136. 2001, Bethesda, Md: The Council.

98. Preston, R.J., The LNT model is the best we can do—today. J Radiol Prot, 2003. 23(3):263–268.

99. Mossman, K.L., Beyond linearity. Health Phys, 1997. 73(1):270.

100. Mossman, K.L., The linear no-threshold debate: Where do we go from here? Med Phys, 1998. 25(3):279-284; discussion, 300.

101. Tubiana, M., Dose-effect relationship and estimation of the carcinogenic effects of low doses of ionizing radiation: The joint report of the Academie des Sciences (Paris) and of the Academie Nationale de Medecine. Int J Radiat Oncol Biol Phys, 2005. 63(2):317–319.

102. Brenner, D.J., et al., Cancer risks attributable to low doses of ionizing radiation: Assessing what we really know. Proc Natl Acad Sci U S A, 2003. 100(24):13761–13766.

103. Beebe, G.W., Studies of cancer among the Japanese A-bomb survivors. Cancer Invest, 1988. 6(4):417–426.

104. Kellerer, A.M., Risk estimates for radiation-induced cancer—The epidemiological evidence. Radiat Environ Biophys, 2000. 39(1):17–24.

105. Upton, A.C., Radiobiological effects of low doses. Implications for radiological protection. Radiat Res, 1977. 71(1):51–74.

106. Little, M.P., A comparison of the degree of curvature in the cancer incidence dose-response in Japanese atomic bomb survivors with that in chromosome aberrations measured in vitro. Int J Radiat Biol, 2000. 76(10):1365–1375.

107. Little, M.P. and C.R. Muirhead, Derivation of low-dose extrapolation factors from analysis of curvature in the cancer incidence dose response in Japanese atomic bomb survivors. Int J Radiat Biol, 2000. 76(7):939–953.

108. National Research Council (NRC), The effects on populations of exposure to low levels of ionizing radiation. BEIR III. 1980, Washington, DC: National Academy of Sciences, p xiii.

109. Little, M.P. and C.R. Muirhead, Curvilinearity in the dose-response curve for cancer in Japanese atomic bomb survivors. Environ Health Perspect, 1997. 105(Suppl 6):S1505–S1509.

110. Hoel, D.G. and P. Li, Threshold models in radiation carcinogenesis. Health Phys, 1998. 75(3):241–250.

111. Kai, M., E.G. Luebeck, and S.H Moolgavkar, Analysis of the incidence of solid cancer among atomic bomb survivors using a two-stage model of carcinogenesis. Radiat Res, 1997. 148(4):348–358.

112. Pierce, D.A. and M.L. Mendelsohn, A model for radiation-related cancer suggested by atomic bomb survivor data. Radiat Res, 1999. 152(6):642–654.

113. Pierce, D.A., Mechanistic models for radiation carcinogenesis and the atomic bomb survivor data. Radiat Res, 2003. 160(6):718–723.

114. Land, C.E. and W.K. Sinclair, The relative contributions of different organ sites to the total cancer mortality associated with low-dose radiation exposure. Ann ICRP, 1991. 22(1):31–57.

115. United Nations Scientific Committee on the Effects of Atomic Radiation (UNSCEAR), Sources and effects of ionizing radiation: UNSCEAR report to the General Assembly with annexes. 1988, New York: United Nations.

116. National Research Council (NRC), Committee on the Biological Effects of Ionizing Radiations (BEIR), Health effects of exposure to low-levels of ionizing radiation. BEIR V. 1990, Washington, DC: NA Press.

117. Webster, E.W., Garland lecture: On the question of cancer induction by small x-ray doses. AJR Am J Roentgenol, 1981. 137(4):647–666.

118. Land, C.E., Estimating cancer risks from low doses of ionizing radiation. Science, 1980. 209(4462):1197–1203.

119. Land, C.E., Low-dose radiation—A cause of breast cancer. Cancer, 1980. 46 (Suppl 4):868–873.

120. Land, C.E., et al., Breast cancer risk from low-dose exposures to ionizing radiation: Results of parallel analysis of three exposed populations of women. J Natl Cancer Inst, 1980. 65(2):353–376.

121. Beebe, G.W. and M. Usagawa, The major atomic bomb casualty commission samples. 1968, Hiroshima, Japan: Atomic Bomb Casualty Commission.

122. Preston, D.L., et al., Effect of recent changes in atomic bomb survivor dosimetry on cancer mortality risk estimates. Radiat Res, 2004. 162(4):377–389.

123. Hennekens, C. and J. Buring, Epidemiology in Medicine. 1987, Boston: Little, Brown.

124. Wing, S., et al., Mortality among workers at Oak Ridge National Laboratory: Evidence of radiation effects in follow-up through 1984. JAMA, 1991. 265(11):1397–1402.

125. Preston, D.L., et al., Dose response and temporal patterns of radiation-associated solid cancer risks. Health Phys, 2003. 85(1):43–46.

126. Preston, D.L., et al., Studies of mortality of atomic bomb survivors. Report 13: Solid cancer and noncancer disease mortality: 1950–1997. Radiat Res, 2003. 160(4):381–407.

127. Shimizu, Y., H. Kato, and W.J Schull, Studies of the mortality of A-bomb survivors. 9. Mortality, 1950–1985: Part 2. Cancer mortality based on the recently revised doses (DS86). Radiat Res, 1990. 121(2):120–141.

128. Shimizu, Y., W.J. Schull, and H. Kato, Cancer risk among atomic bomb survivors: The RERF Life Span Study. Radiation Effects Research Foundation. JAMA, 1990. 264(5):601–604.

129. Preston, D.L., et al., Studies of the mortality of A-bomb survivors. 8. Cancer mortality, 1950–1982. Radiat Res, 1987. 111(1):151–178.

130. Darby, S.C., et al., Long term mortality after a single treatment course with x-rays in patients treated for ankylosing spondylitis. Br J Cancer, 1987. 55(2):179–190.

131. Pierce, D.A. and D. Preston, Joint analysis of site-specific cancer risks for the atomic bomb survivors. 1991, Hiroshima, Japan: Radiation Effects Research Foundation.

132. Little, M.P., et al., Time variations in the risk of cancer following irradiation in childhood. Radiat Res, 1991. 126(3):304–316.

133. Shore, R.E., et al., Skin cancer incidence among children irradiated for ringworm of the scalp. Radiat Res, 1984. 100(1):192–204.

134. Gilbert, E.S., Some effects of random dose measurement errors on analyses of atomic bomb survivor data. Radiat Res, 1984. 98(3):591–605.

135. Pierce, D.A. and M. Vaeth, Cancer risk estimation from the A-bomb survivors: Extrapolation to low doses, use of relative risk models and other uncertainties. 1989, Hiroshima, Japan: Radiation Effects Research Foundation.

136. Pierce, D.A., D.O. Stram, and M. Vaeth, Allowing for random errors in radiation dose estimates for the atomic bomb survivor data. Radiat Res, 1990. 123(3):275–284.

137. Sinclair, W.K. and Herbert. M., Parker Lecture: The risk of radiation-induced cancer: Whence? Whither? J Toxicol Environ Health, 1993. 40(2–3):493–510.

138. Wakeford, R., The cancer epidemiology of radiation. Oncogene, 2004. 23(38):6404–6428.

139. Land, C.E., Uncertainty, low-dose extrapolation and the threshold hypothesis. J Radiol Prot, 2002. 22(3A):A129–A135.

140. Pierce, D.A., D.O. Stram, and M. Vaeth, Allowing for random errors in radiation exposure estimates for the atomic bomb survivor data. 1989, Hiroshima, Japan: Radiation Effects Research Foundation.

141. Preston, D.L. and D.A. Pierce, The effect of changes in dosimetry on cancer mortality risk estimates in the atomic bomb survivors. Radiat Res, 1988. 114(3):437–466.

142. Straume, T., et al., Neutron discrepancies in the DS86 Hiroshima dosimetry system. Health Phys, 1992. 63(4):421–426.

143. Pierce, D.A. and M. Vaeth, The shape of the cancer mortality dose-response curve for the A-bomb survivors. Radiat Res, 1991. 126(1):36–42.

144. Schull, W.J., Y. Shimizu, and H. Kato, Hiroshima and Nagasaki: New doses, risks, and their implications. Health Phys, 1990. 59(1):69–75.

145. Stewart, A., A-bomb data: Detection of bias in the Life Span Study cohort. Environ Health Perspect, 1997. 105(Suppl 6):S1519–S1521.

146. Stewart, A. Induction of cancer in man by external radiation: The role of competing causes of death. In Advances in Medical Oncology, Research and Education, 12th International Cancer Congress. 1978, Oxford: Pergamon Press.

147. Land, C., In A-bomb Survivor Studies, Immunity and the Epidemiology of Radiation Carcinogenesis, J. Dubois, B. Serrou, and C. Rosenfeld, eds. 1981, New York: Raven Press.

148. Jablon, S. and H. Kato, Childhood cancer in relation to prenatal exposure to atomic bomb radiation. Lancet, 1970. 2:1000–1003.

149. Kato, H., Mortality in children exposed to the A-bombs while in-utero. Am J Epidemiol, 1981. 93:435–442.

150. Little, M.P. and M.W. Charles, Bomb survivor selection and consequences for estimates of population cancer risks. Health Phys, 1990. 59(6):765–775.

151. Walter, S.D., J.W. Meigs, and J.F. Heston, The relationship of cancer incidence to terrestrial radiation and population density in Connecticut, 1935–1974. Am J Epidemiol, 1986. 123(1):1–14.

152. Iwasaki, T., et al., Cancer mortality rates in different geographical distribution by levels of natural radiation dose in Japan. In Proceedings of the International Conference on High Levels of Natural Radiation, Ramsar, Iran, 1990. 1991, Vienna: International Atomic Energy Agency.

153. Tirmarche, M., et al., Epidemiologic study of regional cancer mortality in France and natural radiation. Radiat Prot Dosim, 1988. 24:479–482.

154. Jacobson, A., P. Plato, and N. Frigerio, The role of natural radiations in human leukemogenesis. Am. J. Public Health, 1976. 66:31–37.

155. Hickey, R.J., et al., Low level ionizing radiation and human mortality: Multi-regional epidemiological studies: A preliminary report. Health Phys, 1981. 40(5):625–641.

156. Mason, T.J. and R.W. Miller, Cosmic radiation at high altitudes and U.S. cancer mortality, 1950–1969. Radiat Res, 1974. 60(2):302–306.

157. Weinberg, C.R., K.G. Brown, and D.G. Hoel, Altitude, radiation, and mortality from cancer and heart disease. Radiat Res, 1987. 112(2):381–390.

158. Edling, C., et al., Effects of low-dose radiation—A correlation study. Scand J Work Environ Health, 1982. 8(Suppl 1):59–64.

159. High Background Radiation Research Group (HBRRG), Health survey in high background radiation areas in China: HBRRG, China. Science, 1980. 209(4459): 877–880.

160. Wei, L.X., et al., Epidemiological investigation of radiological effects in high background radiation areas of Yangjiang, China. J Radiat Res (Tokyo), 1990. 31(1):119–136.

161. Shimizu, M., et al., Correlation between natural radiation exposure and cancer mortality. J Nihon Univ Sch Dent, 1987. 29:314–320.

162. Court Brown, W.M., et al., Geographical variation in leukaemia mortality in relation to background radiation and other factors. Br Med J, 1960. 5188:1753–1759.

163. Knox, E.G., et al., Background radiation and childhood cancers. J Radiol Prot, 1988. 7:9–18.

164. Darby, S., The contribution of natural ionizing radiation to cancer mortality in the United States. In The Origins of Human Cancer, H. Hyatt, J. Watson, and J. Winsten, eds. 1991, New York: Cold Spring Harbor Laboratory Press.

165. Frigerio, N. and R. Stowe, Carcinogenic and genetic hazard from background radiation. In Proceedings on Biological Effects of Low-level Irradiation Pertinent to Protection of Man and His Environment, vol. 2. 1976, Vienna: International Atomic Energy Agency.

166. Zhai, S., et al., Report of a survey on mortality from malignant tumors. Zhonghua Fangsheyizue Yu Fanghu Zazhi (China), 1982. 2(2):48–51.

167. Sternglass, E.J. and J.M. Gould, Breast cancer: Evidence for a relation to fission products in the diet. Int J Health Serv, 1993. 23(4):783–804.

168. Musolino, S.V., Comments on Breast cancer: Evidence for a relation to fission products in the diet. Int J Health Serv, 1995. 25(3):475–480; discussion, 481–488.

169. Darby, S., et al., Radon in homes and risk of lung cancer: Collaborative analysis of individual data from 13 European case-control studies. BMJ, 2005. 330(7485):223.

170. Krewski, D., et al., Residential radon and risk of lung cancer: A combined analysis of 7 North American case-control studies. Epidemiology, 2005. 16(2):137–145.

171. Lubin, J., J.D. Boice, and C. Edling, Radon and lung cancer risk: A joint analysis of 11 underground miner studies. 1994, Washington, DC: U.S. Department of Health and Human Services.

172. Dionian, J. and S.L. Muirhead, The risks of leukemia and other cancers in Thurso from radiation exposure. 1986, Oxford: National Radiation Protection Board.

173. Darby, S.C., et al., Trends in childhood leukaemia in the Nordic countries in relation to fallout from atmospheric nuclear weapons testing. BMJ, 1992. 304(6833):1005–1009.

174. Wiklund, K., L.E. Holm, and G. Eklund, Cancer risks in Swedish Lapps who breed reindeer. Am J Epidemiol, 1990. 132(6):1078–1082.

175. Lyon, J.L., et al., Childhood leukemias associated with fallout from nuclear testing. N Engl J Med, 1979. 300(8):397–402.

176. Land, C.E., F.W. McKay, and S.G. Machado, Childhood leukemia and fallout from the Nevada nuclear tests. Science, 1984. 223(4632):139–144.

177. Machado, S.G., C.E. Land, and F.W. McKay, Cancer mortality and radioactive fallout in southwestern Utah. Am J Epidemiol, 1987. 125(1):44–61.

178. Stevens, W., et al., Leukemia in Utah and radioactive fallout from the Nevada test site: A case-control study. JAMA, 1990. 264(5):585–591.

179. Stevens, W., et al., A case-control study of leukemia deaths in Utah (1952–1981) and exposure to radioactive fallout from the Nevada test site: Final report. 1990, Bethesda, Md: National Cancer Institute, National Institutes of Health.

180. Kerber, R.A., et al., A cohort study of thyroid disease in relation to fallout from nuclear weapons testing. JAMA, 1993. 270(17):2076–2082.

181. Gilbert, E.S., et al., Thyroid cancer rates and ^{131}I doses from Nevada atmospheric nuclear bomb tests. J Natl Cancer Inst, 1998. 90(21):1654–1660.

182. Caldwell, G.G., D.B. Kelley, and C.W. Heath, Jr., Leukemia among participants in military maneuvers at a nuclear bomb test: A preliminary report. JAMA, 1980. 244(14):1575–1578.

183. Caldwell, G.G., et al., Mortality and cancer frequency among military nuclear test (Smoky) participants, 1957 through 1979. JAMA, 1983. 250(5):620–624.

184. Johnson, C.J., Cancer incidence in an area of radioactive fallout downwind from the Nevada Test Site. JAMA, 1984. 251(2):230–236.

185. Dalager, N.A., H.K. Kang, and C.M. Mahan, Cancer mortality among the highest exposed U.S. atmospheric nuclear test participants. J Occup Environ Med, 2000. 42(8):798–805.

186. Darby, S.C., et al., Further follow up of mortality and incidence of cancer in men from the United Kingdom who participated in the United Kingdom's atmospheric nuclear weapon tests and experimental programmes. BMJ, 1993. 307(6918):1530–1535.

187. Muirhead, C.R., et al., Follow up of mortality and incidence of cancer 1952–98 in men from the UK who participated in the U.K.'s atmospheric nuclear weapon tests and experimental programmes. Occup Environ Med, 2003. 60(3):165–172.

188. Hamilton, T.E., G. van Belle, and J.P. LoGerfo, Thyroid neoplasia in Marshall Islanders exposed to nuclear fallout. JAMA, 1987. 258(5):629–635.

189. Takahashi, T., et al., The relationship of thyroid cancer with radiation exposure from nuclear weapon testing in the Marshall Islands. J Epidemiol, 2003. 13(2):99–107.

190. International Atomic Energy Agency (IAEA), The International Chernobyl Project: Report of an International Committee. 1991, Vienna: IAEA.

191. Chernobyl Forum and International Atomic Energy Agency (IAEA), Chernobyl's legacy: Health, environmental and socioeconomic impacts and recommendations to the governments of Belarus, the Russian Federation and Ukraine. 2005, Vienna: Chernobyl Forum.

192. Mettler, F.A., Jr., et al., Thyroid nodules in the population living around Chernobyl. JAMA, 1992. 268(5):616–619.

193. Prisyazhiuk, A., et al., Cancer in the Ukraine, post-Chernobyl. Lancet, 1991. 338(8778):1334–1335.

194. Kazakov, V.S., E.P. Demidchik, and L.N. Astakhova, Thyroid cancer after Chernobyl. Nature, 1992. 359(6390):21.

195. Ron, E., J. Lubin, and A.B. Schneider, Thyroid cancer incidence. Nature, 1992. 360(6400):113.

196. Davis, S., et al., Risk of thyroid cancer in the Bryansk Oblast of the Russian Federation after the Chernobyl Power Station accident. Radiat Res, 2004. 162(3):241–248.

197. Noschenko, A., et al., Radiation-induced leukemia risk among those aged 0–29 at the time of the Chernobyl accident: A case control study in the Ukraine. Int J Cancer, 2002. 99:609–618.

198. Koshurnikova, N.A., et al., Studies on the Mayak nuclear workers: Health effects. Radiat Environ Biophys, 2002. 41(1):29–31.

199. Kossenko, M.M., et al., Mortality in the offspring of individuals living along the radioactively contaminated Techa River: A descriptive analysis. Radiat Environ Biophys, 2000. 39(4):219–225.

200. Black, D., Investigation of the possible increase incidence of cancer in Western Cumbria. 1984, London: Her Majesty's Stationary Office.

201. Gardner, M.J., et al., Follow up study of children born to mothers resident in Seascale, West Cumbria (birth cohort). Br Med J (Clin Res Ed), 1987. 295(6602):822–827.

202. Gardner, M.J., et al., Follow up study of children born elsewhere but attending schools in Seascale, West Cumbria (schools cohort). Br Med J (Clin Res Ed), 1987. 295(6602):819–822.

203. Gardner, M.J., et al., Results of case-control study of leukaemia and lymphoma among young people near Sellafield nuclear plant in West Cumbria. BMJ, 1990. 300(6722):423–429.

204. Dickinson, H.O. and L. Parker, Leukaemia and non-Hodgkin's lymphoma in children of male Sellafield radiation workers. Int J Cancer, 2002. 99(3):437–444.

205. Doll, R., H.J. Evans, and S.C. Darby, Paternal exposure not to blame. Nature, 1994. 367(6465):678–680.

206. Doll, R. and R. Wakeford, Risk of childhood cancer from fetal irradiation. Br J Radiol, 1997. 70:130–139.

207. Heasman, M.A., et al., Childhood leukaemia in northern Scotland. Lancet, 1986. 1(8475):266.

208. Kinlen, L.J., Can paternal preconceptional radiation account for the increase of leukaemia and non-Hodgkin's lymphoma in Seascale? BMJ, 1993. 306(6894):1718–1721.

209. Kinlen, L.J., K. Clarke, and A. Balkwill, Paternal preconceptional radiation exposure in the nuclear industry and leukaemia and non-Hodgkin's lymphoma in young people in Scotland. BMJ, 1993. 306(6886):1153–1158.

210. Kinlen, L.J., et al., Rural population mixing and childhood leukaemia: Effects of the North Sea oil industry in Scotland, including the area near Dounreay nuclear site. BMJ, 1993. 306(6880):743–748.

211. Urquhart, J.D., et al., Case-control study of leukaemia and non-Hodgkin's lymphoma in children in Caithness near the Dounreay nuclear installation. BMJ, 1991. 302(6778):687–692.

212. Roman, E., et al., Childhood leukaemia in the West Berkshire and Basingstoke and North Hampshire District Health Authorities in relation to nuclear establishments in the vicinity. Br Med J (Clin Res Ed), 1987. 294(6572):597–602.

213. Roman, E., et al., Case-control study of leukaemia and non-Hodgkin's lymphoma among children aged 0–4 years living in West Berkshire and North Hampshire health districts. BMJ, 1993. 306(6878):615–621.

214. Cook-Mozaffari, P.J., et al., Geographical variation in mortality from leukaemia and other cancers in England and Wales in relation to proximity to nuclear installations, 1969–78. Br J Cancer, 1989. 59(3):476–485.

215. Cook-Mozaffari, P., S. Darby, and R. Doll, Cancer near potential sites of nuclear installations. Lancet, 1989. 2(8672):1145–1147.

216. Clarke, E.A., J. McLaughlin, and T.W. Anderson, Childhood leukemia around Canadian nuclear facilities, Phase II. 1991, Ottawa, ON: Atomic Energy Control Board of Canada.

217. Hill, C. and A. Laplanche, Overall mortality and cancer mortality around French nuclear sites. Nature, 1990. 347(6295):755–757.

218. Hatch, M.C., et al., Cancer rates after the Three Mile Island nuclear accident and proximity of residence to the plant. Am J Public Health, 1991. 81(6):719–724.

219. Hatch, M. and M. Susser, Background gamma radiation and childhood cancers within ten miles of a US nuclear plant. Int J Epidemiol, 1990. 19(3):546–552.

220. Jablon, S., Z. Hrubec, and J. Boice, Jr., Cancer in populations living near nuclear facilities. Bethesda, Md: National Institutes of Health, National Cancer Institute.

221. Jablon, S., Z. Hrubec, and J.D, Boice, Jr., Cancer in populations living near nuclear facilities: A survey of mortality nationwide and incidence in two states. JAMA, 1991. 265(11):1403–1408.

222. Michaelis, J., Recent epidemiological studies on ionizing radiation and childhood cancer in Germany. Int J Radiat Biol, 1998. 73(4):377–381.

223. Michaelis, J., et al., Incidence of childhood malignancies in the vicinity of West German nuclear power plants. Cancer Causes Control, 1992. 3(3):255–263.

224. Draper, G.J., et al., Cancer in the offspring of radiation workers: A record linkage study. BMJ, 1997. 315(7117):1181–1188.

225. Yoshimoto, Y., Cancer risk among children of atomic bomb survivors: A review of RERF epidemiologic studies. Radiation Effects Research Foundation. JAMA, 1990. 264(5):596–600.

226. Yoshimoto, Y., et al., Frequency of malignant tumors during the first two decades of life in the offspring (F₁) of atomic bomb survivors. 1990, Hiroshima, Japan: Radiation Effects Research Foundation.

227. Yoshimoto, Y., et al., Malignant tumors during the first two decades of life in the offspring of atomic bomb survivors. Am J Hum Genet, 1990. 46(6):1041–1052.

228. Akahoshi, M., et al., Effects of radiation on fatty liver and metabolic coronary risk factors among atomic bomb survivors in Nagasaki. Hypertens Res, 2003. 26(12):965–970.

229. Izumi, S., et al., Cancer incidence in children and young adults did not increase relative to parental exposure to atomic bombs. Br J Cancer, 2003. 89(9):1709–1713.

230. Izumi, S., A. Suyama, and K. Koyama, Radiation-related mortality among offspring of atomic bomb survivors: A half-century of follow-up. Int J Cancer, 2003. 107(2):292–297.

231. Shleien, B., A.J. Ruttenber, and M. Sage, Epidemiologic studies of cancer in populations near nuclear facilities. Health Phys, 1991. 61(6):699–713.

232. Kinlen, L.J., Childhood leukemia and population mixing. Pediatrics, 2004. 114(1):330–331.

233. Kinlen, L.J., Infection and childhood leukemia. Cancer Causes Control, 1998. 9(3):237–239.

234. Balter, M., Studies set to test competing theories about early infection. Science, 1992. 256(5064):1633.

235. Brues, A.M., Carcinogenic effects of radiation. Adv Biol Med Phys, 1951. 2:171–191.

236. Upton, A.C., et al. (eds), Historical Perspectives on Radiation Carcinogenesis in Radiation Carcinogenesis. 1986, New York: Elsevier, pp. 1–10.

237. Mancuso, T.F., A. Stewart, and G. Kneale, Radiation exposures of Hanford workers dying from cancer and other causes. Health Phys, 1977. 33:369–385.

238. Kneale, G.W., A. Stewart, and T. Mancuso, Reanalysis of Data Relating to the Hanford Study of the Cancer Risks of Radiation Workers: Late Biological Effects of Ionizing Radiation. 1978, Vienna: International Atomic Energy Agency.

239. Beral, V., et al., Mortality of employees of the United Kingdom Atomic Energy Authority, 1946–1979. Br Med J (Clin Res Ed), 1985. 291(6493):440–447.

240. Kendall, G.M., et al., Mortality and occupational exposure to radiation: First analysis of the National Registry for Radiation Workers. BMJ, 1992. 304(6821):220–225.

241. Carpenter, L., et al., Combined analysis of mortality in three United Kingdom nuclear industry workforces, 1946–1988. Radiat Res, 1994. 138(2):224–238.

242. Wilkinson, G.S., et al., Mortality among plutonium and other radiation workers at a plutonium weapons facility. Am J Epidemiol, 1987. 125(2):231–250.

243. Checkoway, H., et al., Radiation doses and cause-specific mortality among workers at a nuclear materials fabrication plant. Am J Epidemiol, 1988. 127(2):255–266.

244. Gilbert, E.S., Mortality of workers at the Oak Ridge National Laboratory. Health Phys, 1992. 62(3):260–264.

245. Wiggs, L.D., et al., Mortality among workers exposed to external ionizing radiation at a nuclear facility in Ohio. J Occup Med, 1991. 33(5):632–637.

246. Hutchison, G.B., et al., Review of report by Mancuso, Stewart and Kneale of radiation exposure of Hanford workers. Health Phys, 1979. 37(2):207–220.

247. Najarian, T. and T. Colton, Mortality from leukaemia and cancer in shipyard nuclear workers. Lancet, 1978. 1(8072):1018–1020.

248. Rinsky, R.A., et al., Cancer mortality at a naval nuclear shipyard. Lancet, 1981. 1(8214):231–235.

249. Boice, J., Study of health effects of low-level radiation in USA nuclear shipyard workers. J Radiol Prot, 2001. 21:400–403.

250. Gilbert, E.S., G.R. Petersen, and J.A. Buchanan, Mortality of workers at the Hanford site: 1945–1981. Health Phys, 1989. 56(1):11–25.

251. Gilbert, E.S., et al., Analyses of combined mortality data on workers at the Hanford Site, Oak Ridge National Laboratory, and Rocky Flats Nuclear Weapons Plant. Radiat Res, 1989. 120(1):19–35.

252. Gilbert, E.S., D.L. Cragle, and L.D Wiggs, Updated analyses of combined mortality data for workers at the Hanford Site, Oak Ridge National Laboratory, and Rocky Flats Weapons Plant. Radiat Res, 1993. 136(3):408–421.

253. Gilbert, E.S., et al., Mortality of workers at the Hanford site: 1945–1986. Health Phys, 1993. 64(6):577–590.

254. Cardis, E., et al., Effects of low doses and low dose rates of external ionizing radiation: Cancer mortality among nuclear industry workers in three countries. Radiat Res, 1995. 142(2):117–132.

255. Baisogolov, G.D., et al., Malignant neoformations of the hematopoietic and lymphoid tissues in the personnel of the first plant of the atomic industry. Vopr Onkol, 1991. 37(5):553–559.

256. Buldakov, L.A., et al., The irradiation of the personnel of industrial and power-generating atomic reactors. Med Radiol (Mosk), 1991. 36(3):38–43.

257. Nikipelov, B., A. Lizlov, and N.A. Koshurnikova, Experience with the first Soviet nuclear installation: Radiation doses and health. Priroda, 1990. 2:28–30.

258. Koshurnikova, N.A., et al., Mortality from malignancies of the hematopoietic and lymphatic tissues among personnel of the first nuclear plant in the USSR. Sci Total Environ, 1994. 142(1–2):19–23.

259. Doshenko, V., Causes of mortality after considerable occupational chronic total gamma irradiation. J Med Radiol, 1991. 8:40.

260. Hohryakov, V.F. and S.A. Romanov, Lung cancer in radiochemical industry workers. Sci Total Environ, 1994. 142(1–2):25–28.

261. Howe, G.R., et al., Analysis of the mortality experience amongst U.S. nuclear power industry workers after chronic low-dose exposure to ionizing radiation. Radiat Res, 2004. 162(5):517–526.

262. Zablotska, L.B., J.P. Ashmore, and G.R. Howe, Analysis of mortality among Canadian nuclear power industry workers after chronic low-dose exposure to ionizing radiation. Radiat Res, 2004. 161(6):633–641.

263. Cardis, E., et al., Risk of cancer after low doses of ionising radiation: Retrospective cohort study in 15 countries. BMJ, 2005. 331(7508):77.

264. Cardis, E., M, Vrijheid, M, Blettner, et al., The 15-country collaborative study of cancer risk among radiation workers in the nuclear industry: Estimates of radiation-related cancer risks. Radiat Res, 2007. 167:396–416.

265. Wakeford, R., Cancer risk among nuclear workers. J Radiol Prot, 2005. 25(3):225–228.

266. Smith, P.G. and R. Doll, Mortality from cancer and all causes among British radiologists. Br J Radiol, 1981. 54(639):187–194.

267. Nambi, K.S. and Y.S. Mayya, Pooled analysis of cancer mortality cases among the employees in five units of the Department of Atomic Energy in India. Indian J Cancer, 1997. 34(3):99–106.

268. Jablon, S. and R.W. Miller, Army technologists: 29-year follow up for cause of death. Radiology, 1978. 126(3):677–679.

269. Wang, J.X., et al., Cancer among medical diagnostic x-ray workers in China. J Natl Cancer Inst, 1988. 80(5):344–350.

270. Ennow, K., et al., Epidemiological assessment of the cancer risk among the staff in radiotherapy departments in Denmark. In Low Dose Radiation: Biological Basis of Risk Assessment, K. Baverstock and J. Stather, eds. 1989, London: Taylor and Francis.

271. National Council on Radiation Protection and Measurements (NCRP), Guidance on radiation received in space activities. NCRP report no. 98. 1989, Bethesda, Md: NCRP, p. x.

272. National Council on Radiation Protection and Measurements (NCRP), Radiation protection guidance for activities in low-earth orbit: Recommendations of the NCRP Report no. 132. 2000, Bethesda, Md: The Council, p. viii.

273. National Council on Radiation Protection and Measurements (NCRP), Operational radiation safety program for astronauts in low-earth orbit: A basic framework. Recommendations of the NCRP Report no. 142. 2002, Bethesda, Md: NCRP, p. ix.

274. Boice, J.D. Jr., M. Blettner, and A. Auvinen, Epidemiologic studies of pilots and aircrew. Health Phys, 2000. 79(5):576–584.

275. Stewart, A., D. Webb, and B. Hewitt, A survey of childhood malignancies. Br Med J, 1958. 1:1495.

276. Stewart, A. and G.W. Kneale, Radiation dose effects in relation to obstetric x-rays and childhood cancers. Lancet, 1970. 1(7658):1185–1188.

277. Bithell, J.F., Epidemiological studies of children irradiated in-utero. In Low Dose Radiation: Biological Basis of Risk Assessment, K. Baverstock and J. Strather, eds. 1989, London: Taylor and Francis.

278. Muirhead, C. and G.W. Kneale, Prenatal irradiation and childhood cancer. J Radiat Prot, 1989. 9:209–212.

279. MacMahon, B., Some recent issues in low-exposure radiation epidemiology. Environ Health Perspect, 1989. 81:131–135.

280. Miller, R.W., Effects of prenatal exposure to ionizing radiation. Health Phys, 1990. 59(1):57–61.

281. Mole, R.H., Antenatal irradiation and childhood cancer: Causation or coincidence? Br J Cancer, 1974. 30(3):199–208.

282. Mole, R.H., Childhood cancer after prenatal exposure to diagnostic x-ray examinations in Britain. Br J Cancer, 1990. 62(1):152–168.

283. Harvey, E.B., et al., Prenatal x-ray exposure and childhood cancer in twins. N Engl J Med, 1985. 312(9):541–545.

284. Yoshimoto, Y., H. Kato, and W.J. Schull, Risk of cancer among children exposed in utero to A-bomb radiations, 1950–84. Lancet, 1988. 2(8612):665–669.

285. Yoshimoto, Y., et al., Studies of children in utero during atomic bomb detonation. In 203rd National Meeting of the American Chemical Society, April 5–10, 1992. 1993, San Francisco: American Chemical Society Press.

286. Yoshimoto, Y., R. Delongchamp, and K. Mabuchi, In-utero exposed atomic bomb survivors: Cancer risk update. Lancet, 1994. 344(8918):345–346.

287. Court Brown, W.M., R. Doll, and R.B. Hill, Incidence of leukaemia after exposure to diagnostic radiation in utero. Br Med J, 1960. 5212:1539–1545.

288. Oppenheim, B.E., M.L. Griem, and P. Meier, Effects of low-dose prenatal irradiation in humans: Analysis of Chicago lying-in data and comparison with other studies. Radiat Res, 1974. 57(3):508–544.

289. Inskip, P.D., et al., Incidence of childhood cancer in twins. Cancer Causes Control, 1991. 2(5):315–324.

290. Rodvall, Y., et al., Childhood cancer among Swedish twins. Cancer Causes Control, 1992. 3(6):527–532.

291. Davis, F.G., et al., Cancer mortality in a radiation-exposed cohort of Massachusetts tuberculosis patients. Cancer Res, 1989. 49(21):6130–6136.

292. Boice, J.D., Jr. and R.R. Monson, Breast cancer in women after repeated fluoroscopic examinations of the chest. J Natl Cancer Inst, 1977. 59(3):823–832.

293. Boice, J.D., Jr., et al., Frequent chest X-ray fluoroscopy and breast cancer incidence among tuberculosis patients in Massachusetts. Radiat Res, 1991. 125(2):214–222.

294. Miller, A.B., et al., Mortality from breast cancer after irradiation during fluoroscopic examinations in patients being treated for tuberculosis. N Engl J Med, 1989. 321(19):1285–1289.

295. da Silva Horta, J., et al., Malignancies in Portuguese Thorotrast patients. Health Phys, 1978. 35(1):137–151.

296. Van Kaick, G., et al., Report on the German Thorotrast study. Strahlentherapie, 1986. 80(Suppl):S114–S118.

297. Mori, T., et al., Current status of the Japanese follow-up study of the Thorotrast patients and its relationships to the statistical analysis of the autopsy series. In Risks from Radium and Thorotrast, D. Taylor, ed. 1989, London: British Institute of Radiology.

298. Mori, T., et al., Present status of the medical study on Thorotrast administered patients in Japan. Strahlentherapie, 1986. 80:123–134.

299. Olsen, J.H., M. Andersson, and J.D. Boice, Jr., Thorotrast exposure and cancer risk. Health Phys, 1990. 58(2):222–223.

300. Andersson, M. and H.H. Storm, Cancer incidence among Danish Thorotrast-exposed patients. J Natl Cancer Inst, 1992. 84(17):1318–1325.

301. Hoffman, D.A., et al., Breast cancer in women with scoliosis exposed to multiple diagnostic x-rays. J Natl Cancer Inst, 1989. 81(17):1307–1312.

302. Boice, J.D., Jr., et al., Diagnostic x-ray procedures and risk of leukemia, lymphoma, and multiple myeloma. JAMA, 1991. 265(10):1290–1294.

303. Holm, L.E., Cancer risks after diagnostic doses of ^{131}I with special reference to thyroid cancer. Cancer Detect Prev, 1991. 15(1):27–30.

304. Little, M.P., Comparison of the risks of cancer incidence and mortality following radiation therapy for benign and malignant disease with the cancer risks observed in the Japanese A-bomb survivors. Int J Radiat Biol, 2001. 77(4):431–464.

305. Ron, E., B. Modan, and J.D. Boice, Jr., Mortality after radiotherapy for ringworm of the scalp. Am J Epidemiol, 1988. 127(4):713–725.

306. Ron, E., et al., Thyroid neoplasia following low-dose radiation in childhood. Radiat Res, 1989. 120(3):516–531.

307. Shore, R.E., et al., Thyroid tumors following thymus irradiation. J Natl Cancer Inst, 1985. 74(6):1177–1184.

308. Hildreth, N.G., R.E. Shore, and P.M. Dvoretsky, The risk of breast cancer after irradiation of the thymus in infancy. N Engl J Med, 1989. 321(19):1281–1284.

309. Mettler, F.A., Jr., et al., Breast neoplasms in women treated with x-rays for acute postpartum mastitis: A pilot study. J Natl Cancer Inst, 1969. 43(4):803–811.

310. Mattsson, A., et al., Radiation-induced breast cancer: Long-term follow-up of radiation therapy for benign breast disease. J Natl Cancer Inst, 1993. 85(20):1679–1685.

311. Smith, P.G. and R. Doll, Mortality among patients with ankylosing spondylitis after a single treatment course with x-rays. Br Med J (Clin Res Ed), 1982. 284(6314):449–460.

312. Wick, R.R. and W. Gossner, Follow-up study of late effects in ^{224}Ra treated ankylosing spondylitis patients. Health Phys, 1983. 44 (Suppl 1):S187–S195.

313. Wick, R., Recent results of the follow-up of radium-224 treated ankylosing spondylitis patients. In Risks from Radium and Thorotrast, D. Taylor, ed. 1989, London: British Institute of Radiology.

314. Wick, R., D. Chmelevsky, and W. Gossner, Radium-224: Risk to bone and hematopoietic tissue in ankylosins spondylitis patients. In The Radiobiology of Radium and Thorotrast, W. Gossner, ed. 1986, Munich: Urban and Schwartzenberg.

315. Griem, M.L., et al., Cancer following radiotherapy for peptic ulcer. J Natl Cancer Inst, 1994. 86(11):842–849.

316. Carr, Z.A., et al., Malignant neoplasms after radiation therapy for peptic ulcer. Radiat Res, 2002. 157(6):668–677.

317. Inskip, P.D., et al., Cancer mortality following radium treatment for uterine bleeding. Radiat Res, 1990. 123(3):331–344.

318. Inskip, P.D., et al., Leukemia following radiotherapy for uterine bleeding. Radiat Res, 1990. 122(2):107–119.

319. Ryberg, M., et al., Malignant disease after radiation treatment of benign gynaecological disorders: A study of a cohort of metropathia patients. Acta Oncol, 1990. 29(5):563–567.

320. Modan, B. and A.M. Lilienfeld, Polycythemia vera and leukemia—The role of radiation treatment: A study of 1222 patients. Medicine (Baltimore), 1965. 44:305–344.

321. Berk, P.D., et al., Increased incidence of acute leukemia in polycythemia vera associated with chlorambucil therapy. N Engl J Med, 1981. 304(8):441–447.

322. Mays, C.W., Alpha-particle-induced cancer in humans. Health Phys, 1988. 55(4):637–652.

323. Speiss, H., C.W. Mays, and D. Chmelevsky. Radium 224 in humans. In Risks from Radium and Thorotrast. 1988, London: British Institute of Radiology.

324. Furst, C.J., et al., Cancer incidence after radiotherapy for skin hemangioma: A retrospective cohort study in Sweden. J Natl Cancer Inst, 1988. 80(17):1387–1392.

325. Furst, C.J., M. Lundell, and L.E. Holm, Tumors after radiotherapy for skin hemangioma in childhood: A case-control study. Acta Oncol, 1990. 29(5):557–562.

326. Goldman, M.B., et al., Radioactive iodine therapy and breast cancer. A follow-up study of hyperthyroid women. Am J Epidemiol, 1988. 127(5):969–980.

327. Holm, L.E., et al., Cancer risk after iodine-131 therapy for hyperthyroidism. J Natl Cancer Inst, 1991. 83(15):1072–1077.

328. Saenger, E.L., G.E. Thoma, and E.A. Tompkins, Incidence of leukemia following treatment of hyperthyroidism: Preliminary report of the Cooperative Thyrotoxicosis Therapy Follow-Up Study. JAMA, 1968. 205(12):855–862.

329. Dobyns, B.M., et al., Malignant and benign neoplasms of the thyroid in patients treated for hyperthyroidism: A report of the cooperative thyrotoxicosis therapy follow-up study. J Clin Endocrinol Metab, 1974. 38:976–998.

330. Hoffman, D.A., et al., Cancer incidence following treatment of hyperthyroidism. Int J Epidemiol, 1982. 11(3):218–224.

331. Chauveinc, L., et al., Radiotherapy-induced solid tumors: Review of the literature and risk assessment. Cancer Radiother, 1998. 2(1):12–18.

332. Little, M.P., et al., Relative risks of radiation-associated cancer: Comparison of second cancer in therapeutically irradiated populations with the Japanese atomic bomb survivors. Radiat Environ Biophys, 1999. 38(4):267–283.

333. Little, M.P., et al., Risks of leukemia in Japanese atomic bomb survivors, in women treated for cervical cancer, and in patients treated for ankylosing spondylitis. Radiat Res, 1999. 152(3):280–292.

334. Boice, J.D., Jr., et al., Second cancers following radiation treatment for cervical cancer: An international collaboration among cancer registries. J Natl Cancer Inst, 1985. 74(5):955–975.

335. Boice, J.D., Jr., et al., Radiation dose and second cancer risk in patients treated for cancer of the cervix. Radiat Res, 1988. 116(1):3–55.

336. Mettler, F.A., et al., Benefits versus risks from mammography: A critical reassessment. Cancer, 1996. 77(5):903–909.

337. Arai, T., et al., Second cancer after radiation therapy for cancer of the uterine cervix. Cancer, 1991. 67(2):398–405.

338. Hay, J.H., W. Duncan, and G.R. Kerr, Subsequent malignancies in patients irradiated for testicular tumours. Br J Radiol, 1984. 57(679):597–602.

339. Fossa, S.D., et al., Second non-germ cell malignancies after radiotherapy of testicular cancer with or without chemotherapy. Br J Cancer, 1990. 61(4):639–643.

340. Steinfeld, A.D. and R.E. Shore, Second malignancies following radiotherapy for testicular seminoma. Clin Oncol (R Coll Radiol), 1990. 2(5):273–276.

341. Boice, J.D., Jr., et al., Cancer in the contralateral breast after radiotherapy for breast cancer. N Engl J Med, 1992. 326(12):781–785.

342. Storm, H.H., et al., Adjuvant radiotherapy and risk of contralateral breast cancer. J Natl Cancer Inst, 1992. 84(16):1245–1250.

343. Curtis, R.E., et al., Risk of leukemia after chemotherapy and radiation treatment for breast cancer. N Engl J Med, 1992. 326(26):1745–1751.

344. Tucker, M., et al., Therapeutic radiation at young age linked to secondary thyroid cancer. Proc Am Soc Clin Oncol, 1986. 5:827.

345. Tucker, M.A., et al., Bone sarcomas linked to radiotherapy and chemotherapy in children. N Engl J Med, 1987. 317(10):588–593.

346. Tucker, M.A., et al., Leukemia after therapy with alkylating agents for childhood cancer. J Natl Cancer Inst, 1987. 78(3):459–464.

347. Holm, L.E., Radiation-induced thyroid neoplasia. Soz Praventivmed, 1991. 36(4):266–275.

348. Edmonds, C.J. and T. Smith, The long-term hazards of the treatment of thyroid cancer with radioiodine. Br J Radiol, 1986. 59(697):45–51.

349. Brincker, H., H.S. Hansen, and A.P. Andersen, Induction of leukemia by iodine 131 treatment of thyroid carcinoma. Br J Cancer, 1973. 28:232–237.

350. Teppo, L., E. Pukkala, and E. Saxen, Multiple cancer—An epidemiologic exercise in Finland. J Natl Cancer Inst, 1985. 75(2):207–217.

351. Tucker, M.A., J. Boice, and D.A. Hoffman, Second cancer following cutaneous melanoma and cancers of the brain, thyroid, connective tissues, bone and eye in Connecticut, 1935–1982. Nat Cancer Inst Monograph, 1985. 68:161–189.

352. Hall, P., et al., Tumors after radiotherapy for thyroid cancer: A case-control study within a cohort of thyroid cancer patients. Acta Oncol, 1992. 31(4):403–407.

353. Goffman, J., Radiation and Human Health, 1981. San Francisco: Sierra Club.

LEUKEMIA

General

Leukemia is the type of malignancy most frequently recognized after whole-body radiation doses on the order of several grays (Gy). Even though it may be a common radiation-induced malignancy following significant absorbed red bone marrow doses, it does not account for the majority of radiogenic malignancies; leukemia often appears to be disproportionately increased because it otherwise is a relatively rare cause of death. The four major types of leukemia are acute lymphatic leukemia (ALL), acute myeloid leukemia (AML), chronic myeloid leukemia (CML) and chronic lymphocytic leukemia (CLL). Most leukemias of childhood are ALL whereas CML and CLL are a higher percentage in adults. ALL, AML, and CML have clearly been associated with radiation exposure but CLL has not.

Leukemia was initially suspected of being increased in incidence by exposure to radiation as early as 1911. Since that time, there have been reports of excess leukemia in early radiologists,[1,2] but this has not been seen after the advent of modern radiation protection measures. The most substantial human experience arises from three major population groups: atomic bomb survivors, persons exposed to high doses of pelvic radiation therapy, and those treated for ankylosing spondylitis and other diseases using x-ray therapy. The Committee on the Biological Effects of Ionizing Radiations (BEIR)[3] has indicated that leukemia mortality is statistically significant above 0.4 Gy but not at lower doses, therefore, the exact nature of leukemia risk at low doses remains unclear and risk estimates below 0.4 Gy are usually derived from mathematical models. Issues regarding an increase in childhood leukemia as a result of preconception parental and intrauterine exposure have been discussed in Chapters 3 and 8.

Leukemia has genetic overtones because certain heritable disorders that carry an increased risk of leukemia have also been associated with faulty repair of genetic damage. Other risk factors include gene rearrangements, Down syndrome, ataxia-telangiectasia (A-T), alkylating chemotherapeutic agents, pesticides, benzene, infective agents, and cigarette smoking (myeloid leukemia).

A number of genetic studies have been done on 75 atomic bomb survivors who have developed leukemia.[4,5]

These have been compared with a nonexposed group. No significant difference was identified between the groups in terms of mutations or sites of base substitution in the N- or K-RAS oncogene sequences. This information is important because the RAS oncogenes are dominantly acting point mutations that have been associated with some leukemias. Even with the advances in this field, at the present time it is not feasible to determine whether a particular non–CLL has been radiation-induced.

Modifying Factors

Leukemia induced by radiation may be any one of several types (with the exception of CLL, which does not appear to be caused by radiation exposure), depending on several factors, such as the age of the person at the time of the exposure and the conditions of irradiation. There are human studies that demonstrate decreasing risk at quite high doses. These incude an analysis of radiation-induced leukemia in patients treated for cervical cancer with radiation therapy. As the dose exceeded 4 Gy, the risk decreased.[6]

Dose also is a modifying factor in regard to risk in a manner that is different from that for solid tumors. The dose-response curve appears to have a better fit to a linear-quadratic model rather than a linear one. This means that risk estimation at low doses based on a linear extrapolation from risk at 1 Gy will likely be an overestimation. A report on leukemia mortality among the atomic bomb survivors reported that the leukemia dose response for survivors suffering from epilation was steeper than for persons receiving lower doses.[7] In the report on mortality up through 1990 the curvature of the dose response fitted a linear-quadratic model such that the excess risk per unit dose was three times higher at 1 sievert (Sv) than at 0.1 Sv.[8] The risk at 0.1 Sv was only based on modeling and not seen in the actual data. In the report on the potential effect of the DS02 dosimetry, leukemia risk estimates appeared to be best reflected by a model which was linear quadratic with curvature independent of age at exposure and the risks were about 8% less than based on prior dosimetry.[9]

In the Life Span Study (LSS) on mortality of atomic bomb survivors through 1985, the excess absolute risk (EAR) was 74% higher in males than in females, and the difference was statistically significant. There was no difference when relative risk (RR) was examined.[10] No major difference in excess relative risk (ERR) by sex is found in the LSS incidence data through 1987 reported by Preston et al.[11,12] In age-adjusted studies, there is an increased absolute risk of all types of leukemia in males versus females by a factor of about 1.5.[13] Age at exposure is a significant modifying factor of the risk estimates, with the absolute frequency of induction for each unit dose increasing with age from early adult life, although it is also relatively high in childhood. Beebe et al.[14] indicated that the induction rate changes with age and is highest in those groups aged 1 to 10 years and over 50 years at exposure. The incidence data from Japan suggest that risks were highest for the youngest survivors. Data from the Israeli tinea capitis study seem to suggest that there is increased RR in young children as opposed to older children. There was an RR of leukemia of 3.3 for 0 to 5 years of age at exposure, 2.6 for the 6- to 8-year-old group, and lower for the group that was 9 to 15 years old at exposure.[15]

Age at exposure not only modifies the magnitude of the risk but the latent period as well. The mean latent period for induction of leukemia by radiation is shorter than for the solid tumors, with mean latency to diagnosis generally averaging about 10 years, although the minimal latent period may be as short as 2 to 3 years. There appears to be no significant difference in the latency period between the types of acute leukemia, although AML may be seen slightly earlier than other types. There is a variation in the length of the latent period with age at exposure for the acute leukemias and possibly for the chronic granulocytic type as well. In general, the older the individual at exposure, the longer is the mean latency period,[16] but no evidence suggests that higher doses cause the minimal latent period to be shortened. The increased risk of developing leukemia is markedly reduced or almost gone 30 years following exposure. The excess risk in the youngest survivors of the atomic bomb was no longer apparent 15 years after exposure, whereas in older cohorts, it began later, increased more slowly over time, and lasted longer. Mortality for radiation-induced types of leukemia is almost 100%, so that excess risk due to radiation, whether expressed as cases induced or deaths, is almost interchangeable.

External Exposure

Atomic Bomb Survivors

A vast literature concerns the incidence of leukemia in atomic bomb survivors both at Hiroshima and Nagasaki. A general review of leukemia encountered in this population has been published by Moriyama and Kato.[17] This report indicates that the annual frequency of deaths from leukemia had returned to about the level observed in the unexposed population by the end of 1972. Although the

information is not separately reported, it appears that the leukemia incidence is minimally higher in males than in females and that although the incidence of acute leukemia appears to be equal for the sexes, chronic granulocytic leukemia (CGL) may be higher in males. It should also be noted, however, that the natural incidence rate of leukemia in Japan appears to be somewhat lower in females than in males. The ERR at 1 Sv derived from the atomic bomb survivor incidence data for all ages and both sexes is 4.4, while the EAR is 2.7 $(10^4 PYSv)^{-1}$. The actual number of leukemia cases observed in the LSS from 1958 to 1987 was 141 versus 67 cases expected.

From the mortality data up to 1985 the values are an ERR at 1 Sv of 5.2 and an EAR of 2.9 $(10^4 PYSv)^{-1}$. The excess number of leukemia deaths observed was 87 up to the end of 1990[8] and 93 up to the end of 2000[9] among the cohort of 86,955 survivors. Some authors have estimated that about 45% of leukemia deaths occurring in survivors who received more than 0.005 Sv were due to radiation exposure.[18] In an analysis of the potential effect of DS02 dosimetry, Preston et al.[9] extended the analysis to include data through 2000. At this time there were a total of 296 leukemia deaths with an expected background of 203 cases and a fitted excess of 93 cases. The EAR for all ages was 12% less than by using the DS86 dosimetry. The EAR by age at exposure for all leukemia mortality is 0.66 (90% CI [confidence interval] 0.13, 1.3) for 0 to 19 years, 1.3 (0.3, 2.5) for 20 to 39 years, and 1.9 (0.4, 3.9) for 40 and over. The linear-quadratic dose-response function appears to fit the atomic bomb survivor data best with the excess risk per unit dose at 1.0 Sv about three times that at 0.1 Sv. It has also been noted that the risk for those exposed early in life decreased more rapidly than those exposed later in life.

The expression of radiation effects differs depending on the leukemia type (Table 5-1).[19] This is not surprising because molecular biology has established that the four spontaneously occurring leukemia types (AML, ALL, CML, and CLL) have at least part of their origin in different genetic abnormalities. The atomic bomb survivor data indicate that the effects of radiation exposure are significantly greater for ALL and CML than for AML. ALL and CML were also observed earlier than AML (Table 5-2). It also appears that the type of leukemia most characteristic of the atomic bomb survivors is CML.[20] In spite of the differences, there does not appear to be a difference in the shape of the dose-response curve.

Table 5-1 • Radiogenic Risk of Various Types of Leukemia

Leukemia Subtype	Excess Relative Risk at 1 Sv	Comparison to ERR for AML
AML	3.3	1
ALL	9.1	9.1/3.3 = 2.76
CML	6.2	6.2/3/3 = 1.88

Table 5-2 • Ratio of Relative Risks* Between Acute Myeloid (AML), Acute Lymphoid (ALL), Chronic Myeloid (CML), and Other Types of Leukemia

Type	Dose (mGy)[†]	1945–1950	1951–1955	1956–1960	1961–1965
ALL	0	1.00	1.00	1.00	1.00
	1–49	10.92	7.49	5.14	3.53
	50–499	9.99	5.82	3.39	1.97
	500–1499	3.32	3.00	2.70	2.44
	> 1499	20.70	12.25	7.25	4.29
CML	0	1.00	1.00	1.00	1.00
	1–49	12.10	7.21	4.30	2.56
	50–499	6.91	5.52	4.90	4.12
	500–1499	9.88	6.97	4.92	3.47
	> 1499	11.68	5.47	2.56	1.20
Other	0	1.00	1.00	1.00	1.00
	1–49	0.14	0.20	0.30	0.45
	50–499	0.14	0.24	0.42	0.74
	500–1499	2.44	1.52	0.95	0.59
	> 1499	2.03	1.43	1.01	0.71

*A relative risk ratio greater than 1.0 indicates a greater radiogenic effect on that leukemia type than on AML. Most RR ratios are statistically different at levels above 2.5.
[†]Dose in shielded kerma.
From Tomonaga M, Matsuo T, Carter R: A-bomb irradiation and leukemia types: An update. RERF Technical Report 9-91, Hiroshima, Japan, Radiation Effects Research Foundation, 1991.

Natural Background

At least 13 studies have tried to relate leukemia to natural background radiation and have found no significant association.[21–31] A paper by Sun et al.[32] used a high-background area and a neighboring control area in Guangdong, China, and has 1.7 million person-years of study from 1979–1995. Dose rate in the high-background area was 4.3 mSv per year and in the control areas it was about 1.6 mSv per year. The RR of leukemia compared to the control area was nonsignificantly elevated at 1.12 (95% CI 0.56, 2.22). Another paper on the same area of China was published in 2000 by Tao et al.[33–35] and had 1.7 million person-years of study from 1979–1995. The authors did not find a radiation effect and the RR of leukemia was 1.00 (95% CI 0.35, 2.81). In the United Kingdom a study was done examining the gamma dose rate in the dwellings occupied prior to a diagnosis of childhood leukemia; no association was found.[36] Axelson et al.[37] reported a marginally significant association with gamma radiation from uranium-containing alum shale concrete dwellings; however, the statistical power of the study is low due to low doses and possible misclassification of the exposures.

Increased natural cosmic irradiation occurs in airline crews. While there has been one report by Gundestrup and Storm[38] of an increase in leukemia (three cases) in airline crews purportedly as a result of cosmic x-ray exposure, this has not been borne out in other larger Nordic studies.[39] Band et al., in a study of 2740 pilots at doses of 6 mSv per year and average 20 years worked (for total average dose of about 120 mSv), found a nonsignificantly elevated SIR for leukemia of 1.65 (90% CI 0.86, 2.88) and a nonsignificantly reduced SMR of 0.86

(90% CI 0.23, 2.22).[40] Blettner et al. also reviewed additional studies with mixed findings.[41,42] Large European cohorts including more than 44,000 cabin crew[43] and 12,000 pilots[44] have not provided evidence of an increased leukemia risk.

Persons Exposed to Fallout

Fallout in the Marshall Islands caused a substantial bone marrow dose to the native islanders. However, AML developed in only one inhabitant of the Marshall Islands.[45] It is possible that this single case may be due to chance, although the possibility of radiation induction cannot be excluded. A study in French Polynesia[46] indicated higher rates of childhood leukemia from 1985–1989 compared to 1990–1995 but these rates were similar to those in Hawaii and, given the time lag between atmospheric weapons testing and these rates, there is not likely to be a connection. Some authors have reported an increase in childhood leukemia in Utah following testing of nuclear weapons. Land et al. have reviewed these data from a statistical viewpoint and demonstrated that the increase reported was artifactual and due to use of control groups who had an unusually low rate of leukemia compared to normal populations.[47] A later leukemia case-control study was performed with specific reference to leukemia.[48,49] This involved 1177 individuals who died of leukemia and 5330 controls. Although the study showed a weak association with estimated bone marrow dose, it was not statistically significant. Studies of the U.S. military who took part in weapons tests in Nevada or the Pacific showed less leukemia mortality than national rates while the RR compared to control groups was nonsignificantly elevated.[50]

Weapons fallout studies have been published by the British National Radiological Protection Board and by the Nordic countries. No consistent increase in leukemia was observed after the period of high fallout during 1964–1965.[51] There have been multiple analyses of U.K. atomic test veterans by Darby et al.,[52] Doll et al.,[53] and Muirhead et al.[54] In the latest 2004 review Muirhead et al. have a cohort of 21,357 test participants and reported a nonsignificant SMR of 1.06 (95% CI 0.77, 1.46) for non–CLL in test participants but a significantly increased motality risk compared to controls.[55] The RR compared to controls for incidence was nonsignificantly elevated at 1.41.

Studies of the Swedish Lapps who breed and eat reindeer have been reported by Wiklund et al.[56] The supposition is that these individuals may have higher rates of tumors because of the known concentration mechanisms of fallout products in the lichen-reindeer food pathway. No increased risk of tumors was detected in organs considered to be most sensitive to radiation carcinogenesis.

To date, studies on the populations exposed to fallout from the Chernobyl accident have shown no increase in leukemia.[57] Studies of adults living in the Bryansk area of Russia have been published by Osechinsky et al.[58] and Gapanovich et al.[59] with negative results. Studies in the most contaminated areas of the Russian Kaluga oblast by Ivanov in 1997[60] and 2003[61] also yielded negative results. Both Bebeshko[62] and Prisyazhniuk[63] evaluated contaminated areas of the Ukraine and Belarus for increases in leukemia and both were negative, although Noshchenko et al.[64] reported a raised risk but only among children born in 1986. Fallout from the Chernobyl accident has been related in some articles to childhood leukemia. Steiner et al.[65] as well as Parkin et al.[66,67] have also observed an increase in infant leukemia in Western Europe but it was not related to radiation exposure as determined by measured contamination. Also no increase in infant or childhood leukemia has been found in Belarus, Russia, or the Ukraine related to the Chernobyl accident according to the United Nations Scientific Committee on Effects of Atomic Radiation (UNSCEAR) 2000 report.[57] While at least one article exists by Noshchenko et al.[64,68] indicating an increase in acute leukemias in males exposed to more than 10 mSv, these results have not been confirmed by many other studies summarized the 2005 Chernobyl Forum report.[69]

Evaluations at greater distances from Chernobyl are unlikely to yield additional useful information due to lower doses. Studies in Hungary have been negative[70] and, while there was a suggested increase in infant leukemia in Scotland and Wales,[71] this was not confirmed in a larger study of the United Kingdom.[72] Cardis et al.[73] have estimated the potential impact of Chernobyl fallout in Europe. They estimate that the accident might result in 2400 excess leukemia cases and 1650 excess leukemia deaths or an attributable fraction of 0.04%. Of course, this small of a hypothetical increase would not be possible to detect. The 2000 UNSCEAR report,[57] the 2005 Chernobyl Forum report,[69] as well as the 2005 BEIR VII report[18] have summarized studies relative to leukemia in children and adults living in areas contaminated by the Chernobyl accident and indicated that, on balance, the existing evidence does not support the conclusion that rates of either childhood or adult leukemia have increased as a result of radiation exposure.

A case-control study conducted in Kazakhstan of a population downwind from the Semipalatinsk nuclear test site showed a nonsignificantly elevated risk in those who had estimated doses above 2 Sv, compared to those with doses of less than 0.5 Sv.[74] Data concerning the environmental contamination of the Techa River in the eastern part of Russia were released in 1992. Leukemia incidence over 422,000 person-years was studied in the over 28,000 persons who were exposed. Results were compared for a population of 394,000 unexposed persons.[75] A statistically significant increase in leukemia was found, although the ERR per unit dose was about 20% to 50% of that reported from the atomic bomb survivors. This may be a result of a dose-rate effect, the difficulty in accurately estimating bone marrow doses, or of inadequate ascertainment of cases. Strengths of this study are a wide range of doses, long follow-up, an unselected population, and a large number of persons. Krestinina et al.[76] have reported on cancer and leukemia mortality in a population of 29,873 persons living in rural villages on the Techa River and exposed to protracted radioactive releases from the Mayak plutonium production plant. Mean bone marrow doses were about 0.3 Gy, but some doses were as high as 2 Gy. The ERR per Gy for non–CLL was estimated to be 6.5 (95% CI 1.8, 24) and 63% of the leukemia deaths were felt to be associated with radiation exposure. Ostroumova et al.[77] conducted a case-control study from the same population and obtained similar results with an ERR of 4.6 (95% CI 1.7, 12.3) for non–CLL.

Public around Nuclear Installations

Studies of potential leukemia in populations living around nuclear power plants in the United States have been discussed in detail by Jablon et al.[78] To date, no consistently significant increase in leukemia attributable to radiation has been found in the United States, Canada,[79] or Israel.[80] There are several articles concerning the possibility of increased leukemia around a number of specific nuclear installations in Europe, including Sellafield, Dounray, and Le Hague. A report from the United Kingdom did not show excess leukemia at other U.K. sites.[81] Reviews of these findings have been presented by Laurier et al.[82–85] as well as in UNSCEAR 2006.[86] They have concluded that there is no relationship to radiation exposure although an infectious etiology could not be excluded. An updated analysis of mortality around the Three Mile Island nuclear plant did not indicate clear patterns of leukemia risk related to the accident.[87] A recent review of leukemia around Japanese nuclear plants by Yoshimoto et al.[88] also does not support an association.

There are three papers concerning potential uranium contamination and the possibility of leukemia in the public. The papers by Boice et al. indicated a nonsignificant elevation of leukemia with an RR of 1.15 (95% CI 0.9, 1.6) around a uranium mining and milling facility in Texas, a nonsignificant decrease near a uranium facility in Pennsylvania, and a significant reduction in SMR near a uranium facility in Colorado.[89,90,90a] No difference in leukemia was found by Boice et al. in a study of persons residing near the Hanford, Washington site.[91] A paper by Bithell et al. examined contamination by uranium 235 and found no evidence of an association with childhood leukemia.[92] Leukemia incidence also has been studied by Grosche et al. around two tritium-releasing nuclear facilities.[93] The results were contradictory to radiation causation. At the facility with the highest releases there was a nonsignificantly decreased rate of childhood leukemia while at another facility with several orders of magnitude smaller releases, there was a significant increase in childhood leukemia.

Medical Occupational Exposure

Early radiologists in the United States incurred a significant increase in leukemia mortality in the period 1920–1939. No excess has been identified in those who began to practice after that time.[2] No risk estimates have been derived because the doses were uncertain, and the normal incidence in the population was also uncertain. Rough estimates of bone marrow dose in the range of 2 to 6 Gy have been given, and a rough estimate of risk is 0.7 leukemia deaths annually in 1 million persons for 0.01 Gy (0.7 deaths year^{-1}). There have been a number of recent updates and papers concerning medical occupational radiation exposures. Berrington et al. have reported on 100 years of U.K. radiologists and reported a nonsignificantly increased SMR for leukemia of 2.50 for those employed from 1897–1920 and a nonsignificantly increased SMR for leukemia of 1.88 for those employed after 1920.[94]

Aoyama et al. have reported on Japanese radiologic technologists employed during 1969–1993 and found a nonsignificantly increased SMR for leukemia of 1.31 (5% CI 0.80, 2.02).[95] Burnett et al. studied the mortality of health and science technicians and found a nonsignificantly decreased proportional leukemia mortality ratio of 0.86 (95% CI 0.43, 1.54).[96] Doody et al. studied mortality among U.S. radiologic technologists from 1926–1990.[97] The study included 143,517 technologists and 7345 deaths whose doses were not evaluated. The SMR for leukemia was nonsignificantly reduced at 0.93 (95% CI 0.76, 1.13).

Mohan et al. studied cancer and other causes of mortality among 146,022 radiologic technologists employed from 1940 and later.[98,99] The SMR for leukemia in males was nonsignificantly reduced at 0.95 (95% CI 0.7, 1.2) and for females it was also nonsignificantly reduced at

0.92 (95% CI 0.8, 1.1). Linet et al. have reported on follow-up of 71,894 radiologic technologists.[100] Neither length of work or first year of certification was related to non–CLL risk; however, there was a trend of increasing risk with longer employment in those who worked before 1950. Sigurdson et al. studied cancer incidence in 90,305 U.S. radiologic technologists and found that the SIR for leukemia was nonsignificantly elevated at 1.09 (95% CI 0.87, 1.32).[101] Wang et al. studied cancer in a cohort of 27,011 Chinese medical diagnostic x-ray workers.[102,103] Cumulative doses were 0.55 Sv for those employed before 1970 and 0.082 Sv for those employed after 1970. The RR for leukemia was significantly elevated with an RR of 2.37 for those employed before 1960 but nonsignificantly elevated at 1.73 for those employed later.

Medical Diagnostic Exposure

Boice et al. have examined the risk of leukemia in two prepaid health plans in which the number of diagnostic x-rays could be retrospectively assessed by case.[104] There was a slight elevation in non–CLL risk (RR 1.17) but no dose-response relationship was found when x-ray procedures performed near the time of leukemia diagnosis were excluded. No statistically significant increase was demonstrated in the Massachusetts tuberculosis (TB) fluoroscopy study.[105] Risks associated with intrauterine exposure are discussed in Chapter 8.

Radiation Therapy

There are many studies of populations that have received radiotherapy for a wide variety of benign conditions, including acne, peptic ulcer, and ringworm. Court Brown and Doll observed an excess of mortality from both leukemia and aplastic anemia in 14,111 patients treated for ankylosing spondylitis between 1935 and 1954.[106] Initially, it was not known whether leukemia was associated with radiation exposure or with the primary disease. Studies by Smith et al. have indicated that leukemia is probably not increased in patients who were not treated with x-rays.[107,108] In general, these patients were given an average of 10 x-ray treatments over a period of 5 to 6 weeks, with an estimated mean marrow dose of 2.2 to 3.2 Gy. Twenty-nine excess leukemia deaths were identified, corresponding to a risk factor of between 0.8 and 1.2 leukemia deaths in 1 million persons annually for 0.01 Gy. Acute leukemia showed the most marked increase, with a smaller increase in CGL. The mean interval from irradiation to death was approximately 7.4 years, contrasted with that of Hiroshima and Nagasaki, where it was about 12.5 years. A follow-up of 14,106 of ankylosing spondylitis patients treated with external beam therapy during 184,000 person-years of study has confirmed the increases in leukemia.[109] In 1995 Weiss et al. studied 14,767 ankylosing spondylitis patients following x-ray treatment.[110] The mean red marrow dose was about 5 Gy. The ratio of observed compared to expected deaths for non–CLL was greatest in the first five years after treatment and decreased to being nonsignificantly elevated after 25 years. The average RR for the period 1 to 25 years posttreatment was 7 for a uniform dose of 1 Gy.

Lundell et al. have studied 14,624 infants who were given radiotherapy in infancy to treat skin hemangiomas.[111] There were no significant associations between childhood leukemia and radiation dose.

Griem et al. have followed a population of patients who received radiotherapy for peptic ulcer treatment, 1831 exposed persons and 1778 controls were studied over 78,000 person-years at risk.[112] A statistically significant increase was identified for leukemia with an RR of 3.3 (95% CI 1.0, 10.6). Individual dosimetry, 50-years follow-up, and a control group of nonexposed patients with peptic ulcer are strengths of this study. Unfortunately, a standardized radiotherapy regimen precludes dose-response analysis. Carr et al. performed a follow-up study of 3719 patients of the same group with doses to the abdomen of about 15 Gy.[113] The RR for leukemia after radiotherapy was 0 in the period 0 to 10 years postexposure and nonsignificantly elevated, with an RR of 2.46 (95% CI 0.75, 8.01) in the follow-up period of 11 to 62 years postexposure. Mattsson et al. have reported on cancer incidence among 3090 women who received radiation therapy for benign breast disease.[114] The RR for leukemia was nonsignificant at 0.67.

Radiation therapy has been used in the treatment of metropathia hemorrhagica after which Smith and Doll observed an excess death rate from leukemia.[115] The mean marrow dose was 1.34 Gy, with a mean follow-up time from treatment of 19 years. The estimated lifetime leukemia risk is 17 in 1 million (CI 3 to 36/1 million) for 0.01 Gy. A similar study by Darby et al.[116] did not find a significant risk of leukemia and reported an ERR per Sv of 0.74 (95% CI −0.11, 1.59). Follow-up of patients who received intrauterine radium radiotherapy for benign uterine bleeding has been performed by Inskip et al.[117,118] Mortality due to leukemia was twice as high as expected in the general population. The average bone marrow dose was 0.53 Gy. A study of women with x-ray-induced menopause receiving a mean pelvic dose of about 7.35 Gy was reported by Brinkley and Haybittle.[119] They followed 277 women for a mean time of 16 years, observing no deaths from leukemia; however, in this study less than one death was expected on the basis of normal incidence.

A small excess incidence of leukemia was reported in children who were treated with radiotherapy for tinea capitis. One series involved 2872 children; however, risk estimates were difficult to make from these data, because the actual marrow dose was uncertain.[120] In another report on tinea capitus patients by Ron et al., the ERR per Sv was significantly elevated at 4.44 (95% CI 1.7, 8.7).[121] Damber et al. reported a cohort follow-up study

of patients treated for benign lesions of the locomotor system. The ERR for leukemia was nonsignificant.[122]

There are many follow-up reports of patients who received radiotherapy for treatment of malignant conditions. A case-control study of leukemia in a cohort of 150,000 women treated for cervical carcinoma showed a twofold excess of non–CLL but not of CLL. The estimated RR at 1 Gy was 1.7.[123] Boice et al. also conducted an incidence study for women treated for cervical cancer: 82,616 exposed women were compared with 99,424 unexposed controls.[124] The women were from Canada, Denmark, Finland, Norway, Sweden, Yugoslavia, the United Kingdom, and the United States. The study covered 1.28 million person-years at risk. Excess risk was found for leukemia in the first five years but not thereafter (Fig. 5-1). Kleinerman et al. reported a study that evaluated second cancers in 86,193 patients with cervical cancer reported to 13 cancer registries in 5 countries.[125] The observed/expected (O/E) ratio was slightly elevated for all leukemia in those who received radiotherapy at 1.2 (95% CI 1.0, 1.4) for all leukemias and 1.4 (95% CI 1.1, 1.7) for non–CLLs. The average dose was 7 Gy to the active marrow. The O/E was nonsignificantly raised for those with no radiotherapy at 1.2 (95% CI 0.7, 1.7) for all leukemias and 1.1 (95% CI 0.6, 1.0) in those who had received radiotherapy. In another study that matched 4188 women treated for cervical cancers and second cancers with 6880 controls, excess risk was again seen

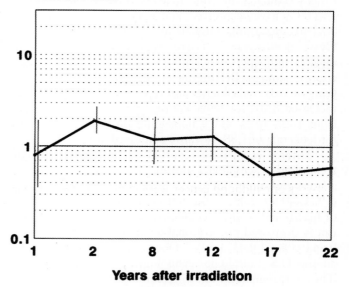

Acute and non-lymphocytic leukemia

Figure 5-1 • Relative risk (RR) of leukemia by time after treatment for cervical carcinoma with radiation therapy. Error bars indicate 95% CI (confidence interval). (From Boice JD, Jr, et al: Second cancers following radiation treatment for cervical cancer: An international collaboration among cancer registries. J Natl Cancer Inst 1985;74:955–975.)

for leukemia.[126] A case-control study, with a smaller number of persons, found no statistically significant excess risks for leukemia.[127] A Japanese study of cervical cancer patients reported on 5725 patients treated only with radiotherapy and 4161 patients treated only with surgery.[128] A significant excess was noted for cancer of the rectum and bladder, as well as for leukemia, in the radiotherapy group. Curtis et al. reviewed cancer after treatment for cancer of the uterine corpus. The ERR at 1 Sv for leukemia was nonsignificant at 0.10 (95% CI < 0.0, 0.23).[129]

Three follow-up studies of women treated for breast cancer were primarily directed at determining the risk of cancer in the other breast and the incidence of leukemia.[130–132] No statistically significant excess of leukemia was found. An additional 2004 report by Kaplan et al. indicated eight cases of leukemia were observed versus nine expected in 2866 patients.[133] Many of these studies are complicated by the use of chemotherapeutic agents (melphalan, and possibly cyclophosphamide) associated with leukemia induction. There have been reports of an increased incidence of acute leukemia in patients after treatment of Hodgkin's disease, multiple myeloma, breast cancer, and other neoplasms.[134–136] The etiology of the increased risk is unclear, and it may be related to radiation, chemotherapy, the primary disease, or even an underlying immunodeficiency. Brenner et al. have studied second malignancies in prostate carcinoma patients treated with radiotherapy or surgery and reported no significant increase in risk of leukemia after radiotherapy.[137]

A number of studies have examined the risk of second tumors after treatment for childhood cancers have been conducted but leukemia was not increased.[138,139] There was, however, a strong dose-response relationship between leukemia risk and the dose of alkylating agents. The RR of leukemia reached 23 in the highest chemotherapy dose group. A lower risk was seen for doxorubicin. The radiation dose had no influence on leukemia risk. Another study by Rosenberg et al. examining leukemia risk after MOPP chemotherapy showed an enhanced leukemia risk, but this was largely independent of radiation dose.[140] A report by Hawkins et al., in which over 16,000 survivors of childhood cancer were studied, indicated that radiation, as well as specific chemotherapies involving alkylating agents or epipodophyllotoxins, can induce secondary leukemias.[141] Follow-up of Hodgkin's disease survivors and leukemia incidence was reported by Kaldor et al., who found a marginally significant increase in ERR per Sv of 0.24 (95% CI 0.04, 0.43).[142]

The BEIR VII report has summarized risk factors for leukemia from a number of medical studies.[18] The ERRs per Gy range from 0.88 per Gy in women who received an average dose to the active bone marrow of 7 Gy from radiotherapy for cervical cancer to 12.4 per Gy in subjects treated with radiotherapy for ankylosing spondylitis (average dose 4.4 Gy). All other estimates of ERR per Gy, with average doses ranging from 0.1 to 2.0 Gy, are relatively close (in the range of 1 to 2.6).

Occupational Nuclear Workers

A large number of studies of leukemia in the occupational setting have been performed and most results are nonsignificant. There have been two large studies of nuclear workers in the United Kingdom. A study by Beral et al. included an analysis of 3373 deaths among 39,546 atomic energy workers during 1946–1979.[143] In a study of 22,552 atomic weapons workers, Beral et al. reported a rate ratio of 0.38 (95% CI 0.08, 3.36) for leukemia, indicating no excess.[144] Leukemia was above the national average but not at a statistically significant level. Another cohort analysis of the U.K. Registry of Radiation Workers by Kendall et al. included 95,217 workers over 1.2 million person-years at risk.[145] The report studied leukemia and did not find a significant excess of leukemia. A second analysis by Muirhead et al. in 1999 gave a nonsignificantly reduced SMR for non–CLL of 0.98 (95% CI 0.79, 1.20).[146]

Douglas et al. studied cancer mortality and morbidity among 14,282 workers with an average dose of 128 mSv per worker at the Sellafield plant of British Nuclear Fuels in which the SMR for leukemia was 0.81.[147] Another report on Sellafield by Omar et al. of nonplutonium workers had an insignificant decrease with an SMR for leukemia of 0.88 and a nonsignificant increase in incidence with a rate ratio of 1.25.[148] McGeoghegan et al. have studied the mortality and cancer morbidity experience of employees at the Chapelcross plant of British Nuclear Fuels from 1955–1995[149]; the cohort included 2628 workers with median doses of 39 mSv. The mean follow-up was 24.3 years and there were 63,967 person-years of study and the SMR for leukemia for radiation workers was nonsignificantly reduced at 0.98. No leukemia cases were found in the nonradiation workers.

Iwasaki et al. conducted a second analysis of mortality of nuclear industry workers in Japan.[150] The study included 176,000 male workers and 5527 deaths. Average annual doses were 3.5 mSv before 1982 and 1.2 mSv after 1982. For leukemia the SMR was nonsignificantly decreased at 0.89 (95% CI 0.68, 1.14). Artalejo et al. reported on mortality among 5657 workers of the former Spanish Nuclear Energy Board with mean exposure of 11.4 mSv.[151] The SMR for leukemia was nonsignificantly decreased with an SMR of 0.70 (95% CI 0.19, 1.80). Habib et al. have reported on cancer incidence among Australian nuclear industry–monitored radiation workers and indicated a nonsignificantly increased SIR of 1.38 for all leukemias.[152]

There are several Canadian occupational studies. In 2001, Sont et al. published the first analysis of cancer incidence and occupational radiation exposure based on the National Dose Registry of Canada.[153] It contained a cohort of 191,333 persons and had an average dose for males of 11.5 mSv and an average dose for the cohort of 6.64 mSv. The SIR for all leukemias for both males and females was significantly reduced at 0.69 (90% CI 0.53, 0.88) and 0.70 (90% CI 0.51, 0.96), respectively. In 1998 Ashmore et al. reported an analysis of mortality and occupational radiation exposure based on the National Dose Registry of Canada with a cohort of 206,620 individuals and with 5426 deaths.[154] The average exposure for males was 10.6 mSv and the SMR for leukemia was also significantly decreased at 0.77 (90% CI 0.61, 0.96). This study was updated and reported in 2004 by Zablotska et al., who concluded that there was a statistically significant ERR of non–CLL of 0.52 (95% CI 0.205, 291).[155] The authors noted, however, that the results were based on only eight cases of leukemia in workers at 1 or more mSv and indicated these risks are higher than those reported in other studies. Further, the difference could be due to chance and that additional follow-up could produce more stable risk estimates. It should also be noted that although the ERR for all leukemia was elevated, the SMR for non–CLL was nonsignificantly reduced at 0.80 (95% CI 0.47, 1.26).

There have been many occupational studies conducted in the United States. A study of workers at the Mound Facility in Ohio during 1947–1979 showed no significant increase for all tumors. An increase in leukemia was detected only when CLL was included.[156] Wiggs et al. pointed out that when CLL, which is not known to be related to radiation, was eliminated from the analysis, the strength of the association with dose was removed. This is another example of how results should be carefully analyzed. A combined cohort analysis of workers at Hanford, Rocky Flats, and Oak Ridge National Laboratory has been performed by Gilbert et al.[157] The Hanford cohort included 23,704 workers with 492,000 person-years at risk, the Rocky Flats cohort included 5897 persons and 83,000 person-years at risk, and the Oak Ridge cohort included 6332 persons over 130,000 person-years at risk. In each cohort there was an analysis for excess risks of leukemia. No statistically significant excess was identified in the combined analysis of all three facilities. In a 1993 update, Gilbert et al. found that the combined ERR estimate for leukemia was negative.[158] This ERR was −1.0 (90% CI < 0, 2.2) per Sv. Howe et al. have reported on the mortality of U.S. nuclear power industry workers and found a nonsignificantly increased risk of leukemia with an SMR of 1.07 (95% CI 0.71, 1.53).[159]

In 1997, Frome et al. updated the mortality study in a cohort of 106,020 Oak Ridge employees which included 27,982 deaths.[160] The SMR for all leukemias in white males was nonsignificantly reduced at 0.98, nonsignificantly increased for nonwhite males at 1.11, and nonsignificantly reduced for both white and nonwhite females at 0.82 and 0.57, respectively. Fry et al. conducted a study of mortality and morbidity among persons occupationally exposed to 50 or more mSv in a year.[161] There were 3145 subjects and 588 deaths. The mean external exposure

was 153 mSv. The SMR for all white males for leukemia was nonsignificantly reduced at 0.47 (95% CI 0.05, 1.68). In a separate analysis of U.S. Department of Energy (DOE) white male contractors there was no leukemia found. Study of an expanded cohort at the Portsmouth naval shipyard followed to the end of 1996 showed less leukemia than expected from national statistics although there was an increasing trend with dose.[162] The study had few cases and wide CIs.[163] Wiggs et al. found 44 cases of leukemia compared to 43.6 expected in a follow-up of Los Alamos workers.[164] In addition the trend with dose was negative for both ALL and CML. Groves et al. conducted a 40-year cancer mortality study of 40,581 Korean War Navy veterans with potential exposure to high-intensity radar equipment which also emits ionizing radiation.[165] The SMR for all leukemia was nonsignificantly increased at 1.14 (95% CI 0.90, 1.44).

Some authors have tried to improve on the statistical power of occupational studies by combining cohorts from different countries. Cardis et al. reported on cancer mortality among nuclear industry workers in three countries.[166] This is a large study of 95,673 workers and includes over 2 million person-years at risk and 15,825 deaths. The only statistically significant positive associations were with non–CLL and myeloma. The dose-response trend for all leukemia was 1.43 (P 0.076). The trend for all non–CLLs was 1.85 (P value of 0.046) and the trend for acute leukemias was nonsignificantly positive at 0.82 (P value of 0.206). No increase was identified when analyses were restricted to workers with less than 400 mSv. The largest study of nuclear workers was reported by Cardis et al. in 2005.[167,168] This was a retrospective cohort study involving facilities in 15 countries and included 407,391 workers and the ERR for leukemia (excluding CLL) was nonsignificantly elevated at 1.93 per Sv (95% CI of < 0 to 7.14). This value is intermediate between the values obtained by the linear and linear-quadratic models of atomic bomb survivors exposed between the ages of 20 to 60.

Information is available on radiation doses and the mortality of workers at the reactor and reprocessing plants at Chelyabinsk (Mayak) in Russia.[169–175] In this facility the radiation doses to workers were very large and the dose ranges were very wide. During the period 1949–1953, most workers received over 0.25 Gy annually. There is strong evidence of an increase in non–CLL with increasing dose. In a 40-year analysis of 931 workers who received an average accumulated gamma dose of 3.26 Gy, 6.2% died from leukemia. In the reprocessing plant during 1949–1953, the average gamma dose was 2.45 Gy, and follow-up of 1812 workers over 62,000 person-years revealed 25 leukemias observed versus 7 expected. For the 1479 workers of the period 1954–1958, followed over 44,000 person-years with an average cumulative dose of 7.16 Gy, the results are less dramatic. There were six leukemias observed versus

3.6 expected. In the most recent analysis by Shilnikova et al., it is estimated that of the 66 non–CLL deaths, 40% might be associated with occupational exposure.[175]

There have been recent reports on Chernobyl workers from the former Soviet Union but they only come from the Russian Federation, Latvia, and Estonia. Neither the Ukraine nor Belarus have worker registries that have provided useful follow-up. Ivanov et al. have reported that while there is an increase in registrations for leukemias among the workers, this is not likely due to radiation since there is no relationship to dose.[176] The estimated RR per Gy for all leukemia was insignificantly elevated at 0.24 (95% CI −3.89, 4.36) and as well for all non–CLLs at 1.67 (95% CI −5.90, 9.23). Konogorov et al. reported similar results with an ERR per Sv of 15.6 (95% CI −24.9, 56.1).[177] Rahu et al. have reported on cancer incidence of 5446 male Latvian and Estonian cleanup workers and indicate a nonsignificant SIR for leukemia and all non–CLL subtypes of leukemia.[178]

Internal Exposure

Radon

A number of studies have examined the potential relationship between radon and leukemia. Most all of the studies have been negative or nonsignificant. Kaletsch et al. concluded that there was no association between indoor residential radon exposure and childhood leukemia.[179] Lubin et al. conducted a case-control study relative to indoor radon and acute lymphoblastic leukemia.[180] There was no evidence for an association. A similar conclusion was reached by Law et al. in the United Kingdom regarding adult acute leukemia.[181] Steinbuch et al. studied the risk of childhood AML and radon exposure and concluded there was no association.[182]

Since miners are exposed to increased levels of radon, a number of studies have focused on these cohorts. Darby et al. studied the effect of radon on Swedish iron miners and found a nonsignificant increase in leukemia with an O/E ratio of 1.05 (95% CI 0.39, 2.30) and no evidence of a trend with increasing radon exposure.[183] Studies of other underground miners (including uranium miners) have been collated by Darby et al. and a review of these reveals an increase in leukemia in the first 10 years of employment but no association once CLL is excluded.[184] A review of the epidemiological evidence of radon and leukemia has been published by Laurier et al. which indicated no significant association between leukemia risk and cumulative exposure to radon decay products.[185] A 2004 update of French uranium miners by Laurier et al. reported a nonsignificant SMR of 1.7 for leukemia.[186] There has been a report by Tomasek on Czech miners that indicates an excess of leukemia after 20 years of exposure which was not thought to be related to radon or radon progeny but to uranium dust.[187] Comments by Laurier et al.[188] as well as Eatough[189] have questioned

the findings at long exposure times, and if there is such an association, the importance is slight. The BEIR VI Committee agreed with the findings of Darby that there is no need to consider cancers other than lung cancer in setting radiation protection standards and guidelines for underground miners.[190]

Occupational Exposure

Carpenter et al. examined workers in the United Kingdom who were occupationally exposed to tritium, plutonium, and other radionuclides.[191] The SMRs for leukemia in each group were all nonsignificant. Ritz et al. have reported on cancer mortality in uranium processing workers at the Fernald Plant in Ohio.[192] The SMR for leukemia was nonsignificantly increased at 1.16. Dupree-Ellis et al. have reported on mortality in a cohort of 2514 uranium processing workers employed between 1942 and 1966 at the Mallinkrodt Chemical Works.[193] The SMR for leukemia was nonsignificantly elevated at 1.11.

Medical Exposure

Each year, a large number of patients are treated with iodine 131 in whom the potential carcinogenic effects of therapeutic and diagnostic doses of radioiodine administered to perform thyroid scanning have been studied. There is a report of two cases of AML developing after the treatment of thyroid carcinoma by Roldan et al.[194] and two cases of CML after iodine 131 treatment for thyroid carcinoma have been reported by Shimon et al.[195] The significance of two case reports is doubtful, however, given the large number of patients treated and the nonsignificant results of large, controlled epidemiological studies.[196,197] One of the largest of these studies included 35,074 patients who were matched with the Swedish Cancer Registry, in which there was only a questionable increase in leukemia.[198] In the United States, in a Cooperative Thyrotoxicosis Therapy Follow-up Study of 19,200 patients, the subjects were followed for 8 years, and no increase in leukemia was found.[199,200] Ron et al.[201] reported on 35,593 hyperthyroid patients treated by different methods. The SMR for non–CLL in patients treated with any iodine 131 was nonsignificantly increased at 1.12 and in patients treated only with iodine 131 the SMR was nonsignificantly increased at 1.22. Another study followed 1000 patients treated at Mayo Clinic for an average of 15 years and compared them with surgically treated patients finding no increase in leukemia.[202] There are five follow-up studies in which patients treated with radioactive iodine for thyroid cancer were followed in Sweden,[203] the United Kingdom,[204] Denmark,[205] and Finland.[206] The study in Sweden followed 834 patients, and the SIR was above unity (1.0) for leukemia, but the difference was not statistically significant. The United Kingdom study had 258 patients and showed statistically significant excesses of leukemia. In a much larger subsequent study,[207] 47,000 Swedish patients who had received radioiodine for thyroid cancer, hyperthyroidism, and diagnostic purposes failed to show a statistically significant increased risk of leukemia. Rubino et al. have pooled data from Swedish, Italian, and French thyroid cancer survivors and found an increased EAR of 0.8 leukemia cases per GBq of iodine 131 with a RR of iodine compared to no-iodine therapy that was marginally significant at 2.5 (95% CI 1.0, 7.4).[208] Whether there was indeed a radiation contribution to leukemia was not possible to ascertain, however, because there was no analysis of dose response, due to the small number of leukemias and no analysis excluding CLL.

Thorotrast (thorium 232 dioxide) was used in the 1940s and 1950s as a contrast agent for diagnostic radiology and many of the follow-up studies show an increase in leukemia. In the case of thorium, the radiation is high-LET radiation and absorbed doses might be converted to equivalent dose using a radiation weighting factor of 20, although Harrison and Muirhead suggest that the relative biological effectiveness of alpha radiation relative to external low-LET radiation might be around only 2 to 3 in the case of leukemia.[209] An initial series including 3772 patients was followed over 30 years after an average dose of 25 mL of Thorotrast, and 44 cases of leukemia were identified.[210] The estimated bone marrow exposure was 2.7 Gy. It is of interest in this regard that only 7 of the 44 cases were CGL, and it is possible that this disease may have a different induction mechanism from that of the acute leukemias. Lifetime excess risk was estimated to be approximately 40 cases in 1 million persons for 0.01 Gy of alpha radiation. A number of more recent publications also indicate an association of Thorotrast with leukemia.[211–221] There is a 2003 report by dos Santos Silva et al. on the 50-year follow-up of mortality in Portuguese Thorotrast patients.[220] The cohort included 1096 systemically exposed and 240 locally exposed. The SMR for leukemia in the systemically exposed was significantly increased at 8.17 and the RR of systemically exposed versus locally exposed was also significantly increased at 10.2. Nyberg et al. reported on cancer incidence after a 40-year follow-up among Swedish patients exposed to radioactive Thorotrast.[222] The SIR for leukemia was significantly elevated at 6.1 (95% CI 2.9, 11.2).

Intravenous treatment with radium 224 has been given in Germany for various ailments, and Speiss et al. have reported a follow-up of some patients treated.[223] The average skeletal dose was estimated to be 1.8 to 2.8 Gy in the 816 traced patients. Two cases of leukemia were identified. A study by Nekolla et al. of 455 patients treated with radium 224 for TB, ankylosing spondylitis, and a few other diseases indicated that leukemias occurred in 8 patients compared to 3.8 expected; however, if the usual latent period or lag period was used, the statistical significance was lost.[224] Wick and Nekolla also reported

on late effects in ankylosing spondylitis patients treated with radium 224.[225] There were 626 exposed and 725 control patients with a mean follow-up time of 21 years. The mean injected activity was 0.17 megabequerel per kilogram (MBq/kg) and the mean alpha skeletal dose was 0.67 Gy. The study showed a statistically significant increase in the rate ratio for leukemia of 3 and an O/E ratio for those exposed of 13/4.2. The largest increase was for myeloid leukemia (P < 0.001). Radium treatment of ankylosing spondylitis in about 2000 children and adults with the disease from Germany has shown increased risk of leukemia.[226–228] Radium has been used in Europe for the treatment of tuberculosis. This ultimately proved ineffective and was discontinued; however, the intravenous radium led to an increased risk of leukemia.[229,230]

Radium 226 dial painters in the United States who were exposed between 1915 and 1929 have demonstrated a very large excess of bone cancers; data on those individuals have been reviewed by Polednak.[231] The number of deaths from leukemia[4] was greater than expected.[1] Unfortunately, risk coefficients could not be calculated because of uncertainties in the dosimetry. These findings have been contradicted by the more recent review of these workers by Spiers et al.[232] They indicate that, as of 1983, in 2940 radium dial painters, 10 leukemias were observed versus 9.24 expected, and no excess was identified. Of the 10 cases of leukemia, 3 were classified as AML, 3 as CLL, 2 as CGL, 1 as splenic, and 1 as chronic lymphatic. Reviews of older radium and leukemia studies by Rowland and Stebbings point to the difficulties encountered due to the differences in the classification of leukemias in the 1920s through the 1940s and currently.[233,234]

There have been several studies of patients treated with encapsulated radium for uterine hemorrhage. The combined studies examined over 6000 women, and no increase in incidence in leukemia was identified.[235,236] The studies are difficult to compare with other epidemiologic studies because of nonuniform radiation exposure of the marrow from radium. Hutchison suggested that the much higher doses used in treatment of cancer of the cervix resulted in cell killing rather than in induction of leukemia.[237] Recently there was a report by Kossman and Weiss of two cases of AML occurring after high-dose therapy with beta-emitting strontium 89 for prostate cancer.[238] The significance of this is unclear.

Polycythemia vera is an overproduction of red blood cells. If severe, it is treated by phlebotomy, radiation therapy, or chemotherapy. The radiation treatment is usually an intravenous injection of phosphorus 32. In a study by Modan et al., patients treated with phosphorus 32 had a cumulative incidence of leukemia of 15% versus 2% in nonirradiated patients.[239] In a study by Berk, the incidence was 6% in irradiated patients versus 1% in those treated by phlebotomy.[240] Sulfur 35 has been used in the treatment of chordomas and chondrosarcomas.

One small study reported that three out of nine patients developed leukemia.[241]

Occupational Exposure

Results of studies involving leukemia and occupational exposure to uranium, plutonium, and some other radionuclides have been largely nonsignificant. McGeoghegan et al. have studied the mortality of workers at two uranium-processing facilities. The mortality and cancer morbidity experience of workers at the Capenhurst uranium enrichment facility was studied from 1946–1995.[242] The cohort included 12,540 workers including 3244 radiation workers with mean doses of 9.8 mSv. The SMR for all leukemia was nonsignificantly reduced in both nonradiation workers and radiation workers at 0.67 and 0.69, respectively. The RR for radiation workers also was nonsignificantly reduced at 0.83. Their study of the mortality and cancer morbidity experience of workers at the Springfields uranium production facility, 1946–1995, included a cohort of 19,454 workers including 13,960 radiation workers with a mean external dose of 22.8 mSv and a mean follow-up period of 24.6 years or 479,146 person-years.[243] The SMR for all leukemia was nonsignificantly elevated in nonradiation workers at 1.12, and in radiation workers it was 1.00. The RR for radiation workers also was nonsignificantly reduced at 0.98. Recent reviews of the potential relation of enriched, natural, and delpleted uranium to leukemia risk have been published.[244,245] It was concluded that any possible leukemia risk would be significantly less than from lung cancer and that any risk from depleted uranium was not likely ever to be detectable. A meta-analysis of 14 studies including 120,000 uranium workers found a nonsignificantly reduced RR of 0.90 (95% CI 0.67, 1.14) for leukemia.[245] As mentioned earlier, multiple studies of populations living near uranium processing facilities have not shown an increase in leukemia.[89,90,90a] A Finnish study of radionuclides including uranium and radium in drinking water did not reveal an association with leukemia at levels assessed.[246]

A report on the Sellafield plant by Omar et al. reported an insignificant decrease with an SMR in plutonium workers for leukemia of 0.71 and the incidence was also reduced with a rate ratio of 0.58.[148] Carpenter et al. examined workers in the United Kingdom who were occupationally exposed to various radionuclides and the SMRs were all nonsignificant.[191] The SMR for leukemia was 0.55 for tritium exposures, 0.62 for plutonium, and 0.72 for other radionuclides. UNSCEAR 2006 has indicated that studies of groups exposed to uranium or plutonium have generally provided little indication, if any, of raised leukemia risks.[86]

Neutron Exposure

The neutron component of dose in the A-bomb LSS has been difficult to assess as it is small enough that a risk estimate for neutron induction of leukemia is not possible. There are only a few instances in which neutron exposure is known to be large. One of these was in the early criticality accidents at Los Alamos National Laboratories. Two of the seven long-term survivors died from AML 19 and 33 years after exposure.[247]

Summary

There is little doubt that non–CLL is induced by radiation, with a mean latency period of approximately 10 years in the atomic bomb survivors and shorter in persons with higher doses from radiotherapy. The tumors induced are either acute forms or CGL, with the acute forms tending to predominate. The 1990 International Commission on Radiological Protection (ICRP) Recommendations estimate the lifetime fatal probability coefficient to be 50 per 10^4 Sv^{-1} among a population of all ages from non–CLLs after exposure to low doses.[248] The risk at low doses is based on mathematical models since the large studies have not shown a statistically significant increase in leukemia at marrow doses of less than 400 mSv. Risk decreases at long times after exposure. The linear-quadratic dose-response model appears to be more appropriate than the linear nonthreshold model and has been used by ICRP 1990,[248] BEIR V[3] and VII[18] Committees, and the UNSCEAR 2006 Committee[86,249] with allowances for dependencies on sex, age at exposure, and time since exposure. Estimates of excess leukemia deaths estimated for a population of 100,000 of all ages and both sexes exposed to 0.1 Gy by different groups are quite similar as follows: BEIR V, 95[3]; ICRP, 50[250]; UNSCEAR 2000, 50[57]; and BEIR VII, 61.[18] Studies that have large enough doses, numbers of people, and statistical power to derive leukemia risks are shown in Table 5-3.

HODGKIN'S DISEASE

General

Hodgkin's disease (HD) is distinguished from other lymphomas by the presence of Reed-Sternberg cells. Incidence rates are higher in white rather than Asian populations. It is typically a disease of teenagers and young adults and is thought to be associated with viral infections such as the Epstein-Barr virus and with immunosuppression in HIV, AIDS, and allogenic bone marrow transplant patients. There also appears to be a significant genetic component with an elevated risk among identical versus fraternal twins.

External and Internal Exposure

There are three papers concerning potential environmental uranium contamination and the possibility of an increased risk of HD in the public. The papers by Boice et al. indicated a nonsignificant elevation of HD around a uranium mining and milling facility in Texas, a nonsignificant decrease near a uranium facility in Pennsylvania, and a nonsignificantly elevated SMR near a Colorado facility.[89,90,90a] A nonsignificant decrease was found by

Table 5-3 • Risk Estimates for Cancer Incidence and Mortality from Studies of Radiation Exposure: Leukemia*

Study	Average Excess Relative Risk at 1 Sv	Average Excess Absolute Risk $(10^4 PYSv)^{-1}$
External Low-LET Exposures		
Incidence		
A-bomb Life Span Study[12]		
Males	4.66 (3.07–6.88)	4.14 (3.06–5.39)
Females	5.05 (3.24–7.61)	2.41 (1.71–3.23)
Age at exposure		
<20	8.27 (4.95–13.66)	2.79 (1.99–3.74)
0–40	3.59 (2.01–5.97)	2.69 (1.7–3.9)
>40	3.98 (2.32–6.45)	4.68 (3.1–6.57)
Time since exposure		
5–15	13.78 (8.67–22.24)	5.19 (3.97–6.60)
15–30	4.37 (2.53–7.16)	2.41 (1.55–3.45)
>30	0.88 (0.17–2.02)	1.09 (0.33–2.19)
All	4.84 (3.59–6.44)	3.08 (2.47–3.77)
Cervical cancer case control[6]	0.74 (0.1–3.8)	0.50 (0.1–2.6)
Cancer of the uterine corpus[129]	0.10 (<0.0–0.23)	NA
Benign lesions in the locomotor system[122]	0.70 (−0.43–3.48)	1.14
Hodgkin's disease[142]	0.24 (0.04–0.43)	NA
Breast cancer therapy[132]	0.19 (0.00–0.6)	0.89 (0.00–3.0)
Techa River population[251]	1.84 (0.9–3.1)	0.91 (0.4–5)
U.K. childhood cancers[141]	0.24 (0.01–1.28)	NA
International childhood cancer[139]	0.0 (0.0–0.004)	NA
Chernobyl recovery operation workers in Russian Federation[177]	15.6 (−24.9–56.1)	NA
Testicular cancer[252]	0.37 (0.12–1.3)	NA
Canada National Dose Registry[153]	2.7 (<0–18.8)	NA
China medical x-ray workers[253]		
Employed before 1970	2.5 (1.2–4.1)	1.0 (0.5–1.6)
Employed only 1970–1980	8.9 (−1.1–25)	1.7 (−0.2–4.6)
Mortality		
A-bomb Life Span Study[9]		
Males	4.07 (2.75–5.84)	3.23 (2.41–4.18)
Females	3.96 (2.57–5.87)	<0 (<0–291.33)
Age at exposure		
<20	6.63 (4.21–10.26)	<0 (<0–271.86)
20–40	3.07 (1.81–4.87)	2.39 (1.56–3.39)
>40	3.15 (1.74–5.24)	3.46 (2.12–5.09)
Time since exposure		
5–15	10.24 (6.34–16.59)	3.92 (2.90–5.13)
15–30	3.82 (2.13–6.40)	1.87 (1.19–2.69)
>30	1.97 (1.09–3.18)	<0 (<0–396.31)
All	4.02 (3.02–5.26)	2.31 (1.85–2.82)
Benign lesions in the locomotor system[122]	0.52	1.14
Ankylosing spondylitis[110]	0.02 (−0.07–0.29)	NA
Benign gynecological disease[117]	2.97	1.25 (0.9–1.7)
Massachusetts TB fluoroscopy[105]	< −0.2 (< −0.2–4.5)	< −0.2 (< −0.2–5.1)
Israeli tinea capitis[121]	4.44 (1.7–8.7)	0.95 (0.4–1.9)
Stockholm skin hemangioma[111]	1.6 (−0.6–5.5)	NA
Metropathia hemorrhagica[116]	0.74 (−0.11–1.59)	0.85
Peptic ulcer[113]	0.91 (<0–4.38)	NA
IARC 15-country nuclear workers study[167,168]	1.93 (<0–7.14)	NA
Nuclear workers in Canada, United Kingdom, United States[166]	2.18 (0.13–5.7)	NA
U.K. National Registry for Radiation Workers[146]	2.55 (−0.03–7.16)	NA
Nuclear power industry workers in the United States[159]	5.67 (−2.56–30.4)	NA
Mayak workers[175]	1.0 (0.5–2.0)	NA
U.S. Oak Ridge X-10 and Y-12[160]	<0 (<0–6.5)	NA
U.S. Los Alamos Laboratory workers[164]	~0	NA
U.S. Portsmouth shipyard workers[162,163]	10.88 (−0.90–38.77)	33.8 (16.8–50.7)
Nuclear industry workers in Japan[150]	0.01 (−10.0–10.0)	NA
Japanese radiological technologists[95]	0.7 (−0.4–2.1)	0.4 (−0.2–1.2)
Yangjiang background radiation[34,35]	1.61 (<0–28.4)	NA

*The studies listed are those for which quantitative estimates of risk could be made.

Table 5-3 • Risk Estimates for Cancer Incidence and Mortality from Studies of Radiation Exposure: Leukemia*—cont'd

Study	Average Excess Relative Risk at 1 Sv	Average Excess Absolute Risk $(10^4 PYSv)^{-1}$
Internal Low-LET Exposures		
Incidence		
Chernobyl-related exposure in Belarus, Russian Federation and Ukraine[254]	32.4 (9.78–84.0)	NA
Chernobyl-related exposure in Ukraine[68]	2.5 (1.1–5.4)	NA
Mortality		
Extended Techa River cohort[76,255]	6.5 (1.8–24)	2.9 (0.8–4.4)
Extended Techa River cohort: leukemia case-control study[77]	4.6 (1.7–12.3)	NA
Semipalatinsk: leukemia case-control study[74]	~0.1	NA
Thyroid cancer patients[208]	0.39 per GBq (?–1.54)	8 per GBq per 10^4 PY
U.S. thyrotoxicosis[201]	−1.0	NA
Internal High-LET Exposures	**Average Relative Risk**	
Incidence		
Danish and Swedish Thorotrast patients[219]	15.2 (4.4–149.6)	
^{224}Ra ankylosing spondylitis patients[225]	2.4	
Uranium in drinking water in Finland[246]	0.91 (0.73–1.13)	
Mortality		
Radon-exposed miners[184]	NA	
German Thorotrast patients[221]	4.9	
Japanese Thorotrast patients (combined data)[214]	12.5 (4.5–34.7)	
U.S. Thorotrast patients[219]	16.8 (0.6–211.7)	
Portuguese Thorotrast patients[220]	10.2 (1.24–471)	

*The studies listed are those for which quantitative estimates of risk could be made.
Adapted from United Nations Scientific Committee of the Effects of Atomic Radiation (UNSCEAR): Sources and effects of ionizing radiation: 2006 report to the General Assembly with annexes. New York, United Nations, 2007.

Boice et al. in a study of persons residing near the Hanford National Laboratory site.[91]

Ashmore et al. reported the first analysis of mortality and occupational radiation exposure based on the National Dose Registry of Canada which included a cohort of 206,620 individuals and 5426 deaths.[154] The average exposure for males was 10.6 mSv. The SMR for HD was nonsignificant at 0.79 (90% CI 0.50, 1.16). Frome reported a mortality study of 106,020 employees in the nuclear industry at Oak Ridge, Tennessee, and the SMR for HD in black and white males and females was nonsignificantly different from unity.[160] Wiggs et al. found a nonsignificant SMR for HD of 0.94 in a follow-up of Los Alamos workers.[164] McGeoghegan et al. reported on the mortality and cancer morbidity experience of employees at the Chapelcross plant of British Nuclear Fuels during 1955–1995.[149] The cohort included 2628 workers with median doses of 39 mSv and among the radiation workers, no cases of HD were found. A second analysis in 1999 of 124,743 workers in the United Kingdom National Registry of Radiation Workers by Muirhead et al., using a lagged analysis, reported a nonsignificantly reduced SMR for HD of 0.89 (95% CI 0.52, 1.42).[146] A report on the Sellafield plant by Omar et al. found a significant decrease in HD among nonplutonium workers with an SMR of 0.30.[148] In plutonium workers

there was an insignificant increase with an SMR of 2.95. Incidence in both groups of workers was nonsignificantly increased.

Artalejo et al. reported on mortality among 5657 workers of the former Spanish Nuclear Energy Board with mean exposure of 11.42 mSv.[151] The SMR for HD was nonsignificant at 1.26 (95% CI 0.41, 4.53). Habib et al. have reported on cancer incidence among Australian nuclear industry–monitored radiation workers and indicated a nonsignificant SIR of 1.62 for HD.[152] Sont et al. performed an analysis of cancer incidence and occupational radiation exposure based on the National Dose Registry of Canada and included a cohort of 191,333 persons with an average dose for males of 11.5 mSv and an average dose for the cohort of 6.64 mSv.[153] The SIR for HD in males was significantly reduced at 0.76 and in females it was nonsignificantly decreased at 0.97. Rahu et al. reported on cancer incidence of 5446 male Latvian and Estonian Chernobyl cleanup workers and indicated a nonsignificant SIR of 1.29 for HD.[178] Cardis et al. reported on cancer mortality among nuclear industry workers in three countries in a large study of 95,673 workers, which included over 2 million person-years at risk with 15,825 deaths.[166] The trend for HD was nonsignificant at 0.28 with a P value of 0.39. Cardis et al. have reported the cancer mortality results from a 15-country collaborative study of nuclear workers.[168] This is the largest occupational study to date and included a cohort of 407,391 workers with 18,993 deaths and 5.2 million person-years of follow-up. The ERR per Sv for HD was nonsignificantly negative at −0.18 (90% CI < 0, 7.25).

McGeoghegan et al. have reported on the mortality of 12,540 workers (including 3244 radiation workers) at the Capenhurst uranium enrichment facility during 1946–1995.[242] The SMR for HD was nonsignificantly elevated in radiation workers at 1.77. They also studied cancer mortality experience of 19,454 workers (including 13,960 radiation workers) at the Springfields uranium production facility during 1946–1995 and the SMR for HD was nonsignificantly elevated in radiation workers at 1.24.[243] Darby et al. studied cancers in Swedish iron miners and found a nonsignificant increase in HD with an O/E ratio of 2.70 (95% CI 0.74, 6.92).[183] Carpenter et al. examined workers in the United Kingdom who were occupationally exposed to tritium, plutonium, and other radionuclides.[191] The SMRs for HD in each group were all nonsignificantly reduced. Ritz et al. have reported on cancer mortality in uranium processing workers at the Fernald Plant in Ohio.[192] The SMR for was nonsignificantly increased at 2.04. Dupree-Ellis et al. have reported on mortality in a cohort of 2514 uranium processing workers employed between 1942 and 1966 at the Mallinkrodt Chemical Works.[193] The SMR for HD was nonsignificant at 0.92. Damber et al. reported a cohort follow-up study of patients treated for benign lesions of the locomotor system. The ERR at 1 Sv for HD was nonsignificant at 0.30 for incidence and 0.93 for mortality.[122]

Doody et al. reported on mortality among 143,517 U.S. radiologic technologists during 1926–1990 whose doses were not evaluated.[97] The SMR for HD was nonsignificantly reduced at 0.87 (95% CI 0.58, 1.26). Sigurdson et al. studied cancer incidence in 90,305 U.S. radiologic technologists and found that the SIR for HD was nonsignificantly elevated at 1.40 (95% CI 0.96, 1.98).[101] Mohan et al. studied cancer and other causes of mortality among 146,022 radiologic technologists employed from 1940 and later.[98,99] The SMR for HD in males was nonsignificantly reduced at 0.61 (95% CI 0.3, 1.2) and for females it was nonsignificantly increased at 1.06 (95% CI 0.7, 1.6). Carr et al. performed a follow-up study of 3719 patients treated with radiotherapy for peptic ulcer with doses to the abdomen of about 15 Gy.[113] No cases of HD were found after radiotherapy in the period 0 to 10 years postexposure or in the follow-up period of 11 to 62 years postexposure.

Summary

With the exception of what are thought to be statistical chance associations, radiation has not been associated with the development of Hodgkin's disease.[158,243] The wide confidence limits are due to the small number of cases or in many instances only a single case of HD occurring. UNSCEAR 2000 concluded that the available data did not indicate an association between HD and external or internal radiation exposure, but that the data were limited.[256] The UNSCEAR 2006 report summarized radiation risk factors for HD (Table 5-4) and concluded that there is no clear indication of an excess of the disease associated with radiation exposure; however, the data remain sparse and lack dose-response analysis.[86] The U.K. Compensation Scheme for Radiation-linked Diseases does not include HD because it was concluded that there was no association with radiation exposure. Hodgkin's disease also is not compensable under the U.S. radiation compensation acts (RECA 1990, REVCA 1988, and EEOICPA 2000). A 2006 U.S. National Academy of Sciences Committee was asked to reevaluate the scientific literature and concluded that epidemiologic studies failed to show any significant association between Hodgkin's disease and radiation exposure and that it should not be listed as a radiation compensable disease.[257]

NON-HODGKIN'S LYMPHOMA

External Exposure

Background and Populations Near Nuclear Facilities

For non-Hodgkin's lymphoma (NHL) the data regarding possible radiogenic induction are variable but generally negative.[3,18] Boice has indicated that any association between radiation exposure and NHL is weak and inconsistent.[258] A paper on a high natural background area of China was published in 2000 by Tao et al. and had 1.7 million person-years of study from 1979–1995.[33] The authors did not find a radiation effect and the RR of lymphoma was 0.98. There are two papers concerning potential environmental uranium contamination and the possibility of NHL in the public. The papers by Boice et al. indicated no increase around a uranium mining and milling facility in Texas and a nonsignificant increase near a uranium facility in Pennsylvania.[89,90] Additionally, no difference was found by Boice et al. in a study of persons residing near the Hanford, Washington site.[91] Increased exposure to natural cosmic irradiation occurs in airline crews and one study reported on lymphoma incidence. Band et al., in a study of 2740 pilots at doses of 6 mSv per year for an average of 20 years and total average dose of about 120 mSv, found a nonsignificantly decreased SIR for NHL and a nonsignificantly decreased SMR.[40]

Atomic Bomb Survivors

The 1950–1987 LSS incidence study by Preston et al. found no significant increase of NHL. In this study,

Table 5-4 • Risk Estimates for Cancer Incidence and Mortality from Studies of Radiation Exposure: Hodgkin's Disease*

Study	Average Excess Relative Risk at 1 Sv	Average Excess Absolute Risk $(10^4 PYSv)^{-1}$
External Low-LET Exposures		
Incidence		
Life Span Study[11]	0.43 (1.6–3.5)	0.04 (–0.1–0.3)
Cervical cancer cohort[125]	–0.005 (–0.06–0.08)	–0.001 (–0.02–0.02)
Benign lesions in the locomotor system[122]	0.30 (–1.01–7.38)	NA
Canada National Dose Registry[153]	64.8 (<0–591.3)	NA
Mortality		
Benign lesions in the locomotor system[122]	0.93	0.33
Ankylosing spondylitis[110]	0.15	0.04
Benign gynecological disease[117]	0.43	0.2
U.K. National Registry for Radiation Workers[146]	<–1.95 (<–1.95–2.84)	NA
IARC 15-country nuclear workers study[167,168]	–0.18 (<0, 7.25)	
Internal Low-LET Exposures		
Mortality		
U.S. thyrotoxicosis[201]	–1.0	NA
Internal High-LET Exposures		
Incidence		
Danish Thorotrast patients[213]	1.6 (0.06–40.4)	NA
Danish and Swedish Thorotrast patients[219]	1.5 (0.1–81.8)	NA
Mortality		
German Thorotrast patients[221]	0.8	NA
U.S. Thorotrast patients[219]	∞ (0.0–∞)	NA

*The studies listed are those for which quantitative estimates of risk could be made.
Adapted from United Nations Scientific Committee of the Effects of Atomic Radiation (UNSCEAR): Sources and effects of ionizing radiation: 2006 report to the General Assembly with annexes. New York, United Nations, 2007.

76 cases of NHL were observed versus 72 expected, which was not statistically significant even at the 90% confidence level.[11]

Occupational Exposure

Cancer incidence among medical diagnostic workers in China has been reviewed by Wang et al. who compared 27,011 workers with 25,782 persons in other medical specialties.[102] The x-ray workers had a 50% higher risk of developing cancer (RR 1.5, 95% CI 1.3, 1.7); however, there was no excess of lymphoma. The doses to the workers were likely to be on the order of 1 Gy or more. Berrington et al. have reported on 100 years' experience in U.K. radiologists and reported a significantly increased SMR for NHL of 2.41 for those employed after 1920.[94] Burnett et al. studied the mortality of health and science technicians and found a nonsignificantly decreased proportional mortality ratio for NHL of 0.83 (95% CI 0.41, 1.48).[96] Mohan et al. studied cancer and other causes of mortality among 146,022 radiologic technologists employed from 1940 and later among whom the SMR for NHL in males was nonsignificantly different from unity at 1.01 (95% CI 0.7, 1.6) and, for females, at 0.98 (95% CI 0.7, 1.1).[98,99] Sigurdson et al. studied cancer incidence in 90,305 U.S. radiologic technologists and found that the

SIR for NHL was nonsignificantly elevated at 1.14 (95% CI 0.95, 1.34).[101]

Several large studies of nuclear workers in the United Kingdom have been performed. A study by Beral et al. of atomic energy workers found NHL was above the national average but not at a statistically significant level.[143] In another study, Beral et al. examined deaths among a group of 22,552 atomic weapons workers. No excess was found for NHL with a rate ratio of 0.90 (95% CI 0.16 to 12.43).[144] A cohort analysis of the U.K. National Registry of Radiation Workers by Kendall et al. did not find a significant excess of NHL.[145] A second analysis in 1999 of 124,743 workers in the U.K. National Registry of Radiation Workers by Muirhead et al. using a lagged analysis reported a nonsignificantly increased SMR for NHL of 1.05 (95% CI 0.83, 1.30).[146] McGeoghegan et al. reported on the mortality and cancer morbidity experience of employees at the Chapelcross plant of British Nuclear Fuels during 1955–1995.[149] The cohort included 2628 workers with median doses of 39 mSv. In radiation workers the SMR for NHL was nonsignificant and decreased at 0.89. A report on the Sellafield plant by Omar et al. of nonplutonium workers had an insignificant decrease of NHL with an SMR of 0.98 and for plutonium workers there was an insignificant increase of 1.47.[148] For incidence of NHL there was a significant decrease in nonplutonium workers and a nonsignificant decrease in plutonium workers. Carpenter et al. studied workers in the United Kingdom who were occupationally exposed to tritium, plutonium, and other radionuclides and the SMRs for NHL in each group were all nonsignificant.[191] Habib et al. have reported on the cancer incidence among Australian nuclear industry–monitored radiation workers and indicated a nonsignificant SIR of 0.51 for NHL.[152] Iwasaki et al. conducted a second analysis of mortality of nuclear industry workers in Japan.[150] The study included 176,000 male workers with 5527 deaths. Average annual doses were 3.5 mSv before 1982 and 1.2 mSv after 1982 and for NHL the SMR was nonsignificantly decreased at 0.80 (95% CI 0.59, 1.07).

Large additional studies of United States and Canadian nuclear workers did not find an excess of lymphoma.[157,158,259,260] In the latter study there were seven cases observed versus 8.5 expected. Ashmore et al. reported the first analysis of mortality and occupational radiation exposure based on the National Dose Registry of Canada which included a cohort of 206,620 individuals and 5426 deaths.[154] The average exposure for males was 10.6 mSv. The SMR for NHL was nonsignificantly reduced at 0.87 (90% CI 0.68, 1.10). Sont et al. also reported on incidence and occupational radiation exposure based on the National Dose Registry of Canada and included a cohort of 191,333 persons with an average dose for males of 11.5 mSv and an average dose for the cohort of 6.64 mSv.[153] The SIR for NHL in males was significantly decreased at 0.71 and in females it was also significantly reduced at 0.71. In 2004, Zablotska et al. reported on mortality of Canadian nuclear workers and concluded that for NHL there was nonsignificantly decreased SMR of 0.71 (95% CI 0.43, 1.11).[155] Frome reported a mortality study of 106,020 employees in the nuclear industry at Oak Ridge, Tennessee.[160] The SMR for lymphosarcoma in black and white males and females was nonsignificant. Groves et al. conducted a 40-year cancer mortality study of 40,581 Korean War Navy veterans with potential exposure to high-intensity radar equipment, which also emits ionizing radiation, among whom the SMR for NHL was nonsignificantly decreased at 0.89 (95% CI 0.72, 1.09).[165]

Cardis et al. reported on cancer mortality among nuclear industry workers in three countries.[166] This is a very large study of 95,673 workers and includes over 2 million person-years at risk and 15,825 deaths. The trend for NHL was nonsignificant at −0.25 with a P value of 0.60. Cardis et al. have reported the cancer mortality results from a 15-country collaborative study of nuclear workers.[168] This is the largest occupational study to date and included a cohort of 407,391 workers with 18,993 deaths and 5.2 million person-years of follow-up. The ERR per Sv for NHL was nonsignificantly positive at 0.44 (90% CI < 0, 4.78).

McGeoghegan et al. have reported on the mortality of 12,540 workers (including 3244 radiation workers) at the Capenhurst uranium enrichment facility during 1946–1995.[242] The SMR for NHL was nonsignificantly elevated in radiation workers at 1.09. They also studied cancer mortality experience of 19,454 workers (including 13,960 radiation workers) at the Springfields uranium production facility during 1946–1995.[243] The SMR for NHL was nonsignificantly reduced for radiation workers at 0.63. Ritz et al. reported on cancer mortality in uranium processing workers at the Fernald Plant in Ohio and the SMRs for lymphosarcoma and lymphopoietic cancers were nonsignificantly different from unity.[192] Dupree-Ellis et al. have reported on mortality in a cohort of 2514 uranium processing workers employed between 1942 and 1966 at the Mallinkrodt Chemical Works and the SMR for lymphosarcoma was nonsignificant at 0.28.[193] A meta-analysis of 14 studies, which included 120,000 uranium workers, found a statistically significant reduced RR of 0.82 (95% CI 0.71, 0.92) for NHL.[245] Rahu et al. have reported on cancer incidence of 5446 male Latvian and Estonian Chernobyl cleanup workers and indicated a nonsignificant SIR of 1.57 for NHL among these workers.[178]

Medical Exposure

Data on in utero diagnostic x-ray exposure from the Oxford Study suggested an elevated risk of lymphoma,[261] while a study of twins in the United States did not show an excess.[262] A slight risk of NHL was reported by Darby et al. in patients treated for ankylosing spondylitis.[109] Follow-up of patients who received intrauterine radium radiotherapy for benign uterine bleeding has been performed by Inskip et al. who found there was no increase in hematopoietic cancer other than leukemia.[118] A more recent update apparently indicated a statistically significant increase in lymphoma.[117] This finding is inconsistent with most other studies including the LSS. Griem et al. followed a population of patients who had radiotherapy treatment for peptic ulcer and reported a nonsignificant increase in RR of 1.9 (95% CI 0.7 to 5.0) for NHL.[112] Carr et al. performed a follow-up study of the same group of 3719 patients treated with radiotherapy for peptic ulcer with doses to the abdomen of about 15 Gy.[113] The RR for NHL in the period 0 to 10 years postexposure was nonsignificantly elevated at 3.2, and in the follow-up period of 11 to 62 years postexposure the RR was also nonsignificant at 2.0. In the group of Massachusetts TB patients treated using repeated fluoroscopy, there was no evidence of an increased risk of NHL.[105] Mattsson et al. have reported on cancer incidence among 3090 women who received radiation therapy for benign breast disease and the RR for lymphoma was nonsignificant at 0.68.[114] Damber et al. reported a cohort follow-up study of patients treated for benign lesions of the locomotor system among whom the ERR at 1 Sv for NHL was nonsignificantly elevated at 0.02.[122]

In an international incidence study of women treated for cervical cancer, there were 82,616 exposed women compared with 99,424 unexposed controls, and no excess was identified for lymphoma.[124] In another study, 4188 women treated for cervical carcinoma who developed subsequent second cancers were compared with 6880 controls, a nonsignificant EAR of NHL was seen.[126]

Internal Exposure

Ron et al. reported on 35,593 hyperthyroid patients treated by different methods.[201] The SMR for lymphoma in patients treated with any iodine 131 was nonsignificantly increased at 1.16 and in patients only treated with iodine 131, it was nonsignificantly decreased at 0.85. An increased incidence of malignant neoplasms of the lymphatic system (other than leukemia) was identified by Archer et al. in U.S. uranium workers, with four such neoplasms versus the one that was expected.[263] This is unexpected given the biodistribution of uranium, radon, and radon daughter products. Darby et al. studied radon and cancers in Swedish iron miners and found a nonsignificant decrease in NHL with an O/E ratio of 0.76 (95% CI 0.16, 2.22).[183] Elevated lymphoma risks (15 cases) were reported in the German Thorotrast Study.[211] In the Danish Thorotrast Study, four cases of NHL were observed, however, expected values were not given.[264]

Summary

Risk estimates that can be derived from epidemiological studies were summarized in the UNSCEAR 2006 report (Table 5-5).[86] Inspection of the table shows that the vast majority of scientific studies in which risk factors can be obtained do not show evidence of an association of NHL with radiation exposure. There remains little data with regard to internal low-LET or high-LET radiation. UNSCEAR 2000[256] and 2006[86] Committee reports concluded that "the results from studies of NHL among groups exposed to external low-LET radiation are mixed, with little evidence of an association overall."[86] In spite of the large body of scientific evidence showing little, if any, association of NHL with low-LET radiation, the U.S. radiation compensation programs (RECA 1990, REVCA 1988, and EOICPA 2000) do list NHL as a compensable disease.

MULTIPLE MYELOMA

External Exposure

Until about 1990, the risk of multiple myeloma was thought to be increased by radiation exposure[3]; although, as more evidence has accumulated, this seems unlikely to be the case.

Fallout and Populations Near Nuclear Facilities

There have been multiple analyses of U.K. atomic test veterans by Darby et al.,[52] Doll et al.,[53] and Muirhead et. al.[54] In the latest 2004 review Muirhead

et al. studied a cohort of 21,357 test participants and reported a nonsignificantly decreased SMR of 0.96 (95% CI 0.61, 1.47) for myeloma in test participants but a nonsignificantly increased risk compared to controls.[55] The RR compared to controls for incidence was nonsignificantly elevated at 1.14. There are two papers concerning potential uranium environmental contamination and the possibility of multiple myeloma in the public. The papers by Boice et al. reported a nonsignificant increase surrounding a uranium mining and milling facility in Texas and a nonsignificant decrease near a uranium facility located in Pennsylvania.[89,90] No difference was found by Boice et al. in a study of persons living near the Hanford National Laboratory site.[91]

Atomic Bomb Survivors

The LSS mortality study data as of 1985 demonstrated statistically significant increases in multiple myeloma.[10] A more recent LSS incidence study by Preston et al. did not find an increase of multiple myeloma.[11] For the 41,000 persons who received 0.01 Sv or more and a mean dose of 0.23 Sv, there were 30 cases observed and 29 expected in over 1 million person-years of study. This study has included a large number of new cancer cases. Several of the incidence cases used in earlier reports were excluded from the new analysis as a result of dose-range restrictions or because of rejection in recent review of the actual cases. Consequently, in the LSS there is no longer a significant association between radiation exposure and myeloma.

Occupational Exposure

Cancer incidence among medical diagnostic workers in China has been reviewed by Wang et al. who compared 27,011 workers with 25,782 persons in other medical specialties.[102] The x-ray workers had a 50% higher risk of developing cancer (RR 1.5, 95% CI 1.3, 1.7); however, there was no excess of multiple myeloma. Doody et al. reported on mortality among 143,517 U.S. radiologic technologists during 1926–1990.[97] Doses were not evaluated. The SMR for myeloma was nonsignificantly reduced at 0.71 (95% CI 0.45, 1.06). Berrington et al. have reported on 100 years of U.K. radiologists and a nonsignificantly increased SMR for myeloma of 1.72 for those employed after 1920.[94] Mohan et al. studied cancer and other causes of mortality among 146,022 radiologic technologists employed from 1940 and later.[98,99] The SMR for myeloma in males was nonsignificantly increased at 1.13 (95% CI 0.7, 1.7) and for females it was nonsignificantly reduced at 0.91 (95% CI 0.6, 1.3). Sigurdson et al. studied cancer incidence in 90,305 U.S. radiologic technologists and found that the SIR for myeloma was nonsignificantly reduced at 0.90 (95% CI 0.57, 1.36).[101]

One of the largest occupational groups studied comprises those persons who have worked at atomic energy

Table 5-5 • Risk Estimates for Cancer Incidence and Mortality from Studies of Radiation Exposure: Non-Hodgkin's Lymphoma*

Study	Average Excess Relative Risk at 1 Sv	Average Excess Absolute Risk $(10^4 PYSv)^{-1}$
External low-LET Exposures		
Incidence		
A-bomb Life Span Study[12]		
Males	0.44 (−0.16–1.42)	0.46 (0.04–1.16)
Females	−0.22 (< −0.22–0.40)	0.00 (<−0.28)
Age at exposure		
<20	0.45 (<0–2.16)	0.18 (<0–0.61)
20–40	−0.12 (< −0.12–0.73)	0.03 (<0–0.63)
>40	0.09 (<0–1.04)	−0.11 (< −0.11–1.72)
Time since exposure		
5–15	0.33 (<0–2.14)	0.24 (−0.01–0.70)
15–30	0.33 (<0–1.44)	0.09 (<0–0.71)
>30	−0.22 (< −0.22–0.45)	−0.17 (< −0.17–2.28)
All	0.08 (<0–0.62)	0.12 (<0–0.40)
Cervical cancer case control[6]	0.21 (−0.03–0.93)	NA
Benign lesions in the locomotor system[122]	0.02	0.05
Canada National Dose Registry[153]	6.6 (<0–28.3)	NA
U.S. case control–occupational exposure[265]	(P = 0.66)	NA
U.K. Springfields uranium workers[243]	20.62 (< −5.69–86.62)	NA
Mortality		
A-bomb Life Span Study[8]		
Males	0.25 (<0–6.41)	0.18 (<0–0.81)
Females	−0.06 (<0–0.22)	−0.12 (<0–0.47)
Total	0.01 (<0–0.42)	0.01 (<0–0.23)
Benign lesions in the locomotor system[122]	−0.31	−0.40
Ankylosing spondylitis[266]	0.17	0.77
Benign gynecological disease[117]	−0.05 (< −0.2–0.2)	−0.08 (< −0.3–0.3)
Massachusetts TB fluoroscopy[105]	−0.05 (< −0.2–6.5)	−0.04 (< −0.2–5.4)
Peptic ulcer[113]	0.65 (<0–3.28)	NA
Nuclear workers in Canada, United Kingdom, and United States[166]	<0	<0
U.K. National Registry for Radiation Workers[146]	0.03 (−1.33–3.06)	NA
Nuclear power industry workers in the United States[159]	61.3 (−2.51–313)	NA
U.S. Oak Ridge workers, 1943–47[267] (Lymphosarcoma, reticulosarcoma, ICD8-200)	<0	<0
U.S. Los Alamos Laboratory workers[164]	>0	NA
Nuclear industry workers in Japan[150]	<0	<0
IARC 15-country nuclear workers study[167,168]	0.44 (<0, 4.78)	
Internal Low-LET Exposures		
Mortality		
U.S. thyrotoxicosis[201]	0.6	
Internal High-LET Exposures	**Average Relative Risk**	
Incidence		
Danish and Swedish Thorotrast patients[219]	1.6 (0.3–11.4)	
^{224}Ra ankylosing spondylitis patients[268]	~2	
Mortality		
German Thorotrast patients[221]	~2.5	

*The studies listed are those for which quantitative estimates of risk could be made.
Adapted from United Nations Scientific Committee of the Effects of Atomic Radiation (UNSCEAR): Sources and effects of ionizing radiation: 2006 report to the General Assembly with annexes. New York, United Nations, 2007.

facilities or nuclear installations. Initially, a number of reports suggested increases, in the United States, of multiple myeloma. More recent, larger, and better-designed studies have not confirmed these findings. In the United Kingdom, a study by Beral et al. included an analysis of 3373 deaths among 39,546 atomic energy workers during

1946–1979 and did not find an excess of multiple myeloma.[143] A study of 22,552 atomic weapons workers yielded a rate ratio of 0.97 for multiple myeloma.[144] A cohort analysis of the U.K. National Registry of Radiation Workers by Kendall et al.,[145] as well as very large studies in the United States[157,158,259] did not find excess multiple myeloma. A second analysis in 1999 of 124,743 workers in the U.K. National Registry of Radiation Workers by Muirhead et al. using a lagged analysis reported a nonsignificantly reduced SMR for myeloma of 0.76 (95% CI 0.53, 1.06).[146] McGeoghegan et al. reported on the cancer mortality and morbidity experience of employees at the Chapelcross plant of British Nuclear Fuels during 1955–1995 with a cohort that included 2628 workers with median doses of 39 mSv.[149] In radiation workers, the SMR for myeloma was nonsignificant and increased at 1.11 based on only two cases. A report on the Sellafield plant by Omar et al. found an insignificant decrease in myeloma among nonplutonium workers with an SMR of 0.67 and incidence was also insignificantly reduced.[148] For plutonium workers the SMR for myeloma was insignicantly elevated at 1.08 and the incidence was insignificantly decreased at 0.94. Carpenter et al. examined workers in the United Kingdom who were occupationally exposed to tritium, plutonium, and other radionuclides and the SMRs for myeloma in each group were all nonsignificantly reduced.[191]

Artalejo et al. reported on mortality among 5657 workers of the former Spanish Nuclear Energy Board with mean exposure of 11.42 mSv and the SMR for myeloma was nonsignificantly reduced at 0.92 (95% CI 0.19, 2.7).[151] Habib et al. have reported on cancer incidence among Australian nuclear industry–monitored radiation workers and indicated no cases of myeloma were identified.[152] Iwasaki et al. conducted a second analysis of mortality of nuclear industry workers in Japan which included 176,000 male workers and 5527 deaths.[150] Average annual doses were 3.5 mSv before 1982 and 1.2 mSv after 1982 and the SMR for myeloma was nonsignificantly increased at 1.12 (95% CI 0.69, 1.74).

In one Canadian study there were two cases observed versus 3.5 expected.[260] Ashmore et al. reported the first analysis of mortality and occupational radiation exposure based on the National Dose Registry of Canada which included a cohort of 206,620 individuals and 5426 deaths.[154] The average exposure for males was 10.6 mSv. The SMR for myeloma was nonsignificant at 0.73 (90% CI 0.47, 1.10). Sont et al. studied the relationship between cancer incidence and occupational radiation exposure based on the National Dose Registry of Canada and included a cohort of 191,333 persons with an average dose for males of 11.5 mSv and an average dose for the cohort of 6.64 mSv.[153] The SIR for myeloma in males was nonsignificantly reduced at 0.73 and in females it was nonsignificantly reduced at 0.54. In 2004, Zablotska et al. reported on mortality of Canadian nuclear workers and concluded that for myeloma there was a nonsignificantly decreased SMR of 0.97 (95% CI 0.47, 1.79).[155] Howe et al. have reported on the mortality of U.S. nuclear power industry workers and found a nonsignificantly decreased risk of myeloma with an SMR of 0.63 (95% CI 0.23, 1.37).[159]

Cardis et al. reported on cancer mortality among nuclear industry workers in three countries in a large study of 95,673 workers which included over 2 million person-years at risk and 15,825 deaths.[166] The trend for myeloma was significant at 1.87 with a P value of 0.037. Cardis et al. also have reported the cancer mortality results from a 15-country collaborative study of nuclear workers.[168] This is the largest occupational study to date and included a cohort of 407,391 workers with 18,993 deaths and 5.2 million person-years of follow-up. The ERR per Sv for myeloma was nonsignificantly positive at 6.15 (90% CI <0, 20.6). Rahu et al. have reported on cancer incidence of 5446 male Latvian and Estonian Chernobyl cleanup workers and indicate a nonsignificant SIR of 1.0 for myeloma.[178]

McGeoghegan et al. have reported on the mortality of 12,540 workers (including 3244 radiation workers) at the Capenhurst uranium enrichment facility during 1946–1995 among whom the SMR for myeloma was nonsignificantly elevated in radiation workers at 1.15.[242] They also studied cancer mortality experience of 19,454 workers (including 13,960 radiation workers) at the Springfields uranium production facility during 1946–1995 and the SMR for myeloma was nonsignificantly reduced for radiation workers at 0.80.[243] Darby et al. studied radon and cancers in Swedish iron miners and found a nonsignificant increase in myeloma with an O/E ratio of 1.92 (95% CI 0.77, 3.96).[183]

Medical Exposure

Boice et al. have examined the risk of leukemia, NHL, and multiple myeloma in two prepaid health plans in which the number of diagnostic x-rays could be retrospectively determined.[104] An increase in multiple myeloma was seen but was not dose-related or consistent with other epidemiologic studies; therefore, it was not thought to be radiation-related. Mattsson et al. have reported on cancer incidence among 3090 women who received radiation therapy for benign breast disease.[114] The RR for myeloma was nonsignificant at 0.38. Griem et al. have followed a population of patients who had radiotherapy for peptic ulcer disease in whom there was no significant excess of myeloma (RR 1.38, 95% CI 0.1 to 15).[112] Carr et al. performed a follow-up study of the same group with doses to the abdomen of about 15 Gy.[113] No cases of myeloma were found after radiotherapy in the period 0 to 10 years postexposure and in the follow-up period of 11 to 62 years postexposure, the RR was nonsignificantly reduced at 0.03. A nonsignificant excess of myeloma was reported in patients treated with radiation for ankylosing spondylitis.[109] In an international incidence study of women treated for cervical cancer, 82,616 exposed women were compared with 99,424 unexposed controls, and no excess was identified for myeloma.[124] In another similar study myeloma again was not increased.[126]

Internal Exposure

Ron et al. reported on 35,593 hyperthyroid patients treated by different methods.[201] The SMR for myeloma in patients treated with any iodine 131 was nonsignificantly increased at 1.02 and in patients treated with iodine 131 only, it was nonsignificantly decreased at 0.81.

Summary

Radiation risk estimates for multiple myeloma that can be derived from epidemiologic studies were summarized by the 2006 UNSCEAR Committee and are shown in Table 5-6.[86] UNSCEAR 2006 concluded that there is only weak evidence linking myeloma to radiation exposure and that the better quality of diagnostic information from atomic bomb survivor incidence data would suggest that there is little evidence of an association with low-LET radiation and that while there is some evidence from a few high-LET studies these are based on very few cases. The 2006 National Academy of Sciences Committee on Radiation Screening and Compensation Programs Report concluded that multiple myeloma is classified as having very low or no susceptibility to radiation induction and that there is no convincing epidemiologic evidence to warrant inclusion of myeloma as a radiation compensable

Table 5-6 • Risk Estimates for Cancer Incidence and Mortality from Studies of Radiation Exposure: Multiple Myeloma*

Study	Average Excess Relative Risk at 1 Sv	Average Excess Absolute Risk $(10^4 PYSv)^{-1}$
External Low-LET Exposures		
Incidence		
A-bomb Life Span Study[12]		
Male	0.17	0.26
Female	0.28	0.08
Age at exposure		
<20	1.07	0.07
>20	0.09	0.04
All	0.20 (<0–21.7)	0.05 (<−0.05–0.4)
Cervical cancer case control[6]	−0.10 (<0–0.23)	NA
Benign lesions in the locomotor system[122]	−0.09	−0.16
U.K. Springfields uranium workers[243]	7.66 (<−17.18–109.52)	NA
Mortality		
A-bomb Life Span Study[8]		
Male	1.13 (<0–6.41)	0.15 (<0–0.51)
Female	1.16 (0.01–3.9)	0.19 (0.001–0.5)
All	1.15 (0.12–3.27)	0.17 (0.02–0.4)
Benign lesions in the locomotor system[122]	0.65	0.95
Ankylosing spondylitis	NA	NA
Benign gynaecological disease[117]	0.11 (<−0.2–0.6)	0.05 (<−0.1–0.3)
Peptic ulcer[113]	−0.61 (<−0.61–1.38)	NA
Metropathia haemorrhagica[116]	1.23 (0.3–2.7)	0.90 (0.2–2.0)
Nuclear workers in Canada, United Kingdom, and United States[166]	4.2 (0.3–14.4)	NA
U.K. National Registry for Radiation Workers[146]	4.1 (0.03–14.8)	NA
Nuclear industry workers in Japan[150]	NA	NA
U.S. 4-cohort analysis[269]	0.66 (−2.35–3.67)	NA
IARC 15-country nuclear workers study[167,168]	6.15 (<0, 20.6)	
Internal Low-LET Exposures		
Incidence		
Diagnostic ^{131}I[270]	NA	NA
Swedish ^{131}I hyperthyroid[271]	NA	NA
Mortality		
U.S. thyrotoxicosis[201]	11.0	NA
Internal High-LET Exposures	**Average Relative Risk**	
Incidence		
Danish Thorotrast patients[272]	4.34 (0.85–31.3)	
Danish and Swedish Thorotrast patients[219]	3.7 (0.5–30.9)	
Mortality		
U.S. Thorotrast patients[219]	1.8 (0.1–51.6)	

*The studies listed are those for which quantitative estimates of risk could be made.
Adapted from United Nations Scientific Committee of the Effects of Atomic Radiation (UNSCEAR): Sources and effects of ionizing radiation: 2006 report to the General Assembly with annexes. New York, United Nations, 2007.

disease.[257] In spite of the contrary body of scientific evidence, myleoma has been included in some of the (presumably politically motivated) U.S. radiation compensation programs.

APLASTIC ANEMIA AND POLYCYTHEMIA

Although aplastic anemia was initially reported in atomic bomb survivors in Japan, subsequent analysis has demonstrated no association of exposure and incidence in the confirmed cases.[273] The British series of patients treated with radiation for ankylosing spondylitis showed an increased incidence of deaths from cancers of both lymphatic and hematopoietic tissues. Aplastic anemia was originally reported in this series, although later this was thought to be aleukemic leukemia.[106,109] There are several occupational studies of mortality that have looked at diseases of blood (International Classification of Diseases [ICD] codes 280 to 289) as well as benign and unspecified neoplasms (ICD codes 210 to 239). The ICD code for aplastic anemia is 284, for primary polycythemia vera it is 238, and for acquired polycythemia it is 289. The study by Beral et al. of atomic energy workers gives an SMR of 0.96 (95% CI 0.52, 1.61) for ICD codes 210 to 239.[143] In another study of atomic workers by Beral et al., the ratio for the same codes was 0.97 (95% CI 0.03, 17.23) and for ICD codes 280 to 289 the rate ratio was 0 (95% CI 0, 28.26).[144] In the series of U.S. radiologists, excess deaths to aplastic anemia were reported, however, the data are difficult to evaluate in terms of risk because no reliable estimates of the absorbed dose have been made.[274] In 1982 the public media drew attention to the "possible" identification of 25 cases of polycythemia rubra vera near a nuclear facility. This was unusual because such a finding was not identified in Hiroshima or Nagasaki, and the dose levels to the individuals were essentially background. At present, the only association known between polycythemia rubra vera and radiation is an increase in leukemia identified in those patients treated for the disease by administration of phosphorus 32.[275]

MYELODYSPLASIA

The terms *myelodysplasia* and *myelodysplastic syndrome* (MDS) refer to clonal hematologic disorders characterized by ineffective hematopoiesis. In about 30% to 40% of cases there is subsequent development of AML. Some authors feel that MDS is one step in the multistep process leading to AML while others feel MDS is a distinct clinical entity and should not always be considered early AML. The reader is referred to a review article by Heaney and Gold[276] and a recent article by Finch[277] which address radiation causation specifically.

There are a quite a number of Web and literature sources that suggest possible etiological factors for MDS, including benzene, hair dye, pesticides, organic solvents, petroleum products, chemotherapeutic agents, and ionizing radiation. Unfortunately, most of these secondary literature sources rarely provide definitive references that have statistical significance. In addition, the criteria for the diagnosis of MDS keeps evolving and the definitions used are somewhat imprecise. As a result, in the older radiation effects literature, it is not clear whether the terms *aplastic anemia*, *pernicious anemia*, and *preleukemic changes* actually refer to MDS or some other condition.

In the more recent literature, follow-up of Thorotrast-exposed persons did not demonstrate an increase in MDS, but there was an increase in clonal chromosomal aberrations. In the atomic bomb survivors there was a clear increase in non–CLL, but only 2 of 50 persons who developed AML (and for whom adequate preleukemia data are present) appear to have had a preleukemic phase with MDS. In a review of the pathological slides of 190 atomic bomb survivors who were thought to have developed AML, 11 cases were reclassified as MDS.[277]

There are several recent papers dealing with long-term health effects resulting from occupational exposure of radiologists and radiologic technologists. A 100-year study of U.K. radiologists does not specifically address MDS but it does address total mortality, cancer, and leukemia. The study found that the SMR of radiologists employed after 1920 was similar to that of other medical practitioners (SMR 1.04, 95% CI 0.89, 1.21) and that cancer mortality rates were not elevated for those radiologists employed after 1954. Leukemia was elevated in radiologists employed prior to 1954, but was not statistically significantly increased after 1954, when radiation protection was presumably better.[94] A study of over 146,000 radiologic technologists employed after 1940 reported on deaths due to both leukemia as well as "diseases of blood and blood forming organs" (ICD-8 codes 280 to 289 which presumably included MDS). In neither case was there a statistically significant elevation of mortality.[99]

In the last four decades, probably as a result of radiation protection, there is no evidence that the incidence of leukemia and particularly AML is statistically significantly increased in radiologists. There is also no evidence that MDS is increased in radiologists. The risk of MDS as a result of radiation exposure, if present, appears to be quite low in spite of the perception that one may get from secondary literature. The rarity of the syndrome and the difficulty in making the diagnosis leave the question of whether radiation can induce MDS at all a matter of conjecture.

BRAIN AND CENTRAL NERVOUS SYSTEM TUMORS

General

The potential induction of brain tumors by radiation has been examined in a large number of epidemiologic studies.

Most studies indicate that the risk in adults is low relative to that of other tissues. Most studies also report no excess risk or a nonstatistically significant excess, particularly when exposures are less than 1 Gy. When radiotherapy situations are encountered with much higher doses directly to the head of children, the findings are usually positive.

The reported radiogenic tumor types are often mesenchymal (sarcomas, meningiomas) but have also included malignant glioma, astrocytoma, hemangioblastoma, and acoustic neuroma.[278] It is often difficult to separate brain tumors into either strictly malignant or nonmalignant categories because many (particularly astrocytomas) may be very slow-growing. Additionally, very few brain tumors metastasize in the way that other malignancies do, and, for this reason, many of the published reports give a total brain tumor induction rate rather than indicating a separate malignant brain tumor rate.

External Exposure

Atomic Bomb Survivors

Recent data from the atomic bomb survivors reveal a small excess of brain cancers; however, the CIs of RR usually encompass unity. The incidence data reveal an ERR at 1 Sv of 0.26 (95% CI −0.2, 1.3) and an EAR of 0.2 $(10^4 PYSv)^{-1}$.[279,280] Mortality data give the same quantities as 0.4 and 0.1, respectively. The actual number of cases observed in the 41,000 persons studied who received over 0.01 Sv, and an average dose of 0.23 Sv, was 71 versus the 67 expected, or an excess of 4 cases. This increase is not statistically significant. The incidence data by dose are graphically shown in Figure 5-2. Analysis of the LSS incidence data reveals no definite sex difference or age-at-exposure effect.

In the 2003 update, studies of mortality of atomic bomb survivors during 1950–1997, Preston et al. had a cohort of 86,572 persons with an average external dose of 0.23 Sv.[281] In males there was a statistically significant excess of brain cancer at dose levels of 1 Sv, with an ERR of 5.3 (90% CI 1.4, 16.0). In females there was a nonsignificant excess at dose levels of 1 Sv, with an ERR of 0.51 (90% CI < −0.3, 3.9).

Natural Background

There has been no excess of brain cancer in regions of naturally occurring high-background radiation.[29,30] A paper from China was published in 2000 by Tao et al. with 1.7 million person-years of study from 1979 to 1995.[33] The authors did not find a radiation effect and the RR of brain cancer was 1.84 (95% CI 0.40, 8.52). Increased exposure to natural cosmic radiation occurs in airline crews and there have been a number of studies of brain and central nervous system (CNS) cancer incidence in such workers. Pukkala et al. studied over 10,000 Nordic airline pilots and found a nonsignificant decrease in brain

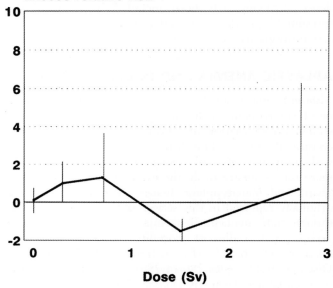

CNS cancer incidence (A-bomb)

Figure 5-2 ● Excess relative risk (ERR) of cancer of the central nervous system in atomic bomb survivors at different dose levels. Error bars indicate 95% CI. (From Thompson D, Mabuchi K, Ron E, et al: Cancer incidence in atomic bomb survivors. II: Solid tumors, 1958–1987. RERF Technical Report 5-92, Hiroshima, Japan, Radiation Effects Research Foundation, 1992.)

and CNS cancers.[39] Band et al., in a study of 2740 pilots exposed at doses of 6 mSv per year over an average 20 years for a total average dose of about 120 mSv, found a nonsignificantly increased SIR and a nonsignificant increase in SMR.[40]

Public Near Nuclear Facilities

Forman et al. examined persons living near nuclear facilities and found no increase in primary CNS tumors.[282] There are three papers concerning potential uranium contamination and the possibility of brain and CNS cancer in the public. The papers by Boice et al. indicated a nonsignificant decrease around a uranium mining and milling facility in Texas, a nonsignificant decrease near a facility in Pennsylvania, and a nonsignificant decrease near a Colorado facility.[89,90,90a] A nonsignificant decrease was found by Boice et al. in a study of persons residing near the Hanford National Laboratory site.[91] Lopez-Abente et al. reported on solid tumor mortality near Spain's four nuclear power plants and four uranium fuel cycle facilities finding the RR for brain cancer was nonsignificantly reduced at 0.83.[283]

Occupational Exposure

In a controversial paper, Checkoway et al. indicated that there was an excess mortality from CNS cancers in men who worked in a nuclear weapons fabrication plant.[284] In fact, the SMR relative to the state of Tennessee for death from this cause was 1.4, but the 95% confidence limits ranged from 0.8 to 2.38. In addition, the RR was not dose-related, and no cases of brain cancer were present when a biologically plausible latent period of 10 years was used. In two other controversial papers on workers at the Oak Ridge National Laboratory[285] and at the Rocky Flats plant,[286] no excess of brain cancer was identified. A study of over 44,000 Hanford workers by Gilbert et al.,[287] as well as a combined study of several large nuclear facilities,[157,158] failed to show an excess risk of brain cancer. Howe et al. have reported on the mortality of U.S. nuclear power industry workers in whom they found a nonsignificantly decreased risk of brain cancer with an SMR of 0.85 (95% CI 0.54, 1.28).[159] No excess of brain cancer was found by Cragle et al. in a study of workers at the U.S. Department of Energy Savannah River plant.[288] Frome reported a mortality study of 106,020 employees in the nuclear industry at Oak Ridge, Tennessee.[160] The SMR for cancer of the brain in black and white males and females was nonsignificantly different from unity. Wiggs et al. found a reduced SMR of 0.68 in a follow-up of Los Alamos workers.[164] Groves et al. conducted a 40-year cancer mortality study of 40,581 Korean War Navy veterans with potential exposure to high-intensity radar sources, which also emit ionizing radiation, and found the SMR for brain cancer was significantly decreased at 0.71 (95% CI 0.51, 0.98).[165]

A number of large studies have been performed in the United Kingdom. A study of 22,347 men who participated in atmospheric nuclear weapons tests has been reported by Darby et al.[52] A nonsignificant increase in tumors of the CNS was reported, with an RR of 1.3 and 90% CI of 0.8 to 2.2. A study by Beral et al. included an analysis of 3373 deaths among 39,546 workers during 1946–1979.[143] No excess of brain cancer was seen among the employees, and there were no cases in the greater-than-10-mSv cumulative-dose group. A study of the U.K. National Registry of Radiation Workers by Kendall et al. included 95,217 workers over 1.2 million person-years at risk.[145] The report studied leukemia and all cancers and did not find a significant excess. A second analysis in 1999 of 124,743 workers in the U.K. National Registry of Radiation Workers by Muirhead et al. using a lagged analysis reported nonsignificantly reduced SMR for brain and CNS cancers of 0.97 (95% CI 0.80, 1.17).[146] Brain cancer was specifically studied by Carpenter et al. in a study of 27 cases and 90 matched controls from workers in a nuclear facility.[289] No association was found with radiation exposure. McGeoghegan et al. reported on the mortality and cancer morbidity experience of employees at the Chapelcross plant of British Nuclear Fuels during 1955–1995.[149] The cohort included 2628 workers with median doses of 39 mSv. In radiation workers the SMR for cancer of the brain was nonsignificant and increased at 1.70. Nonplutonium workers at the Sellafield plant were reported by Omar

et al. to have a nonsignificant decrease in brain cancer with an SMR of 0.76 and the incidence of such tumors was also nonsignificantly decreased.[148]

Ashmore et al. reported the first analysis of mortality and occupational radiation exposure based on the National Dose Registry of Canada which included a cohort of 206,620 individuals and 5426 deaths.[154] The average exposure for males was 10.6 mSv. The SMR for brain cancer was nonsignificantly reduced at 0.73 (90% CI 0.57, 0.91). Sont et al. also reported on incidence and occupational radiation exposure based on the National Dose Registry of Canada which included a cohort of 191,333 persons with an average dose for males of 11.5 mSv and an average dose for the cohort of 6.64 mSv.[153] The SIR for brain cancer in males was nonsignificantly reduced at 0.86 and in females it was significantly reduced at 0.65. In 2004 Zablotska et al. reported on the mortality of Canadian nuclear workers and concluded that for brain cancer there was a nonsignificantly decreased SMR of 0.85 (95% CI 0.55, 1.26).[155]

Artalejo et al. reported on mortality among 5657 workers of the former Spanish Nuclear Energy Board with mean exposure of 11.42 mSv.[151] The SMR for brain cancer was nonsignificantly elevated at 1.33 (95% CI 0.61, 2.52). Habib et al. have reported on cancer incidence among Australian nuclear industry–monitored radiation workers in whom they found a nonsignificantly increased SIR of 1.21 for brain and CNS cancer.[152]

Fry et al. reported a study of mortality and morbidity among 3145 persons occupationally exposed to 50 or more mSv in a year.[161] The mean external exposure was 153 mSv. The SMR for brain cancer was nonsignificantly different from unity. Iwasaki et al. conducted a second analysis of mortality of nuclear industry workers in Japan which included 176,000 male workers and 5527 deaths.[150] Average annual doses were 3.5 mSv before 1982 and 1.2 mSv after 1982. For brain cancer the SMR was nonsignificantly decreased at 0.69 (95% CI 0.45, 1.01).

Cardis et al.[166] reported on cancer mortality among nuclear industry workers in three countries in a large study covering 95,673 workers and over 2 million person-years at risk and 15,825 deaths. The trend for brain cancer was nonsignificantly reduced at −0.24 with a P value of 0.59. Cardis et al. have reported the cancer mortality results from a 15-country collaborative study of nuclear workers. This is the largest occupational study to date and included a cohort of 407,391 workers with 18,993 deaths and 5.2 million person-years of follow-up. The ERR per Sv for brain and CNS cancer was nonsignificantly negative at less than 0.[168]

Cancer incidence among medical diagnostic workers in China has reported by Wang et al. who compared 27,011 workers with 25,782 persons in other medical specialties.[102] There was no excess of cancer of the brain, even though cumulative doses were probably on the order of 1 Gy. In a follow-up Wang et al. reported that the RR for cancer of the brain was nonsignificantly decreased at 0.8.[253] Aoyama et al. conducted a mortality survey of over 12,000 male Japanese radiological technologists during 1969–1993.[95] The cohort had an average dose of 466 mSv. The SMR for brain cancer was significantly increased at 3.58 (95% CI 1.64, 6.79). Rahu et al. have reported on cancer incidence of 5446 male Latvian and Estonian Chernobyl cleanup workers and indicate a borderline significantly increased SIR of 7.06 (95% CI 2.84, 14.55) for brain cancer, however, the authors point out that this finding is at variance with other studies and may be due to chance or misdiagnosis of brain metastases from cancer at other sites.[178]

Burnett et al. studied the mortality of health and science technicians and found a nonsignificantly decreased proportional mortality ratio for brain cancer of 0.73 (95% CI 0.32, 1.44).[96] Doody et al. reported on mortality among 143,517 U.S. radiologic technologists during 1926–1990.[97] Doses were not evaluated. The SMR for brain cancer was nonsignificantly reduced at 0.83 (95% CI 0.65, 1.03). Sigurdson et al. studied cancer incidence in 90,305 U.S. radiologic technologists and found that their SIR for brain cancer was nonsignificantly reduced at 0.95 (95% CI 0.75, 1.16).[101] Mohan et al. studied cancer and other causes of mortality among 146,022 radiologic technologists employed from 1940 and later.[98,99] The SMR for brain cancer in males was nonsignificantly reduced at 0.77 (95% CI 0.6, 1.0) and for females it was nonsignificantly reduced at 0.92 (95% CI 0.7, 1.1).

Ritz et al. have reported on cancer mortality in uranium processing workers at the Fernald Plant in Ohio.[192] The SMR for brain and CNS cancer was nonsignificantly increased at 1.24. Dupree-Ellis et al. have reported on mortality in a cohort of 2514 uranium processing workers employed between 1942 and 1966 at the Mallinkrodt Chemical Works.[193] The SMR for brain cancer was nonsignificantly increased at 1.57. McGeoghegan et al. have reported on the mortality of 12,540 workers (including 3244 radiation workers) at the Capenhurst uranium enrichment facility during 1946–1995 and the SMR for brain cancer was nonsignificantly elevated in radiation workers at 1.39.[242] They also studied cancer mortality experience of 19,454 workers (including 13,960 radiation workers) at the Springfields uranium production facility during 1946–1995.[243] The SMR for brain cancer was nonsignificantly reduced for radiation workers at 0.67. A meta-analysis of 14 studies, which included 120,000 uranium workers, found a nonsignificantly decreased RR of 0.91 (95% CI 0.65, 1.17) for brain cancer.[245]

Medical Exposure

In an unusual paper, Preston-Martin et al. indicate that dental x-rays are a risk factor for some types of brain tumors.[290] The paper also claims that the incidence of meningioma is related to the incidence of previous severe head injuries and that vitamin C was protective against gliomas. Careful analysis reveals that all of the odds ratios (ORs) include 1.0 within the 95% CIs. In addition, this was a retrospective interview study, raising the question of recall bias. It should also be noted that there is another study of gliomas in adults that failed to find a correlation with dental x-rays.[291] Longstreth et al. have discussed other potential etiologic agents and the occurrence of meningiomas.[292] In a follow-up study of patients exposed to repeated fluoroscopy for TB management, there was no excess of brain cancers. In fact, the control group had more brain cancers, with an SMR of 1.5 compared with 0.7 for the exposed group.[105]

The effects of radiation therapy for childhood tinea capitis in New York patients has been reported by Shore et al.[293] and in Israeli patients by Ron and coauthors.[121] The mean dose to the brain in both studies was between 1.4 and 1.5 Gy. The Israeli tinea capitis studies by Ron et al. include 10,834 exposed persons and 16,226 controls.[294,295] The exposure involved direct irradiation of the scalp with doses in excess of several Gy. An excess incidence of brain cancers (meningiomas, gliomas, nerve sheath tumors, and others) was found in this study as well as in a New York series.[293] In the New York study, eight brain tumors were found in the irradiated group versus none in the controls; in the Israeli group, 16 brain tumors were found in the irradiated group and 3 among the controls. The tumors appeared as early as 5 years after irradiation, but many occurred more than 25 years later. The absolute risk estimate for both studies was between 0.7 and 1.3 cases annually in 1 million persons exposed for each 0.01 Gy.

An excess of brain neoplasms has been reported in subjects who received childhood radiation for the prevention of deafness. In those circumstances, a radium applicator was applied to the nasopharynx to reduce the size of the adenoid tissue. The dose at 1 cm from the applicator was estimated to be 7.2 Gy, dropping to 0.78 Gy at 3 cm. The series included 904 irradiated subjects and 2021 controls who were treated surgically. Three brain tumors were identified in the irradiated population compared to none in the controls.[296]

After radiotherapy for ankylosing spondylitis, Darby et al. have reported a significant excess of brain tumors; however, the authors themselves point out the dubious nature of a radiation relationship and indicate that lung tumor metastases may have been erroneously classified as brain tumors.[109] Griem et al. have followed a population of patients who received radiotherapy for peptic ulcer treatment. There was no excess of cancer of the brain (RR 0.83).[112] Carr et al. performed a follow-up study of the same group with doses to the abdomen of about 15 Gy finding no cases of brain cancer after radiotherapy in the period 0 to 10 years postexposure and, in the follow-up period of 11 to 62 years postexposure, the RR was nonsignificantly elevated at 1.08.[113]

There are several studies of treatment for benign gynecologic conditions. Most found no increase in brain cancers, while a study by Ryberg et al. reported nonsignificant increases in tumors of the nervous system.[297] In another study, of over 5000 persons who received x-ray therapy to the head and neck for various reasons, 14 intracranial tumors were observed versus 1.6 expected.[298] This study is somewhat difficult to assess for absolute risk because the dose to the midplane of the neck was calculated rather than dose to the brain. Munk et al. suggest that for at least some brain tumors, the latent period may have a mean value of about 27 years.[299] An increase in the frequency of brain tumors has also been reported in a British series after therapy for pituitary adenomas.[300]

Furst et al. have followed patients in Sweden who were treated with external beam radiotherapy for childhood skin hemangiomas.[301] This study of 144 exposed persons and 314 controls showed an excess risk of thyroid and brain cancer but not of cancers of the bone, soft tissue, or breast. In another report by Furst et al., a cohort of 14,647 children who were treated between 1920 and 1959 was compared with 2694 patients who were not treated with radiotherapy.[302] In this study RRs of brain cancer in the irradiated group were less than unity. In a study of survivors of childhood cancer, Neglia et al. reported that radiation exposure was associated with increased risk of glioma and meningioma, with odds ratios of 6.78 (1.54–29.7) and 9.94 (2.17–45.6), respectively. For glioma, the ERR/Gy was highest among children exposed at less than 5 years of age.[302a] In a study that matched 4188 women treated with radiotherapy for cervical carcinoma and who developed second cancers with 6880 controls, a deficit of brain cancer was observed.[126] There are a number or studies linking gliomas to previous cranial radiation for childhood leukemia (usually ALL).[303–306] A number of authors have indicated the possibility of genetic predisposition, intrathecal methotrexate, and radiation as possible causes.[307,308] In one study of 981 children in Nordic countries, the incidence of brain tumor was 27 times greater than expected.[309] No increase was seen after chemotherapy alone. There are several isolated case reports of meningioma occurring after cranial radiotherapy.[310,311]

Internal Exposure

There have been studies of the potential carcinogenic effects of internal irradiation from diagnostic doses of radioiodine administered to perform thyroid scanning. The largest and most recent of these studies included 35,074 patients who were matched with the Swedish cancer registry. A questionable increase in leukemia and cancers of the CNS was found.[270] With regard to the latter tumors, there is no reason to expect that CNS tumors should be increased by radioiodine in this study. Much larger doses are received by organs that are more sensitive to radiogenic tumor induction, and increases in those tumors were not seen. In addition, CNS tumors have not been seen following higher dose therapy with radioiodine for thyroid cancer.

There are a very large number of patients treated each year with iodine 131 for hyperthyroidism. In one study of 1762 women, there was no increase in the SIR when all malignant neoplasms were considered together. Analysis of cancers of the breast, digestive organs, pancreas, brain, or all other sites failed to show either a significant or dose-related increase.[199] In another study of 10,552 patients treated in Sweden there was no significant increase in all tumors considered together.[271] Increases in cancers of the brain, kidney, and stomach were detected, but these were not significantly related to iodine dose. Ron et al. reported on 35,593 hyperthyroid patients treated by different methods.[201] The SMR for brain cancer in patients treated with any iodine 131 was nonsignificantly increased at 1.06, and in patients treated with iodine 131 only it was nonsignificantly decreased at 0.98.

There is a 2003 report by dos Santos Silva et al. on the 50-year follow-up of mortality in Portuguese Thorotrast patients.[220] The cohort included 1096 systemically exposed and 240 locally exposed. The SMR for brain cancer in the systemically exposed was significantly increased at 13.2. The RR of systemically exposed versus locally exposed was nonsignificantly increased at 2.94. The authors pointed out that the increased risk of CNS lesions was almost certainly due to the intial diagnosis for which they were receiving cerebral angiography and that the risk was not related to radiation dose and decreased over time. Nyberg et al. reported on cancer incidence after a 40-year follow-up among Swedish patients exposed to radioactive Thorotrast. The SIR for brain cancer was marginally elevated at 3.1 (95% CI 1.0, 7.4).[222]

A report by Goss indicates a fourfold excess of tumors of the CNS in patients exposed to radium.[312] This may be artifactually high because radon is known to cause cancers of the cranial sinuses that can invade the brain and, thus, be misclassified as primary brain tumors. There are reports of increased brain cancer in the German and Danish Thorotrast studies.[213,313,314] As the authors point out, many patients received Thorotrast injections for cranial arteriograms, and a large number of these persons had brain tumors that caused subsequent mortality. Therefore, it is extremely unlikely that radiation was the cause of the increase.

A 2004 update of French uranium miners by Laurier et al. reported a nonsignificantly elevated SMR of 1.7 for brain cancer.[186] Darby et al. studied radon and cancers in Swedish iron miners and found a nonsignificant increase in brain cancer with an O/E ratio of 2.22 (95% CI 0.89, 4.58).[183] A report on the Sellafield plant by Omar et al. indicated a nonsignificant decrease in brain cancer among plutonium workers with an SMR of 0.96 and incidence was also nonsignificantly decreased.[148] Carpenter et al. studied workers in the United Kingdom who were occupationally exposed to tritium, plutonium, and other radionuclides and found the SMRs for brain and CNS cancer in each group were all nonsignificantly reduced.[191] Wiggs et al. found a nonsignificant elevation of the RR of brain cancer in a follow-up of Los Alamos plutonium workers.[164]

Prenatal Exposure

Another large group of patients in whom brain tumors have been reported received intrauterine radiation. These studies are of particular importance because it appears that the fetal brain may have a relatively high sensitivity to tumor induction. MacMahon indicated that tumors of the CNS accounted for approximately one quarter of all malignancies apparently induced by in utero irradiation.[315] Of 120 CNS cancer deaths identified, 19 had received prenatal radiation, with an RR of 1.6. The absolute radiogenic risk estimate for brain tumors of the adjusted data is 6.3 excess deaths annually in 1 million persons exposed for 0.01 Gy. UNSCEAR indicated that from these data, the absolute risk factor on a lifetime basis may be 50 excess cases in 1 million persons exposed to 0.01 Gy.[316] There are, however, wide confidence limits on these estimates. Bithell et al. examined the radiation history in 1332 deaths from malignancy before the age of 14 years: 13.4% of the children with CNS tumors had a history of prenatal irradiation versus 9.9% in the controls.[261] When matched controls were included, the RR was approximately 1.3. The 1980 BEIR Committee reviewed these findings and indicated an estimate of 8 mGy as the average dose, with an absolute risk factor of 4 to 8 deaths annually per 10^6 persons exposed for 0.01 Gy.[13] Atomic bomb survivors have been studied by Jablon and Kato; 740 children were exposed in utero to 10 mGy or more.[317] No brain tumors were identified; however, using the risk factors from the previously mentioned studies, one would have expected less than one case. Therefore, the data only serve to indicate that the risk factor is not substantially higher than that indicated by other studies. Another study, performed by Diamond et al., included 20,000 irradiated children in whom three CNS deaths were identified before the age of 9 years.[318] Eight similar deaths were observed among 35,000 nonirradiated children. Although the number of cases studied was large, the number of observed cancers was too small to allow statistical analysis.

Summary

Ionizing radiation can induce tumors of the CNS although the relationship is not as strong as for some other tumors and there appear to be strong age-at-exposure and different-dose-response relationships. The UNSCEAR 2006 report points out that malignant tumors of the CNS are seen only after very high doses from radiotherapy and the risk is predominantly after exposure in childood.[86] Risk from lower dose exposure and during exposure as an adult is essentially limited to benign tumors, particularly meningioma, schwannoma, and neurilemmoma.

Radiation risk estimates for induction of brain tumors that can be derived from epidemiological studies were summarized in the UNSCEAR 2006 report (Table 5-7).[86]

Table 5-7 • Risk Estimates for Cancer Incidence and Mortality from Studies of Radiation Exposure: Brain and CNS*

Study	Average Excess Relative Risk at 1 Sv	Average Excess Absolute Risk $(10^4 PYSv)^{-1}$
External Low-LET Exposures		
Incidence		
A-bomb Life Span Study[319]		
Males	1.54 (0.66–2.87)	1.21 (0.58–2.03)
Females	<0 (<0–0.46)	0.01 (<0–0.50)
Age at exposure		
<20	0.88 (0.28–1.78)	0.68 (0.24–1.28)
20–40	0.64 (<0–1.82)	0.48 (<0–1.43)
>40	<0 (<0–0.51)	<0 (<0–0.28)
Time since exposure		
12–15	2.20 (<0–11.11)	<0 (<0–226.13)
15–30	0.42 (<0–1.44)	<0 (<0–357.41)
>30	0.57 (0.10–1.24)	0.96 (0.26–1.83)
All	0.55 (0.16–1.07)	0.57 (0.23–1.01)
Life Span Study[320]		
All nervous system tumours	1.2 (0.6–2.1)	NA
Glioma	0.56 (−0.2–2.0)	NA
Meningioma	0.64 (−0.01–1.8)	0.14 (0.00–0.45)
Schwannoma	4.5 (1.9–9.2)	0.67 (0.3–1.1)

*The studies listed are those for which quantitative estimates of risk could be made.

Table 5-7 • Risk Estimates for Cancer Incidence and Mortality from Studies of Radiation Exposure: Brain and CNS*—cont'd

Study	Average Excess Relative Risk at 1 Sv	Average Excess Absolute Risk $(10^4 PYSv)^{-1}$
External Low-LET Exposures—cont'd		
Incidence—cont'd		
Life Span Study[320]—meningioma		
Male	1.6 (−0.04–7.1)	NA
Female	0.4 (−0.2–1.7)	NA
Age at exposure		
<20	1.3 (0.01–4.5)	NA
20–39	0.5 (−0.05–2.8)	NA
≥40	0.3 (<−0.1–2)	NA
Life Span Study[320]—schwannoma		
Male	8 (2.7–21)	NA
Female	2.3 (0.3–7)	NA
Age at exposure		
<20	6.0 (2.1–14)	NA
20–39	2.6 (< −0.2–10)	NA
≥40	3.3 (0.33–11)	NA
Israel tinea capitis [294]	4.9	NA
Glioma	1.6	NA
Meningioma	5.7	NA
Schwannoma	21.4	NA
Israel tinea capitis[321]		
Malignant brain tumors	1.98 (0.73–4.69)	0.31 (0.12–0.53)
Benign meningioma	4.63 (2.43–9.12)	0.48 (0.28–0.73)
New York tinea capitis[322]		
Brain cancer	1.1 (0.1–2.8)	NA
All intracranial tumors	5.6 (3–9.4)	NA
Swedish pooled skin hemangioma[323]	2.7 (1–5.6)	2.1 (0.3–4.4)
Childhood cancer survivors[324]		
All brain tumors	0.19 (0.03–0.85)	NA
Malignant tumors	0.07 (<0–0.62)	NA
Benign tumors		NA
U.K. Springfields uranium workers[243]	−1.96 (< −2–9.31)	NA
Mortality		
A-bomb Life Span Study[281]		
Males	5.87 (1.55–17.94)	<0 (<0–46.43)
Females	0.78 (<0–4.62)	<0 (<0–29)
Age at exposure		
<20	5.72 (1.56–17.04)	<0 (<0–<0)
>20	0.77 (<0–4.88)	<0 (<0–35.7)
Time since exposure		
5–30	<0 (<0 – >10,000)	<0 (<0–14.96)
>30	2.56 (0.54–6.89)	<0 (<0–72.6)
All	2.86 (0.83–6.76)	<0 (<0–35.75)
Pituitary adenoma (U.K.)[300]	0.2 (0.07–0.45)	0.27 (0.09–0.59)
Nuclear workers in Canada, United Kingdom, United States[166]	<0	NA
U.K. National Registry for Radiation Workers[146]	−0.54 (< −1.95–4.26)	NA
Nuclear power industry workers in the U.S.[159]	−2.5 (< −2.51–27.1)	NA
Canada National Dose Registry[153]	<0	<0
IARC 15-country nuclear workers study[167,168]	<0	
Internal High-LET Exposures		
Mortality		
United States Thorotrast patients[219]	1.3 (0.6–3.7)	NA

*The studies listed are those for which quantitative estimates of risk could be made.
Adapted from United Nations Scientific Committee of the Effects of Atomic Radiation (UNSCEAR): Sources and effects of ionizing radiation: 2006 report to the General Assembly with annexes. New York, United Nations, 2007.

It should be noted that in the following text, many of the studies mentioned do not show an excess of brain cancer and, hence, are not included in the table.

CRANIAL SINUS TUMORS

In contrast to CNS neoplasms, radiogenic tumors of the cranial sinuses have been reported only as a result of internal irradiation by radium and thorium and not as a result of external irradiation. Carpenter et al. examined workers in the United Kingdom who were occupationally exposed to tritium, plutonium, and other radionuclides and found that the SMRs for sinus and nasal cavity tumors in each group were all nonsignificantly different from unity.[191] Cardis et al. have reported the cancer mortality results from a 15-country collaborative study of nuclear workers.[168] This is the largest occupational study to date and included a cohort of 407,391 workers with 18,993 deaths and 5.2 million person-years of follow-up. The ERR per Sv for cancer of the nasal cavity was negative at less than 0.

The metabolism of radium and its decay scheme produce a unique situation in which radon 222 accumulates in the paranasal and mastoid cavities, causing irradiation of the mucosal lining. The tumors (Fig. 5-3) have been observed only in those persons internally contaminated with radium 226, because it is the only isotope of radium that has radon 222 gas as its daughter product. Several researchers have studied persons internally contaminated with radium 228 and radium 224 (which do not produce radon 222 as a daughter product),[325–327] and have found no sinus tumors.

In general, the carcinomas of the sinuses occur with about one half the frequency of the bone sarcomas. This relationship may be artifactual because the carcinomas of the sinuses may have a longer latent period. In the radium

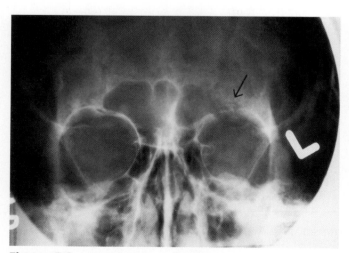

Figure 5-3 ● Frontal sinus carcinoma in a radium dial painter. The arrow indicates destruction of the superior orbital rim. (Case courtesy of the Argonne National Laboratory Radium Registry, Argonne, Ill.)

dial painters in the United States, the latent periods for sinus and paranasal tumors are quite long, ranging from 19 to 52 years and possibly longer. Through 1980, 35 tumors of the cranial sinuses developed in the 4059 radium dial painters studied by Rowland et al.[328] They have indicated the following risk for induction of paranasal and mastoid carcinomas by radium 226: 16 excess carcinomas annually in 1 million persons each with 37 kBq (1μCi) of radium 226, with the cumulative risk to the end of lifespan being 64 excess carcinomas in 1 million persons exposed for each 0.01 Gy. Thorotrast (colloidal thorium 232 dioxide) has been used not only for angiographic purposes and retrograde pyelograms, but also for diagnosing diseases of the maxillary sinuses. For these purposes, there has been actual injection into the sinus cavities themselves, often with the Thorotrast being left in place after the radiographs were obtained. Ten cases of neoplasms occurring in this setting have been described by Fabrikant.[329] In patients in whom the Thorotrast was removed shortly after instillation, no such tumors were observed.[330]

SALIVARY GLAND TUMORS

General

Salivary gland tumors are uncommon, with incidence rates below 0.1 per 100,000. Much higher rates have been seen in Eskimos. About 80% of the malignant salivary tumors involve the parotid glands.

External Exposure

Atomic Bomb Survivors

Benign and malignant tumors of the salivary, and particularly parotid, glands have been reported to follow external exposure in the atomic bomb survivors and in children who have received radiation therapy. These are easily detected because spontaneous salivary gland tumors are rare. The risk rates are usually reported in numbers of cases rather than mortality. The 15-year survival rate of naturally occurring cancers of the salivary glands is approximately 70%; if this survival figure is applied to radiation-induced salivary tumors, the average risk rate for fatal salivary gland cancers is approximately 5 deaths in 1 million persons for each 0.01 Gy. Latent periods for both benign and malignant tumors appear to be in the range of 13 to 25 years following irradiation. Presently, data are insufficient for assessing the effect of age at irradiation or the possible difference in induction rates between males and females. Studies of survivors at Hiroshima and Nagasaki have been performed by Belsky et al.[331,332] and Takeichi et al.[333,334] On the basis of the T65 dosimetry, it appears that the radiation risk estimate is between 1 and 8 excess salivary gland tumors in 1 million persons exposed for each 0.01 Gy over a 15-to-20-year follow-up period. A report by Wakabayaski et al. based only on research in Nagasaki failed to find an increase in salivary gland tumors.[335] However, in Hiroshima, the RR of atomic bomb survivors was significantly increased over that of nonexposed persons.[334] More recent updates of mortality in the LSS have not reported on salivary gland tumors, but the incidence data indicate an ERR at 1 Sv of 1.8 (90% CI 0.15 to 6.04). The EAR was not given.[279]

Occupational Exposure

Ashmore et al. reported the first analysis of mortality and occupational radiation exposure based on the National Dose Registry of Canada which included a cohort of 206,620 individuals and 5426 deaths.[154] The average exposure for males was 10.6 mSv. The SMR for salivary gland tumors was nonsignificantly increased at 1.09 (90% CI 0.29, 2.81). McGeoghegan et al. reported on the cancer mortality and morbidity experience of employees at the Chapelcross plant of British Nuclear Fuels during 1955–1995 and the cohort included 2628 workers with median doses of 39 mSv.[149] No case of salivary gland cancer was found among radiation workers. Sont et al. studied the relationship of cancer incidence and occupational radiation exposure based on the National Dose Registry of Canada which included a cohort of 191,333 persons with an average dose for males of 11.5 mSv and an average dose for the cohort of 6.64 mSv.[153] The SIR for salivary gland cancer in males was nonsignificantly reduced at 0.83 and in females it was nonsignificantly reduced at 0.98. McGeoghegan et al. reported on the mortality of 12,540 workers (including 3244 radiation workers) at the Capenhurst uranium enrichment facility during 1946–1995 and no case of salivary cancer was identified in radiation workers.[242] They also studied cancer mortality experience of 19,454 workers (including 13,960 radiation workers) at the Springfields uranium production facility during 1946–1995.[243] The SMR for salivary cancer was nonsignificantly reduced for radiation workers at 0.66.

Medical Exposure

Dental x-rays have been associated by Preston-Martin et al. with an increase in salivary gland tumors.[336] This seems unlikely to be causally related in view of the risk estimates derived from other studies, particularly in relation to the comparative sensitivity of the thyroid gland. In addition, a dose-response relationship could not be obtained. Studies involving children who received radiotherapy for benign diseases have been performed by Saenger et al.,[337] Pifer et al.,[338] Janower et al.,[339] Shore et al.,[293] and Modan et al.[340] The series yields absolute risk factors in the range of 5 to 16 excess salivary gland tumors in 1 million exposed children for each 0.01 Gy over a follow-up of approximately 20 years. Annual risk estimates are in the range of 0.06 to 0.25 cases of malignant and benign tumors in 1 million persons annually for 0.01 Gy. If there were a longer follow-up period, the absolute risk factor might be somewhat greater. Although the data concerning adults and children are limited and from fairly different exposure circumstances and populations, it appears that exposure may involve a higher risk in children than in adults. A paper by Schneider et al. reports an increase in salivary gland tumors after head and neck therapy following childhood irradiation.[341] The imaging appearance of these tumors has been reported by Kaste et al.[342]

Internal Exposure

At least two cases of lymphoma have been described in the parotid gland in individuals who had received ablative thyroid therapy with radioiodine.[343] The administered activities of iodine were extremely high: 14 GBq to 27 GBq. Such reports seem to implicate radiation as the etiology because of the extreme rarity of such tumors on a natural basis. No increase in salivary neoplasms was reported by Holm et al. after radioiodine therapy for hyperthyroidism, but this is refuted by the previous discussion related to the lack of radiation-induced lymphomas elsewhere in the body.[271] However, the same group reported an increased risk after thyroid cancer therapy, with three cases noted in 1955 patients.[203]

Summary

The UNSCEAR 2006 Committee has summarized radiation risk factors for salivary gland cancer from the epidemiological studies where they could be derived (Table 5-8) and concluded that the salivary gland is susceptible to the induction of cancer by ionizing radiation.[86] The evidence for this comes almost exclusively from studies of external low-LET exposure. There appears to be little modifying effect of sex, age at exposure, or time since exposure.[86]

PARATHYROID GLAND TUMORS

General

Radiation has been reported to cause increases in the risks of both benign and malignant parathyroid tumors. In analysis of radiation causation, the situation is often complicated in that some patients have other endocrine abnormalities as well. The diagnosis of multiglandular endocrine neoplasia (MEN) needs to be excluded.[345] MEN Type I includes features of hyperparathyroidism, pancreatic islet cell tumors, and pituitary adenoma. Type II includes medullary thyroid carcinoma, pheochromocytoma, hyperparathyroidism, and C-cell hyperplasia. They may also be associated with carcinoid tumors.[346] Most of these syndromes appear to have a genetic basis. Another complicating factor is the association of thyroid abnormalities with parathyroid adenomas in nonirradiated patients.[347]

Table 5-8 • Risk Estimates for Cancer Incidence and Mortality from Studies of Radiation Exposure: Cancer of the Salivary Gland*

Study	Average Excess Relative Risk at 1 Sv	Average Excess Absolute Risk $(10^4 PYSv)^{-1}$
External Low-LET Exposure		
Incidence		
Life Span Study[319]		
Males	4.50 (1.32, 12.68)	<0 (<0, 105.57)
Females	0.95 (<0, 4.09)	<0 (<0, 46.27)
Age at exposure		
<20	11.12 (3.40, 43.32)	<0 (<0, 64.40)
20–40	<0 (<0, 0.46)	<0 (<0, 0.05)
>40	1.39 (<0, 8.30)	<0 (<0, 63.69)
Time since exposure		
12–15	1.91 (<0, 25.28)	<0 (<0, 81.44)
15–30	1.42 (0.01, 5.76)	<0 (<0, 55.01)
>30	3.81 (0.99, 10.65)	<0 (<0, 85.38)
All	2.55 (0.87, 5.72)	<0 (<0, 73.21)
Mortality		
Life Span Study[344]		
Mucoepidermoid carcinoma	8.30 (2.56–29.6)	0.21 (0.10–0.37)
Other malignant neoplasm	1.36 (–0.01–4.73)	0.12 (0.01–0.28)
Warthin's tumor	3.05 (0.58–10.3)	0.10 (0.01–0.25)
Other benign neoplasm	0.30 (–0.10–1.18)	0.08 (<0–0.26)
Childhood benign head and neck tumor cohort		
Benign tumors	19.6 (0.16–∞)	NA
Malignant tumors	–0.06 (–∞–4.0)	NA

*The studies listed are those for which quantitative estimates of risk could be made. Adapted from United Nations Scientific Committee of the Effects of Atomic Radiation (UNSCEAR): Sources and effects of ionizing radiation: 2006 report to the General Assembly with annexes. New York, United Nations, 2007.

External Exposure

Hyperparathyroidism has been identified in atomic bomb survivors.[348-350] Of the original cohort, 4675 persons were screened with blood chemistry, and 22 hyperparathyroid persons were detected. The latent period was 41 years. In these studies of subclinical hyperparathyroidism, the data fit a linear model with an ERR of about 4 at 1 Gy. In an autopsy study of 4136 atomic bomb survivors, Fujiwara et al. found 16 cases of parathyroid adenoma.[351] The time of autopsy was 20 to 27 years after exposure, and the normal incidence in the Japanese population is unknown.

A number of reports have retrospectively questioned hyperparathyroid patients about prior radiotherapy. In 1977, Prinz et al. reported 89 patients, 27 of whom (30%) had received prior radiotherapy with estimated doses of 3 to 7 Gy to the neck.[352] The mean latent period was 30 years, with about one half of the patients

having adenomas and the other half hyperplasia. Russ et al. shortly followed with another series of 74 patients with documented parathyroid adenomas.[353] Twenty-five percent gave a history of prior radiation exposure, compared with a matched control incidence of 8%. Beard et al. have reported a case-control study of 51 cases of hyperparathyroidism and indicated an association with radiation.[354] Most patients had parathyroid adenomas, and a few had parathyroid hyperplasia. The mean estimated dose was 0.32 Gy, and the mean time of appearance was 29 years postexposure. In a retrospective review of 1550 cases of hyperparathyroidism, Christmas et al. found a past history of neck irradiation in 0.7% (10 cases). The mean latent period was 32 years, with a range of 3 to 63 years.[355] In addition to the above reviews, a number of authors have followed radiotherapy patients to assess the development of hyperparathyroidism. Tisell et al. followed 444 persons treated for tuberculous adenitis; 14% developed hyperparathyroidism[356] The estimated doses ranged from 0.6 to 45 Gy. The risk was judged to be three times as high in females as with males. The mean latent period was 44 years (range 28 to 62). Cohen et al. performed a study of 2923 children who had received irradiation for tonsillar hypertrophy at an average age of 4 years; 32 cases with a mean dose of 7.8 Gy and a latent period of 19 to 45 (mean 35) years were detected.[357] In our review of 10 external exposure epidemiologic studies of hyperparathyroidism and parathyroid adenoma, the latent period ranges from 10 to 63 years with a mean of 38 years.

Internal Exposure

After radioiodine therapy for hyperthyroidism, Holm et al. have reported a statistically significant increase in the frequency of parathyroid cancer, with 27 cases found in 10,552 patients.[271]

LARYNX CANCER

Cancer of the larynx was reported to be increased in the German Thorotrast Study,[211,212] however, in the Danish series[213] a nonsignificantly elevated SIR of 1.3 (95% CI 0.3, 3.9) was found. Residual Thorotrast can give high doses to tissues of the neck (Fig. 5-4). At least 20 other epidemiologic studies have examined cancer of the larynx, with nonsignificant results relative to radiation causation. These deal with persons exposed to fallout,[52] nuclear workers in the United Kingdom,[143,145,146,148,191] United States,[164,287] and Australia,[152] radiologic technologists,[97-99,101] and patients exposed for treatment of TB,[105] peptic ulcer treatment,[113] ankylosing spondylitis patients,[109] Chernobyl cleanup workers,[178] hyperthyroid patients receiving radioiodine,[201] uranium workers,[193] and uranium miners.[186] Cardis et al. have reported the cancer mortality results from a 15-country collaborative study of nuclear workers.[168] This is the largest occupational study to date and

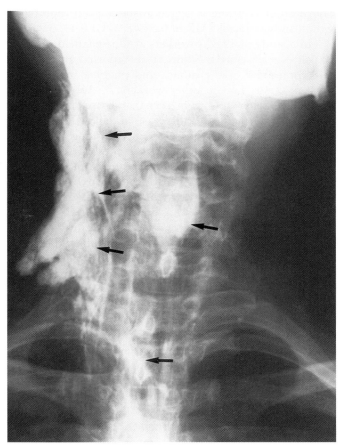

Figure 5-4 • Thorotrast in the soft tissues of the neck. This occurred as a result of extravasation of contrast during a direct puncture carotid arteriogram in the 1950s.

included a cohort of 407,391 workers with 18,993 deaths and 5.2 million person-years of follow-up and the ERR per Sv for larynx cancer was nonsignificantly negative at less than 0.

ORAL CAVITY AND PHARYNX CANCER

General

The oral cavity, pharynx, and larynx are generally regarded as tissues of low risk in radiation carcinogenesis. Tumors of these sites represent a subject in which careful analysis of confounding factors must be performed prior to reaching a conclusion that radiation is a possible cause. Tobacco and alcohol use are known to be major causes of these tumors. In nondrinking male cigarette smokers, the risk is double that of nondrinking nonsmokers. The risk is 10-fold or more for cancer of the larynx.[358]

Cancer of the oral cavity and pharynx is the sixth most common cancer in males and twelfth most common in females. Rates tend to be highest in fair-skinned populations and in Canada. Risks are clearly higher in smokers and persons with high consumption of alcohol. Cancer of

the nasopharynx is rare except in parts of China and southeast Asia. Factors that may be involved in the causation of this tumor are the Epstein-Barr virus and diets with high-nitrate content, such as salted fish. Essentially, all epidemiologic studies searching for an association between radiation and oral and pharyngeal cancer are negative. Most studies have smoking and alcohol consumption as confounding factors.

External Exposure

Natural Background and Population Near Nuclear Facilities

In a very large study conducted in China, where there are areas of high natural background radiation, no increase in nasopharyngeal cancer was found.[29,30] A paper by Sun et al. compared a high-background area and a neighboring control area in Guangdong, China, evaluating 1.7 million person-years of study from 1979–1995.[32] The dose rate in the high-background area was 4.3 mSv per year and in the control areas it was about 1.6 mSv per year. The RR of nasopharynx cancer compared to the control area was nonsignificantly elevated at 0.10 ERR per Sv (95% CI −1.21, 3.28). No increase has been found in populations living near nuclear plants in the United States.[78]

Atomic Bomb Survivors

Slightly increased risks were found for oral cavity tumors in the atomic bomb survivors. Incidence studies report data for tumors of the oral cavity and pharynx as a group. The studies do not provide evidence of a statistically significant dose response, and the EAR was estimated to approximate 0.2 $(10^4 PYSv)^{-1}$ (95% CI < 0.01, 0.7).[279] The earlier mortality studies did not report data relative to these tumor types.[10] In a later mortality report covering 1958–1987, Ron et al. indicated an ERR at 1 Sv of −0.2 (95% CI < −0.2, 0.3) and EAR of −0.1 $(10^4 PYSv)^{-1}$ (95% CI < 0.05, 0.08).[359] The incidence data indicate an ERR of 0.29 at 1 Sv; however, examination of the graph (Fig. 5-5) indicates that the confidence limits for all points, even up to 3 Sv, include 0 as a possibility. On the basis of the incidence data, tumors of the oral cavity appear to have only a weak association with radiation exposure.

The initial mortality data from Japan actually indicated a slightly negative association with radiation. In the 2003 update studies of mortality of atomic bomb survivors during 1950–1997, Preston et al. studied a cohort of 86,572 persons with an average external dose of 0.23 Sv.[281] In males there was a statistically nonsignificant decrease of buccal cancer at dose levels of 1 Sv, with an ERR of −0.20 (90% CI < −0.3, 0.45). In females there was a statistically nonsignificant decrease at dose levels of 1 Sv, with an ERR of −0.20 (90% CI < −0.3, 0.75). For oral cavity and pharynx cancer incidence, the ERR per Gy was 0.39 (90% CI 0.11 to 0.79).[319]

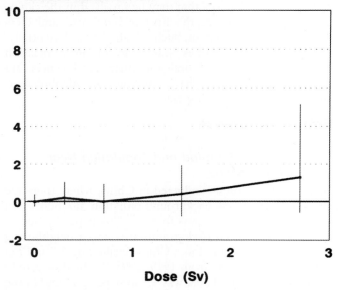

Excess relative risk

Oral cavity cancer incidence (A-bomb)

Figure 5-5 ● ERR of cancer of the oral cavity in atomic bomb survivors at different dose levels. Bars indicate 95% CI. (From Thompson D, Mabuchi K, Ron E, et al: Cancer incidence in atomic bomb survivors. II: Solid tumors, 1958–1987. RERF Technical Report 5-92, Hiroshima, Japan, Radiation Effects Research Foundation, 1992.)

Occupational Exposure

A large number of occupational studies are predominantly negative with respect to radiation induction of oropharyngeal cancer. There have been multiple analyses of UK atomic test veterans by Darby et al.,[52] Doll et al.,[53] and Muirhead et al.[54] The latest 2004 review by Muirhead et al. included a cohort of 21,357 test partipants and reported a nonsignificantly increased SMR of 1.18 (95% CI 0.82, 1.69) for cancers of the mouth and pharynx in test participants but a significantly decreased risk compared to controls.[55] The RR compared to controls for incidence was nonsignificantly decreased at 0.86.

A study by Beral at al. included an analysis of 3373 deaths among 39,546 United Kingdom atomic energy workers during 1946–1979.[143] Beral et al. also studied atomic weapons workers and reported a rate ratio of 0.31 (95% CI 0.01 to 3.64) for neoplasms of oral cavity and pharynx.[144] In this study the ratio rate for cancer of buccal cavity and pharynx, comparing the exposed to nonexposed employees, was 0.31 (95% CI 0.01 to 3.64). A cohort analysis of the U.K. National Registry of Radiation Workers by Kendall et al. included 95,217 workers with over 1.2 million person-years at risk.[145] A statistically significantly low SMR of 0.59 was reported for cancer of the tongue, mouth, and pharynx. A second analysis in 1999 of 124,743 workers in the U.K. National Registry of Radiation Workers by

Muirhead et al. using a lagged analysis again reported a significantly reduced SMR of 0.64 (95% CI 0.44, 0.90).[146]

In a study of 14,327 workers at the Sellafield plant of British Nuclear Fuels, Smith et al. reported an SMR of 0.48 for cancer of the mouth and pharynx in radiation workers versus 1.73 in other workers.[360] Another report on the Sellafield plant by Omar et al. indicated no evidence of a significant increase or decrease in the SMR or SIR of lip, tongue, mouth, or pharynx cancer among nonplutonium workers.[148] McGeoghegan et al. reported on the mortality and cancer morbidity experience of employees at the Chapelcross plant of British Nuclear Fuels during 1955–1995.[149] The cohort included 2628 workers with median doses of 39 mSv and, among radiation workers, the SMR for buccal cancer was nonsignificantly reduced at 0.90. The SMRs for larynx cancer in both studies were nonsignificantly reduced at 0.53 and 0.76, respectively.

Artalejo et al. reported on mortality among 5657 workers of the former Spanish Nuclear Energy Board with mean exposure of 11.42 mSv.[151] The SMR for buccal cancer was nonsignificant at 0.98 (95% CI 0.39, 2.01). Iwasaki et al. conducted a second analysis of mortality of nuclear industry workers in Japan.[150] The study included 176,000 male workers and 5527 deaths. Average annual doses were 3.5 mSv before 1982 and 1.2 mSv after 1982. For buccal cancer the SMR was nonsignificantly decreased at 0.79 (95% CI 0.56, 1.08). Habib et al. have reported on cancer incidence among Australian nuclear industry–monitored radiation workers and indicated a significantly decreased SIR of 0.36 for buccal and pharynx cancer.[152] Cardis et al. reported on cancer mortality among nuclear industry workers in three countries.[166] This is a very large study of 95,673 workers and includes over 2 million person-years at risk and 15,825 deaths. The trend for buccal cancer was nonsignificantly increased at −1.10 with a P value of 0.864. Cardis et al. also have reported the cancer mortality results from a 15-country collaborative study of nuclear workers.[168] This is the largest occupational study to date and included a cohort of 407,391 workers with 18,993 deaths and 5.2 million person-years of follow-up. The ERR per Sv for buccal and pharynx cancer was nonsignificantly positive at 0.40 (90% CI < 0, 5.99). Rahu et al. have reported on cancer incidence of 5446 male Latvian and Estonian Chernobyl cleanup workers and indicated a nonsignificantly elevated SIR of 1.27 for mouth and pharynx cancer in these workers.[178]

Large occupational studies have been carried out in the United States and Canada. Gilbert et al. have reported on workers at Hanford in which they found an SMR for buccal cavity and pharynx cancer of 0.76.[361] Frome reported a mortality study of 106,020 employees in the nuclear industry at Oak Ridge, Tennessee, and the SMR for buccal cancer in black and white males and females was nonsignificantly different from unity.[160] Fry et al. reported a study of mortality and morbidity among

3145 persons occupationally exposed to 50 or more mSv in a year.[161] The mean external exposure was 153 mSv and the SMR for buccal cancer was nonsignificantly elevated.

Cragle et al., reporting on 9860 white male workers at the Savannah River plant, indicated that there were consistently fewer than expected cases of cancer of the buccal cavity and pharynx.[288] Wiggs et al. found a reduced SMR in a follow-up of Los Alamos workers.[164] At the Mound Facility in Ohio the SMR for oral cancer was 0.79 (95% CI 0.10, 2.87)[156] and in a Canadian study of 8977 workers there was an SMR of 1.04 (95% CI 0.45, 2.06).[260] Ashmore et al. reported the first analysis of mortality and occupational radiation exposure based on the National Dose Registry of Canada which included a cohort of 206,620 individuals and 5426 deaths.[154] The average exposure for males was 10.6 mSv and the SMR for buccal cancer was nonsignificantly reduced at 0.62 (90% CI 0.37, 0.97). In addition it was reported that the SMR for pharyngeal cancer was also nonsignificantly reduced at 0.75 (90% CI 0.50, 1.09). Sont et al. studied the relationship of cancer incidence and occupational radiation exposure based on the National Dose Registry of Canada and included a cohort of 191,333 persons with an average dose for males of 11.5 mSv and an average dose for the cohort of 6.64 mSv.[153] The SIR for tongue and mouth cancer in males was nonsignificantly reduced at 0.52 and in females it was nonsignificantly reduced at 0.56. For cancer of the pharynx, there was a significant reduction in males (SIR 0.61) and a nonsignificant reduction in females (SIR 0.66). In 2004 Zablotska et al. reported on mortality of Canadian nuclear workers and concluded that for buccal cancer there was a nonsignificantly decreased SMR of 0.61 (95% CI 0.32, 1.04).[155]

Groves et al. conducted a 40-year cancer mortality study of 40,581 Korean War Navy veterans with potential exposure to high-intensity radar sources which also emit ionizing radiation.[165] The SMR for buccal cancer was significantly decreased at 0.49 (95% CI 0.32, 0.76). A somewhat more controversial study also yielded negative results for an association with occupational exposure and buccal and oral cavity cancer. Wilkinson et al. found an SMR of 0.22 (90% CI 0.01, 1.04) at the Rocky Flats plant.[286]

Studies in uranium miners have not shown an increase in these cancers. Waxweiler et al. did not observe any of these tumors, as compared with four cases expected.[362] A 2004 update of French uranium miners by Laurier et al. reported a nonsignificant SMR of 0.6 for buccal cancer.[186] A study of uranium enrichment workers by Brown et al. did not find an excess of tumors of the buccal cavity or pharynx and reported an SMR of 0.80 (95% CI 0.22 to 2.05).[363] Ritz et al. have reported on cancer mortality in uranium processing workers at the Fernald plant in Ohio among whom the SMR for buccal was nonsignificantly increased at 1.03.[192] McGeoghegan et al. have reported on the mortality of 12,540 workers (including 3244

radiation workers) at the Capenhurst uranium enrichment facility during 1946–1995 and found that the SMR for buccal cancer was nonsignificantly reduced in radiation workers at 0.98.[242] They also studied cancer mortality experience of 19,454 workers (including 13,960 radiation workers) at the Springfields uranium production facility during 1946–1995 and again found the SMR for buccal cancer was nonsignificantly reduced for radiation workers at 0.96.[243]

Cancer incidence among medical diagnostic workers in China was reported by Wang et al. in 1988 who compared 27,011 workers with 25,782 persons in other medical specialties.[102] The x-ray workers had a 50% higher risk of developing some form of cancer. However, there was no evidence (RR of 0.7) of an excess of cancer of the oral cavity or pharynx as a result of radiation exposure. In 2002 Wang et. al reported a follow-up and the RR for buccal cancer was nonsignificantly decreased at 0.75.[253] Doody et al. reported on mortality among 143,517 U.S. radiologic technologists during 1926–1990 whose doses were not evaluated.[97] The SMR for buccal cancer was significantly reduced at 0.67 (95% CI 0.45, 0.95). Sigurdson et al. studied cancer incidence in 90,305 U.S. radiologic technologists and found that the SIR for buccal cancer was significantly reduced at 0.73 (95% CI 0.55, 0.90).[101] Mohan et al. studied cancer and other causes of mortality among 146,022 radiologic technologists employed from 1940 and later and found the SMR for buccal cancer in males was significantly reduced at 0.59 (95% CI 0.4, 0.9) while for females it was nonsignificantly reduced at 0.89 (95% CI 0.6, 1.3).[98,99]

Medical Exposure

Buccal cancer has been studied in patients after external exposures in diagnostic radiology. Massachusetts TB patients treated with multiple fluoroscopies have been followed by Davis et al.[105] They have indicated an SMR of 0.4 for this cancer in exposed females and 1.9 in unexposed females. The SMR for exposed males was elevated at 2.2 but was even higher (3.3) for unexposed male controls. In another study of Massachusetts TB patients, the SMR for cancer of the buccal cavity and pharynx in male controls was significantly elevated at 2.4, but in the exposed males the SMR was 0.9.[364] In the females the SMR for the exposed persons was 0.0, and for controls it was 2.1 (the data on females are based on very few cases). Radiation therapy can give quite high doses to specific organs, and patients have been followed after therapy for benign as well as malignant conditions. It is of interest that patients treated with radiotherapy for tinea capitis did not appear to develop oral cavity tumors.[293] In patients who were treated for ankylosing spondylitis, cancer of the mouth and pharynx were both nonsignificantly elevated with O/E ratios of 1.58 and 1.56, respectively.[109] Interestingly, even though there was a small number of cases, cancer of the pharynx was elevated (two cases vs. 0.12 expected) in patients with ankylosing spondylitis not given x-ray therapy.[365] In women given x-ray therapy for benign uterine bleeding, the reported O/E ratio for cancer of the oral cavity was 0.7, based on three cases.[118] Mattsson et al. have reported on cancer incidence among 3090 women who received radiation therapy for benign breast disease.[114] The RR for mouth cancer was nonsignificantly increased at 1.05. Carr et al. performed a follow-up study of 3719 patients treated with radiotherapy for peptic ulcer with doses to the abdomen of about 15 Gy.[113] No cases of buccal cancer were found after radiotherapy in the period 0 to 10 years postexposure and in the follow-up period of 11 to 62 years postexposure the RR was nonsignificantly reduced at 0.38.

In an incidence study of women treated with radiation for cervical cancer, 82,616 exposed women were compared with 99,424 unexposed controls.[124] Women from Canada, Denmark, Finland, Norway, Sweden, Yugoslavia, the United Kingdom, and the United States were studied over 1.28 million person-years at risk. No evidence of a radiation-related excess risk was found for tumors of the oral cavity and pharynx. In patients treated for invasive cervical cancer, the O/E ratio was 1.3 for those treated with radiotherapy and 1.5 for those treated without radiotherapy. In patients who were followed for 10 years or more, the O/E ratio was 1.7 for both groups. In general, no increase in oral cavity or pharyngeal tumors has been identified in children who were treated for childhood malignancies such as Wilms' tumors and HD. Reviews of other series of radiotherapy patients have reported some carcinomas of the pharynx.[366–368]

Internal Exposure

Among studies of the potential carcinogenic effects of diagnostic doses of radioiodine administered to perform thyroid scanning, the largest and most recent included 35,074 patients who were matched with the Swedish cancer registry.[270] No increase in the grouped category of oral cavity, pharynx, and digestive cancers was noted, the SIR being reported as 0.97 (95% CI 0.91 to 1.04). After treatment for hyperthyroidism, Holm et al.[271] indicated an SIR for oral cavity and pharynx of 1.02 (95% CI 0.63 to 1.55), and Hoffman et al.[202] indicated an RR of 2.1 based on one case being observed (95% CI 0.2 to 16.1). The studies examining risk after large radioiodine treatments for thyroid cancer have not reported on these tumor types. Ron et al.[201] reported on 35,593 hyperthyroid patients treated by different methods. The SMR for buccal cancer in patients treated with any iodine 131 was nonsignificantly increased at 1.12 and in patients treated with only iodine 131 it was also nonsignificantly increased at 1.12.

A report on the Sellafield plant by Omar et al. indicated no significant increase or decrease in SMR or SIR for lip, tongue, mouth, or pharynx cancer among plutonium workers.[148] Carpenter et al. examined workers in the United Kingdom who were occupationally exposed to tritium, plutonium, and other radionuclides.[191] The SMRs for buccal and pharynx cancer in each group were reduced (significantly so for plutonium exposures). Wiggs et al. found nonsignificantly increased RR in a follow-up of Los Alamos plutonium workers.[164]

Summary

Epidemiologic studies show no consistent or statistically significant increase in cancer of the oral cavity or pharynx following internal or external radiation exposure. Neither the 1988 or 1994 UNSCEAR reports[369,370] nor the 1990 ICRP report[248] give radiation risk estimates for this category of tumors.

THYROID CANCER

General

Thyroid cancer causes approximately 1000 deaths annually in the United States. There are approximately 13,000 new thyroid cancer cases annually in the United States. Thyroid cancer represents about 1% to 2% of all cancers. High rates are found in Hawaiian Islanders, Filipino immigrants of Hawaii and California, native Alaskan women, and the population of Iceland. Thyroid cancer is approximately twice as common in females as in males, with the incidence increasing with age. The overall age-adjusted incidence is 3.9 in 100,000 members of the population. Incidence rates for both sexes are increasing in the United States and Nordic countries, especially in the younger age groups. In Connecticut, for example, the age-adjusted incidence rates for females rose from 1.7 per 100,000 in 1945 to 5.5 per 100,000 in 1985.

In Europe, the incidence of thyroid cancer has also been rising, which has prompted a number of authors to question the potential impact of the Chernobyl accident as a cause. The matter has been examined by Catelinos et al. who have pointed out that if the normal increase in spontaneous incidence/detection is not taken into account, there can be substantial variation in potential radiation risk estimates.[371] Despite this rise in incidence, mortality rates have been declining. The reason for the increased incidence may be increased diagnosis of clinically occult lesions.

The 5-year survival for all types of thyroid tumors is approximately 85%, with the majority of these being well-differentiated carcinomas. It should be noted that about 25% of cases of medullary carcinoma occur on a familial basis in persons with multiple endocrine neoplasia type 2a. Robbins et al.[372] have estimated that 9% of thyroid cancers may be attributable to radiation.[372]

Because radiation-induced thyroid cancers do not usually include the anaplastic and medullary types, the ultimate fatality rate of radiation-induced thyroid tumors is between 3% and 9%. For many years, the thyroid has been the subject of many investigations concerning induction of neoplasms, both malignant and benign. X-ray and gamma radiation, as well as internally deposited radionuclides (particularly radioiodines), may induce thyroid carcinoma. Radiogenic thyroid tumors were first detected by Duffy in 1950.[373] As with other types of tumors, the risk estimates given generally are based on the linear-nothreshold model, although at very high absorbed doses these estimates are not valid (because of cell killing).

The risk factors derived in various epidemiologic studies are not always easy to compare because they include different age groups, ethnic backgrounds, primary diseases, and ratios of males to females in the population examined. Excellent sources of information regarding radiation induction of thyroid cancer include an NCRP report,[374] the BEIR reports of 1990[3] and 2005,[18] the 1991 ICRP report,[248] the UNSCEAR reports of 2000[375] and 2006,[86] a review article by Shore,[376] and a monograph edited by Nagataki.[377]

In general, the majority of thyroid cancers induced by radiation are well-differentiated papillary adenocarcinomas, with a lesser percentage being follicular. For the most part, these tumors are associated with long survival periods. In one study performed at the Mayo Clinic (including more than 1100 patients), the 25-year survival of patients with papillary carcinomas was in excess of 90%, whereas the 25-year survival for follicular carcinoma was only 45%.[378] Data from the American Cancer Society indicate that only 11% of patients with well-differentiated thyroid carcinoma will eventually die of their disease.[379] United States data from 1981–1986 indicate that 5-year survival rates for all forms of thyroid cancer are about 95%.

The so-called occult carcinoma, which is usually of a nonsclerosing papillary type, is not considered in radiogenic risk estimates because these occult tumors are of doubtful clinical significance and are usually discovered incidentally by pathologists. Martinez-Tello et al. have indicated that in an autopsy study of a nonexposed Spanish population, up to 22% of completely sectioned thyroids contained occult papillary carcinomas.[380] An incidence of 8.8% occult papillary carcinoma has been reported by Furmanchuk et al. in a Belarussian autopsy series.[381]

It should be noted that at least several cases of anaplastic thyroid tumors have been reported as following radiation exposure,[382,383] but it is uncertain whether these were fortuitous or whether they were indeed radiation-induced. It is possible that they may have resulted from degeneration of better differentiated radiogenic tumors.

Since the Chernobyl accident there has been great interest in a possible genetic or mutational signature (a genomic fingerprint) that might be associated with radiation-induced thyroid cancers. A large proportion of the childhood cancers occurring after Chernobyl were reported to be aggressive. Initial reports indicated that rearrangements of the tyrosine kinase domain of the *RET* proto-oncogene were found at a higher than expected rate for these rearrangements in thyroid tumors in the general population.[384–386] The most frequently observed were *RET/PTC1* and *RET/PTC3* rearrangements; however 30% to 50% of the papillary cancers did not have these findings. At the present time, it appears that the genomic differences and aggressive nature of the tumors reported may represent the type of thyroid cancer that occurs in childhood rather than a radiation signature per se.[387–389]

The cell type of childhood thyroid cancers occurring after Chernobyl was also initially felt to be rather specific, with a solid-follicular variant of papillary cancer being predominant from 1990–1995. This cell type, however, has decreased with time since exposure, and the proportion of papillary cancers composed mainly of papillae has been increasing with time.[390] As of 2000–2001 the percentage of each type of papillary cancer was almost equal. It also appears that RAS, p53, *BRAF*, B-raf, and *NTRK1* mutations are not characteristic of the Chernobyl or radiation-associated thyroid tumors.[391–395]

Modifying Factors

Several modifying factors are associated with radiation-induced thyroid neoplasms. The first of these is the type and duration of exposure. Acute external radiation appears to be more effective in causing radiogenic thyroid tumors than is iodine 131 for each unit of absorbed dose (Gy). Other radionuclides such as iodine 125 and 123 probably have an intermediate effectiveness. This may be due to a dose-rate effect since the absorbed dose from iodine 131 is delivered over days to weeks.

The latent period from radiation exposure to clinical development of thyroid neoplasms varies widely among the human clinical studies. Following external radiation, the latent period has been reported to be anywhere between 4 or 5 and 40 or more years. The reported mean latent period appears to be a function of the follow-up time of the particular study, with several authors indicating an excess number of cancer cases occurring 30 to 40 years after irradiation. Schneider et al. have reported that for children who received radiation therapy to the head and neck for benign conditions, the ERR per 10 mGy was about 0.02 at less than 10 years postexposure, 0.04 at 10 to 25 years, rose to a maximum (0.084) at 25 to 29 years postexposure, and then declined to about 0.04 at 40 or more years.[396] Any epidemiologic study that is not conducted with a long enough follow-up period will give an estimate of the mean latency period that is likely to be short. It also appears that the latent period may increase with the age at irradiation.[397,398]

In a study of children irradiated for skin angiomas by DeVathaire et al., radiation therapy was delivered from various sources at substantially different rates.[399] These included x-ray, strontium, radium 226, yttrium 90, and phosphorus 32. With exposures of short duration an ERR per Gy of 10 was found but not with exposures of long duration. This data as well as the studies by Lundell et al. of risks with radium 226 applicators for skin hemangiomas tend to confirm the data relative to reduced effectiveness with lower dose rate when thyroid cancer is studied.[400] Similar conclusions have been reached when the effects of diagnostic uses of iodine 131 have been studied. This is discussed later in the section on internal exposure.

Various studies reviewed later indicate that the thyroid is more radiosensitive in children and adolescents than in adults. Whether this is due to differences in metabolism or concentration of radionuclides is unknown. Certainly, inhalation of a fixed amount of radioiodine results in greater concentration by the infant thyroid than by the adult thyroid.[401] It is certain that the younger a person is at the time of exposure, the higher the future risk of developing radiation-induced thyroid cancer. Except at high therapeutic doses, exposures over the age of 20 years from external radiation have not been found to significantly increase the risk of thyroid cancer. The best estimate of risk for persons exposed to external radiation at ages of less than 20 comes from a pooled analysis by Ron et al.[402] The ERR at 1 Gy is estimated to be 8.7 following exposures in childhood. The risks from iodine 131 exposure have been best elucidated in a recent report by Cardis et al. in a study of childhood cancer following the Chernobyl accident.[403] Excess risk was identified at all doses above 0.2 Gy. At thyroid doses in excess of 2.0 Gy the risk plateaued. At 1 Gy the OR was between 5.5 (95% CI 3.1, 9.5) to 8.4 (95% CI 4.1, 17.3) depending on the risk model used. The risk therefore was slightly smaller than that seen with external exposure. Ronckers et al. studied subsequent thyroid cancer risk among 14,054 childhood cancer survivors and reported an ERR per Gy of 1.3 (95% CI 0.4, 4.1), but which decreased by 53% at 20 Gy and 95% at 40 Gy.[403a] This strong downturn in risk at high doses had not been previously quantified for thyroid cancer.

The National Cancer Institute has developed a program for estimation of thyroid cancer probability following radiation exposure. The ERR per Gy for various ages that is used in the program as well as the statistical uncertainty, are shown in Table 5-9.

Sex also appears to be a modifying factor. Several epidemiologic studies indicate that females are more sensitive than males to radiogenic thyroid adenomas and cancers. The absolute risk in females may be 2 to 4 times that in males, but the ERR per Sv is about the same for both sexes.[105,404,405] In the U.S. population, spontaneous thyroid carcinoma occurs in females approximately two and a half times more commonly than in males. Ethnic background also appears to be a significant modifying factor. This has been noted particularly in the studies of

Table 5-9 •	Excess Relative Risk per Gy for Thyroid Cancer at Various Ages of Exposure	
Exposure Age	Geometric Mean	Geometric Standard Deviation
0	9.463	2.183
5	6.262	1.924
10	4.136	1.976
15	2.732	2.160
20	1.804	2.301
25	1.192	2.367
30	0.788	2.365
35	0.521	2.379
40	0.345	2.732
45	0.228	3.140
50	0.151	3.611

individuals of Jewish ancestry.[120,376] Risk factors for those with Jewish ancestry appear to be 2 to 8 times higher than for non-Jewish populations. Persons of Jewish ancestry from Morocco and Tunisia appear to be 10 times more sensitive than non-Jewish populations. Whether this is due to a high prevalence of A-T heterozygosity is unknown. A report of Momani et al. involving a study of siblings who were irradiated did not identify familial factors that modified the effects of radiation exposure.[405]

Some authors have suggested that iodine deficiency may be a promoting factor in radiation-induced thyroid carcinogenesis because of a reduction in level of thyroid hormone and resulting stimulatory effect on the cells. While this has been suggested in animal studies, at least two human studies indicate the opposite: that thyroid cancer can be associated with high iodine intake.[406,407] Whether there is an association between thyroid cancer and goiter was previously unclear.[408] The study of Cardis et al., discussed above, indicates that in areas of iodine deficiency the risk of cancer may be threefold higher than in areas of normal iodine levels and that with iodine prophylaxis the risk can be reduced at least threefold.[403] Some authors believe that Graves' disease influences the development and behavior of thyroid carcinoma.[409]

Many workers have suggested that one reason for the sensitivity of the thyroid to radiation carcinogenesis may be that thyroid-stimulating hormone (TSH) enhances the effect of ionizing radiation.[410] They have also suggested that patients at risk be given prophylactic exogenous thyroxine. In at least a few cases, however, this treatment seems to have had little effect.[411] Shore has reviewed information related to reproductive history as a potential modifying factor.[376] In the Marshall Islands all the cancers occurred in multiparous women. It appears that in some studies, parity may raise risk, but whether it affects sensitivity to radiation remains unclear.

External Exposure

High Natural Background

Excess relative risk of solid cancer mortality after prolonged exposure to naturally occurring high-background radiation in Yangjiang, China, has been published. Tao et al. reported on a population living in a high-background area and a neighboring control area in Guangdong, China, and had 1.7 million person-years of study from 1979–1995.[33] The mortality due to thyroid cancer was nonsignificantly elevated in the high-background high-dose group with an RR of 1.47 (95% CI 0.21, 10.47). Increased exposure to cosmic ray radiation occurs among airline crews; in a report from Pukkala et al., a five-decade study of over 10,000 Nordic pilots found only three cases of thyroid cancer and no relationship to cumulative dose.[39] Another report of over 28,000 European airline pilots by Blettner et al. found a nonsignificant increase in thyroid cancer mortality, with an SMR of 1.48 (95% CI 0.47, 3.48) based on only five cases.[412]

Atomic Bomb Survivors

Thyroid cancer induction has been apparent in the survivors of the atomic bomb at Hiroshima and Nagasaki (Fig. 5-6).[413,414] The rate of induction of thyroid tumors, as in other series, was higher in females than males by a factor of slightly greater than 2. The exact risk is difficult to calculate because of the uncertainties in dosimetry; however, the rates appear to be between 5 and 20 cases in 1 million persons exposed for each 10 mGy. Wakabayashi et al. indicated an annual absolute risk of about 1.4 excess cases annually in 1 million persons for each 10 mGy and an RR of between 3.2 and 5.1.[335] Parker et al. identified 74 thyroid cancers in the population, although only 40 were diagnosed during life.[415] Those diagnosed at autopsy were usually of the occult papillary sclerosing type. The 1977 UNSCEAR report indicated that these occult tumors were found in about 16% of autopsies of nonirradiated subjects, although in the atomic bomb survivors, they were found at approximately 23% of autopsies of females.[316] The LSS mortality studies have not reported on thyroid cancer. A 1994 report on the incidence of thyroid cancer in the 75,493 subjects of the LSS revealed about 130 cases of thyroid cancer with an estimated ERR at 1 Gy of 1.2. The elevated risk was confined to women, and there was an increasing risk with decreasing age at exposure and attained age.[359,416,417] Of particular interest is that, at autopsy, latent or occult thyroid cancer was found in 2.5% of males and 4.5% of females. In the 1958–1998 LSS incidence report, the ERR at 1 Gy was 0.57 (95% CI 0.24–1.1), and the EAR was 1.2 (95% CI 0.48–2.2).[319] The increase in risk was statistically significant at a dose of about 0.3 Gy.

There was no significant difference in the ERR between males and females, although risk decreased with age at exposure. At 0 to 9 years of age at exposure, the ERR per Gy was 1.5; at 10 to 19 years of age it was 1.2; at 20 to 29 years of age it was 0.46; and at 40 or more years of age it was 0.31. The sex ratio (F:M) was 1.3 for ERR and 3.6 for EAR. The percentage change per decade increase for age at exposure was −31% for ERR and −46% for EAR.[319]

Populations Near Nuclear Facilities

Bowlt et al. examined the incidence of thyroid cancer in Cumbria of the United Kingdom, an area near the Sellafield nuclear plant, which discharged both iodine 131 and 129.[418] Measurements were made of iodine 129 in the thyroids of adults dying from various causes, and levels of activity were found to decrease with distance from the plant. Age-standardized cancer rates showed an increase in thyroid cancer with increasing distance from the plant, which is the opposite of what would be expected if a carcinogenic effect were present from the iodine releases. Lopez-Abente et al. have reported on solid tumor mortality near Spain's four nuclear power plants and four uranium fuel cycle facilities finding that the RR for thyroid cancer was nonsignificant at 0.54.[283] A comprehensive study in the United States of populations living near nuclear facilities has failed to find an increase in thyroid cancer.[78] There are three papers concerning potential uranium contamination and the possibility of increased risk of thyroid cancer in the public.

Excess relative risk

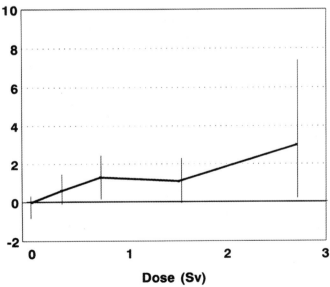

Thyroid cancer incidence (A-bomb)

Figure 5-6 ● ERR of thyroid cancer in atomic bomb survivors at different dose levels. Bars indicate 95% CI. (From Thompson D, Mabuchi K, Ron E, et al: Cancer incidence in atomic bomb survivors, II: Solid tumors, 1958–1987. RERF Technical Report 5-92, Hiroshima, Japan, Radiation Effects Research Foundation, 1992.)

The papers by Boice et al. indicated a nonsignificant decrease around a uranium mining and milling facility in Texas, a nonsignificant increase near a uranium facility in Pennsylvania, and a nonsignificant decrease near a Colorado facility.[89,90,90a] A nonsignificant decrease was found by Boice et al. in a study of persons residing near the Hanford National Laboratory.[91]

Occupational Exposure

Several studies of occupationally exposed workers have examined thyroid cancer specifically. The results are generally nonsignificant. This is because the workers are all adults, the doses tend to be relatively low, and many of the studies are based on mortality statistics. Four early studies predominantly from the United Kingdom yielded negative results.[52,143–145] More recent studies of U.K. workers have been published by Muirhead et al.[54,146] The first study of over 130,000 workers showed a nonsignificantly increased SMR for thyroid cancer of 1.8 (95% CI 0.8, 1.17) and the second study of over 22,000 servicemen and civilians exposed to atmospheric nuclear tests and experimental programs had similar results with an RR of 1.92 (95% CI 0.5, 8.0). A second analysis in 1999 of 124,743 workers in the U.K. National Registry of Radiation Workers by Muirhead et al. using a lagged analysis reported a nonsignificantly increased SMR for thyroid cancer of 1.80 (95% CI 0.90, 3.21).[146] A mortality study of 2628 U.K. workers working at British Nuclear Fuels and reported by McGeoghegan et al. did not identify any deaths due to thyroid cancer.[149] A report on the Sellafield plant by Omar et al. indicated a significant increase among nonplutonium workers in thyroid cancer with an SMR of 4.29 (based on only three cases).[148] Incidence was also significantly increased (based on three cases). A mortality study of over 200,000 Canadian nuclear workers reported by Ashmore et al. had a nonsignificantly raised SMR of 1.5 (95% CI 0.6 to 3.1) based on five cases.[154] Habib et al. have reported on cancer incidence among Australian nuclear industry–monitored radiation workers and indicated a nonsignificant SIR of 1.21 for thyroid cancer.[152]

One study of atomic weapons workers showed what appeared to be a large increase with a rate ratio of 11.05; however, the number of cases was small and the large 95% CI (0.22 to 1311.8) encompasses unity.[287] An additional study had an increased risk but it was not dose-related.[158] A mortality study by Fry et al. of over 3000 Department of Energy workers and contractors who received doses equal to or greater than 50 mSv did not find any cases of thyroid cancer.[161] Sont et al. reported on the first analysis of cancer incidence and occupational radiation exposure based on the National Dose Registry of Canada; the cohort contained 191,333 persons with an average dose for males of 11.5 mSv and an average dose for the cohort of 6.64 mSv.[153] The SIR for cancer of the thyroid was nonsignificantly elevated at 1.32 (90% CI 0.97 to 1.75) and the SIR for females was significantly elevated at 1.42 (90% CI 1.19 to 1.69). Frome reported a mortality study of employees in the nuclear industry at Oak Ridge, Tennessee, which included a cohort of 106,020 employees with 27,982 deaths.[160] The SMR for cancer of the thyroid in white males was 0.33 and 0.52 for white females. Cardis et al. reported on cancer mortality among nuclear industry workers in three countries in a large study of 95,673 workers, which included over 2 million person-years at risk, with 15,825 deaths.[166] The dose-response trend for cancer of the thyroid was negative at 0.58 with a P value 0.281. Cardis et al. have reported the cancer mortality results from a 15-country collaborative study of nuclear workers.[168] This is the largest occupational study to date and included a cohort of 407,391 workers with 18,993 deaths and 5.2 million person-years of follow-up. The ERR per Sv for thyroid cancer was nonsignificantly negative at −0.06.

A study of 27,011 Chinese x-ray workers who had received total cumulative doses in excess of 1 Gy found seven cases of thyroid cancer, for a nonsignificant ERR per Gy of 0.7 (95 CI < 0 to 3.7). A follow-up study of the same group by Wang et al. extending findings through 1995 reported 14 cases and a nonsignificantly increased RR of about 1.7.[253] There are two studies of occupationally exposed x-ray technologists in the United States. A study by Mohan et al. of 146,000 workers reported a nonsignificantly reduced SMR based on seven cases of 0.36 for males and 0.79 for females.[99] Sigurdson et al. studied over 90,000 technologists, and with 125 cases of thyroid cancer, the SIR was statistically significantly elevated at 1.61 (95% CI 1.34 to 1.88).[101]

Medical Diagnostic Exposure

No increased risk of thyroid cancer was found in 13,385 Massachusetts adult TB patients treated using multiple fluoroscopic procedures.[105] Kaplan et al. also reported on a similar group of patients, in which none of the patients reported past or present history of thyroid cancer, nor was any found at examination.[419]

Radiation Therapy

In several major epidemiologic studies external radiation thyroid doses were below 15 Gy. Hempelmann et al., at the University of Rochester, compared 2872 individuals who had x-ray therapy for presumed thymic enlargement.[420] The treatment was given in infancy, and the study population was compared to 5055 nonirradiated siblings. The mean thyroid dose was 1.19 Gy. The absolute risk derived was 2.7 cases annually in 1 million persons exposed for each 10 mGy. With Jewish subjects excluded, the absolute risk was lower, 1.7 cases annually in 1 million for 10 mGy (48 cases/1 million for 10 mGy). In 1993, Shore et al. reported on this group at a mean follow-up time of 37 years.[421] There were 37 thyroid cancers in the exposed group and 5 in the sibling controls. In the irradiated group, 33 cancers were papillary, and 4 were follicular. There were no other cell types. The earliest cancer in this group was found 6 years after exposure, and the latest was at 49 years after irradiation. The ERR was 9.5 at 1 Gy (95% CI 6.9, 12.7). An excess of cancers was statistically significant only at doses over 2 Gy although some excess was present at lower doses. This study is important because it includes a wide range of doses, from 0.01 to greater than 6.0 Gy. The risk ratio was 5.0 in the 0.01 to 0.25 Gy group; however, the confidence limits included unity. The confidence limits for the 0.5 to 1.99 Gy group also included unity; although, for all the data a linear fit appears appropriate. Jewish subjects, again, were noted to be at higher risk, as were women with older ages at menarche or at first childbirth.

Maxon et al., at the University of Cincinnati, examined 1266 patients who had received external radiotherapy for an assortment of benign diseases.[404] The mean thyroid dose was approximately 2.9 Gy. The male-female ratio in those who developed thyroid cancer was 0.6, and the mean latent period was 15.7 years in men and 22.7 years in women. The absolute risk factor derived from this study was 1.5 cases annually in 1 million persons for each 10 mGy.

Ron and Modan examined 10,902 Israeli patients who had been treated with x-ray between 1949 and 1960 for tinea capitis; the estimated thyroid dose was 90 mGy.[120] During irradiation, parts of the head, face, and neck were shielded with lead rubber sheeting, and the estimate of the dose depended critically on the children maintaining a constant position. The ethnic background of this group was almost exclusively Jewish, and the absolute risk determined in this study was 13 cases annually in 1 million persons for each 10 mGy. A higher risk factor was found in patients of Moroccan or Tunisian descent. There were 5420 such subjects included, and, if the groups are separated and their risks determined, the Moroccan and Tunisian subjects had an absolute risk factor of 15 cases annually in 1 million persons for each 10 mGy and a lifetime risk of 140 cases in 1 million persons for each 10 mGy, whereas subjects from Israel, Asia, and other countries in North Africa had an absolute risk factor of 7 cases annually in 1 million persons for each 10 mGy and a lifetime risk of 70 cases in 1 million persons for each 10 mGy. In another report on the Israeli tinea capitis group, Ron et al. estimated the ERR as 0.3 per 0.01 Gy for childhood exposure.[396,422] The absolute excess risk was 13 per 10^6PYcGy. A statistically significant excess risk for thyroid cancer was found at doses between 50 and 100 mGy. A report by Shore et al. of a group of 2224 patients treated in New York with a median follow-up of 39 years and an average thyroid dose of about 60 mGy found two thyroid cancers in the exposed group and none in the controls.[322] The numbers are small but the results are consistent with risks estimated from the Israeli study. The risk coefficient is higher than for many other studies.

Whether it is due to patient movement during radiotherapy, statistical fluctuations, or an unusual sensitivity of this particular population is unclear. Risk factors from this study should not be used out of context from other available epidemiologic studies. The study of tinea capitis patients in New York, for example, yields an absolute excess risk estimate six times lower than the Israeli study. The Israeli study did indicate a higher RR of younger children compared with older children. Another study by Shore et al. included 2215 patients who were treated for tinea capitis and compared to 1395 nonirradiated subjects.[293] The mean thyroid dose in the exposed group was about 80 mGy and, in this group, no thyroid carcinomas were identified.

A study performed in Chicago at Michael Reese Hospital followed 2189 individuals who had received external radiation therapy to the head, neck, or chest prior to or during adolescence, predominantly for tonsillar hypertrophy.[423] The absolute risk of cancer in this group was determined to be three to four cases annually in 1 million persons for each 10 mGy. The population included in this group may have a relatively high proportion of Jewish patients. If a composite risk derived from these studies is valid, it would appear that the absolute risk in children and adolescents exposed to external radiation is three to four cancers annually in 1 million persons for each 10 mGy. Refetoff et al. reported the results of approximately 100 patients who had presented themselves to physicians' offices after becoming aware of the possible consequences of irradiation to the neck region during their childhood or adolescence.[424] Fifteen of these patients were subsequently subjected to operation, and seven cases of thyroid carcinoma were found. None of these were of the occult sclerosing papillary type; all were either papillary follicular or mixed in character. Paloyan et al. reported histologic findings in 38 cancers found at operation in 70 such patients.[425] Thirteen of the carcinomas were papillary, 8 were follicular, and 17 were mixed papillary and follicular. DeGroot reported that among 50 patients seen for thyroid cancer, 20 had a prior history of neck irradiation.[426] In addition, two thirds of patients who had a history of neck irradiation and who had clinical thyroid abnormalities were later shown to have cancer. The ERR for the Chicago tonsillar radiation study was 3.0 (95% CI 2.6, 3.5) and an excess of cancers was seen at doses of about 0.5 Gy.

In a prospective study, DeGroot et al. examined 263 patients who were irradiated at a mean age of 7 years and a mean thyroid dose of 4.51 Gy.[427] Mean age at examination was 33.5 years and 41 thyroid carcinomas were detected. The average size was 1.7 cm, with 37% being less than 1 cm in size. Fifty-nine percent of tumors were multifocal, and 10 of 38 patients with cancer had normal radionuclide thyroid scans. Carcinoma occurred in 37% of single nodules and in 18% of multinodular glands in this population.

The Boston questionnaire study reported by Pottern et al. of over 1100 patients treated for lymphoid hyperplasia revealed an ERR per Gy of 5.9 (95% CI 1.8, 12) for thyroid cancer.[428] There were only a small number of thyroid cancers, and none in the control group. Radium applicators were used in some countries for nasopharyngeal irradiation to reduce the size of adenoid tissue. This was often used in children to reduce the incidence of otitis media and for submariners to reduce the potential for barotraumas.[429] A report by Ronckers et al. on mortality in 5358 subjects included no deaths due to thyroid cancer.[430] A study of 904 children treated with radium for adenoid hypertrophy by Yeh et al. found a nonsignificant excess of thyroid cancer based on two cases with an RR of 4.2 (95% CI 0.38, 45).[431]

Thyroid nodules, both benign and malignant, have been reported after high-dose external radiotherapy. Hallquist et al. reviewed 1056 cases of thyroid cancer.[432] Thirty-seven of these had a previous cancer and 10 of these had received radiation therapy. The OR was nonsignificantly increased at 1.1 (95% CI 0.5 to 2.8) and the thyroid doses ranged from 3 to 40 Gy. Van Daal et al. have followed 605 persons treated with radiotherapy for benign diseases of the head and neck 16 to 46 years earlier.[433] Seven thyroid carcinomas were found in this group, with a mean latency of 37 years. The mean dose to the thyroid was 11.1 Gy. The female-male ratio was 2.5, and average age at irradiation was 10 years. On the basis of UNSCEAR 1977 risk factors, 10.3 cases of thyroid cancer were expected versus the seven found.[316]

No increase of thyroid cancer was found by Griem et al. in adult patients treated with radiation for peptic ulcer disease.[112] A mortality follow-up of the same group by Carr et al. reported a nonsignificant increase in the RR for thyroid cancer of 2.4 (95% CI 0.2 to 27) at 11 to 62 years postexposure.[113] Thyroid dose was estimated to be 0.2 Gy and no cases of thyroid cancer deaths were found at less than 10 years. De Jong et al. have reported on retrospective analysis of thyroid surgery of 110 persons who had received childhood radiotherapy for acne.[434] Of this highly select sample, 31% were found to have thyroid cancer. Such studies, unfortunately, cannot be used to develop risk estimates, due to patient selection by a number of unknown factors.

Mattsson et al. have reported on the incidence of various second malignancies in 1216 women treated with radiation therapy for benign breast disease.[114] Based on four cases the RR for thyroid cancer was nonsignificantly increased at 1.33 (95% CI 0.26, 6.2). Boice et al. have reported on second cancers in 182,040 women treated for cervical cancer.[124] Large local radiation doses were received by 82,616 women, and this group was compared with 99,424 women who were not treated with radiation. Thirty-seven thyroid cancers were observed versus 35 expected, for an RR of 1.1, which is not significantly increased. Doses to the thyroid gland from pelvic radiotherapy were not calculated but should have been quite low. In a case-control study of a similar group of women, Boice et al. found an RR of 2.3 (95% CI 0.6, 8.7). The authors indicate this increase was not statistically significant. Higher thyroid doses are received by patients who receive mediastinal or neck radiotherapy.

Several reports of late effects after childhood radiation therapy reveal that the frequency of thyroid cancer ranks second or third behind bone and soft-tissue sarcomas. Mike et al. found 17 thyroid cancers in 15,000 children who received radiotherapy for other cancers.[435] Increases were noted mostly for patients who had been treated for HD, neuroblastoma, or Wilms' tumor.[436,437] Hancock et al. have reviewed 1677 patients who received radiation therapy for HD.[438] Forty-four patients developed thyroid nodules, and six of these proved to be papillary cancers. The actuarial risk of thyroid cancer was 1.7%, and the risk was 15.6 times that expected in a normal population. In more recent reports of the Late Effects Study Group (LESG), there was a 53-fold increased risk of thyroid cancer in the 9170 children who survived more than 2 years after treatment of another cancer.[439] Sixty-eight percent of the cancers arose within the radiation field. The risk increased with dose and did not decrease even at doses as high as 60 Gy. The ERR per Gy was estimated to be 4.5 (95% CI 3.1, 6.4). The Stanford HD follow-up study of over 1700 adults yielded an ERR per Gy of 0.3 (95% CI 0.1, 0.7).[140] A Nordic study by Sankila et al. of over 1600 patients treated for HD estimated an almost identical ERR per Gy of 0.8 (95% CI 0.4, 1.5).[440]

In a study of over 19,200 patients who received allogenic bone marrow transplants reported by Curtis et al., the absorbed whole-body dose was about 1.2 Gy and the median age was 25 years.[441] There was a statistically significant increase in thyroid cancer with an O/E ratio of 6.6, mostly occurring more than 10 years after treatment. An O/E ratio of 10 was found by Bhatia et al., which, considering their absorbed doses are in the range of 10 to 12 Gy, would yield an ERR of about 1.0 per Gy.[442] Socie et al. reported on over 3100 children following bone marrow transplantation and reported five cases of papillary carcinoma, with four of five occurring more than 5 years postirradiation.[443]

A study reported by De Vathaire et al. of 4096 children treated for cancer in France and the United Kingdom with a mean follow-up of 15 years was also consistent with an ERR per Gy in the range of 4 to 8.[444] In a small study by Cohen et al. there was a high incidence of thyroid cancer (8 cases among 113 children).[445] Six were papillary and two were follicular, and they appeared 3.1 to 15.7 years post-treatment. The study employed ultrasound and annual palpation as screening methodology which probably influenced the results. A similar risk estimate with an ERR per Gy of 0.6 (95% CI 0.0 to 1.4) was obtained from the adult Swedish cervical spine radiotherapy study of over 8100 patients (with an average thyroid dose of about 1 Gy) reported by Damber et al.[446] Most (15 of 22) of the thyroid cancers were diagnosed more than 15 years postexposure.

Internal Exposure

The major sources of human data concerning internal thyroid irradiation are (1) patients receiving iodine 131 (and occasionally iodine 125) for therapeutic purposes, (2) those receiving iodine 131 for diagnostic purposes, and (3) individuals receiving mixtures of radioiodines under fallout circumstances.

Occupational Exposure

Reports of internal occupational exposure and subsequent risk of thyroid cancer are few. Ritz reported on cancer mortality among 4014 uranium-processing workers in whom no cases of thyroid cancer were found.[447] Ritz et al. have reported on cancer mortality in uranium processing workers at the Fernald plant in Ohio.[192] No thyroid cancer cases were found. Dupree-Ellis et al. have reported on mortality in a cohort of 2514 uranium processing workers employed between 1942 and 1966 at the Mallinkrodt Chemical Works.[193] Again, no cases of thyroid cancer were identified. McGeoghegan et al. reported on mortality and cancer morbidity experience of workers at the Capenhurst uranium enrichment facility from 1946–1995 with a cohort that included 12,540 workers, including 3244 radiation workers with mean doses of 9.85 mSv.[242] No thyroid cancers were identified. McGeoghegan et al. also reported on mortality and cancer morbidity experience of workers at the Springfields uranium production facility during 1946–1995.[243] They comprised a cohort of 19,454 workers, including 13,960 radiation workers with a mean external dose of 22.8 mSv and a mean follow-up period of 24.6 years (or 479,146 person-years) and the SMR for cancer of the thyroid in this group was nonsignificantly elevated at 2.15 (based on only four cases). A meta-analysis of 14 studies that contained 120,000 uranium workers found a statistically significant decrease with an RR of 0.38 (95% CI 0, 0.81) for thyroid cancer.[245] A report on the Sellafield plant by Omar et al. indicated a nonsignificant increase in thyroid cancer among plutonium workers with an SMR of 1.50 (based on only one case) but the incidence study reported no case of thyroid cancer.[148] Carpenter et al. studied workers in the United Kingdom who were occupationally exposed to tritium, plutonium, and other radionuclides and found that the SMRs for thyroid cancer in each group were all reduced and significant for exposure to plutonium and other radionuclides.[191] Darby et al. studied radon and cancers in 1415 Swedish iron miners and did not find a single case of thyroid cancer.[183]

Medical Exposure

Patients are sometimes administered radioactive iodine for diagnostic purposes. Hahn et al. followed up over 2000 children who had received iodine 131 and had an average thyroid dose of 1 Gy.[448] There was no increase in thyroid cancer later in life and the reported RR was 0.86 (95% CI 0.14, 5.13).[13] Major epidemiologic studies in this category included Swedish individuals who received iodine 131 for diagnostic purposes.[449,450] The diagnostic administrations of iodine 131 were all less than 37MBq, and the study population included 10,133 subjects. The mean calculated thyroid dose was 0.58 Gy in adults and 1.59 Gy in children and adolescents. Eight thyroid cancers were identified, all in adults. As in other studies, there were more cases in the female population (six out of eight). This cancer incidence did not represent an increase from that expected in a normal population. Holm et al. studied even larger groups, numbering over 35,000, and no statistically significant increase in thyroid carcinoma was found.[198,270,451]

In general, patients who have received very large administered activities of iodine 131 for treatment of hyperthyroidism have not demonstrated radiogenic thyroid neoplasms. Certainly, there is substantial cell killing at these high levels of radiation exposure. Dobyns et al. have reviewed over 16,000 patients with hyperthyroidism treated with radioiodine therapy.[199] In this study, the patients were followed for an average of 10 years; no excess of thyroid carcinoma was observed. The radiation dose to the thyroid in these patients was more than 20 Gy, with the mean being over 85 Gy. This is based on an assumed 6-day effective half-life of iodine 131 in these patients. Holm et al. studied 4557 people treated for hyperthyroidism with iodine 131 with a mean follow-up time of 9.5 years, and with thyroid doses in the range of 60 to 100 Gy.[452] Four thyroid carcinomas were identified, which did not represent a statistically significant increase over the number expected. Thyroid cancer risk was also examined in 10,552 patients who received iodine 131 therapy for hyperthyroidism.[271] The average thyroid dose was over 100 Gy, and the SIR was nonsignificantly elevated at 1.26 (95% CI 0.76, 2.03). Similar results were reported by Goldman et al.[196] With doses high enough to treat hyperthyroidism, cell killing is the predominant effect. Choice of an appropriate control group for these studies is difficult because persons with thyrotoxicosis may have a thyroid cancer incidence as much as 10 times that of the general population.[366,409] The lower risk from radioiodine compared with acute external exposure has been interpreted by many authors as indicating that protracted radiation of the thyroid has substantially less effect than acute doses. Also, these studies were conducted on adults, which are less radiosensitive than children.

Safa et al. and the Cooperative Thyrotoxicosis Follow-up Study Group have examined patients aged 1 to 20 years who were treated for Graves' disease with iodine 131.[453] Estimates of the mean thyroid dose are approximately 90 Gy and two cases of cancer were observed, which was not a statistically significant deviation from the expected number. With the extent of cell killing occurring at doses above 15 Gy of external irradiation, cell killing can be expected to predominate in the dose range of approximately 100 Gy found in most of the therapeutic radioiodine series. A follow-up mortality report of 35,593 adult patients was published in 1998 by Ron et al. after over half of the study cohort had died.[201] While there was an increase in thyroid cancer following iodine 131 treatment, no statistically significant increase in mortality from thyroid cancer was associated with either hyperthyroidism or iodine 131 treatment. Many cases occurred in less than 4 years after exposure and may have been related to underlying disease.

The most recent report on the same group by Dickman et al. also found no increase (SIR 0.91) except on the subgroup of patients who had prior external beam radiotherapy (SIR 9.8).[454] The report also suggests a lower risk per unit dose for iodine 131 compared to brief x-ray exposures.

No significant increase of thyroid cancer was reported in the 1095 Danish Thorotrast patients in whom there was one case of thyroid cancer, yielding a nonsignificantly elevated SIR of 2.4 (95% CI 0.1, 14).[213] A study by Nekolla et al. of 455 patients treated with radium 224 for TB, ankylosing spondylitis, and a few other diseases indicated that thyroid cancer occurred in five patients, which was a statistically significant excess.[224] Nyberg et al. reported on cancer incidence after a 40-year follow-up among Swedish patients exposed to radioactive Thorotrast among whom the SIR for thyroid cancer was nonsignificantly elevated.[222]

Unfortunately, most of the diagnostic follow-up studies have been conducted for mean follow-up times of less than 20 years. Longer follow-up studies might identify some thyroid cancers, but, if the risk estimates for external radiation were applicable to iodine 131, some thyroid tumors should have been identified in these groups. The failure to identify such tumors indicates a relatively reduced efficiency of iodine 131 compared with external radiation for tumor induction.

Fallout

NUCLEAR WEAPONS FALLOUT

Rallison et al. examined 5179 children exposed to fallout in the western United States, with a mean thyroid dose of 0.46 Gy.[455] No significant difference between irradiated and nonirradiated subjects was identified. In a subsequent report by Machado et al. thyroid cancer mortality in southwestern Utah was compared with that in the rest of Utah and the rest of the United States.[456] The OR in both cases was nonsignificantly reduced at 0.4 (90% CI 0.08, 2.00), indicating less thyroid cancer mortality in the areas receiving fallout. In a 1993 paper, Kerber et al. studied 2500 children exposed to fallout who had an average thyroid dose of 0.17 Gy.[457] There were 19 cases

of thyroid cancer found and about 13 expected. This leads to an ERR of about 7 per Gy, which is substantially higher than risks obtained from the Swedish diagnostic iodine 131 studies in which the average thyroid dose was 0.56 Gy and the ERR per Gy was 0.4. Kerber's study may have significant error in the dose reconstruction since it relied on dietary recall.

More recently, Gilbert et al. examined mortality from thyroid cancer across the continental United States compared to areas felt to have been affected by fallout from Nevada nuclear weapons tests.[458] The result was a negative ERR in the latter group, which was not statistically significant, and the risk did not increase with cumulative dose or dose received at ages 1 to 15 years. Nonsignificant associations were suggested for those exposed at less than 1 year of age with a mortality ERR per Gy of 10.6 (95% CI −1.1, 29) and incidence ERR per Gy of 2.4 (95% CI −0.5 to 5.6).

In 1954, the residents of the Marshall Islands were exposed to fallout that resulted in both external irradiation and ingestion of radioiodines. Nine thyroid tumors were identified in 243 exposed subjects. The estimated risk was 145 (70 to 270) cases in 1 million for each 10 mGy. An increased sensitivity in childhood could not be supported by the data, although the confidence limits of the statistics were quite wide. All the cancers occurred in females, again suggesting a higher induction rate in females than males. No thyroid tumors were observed in 504 unexposed subjects.[459] The major contributions to dose were from the short-lived iodines (132, 133, and 135) with only about 10% to 15% of the dose from iodine 131. Conard has suggested that the effects of shorter-lived isotopes of iodine appear to be more like those predicted from external radiation exposure than from iodine 131, although the exact types of exposures and amount of exposure in the Marshall Islands is somewhat difficult to ascertain. Other radioisotopes of iodine (particularly iodine 125) are more frequently used for research purposes, although in the past, iodine 125 was used occasionally for treatment of hyperthyroidism.

A Scandanavian study of thyroid cancer by Lund et al. appears on initial inspection to indicate an increase in thyroid cancer due to atomic weapons fallout.[460] The authors themselves indicate that the birth cohorts had "presumably" different levels of exposure. In fact, only one of the groups had "borderline significant risk" (RR 1.7, 95% CI 1.0, 3.0)—and that was comparing the 1951–1962 birth cohort with the 1963–1970 group—but this occurred with results "estimated in a model" and only at ages 7 to 14 years old at diagnosis. Under the same model there was no increase when ages 7 to 19 years, with an RR 5.8 (95% CI 3.7, 9.2) versus 4.9 (95% CI 2.8, 8.4), were compared. When the groups were compared at ages of 7 to 24 years at the time of diagnosis, the RR was nonsignificantly higher for those with no exposure, that is, RR 11.4 (95% CI 6.9, 19.0), compared to those with presumed higher exposure of an RR of 10.3 (95% CI 6.5, 16.4).

There exist few human data concerning effects of iodine 125, with the exception of some material published by McDougall et al.[461] and Weidinger et al.[462] These studies indicate that iodine 125 is quite similar to iodine 131 in terms of the induction of hypothyroidism in humans. It might be expected on a theoretical basis that irradiation by iodine 125 would produce less hypothyroidism. Iodine 125 has a decay scheme that produces electrons that travel less than 1 μm in tissue. Although this process could interfere with the interface between the thyroid cell and the thyroid follicle, much of the radiation should not reach as far as the nucleus of the thyroid cell. There is literature comparing the relative carcinogenicity of iodine 125 and iodine 131 in animals; it has been generally concluded from such studies that iodine 125 is not substantially different from iodine 131 in regard to carcinogenesis. For the present time, it would probably be conservative to assume that exposure to short-lived radioiodines (iodine 132, 133, and 135) carries risk factors close to those for external radiation exposure and that the risk of the longer-lived iodine 125 is close to that of iodine 131.

Presently, there are few research findings available on thyroid tumors due to placental transfer of radioiodine during pregnancy. It is known, however, that the fetal thyroid does not accumulate iodine until after the 12th week of gestation.[463]

HANFORD

A recent analysis of the effects of releases of radioiodine from the Hanford nuclear facility in Richland, Washington, included 3447 subjects who were born between 1940 and 1946 and resided near the Hanford plant. The study reported by Davis et al. did not find a significant increase in thyroid cancer.[105,364] The estimated slope per Gy was 0.002 (95% CI < 0.001, 0.017) and the RR detectable with an 80% or better power at 170 mGy was 2.14. One group has suggested that the confidence limits should be wider and the results interpreted as inconclusive.[364a]

CHERNOBYL

After the Chernobyl accident, there was an examination of thyroid cancer in the areas affected by fallout. The four components of the thyroid doses were (1) internal irradiation from intakes of iodine 131, (2) the dose from internal irradiation from intakes of short-lived radioiodines (132, 133, and 135) and of short-lived radiotelluriums (^{131m}Te and ^{132}Te), (3) the external dose from radionuclides deposited on the ground (predominantly ^{137}Cs and ^{134}Cs), and (4) the dose from internal intakes of long-lived radionuclides (including radiocesiums). The dose from iodine 131 represents more than 80% of the total thyroid dose and was predominantly due to

ingestion of fresh cow's milk. The estimated release of iodine 131 was about 1.8 EBq (about 45 million curies). The median thyroid dose in the most contaminated regions of both Belarus and the Ukraine was about 0.3 Gy with a substantial fraction of doses exceeding 1 Gy.

As of 1989, no definite increase in thyroid cancer rates was seen, in part, perhaps, due to the lack of a reliable preaccident tumor registry.[464] In 1991 and 1992 several reports appeared of markedly increased thyroid cancer in children in Belarus and to some extent in the Ukraine (Fig. 5-7).[465,466] These reports were unusual because the latent period was shorter than reported in other studies of thyroid cancer and because no increase had been found at that time in contaminated areas of the Russian Federation. As of the year 2000, however, many additional descriptive studies,[467–472] two ecological studies by Jacob et al.,[473,474] and one case-control study by Astakhova et al.[475] had indicated a clear increase in childhood thyroid cancer. More than 2000 cases were diagnosed in the three affected countries in those under the age of 18 at the time of exposure. Many of the studies published after 2000 continue to report an increased SIR. Evaluation of the dose-response relationship is complicated in that very few of the persons who developed thyroid cancer had actual thyroid radioactivity measurements made shortly after the accident. As a result, most estimates to come from dose reconstruction based on the relationship of radioiodine exposure and cesium deposition.

The risks from iodine 131 exposure have been best elucidated in a recent report by Cardis et al. in a study of childhood cancer following Chernobyl.[403] The study included 276 patients and all have had individual dose estimates performed. Excess risk was identified at all doses above 0.2 Gy. At thyroid doses in excess of 2.0 Gy the risk plateaued. At 1 Gy the OR was between 5.5 (95% CI 3.1, 9.5) and 8.4 (95% CI 4.1, 17.3), depending on the risk model used. The risk is similar to that reported by Davis et al. and slightly less than that reported from external radiation exposure.[476] The results of two large and

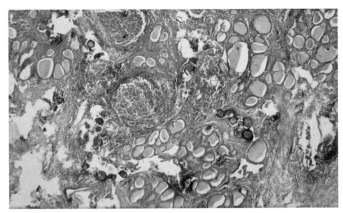

Figure 5-7 • Pathological specimen of a thyroid cancer which occurred in a child after exposure to radioiodine as a result of the Chernobyl accident.

most important studies (the Ukrainian-American and the Belarus-Russia-International Agency for Research on Cancer [IARC]) have yet to be published.

The roles of iodine deficiency, iodine prophylaxis (for the accident and public health measures due to the area being an endemic goiter area), and screening bias remain confounding issues.[477] Ultrasound and physical screening of the general population appear to have had minimal impact in studies of the general population. During the period of 1996–2000, screening found only 15% of the thyroid cancer cases that occurred in the most contaminated regions of the Ukraine. Shakhtarin et al. have indicated that the ERR at 1 Gy was twofold higher in areas of severe iodine deficiency.[478] The risk in children under the age of 10 has been reported by Heidenreich et al. to be about threefold higher than in older children.[479] In addition, girls were found to be more sensitive than boys by a factor of 5:1.

Thyroid cancer in Russian recovery workers and in adults in contaminated areas has been studied by Ivanov et al.[480,481] A statistically significant increase in thyroid cancer incidence was found in recovery workers, as compared to the baseline male population of Russia. The SIR was 4.3 (95% CI 3.3, 5.5) but there was no relation to external dose with an ERR per Gy of 2.2 (95% CI −4.7, −0.2). The increased incidence in the recovery workers may be an effect of screening or poor ascertainment of the normal risk of thyroid cancer in the general population. No radiation-related increase was found in the general population of contaminated areas of Bryansk. Rahu et al. have reported on cancer incidence of 5446 male Latviana and Estonian Chernobyl cleanup workers and indicated a significantly elevated SIR of 7.06 (95% CI 2.84, 14.55) for thyroid cancer among these workers.[178] There is a nested case-control study conducted by Kesniiniene and the IARC of thyroid cancer incidence in recovery workers from several countries but the results are not available yet.[482]

THYROID ADENOMAS AND NODULES

General

Benign thyroid neoplasms can occur after irradiation. Presently, these benign adenomas do not appear to have a malignant potential and in the induction process they appear to be parallel, but independent from, thyroid carcinogenesis. Epidemiologic studies of thyroid nodules or adenomas are complicated by a number of issues that must be resolved before the studies can be compared. In the older literature, the presence of nodules typically refers to results of palpation. Palpation can be difficult, especially in overweight adults, and there is often considerable interobserver variability. In the last two decades there has been development of high-resolution ultrasound imaging to examine the thyroid gland. With this technology many more nodules are visualized than can be palpated.

In addition, the term *nodule* is not always defined in the same way, particularly relative to the diameter of the visualized abnormality.

Another problem is that some reports indicate the presence of "goiter," and whether this means an enlarged gland or a normal-sized gland with a nodule is often unclear. In the final analysis, either surgical specimens or autopsy can give the true number of thyroid nodules in the population. The prevalence of thyroid nodules in nonexposed populations varies widely (<1 to 50%) depending on the age and sex of the population studied as well as the nodule-definition criteria used. Thyroid nodules are more common in adults than children and about twice as common in females as in males. The prevalence of palpable nodules in nonexposed children ranges between 0.2% and 1.5%.[464,483,484] In adults, palpable nodules are present in 4% to 7% of the population.[485] In the Framingham study by Vander et al. palpable nodules were detected in 6.4% of females and 1.5% of males.[486] These were followed for about 15 years, and none showed evidence of malignancy during that time. The prevalence of nodules detected by ultrasound is much greater than by palpation.

Depending on what criteria are used, nodules are detected in 4% to 40% of adult studies.[464,487–492] The prevalence of nodules detected by ultrasound rises with age and is about 60% in persons over 70 years of age. Mortensen et al. examined 821 clinically normal thyroid glands at autopsy and indicated that visible lesions 2 mm to 7.5 cm were present in up to 50% of adults.[493] These were solitary in 12% and multiple in 38% of the glands. A large number of reports are concerned with thyroid nodule induction in areas of high natural background radiation, atomic bomb survivors, fallout situations, and background radiation after medical diagnosis and therapy.

External Exposure

Natural Background Radiation

Wang et al. examined 1001 women living in high-background areas of China (330 mR/year) with 1005 women living in an area of lower radiation (114 mR/year).[494] Cumulative thyroid doses were estimated to be 0.14 Gy and 0.05 Gy, respectively. The thyroids were examined by palpation. For all nodular disease the prevalences were 9.5% and 9.3%, respectively, in the two groups. For single nodules the prevalences were 7.4% and 6.6%, which was a nonsignificant difference. The RR of the exposed group was 1.02 (95% CI 0.76 to 1.35). This study was designed to test the conclusions of a smaller, more poorly conducted study reported by Radford, in which thyroid nodularity was alleged to be increased in residents living near a uranium waste disposal site in Pennsylvania.[495] The conclusion of this latter study can be rejected with a high degree of confidence.

The Chinese study also excludes a doubling dose of 0.09 Gy reported in the Israeli tinea capitis study mentioned previously.

Atomic Bomb Survivors

Thyroid nodules and adenomas have been reported to be increased in some atomic bomb survivors in Nagasaki.[496] The persons were chosen from a very specific area (the Nishiyama district) where there was substantial radioactive fallout, and, thus, the results may be nontypical for other atomic bomb survivors. Nodular goiter was reported in 1.1% of the controls, 1.5% of the 0.01 to 0.49 Gy group, and 3.9% in the 0.5 to 1.0 Gy group. Because the study used high-resolution ultrasound, it is unusual that the incidence in both groups is much lower than is reported by most other authors in palpation or ultrasound studies of nonexposed populations. A later study also of Nagasaki survivors confirmed an increase in nodules but strangely enough there was no relation of thyroid cancer to radiation dose.[497]

Medical Exposure

Analysis of patients exposed to multiple fluoroscopies during treatment of TB has been published by Kaplan et al.[419] One hundred and sixty-three women participated in a recall study. Thyroid dose was difficult to estimate but was thought to be between 0.11 and 1.2 Gy. Palpation was performed but not ultrasound. Thyroid nodules were present in 7.7% of the exposed and 4.2% of the controls. The prevalence ratio was 1:8, which is not significantly elevated because the 90% CI was 0.6 to 5.7.

A number of studies report on nodule induction after childhood radiation therapy for benign entities. Shore et al. in quite strong and well-designed studies have studied the occurrence of thyroid adenomas in children who received radiation for presumed thymic enlargement.[293,498] In the most recent report a cohort of 2657 irradiated children was compared with 4833 siblings. The study was performed using a questionnaire. There were 86 cases in the irradiated group and 11 in the sibling controls. The ERR was 6.3 per Gy (90% CI 3.7 to 11.2). Elevation in risk was seen even in the dose group of less than 0.25 Gy. There was no increase in risk in less than 13 years after exposure, and the mean latency was 38 years.

Studies of Israeli children who received radiation therapy for tinea capitis have been reported by Ron et al.[120] These children were typically irradiated over a 5-day period with 70 to 100 kVp x-rays. As mentioned earlier these are strong studies from the aspect of ascertainment and population size, but there is a question about the large risk factors obtained for thyroid and brain cancer relative to almost all other studies. Perhaps dosimetry was a problem secondary to patient motion during treatment. Of interest in these studies is that during the first 10 years postexposure, the incidence of adenomas in the control population was greater than in the exposed population.

For the first 10 years after exposure the RR was 0.8. The mean latent period for adenomas was 17.9 years with a minimum of 5.1 years, while for thyroid nodules the mean latent period was 21.4 years and a minimum of 5.7 years. An estimated thyroid dose of 0.09 Gy was linked to a two-fold increase in benign tumors. The estimated ERR for benign tumors was 10 per Gy, and the absolute risk was 1500 cases per million person-years per Gy.

Children who had been irradiated for lymphoid hyperplasia between 1938–1969 were followed up by Pottern et al. and compared with surgically treated subjects.[428] The mean thyroid dose was estimated to be 0.24 Gy. This was a very interesting study in that results were obtained both by questionnaire and by clinical examination. A much higher RR of thyroid nodules was estimated from the questionnaire (RR 15.8) than from clinical examination (RR 2.7). This study indicates that there are major differences in risk estimates that can be obtained based solely on the study design and that questionnaire studies may substantially overestimate true risk. Palpation by two physicians was used for clinical evaluation, and nodules were found in 10.3% of exposed persons compared with 4.2% of controls. The ERR was estimated to be 7% per 0.01 Gy. This can be compared with risks of 10% to 30% per 0.01 Gy obtained in the Israeli tinea capitis study.

Treatment of HD with radiotherapy during childhood has been the subject of study relative to thyroid nodules. Hancock et al. have reported on 1787 patients treated at Stanford University with radiation alone (810 patients), radiation and chemotherapy (920 patients), and chemotherapy alone (57 patients).[438] Palpable abnormalities were found in 48 patients 1.5 to 25 years after therapy. Thyroidectomy was performed on 26 patients. The patients had benign adenomas, six had adenomatous nodules, four had multinodular goiters, and six had cancer. The cancers occurred 9 to 19 years after therapy. No risk estimates for nodule induction are given. In a limited thyroid ultrasound study of 30 patients who had previous treatment for HD, abnormalities were described in 24 patients[499] who had received mantle radiotherapy. Nine of these appeared to have nodular lesions that would fit usual criteria. Other abnormalities included such things as atrophy of the gland. An unusual part of this study is that 30 volunteers also had ultrasound performed, and none showed an abnormality. Given the prevalence of ultrasound findings reported in many other studies of nonexposed populations, this would seem to raise the question of whether the sample size in this study is adequate for other than anecdotal information.

Internal Exposure

Medical Exposure

Hall et al. examined the issue of thyroid nodularity after diagnositic administration of iodine 131.[500] The study included 1005 women referred for diagnostic reasons and who received iodine 131 with a mean thyroid dose of 0.54 Gy. The prevalence of thyroid nodularity was 10.6% among women who had received iodine 131 and 11.7% in controls for an RR of 0.9 (95% CI 0.6 to 1.4). There was however a positive association with dose with an ERR per Gy of 0.9 (95% CI 0.2 to 1.9). The authors indicated it was unclear whether this was causal or due to confounding factors. Rosen et al. have reported on thyroid nodular disease in a heterogeneous group of patients in essentially a collection of cases who developed disease.[501] No risk estimates are obtainable from this study.

Fallout

NUCLEAR WEAPONS

The 1954 BRAVO thermonuclear test exposed residents of the Marshall Islands to fallout. A number of reports indicate a higher-than-expected incidence of thyroid cancer and thyroid nodules.[502,503] Data through 1986 indicated that 51 patients had nodules in the exposed group and 10 in the control group. The first nodule was found in a girl 9 years after the accident. Nodules were palpated in 2.6% of control children under the age of 10 and in 7.8% of persons over the age of 10. On Rongelap atoll nodules were palpated in over 60% of persons exposed at age 10 years or less and in 13% of those over age 10 at exposure. The percentages were smaller for the Ailingae and Utirik atolls. Analysis of these data reveals virtually no excess of nodules at doses of less than 3 Gy. The risk in females was about 3.7 times that in males. Pathologic diagnosis of the nodules indicates that most were adenomatous and frequently multiple.

In another study Hamilton et al. screened 2273 Marshall Islanders using palpation, defining a nodule as being 1 cm or greater.[504] The prevalence of thyroid nodules ranged from 0.9% to 10.6% and decreased with distance from the test site. A risk estimate was reported of 1100 cases per Gy per million person-years. This risk factor is complicated in that there are wide variations in the natural incidence of thyroid cancer in Polynesian populations, and the spontaneous prevalence of thyroid nodules is not well known. Given these factors the risk estimates from this population should be used with caution. An analysis of thyroid nodules in Utah has been conducted to examine the potential effect of fallout from the Nevada test site. Using palpation, Rallison et al. did not find any significant difference between 5179 children in Utah and Nevada exposed to fallout and 3453 in a control group.[455] Cumulative thyroid dose to the exposed groups was estimated to be in the range of 0.5 to 1.0 Gy. An increase in thyroid nodules associated with protracted childhood exposure to iodine 131 from atmospheric emissions from the Russian Mayak facility was reported. The prevalence was 20.7% in the exposed group and 14.4% in the non-exposed group, with an RR of 1.4 (95% CI 1.1, 1.9).[504a]

HANFORD

As noted above, a recent analysis of the effects of releases of radioiodine from the Hanford nuclear facility in Richland, Washington, included 3447 subjects who were born between 1940 and 1946 and resided near the Hanford plant.[505–507] The study did not find an increased incidence of benign nodules and, in fact, the estimated slope per Gy was actually negative at −0.008 (95% CI < 0.022, 0.041). The RR detectable with an 80% or greater power at 170 mGy was 1.37.

CHERNOBYL

The population living in the fallout-contaminated areas around Chernobyl were studied as part of the International Chernobyl Project,[464] and additional results were reported by Mettler et al.[492] Both palpation and high-resolution ultrasound were performed in seven highly contaminated villages and compared with results from five clean villages. At ages 5 and 10 both methods in contaminated and control populations yielded less than 1.2% of children with a thyroid nodule. In 40-year-old persons nodules were palpated in 3.7% and 1.7% in the contaminated and control areas, respectively. Sonographic nodules were seen in the same group in 15.7% and 12.8%, respectively. In 60-year-old persons nodules were palpated in 4.9% and 7.2% in the contaminated and control areas, respectively. Sonographic nodules were seen in the same group, in 17.9% and 19.0%, respectively. Nodules were more common in females. Of interest was relatively poor agreement between the palpation and ultrasound findings. Based on the latent periods indicated for thyroid nodules in other studies, it is not surprising that no difference was found 5 years after the accident.

Summary

There are a number of studies showing increased risk of thyroid cancer and nodules, particularly in children, after radiation therapy of the head and neck. In general, children may be considered to be substantially more sensitive than adults. The ERR per Gy for those irradiated in childhood is mostly derived from studies of external irradiation and range from 0.6 to 9.5. A pooled analysis indicates a risk of about 7.7 per Gy. There are several studies that indicate that fractionation or low-dose rate is associated with less risk per unit dose. For adults many of the risk factors derived encompass unity, particularly those from studies of occupational exposure. Studies from which risk estimates for thyroid cancer can be derived have been summarized by the UNSCEAR 2006 Committee (Table 5-10).[86]

For the available data above 50 mGy and below 4 to 5 Gy, a linear model provides a good fit to the data on cancer and nodules; however, due to the inherent difficulties in ascertainment for this category of tumors and the potential uncertainties and biases in a number of

Table 5-10 • Risk Estimates for Cancer Incidence and Mortality from Studies of Radiation Exposure: Thyroid Cancer*

Study	Average Excess Relative Risk at 1 Sv	Average Excess Absolute Risk $(10^4 PYSv)^{-1}$
External Low-LET Exposures		
Incidence		
A-bomb Life Span Study[319]		
Males	0.78 (0.15–1.77)	1.03 (0.46–1.79)
Females	1.89 (1.28–2.65)	3.75 (2.73–4.89)
Age at exposure		
<20	3.93 (2.57–5.81)	3.07 (2.14–4.14)
20–40	0.99 (0.34–1.93)	1.46 (0.49–2.69)
>40	0.29 (<0–0.95)	0.86 (<0–2.84)
Time since exposure		
12–15	3.24 (1.1–7.28)	2.85 (1.17–5.22)
15–30	1.35 (0.69–2.23)	2.04 (1.18–3.07)
>30	1.61 (0.93–2.52)	2.31 (1.34–3.48)
All	1.59 (1.1–2.19)	2.3 (1.67–3.02)
Tuberculosis, adenitis screening[376]		
Age at exposure		
<20	36.5 (16–72)	7.7 (3.3–15)
>20	1.2 (0.1–3.7)	0.7 (0.1–2.4)
Cohort Studies of Children		
Israeli tinea capitis[422]	34 (23–47)	13 (9–18)
New York tinea capitis[376,322]	7.7(<0–60)	1.3 (<0–10.3)
Rochester thymic irradiation[421]	9.5 (6.9–12.7)	3 (2.2–4)
Childhood cancer[439]	4.5 (3.1–6.4)	0.4 (0.2–0.5)
Stockholm skin hemangioma[400]	4.9 (1.3–10.2)	0.9 (0.2–1.9)
Gothenburg skin hemangioma[508]	7.5 (0.4–18.1)	1.6 (0.09–3.9)
Screening Studies of Children		
Lymphoid hyperplasia screening[428,376]	5.9 (1.8–11.8)	9.1 (2.7–18.3)
Thymus adenitis screening[404,376]	4.5 (2.7–7)	1.2 (0.7–1.8)
Michael Reese, tonsils[396]	3 (2.6–3.5)	37.6 (32–43)
Tonsils/thymus/acne screening[427,376]	12 (6.6–20)	3.5 (2–5.9)
Pooled Analysis of Five Studies of Children		
Life Span Study		
Israeli tinea capitis		
Rochester thymic irradiation		
Lymphoid hyperplasia screening Michael Reese tonsil[402]	7.7 (2.1–28.7)	4.4 (1.9–10.1)
Studies of Adults		
Cervical cancer case control[6]	12.3 (<0–76)	6.9 (<0–39.2)
Cervical cancer cohort[124]	2.5 (<0–6.8)	0.9 (<0–2.5)
Stanford thyroid[438]	0.3 (0.1–0.7)	0.07 (0.03–0.1)
Canada National Dose Registry[153]	5.9 (2.5–9.9)	2.1 (0.9–3.4)
China medical x-ray workers[253]		
Employed before 1970	1.9 (0.3–4.4)	0.3 (0.15–0.8)
Employed only 1970–1980	<0	<0
Internal Low-LET Exposures		
Incidence		
Diagnostic ^{131}I[454]	<0	<0
RSFSR-Belarus Chernobyl case control study[403]	4.9 (2.2–7.5)	NA
Ukraine-Belarus Chernobyl cohort study[509]	18.9 (11.1–26.7)	2.66 (2.19–3.13)
External Low-LET Exposures		
Mortality		
A-bomb Life Span Study[281]		
Males	0.46 (<0–2.96)	<0 (<0–24.9)
Females	<0 (<0–0.22)	<0 (<0–0.09)
Age at exposure		
<20	1.67 (<0–7.67)	<0 (<0–12.88)
20–40	<0 (<0–0.87)	<0 (<0–0.23)
>40	<0 (<0–<0)	<0 (<0–0.01)

*The studies listed are those for which quantitative estimates of risk could be made.

Continued

Table 5-10 • Risk Estimates for Cancer Incidence and Mortality from Studies of Radiation Exposure: Thyroid Cancer*—cont'd

Study	Average Excess Relative Risk at 1 Sv	Average Excess Absolute Risk $(10^4 PYSv)^{-1}$
External Low-LET Exposures—cont'd		
Mortality—cont'd		
Time since exposure		
5–15	<0 (<0–2.03)	<0 (<0–<0)
15–30	<0 (<0–3.17)	0.12 (<0–0.41)
>30	<0 (<0–0.45)	<0 (<0–97.9)
All	<0 (<0–0.42)	<0 (<0–43.97)
IARC 15-country nuclear workers study[167,168]	<0	

*The studies listed are those for which quantitative estimates of risk could be made.
Adapted from United Nations Scientific Committee of the Effects of Atomic Radiation (UNSCEAR): Sources and effects of ionizing radiation: 2006 report to the General Assembly with annexes. New York, United Nations, 2007.

the studies, it is difficult to decide which model is most appropriate for risk projection.

Females have two to three times more spontaneous thyroid cancer and nodules than males and have a higher absolute excess risk after radiation exposure. The RR for both sexes is about the same. The induced cancers are papillary, follicular, or mixed. Epidemiological studies are often difficult to perform, due to the low mortality from thyroid cancer, the presence of occult cancers, and screening bias. Radiogenic thyroid cancer appears to have a minimum latent period of about 4 years, and the risk continues for up to 40 years. The mean latency time reported for cancers is about 25 to 30 years. No excess risk has been consistently identified for radioiodine uses in medicine although there was a clear increase in thyroid cancer resulting from iodine 131 releases at Chernobyl. Overall, it appears that iodine 131 is less effective in causing thyroid cancer than is external radiation.

BREAST CANCER

General

Breast cancer accounts for 32% of all malignancies in women and less than 0.2% of all malignancies in men. It is the third most common cancer in the world and represents 9% of the global cancer burden. It is the most common cancer in females. The incidence of cancer varies considerably in different geographical areas. The highest incidence is seen in Hawaiian women (94 per 100,000) and in U.S. white women (70 to 90 per 100,000). Low incidence rates are found in American Indians. China and Japan are low-risk areas. Overall, incidence increases with age from 30 to 70 years with a relative plateau of the rise after age 45 to 50. In the United States there are about 183,000 cases diagnosed annually and about 46,000 deaths from breast cancer. The disease is now projected to strike about one out of every eight women in the United States at some time during her

life. Approximately 12% of U.S. women will develop breast cancer. In the white race, the annual incidence rate is 108 cancers of the breast in 100,000 women and 7 in 1 million men. In blacks, it is 58 in 100,000 women and 1 in 100,000 men. The 5-year survival rate for patients with all stages of disease is 53% in white men and 74% in white women. Localized disease has a better prognosis, with the 5-year survival being 93% in white females. Ductal adenocarcinoma accounts for 52% of all tumors, carcinoma not otherwise specified (NOS) 26%, and adenocarcinoma 15%. The average age at occurrence is 59 years. Of all tumor types, 49% are localized at diagnosis, 41% have regional spread, and 8% have distant spread.

Even within countries, there is considerable variation in the incidence of breast cancer. This occurs by age, race, marital status, age at first pregnancy, breast-feeding, hormonal status, and diet. To illustrate the variations that occur within a country, in Israel there are three- to fourfold differences in incidence between Jews (high) and non-Jews (low). There is clearly a genetic component to female breast cancer, and if a cancer occurs in a premenopausal sister and a mother, the risk to another sister approaches 50%. Some authors also suggest that up to 5% of breast cancer may occur as a result of an A-T trait. Breast cancer is more common in single than in married women. Ovarian function seems to play a role in the development of breast cancer, and castration by surgery or radiation substantially reduces risk. Breast cancer is less common in women who are younger at age of first pregnancy and who breast-feed. Age at first pregnancy may be one of the strongest associations found. Women who have a full-term pregnancy under the age of 18 years have one third the breast cancer risk of women who delay pregnancy until age 30. Positive correlations also have been reported between breast cancer incidence and dietary fat, animal protein, and total calories, although some of these associations remain controversial.[358,296]

Data concerning risk factors for breast cancer following radiation exposure come from three major population groups. These groups have been extensively studied and include atomic bomb survivors, patients who have had exposure to diagnostic radiology, and individuals who have had radiotherapy to the breast. Epidemiologic studies of radiogenic breast cancer are of special interest with regard to the more general effect of dose rate on the process of radiation carcinogenesis. The atomic bomb survivors received an essentially instantaneous exposure, whereas the patients receiving therapeutic exposure received it over several weeks, and those receiving diagnostic exposure received it over several years. In spite of these very large dose-rate differences, the risk estimates from the three groups are remarkably similar. Even though the three population groups have relatively large numbers of people, the total absorbed doses were either intermediate or high, and the precise levels of risk associated with low-dose levels (such as those that occur during mammography) remain uncertain. As with other types of tumors, it is possible that the incidence rate following radiation exposure may change with different dose-fractionation schemes, age of patients, and other factors. All the studies, however, do indicate that breast cancer may be induced with a reasonably high frequency after radiation exposure of women who are under the age of 40 at exposure. The tumors generally arise from the duct cells but quickly infiltrate surrounding tissue. The types of breast tumors that are induced by radiation show the same distribution that occurs spontaneously. It is estimated that about 60% of radiation-induced breast cancers are fatal. Land et al. have analyzed the dose-response relationship for three groups of patients, taking into account the age at exposure.[510] The authors indicated that they thought the best statistical fit to the available data was a dose-response curve of approximate linearity. Although there may be a small element of curvilinearity, with the available data, it appears that risk estimates based on linearity of the dose-response curve are not likely to be far off.

Modifying Factors

In general, the results of population studies provide only suggestions about modifying factors rather than specifics. Radiogenic tumors generally do not appear until the women reach the age when spontaneous breast cancers usually occur; that is, in terms of the distribution of cases in time after exposure, the radiation-related cancers are indistinguishable from spontaneous cancers. It is possible that radiation-induced breast cancer, particularly with respect to its appearance time, may be determined by hormonal or other factors, such as those mentioned by MacMahon in his review of the etiology of human breast cancer.[511] Genetic issues related to spontaneously occurring breast cancer have been mentioned in the introductory paragraphs, and similar issues might be of concern with radiation-induced breast cancer. Increased cancer risk has been reported in families affected by A-T. The persons who are homozygous usually have a high risk of leukemia and lymphoma but not of breast cancer. Swift et al. have indicated that female heterozygotes in their study were predisposed to breast cancer, and there was a fivefold excess risk of breast cancer in those who had been exposed to diagnostic fluoroscopic examinations compared with nonexposed females.[512] Initially, this study would seem to be important; however, there are a number of significant flaws. The diagnostic radiology involved was almost always of the abdomen, which would only give scattered radiation to the breast at very low doses (less than the annual dose from natural background radiation). This would then imply that natural background radiation would be responsible for a huge number of breast cancers, which clearly is not the case. In addition, the exposed and control groups were of very different ages so that an adjustment for this would not be possible.[513] This type of report illustrates that each study needs to be carefully evaluated rather than simply accepting the authors' conclusions at face value. In a 1993 LSS report by Land, there was a markedly higher ERR in early onset breast cancers than in those that occur later.[514,515] It has been postulated that this may be due to a genetic subgroup with high sensitivity to radiation-induced breast cancer. The same report concluded that a lower age at first pregnancy is protective, not only of spontaneous breast cancers, but also of radiation-induced cancers.

Age at exposure and its relation to breast cancer incidence has been carefully examined. Scattered reports in the literature have indicated that radiation exposure during infancy may result in breast cancer in very young women, and, in most studies of breast cancer, risk decreases markedly with increasing age at exposure.[516,517] In fact, the LSS of atomic bomb survivors and studies of patients receiving multiple fluoroscopies in Massachusetts and Canada show little if any detectable risk in women exposed over the age of 40.[518,519] The LSS incidence and mortality studies indicate a 3- to 10-fold higher ERR at 1 Gy when women were exposed at an age less than 20 compared with an age over 20. Excess relative risk did not significantly rise until 20 to 30 years after exposure. Similar findings were reported for average EAR. The LSS data also indicate that for survivors exposed before age 20, a 13-fold ERR at 1 Sv was found for cancers occurring before age 35 compared to a twofold ERR for cancers occurring after age 35. In the postpartum mastitis series, RR was not significantly affected by age at exposure, and EAR may have increased with age at exposure. Time after exposure affects expression of risk. The RR appears to increase for 15 years after exposure and then to decrease.[520]

The total dose can affect breast cancer risk. As mentioned later in this section, acute doses up to 3 Gy appear linearly related to risk. However, in a study of women treated for postpartum mastitis, risk of breast cancer flattened at about 3 Gy and decreased at doses over 5 Gy.[521] In general, most tumors show a decreasing risk as the radiation dose is fractionated or spread out over time. While this effect appears evident for lung and thyroid cancer, it does not appear to hold true for breast cancer. The risk estimates derived from treatment of TB patients using multiple fluoroscopies is quite similar to risks derived from high dose-rate exposures. The study of acute postpartum patients also did not show an effect of fractionation.

The mortality data on the atomic bomb survivors reported by Shimizu et al. indicate that the minimum latent period is 20 to 24 years for cancer of the breast.[522] The incidence data on the same population indicates that excess risk began between 12 and 16 years after exposure.[523] If age at exposure is not considered, there does appear to be a relationship between the radiation dose and latent period, apparently on an artifactual basis. The initial reports of a relationship between latent period and dose were published by Shore et al.[524] and Baral et al.[525] In the New York postpartum mastitis series, dose did not appear to affect latent period. In the patients treated for HD the addition of chemotherapeutic agents (mechlorethamine, vincristine, procarbazine, and prednisone) increased the risk of breast cancer within the first 15 years.[526] Thus, it appears that some of these agents may be able to shorten the latent period.

External Exposure

Many epidemiological studies are limited in stastical power and a number of authors have pooled results from different studies to achieve better precision. Preston et al. have performed a pooled analysis of incidence data from eight major breast cancer cohorts including the A-bomb LSS subjects, TB patients who received multiple fluoroscopies, patients treated with radiotherapy for benign breast disease, skin hemangioma, and presumed enlarged thymus.[527] There were significant variations among the findings in different studies. The RRs were higher in the Japanese than in the United States or European populations, there was a rapid decrease with age at exposure in the Swedish benign breast group and little or none in some other cohorts, and risk per unit dose was low in the hemagioma cohort. As a result, it is clear that pooling data may mask important risk differences among the groups.

Atomic Bomb Survivors

Wanebo identified a statistically significant excess of breast carcinoma in Hiroshima and Nagasaki.[528] This was further studied and reported in 1972 by Jablon and Kato.[529] For females of all ages from both cities, the excess mortality was reported as 19 (6 to 35) cases in 1 million persons exposed for each 10 mGy. Wakabayashi et al. estimate *annual* absolute risk to be about 3.4 excess

cases in 1 million persons for each 10 mGy.[335] Tokunaga et al. reported an excess risk of breast cancer among Japanese women who were less than 10 years of age when exposed to the atomic bombs.[530] In a follow-up report of the same study, it was reported that both RR and absolute excess risk tended to decrease with increasing age at exposure.[523] There was no tendency for one or more histologic types of breast cancer to preferentially be induced by radiation. The 1958–1998 incidence data from the LSS indicate that the ERR at 1 Gy was 0.87, and the EAR was 9.2 $(10^4 PYSv)^{-1}$. For ERR, the data fit a linear model best. Some earlier dose-response data are shown in Figure 5-8. The actual number of cases observed for the 41,000 persons who received 0.01 Sv or more and a mean dose of 0.23 Sv was 1073 versus 926 expected in the 1.7 million person-years of study. In the entire LSS sample there were 147 excess cases diagnosed from 1950–1998. Tokunaga et al. and Preston et al. reported that the data from 1950–1985 on breast cancer incidence show a strongly linear dose response.[319,531] They also postulate the existence of a susceptible genetic subgroup with early expression of breast cancer. The same authors also have speculated that women who are exposed at older ages may receive too little hormonal promotion to allow full expression of potential radiogenic cancers.[532]

The LSS mortality data on the same group yield an ERR at 1 Sv of 1.3 and an absolute excess risk of 1.3 $(10^4 PYSv)^{-1}$. In this study there were 105 deaths from breast cancer versus the 74 expected in 731,300

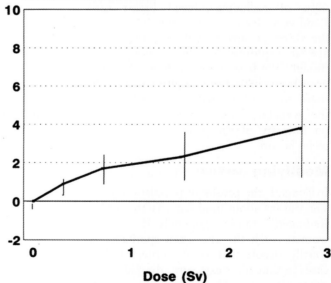

Excess relative risk

Breast cancer incidence (A-bomb)

Figure 5-8 ● ERR of breast cancer in atomic bomb survivors at different dose levels. Bars indicate 95% CI. (From Thompson D, Mabuchi K, Ron E, et al: Cancer incidence in atomic bomb survivors. II: Solid tumors, 1958–1987. RERF Technical Report 5-92, Hiroshima, Japan, Radiation Effects Research Foundation, 1992.)

person-years of study.[10,359] It is of interest that the LSS studies are the largest breast cancer epidemiologic studies that have been performed in regard to person-years, and the mortality study does not show a statistically significant increased RR at doses below 0.5 Gy. In the 2003 update studies of mortality of atomic bomb survivors during 1950–1997, Preston et al. reported on a cohort of 86,572 persons with an average external dose of 0.23 Sv.[281] In females there was a statistically significant excess of breast cancer at dose levels of 1 Sv, with an ERR of 0.79 (90% CI 0.29, 1.5).

Background Radiation, Fallout, and Populations Living Near Nuclear Plants

A paper on the high natural background area of Guangdong, China, was published in 2000 by Tao et al. and had 1.7 million person-years of study from 1979–1995.[33] The authors did not find a radiation effect and the RR of breast cancer was 0.92 (95% CI 0.23, 3.68). A few studies have examined the risk of breast cancer in populations exposed to fallout. A Swedish study found that Lapps who are presumed to have more fallout (especially cesium) in their diets did not show increased risk.[56] Studies of fallout within the United States as a result of weapons testing at the Nevada test site have not shown an increase in breast cancer. In fact, the OR of exposed persons in southwest Utah was statistically significantly lower than for the United States (OR 0.59) or the remainder of Utah (OR 0.72).[456] A very extensive study of U.S. populations living near nuclear installations has failed to show evidence of a consistent increase in breast cancer.[78] There are papers concerning potential environmental uranium contamination and the possibility of breast cancer in the public. Papers by Boice et al. indicated a nonsignificant increase around a uranium mining and milling facility in Texas, a nonsignificant decrease near a facility in Pennsylvania, and a statistically significant decrease near a Colorado facility.[89,90,90a] A nonsignificant decrease was found by Boice et al. in a study of persons residing near the Hanford site.[91] Lopez-Abente et al. have reported on solid tumor mortality near Spain's four nuclear power plants and four uranium fuel cycle facilities and found that the RR for female breast cancer was nonsignificantly increased at 1.07.[283] Bauer et al. have reported on cancer mortality due to local fallout from Soviet atmospheric nuclear weapons testing at the Semipalatinsk test site in Kazakhstan.[533] Effective doses ranged from 20 mSv to about 4 Sv. The dose-response likelihood ratio test (LRT) for female breast cancer was nonsignificantly increased at a P value of 0.0047 and the estimated ERR per Sv for the exposed cohort was 1.09 (95% CI −0.05, 15.8).

Occupational Exposure

Occupational studies of workers at atomic energy facilities or nuclear installations are often limited by the small number of women employed in these fields. A second analysis in 1999 of 124,743 workers in the U.K. National Registry of Radiation Workers by Muirhead et al. using a lagged analysis reported a significantly reduced SMR for female breast cancer of 0.64 (95% CI 0.41, 0.95).[146] A report on the Sellafield plant by Omar et al. indicated a significant decrease in breast cancer with an SMR of 0.34 (based on only two cases) among nonplutonium radiation workers.[148] Incidence was nonsignificantly decreased. No significant increase in breast cancer has been reported in some of the larger studies in the United Kingdom,[143–145] or in the United States.[157,361] Ashmore et al. reported the first analysis of mortality and occupational radiation exposure based on the National Dose Registry of Canada which included a cohort of 206,620 individuals and 5426 deaths.[154] The average exposure for males was 10.6 mSv and the SMR for breast cancer was nonsignificantly elevated at 2.5 (90% CI 0.99, 5.5). Sont et al. also reported on incidence and occupational radiation exposure based on the National Dose Registry of Canada and analyzing a cohort of 191,333 persons with an average dose for males of 11.5 mSv and an average dose for the cohort of 6.64 mSv.[153] The SIR for breast cancer in males was nonsignificantly reduced at 0.67 and in females it was also nonsignificantly reduced at 0.93.

Habib et al. have reported on cancer incidence among Australian nuclear industry–monitored radiation workers in whom they observed a nonsignificantly elevated SIR of 1.53 for female breast cancer.[152]

Frome reported on a mortality study of 106,020 employees in the nuclear industry at Oak Ridge, Tennessee, in whom the SMR for cancer of the breast in black and white females was nonsignificantly reduced.[160] Groves et al. conducted a 40-year cancer mortality study of 40,581 Korean War Navy veterans with potential exposure to high-intensity radar sources which also emit ionizing radiation.[165] The SMR for breast cancer was nonsignificantly increased at 1.05 (95% CI 0.26, 4.20).

Cardis et al. reported on cancer mortality among nuclear industry workers in three countries in a large study including 95,673 workers followed over 2 million person-years at risk with 15,825 deaths.[166] The trend for breast cancer was nonsignificantly positive at 0.50 with a P value of 0.31. Cardis et al. have reported the cancer mortality results from a 15-country collaborative study of nuclear workers[168] This is the largest occupational study to date and included a cohort of 407,391 workers with 18,993 deaths and 5.2 million person-years of follow-up. The ERR per Sv for female breast cancer was nonsignificantly negative at −0.47.

Cancer incidence among medical diagnostic workers in China was reported by Wang et al. in 1988 who compared 5443 female x-ray workers with 8088 women in other medical specialties.[102] There was a higher risk for cancer of the breast, with 11 cancers found versus

8 expected. The risk was concentrated in women who had worked with x-rays for over 20 years. As mentioned earlier, China has a low spontaneous incidence of breast cancer. The doses to the workers were likely to be on the order of 1 Gy or more because the workers often had depressed white blood cell counts. When this was noted they were given time off from work so that their marrow could recover. Lack of knowledge of individual doses precludes quantitative estimation of risk from this study. In a 2002 follow-up, Wang et al. reported that for those employed before 1970 cumulative doses were 551 mSv and the RR for cancer of the breast was nonsignificantly increased at 1.34 and that for those employed after 1970 with a cumulative mean dose of 82 mSv, the RR was also nonsignificantly increased at about 1.33.[253]

Burnett et al. studied the mortality of health and science technicians and found a nonsignificantly increased proportional mortality ratio for breast cancer of 1.05 (95% CI 0.84, 1.30).[96] Doody et al. reported on mortality among 143,517 U.S. radiologic technologists during 1926–1990 whose doses were not evaluated.[97] The SMR for breast cancer was nonsignificantly reduced at 0.99 (95% CI 0.90, 1.3). Sigurdson et al. studied cancer incidence in 90,305 U.S. radiologic technologists and found that the SIR for breast cancer was significantly elevated at 1.16 (95% CI 1.09, 1.23).[101] Mohan et al. studied cancer and other causes of mortality among 146,022 radiologic technologists employed from 1940 and later.[98,99] The SMR for breast cancer in males was nonsignificantly increased at 1.06 (95% CI 0.1, 3.8) and for females it was nonsignificantly increased at 1.01 (95% CI 0.9, 1.1).

McGeoghegan et al. have reported on the mortality of 12,540 workers (including 3244 radiation workers) at the Capenhurst uranium enrichment facility during 1946–1995 and the SMR for breast cancer was nonsignificantly elevated in radiation workers at 1.35.[242] They also studied the cancer mortality experience of 19,454 workers (including 13,960 radiation workers) at the Springfields uranium production facility during 1946–1995 and the SMR for breast cancer was nonsignificantly reduced for radiation workers at 0.81.[243]

Diagnostic Radiology

There has been a report of increased breast cancer in patients who received diagnostic x-rays for scoliosis.[534] Eleven cancers were observed versus six expected. This yielded an SIR of 1.82 (90% CI 1.0, 3.0). Only the SIR in the group with greater than 0.2 Gy achieved statistical significance. The estimated mean dose to the breast was 0.13 Gy. Risk estimates from this report should be viewed with skepticism because some cancers were found as a result of an intensive screening process, and many of the women were nulliparous, which is known to increase the risk of breast cancer. Thomas et al. suggested in 1994 that male breast cancer can be increased by chest x-rays.[416]

This study cannot be taken seriously since "exposure" was determined by personal interview and such studies are subject to significant recall bias. In addition, given the risk factors from major epidemiological studies, a sample size much greater than 277 cases and 300 controls is needed.

In 1965, MacKenzie reported the occurrence of excess breast cancer among female patients exposed to multiple fluoroscopic examinations for treatment of pulmonary TB by artificial pneumothorax.[535] The patients studied were treated in a Nova Scotia sanatorium. The dose to the breast was generally higher than that to the rest of the body because the patients receiving fluoroscopy in Nova Scotia were turned to face the x-ray tube. When the pneumothorax treatment was unilateral (and therefore the majority of the radiation exposure), the cancer usually developed on that side.[536] An additional follow-up of this group was reported somewhat later by Myrden and Quinlan.[537] There were 256 patients exposed during pneumothorax treatment (who developed 32 breast cancers) and a control group of 535 patients with pulmonary TB who were not treated with pneumothorax (who developed only 7 breast cancers). The dose rates were estimated to be between 0.04 and 0.20 Gy for each examination, and the numbers of fluoroscopic examinations often exceeded 100. The average breast dose estimated for the Nova Scotia series was 6 to 12 Gy. The 1977 UNSCEAR report estimated the excess cancer incidence rate to be between 20 and 200 cases in 1 million persons for each 10 mGy.[316] A similar study was performed by Boice and Monson on former patients of a Massachusetts TB sanatorium.[538] The study included 1047 patients treated with pneumothorax and 717 controls. Approximately 60% to 75% of the exposures were made with the patient's back facing the x-ray tube, in contrast to the positioning used in the Nova Scotia series. The dose for each examination was estimated to be 15 mGy, with an average cumulative breast dose of 1.5 Gy. Statistically significant increases in breast cancer began to appear approximately 15 years after exposure and continued for at least 40 years; 41 cancers were observed versus 23.3 expected. Most of the observed excess cases occurred in women who were less than 20 years at the time of exposure. The mean interval between exposure and diagnosis was 27 years. The estimated excess cancer rate was 162 (74 to 285) cases in 1 million persons for each 10 mGy for those under the age of 20 at exposure, and 78 cases (8 to 189) cases in 1 million persons for each 10 mGy in those over 20 years. There is clearly a wide CI associated with these numbers, but they do suggest higher risk in women exposed before the age of 20 years. The best fit to the dose-incidence data appears to be nearly linear.[539]

An initial report of a group of about 2000 Massachusetts patients appeared in 1987.[364] In a 1989 report of the Massachusetts group, risk was consistent with a linear risk up to 4 Gy, and the ERR at 1 Sv was

0.7. As of 1980, in the 1044 women examined an average of 101 times with fluoroscopy, there were 55 breast cancers compared with 36 expected. No excess risk was identified until 15 years after exposure. As with the atomic bomb survivors, risk decreased with increasing age at exposure.[540] In a later 1991 report of a larger number of Massachusetts patients, the conclusions were essentially the same. The ERR at 1 Sv was 0.61.[518] In a much larger report of about 30,000 Canadian patients, Miller et al. reported similar findings, but they indicated that when the females were between 10 and 14 years of age at exposure, the ERR was 3.5 per Sv and the absolute risk was 6.1 per $(10^4PYSv)^{-1}$.[519] The radiation effect appeared to peak 25 to 34 years after exposure. Of interest was that patients treated in Nova Scotia (where the women faced the x-ray beam) had a three times higher RR per Gy than women treated in other provinces. One of the major problems associated with these studies is exact determination of the fluoroscopic dose, as well as the effect of disease and nutritional status on the patients.

Radiotherapy for Benign Disease

In 1969 Mettler et al. reported on 606 patients who were treated in 1940–1955 for acute postpartum mastitis by radiation therapy.[541] There were 13 confirmed cases of breast cancer versus 6 expected. The mean exposure to the breast was 3.46 Gy. The induction rate for excess breast cancer was estimated to be 55 (15 to 115) cases in 1 million persons exposed for each 10 mGy. A follow-up of this group was reported in 1977 by Shore et al. who reported that excess breast cancer began to appear at 12 to 15 years after irradiation, with a suggestion of a decrease in the latency period with increasing dose.[524] The estimated annual incidence rate in the whole exposed group was estimated to be 8.3 cases in 1 million persons exposed for each 10 mGy. In a 1986 update of the postpartum mastitis patients, Shore et al. reported that after an average follow-up of 29 years, 56 breast cancers were identified in the 601 women irradiated.[521] The cancer risk increased in a relatively linear fashion up to 3 Gy, reached a plateau from 3 to 5 Gy, and actually decreased from 5 to 8 Gy. This may have been the result of cell killing at higher doses or chance. In the multiple fluoroscopy TB series, there was no downward trend in risk at high doses. Perhaps this may be a result of multiple low doses. The median latent period was reported to be about 24 years, and the minimum latent period was about 15 years. A Swedish group investigated 1115 women who received radiotherapy for benign diseases of the breast, particularly fibroadenomatosis but also acute mastitis.[525] In that study, 115 breast cancers were identified, compared with 28.7 expected. The risk rate estimated was approximately 87 cases in 1 million persons for each 10 mGy; however, interpretation of this estimate is complicated in that the study lacked an appropriate control group, with the result that the observed excess may have been due in large measure to the influence of fibroadenomatosis and other confounding risk factors. In the study, the patients receiving higher doses had shorter mean latent periods. Those with doses above 15 Gy to the breast had mean latent periods of 25.8 years. Analysis of these data suggest that the mean latent period–dose effect observed here is confounded by the ages of the patients treated.

In a 1987 report of ankylosing spondylitis patients by Darby et al., a significant increase in breast cancer was identified when 26 cases were observed versus 16 expected.[109] The O/E ratio was about 1.6 from the beginning of the study and did not rise above this except in the greater than 25 years after exposure group. In another radiotherapy group Griem et al. reported on a population of patients who received radiotherapy for peptic ulcer treatment; 1831 exposed persons and 1778 controls were studied over 78,000 person-years at risk.[112] The breast dose was 0.10 to 0.17 Gy. A statistically significant increase was not identified for cancer of the female breast (RR 1.82, 95% CI 0.5 to 6.3). Carr et al. performed a follow-up study of 3719 patients treated with radiotherapy for peptic ulcer with doses to the abdomen about 15 Gy.[113] No cases of breast cancer were found after radiotherapy in the period 0 to 10 years postexposure and in the follow-up period of 11 to 16 years postexposure the RR was nonsignificant at 1.02.

Follow-up of patients who received intrauterine radium radiotherapy for benign uterine bleeding has been reported by Ryberg et al.[297] The study showed a decreased risk for cancer of the breast. Mattson et al. have studied 1216 women who received radiation therapy when they were 40 years or older.[542] Their mean breast dose was 5.8 Gy. An excess risk was demonstrated in this group, with a ratio rate of 3.6 (95% CI 2.8, 4.6).

An increased risk of breast cancer in children treated for presumed thymic enlargement in infancy has been reported by Hildreth et al.[543] The 2872 children treated were compared with their 5055 nonirradiated siblings. An increased risk was identified even in the group who received doses of 0.01 to 0.49 Gy. In a 1989 update report on this same group, there were 2652 exposed persons and 4823 unexposed sibling controls. The strengths of this study are that individual dosimetry was available, there was a long follow-up, and there was a sibling control group. The study also was able to evaluate dose-fractionation effects, and a dose-response analysis could be performed. The weaknesses are that the size of the treatment fields varied; so dosimetry for some sites is uncertain and the questionnaire follow-up may have caused some underascertainment of cases. There were 221,000 person-years of study, again demonstrating increased risks of thyroid and breast cancer.[544] Furst et al. have followed patients in Sweden who were treated with external beam radiotherapy for childhood skin hemangiomas.[301] This study of 144 exposed persons and 314 controls showed an excess risk of thyroid and brain cancer but not of cancers of the breast. Another report by Furst et al. included a cohort of 14,647 children who were treated between 1920 and 1959.[302] The findings were the same. The Israeli tinea capitis study by Ron et al. includes 10,834 exposed persons and 16,226 controls.[121] This study has the advantage of a large number of patients and two control groups. There were 686,000 person-years of study, and no statistically significant excess of breast cancer was reported. Male breast cancer following therapeutic radiation for benign conditions has occasionally been reported as individual cases.[545,546]

Radiotherapy of Malignant Disease

In a cohort study of women treated for cervical cancer, 82,616 exposed women were compared with 99,424 unexposed controls.[124] The women were from Canada, Denmark, and Finland. No excess was identified for breast cancer (RR 0.7). In a case-control study that matched 4188 women with second cancers with 6880 controls, cancer of the breast was not increased (RR 0.88, with 90% CI 0.7 to 1.1).[126] The authors inferred that this low risk was possibly secondary to hormonal factors related to ovarian sterilization from pelvic radiation. In a smaller case-control study of those who were treated for cervical cancer and also developed breast cancer, the same RR was reported. The low risk of breast cancer was also thought to be due to the number of patients over the age of 35 at irradiation.[127]

There have been several follow-up studies of women treated for breast cancer.[130,131] Typical radiation doses to the contralateral breast are on the order of 3 Gy. These studies were primarily directed at the risk of breast cancer in the other breast and leukemia. These studies are strong because there is individual dosimetry, a wide range of high doses, and a large number of incident cases. The first study found a statistically significant increase in contralateral breast cancer only in women less than 45 years of age at exposure. Other studies have found no effect. The first study also indicated that there was virtually no risk in the older women and that radiotherapy for breast cancer contributes little to the already high risk of a second cancer in the opposite breast. Less than 3% of second breast cancers found in the study were thought to be due to radiation exposure. These studies support similar findings in a number of earlier reports.

A number of studies examining the risk of second tumors after treatment for childhood cancers have been performed, including some that indicate increased risks after therapy for Wilms' tumors, but the number of excess cases is small.[547] These studies have strengths in that there is individual dosimetry, but cell killing and effects of chemotherapy make analysis complex. Li et al. have reviewed breast carcinoma following therapy for childhood malignancies: 4 carcinomas were identified versus 0.3 expected in the 910 patients studied. No risk estimates were reported.[548]

Follow-up studies after treatment for HD with mantle radiotherapy have indicated a fourfold increase of breast cancer risk, with breast doses varying from 4 to 40 Gy, depending on the technical factors and positioning. Janjan et al. have indicated a dose response that is between a linear and cell-killing model.[549] Some authors believe that the increased risk in young females receiving treatment justifies routine mammographic screening before the age of 35.[550] In general, the increased risk increases dramatically more than 15 years after therapy. In a study of 885 women treated for HD, Hancock et al. found 25 patients who developed breast cancer.[526] The estimated RR was 4.1 (95% CI 2.5 to 5.7). The RR in women treated under 15 years of age was extremely high (RR 136, 95% CI 34 to 371). For women who were over 30 years of age at exposure, there was no elevation of risk (RR 0.7, 95% CI 0.2 to 1.8). A U.S. study by Bhatia et al. of childhood HD survivors found an SIR for breast cancer of 52 (95% CI 40, 76).[551] A Dutch cohort study by van Leeuwen et al. reported an SIR of 17 (95% CI 8, 32) for pediatric cases but this was reduced to about 4 for those women treated after the age of 20.[552,553] This study is also of interest because it suggests that known protective factors for breast cancers (e.g., multiple births) also reduces the risk of radiogenic breast cancers to the same degree as for nonradiogenic cancers. A pooled study of European and U.S. pediatric HD survivors by Metayer et al. found an SIR of 14 for women treated prior to age 25 while for women treated at ages 25 to 55, the SIR was 2 (and nonsignificantly different from unity).[554] This study also suggested that the risk of breast cancer might increase with the presence of benign breast disease.

Internal Exposure

There have been studies of breast cancer risk following radioiodine exposure.[196,270] After diagnostic doses no excess was reported. In one study, 38,701 patients (79% of whom were female) were exposed.[198] Four hundred fifty-nine cancers were observed for an SIR of 0.86 (95% CI 0.78 to 0.94). A very large number of patients are treated each year with iodine 131 for hyperthyroidism, and reported results differ slightly. In one study of 1762 women, followed for a mean time of 17 years, analysis of cancers of the breast failed to show a significant or dose-related increase.[196] The SMR was 1.2 (95% CI 0.9, 1.5). When age at treatment and year of treatment were controlled, women who were treated with radioactive iodine had a nonsignificantly elevated standardized rate ratio (SRR) for breast cancer of 1.9 (95% CI 0.9, 4.1) compared with those who were never treated with radioactive iodine. It should be noted that all of these CIs encompass unity. In women who developed hypothyroidism as a result of iodine treatment, the SIR was nonsignificantly elevated at 1.1 (95% CI 0.8, 1.6). In another and much larger study of 10,500 patients treated in Sweden, there was no significant increase in cancer of the female breast and the SIR was nonsignificantly different from unity at 1.02 (95% CI 0.90, 1.15).[271] The average dose to the breast was estimated to be 0.06 Gy. Another study of 1000 patients treated at Mayo Clinic and followed for an average of 15 years, and compared with surgically treated patients, showed no increase in leukemia or cancers other than an increased RR for cancer of the thyroid.[202] Ron et al. reported on 35,593 hyperthyroid patients treated by different methods. The SMR for breast cancer among thyroid cancer patients treated with any iodine 131 was nonsignificantly increased at 1.08, and in patients treated with iodine 131 only, it was nonsignificantly increased at 1.10.[201]

A United Kingdom study of 258 thyroid cancer patients showed a statistically significant excess of breast cancer.[204] However, a larger study in Sweden followed 834 thyroid cancer patients who were treated with radioiodine.[203] The SIR for radioiodine treated patients was 0.74 (95% CI 0.34, 1.40). The SIR for patients treated with other methods was higher (1.37) but the confidence limits of the SIRs for the two groups overlapped.

An increased risk of breast cancer has been reported in two small series of radium dial painters.[555,556] Adams et al. reported that there was a breast cancer excess in radium dial painters who had a radium intake of 2 MBq (50 μCi) or greater.[557] As of 1980 there were 36 deaths from breast cancer among the located 1180 female dial workers who were employed before 1930. Radium treatment of about 2000 children and adults from Germany with ankylosing spondylosis has shown increased risk of bone sarcomas, breast cancer, liver cancer, and leukemia.[226–228,558] A study by Nekolla et al. of 455 patients treated with radium 224 for TB, ankylosing spondylitis, and a few other diseases indicated that male and female breast cancer were both significantly increased although there were only two cases of male breast cancer.[224] Wick and Nekolla also reported on late effects in ankylosing spondylitis patients treated with radium 224.[225] There were 626 exposed and 725 control patients with a mean follow-up time of 21 years. Mean injected activity 0.17 MBq/kg and the mean alpha skeletal dose was 0.67 Gy. The study showed a decrease in the O/E ratio for breast cancer in those exposed of 3:4.5.

A significant excess of breast cancer was reported among Danish Thorotrast patients.[213] The SIR was 1.8 (95% CI 1.1 to 2.8). There was no relationship between the SIR and the volume of Thorotrast injected or time since injection. In contrast, no increase was found in the German Thorotrast patient series reported by van Kaick et al.[212] There is a 2003 report by dos Santos Silva et al. on the 50-year follow-up of mortality among Portuguese Thorotrast patients.[220] The cohort included 1096 systemically exposed and 240 locally exposed among whom the SMR for breast cancer in the systemically exposed was nonsignificantly increased at 2.22. The RR of systemically exposed versus locally exposed was nonsignificantly increased at 1.93. A report on the Sellafield plant by Omar et al. indicated a significant increase in breast cancer among plutonium workers with an SMR of 2.36 (based on six cases).[148] Incidence was nonsignificantly increased. A significantly increased risk of breast cancer has been reported in women exposed to fallout in the Semipalatinsk area of Kazakhstan.[533]

Summary

Female breast cancer can be induced by radiation under certain conditions. Male breast cancer has not been shown to be increased as a result of radiation exposure in the epidemiologic studies to date. Age at exposure is an important factor in determining risk of radiation-induced breast cancer. The highest risk occurs when age at exposure is less than 15 years. At ages over 40 at exposure, the risk appears to be minimal or small enough to be undetectable in most low-dose studies. The mean latent period depends on the age at exposure, with longer latent periods in the groups exposed at younger ages. This is the result of the tumors generally occurring at the time of high spontaneous risk. The mean latent period appears to be about 24 years and the minimum about 15 years.

Most data support a linear dose-incidence model up to breast doses of 3 Gy. At higher doses the risk reaches a plateau and then decreases. There are a number of confounding variables that must be considered in analysis of data, including length of follow-up, potential for cell killing, age at first pregnancy, genetic history, hormonal status, and dietary factors. Many studies of groups exposed to doses less than 0.2 Gy do not show an increased risk. On the other hand, higher dose levels do clearly increase the risk of breast cancer in females exposed at young ages but show little effect at older ages. There is some evidence that radiation may act additively with respect to baseline rate differences between Japanese and Western populations and there is some limited data that radiation may act multiplicatively with respect to reproductive factors and perhaps benign breast disease.[86]

The effect of fractionation does not appear to be large except, perhaps, in the radioiodine studies, in which no consistent risk increase is noted. Risk estimates for population exposure have been summarized by both UNSCEAR and ICRP. The 1988 UNSCEAR Report gave estimates of 6.0 (90% CI 2.8 to 10.5) excess fatal cancers in a population of 1000 persons exposed to 1 Gy of low-LET radiation at high-dose rate.[370] This value potentially could be reduced by a factor of 1.5 to 2 for chronic radiation, and ICRP gives an estimate of lifetime mortality after exposure of a population of all ages as 20 $(10^{-4}\text{Sv})^{-1}$.[248] As pointed out previously in the text, risk factors for a given individual may differ markedly from the numbers given here for general population exposure. Radiation risk factors for breast cancer have been summarized in the 2006 UNSCEAR report (Table 5-11).[86]

Table 5-11 • Risk Estimates for Cancer Incidence and Mortality from Studies of Radiation Exposure: Female Breast Cancer*

Study	Average Excess Relative Risk at 1 Sv	Average Excess Absolute Risk $(10^4 PYSv)^{-1}$
External Low-LET exposures		
Incidence		
A-bomb Life Span Study[319]		
Age at exposure		
<20	1.89 (1.38–2.5)	8.78 (6.54–11.28)
20–40	1.31 (0.86–1.87)	6.97 (4.71–9.54)
>40	0.62 (0.04–1.51)	2.49 (0.02–5.82)
Time since exposure		
12–15	1.45 (0.09–4.18)	<0 (<0–3.01)
15–30	1.94 (1.3–2.77)	6.07 (4.29–8.09)
>30	1.3 (0.94–1.73)	11.08 (8.36–14.05)
All	1.49 (1.17–1.85)	7.55 (6.08–9.14)
Pooled analysis: 8 cohorts[527]	0.86 (0.7–1.04)	13.4 (9.5–17)
Massachusetts TB fluoroscopy[518]	0.4 (0.2–0.7)	7.98 (3.6–13)
New York acute post-partum mastitis[521]	0.43 (0.3–0.6)	9.14 (6–13)
Swedish benign breast disease[542,559]	0.35 (0.3–0.4)	2.72 (2.2–3.3)
Cervical cancer case control[127]	−0.2 (<−0.2–0.3)	<−0.3 (<−0.3–0.2)
Without ovaries	0.33 (<−0.2–5.8)	NA
Contralateral breast		
Denmark[131]	0.02 (<−0.1–0.2)	NA
United States[130]	0.07 (<−0.1–0.2)	NA
Rochester thymic irradiation[544]	2.39 (1.2–4)	4.89 (2.4–8.1)
Childhood skin hemangioma[560]	0.35 (0.18–0.59)	1.44 (0.78–2.28)
Hodgkin's disease (Stanford)[526]	0.07 (0.04–0.11)	0.04 (0.03–0.07)
Hodgkin's disease (Netherlands)[553]	0.06 (0.01–0.13)	NA
Hodgkin's disease (international)[561]	0.15 (0.04–0.73) (RT alone)	NA
Canada National Dose Registry[153]	<0	<0
China medical x-ray workers[253]		
Employed before 1970	0.62 (−0.16–1.6)	0.37 (−0.09–1)
Employed only 1970–1980	4 (−2.4–13)	1.5 (−0.9–5)
Mortality		
A-bomb Life Span Study[281]		
Males	2.94 (1.63–4.86)	<0 (<0–437.6)
Females	1.01 (0.31–2.06)	<0 (<0–556.08)
Age at exposure		
<20	<0 (<0–0.99)	<0 (<0–622.72)
20–40	0.04 (<0–1.61)	<0 (<0–279.27)
>40	1.33 (0.46–2.68)	1.13 (0.3–2.23)
Time since exposure		
12–15	1.82 (0.98–2.98)	3.28 (1.97–4.83)
15–30	1.39 (0.83–2.1)	<0 (<0–513.45)
Scoliosis patients[562]	5.4 (1.2–14.1)	12.9 (4.0–21)
Ankylosing spondylitis[266]	0.08 (−0.3–0.65)	NA
Canadian TB fluoroscopy[563]	0.9 (0.55–1.39)	3.16 (1.97–4.78)
Peptic ulcer[113]	0.1 (<0–10.4)	NA
Nuclear workers in Canada, United Kingdom, United States[166]	>0	NA
U.K. National Registry for Radiation Workers[146]	0.12 (<−1.95–40.5)	NA
IARC 15-country nuclear workers study[167,168]	<0	
Internal Low-LET Exposures		
Mortality		
Semipalatinsk Study[533]	1.09 (−0.05, 15.8)	NA
Internal High-LET Exposures		
Incidence		
^{224}Ra TB and ankylosing spondylitis patients[224]	0.9	NA
Danish and Swedish Thorotrast patients[219]	1.6 (0.9–2.8)	NA
Mortality		
U.S. Thorotrast patients[219]	0.9 (0.3–7.2)	NA

*The studies listed are those for which quantitative estimates of risk could be made.
Adapted from United Nations Scientific Committee of the Effects of Atomic Radiation (UNSCEAR): Sources and effects of ionizing radiation: 2006 report to the General Assembly with annexes. New York, United Nations, 2007.

It should be remembered that there are a large number of negative and positive epidemiologic studies for which no risk factor could be derived but which do add to our knowledge about specific exposure circumstances.

LUNG CANCER

General

In the United States, cancers of the lung and bronchus account for 17% of all malignancies in males and 12% of malignancies in females. The 5-year survival of patients with these tumors averages about 13%. Survival at 15 years after diagnosis is 3% to 4%. The fatality rate for radiation-induced lung cancer is between 95% and 100%. Squamous cell carcinoma accounts for 35% of the tumors; carcinoma NOS, 33%; adenocarcinoma, 15%; and small-cell carcinoma, 8%. The annual rate per 100,000 population is approximately 74 for males and 41 for females. There are about 172,000 new cases and 153,000 deaths annually in the United States due to lung cancer.

Lung cancer was one of the earliest cancers identified as possibly being related to radiation exposure. The relationship was initially suggested in a study of Bohemian miners. To date, several other major population groups have been studied, including those exposed to natural background, fallout, and occupational radiation, atomic bomb survivors, patients exposed to radiation therapy, and those exposed to radon daughter products in homes and underground mines. These sources of information used for risk estimates are rather discordant for several reasons: uncertainties in dosimetry at Hiroshima and Nagasaki, problems of comparison of external radiation exposure with internal exposure from radon daughter products, and confounding of the data by other associated carcinogenic agents (such as cigarette smoking).

A book on the epidemiology of lung cancer has been published by Samet.[564] The most common histologic types of lung cancer are squamous cell, small-oat cell, adenocarcinoma, and large cell tumors. There is a strong association between smoking and squamous cell cancer and small-cell cancers but adenocarcinoma also is increased. In fact, over 90% of adenocarcinomas arise in smokers. Studies relating cell type are often complicated by poorly differentiated tumors or tumors that are a mixture of cell types. The cell type reported also is significantly affected by the type of specimen examined, stain used, and interobserver variability.

Modifying Factors

The various portions of the respiratory tract do not appear to be equally radiosensitive. The most proximal portions of the bronchial tree appear to be the most sensitive to induction of neoplasms by radiation as well as other agents. Estimates of the risk of radiation induction of lung cancer depend on the age of the subjects at the time of exposure. Relative risk appears to differ in expression between the atomic bomb survivors and the uranium miners. In the uranium miners the ERR declines over time, following cessation of exposure, while among the atomic bomb survivors, if this trend exists at all, it is much less marked.[565] The risk from radiation-induced lung cancer at later ages rises steeply, as it does from normally occurring lung cancers.

The latent period (as with most solid tumors) is generally more than 10 years from the time of exposure, and excess cases have been identified in some populations as long as 50 years after the beginning of the exposure. The mortality data on the atomic bomb survivors reported by Shimizu et al. indicate that the minimum latent period is 20 to 24 years for cancer of the lung.[10] Latent period related to lung cancer and radon exposure in uranium miners has been discussed by Archer et al. and they have concluded that the latency period is likely in the range of 25 years regardless of magnitude of exposure and about 19 years among cigarette smokers.[566]

There has been a question as to whether the cell type of radiation-induced lung cancer may vary by radiation type. The atomic bomb survivor data (low-LET radiation) have indicated an increase in squamous, small-cell, and adenocarcinoma, whereas small-cell carcinoma appears to have disproportionately increased (about 55% of cases in uranium miners exposed to high-LET radiation vs. 20% in the general population of smokers and nonsmokers). In a recent review of lung cancer slides from 92 uranium miners and 108 atomic bomb survivors, Land et al. indicate that the proportions of squamous cell cancers were related to smoking, as expected.[565] Radiation-induced cancers were more likely to be of a small-cell subtype and less likely to be adenocarcinomas. Tokarskaya et al. have examined the cell types of lung cancer in plutonium workers and concluded that adenocarcinoma was most commonly associated with radiation.[567,568] Squamous and small-cell carcinoma are most closely linked with smoking.

The issue of acute versus fractionated exposure on the induction of lung cancer has been examined for low-LET radiation by Howe comparing a TB chest fluoroscopy cohort to the atomic bomb survivors. In the fluoroscopy study based on 1178 lung cancer deaths there was no evidence of a positive association between risk and dose with the RR at 1 Sv being 1.00 (95% CI 0.94, 1.07) and the mean lung dose of 1.02 Sv. No excess lung cancer was identified in the U.S. Massachusetts TB cohort either. This implies that extrapolation of high-dose risk factors to fractionated low-LET exposure would result in an overestimate.

The type of radiation (alpha vs. gamma) has been examined regarding lung cancer risk and dose, particularly with regard to comparison of plutonium workers at Mayak and atomic bomb survivors and with studies of the Mayak workers and their external doses. Assuming a radiation weighting factor of 20 for alpha particles, the estimates of lung cancer risk per unit dose overlap. This issue is discussed later in the descriptions of the Mayak studies. Some authors have attempted to find a unique genetic change associated with radon-associated lung cancers but to date no consistent radiation signature has been confirmed.[570]

There is a well-documented association between smoking and lung cancer. The American Cancer Society estimates that smoking is responsible for about 83% of lung cancer cases in men and 43% among women, accounting for an overall total of more than 75% of all lung cancers. The 1989 report of the U.S. Surgeon General indicated that in 1985 cigarette smoking was responsible for 90% of lung cancer in males and 79% in females. It also indicated that the estimated RR for male smokers during 1982–1986 was 22.3. Several studies indicate that the age at which an individual began smoking substantially affects the mortality ratio and that the RR of lung cancer is related to the number of cigarettes smoked each day.

The interaction between smoking and radiation continues to be a subject of intense interest. Early studies of uranium miners have suggested a multiplicative interaction. For example, a given exposure to radon may double the risk in a nonsmoker, and the same exposure would also double the 10-fold higher risk in a smoker to 20-fold.[571] Lubin et al. have performed a very large joint analysis of 11 underground miner studies.[572] A clear pattern of risk for the joint association of smoking and exposure to radon progeny did not emerge, although the data were consistent with a relationship which was intermediate between additive and multiplicative. The data do show that even with the levels of radon in mines, lung cancer in smoking miners is more likely due to smoking than to radon (attributable risk of 0.39 for radon). Lubin et al. also estimated the lung cancer attributable to radon in the United States and concluded that the attributable percentage of lung cancer deaths from residential radon may be twofold greater in nonsmokers than in smokers.[573] The 1998 BEIR VI report on health effects of radon indicated that although it was difficult to precisely characterize the joint effect of smoking and radon exposure, the submultiplicative relation was most consistent with available data.[190]

The atomic bomb survivor data suggest a more nearly additive relationship,[574] although a multiplicative relationship is also consistent with the early data.[575] Two more recent articles by Travis et al.[576] and Pierce et al.[577] indicate that the relationship is not synergistic and is significantly submultiplicative and quite consistent with additivity. They also point out that the ERR per Sv decreases substantially as smoking increases. For example, the ERR for nonsmokers is about 0.6 per Sv while for those who smoke in excess of 16 cigarettes per day the ERR per Sv is not statistically significantly different from zero. In other words, the smoking risk dominates so much that any ERR from radiation becomes difficult to detect.

Long times since radiation exposure appear to be associated with a decreased risk of lung cancer. This has been seen in the Czech studies of uranium miners published by Tomasek et al., in the atomic bomb survivor studies, and in the Russian workers at Mayak.[578,579] The issue of risk versus exposure rate is discussed later; however, in the radon progeny studies, there may be a decreasing risk with higher exposures but this issue is intertwined with the decrease in risk with time since exposure.

External Exposure

Atomic Bomb Survivors

Findings on the survivors of Hiroshima and Nagasaki through 1974 have been based on mortality follow-up. Unfortunately, autopsy studies indicated that lung cancer was often underdiagnosed on the Japanese death certificates, indicating that risk estimates for lung cancer from Japan are possibly low.[580] The additional problems with dosimetry at Hiroshima and Nagasaki (as discussed elsewhere) have caused difficulties in interpretation of the risk estimates.

The 1958–1998 incidence study of atomic bomb survivors published by Preston et al. in 2007 has yielded incidence risk estimates of 0.81 ERR at 1 Gy and absolute excess risk of 7.5 $(10^4 PYSv)^{-1}$.[319] Current and earlier dose response data are linear (Fig. 5-9).[279] As of 1998, there

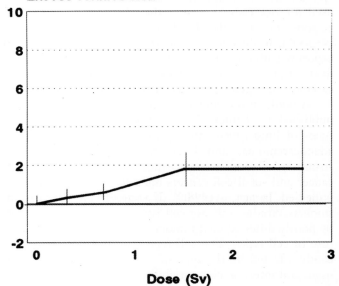

Lung cancer incidence (A-bomb)

Figure 5-9 • ERR of lung cancer in atomic bomb survivors at different dose levels. Bars indicate 95% CI. (From Thompson D, Mabuchi K, Ron E, et al: Cancer incidence in atomic bomb survivors. II: Solid tumors, 1958–1987. RERF Technical Report 5-92, Hiroshima, Japan, Radiation Effects Research Foundation, 1992.)

was an estimated excess of 117 lung cancer cases out of 1759 total cases. The mortality data up to 1985 published by Shimizu et al. found 638 lung cancer deaths and indicated an RR at 1 Gy of 1.46 (90% CI 1.25, 1.72) and an EAR per 10,000 PYGy of 1.25 (90% CI 0.70, 1.89).[10] The attributable risk was estimated to be 11.4% (90% CI 6.4, 17.1). The paper also has data on ERR by dose level, and age at exposure for lung cancer and indicates a significant ERR for lung cancer at less than 0.5 Gy. A later mortality study up to 1990 published by Pierce et al. in 1996 indicated an ERR per Sv in males of 0.33 (95% CI 0.03, 0.69), an ERR in females of 0.75 (95% CI 0.30, 1.33), and for both sexes an ERR of 0.42 per Gy (95% CI 0.24, 0.63).[8]

The latest mortality study contains data up through 1997 and was published by Preston et al. in 2003.[281] There are a total of 86,572 persons in the study with 9335 solid cancer deaths versus 8895 expected for an excess of 440 solid cancer deaths. Additionally, 48% of the atomic bomb survivor population was still alive. Other causes of death were 582 hematopoietic tumors, 447 other tumors, 222 deaths from noncancer blood diseases, 31,881 from other diseases, 2200 from external causes, and 104 from unknown causes. There was a statistically significant relationship between radiation dose and cancers of the lung. For males the ERR was 0.48 at 1 Sv organ dose (90% CI 0.23, 0.78), the EAR was 2.7 per 10,000 PYSv (90% CI 1.4, 4.1), and the attributable risk (%) was 9.7 (90% CI 4.9, 15). For females the ERR was 1.1 at 1 Sv organ dose (90% CI 0.68, 1.6), the EAR was 2.5 per 10,000 PYSv (90% CI 1.6, 3.5), and the attributable risk (%) was 16 (90% CI 10, 22).

Natural Background Radiation

There is no consistent evidence of an increase in lung cancer as a result of terrestrial or cosmic background radiation exposure. One study has examined background radiation and lung cancer incidence in Connecticut.[21] In this study lung cancer had no relation to radiation level. Another analysis by different states indicated a significantly negative correlation.[25,26] An ecological study comparing cancer rates in Gulf Coast states (with lower background radiation) with Rocky Mountain states (which had 3.2 times higher natural radiation levels) was published by Jagger in 1998.[581] It showed that lung cancer was in fact higher in the states with the lower background radiation. The study, however, could not easily deal with the confounding issues of more smoking in Gulf Coast states pointed out by Archer.[582]

Excess relative risk of solid cancer mortality after prolonged exposure to naturally occurring high-background radiation in Yangjiang, China, has been published in a paper by Sun et al.[32] The paper used a high-background area and a neighboring control area in Guangdong, China, and covered 1.7 million person-years of study from 1979–1995. Dose rate in the high-background area was 4.3 mSv per year and in the control areas it was about

1.6 × 10 mSv per year. The correlation of lung cancer mortality with dose was negative with an ERR per Sv of −0.68 (95% CI −1.58, 1.66). An additional report on the same areas by Tao et al. covered 1.7 million person-years of study from 1979–1995.[33] The mortality due to lung cancer was again less in the high-background area with an RR of 0.87 (95% CI 0.51, 1.49).

Natural cosmic radiation and its potential effect on lung cancer has been studied in airline crews since they receive more cosmic radiation due to flying at high altitudes. Band et al. have published a study of 2740 pilots with doses of 6 mSv per year over an average of 20 years and total average dose of about 120 mSv and found a significantly reduced risk of respiratory cancers with an SMR of 0.25 (90% CI 0.12, 0.45).[40] Blettner et al. have reviewed additional studies and found nonsignificantly increased lung cancer mortality in two studies and decreased mortality in two other studies.[41] Blettner et al. also have reported on cancer mortality among airline cabin attendants in Germany during 1960–1997 and indicated that the SMR for lung cancer was nonsignificantly reduced for both males and females.[583] Pukkala et al. reported on cancer mortality among 10,032 Nordic pilots over five decades and found a nonsignificant decrease in lung cancer SMR of 0.92 (95% CI 0.55, 14.3).[39]

Fallout and Populations Near Nuclear Facilities

At least two studies have looked for lung cancer as a result of nuclear fallout. In both a Swedish[56] and a U.S. study in Utah[456] there was a negative correlation between fallout and lung cancer. In the Swedish study the SIR was 0.39 (95% CI 0.14, 0.86), and in the Utah fallout study the OR was 0.78 (90% CI 0.64, 0.94). There have been no consistent or statistically significant increases in lung cancer in U.S. populations living near nuclear facilities.[78] When an individual plant is considered, differences may be identified on a chance basis or as a result of other environmental factors and smoking. Such findings should be carefully considered and evaluated with the usual epidemiologic criteria before acceptance of conclusions as to causation. There are three papers by Boice et al. concerning potential environmental uranium contamination and the possibility of lung cancer in the public indicating a nonsignificant decrease around a uranium mining and milling facility in Texas, a nonsignificant decrease near a uranium facility in Pennsylvania, and at a Colorado facility a statistically significant increase (compared to Colorado) and a statistically significant decrease compared to the United States.[89,90,90a] Lopez-Abente et al. have reported on solid tumor mortality near Spain's four nuclear power plants and four uranium fuel cycle facilities and the RR for lung cancer was nonsignificantly decreased at 0.93.[283] A significant decrease was found by Boice et al. in a study of persons residing near the Hanford National Laboratory.[91] Bauer et al. have reported on cancer mortality due to local fallout from Soviet atmospheric nuclear weapons testing at the Semipalatinsk test site in Kazakhstan.[533] Effective doses ranged from 20 mSv to about 4 Sv. The dose-response LRT for lung cancer was significant with a P value of less than 0.0001 in males and 0.0003 in females. The estimated ERR per Sv for the exposed cohort was 1.76 (95% CI 0.48, 8.83).

Nonminer Occupational Exposure

One of the largest occupational groups studied comprises persons who have worked at atomic energy facilities or nuclear installations. A number of large studies have been performed in the United Kingdom. A study by Beral et al. included an analysis of 3373 deaths among 39,546 atomic energy workers during 1946–1979.[143] The SMR was 0.74 for all deaths and 0.79 for all cancer deaths. Lung cancer was less common than expected, with the rate ratio reported at 0.84 (95% CI 0.61, 1.15). Another study of atomic weapons workers by Beral et al. also did not show an increase of lung cancer.[144] They reported a rate ratio of 0.84 (95% CI 0.61, 1.15). A cohort analysis of the U.K. National Registry of Radiation Workers by Kendall et al. included 95,217 workers over 1.2 million person-years at risk.[145] The report studied lung cancer and reported a significant decrease in lung cancer with radiation exposure (SMR of 0.76). In a second expanded analysis of the same group, Muirhead et al. reported on a cohort of 124,743 workers with means doses of 30.5 mSv.[146] The lagged SMR analysis for cancer of the lung was significantly reduced at 0.71 (95% CI 0.66, 0.76) and cancer of the pleura was significantly elevated with an SMR of 1.96 (95% CI 1.38, 2.71). Muirhead also reported on the mortality and incidence of cancer during 1952–1998 in men from the United Kingdom who participated in the United Kingdom's atmospheric nuclear weapons tests and experimental programs.[54] The RR for test participants was nonsignificantly reduced at 0.94 (95% CI 0.85, 1.04). Another paper in 2004 on epidemiological studies of mortality and cancer incidence among U.K. test veterans indicated that their RR for lung cancer mortality was 0.97 (95% CI 0.88, 1.08) and the SMR was significantly reduced at 0.85 (95% CI 0.78, 0.93).[55] Lung cancer incidence was also reduced with an RR of 0.95 (95% CI 0.86, 1.04).

In other U.K. studies, Douglas et al. reported a significantly decreased SMR and SRR for cancer of the lung at 0.84 and 0.86, respectively.[147] Cancer of the pleura was significantly increased with an SMR of 4.25. A report on the Sellafield plant by Omar et al. indicated a significant decrease in lung cancer in nonplutonium radiation workers with an SMR of 0.80 but there was a significantly increased SMR again in cancer of the pleura.[148] Incidence was significantly decreased for lung cancer and significantly increased for pleural cancer. McGeoghegan et al. have reported on the mortality and cancer morbidity experience of employees at the Chapelcross plant of British Nuclear Fuels during 1955–1995, which included a cohort of 2628 workers with median doses of 39 mSv.[149] The mean follow-up was 24.3 years and there were 63,967 person-years of study. The SMR for cancer of the lung for radiation workers and all workers was significantly less than expected at 0.65 and 0.71, respectively, and the SMR for pleural cancer in radiation workers was nonsignificantly elevated at 2.63 but based on only two cases.

In 2003 Iwasaki et al. reported on the second analysis of mortality of nuclear industry workers in Japan.[150] The study included 176,000 male workers and 5527 deaths. Average annual doses were 3.5 mSv before 1982 and 1.2 mSv after 1982. For cancer of the lung the SMR was 0.97 (95% CI 0.87, 1.07). Artalejo et al. studied occupational exposure to ionizing radiation and mortality among workers of the former Spanish Nuclear Energy Board.[151] The cohort mortality study of 5657 workers with mean exposure of 11.42 mSv indicated an SMR for lung cancer of 0.98 (95% CI 0.71, 1.31). Habib et al. have reported on cancer incidence among Australian nuclear industry–monitored radiation workers and indicated a nonsignificantly reduced SIR of 0.46 for lung cancer.[152] SIR for pleural cancer was significantly raised in the radiation workers but it was even higher in the nonradiation workers (probably as a result of asbestos exposures). Rahu et al. have reported on cancer incidence of 5446 male Latvian and Estonian Chernobyl cleanup workers and indicate a nonsignificant SIR of 1.37 for lung cancer.[178]

There are several studies of Canadian radiation workers in whom initial studies by Gribbin et al. failed to find any increase in lung cancer.[260] Ashmore et al. studied a cohort of 206,620 individuals and 5426 deaths.[154] The average exposure for males was 10.6 mSv and the SMR for cancer of the lung was significantly reduced at 0.61 (90% CI 0.55, 0.66). Sont et al. reported on a cohort of 191,222 persons from the National Dose Registry of Canada with an average dose for males of 11.5 mSv and an average dose for the cohort of 6.64 mSv.[153] The SIR for lung cancer was significantly reduced for both males and females, at 0.64 and 0.79, respectively. Zablotska et al. recently reported on the mortality among Canadian nuclear power industry workers after chronic low-dose exposure to ionizing radiation and found a significantly reduced SMR for lung cancer, of 0.79 (95% CI 0.68, 0.91).[155]

A number of studies have been performed in the United States. Some of these have generated a large amount of controversy and merit careful review of their methods before their findings are accepted. Wilkinson et al. studied the mortality of workers at the Rocky Flats nuclear weapons facility and while this report indicates excess cancers in some tables, the excesses have CIs that usually are very wide due to the small number of cases, and an estimate of no risk (unity) is well within the range of estimates.[286] The SMR reported for lung cancer in employees who worked at least 2 years was 0.96. When workers with plutonium body burdens equal to or more than 74 Bq (2 nCi) were compared with unexposed controls, the RR was 1.43 (90% CI 0.33 to 4.65) for a 10-year latent period. When exposure to more than 0.01 Sv of external radiation was considered, the RR was 0.91 (90% CI 0.44 to 1.89).

A paper by Checkoway et al. discussed the mortality of workers at the Oak Ridge Y-12 plant.[284] A statistically significant excess of lung cancer is seen only if a 0-year latent period analysis was used. If an appropriate 10-year latent period was used, there was no statistical excess of lung cancer at any level of radiation. In a report of the mortality of workers from the Oak Ridge National Laboratory, Wing et al. suggest that risk estimates for all cancers are 10 times higher than those reported from a study of the atomic bomb survivors.[285] An increase in lung cancer was found but had little relationship to latent period. The authors themselves indicate that they find their results difficult to explain and indicate that confounding factors such as smoking were not taken into consideration. A later analysis by Gilbert actually implied that the significant associations were largely due to smoking-related cancers.[124] No increase in lung cancer mortality was reported at the Mound Nuclear Facility in Ohio.[156]

In a combined cohort analysis of workers at Hanford, Rocky Flats, and the Oak Ridge National Laboratory by Gilbert et al., no excess of lung cancer was identified.[157] No increase in lung cancer reported by Gilbert et al. in their analysis of Hanford workers from 1945–1986.[158] Frome et al. reported on a mortality study of 106,020 employees and 27,982 deaths in the nuclear industry at Oak Ridge, Tennessee.[160] The SMR for cancers of the respiratory tract in white males was nonsignificantly elevated at 1.16, for nonwhite males it was 0.97, for white females 1.10, and for nonwhite females 0.92. Their respective values for lung cancer were 1.18 (significantly elevated), 0.94, 1.00, and 0.92. Fry et al. reported on a similar group of 3145 DOE contractors exposed to more than 50 mSv with a mean external exposure of 1 mSv in whom the SMR for lung cancer was nonsignificantly elevated at 1.09 (95% CI 0.80, 1.46).[161] Howe et al. analyzed the mortality experience among 53,698 U.S. nuclear power industry workers with chronic low-dose exposure to ionizing radiation.[159] Their mean cumulative dose was 25.7 mSv and the SMR for lung cancer was significantly reduced at 0.59 (95% CI 0.49, 0.71). The mean duration of follow-up was about 12 years which limits the value of this finding. Groves et al. conducted a 40-year cancer mortality study of 40,581 Korean War Navy veterans with potential exposure to high-intensity radar which also emits ionizing radiation.[165] The SMR for lung cancer was significantly decreased at 0.64 (95% CI 0.58, 0.70).

Cardis et al. reported on cancer mortality among nuclear industry workers in three countries in a large study of 95,673 workers followed over 2 million person-years at risk and with 15,825 deaths.[166] The trend for lung cancer was nonsignificantly decreased at −0.28 with a P value of 0.61. The trend for cancer of the pleura was nonsignificantly decreased at −0.18 with a P value of 0.57. Cardis et al. have reported the cancer mortality results from a 15-country collaborative study of nuclear workers.[168] This is the largest occupational study to date and included a cohort of 407,391 workers with 18,993 deaths and 5.2 million person-years of follow-up. The ERR per Sv for lung cancer was significantly positive at 1.86 (90% CI 0.49, 3.63). The ERR per Sv for pleural cancer was nonsignificantly positive at 5.28 (90% CI < 0, 39.9).

Cancer incidence among medical diagnostic workers in China was reported by Wang et al. in 1988 who compared 27,011 workers with 25,782 persons in other medical specialties.[102] The x-ray workers had a 50% higher risk of developing cancers, but there was no excess of cancer of the lung, even though the workers were likely to have been exposed to external doses on the order or 1 Gy or more. The RR reported was 0.87. Wang et al. published a follow-up in 2002 of a cohort of 27,011 medical diagnostic x-ray workers.[253] Cumulative doses were 0.55 Sv for those employed before 1970 and 8.2 Sv for those employed after 1970. The RR for cancer of the lung was 1.10 for those employed before 1970, and, for those employed from 1970–1980 the RR was significantly elevated at 1.57, probably due to smoking as the earlier cohort would have received more radiation dose.

The mortality of British radiologists from lung cancer has been studied by Smith et al. who found a statistically significant increase in those who were employed before 1920 but no increase in those employed later.[584] Uncertainty about smoking histories and radiation dose precludes derivation of risk estimates. Berrington et al. published a follow-up including 100 years of experience in British radiologists with reference to their mortality from cancer and other causes from 1897–1997.[94] For those employed during 1897–1920 the SMR for lung cancer was elevated at 2.46 before radiation protection was used and radiologists were likely exposed to very high doses. For those employed after 1920 the SMR was below that expected at 0.70.

There are at least six studies that have evaluated mortality and cancer incidence in radiologic technologists. Aoyama et al. reported a mortality survey of Japanese radiological technologists during 1969–1993.[95] The SMR for lung cancer was significantly reduced at 0.62 (95% CI 0.47 to 0.80).[80] Burnett et al. indicated a proportional cancer mortality ratio for lung cancer that was nonsignificantly elevated at 1.15 (95% CI 0.92, 1.42).[96] Doody et al. reported on mortality among 143,517 U.S. radiological technologists during 1926–1990.[97] Their doses were not evaluated and the SMR for cancer of the lung was significantly reduced at 0.74 (95% CI 0.67, 0.82). Jablon et al. studied Army technologists in a 29-year follow-up for cause of death, which included 6560 radiological technologists and 6826 controls who were other types of technologists (laboratory, pharmacy, etc).[585] Follow-up was from 1946–1974 for an average of 26.6 years or 174,500 person-years of observation. No statistically significant difference was found between groups. The mortality from lung cancer was the same in both x-ray technicians and controls (0.62% in each). In 2003 Mohan et al. reported a study of 146,022 radiologic technologists employed from 1940 and later.[99] The SMR for cancer of the lung in males was significantly reduced at 0.67 (95% CI 0.6, 0.7) and for females it was also significantly reduced at 0.80 (95% CI 0.7, 0.9). Also in 2003, Sigurdson et al. reported on cancer incidence among 90,305 U.S. radiological technologists; again, the SMR for lung cancer was significantly reduced at 0.77 (95% CI 0.70, 0.85).[101]

Information has become available on radiation doses and the mortality of workers at the reactor and reprocessing plants at Chelyabinsk (Mayak) in Russia. For workers in the Mayak radiochemical plant, the exposure was mostly from inhalation, and in 2346 workers, 45 cases of lung cancer were observed versus 33 expected. There was an increasing trend with dose, although the role of chemicals remains uncertain in the etiology of the lung cancers.[174] Studies of the Mayak plant provide information on the health effects of plutonium as well as chronic external exposure. A 1998 report by Koshurnikova found no evidence of an association of lung cancer with external doses in the range of 0.2 to 5.5 Gy.[586] A later study by Gilbert et al. found that the ERR per unit dose was not substantially different from that of the atomic bomb survivors.[587] The ERR per Sv (equivalent dose) was 0.23 (95% CI 0.16, 0.33) for males at attained age of 60 compared with 0.40 (95% CI 0.032, 0.86) in the male atomic bomb survivors. The results in females were 0.93 (95% CI 0.46, 1.9) in the Mayak workers compared to 1.40 (95% CI 0.76, 2.2) in the female atomic bomb survivors. The sex difference in ERR is probably the result of more cigarette smoking in males which reduces the ERR per unit dose. As with the atomic bomb survivors the relative risk of lung cancer in the Mayak workers decreased with attained age. Risks for internal and external exposure were adequately described by linear functions and there was evidence of risk when the analysis was restricted to internal absorbed doses to the lung of less than 0.5 Gy (or with an RBE of 20, about 10 Sv).

Medical Diagnostic Exposure

Even though some authors have thought that there is a positive relationship between TB and lung cancer without radiation exposure, this has not been borne out in some radiation studies. In the Massachusetts TB patients treated with pneumothorax and multiple fluoroscopies, cancer of the esophagus was statistically significantly increased, but cancer of the lung was not.[105,364] For lung cancer an SMR of 0.8 was reported suggesting that fractionation may have reduced the risk. In this study the mean lung dose was estimated to be 0.84 Gy. As mentioned previously, in a report by Howe no excess lung cancer risk was identified in the Canadian TB fluoroscopy cohort either.[569] The RR per Sv lung dose was 1.00 (95% CI 0.94, 1.07).

Radiation Therapy

Smith and Doll reported the follow-up of some 14,000 patients treated with radiation for ankylosing spondylitis.[588] This group, treated as early as 1935, was followed to 1970. By that time, 124 had died of lung cancer, compared with 87 expected. Smoking histories were unfortunately not available. Estimated total absorbed dose to the bronchial tree was 1.97 Gy, with an annual absolute risk estimate of 2.8 lung cancer deaths in 1 million persons for each 10 mGy. The follow-up has since been extended to 1983 by Darby et al. who observed 224 deaths, as compared to the 184.5 deaths expected (O/E ratio of cancer, 1.42; P value < 0.001).[109] Follow-up studies by Weiss et al. in 1994 of 15,577 patients treated and who received a mean lung dose of 2.54 Gy for ankylosing spondylitis indicated a statistically significant excess of lung cancer; however, the O/E ratio at less than 5 years after treatment was elevated (1.22) and, at 5 to 25 years after treatment, the O/E was 1.37.[266] After 25 years posttreatment the risk decreased with an O/E ratio of 0.97.

In women treated with radiotherapy for benign breast disease, during which parts of the lungs received about 1 Gy, no statistically significant excess of lung cancer was identified by Mattsson et al.[114] The SIR for lung cancer was 0.89 (95% CI 0.43, 1.65) and the RR was 1.79 (95% CI 0.65, 4.99). Griem et al. have followed a population of patients who received radiotherapy for peptic ulcer in whom a statistically significant increase in cancer of the lung was identified with an RR of 1.70 (95% CI 1.2, 2.4).[112] Carr et al. followed up the same group of 3719 patients in whom the dose for the left lung was estimated to be 1.8 Gy.[113] The RR for lung cancer was 0.84 (95% CI 0.28, 2.56) during 0 to 10 years postexposure but statistically significantly increased with an RR of 1.5 (95% CI 1.08, 2.08) during 11 to 62 years postexposure. Lundell et al. reported on the risk of solid tumors in 14,351 infants treated for skin hemangiomas with either photons or radium applicators in whom the ERR per Gy was nonsignificantly increased at 1.4.[589]

In an incidence study of women treated for cervical cancer, 82,616 exposed women were compared with 99,424 unexposed controls.[124] The women were from Canada, Denmark, Finland, Norway, Sweden, Yugoslavia, the United Kingdom, and the United States and the study covered 1.28 million person-years at risk. There was a threefold increase in lung cancer both in the patients treated with radiotherapy and those who received no radiation. Relative risk was highest in the first 15 years after treatment and decreased to normal levels after 20 years, which, of course, does not indicate a radiation effect because of the lack of the usual latent period and no risk at later times when radiation-induced tumors are characteristically seen. The authors conclude that the greatly elevated risk seen in the first 15 years was probably due to cigarette smoking and misclassification of cervical cancer metastases as lung cancer. Kleinerman et al. also evaluated second cancers in 86,193 patients with cervical cancer reported to 13 cancer registries in 5 countries and found the risk of lung cancer to be increased in patients who were treated with radiotherapy (with a mean organ dose of 0.3 Gy) or without radiotherapy.[125] The O/E ratios were 3.0 (95% CI 2.8, 3.2) and 2.2 (95% CI 1.8, 2.5), respectively. A Japanese study reported on 5725 cervical cancer patients treated with radiotherapy alone and 4161 treated with surgery alone.[128] Again, an excess of lung cancer was seen in both the radiotherapy alone and surgery alone groups.

A number of studies have evaluated lung cancer after radiation treatment for breast cancer, and the data are conflicting. Data from the Connecticut Tumor Registry indicated an excess risk of lung cancer more than 5 years after breast radiotherapy.[590] An Israeli study indicated an increase, but this was evenly split between the ipsilateral and contralateral lung (suggesting that this was not radiation-related).[591] In a study of patients treated at M.D. Anderson Cancer Center in Houston, Texas, there was no significant difference between women treated with radiation and those treated with surgery; however, small-cell carcinoma was apparently more frequent in patients treated with radiotherapy.[592]

Another hospital series also did not show an increase in lung cancer after breast-conserving radiation therapy.[593] Neugut et al., using data from the Surveillance, Epidemiology, and End Results Program of the National Cancer Institute, have reported an RR of 2.0 (95% CI 1.0 to 4.3) of cancer developing in the ipsilateral lung as opposed to the contralateral lung, suggesting a true radiation effect.[594] The risk appeared 10 years after breast cancer radiotherapy. Risk was increased for all of the three major histologic subgroups. This report of increased risk is contrary to the other studies discussed earlier and to the postpartum mastitis series discussed earlier.

Inskip et al. also reported on lung cancer risk and radiation dose among women treated for breast cancer.[595] For 10-year survivors the RR for lung cancer associated with initial radiotherapy was 1.8 (95% CI 0.8 to 3.8). For 15 years or more the RR was 2.8 (95% CI 1.0 to 8.2). Mean dose was 15.2 Gy to the ipsilateral lung and 4.6 Gy to the contralateral lung. The ERR was 0.08 per Gy based on the average dose to both lungs and 0.20 per Gy to the highly exposed lung. Zablotska et al. reported an increase in ipsilateral lung cancer 10 or more years after radiotherapy following mastectomy with an RR of 2.06 (95% CI 1.53, 2.78), but no increase was seen after postlumpectomy radiotherapy due to the lower dose to the lung.[596] The average dose to the isplateral lung with postmastectomy radiotherapy was 15.2 Gy.

Several reports discuss second tumors after treatment for testicular cancers. One, a Norwegian study of 876 patients, reported that 65 persons developed a second cancer.[597] There was a statistically significant increase in cancers of the lung which was thought to be radiation-related. Chemotherapy may have played a role in subsequent cancer induction. Brenner et al. have studied second malignancies in prostate carcinoma patients treated with radiotherapy or surgery and reported a significantly increased risk of lung cancer in the radiotherapy group.[137] This is somewhat surprising given that the radiotherapy was to the pelvis. One explanation is that smoking may have been considered a contraindication to surgery and thus there may have been more smokers in the radiotherapy group.

A number of studies have examined the risk of second tumors after treatment for childhood cancers. In one study by van Leeuwen, 14 lung cancers were identified in 744 patients treated for HD.[598] Nine cases were seen in the patients treated with radiotherapy alone (RR 5.4), and none were found in patients treated by chemotherapy alone. Kaldor et al. examined cases of lung cancer occurring in HD survivors and found that lung cancer was twice as common in those treated with chemotherapy as compared to those treated with radiotherapy.[599] They concluded that HD itself may be associated with an increase in lung cancer. This was supported by the fact that three quarters of the cases occurred within 10 years of the treatment. In a 2003 report by Gilbert et al. on 227 patients with lung cancer treated for HD, the ERR for lung cancer was elevated at 0.15 (95% CI 0.06, 0.39).[600] There was no evidence of a departure from linearity even though lung doses exceeded 30 Gy. Also the relationship of radiation to smoking was consistent with a multiplicative and not an additive relationship. Curtis et al. reported on solid cancer incidence in 19,229 patients following bone marrow transplantation.[441] Treatment regimens often included total-body (usually about 10 to 12 Gy) of nodal irradiation and cyclophosphamide. Lung cancer was not found to be increased and the O/E ratio was 0.7. The study is limited by the small number of lung cancer cases. Scattered, nonstatistically significant case reports of mesotheliomas[601–604] after chest wall radiotherapy have been published and even one case of mediastinal osteosarcoma after treatment for HD.[605]

Summary of External Exposure

Several studies have shown an increase in the risk of lung cancer following low-LET external radiation exposure. However, there are also a number of studies involving nuclear workers, populations exposed to fallout, and populations living in areas of high natural background radiation or around nuclear plants that do not show an increase in lung cancer. Many of the positive and negative studies are complicated by the lack of adjustment for factors such as cigarette smoking, other pollutants, and the "healthy worker" effect.

The data from the positive studies are compatible with a linear dose-response relationship. The latent period for lung cancers appears to be at least 10 years, with the mean being on the order of 20 to 30 years. The atomic bomb survivor mortality study indicates that age at exposure has no consistent effect and there does not appear to be significantly decreasing RR with increasing time since exposure. However the opposite is true for

radon. The effect of fractionation is not clear, but the data suggest that the risk decreases with fractionation of low-LET radiation but not with high-LET radiation. The interactive effect of smoking is probably between additive and multiplicative. At low doses, the interaction of smoking and radiation has not been confirmed due to the overwhelming carcinogenicity of smoking which obscures any possible radiation effect.

The ICRP 1990 risk estimate of the fatal probability coefficient for lung cancer is 85 $(10^{-4}Sv^{-1})$, referable to exposure of a general population to low-LET radiation.[248] Risk estimates summarized by UNSCEAR 2006 from the various low-LET radiation epidemiological studies are shown in Table 5-12.[86]

Table 5-12 • Risk Estimates for Cancer Incidence and Mortality from Studies of Radiation Exposure: Lung Cancer*

Study	Average Excess Relative Risk at 1 Sv	Average Excess Absolute Risk $(10^4 PYSv)^{-1}$
External Low-LET Exposures		
Incidence		
A-bomb Life Span Study[319]		
Males	0.32 (0.13–0.55)	0.57 (0.04–1.54)
Females	1.48 (1.04–1.99)	2.38 (1.37–3.53)
Age at exposure		
<20	0.68 (0.28–1.2)	0.64 (0.1–1.38)
20–40	0.65 (0.35–1)	2.65 (1.04–4.6)
>40	0.71 (0.4–1.09)	9.47 (5.75–13.78)
Time since exposure		
12–15	1.41 (0.07–4.09)	5.49 (0–32.06)
15–30	0.96 (0.57–1.44)	0.89 (0.21–1.86)
>30	0.53 (0.31–0.78)	3.35 (1.93–5.02)
All	0.69 (0.49–0.92)	1.55 (0.84–2.37)
Hodgkin's disease—international[576,600,679] (5-year lagged dose > 0)	0.15 (0.06–0.39)	NA
Breast cancer[595]	0.2 (−0.62–1.03)	NA
Swedish benign breast disease[114]	0.38 (<0–0.6)	NA
Stockholm skin hemangioma[589]	1.4 (ns)	0.33
Canada National Dose Registry[153]	3.0 (0.5–6.8)	NA
Capenhurst uranium facility[242]	−1.3 (<−1.3–9.66)	NA
U.K. Springfields uranium workers[243]	1.48 (<−2.43–6.06)	NA
U.K. Chapelcross workers[149]	0.63 (−1.61–5.95)	NA
Mortality		
A-bomb Life Span Study[281]		
Males	0.57 (0.3–0.89)	0.19 (<0–0.85)
Females	1.28 (0.84–1.8)	<0 (<0–1269.1)
Age at exposure		
<20	0.94 (0.42–1.63)	0.11 (<0–0.56)
20–40	0.78 (0.43–1.19)	0.51 (<0–1.83)
>40	0.76 (0.38–1.23)	<0 (<0–4062.9)
Time since exposure		
12–15	0.72 (<0–2.16)	<0 (<0–294.01)
15–30	0.9 (0.43–1.49)	0.24 (<0–0.97)
>30	0.71 (0.44–1.02)	2.56 (1.32–4.03)
All	0.84 (0.59–1.11)	0.37 (0.02–0.87)
A-bomb Life Span Study[563] (adjusted for smoking, and based on additive model for smoking and radiation)	0.9 (S.E. = 0.64) Sex-averaged	NA
Ankylosing spondylitis[266]	0.05 (0.002–0.09)	NA
Canadian TB fluoroscopy[569]	0 (−0.06–0.07)	0 (−0.4–0.4)
Massachusetts TB fluoroscopy[105]	−0.19 (<−0.2–0.04	−0.90 (<−1.8–0.2)

*The studies listed are those for which quantitative estimates of risk could be made.

Table 5-12 • Risk Estimates for Cancer Incidence and Mortality from Studies of Radiation Exposure: Lung Cancer*—cont'd

Study	Average Excess Relative Risk at 1 Sv	Average Excess Absolute Risk $(10^4 PYSv)^{-1}$
External Low-LET Exposures—cont'd		
Mortality—cont'd		
Peptic ulcer[113]	0.24 (0.07–0.44)	NA
Yangjiang background radiation[34,35]	−0.68 (−1.58–1.67)	NA
Male Mayak nuclear workers[680] (external dose; adjusted for plutonium exposure)	0.06 (0.07–0.2)	
Mayak nuclear workers[587] (external dose; adjusted for plutonium exposure)		
Males	0.17 (0.052–0.32)	2.4 (0.56–4.4)
Females	0.32 (<0–1.3)	0.43 (<0–1.6)
Nuclear workers in Canada, United Kingdom, United States[166]	<0	NA
U.K. National Registry for Radiation Workers[146]	−0.11 (−0.72–0.72)	NA
Canadian National Dose Registry[154]	3.6 (0.4–6.9) (males)	NA
Nuclear industry workers in Japan[150]	<0	<0
Nuclear power industry workers in the United States[159]	0.25 (<−2.51–8.44)	NA
IARC 15-country nuclear workers study[167,168]	1.86 (0.49, 3.63)	NA
Internal Low-LET Exposures		
Mortality		
Semipalatinsk[533]	1.76 (0.48–8.83)	NA
Internal High-LET Exposures (Plutonium)		
Mortality		
Male Mayak nuclear workers[680] (dose from plutonium; adjusted for external dose)	4.50 (3.15–6.1)	NA
Mayak nuclear workers[587] (dose from plutonium; adjusted for external dose)		
Males	4.7 (3.3–6.7)	115 (81–156)
Females	19 (9.5–39)	49 (29–78)
Sellafield plutonium workers[148]	1.12 (plutonium workers compared to other radiation workers)	NA
Internal High-LET Exposures (Other than Radon and Plutonium)		
Incidence		
^{224}Ra ankylosing spondylitis patients[225]	1.2	NA
^{224}Ra ankylosing spondylitis patients[224]	0.67	NA
Danish Thorotrast patients[272]	0.7 (0.3–1.7)	NA
Danish and Swedish Thorotrast patients[219]	1.3 (0.7–2.2)	NA
Mortality		
Japanese Thorotrast patients, combined data[214]	2.0 (1–3.9)	NA
German Thorotrast patients[681]	0.75	NA
U.S. Thorotrast patients[219]	3.3 (0.7–14)	NA

*The studies listed are those for which quantitative estimates of risk could be made.
Adapted from United Nations Scientific Committee of the Effects of Atomic Radiation (UNSCEAR): Sources and effects of ionizing radiation: 2006 report to the General Assembly with annexes. New York, United Nations, 2007.

Internal Exposure

The main body of scientific literature on the relationship between lung cancer and internal irradiation concerns radon exposure. The literature has been summarized by a number of scientific groups including the ICRP 1990 Recommendations,[248] NCRP reports,[606] the UNSCEAR 2006 report,[86] and the National Academy of Sciences BEIR Report on radon.[190] The reader is referred to these reports for more complete discussions of the topic.

Given the risk estimates of the National Academy of Sciences (BEIR IV) on radon,[190] the U.S. Environmental Protection Agency has tried to estimate the number of lung cancer deaths in the United States that may be due to radon and radon daughters.[607] The agency estimates the average annual exposure in U.S. homes to be 0.242 WLM, and based on a risk factor of 2.2×10^{-4} lung cancer deaths per WLM, they have calculated 13,600 lung cancer deaths, with a range between 7000 and 30,000 per year. In application of risk estimates obtained from a combination of 11 underground miner studies, Lubin et al. have likewise concluded that residential radon exposure may be responsible for 15,000 lung cancer deaths annually in the United States.[572,573]

Geologic Radon Studies

A large number of studies have examined the incidence or mortality from lung cancer and geologic conditions presumed to lead to increased radon exposure. These studies generally have a number of faults that are hard to overcome; for example, radon exposure is higher indoors than outdoors and varies by orders of magnitude even within small geographic areas. Lack of actual radon measurements and lack of information related to smoking are confounding factors that are extremely difficult, if not impossible, to overcome. As a result, the studies have led to a wide variety of conflicting conclusions and no real consensus.

Studies in Norway indicated positive correlations of assumed radon exposure with lung cancer,[608,609] a study in Italy showed a nonsignificant increase in lung cancer risk,[610] studies in China[611] and Finland showed no relation with exposure, a Japanese study reported a nonsignificant decrease,[612] and, finally, studies in Canada[613] and the United Kingdom[614] showed less lung cancer with increasing exposure.

Similar studies in the United States also give conflicting results. Of three studies done in Florida (where phosphate levels are high), one reported an increase in lung cancer,[615] one reported a positive correlation for male nonsmokers but not for females or male smokers,[616] and one found no association at all.[617] Alavanja et al. reported a positive correlation with residential radon in Missouri but only when surface monitors were used but not standard radon dosimetry.[618] In Iowa, a significantly positive association was found between lung cancer and radium concentration in water for males but not for females,[619] while in Maine a positive association was reported for lung cancer and radon concentration in water.[620]

There is an area of Precambrian granite located in the northern part of New Jersey and extending into New York State that is known as the Reading Prong. Some homes in this area are known to have high radon levels. Fleischer et al. have reported that lung cancer rates were somewhat higher in some, but not all, counties whose boundaries extended into the Reading Prong area.[621] The authors suggested a probable correlation of lung cancer with the geology. Unfortunately, no dose-response data, indoor radon measurements, or smoking histories were available or included. Archer et al. have performed a similar study of lung cancer rates in 16 counties located near the Reading Prong, in which lung cancer rates were elevated compared to nearby control counties; however, the study included no information on smoking habits, and home radon measurements were inadequate.[622]

Finally, studies of various U.S. counties have also produced conflicting results. One study of lung cancer mortality from 1950–1969 found significant excesses of lung cancer in counties with phosphate mills,[623] while another study of 411 counties found an inverse relation between lung cancer rates and the county mean radon concentrations (measured in at least 10 homes).[624] A large study by Cohen based on county radon levels purports to show an inverse relationship between low-dose radon levels and lung cancer risk.[625] This study has been critiqued by many authors, including Heath et al., based on the fact that these are grouped population rates as opposed to individual data especially relating to smoking.[626]

Residential Radon Studies

Case-control studies of radon have the advantage of a smaller number of persons to deal with; thus, smoking histories may be obtained, as well as indoor radon measurements in the person's home. While the resulting data are better than assumptions based on the underlying geology, studies of indoor radon are always complicated in that exposure to radon has occurred over the lifespan of the individual. Also, radon measurements are typically only made in the current residence of a person and at the time of the study. Any of these retrospective measurements has to include assumptions about possible effects due to changes in ventilation, construction, heating, and personal habits. While early studies were somewhat contradictory, later larger pooled studies appear to indicate an increased lung cancer risk with increasing residential radon exposure.

In the United States, population mobility has been a major problem because persons have often lived in three or more homes during their lifetimes. The more mobile a population is, the greater the degree of uncertainty, and the greater the sample size necessary for statistical confidence. As an example, if radon measurements were accurate to plus or minus 50% and the population lived in the same house for 60 years, a sample size of only 365 would be sufficient. If the population lived in 10 houses for 6 years each, the necessary sample size would be over 2000. Of course, given the usual extrapolation of basement radon levels to living areas and the historical issues related to number of homes and constancy of habits and ventilation, it is highly unlikely that the radon exposure estimates are accurate to plus or minus 50%. For true statistical significance at average indoor radon levels, it appears that sample sizes of less than several thousand will not be useful. Alavanja et al. examined residential radon exposure and lung cancer in nonsmoking U.S. women in an attempt to quantify the relationship in the absence of the large confounding factor of smoking.[627] An association between domestic levels of radon and radon was not convincingly demonstrated.

A case-control study of New Jersey women and residential radon was reported by Schoenberg et al.[590] This study included 433 women with lung cancer and 402 controls. Odds ratios increased with increasing exposure, but at all exposure levels the OR 90% CI encompassed unity. This study is in conflict with two cohort studies done in New Jersey and Maryland. The New Jersey study of 752 persons who had lived in homes with documented high exposure levels found a nonsignificant increase in lung cancer,[628] while the Maryland study found no association of lung cancer incidence rates with housing characteristics.[629] Case-control studies from both Canada and China have either found no association or a nonsignificant relationship with residential radon exposure.[630–632] In the case-control study in Shenyang, China, which has one of the world's highest lung cancer rates in women, Blot et al. have measured radon in the homes of 308 women who had lung cancer and compared the levels with those found in homes of 356 controls.[632] There was no association between lung cancer risk and radon level, and no definite cell type was associated with higher radon levels. In 2004, however, Lubin et al.[633] reported on the results of two pooled studies of residential radon in China. The OR increased significantly with greater radon concentration.

A number of Swedish case-control studies report positive results[634–636] but one large study reported that no association was found.[637] In other Swedish studies, one found exposure associated with risk in rural, but not in urban, dwellers,[638] and another found confounding factors due to differences in radon levels; that is, higher radon exposures were found in homes of smokers compared with controls but not in homes of nonsmokers compared with controls.[639] A large study concerning the potential effect of indoor radon, smoking, and lung cancer was reported by Pershagen et al.[636,640] In this countrywide Swedish study, 586 female and 774 male cases of lung cancer were compared with 1380 female and 1467 male controls. Measurements of radon were made using etch track detectors, smoking histories were obtained, and radon exposure was estimated back to 1947. The authors indicate that there was an increasing risk with increasing radon exposure; however, examination of the actual data initially presented indicates that the risk of lung cancer in nonsmokers did not differ significantly regardless of radon level. The risk in smokers was significantly elevated only when radon levels exceeded 400 Bq per m^3 of air.

Most of the residential indoor radon studies are limited by relatively low exposures and many confounding factors. To overcome this, there have been recent attempts to pool data from various studies and increase statistical power. The pooled results of Chinese data were discussed above and the derived excess OR was 0.13 (95% CI 0.01 to 0.36) per 100 Bq per m^3. A combined analysis of residential radon studies in Germany was reported in 2005 by Wichmann et al. and included 2963 incident lung cancer cases.[641] The study showed a nonsignificant increase in the OR with increasing exposure. The odds ratio was 0.97 (95% CI 0.85, 1.11) for radon concentrations of 50 to 80 Bq per m^3, 1.06 (95% CI 0.87, 1.30) for 80 to 140 Bq per m^3, and 1.40 (95% CI 1.03, 1.89) for concentrations in excess of 140 Bq per m^3. Small-cell

carcinoma appeared to be more closely associated with radon than other cell types.

Also in 2005 and 2006, Darby et al. reported the result of pooling of radon data from 13 European studies in which there were 7148 persons with lung cancer, all of whom had information about smoking histories and residential radon measurements.[642,643] There was a clear relationship of radon to lung cancer which fit a linear dose-response relationship with no evidence of a threshold. The ERR after adjusting for confounding factors was 0.08 (95% CI 0.06, 0.16) per 100 Bq per m^3. The ERR after adjusting for confounding factors was 0.16 (95% CI 0.05, 0.31) per 100 Bq per m^3. The estimated risks at 0, 100, and 400 Bq per m^3 for a lifelong nonsmoker were 1.0, 1.2, and 1.6, respectively, and the risks for a lifelong current smoker (15 to 24 cigarettes per day) were 25.8, 29.9, and 42.3, respectively. Krewski et al. have published two reports on a pooled study of North American data, one published in 2005 and the other in 2006.[644,645] The second report covered a slightly larger data set, with 4081 cases of lung cancer. The excess OR was 0.11 (95% CI 0.00, 0.28) per 100 Bq per m^3. Again there was no evidence of a threshold and the dose response was consistent with linearity. The pooled residential studies also show no significant variations on a multiplicative scale for radon effect by gender, age, or smoking status. The results of the pooled studies are in quite good agreement with the risk estimates derived from miner studies of an ERR per WLM of 0.0117 for exposures under 50 WLM. There are some differences, however, in that the residential radon studies do not show either declining radon effects with age or greater radon effects in nonsmokers. The reasons for this are unclear.

Underground Miner Studies

A large body of data concerns the excess of lung cancer mortality in underground miners, particularly uranium miners. As early as the year 1470 there were extensive silver mines near Saxony in southern Germany at the northern edge of the Erzgebirge (Ore Mountains). This region was known as the Schneeberg where mine shafts were as deep as 400 m. In the early 1500s a very high mortality was recognized from lung disease in the miners. During the next two centuries the "Schneeberger Lung Disease" increased as mining expanded to include cobalt and copper. The disease was finally identified as lung cancer by Haerting and Hesse in 1879, and they reported that up to 75% of miners died from lung cancer. After the discovery of radon in 1900, the high radon concentrations in the mines became evident, and in 1913 Muller suggested radon as the cause of the lung cancer. The radon concentrations in these mines ranged from 70 to 500 kBq/m^{-3}.

The underground miner studies suffer from a lack of knowledge of the exact exposure of the miners, particularly in the earlier times when few radon measurements were made and the exposures were at their highest. In addition, radon dosimetry in mines is quite difficult because radon and radon daughter exposure varies as a function of distance from the mine wall, presence of dead-end passages, ventilation, breathing rate, and dust concentration. Another problem that has beset a number of studies is the high number of miners who smoke. The miner data have been used by many to attempt to estimate the number of lung cancer deaths due to residential radon. Lubin et al. have estimated that about 40% of all lung cancer deaths in miners may be due to radon progeny exposure, 70% of lung cancer deaths in nonsmoking miners, and 39% in smokers.[572,646] They also estimate that about 10% of all lung cancer deaths in the United States may be due to radon progeny, 11% of deaths in smokers, and 30% in never smokers. Chen has derived tables for RR at different radon concentrations, age, and duration of exposure.[647]

The exposure received in these mines is from radon 222. Radon 222 levels can be measured in the mines and are normally expressed in working level months (WLM); a WLM is exposure to 1 working level during 170 hrs. Conversion of WLM to an absorbed dose is difficult since the radon may be in free ions (which are inhaled and exhaled) or bound to dust particles (which may be deposited, depending on the particle size). It should be noted that the number of WLM does not equal the number of months worked.

As a rough physics approximation, 1 WLM equals 5 mGy absorbed dose. Multiplication by the radiation weighting factor for alpha particles (W_R of 20) and multiplication by the tissue weighting factor for lung ($W_T = 0.12$), yields an effective dose of 12 mSv (1.2 rem). Epidemiological studies indicate that 1 WLM of radon gives about the same risk as an effective dose of 5 mSv.

Czechoslovakian uranium miners in Joachimsthal who began mining between 1948 and 1952 have been epidemiologically studied by Sevc et al.[648] A great majority of these miners had had no previous hard-rock mining experience. An excess lifetime rate of deaths from lung cancer of 230 in 1 million persons exposed per WLM has been estimated. The rate reported varied with age, being 140×10^{-6} under the age of 30 and rising to 370 in the age group over 40. A random sample of 700 of the miners indicated that 70% were cigarette smokers, a frequency equal to that for the general male population. BEIR 1980 indicated total excess risk in this group on an annual basis as 19 excess cases in 1 million persons per WLM.[13] The exposure of the European miners was quite low, with the concentrations of radon daughters being about 1 WLM (radon levels in U.S. uranium mines before 1960 were substantially higher). Analysis of the types of bronchial cancers identified in the miners indicated that epidermoid and small-cell anaplastic cancer were about equally increased and dose-dependent, with only a small excess of adenocarcinomas.[649] The pattern of risk in these miners has been analyzed by Tomasek et al.[650] At exposure rates of less than 10 WL, ERRs were greater in young men and increased linearly with time-weighted cumulative exposure.

Tirmarche et al. have reported on the mortality of 1785 French uranium miners exposed to low radon concentrations and found an increase in SMR for lung cancer of 0.6% per WLM.[651] A 2004 update of French uranium miners by Laurier et al. reported a significantly increased SMR of 1.9 for lung cancer.[186] The increase persisted even when smoking was taken into account.[651a] Xuan et al. conducted a cohort study in southern China of 17,143 tin miners exposed to radon and radon decay products.[652] The study included 175,143 person-years and reported an RR of 1.0 in those with low radon exposures, 14.4 with medium exposures, and 1.8 in those with high exposures. The study rejected either an additive or multiplicative association with smoking and was consistent with an intermediate effect.

Among 15,094 miners studied in Ontario, 81 deaths from lung cancers were certified.[653] This group received radon exposures that were generally below 1 working level (WL). In spite of this, 81 cancer deaths were identified versus 45 expected (an RR of 1.8). As in the Czechoslovakian study, miners who began working at older ages appeared to be at a somewhat higher risk than those who began mining at younger ages. Because of the nature of the study, it has not been possible to derive absolute risk estimates.

About 1946, extensive uranium ore deposits were discovered in the Colorado plateau area of the United States. Soon there were over 350 small mines in the area. U.S. uranium miners who worked mines in this region have been extensively studied by Archer et al.[654,655] and Waxweiler.[362] The studies included 3366 white miners and 780 nonwhite miners. The U.S. uranium mining experience is somewhat unique in that the concentrations of radon daughter products in the mines were substantially higher than in other studies. Radon levels generally ranged from 10 to 100 or more WLs. Substantial excess lung cancer mortality was identified (437 observed vs. 276.6 expected). It is of interest that the lower-exposure groups had risk estimates two to three times those for the higher-exposure groups. For example, in the range of 120 to 239 cumulative WLM, the absolute annual risk was 8.0 cases in 1 million persons per WLM, whereas in the group with 1800 to 3719 WLM, the risk decreased to 2.8 cases in 1 million persons per WLM annually. These risk estimates are below those calculated for the Czechoslovakian miners, and the difference cannot be explained by smoking experience. A dose-rate effect is possible but certainly has not been proved. The types of cancer found in the United States experience were studied by Archer et al.[656] Not only were small-cell anaplastic-type cancers increased, but epidermoid neo-plasms and adenocarcinomas, as well as mixed types, were present in greater numbers than expected.

If one assumes that U.S. cigarette smokers have an increased risk of lung cancer that is 12 times that of non-smokers and that 30% of the miners were nonsmokers, the relative radiation risk for nonsmoking miners is 10.3, and for smoking miners 6.2. A study by Gilliand et al. of non-smoking U.S. uranium miners indicated that the RR of lung cancer was 29.2 (95% CI 5.1, 167.2) for miners with greater than 1450 WLM, compared to those with less than 80 WLM.[657] There was a slightly decreased slope in risk with increasing WLM.

In the 1950s, lung cancer deaths were reported among Canadian fluorspar miners. Fluorspar (CaF_2) mines have radon, and radon daughter products are con-tained in water that seeps into the mines. Eight hundred Newfoundland fluorspar miners have been followed for an average of 26 years by DeVilliers and Windish.[658] Radon daughter measurements in these mines in Newfoundland varied from approximately 2 to 8 WLs before 1960. After this, ventilation decreased radon levels to 0.5 WLs. Sixty-five deaths from lung cancer occurred among the underground miners, with an average latent period of 22.6 years. The expected number of deaths was only 3.76. The absolute risk has been calculated at 17.7 deaths annually in 1 million persons exposed per WLM. Nearly all of the miners were smokers. There was no evidence of an effect of age at exposure on the length of the latent period. One possible explanation is that smoking caused radiogenic lung cancers of a shorter latent period. A 2007 update reported an SMR of 3.09 (95% CI 2.66, 3.56) and ERR per WLM decreased with attained age and time since exposure.[658a] An inverse dose rate was also observed. Morrison et al. have reported on the mortality experience from 1950 to 1984 of a cohort of 1772 underground fluorspar miners working from 1933 to 1978.[659] The mean cumulative exposure was 383 WLM over 5.7 years. The risk was calculated to be 0.9% per WLM for lung cancer.

A number of reports have documented the Swedish metal miners (particularly zinc miners).[660,661] Overall, the Swedish reports are preliminary or lack complete follow-up. They are, however, of some interest because they indicate that the excess risk for smokers may not be markedly greater than for nonsmokers (22.3 versus 16.3 cases annu-ally in 1 million persons/WLM); in fact, the RR was higher for nonsmokers than for smokers (10.3 vs. 3.8). These data must be treated with caution since they are not age-adjusted and the nonsmokers lived longer. In addition to the earlier studies there have been some other studies of pitchblende miners in Port Radium, Canada, and tin miners in the Yunnan province of China.[662]

While there are problems associated with many mining studies, most do show an excess of lung cancer.

The main problem lies in extracting a risk estimate from the data. These reports include uranium miners in Colorado,[663] New Mexico,[664] Ontario and Saskatchewan, Canada,[665,666] Bohemia, Czechoslovakia,[667] and Fran-ce.[651] There has also been a study of Swedish iron miners that yields risk estimates.[668] These eight studies include over 31,000 miners, with an average of 8 years of employment. The weighted mean exposure is 120 WLM, and the weighted mean length of follow-up is 20 years. It should be noted that the original exposure estimates proposed for the Beaverlodge miners has been reassessed by Chambers et al. and estimated to be twice as high as originally thought.[669] A study by Woodward et al. reported on miners employed at Radium Hill in Australia showed increased lung cancer mortality.[670]

The U.S. National Cancer Institute performed an analysis of 11 miner studies that had individual estimates of radon exposure.[572] The combined data included 67,776 miners, 2736 lung cancer cases, and 1.15 million WLM. The average duration of exposure was 6.8 years, and the individual mean weighted cumulative radon exposure was 162 WLM. The result of the combined data was an estimated ERR of 0.5% per WLM. At 100 WLM the ERR was estimated to be 0.49 (or an RR of 1.49). This was less than the ERR of 1.34% per WLM estimated by the BEIR IV report.[575] This suggests overestimation by the BEIR IV Committee at high exposure levels. The combined data also showed declining risk with attained age and no variation relative to age at first exposure.

The combined miner data also give some information concerning the effect of smoking and radon. In the non-smoker group the ERR per WLM was 1.1%, and for smokers 0.34%. Because smokers begin with an RR of 10 to 15 compared with nonsmokers, even with a higher ERR per WLM, the nonsmokers still had much less increase in the risk of lung cancer when exposed to radon than did smokers.

An interesting aspect of the Czechoslovakian study is that exposures below 100 cumulative WLM appeared to be more effective per WLM than cumulative doses exceeding 100 WLM. The Chinese tin miner study found that there was a decreasing ERR per WLM as expo-sure rate increased. While there may be an increasing risk with lower estimated exposure rates, this does not appear to exceed a factor of 3 or so. The exact magnitude is, of course, very dependent on the original radon expo-sure estimates, which, as pointed out earlier, are subject to considerable uncertainty. The effect of dose rate does not appear to be a major issue when extrapolation is made to lower radon levels (such as those in homes), given the findings of the domestic radon studies recently performed in Sweden and discussed earlier in the chapter.

The suggestion of an inverse dose-rate effect has also been a major subject of interest in the National Cancer Institute's combined data from the 11 miner cohort studies. The inverse dose-rate effect refers to a situation where for a given exposure the effect observed is greater if the exposure is spread out over time. Whether this effect is real or is an artifact due to the increased unattached radon fraction in the newer mines from improved ventilation is unknown. An increase in the unattached fraction would give higher bronchial dose per WLM, and if recent mining data were compared to high exposure data from early mines, this would result in confounding of the data to create an "inverse dose-rate effect."

Uranium Workers

Ritz et al. have reported on cancer mortality in uranium processing workers at the Fernald plant in Ohio.[192] The SMR for lung cancer was nonsignificantly increased at 1.01. There was a statistically significant increase for workers exposed to more than 200 mSv of internal alpha radiation (but this was based on less than three cases). Dupree-Ellis et al. have reported on mortality in a cohort of 2514 uranium processing workers employed between 1942 and 1966 at the Mallinkrodt Chemical Works.[193] The SMR for respiratory system cancer was nonsignificantly elevated at 1.03. McGeoghegan et al. reported on the mortality and cancer morbidity experience of workers at the Capenhurst uranium enrichment facility from 1946–1995; the cohort included 12,540 workers, including 3244 radiation workers, with mean doses of 9.85 mSv.[242] The SMR for lung cancer was decreased for radiation workers at 0.89 and increased slightly in the nonradiation workers at 1.06 for an RR of 0.85. Cancer of the pleura was significantly increased in the radiation workers. McGeoghegan et al. also reported on workers at the Springfields uranium production facility during 1946–1995.[243] The cohort of 19,454 workers included 13,960 radiation workers with a mean external dose of 22.8 mSv, a mean follow-up period of 24.6 years, and 479,146 person-years in whom the SMR for cancer of the lung was significantly reduced for radiation workers at 0.85 and nonsignificantly reduced for the nonradiation workers at 0.88. A meta-analysis of 14 studies, which included 120,000 uranium workers, found a non-significant decrease with a RR of 0.94 (95% CI 0.83, 1.05) for lung cancer.[245]

Plutonium Workers

Although few human data concern lung cancer induction following inhalation of plutonium, the matter is of great public and scientific interest. There has been extensive work in animals, particularly involving inhalation of plutonium 239 oxide ($^{239}PuO_2$) by dogs. Actual distribution of plutonium in the lung is dependent on the particle size, with the larger particles being deposited more centrally in the tracheobronchial tree. If the inhaled plutonium compound is relatively insoluble, the only major accumulation outside the lung is in the tracheobronchial lymph nodes. In such areas, the concentration of plutonium can reach 50 to 100 times that in the lung.

At the present time, there is only limited human experience concerning the inhalation of plutonium. This comes from 25 workers who inhaled substantial amounts of plutonium 239 during the Manhattan Project in Los Alamos, New Mexico, during 1942–1945. Analysis of these workers has confirmed substantial plutonium body burdens, and careful medical follow-up has continued for over 42 years.[671] Three cases of lung cancer in a group of 26 men over a 44-year period is a higher incidence than expected for the general population but still within the statistical limits of expectation for smokers without plutonium inhalation or exposure. The finding is consistent with the known risks of cigarette smoking, particularly given that all three men had long cigarette-smoking histories. Whether there was additional risk due to plutonium inhalation cannot be determined from these data due to the small numbers involved. Wiggs et al. found a nonsignificantly increased RR for lung cancer in a follow-up of Los Alamos plutonium workers.[164]

Wing and Richardson have recently published a report on cancer risks at the Hanford site.[672] Lung cancer risks were significantly lower for workers judged to have potential plutonium exposure. The exception was those aged 50 and above. Since the authors used several alternative age splits, this latter finding may be due to chance. Brown et al. conducted a lung cancer case-control study of workers at the Rocky Flats facility.[673] There was no evidence of increased risk from americium or uranium. Analysis of cumulative dose from plutonium showed either a nonsignificant increase in most dose categories but no consistent increase with increasing dose. Omar et al. studied cancer mortality and morbidity among plutonium and other workers at the Sellafield plant of British Nuclear Fuels.[148] The rate ratio for the SMR for lung cancer deaths of plutonium versus other radiation workers was nonsignificantly elevated at 1.12 and was 0.98 for radiation versus nonradiation workers. The trend for lung cancer with both external dose and plutonium exposure was negative. Carpenter et al. examined workers in the United Kingdom who were occupationally exposed to tritium, plutonium, and other radionuclides.[191] The SMRs for lung cancer in each group were all reduced. The SMR for pleural cancer was significantly elevated (although the RR compared to unmonitored workers was not statistically elevated) in the plutonium exposure group and the SMR for pleural cancer was nonsignificantly elevated for the other two exposed groups.

Internal contamination of the lung with plutonium 239 has sparked a controversy about the effectiveness of this isotope in tumor induction. The controversy was popularly known as the "hot particle problem." The controversy centered about the distribution of the radiation dose in the lung. If plutonium 239 is inhaled as small insoluble particles, there can be very intense doses of radiation to microscopic areas of the lungs. Some authors indicated that the risk of cancer was the same as if the total amount of radiation absorbed were applied uniformly over the lungs, whereas others suggested that the intense radiation in localized areas may cause cell killing and thus result in less cancer than would be expected. Conversely, a third group suggested that the localized intense radiation, which has a spatial distribution similar to the cell size, may cause substantially more damage to the DNA than low-LET radiation and that a much higher number of tumors might thus be induced.

Most scientists now think that very intense doses of radiation to microscopic areas result in either the same or less risk than that incurred from irradiating the lungs uniformly to the same dose level. The population with perhaps the highest exposures from plutonium are the workers at the Russian Mayak production facility. Reports on this population have been published by a number of authors. The Koshurnikova report indicated a statistically significant association between alpha particle radiation and lung cancer, which is best described by a linear nonthreshold function with a lifetime cancer risk in the dose range below 30 Sv lung dose of 0.012 per Sv but no association with external lung dose below 5.5 Gy.[586]

Kreisheimer et al. compared alpha and gamma risk factors, and using a radiation weighting factor of 20 for alpha particles, reported an estimated ERR of 0.6 per Sv organ dose (95% CI 0.39, 1.00) compared to 0.20 per Sv (95% CI −0.04, 0.69) for gamma radiation.[674] In a later and larger study of the same population, Gilbert et al. found that the ERR per unit dose was not substantially different from that of the atomic bomb survivors.[587] The ERR per Sv (equivalent dose) was 0.23 (95% CI 0.16, 0.33) for males at attained age of 60, compared with 0.40 (95% CI 0.032, 0.86) in the male atomic bomb survivors. The results in females were 0.93 (95% CI 0.46, 1.9) in the Mayak workers compared to 1.40 (95% CI 0.76, 2.2) in the female atomic bomb survivors.

Internal Medical Exposure

Several studies of the potential carcinogenic effects of diagnostic doses of radioiodine administered to perform thyroid scanning have been performed. The largest of these studies included 35,074 patients who were matched with the Swedish cancer registry data.[270] No statistically significant increase in lung cancer was found (SIR 1.05, 95% CI 0.93, 1.18).

In another Swedish study of 10,500 patients treated for hyperthyroidism with radioiodine, there was no significant increase in all tumors considered together, but there was a significant increase in cancer of the lung (SIR 1.3, 95% CI 1.1, 1.6).[271] This increase, however, was only due to an increased risk in the first 1 to 4 years after exposure and, therefore, not considered to be due to radiation. In a later paper, the authors suggested that there was the possibility of misclassification of cancers and that

patients with Graves' disease tend to be smokers.[675] This concept is supported by a study by the same authors in which patients treated with radioactive iodine for thyroid cancer were followed up.[203] The lung doses would have been an order of magnitude higher, yet there was no statistically significant elevation of lung cancer. In another study by Hoffman et al. of 1005 women treated with iodine 131 and compared with 2141 treated surgically, there was no significant increase in tumors of the respiratory tract.[202,676] The RR was 1.2 (95% CI 0.3, 4.3). In another study of hyperthyroid patients, Ron et al. reported a reduced SMR for lung cancer of 0.91 for those treated with iodine 131 only and a statistically significantly increased SMR for lung cancer in those treated by surgery only with an SMR 1.17 (95% CI 1.10, 1.35).[201]

There has been interest in Thorotrast patients, thorium plant workers, and lung cancer because internal thorium 232 in the body has radon as a daughter product that is exhaled and theoretically exposes lung tissue. In a Danish study of 1095 Thorotrast patients, Andersson et al. reported that there was a statistically significant increase in lung cancer (SIR 2.3, 95% CI 1.4, 3.4).[213] However, there was no relation between volume of Thorotrast injected and the SIR, nor was there any relation with time since injection. Therefore, the increase was not attributed to radiation exposure. Other known risk factors such as tobacco were not controlled in this study. In a larger study of 2434 Portuguese patients, there was no increase in lung cancer.[216] In a later follow-up reported in 2003 by dos Santo Silva et al., there was a nonsignificant increase in the RR of 9.07 (95% CI 0.90, 447).[220] The wide CIs are due to the small number of lung cancer cases (four in the Thorotrast patients and one in the controls).

No apparent excess of lung cancer was found in the German Thorotrast Study.[212] In a follow-up of 255 Japanese Thorotrast patients, 11 lung cancers were found.[677] Small-cell cancers were increased as a proportion of the total, but overall the lung cancer rate was not significantly different from that of a control population. The authors concluded that the risk from radon was not as high as expected from risk estimates derived from mining studies and that the higher risks from mining studies might include a component from dusts. In 1999 Mori et al. summarized the entire Japanese Thorotrast follow-up study and indicated a marginally significant increase in lung cancer with a rate ratio of 2.0 (95% CI 1.0, 3.9).[214] Travis et al. studied the site-specific cancer incidence and mortality after cerebral angiography with radioactive Thorotrast.[219] There was a nonsignificant increase in lung cancer incidence with an RR of 1.3 (95% CI 0.7, 2.2) and also a nonsignificant increase in lung cancer mortality with an RR of 3.3 (95% CI 0.7, 13.7). Nyberg et al. found no increase in lung cancer in male Swedish Thorotrast patients, with an SMR of 0.9 (95% CI 0.2, 2.7) but a significant increase in females with an SMR of 4.6.[222] In a study of 592 men who worked at a thorium

Table 5-13 • Risk Estimates for Lung Cancer Mortality from Studies of Radon Daughter Exposure in Underground Miners	
Study	**Average ERR at 100 WLM**
Internal High-LET Exposures (Occupational Radon)	
Chinese tin miners[646,652]	0.16 (0.1–0.2)
West Bohemia uranium miners[650]	1.6 (1.2–2.2)
Colorado Plateau uranium miners[646,663]	0.42 (0.3–0.7)
Ontario uranium miners[646,682]	0.89 (0.5–1.5)
Newfoundland fluorspar miners[646,683]	0.70 (0.44–1.14)
Swedish iron miners[646,668]	0.95 (0.1–4.1)
New Mexico uranium miners[646,664]	1.72 (0.6–6.7)
Beaverlodge uranium miners[666,684,646]	3.25 (1.0–9.6)
Port Radium uranium miners[646,662]	0.19 (0.1–0.6)
Radium Hill uranium miners[646,670]	5.06 (1.0–12.2)
French uranium miners[186,646, 651,685]	0.47 (0.0–0.98)
Cornish tin miners[686]	0.045

From United Nations Scientific Committee of the Effects of Atomic Radiation (UNSCEAR): Sources and effects of ionizing radiation: 2006 report to the General Assembly with annexes. New York, United Nations, 2007.

processing plant, 10 lung cancer deaths versus 6 expected were detected, but the SMR of 1.7 had 95% confidence limits of 0.81 to 3.1.[678]

Wick et al.[225] and Nekolla[224] reported on late effects in ankylosing spondylitis patients treated with radium 224. In the first study there were 626 exposed and 725 control patients with a mean follow-up time of 21 years. The mean injected activity was 0.17 MBq/kg and the mean alpha skeletal dose was 0.67 Gy. The study showed a statistically significant decrease in the O/E ratio for lung cancer in those exposed of 25 to 36. In the second study there was also a statistically significant decrease in lung cancer with a rate ratio of 0.64 (P value 0.03).

Summary of Internal Exposure

High-level exposure to radon over a period of years clearly increases the risk of lung cancer (probably small-cell type more than others). The exact level of risk remains somewhat uncertain due to dosimetry issues and confounding factors. In spite of this, most underground miner studies yield risk estimates that agree within a factor of 3 to 4. Pooled studies at lower radon and radon daughter concentrations, such as in homes, have now revealed a reasonably consistent statistically significant increase. Smoking continues to represent a much more potent carcinogen than radon at domestic levels. Even uranium miners who smoke and develop lung cancer are more likely to have had their cancer caused by smoking than by radon. The interaction of smoking and radon exposure appears to be more than additive and less than multiplicative. Medical uses of internally deposited radionuclides have not been linked to an increase in lung cancer.

Table 5-14 • Results from Analyses of Pooled Data from Case-control Studies of Residential Radon Exposure in China,[633] Europe,[642] and North America[644,645]			
Study	**EOR/100 Bq m^{-3}**	**Lower 95% CI**	**Upper 95% CI**
Studies in China			
Shenyang[632]	–0.02	–0.13	0.43
Gansu[687]	0.18	0.02	0.49
Studies in Europe			
Austria[688]	0.46	NA	> 5.00
Czech Republic[689]	0.19	–0.00	2.07
Finland (nationwide)[690]	0.03	NA	0.17
Finland (south)[691]	0.06	–0.08	1.58
France[692]	0.11	–0.01	0.41
Germany (eastern)[641]	0.18	–0.00	0.56
Germany (western)[641]	–0.02	NA	0.36
Italy[693]	0.10	–0.18	1.40
Spain[694]	–0.11	NA	0.59
Sweden (nationwide)[636]	0.11	–0.04	0.46
Sweden (never smokers)[695]	0.24	–0.08	0.95
Sweden (Stockholm)[696]	0.12	–0.14	1.41
United Kingdom[697]	0.04	–0.05	0.22
Studies in North America			
New Jersey[628]	0.56	–0.22	2.97
Winnipeg[631]	0.02	–0.05	0.25
Missouri I[627]	0.01	NA	0.42
Missouri II[618]	0.27	–0.12	1.53
Iowa[698]	0.44	0.05	1.59
Connecticut[699]	0.02	–0.21	0.51
Utah/South Idaho[699]	0.03	–0.20	0.55
Combined Studies			
China[633]	0.13	0.01	0.36
Europe[642]	0.08	0.030	0.16
North America[644,645]	0.11	0.00	0.28

Summary information based on pooled analyses and may differ slightly from original publications.
EOR, excessive odds ratio.
From United Nations Scientific Committee of the Effects of Atomic Radiation (UNSCEAR): Sources and effects of ionizing radiation: 2006 report to the General Assembly with annexes. New York, United Nations, 2007.

Assuming a radiation weighting factor of 20 for alpha particles, risk estimates per unit organ dose overlap with risk estimates from external gamma exposure. Generally, as with external exposure, the ERR for lung cancer appears to decrease with attained age. The exception appears to be the residential radon studies. Radiation risk factors for lung cancer that can be derived from various studies have been summarized in the UNSCEAR 2006 report and are shown in Tables 5-12 to 5-14.[86]

KIDNEY CANCER

General

The incidence of primary renal-cell carcinoma has increased slowly over the last decade. In the United

States roughly 28,000 patients are diagnosed annually.[358] The 5-year survival is about 55%. Primary renal-cell carcinoma accounts for about 85% of primary malignant tumors of the kidney. Other malignant tumors include Wilms' tumor, transitional cell carcinoma, lymphoma, and others. Primary renal-cell carcinoma is 1.8 times more frequent in males than in females. Tumors of the parenchyma are usually adenocarcinomas, and tumors of the collecting system are uroepithelial carcinomas.

The highest rates of tumors of the kidney and renal pelvis are seen in North America and Europe, with rates being almost the same in whites and blacks.[700] Rates tend to be low in Chinese, Japanese, and Indian populations. Migration appears to modify risk, suggesting a role for environmental causation. Both renal adeno-carcinoma and tumors of the renal pelvis have been linked to chewing and smoking tobacco. A clear dose-response relationship has been found in some studies. The RR in smokers is about 2.7 compared with nonsmokers. Depending on the study reviewed, risk factors between 2 and 10 can be found. Assuming a population prevalence of 50% for smoking, 30% to 40% of renal tumors are the result of smoking. Increased risk of renal cancer has also been found in persons working in petroleum-related and dry-cleaning industries. Increased risk is also noted in persons with phenacetin or analgesic nephropathy, end-stage kidneys, renal dialysis, and renal transplantation.

External Exposure

Background Radiation

In a study of the influence of terrestrial radiation in Connecticut, Walter et al. reported an increase in bladder cancer in females living in the higher radiation areas.[21] No difference between the two areas was found for mortality from kidney cancer. Airline crews are exposed to higher than normal levels of cosmic radiation. Band et al. reported on a cohort mortality study of 2740 Air Canada pilots who received doses of 6 mSv per year over an average 20 years (for a total average dose of about 120 mSv).[40] The SIR for kidney cancer was nonsignificantly reduced at 0.51 (90% CI 0.14, 1.32), and the SMR was nonsignificantly increased at 1.22 (90% CI 0.33, 3.15).

Populations Near Nuclear Facilities

There are three papers concerning potential environmental uranium contamination and the possibility of an increased risk of renal cancer in the public. The papers by Boice et al. indicated a nonsignificant decrease around a uranium mining and milling facility in Texas and near facilities in Pennsylvania and Colorado.[89,90,90a] Lopez-Abente et al. have reported on solid tumor mortality near Spain's four nuclear power plants and four uranium fuel cycle facilities and found that the RR for kidney cancer was nonsignificantly reduced at 0.85.[283]

Atomic Bomb Survivors

The incidence study of atomic bomb survivors through 1998 published by Preston et al. yields risk factors that are nonsignificantly elevated with an ERR per Gy of 0.13 (90% CI −0.25, 0.75).[319] There was an estimated excess of 2 cases out of a total 167 cases and an attributable fraction of 2.7% for those with doses in excess of 5 mGy. In the report on mortality through 1997 by Preston et al. on kidney cancer in males, there was a nonsignificantly reduced relationship with radiation dose.[281] The ERR per Sv was −0.02 (90% CI < −0.3, 1.1), the EAR was −0.01 per 10,000 PYSv (90% CI −0.01, 0.28), and the attributable risk (−0.4%) was based on 36 deaths. For kidney cancer in females there was a nonsignificant relationship with radiation dose. The ERR per Sv was 0.97 (90% CI < −0.3, 3.8), the EAR per $(10^4 PYSv)^{-1}$ was 0.14 (90% CI < −0.1, 0.42), and the attributable risk (14%) was based on 31 deaths.

Occupational Exposure

A large number of occupational studies are negative or nonsignificant with respect to radiation induction of kidney cancer. A study of 176,000 nuclear workers in Japan by Iwasaki et al. found a nonsignificantly reduced SMR for kidney cancer of 0.86 (95% CI 0.58, 1.21).[150] A mortality study of 5657 Spanish nuclear energy workers by Artalejo et al. reported a nonsignificantly elevated SMR for kidney cancer of 1.26 (95% CI 0.34, 3.21).[151] Habib et al. have reported on cancer incidence among Australian nuclear industry–monitored radiation workers and indicated a nonsignificantly reduced SIR of 0.96 for kidney cancer.[152]

A study by Darby et al. of 22,347 United Kingdom workers exposed to fallout and other sources reported for kidney cancer that the SMR was 1.76 relative to the general population, but the RR was significantly lower relative to the control groups at 0.30 (90% CI 0.12 to 0.71).[52] A follow-up study, also by Darby et al., reported a nonsignificant reduction in kidney cancer with an SMR of 0.68 (95% CI 0.41, 1.12).[701] In 2003, Muirhead et al. reported that the RR for cancer of the kidney was significantly reduced at 0.74 (90% CI 0.57, 0.96) during 1952–1998 in men from the United Kingdom who participated in the United Kingdom's atmospheric nuclear weapons tests and experimental programs.[54]

A study by Beral et al. included an analysis of 3373 deaths among 39,546 U.K. atomic energy workers during 1946–1979.[143] In this study the ratio rate for cancer of the kidney, comparing exposed with nonexposed employees, was nonsignificantly elevated at 2.39 (95% CI 0.94 to 6.09). A study by Beral et al. of atomic weapons workers did not show significant increase with a rate ratio of 2.39 (95% CI 0.94 to 6.09) for kidney cancer.[144] A cohort analysis of the U.K. National Registry of Radiation Workers by Kendall et al. included 95,217 workers studied over 1.2 million person-years at risk.[145] In these workers an insignificantly low SMR of 0.84 was reported for cancer of the kidney. In a second expanded analysis of the same group, Muirhead et al. reported a cohort of 124,743 radiation workers with mean doses of 30 mSv in whom the lagged SMR for cancer of the kidney was nonsignificantly reduced at 0.92 (95% CI 0.71, 1.16) and the 10-year lagged ERR per Sv for kidney cancer was significantly reduced at less than −1.95 (95% CI < −1.95, −0.96).[146] Fraser et al. studied the cancer mortality and morbidity in employees of the United Kingdom Atomic Energy Authority during 1946–1986 in whom they found the rate ratio for kidney cancer nonsignificantly reduced at 0.51 (95% CI 0.23, 1.10).[702]

There have been several reports relative to specific nuclear facilities in the United Kingdom. Douglas et al. reported on cancer mortality and morbidity among 14,282 workers at the Sellafield plant of British Nuclear Fuels in whom the average dose was 128 mSv.[147] The SMR for kidney cancer was nonsignificant at 1.10. An earlier study of the same population by Smith et al. had found nonsignificant decreases in kidney cancer.[360] A recent report on the Sellafield plant by Omar et al. indicated a nonsignificant increase in kidney cancer among nonplutonium radiation workers with an SMR of 1.13 but the incidence was nonsignificantly decreased.[148] McGeoghegan et al. reported on the mortality and cancer morbidity experience of 2628 employees at the Chapelcross plant of British Nuclear Fuels during 1955–1995 in whom the median dose was 39 mSv and the mean follow-up was 24.3 years.[149] The SMR for kidney cancer was nonsignificantly elevated at 1.67; however, the trend was negative with increasing dose.

In a Canadian study by Gribbin et al. of 8977 male workers, there was an SMR of 0.60 (95% CI 0.16 to 1.54) for kidney cancer.[260] Ashmore et al. reported on the mortality and occupational radiation exposure of a cohort based on the National Dose Registry of Canada.[154] The cohort included 206,620 individuals and 5426 deaths. The average exposure for males was 10 mSv. The SMR for kidney cancer was significantly reduced at 0.63 (90% CI 0.45, 0.87). Sont et al. reported on cancer incidence as well, also using the National Dose Registry of Canada.[153] The cohort included 191,333 persons with an average dose for males of 11.5 mSv and an average dose for the cohort of 6.64 mSv. The SIR for cancer of the kidney in males was significantly reduced at 0.76 (90% CI 0.61, 0.93) and for females it was insignificantly reduced at 0.79 (90% CI 0.53, 1.14).

There have also been very large occupational studies in the United States. Gilbert et al. have reported on workers at Hanford in whom they found an SMR of 0.95 for kidney cancer in all workers (0.94 for radiation workers).[361] Cragle et al., reporting on 9860 white male workers at the Savannah River facility, indicated that there were consistently fewer than expected cases of cancer of the kidney, with SMRs for all groups of workers below unity (0.40).[288] At the Mound Facility in Ohio, Wiggs

et al. reported an SMR for kidney cancer of 1.01 (95% CI 0.12 to 3.63).[156] Frome et al. analyzed the mortality among a cohort of World War II nuclear industry workers and reported a nonsignificantly reduced SMR for cancer of the kidney at 0.84.[267] Frome also performed a mortality study of 106,020 employees in the nuclear industry at Oak Ridge, Tennessee.[160] For kidney cancer the SMR for white males was nonsignificantly reduced at 0.92 and for nonwhite males it was nonsignificantly reduced at 0.31. Fry et al. studied 3145 persons occupationally exposed to 50 or more mSv in a year in whom the SMR for cancer of the kidney was nonsignificantly elevated at 1.31 (95% CI 0.11, 3.41).[161] Howe et al. performed an analysis of the mortality experience among 53,698 U.S. nuclear power industry workers chronically exposed to low-dose ionizing radiation in whom the SMR for cancer of the kidney was nonsignificantly reduced at 0.79 (95% CI 0.43, 1.32).[159]

Other U.S. occupational studies also have yielded generally negative or nonsignificant results for an association between occupational exposure and renal cancer. Acquavella et al. studied mortality of workers at the Pantex nuclear plant, whose SMR for kidney cancer was insignificantly reduced at 0.51 (95% CI 0.01, 2.84).[703] Wilkinson et al. found an SMR of 0.56 (95% CI 0.10 to 1.75) for kidney cancer at the Rocky Flats Plant.[286] Checkoway et al. reporting on workers at Oak Ridge National Laboratory, indicated a nonsignificantly elevated SMR of 1.22 (95% CI 0.45 to 2.66) for kidney cancer.[284] Wiggs et al. found significantly reduced SMR for kidney cancer (0.59) in a follow-up of Los Alamos workers.[164]

Cardis et al. reported on cancer mortality among nuclear industry workers in three countries in a large study which included 95,673 workers followed over 2 million person-years at risk with 15,825 deaths.[166] The trend for kidney cancer was nonsignificantly reduced at −1.03 with a P value of 0.85. Cardis et al. have reported the cancer mortality results from a 15-country collaborative study of nuclear workers.[168] This is the largest occupational study to date and included a cohort of 407,391 workers with 18,993 deaths and 5.2 million person-years of follow-up. The ERR per Sv for kidney cancer was nonsignificantly positive at 2.26 (90% CI < 0, 14.9) with a nonsignificant trend P value of 0.34.

Doody et al. have examined mortality among 143,517 U.S. radiologic technologists, during 1926–1990.[97] The SMR for kidney cancer was nonsignificantly reduced at 0.96 (95% CI 0.71, 1.27). Mohan et al. studied cancer and other causes of mortality among 146,022 radiologic technologists in the United States employed from 1940 and later; the SMR for cancer of the kidney in males was nonsignificantly reduced at 0.89 (95% CI 0.6, 1.2) and for females it was nonsignificantly reduced at 0.94 (95% CI 0.7, 1.3).[99] Sigurdson et al. studied the cancer incidence among 90,305 U.S. radiologic technologists in whom the SIR for kidney cancer was nonsignificantly elevated at 1.18 (95% CI 0.84, 1.52).[101]

Medical Diagnostic Exposure

Kidney cancer and radiation have been studied in patients after external exposures in diagnostic radiology. Massachusetts TB patients treated with multiple fluoroscopies have been followed by Davis et al.[364] They reported, for kidney cancer, an SMR of 0.7 in exposed females and 0.3 in unexposed females. SMRs for both exposed and unexposed males were nonsignificantly elevated at 1.6. In another study also of Massachusetts TB patients, the SMRs for cancer of the kidney in male controls were nonsignificantly elevated at 2.5, but in the exposed males the SMR was 1.1.[105] In the females the SMR for the exposed group was nonsignificantly reduced at 1.5, and for controls it was 0.6 (the data on females are based on very few cases).

Radiation Therapy

Radiation therapy can give quite high doses to specific organs, and patients have been followed after therapy for benign, as well as malignant, conditions. Darby et al. reported a study of patients who were treated for ankylosing spondylitis in whom cancer of the kidney was nonsignificantly elevated, with an O/E ratio of 1.52.[109] A follow-up study by Weiss et al. of 15,577 patients with a mean total-body dose of 2.6 Gy found the RR for kidney cancer was nonsignificantly elevated at 1.69 during 5 to 24.9 years post-treatment and a statistically significant elevation of 1.58 after more than 25 years.[266] The estimated ERR per Gy was 0.10 (95% CI 0.02, 0.20). Cancer following radiotherapy for peptic ulcer has been studied in over 3700 patients by Griem et al.[112] and the series was updated by Carr et al.[113] In such patients the dose to the abdomen was about 15 Gy and the RR for cancer of the kidney was nonsignificantly elevated at 2.68 (95% CI 0.49, 14.76). Mattsson et al. studied the incidence of primary malignancies other than breast cancer among women treated with radiation therapy for benign breast disease in whom the RR for kidney cancer was nonsignificantly reduced at 0.24 (95% CI 0.03, 1.08).[114] In women who received radium therapy for benign gynecologic conditions, the median doses were estimated as 0.21 Gy to the kidney. In a study by Inskip et al. the SMR for kidney cancer was nonsignificantly elevated at 1.4 (95% CI 0.6, 2.4).[118]

Studies of second cancers in women treated for cervical carcinoma with radiotherapy do not reveal a consistent increase in kidney cancer, even though doses are on the order of several Gy (Fig. 5-10). One cohort study of women treated for cervical cancer compared 82,616 exposed women with 99,424 unexposed controls from Canada, Denmark, Finland, Norway, Sweden, Yugoslavia, the United Kingdom, and the United States. The study covered 1.28 million person-years at risk and found no evidence of a radiation-related excess risk for cancer of the kidney.[126] In patients treated for invasive

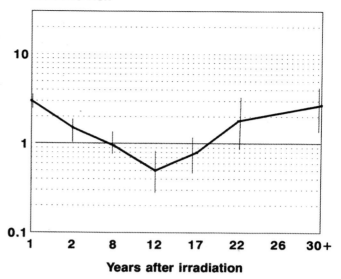

Relative risk

Years after irradiation

Kidney cancer (cervix series)

Figure 5-10 • RR of kidney cancer by time after treatment for cervical carcinoma with radiation therapy. Error bars indicate 95% CI. (From Boice JD, Jr, et al: Second cancers following radiation treatment for cervical cancer: An international collaboration among cancer registries. J Natl Cancer Inst 1985;74:955–975.)

cervical cancer, the O/E ratio for kidney cancer was 1.0 with radiotherapy and 2.1 for those treated without radiotherapy. In patients who were followed for 10 years or more, the O/E ratio was not much different. In a large case-control study 4188 women who developed second cancers after treatment for cancer of the cervix were compared with 6880 matched controls.[124] The estimated dose to the kidney was 2 Gy. The RR for cancer of the kidney was nonsignificantly elevated at 1.23 (90% CI 0.7 to 2.2), the ERR per Sv was 0.71 (90% CI 0.03, 2.24). and the EAR was 1.10 (90% CI 0.05, 3.0). Kleinerman et al. reported on second primary cancer after treatment for cervical cancer in an international registries study.[125] The study evaluated second cancers in 86,193 patients with cervical cancer reported to 13 cancer registries in 5 countries. The O/E ratio for kidney cancer was barely statistically significantly elevated at 1.3 (95% CI 1.0, 1.5), but it was even higher for those who were treated surgically (O/E ratio 1.8 [95% CI 1.2, 2.4]). The risk factors per unit dose for kidney cancer can be derived from this study; the ERR per Gy was 0.14 (95% CI 0.03, 0.26) and the EAR was 0.29 (95% CI 0.07, 0.54) per 10,000 PYGy. In a Japanese study of women also treated for cancer of the cervix, the O/E ratio for kidney cancer was 1.0 in those treated with radiotherapy but significantly elevated in those treated without radiotherapy.[128] A Danish series of 19,470 treated cervical cancer patients was reported by Storm.[704] For kidney cancer the SIR was not elevated and was 1.0 (95% CI 0.7, 1.4). Travis et al. have reported on long-term survival and second cancers in over 40,000 testicular cancer patients almost all of whom received infradiaphragmatic radiotherapy in whom the RR for kidney cancer was significantly increased.[705]

Curtis et al. have studied second cancer following radiation treatment for cancer of the female genital system.[706] For cancer of the kidney the SIR was statistically significantly elevated 2.4 (90% CI 1.3, 4.1). Interestingly, in a study of about 700 patients treated for Wilms' tumors with radiotherapy, there was no report of a subsequent kidney cancer, even though portions of at least one kidney would have received very high doses and the other probably would have received at least several Gy.[547]

Internal Exposure

Weapons Testing Fallout

Wiklund et al. have studied Lapps, who are presumed to have an increased level of cesium 137, and found a significantly reduced SIR for kidney cancer of 0.16 (95% CI 0.00 to 0.88).[56]

Uranium

Waxweiler et al. did not observe any increase of kidney cancer in uranium miners and reported an SMR of 0.33 (95% CI 0.01, 1.84).[362] Similarly, a study of uranium enrichment workers by Brown et al. did not find an excess of tumors of the urinary organs and reported an SMR of 0.85 (95% CI 0.31, 1.85) among workers.[363] Tirmarche et al. studied mortality of a cohort of French uranium miners exposed to relatively low radon concentrations and did not find a statistically significant increase in bladder and kidney cancers (as a group).[651] Laurier et al. followed up the same group and for cancers of the bladder and kidney (as a group) the SMR was nonsignificantly elevated at 1.1 (95% CI 0.5, 2.0).[186]

Ritz et al. have reported on cancer mortality in uranium processing workers at the Fernald plant in Ohio.[192] The SMR for kidney cancer was nonsignificantly reduced at 0.63. Dupree-Ellis et al. have reported on mortality in a cohort of 2514 uranium processing workers employed between 1942–1966 at the Mallinkrodt Chemical Works. The SMR for kidney cancer was nonsignificantly elevated at 1.17.[193] McGeoghegan et al. have examined the mortality and cancer morbidity experience of workers at the Capenhurst uranium enrichment facility during 1946–1995.[242] The cohort included 12,540 workers including 3244 radiation workers with mean doses of 9.85 mSv. For radiation workers the SMR for kidney cancer was nonsignificantly reduced at 0.49. McGeoghegan et al. also studied workers at the Springfields uranium production facility during 1946–1995.[243] There was a cohort of 19,454 workers including 13,960 radiation workers with a mean external dose of 23 mSv and a mean follow-up period of 24.6 years or 479,146 person-years. For radiation workers the SMR for cancer of the kidney was nonsignificantly reduced at 0.60. A meta-analysis of 14 studies, which included 120,000 uranium workers, found a significant decrease with an RR of 0.78 (95% CI 0.59, 0.96) for kidney cancer.[245]

Plutonium

Omar et al. studied cancer mortality of plutonium workers at the Sellafield plant of British Nuclear Fuels and found that the SMR for kidney cancer was insignificantly reduced at 0.69 for plutonium workers and insignificantly elevated at 1.33 for other radiation workers.[148] Wilkinson et al. studied mortality among plutonium and other workers at a plutonium weapons facility (Rocky Flats in Colorado).[286] The SMR for kidney cancer was 0.56 (90% CI −10, 1.75). Wiggs et al. examined mortality through 1990 among white male workers at the Los Alamos National Laboratory considering both exposures to plutonium and external ionizing radiation.[164] The SMR for kidney cancer was statistically significantly reduced at 0.59 (95% CI 0.34, 0.95). The RR of kidney cancer for plutonium workers compared to other radiation workers was nonsignificantly elevated. Carpenter et al. examined workers in the United Kingdom who were occupationally exposed to various radionuclides and the SMRs in such workers were all nonsignificant.[191] The SMR for kidney cancer was 0.65 for tritium exposures, 0.89 for plutonium exposures, and 1.53 for exposures to other radionuclides.

Chernobyl

The exposures from Chernobyl are the result of both external and internal irradiation. The predominant radionuclides are radioiodines and radiocesiums. The data as of 2000 do not indicate any increase in neoplasms in the general public and for the liquidators there may be a slight dose-response trend; however, the SMR for all solid cancers is below that of the general population.[157] There are some reports that are based on a very small series and without any dose estimation or dose-response data published by Romanenko et al. concerning renal-cell carcinomas.[707,708] While no significant differences in renal-cell cancer size, stage, and histological type were found, the authors indicate that there were microscopic differences between the 236 Ukrainian subjects and 112 Spanish controls; however, there was no adjustment for smoking as a potential bias factor and these results also have not been confirmed by other authors. Review of the topic by the 2005 Chernobyl Forum concluded that such studies have too little statistical power.[69] Rahu et al. have reported on cancer incidence of 5446 male Latvian and Estonian Chernobyl cleanup workers and indicate a nonsignificantly reduced SIR of 0.81 for kidney and bladder cancer as a group.[178]

Iron Miners

Darby et al. reported on radon exposure and cancers other than lung cancer in Swedish iron miners.[183] The cohort included only 1415 miners born between 1880 and 1919, and 162 observed deaths. The O/E ratio for kidney cancer was nonsignificantly reduced at 0.85 (95% CI 0.31, 1.85).

Thorotrast

Most studies of Thorotrast patients have not reported on kidney and bladder cancer but in the Danish series of Andersson et al. this category was considered, and in a cohort of 1095 patients a nonsignificantly elevated SIR of 2.1 (95% CI 0.7, 4.8) was reported for kidney cancer.[213] Nyberg reported in the Swedish Thorotrast series that the SIR for kidney cancer was significantly elevated at 3.4 (95% CI 1.4, 7.0) but only based on seven cases.[222] Travis et al. reported on cancer incidence and mortality after cerebral angiography with radioactive Thorotrast and found a significant increase in kidney cancer incidence with an RR of 5.7 (95% CI 1.9, 21.0).[219]

Radioiodine

Studies examining tumors after administration of radioiodine have yielded mixed and inconsistent results. The kidney is of interest because there is a physiologic excretion of radioiodine through the urinary tract. Among studies of the potential carcinogenic effects of diagnostic doses of radioiodine administered to perform thyroid scanning, the largest and most recent of these studies included 35,074 patients who were matched with the Swedish cancer registry.[270] In this study no statistically significant increase in cancer of the kidney or bladder was noted, and there was a combined SIR of 1.08 (95% CI 0.95, 1.22).

After treatment for hyperthyroidism, Hoffman et al. indicated an RR for kidney cancer of 8.6 based on two cases being observed (95% CI 0.1, 752.0).[202] In a much larger study Holm et al. reported a significant elevation in kidney cancer, with an SIR of 1.39 (95% CI 1.07, 1.76).[271] Estimated dose to the kidney was 0.05 Gy. Based on all the other epidemiologic literature and the size of the absorbed dose, it seems extremely unlikely that the detected excess of renal cancer was a result of radiation exposure. Ron et al. have reported on cancer mortality among 35,593 hyperthyroid patients.[201] The SMR for kidney cancer was nonsignificant.

During treatment for thyroid cancer the quantities of radioiodine that are administered are 10 to 20 times higher than for treatment of hyperthyroidism. One would then expect the absorbed doses to be higher by about the same amount. Edmonds et al. reported that in a series of 365 patients, there was no evidence of a significant excess in deaths from cancer of the kidney.[204] In a much larger series, Hall et al. found the SIR for kidney cancer was significantly elevated at 3.0 (95% CI 1.21, 6.19).[203]

Radium

There are several reports of subsequent cancers in patients treated with radium 224 for various conditions. Wick et al. studied late effects in ankylosing spondylitis patients treated with radium 224, among whom there were 626 exposed and 725 control patients with a mean follow-up time of 21 years.[225] The mean injected activity was 0.17 MBq/kg and the mean alpha skeletal dose was 0.67 Gy. The O/E ratio for urinary system cancer was 1.16 for those exposed and 0.73 for the controls. The rate ratio for kidney cancer was marginally significant at 1.8 (P value of 0.05). Nekolla et al. studied malignancies in patients treated with high doses of radium 224 and found statistically significant elevation in the rate ratio for kidney cancer at 2.4 (one-sided 95% CI 1.3).[224]

Summary

The kidney appears to be less sensitive than the bladder relative to radiation induction of cancers. Most occupational studies are negative. Most authoritative reports do not give risk estimates for kidney cancer. The 1990 BEIR V report concluded that radiation can cause cancer of the bladder and, to a lesser extent, cancer of the kidney and suggested use of the atomic bomb survivor risk estimates.[3] The recently released BEIR VII report does not provide any risk factor for kidney cancer.[18] UNSCEAR 2006 has summarized those epidemiological studies that can be used to derive risk estimates for kidney cancer.[86] These are shown in Table 5-15. UNSCEAR 2006 also indicates that there is only weak evidence linking kidney cancer with radiation exposure and it primarily comes from those studies where the kidney dose is high (in the radiotherapy range).[86] The 2006 National Academy of Sciences Committee on Radiation Screening and Compensation Programs Report concluded that there is no epidemiologic evidence that uranium miners are at a greater risk of renal cancer than the general population and also that downwinders and civilian onsite participants at nuclear weapons tests are probably not at risk for increased death from renal cancer.[257]

BLADDER CANCER

General

Bladder cancer represents about 3% to 4% of all cancers in the world. Rates are high in industrialized countries, particularly in Europe and North America. Low rates occur in India and Japan. Males are about three times more frequently affected than females. Squamous cell carcinoma of the bladder is frequent in countries where shistosomiasis is endemic (such as Egypt and the Middle East).

A wide variety of causes of bladder cancer have been identified. The most common causes are occupational, tobacco smoking, and parasitic infection. Early workers in the dye industry had higher rates of bladder cancer due to aromatic amines (benzidine and 2-naphthylamine). Workers in leather, painting, and other industries using organic chemicals also may have higher than expected rates.

Table 5-15 • Risk Estimates for Cancer Incidence and Mortality from Studies of Radiation Exposure: Kidney*

Study	Average Excess Relative Risk at 1 Sv	Average Excess Absolute Risk $(10^4 PYSv)^{-1}$
External Low-LET Exposures		
Incidence		
Life Span Study[319]		
Males	<0 (<0–0.42)	0.18 (0.02–0.61)
Females	1.04 (0.02–2.83)	<0 (<0–244.95)
Age at exposure		
<20	0.75 (<0–2.19)	0.31 (0.08–0.74)
20–40	0.23 (<0–1.94)	<0 (<0–304.44)
>40	<0 (<0–<0)	<0 (<0–<0)
Time since exposure		
12–15	<0 (<0–0.33)	<0 (<0–92.43)
15–30	0.66 (<0–2.38)	0.47 (0.13–0.96)
>30	<0 (<0–0.71)	0.10 (<0–0.69)
All	0.16 (<0–0.78)	0.28 (0.09–0.58)
Cervical cancer cohort[126]	0.3 (–0.1–1.63)	NA
Cervical cancer case control[126]	0.71 (0.03–2.24)	1.10 (0.05–3.5)
U.K. Springfields uranium workers[243]	19.85 (<–14.57–108.3)	NA
Mortality		
Life Span Study[281]		
Males	<0 (<0 – >10,000)	<0 (<0–114.09)
Females	1.17 (<0–4.28)	<0 (<0–71.62)
Age at exposure		
<20	<0 (<0 – >10,000)	<0 (<0–39.84)
20–40	0.86 (<0–4.13)	<0 (<0–106.2)
>40	<0 (<0–<0)	<0 (<0–198.97)
Time since exposure		
5–15	<0 (<0–2.02)	<0 (<0–25.61)
15–30	1.25 (<0–4.6)	<0 (<0–76.09)
>30	<0 (<0–1.29)	<0 (<0–150.04)
All	0.35 (<0–1.51)	<0 (<0–88.31)
Ankylosing spondylitis[110]	0.1 (0.02–0.2)	0.06 (0.01–0.12)
Radiotherapy for peptic ulcer[113]	0.12 (<0–0.97)	NA
Nuclear workers in Canada, United Kingdom, and United States[166]	<0	NA
U.K. National Registry for Radiation Workers[146]	<–1.95 (<–1.95–0.96)	NA
Nuclear power industry workers in the United States[159]	48.8 (–1.77–315)	NA
U.S. Oak Ridge X-10 and Y-12[160]	2.6 (<0–10.9)	NA
U.S. Los Alamos Laboratory workers[164]	>0	NA
Nuclear industry workers in Japan[150]	<0	<0
IARC 15-country nuclear workers study[167,168]	2.26 (< 0, 14.9)	NA
Internal Low-LET Exposures		
Incidence		
Swedish ^{131}I for hyperthyroidism[271]	7.8 (1.7–15)	27 (6–52)
Internal High-LET Exposures		
Incidence		
Danish and Swedish Thorotrast patients[219]	5.7 (1.9–21)	NA
Mortality		
U.S. Thorotrast patients[219]	∞ (0.1–∞)	NA

*The studies listed are those for which quantitative estimates of risk could be made.
Adapted from United Nations Scientific Committee of the Effects of Atomic Radiation (UNSCEAR): Sources and effects of ionizing radiation: 2006 report to the General Assembly with annexes. New York, United Nations, 2007.

In a review article on the etiology and epidemiology of bladder cancer, Cohen and Johansson conclude "cigarette smoking is the most important single cause of bladder cancer."[709] As many as 40% to 50% of bladder cancers are attributed to smoking. The RR in smokers is about 2 compared with nonsmokers. Use of chlorinated water, coffee drinking, and artificial sweeteners has been suggested as being related to bladder cancer, but the evidence is limited.

External Exposure

Background Radiation

In a study of the influence of terrestrial radiation in Connecticut, Walter et al. reported an increase in bladder cancer in females living in the higher radiation areas.[21] No significant increase was found for males living in the same areas. Airline crews are exposed to higher than normal levels of cosmic irradiation. Band et al. reported on a cohort mortality study of 2740 Air Canada pilots who received doses of 6 mSv per year over an average of 20 years (or a total average dose about 120 mSv) in whom the SIR for bladder cancer was significantly reduced at 0.36 (90% CI 0.12, 0.82).[40]

Populations Near Nuclear Facilities

Jablon et al. reported no increase in mortality from bladder cancer in populations living around U.S. nuclear facilities as a result of plant operations.[78] The SMR in study areas was 1.06 before plant operations began and 1.07 after operations. This can be compared with an SMR of 1.09 in the control areas before plant operations and 1.07 afterward. There are three papers concerning potential uranium contamination and the possibility of an increased risk of bladder cancer in the public. The papers by Boice et al. indicated a nonsignificant decrease around a uranium mining and milling facility in Texas and a nonsignificant decrease in bladder cancer near uranium facilities in Pennsylvania and Colorado.[89,90,90a] A nonsignificant decrease in bladder cancer was found by Boice et al. as well in a study of persons residing near the Hanford National Laboratory.[91] Lopez-Abente et al. have reported on solid tumor mortality near Spain's four nuclear power plants and four uranium fuel cycle facilities, and the RR for bladder cancer was nonsignificantly elevated at 1.03.[283]

Atomic Bomb Survivors

The incidence study of atomic bomb survivors through 1998 by Preston et al. yield risk estimates of an ERR per Gy of 1.23 (90% CI 0.59, 2.1) and an EAR per Gy of 3.2 (90% CI 1.1, 5.4) per 10^4PYGy.[319] There was an estimated excess of 35 cases among a total of 469 bladder cancer cases for an attributable fraction of 16.4% (Fig. 5-11). In the report on mortality though 2000 by Preston et al. there

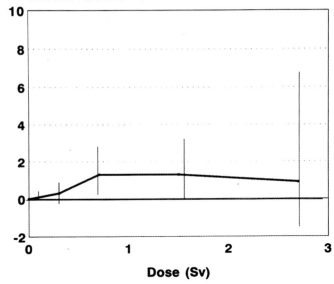

Excess relative risk

Dose (Sv)

Bladder cancer incidence (A-bomb)

Figure 5-11 • ERR of bladder cancer in atomic bomb survivors at different dose levels. Bars indicate 95% CI. (From Thompson D, Mabuchi K, Ron E, et al: Cancer incidence in atomic bomb survivors. II: Solid tumors, 1958–1987. RERF Technical Report 5-92, Hiroshima, Japan, Radiation Effects Research Foundation, 1992.)

was a statistically significant relationship between radiation dose and cancer of the bladder for males.[281] The ERR at 1 Sv was 1.1 (90% CI 0.2, 2.5), the EAR was 0.7 (90% CI 0.1, 1.4), and the attributable risk (17%) was based on 83 deaths. For females there was a statistically significant relationship between radiation dose and cancer of the bladder. The ERR at 1 Sv was 1.2 (90% CI 0.1, 3.1), the EAR was 0.33 (90% CI 0.02, 0.74), and the attributable risk (16%) was based on 67 deaths.

Occupational Exposure

A large number of occupational studies are generally negative with respect to radiation induction of bladder cancer. A study of 176,000 nuclear workers in Japan by Iwasaki et al. found a nonsignificantly elevated SMR for bladder cancer of 1.15 (95% CI 0.76, 1.68).[150] Habib et al. have reported on cancer incidence among Australian nuclear industry–monitored radiation workers and indicated a nonsignificantly decreased SIR of 0.94 for bladder cancer.[152] A study by Darby et al. of 22,347 U.K. workers exposed to fallout and other sources reported a nonsignificantly elevated RR of 2.79 (90% CI 0.94 to 8.94) for cancer of the bladder.[52] A follow-up study, also by Darby et al., reported a statistically significant elevation of bladder cancer with an SMR of 2.69 (95% CI 1.42, 5.20).[701] In 2003, Muirhead et al. reported on the cancer mortality and incidence during 1952–1998 in men from the United Kingdom who participated in the United Kingdom's atmospheric nuclear weapons tests and experimental programs.[54] The RR for cancer of the bladder was nonsignificantly elevated at 1.09 (95% CI 0.89, 1.32).

A study by Beral et al. included an analysis of 3373 deaths among 39,546 United Kingdom atomic energy workers during 1946–1979.[143] In this study the ratio rate for cancer of the kidney, comparing exposed with nonexposed employees, was nonsignificantly elevated at 2.39 (95% CI 0.94 to 6.09). For bladder and other urinary cancers it was nonsignificantly lower, at 0.70 (95% CI 0.25 to 1.98). A study by Beral et al. of atomic weapons workers did not show significant increase with a rate ratio of 2.39 (95% CI 0.94, 6.09) for kidney cancer.[144] A cohort analysis of the U.K. National Registry of Radiation Workers by Kendall et al. included 95,217 workers studied over 1.2 million person-years at risk.[145] In these workers an insignificantly low SMR of 0.84 was reported for cancer of the kidney, and an identical SMR was reported for cancer of the bladder. In a second expanded analysis of the same group, Muirhead et al. reported on a second analysis of the UK National Registry for 124,743 radiation workers with mean doses of 30 mSv.[46] The lagged SMR for cancer of the bladder was nonsignificantly reduced at 0.84 (95% CI 0.69, 1.01). Fraser et al. studied the cancer mortality and morbidity in employees of the United Kingdom Atomic Energy Authority, 1946–1986.[702] The rate ratio for cancer of the bladder was nonsignificantly elevated at 1.98 (95% CI 0.98, 3.97).

There have been several reports relative to specific nuclear facilities in the United Kingdom. Douglas et al. reported on cancer mortality and morbidity among 14,282 workers at the Sellafield plant of British Nuclear Fuels.[147] The average dose was 128 mSv. The SMR for bladder cancer was nonsignificantly reduced at 0.95. An earlier study of the same population by Smith et al. found a nonsignificant decrease in bladder cancer.[360] A more recent report on the Sellafield plant by Omar et al. indicated a nonsignificant decrease in bladder cancer among nonplutonium radiation workers with an SMR of 0.88.[148] McGeoghegan et al. reported on the mortality and cancer morbidity experience of 2628 employees at the Chapelcross plant of British Nuclear Fuels from 1955–1995.[149] The median dose was 39 mSv and the mean follow-up was 24.3 years. The SMR for bladder cancer was nonsignificantly elevated at 1.02.

In a Canadian study by Gribbin et al. of 8977 male nuclear industry workers, a significantly low SMR of 0.15 (95% CI 0.00 to 0.85) for bladder cancer was reported.[260] Ashmore et al. reported on the mortality and occupational radiation exposure based on the National Dose Registry of Canada.[154] The cohort included 206,620 individuals and 5426 deaths. The average exposure for males was 10 mSv and the SMR for cancer of the bladder was significantly reduced at 0.43 (90% CI 0.27, 0.66). Sont et al. reported on cancer incidence also using the National Dose Registry of Canada.[153] The cohort included 191,333 persons

with an average dose for males of 11.5 mSv and an average dose for the cohort of 6.64 mSv. The SIR for cancer of the bladder in males was significantly reduced at 0.76 (90% CI 0.66, 0.87) and for females it was insignificantly reduced at 0.68 (90% CI 0.45, 1.00). The risk per unit dose can be derived for this study relative to bladder cancer and the ERR per Sv was 1.4 (90% CI <0.8, 8.2).

There have also been very large occupational studies in the United States. Gilbert et al. have reported on workers at Hanford in whom they found a nonsignificantly reduced SMR for bladder cancer of 0.69.[361] Cragle et al., reporting on 9860 white male workers at the Savannah River plant, indicated that for bladder cancer, the SMR was lower than expected (0.60) in two groups of workers and nonsignificantly elevated in another group.[288] At the Mound facility in Ohio, Wiggs et al. reported an SMR for bladder cancer at 0.55 (95% CI 0.01, 3.08).[156]

Frome et al. analyzed the mortality among a cohort of World War II nuclear industry workers and reported a nonsignificantly reduced SMR for cancers of the bladder at 0.82.[267] Frome also performed a mortality study of 106,020 employees in the nuclear industry at Oak Ridge, Tennessee.[160] The SMR for cancer of the bladder was nonsignificantly reduced in all groups of males and females. The SMR in white males was 0.76 and in nonwhite males it was 0.98. Fry et al. studied 3145 persons occupationally exposed to 50 or more mSv in a year in whom there were 588 deaths.[161] The mean external exposure was 153 mSv. No deaths from cancer of the bladder were found.

Other U.S. occupational studies also yielded nonsignificant results for an association between occupational exposure and bladder cancer. Acquavella et al. studied mortality of workers at the Pantex nuclear plant.[703] The SMR for bladder cancer was insignificantly reduced at 0.59 (95% CI 0.02, 3.26). Wilkinson et al. found an SMR of 0.93 (90% CI 0.25, 2.40) for bladder cancer at the Rocky Flats plant.[286] Checkoway et al., reporting on workers at Oak Ridge National Laboratory, indicated a less than expected SMR of 0.72 (95% CI 0.15, 2.10) for bladder cancer.[284] Wiggs et al. found significantly reduced SMR for bladder cancer (0.60) in a follow-up of Los Alamos workers.[164]

Cardis et al. reported on cancer mortality among nuclear industry workers in three countries in a large study of 95,673 workers and followed for over 2 million person-years at risk with 15,825 deaths.[166] For bladder cancer the trend with dose was nonsignificant at 0.62 with a P value of 0.26. Cardis et al. have reported the cancer mortality results from a 15-country collaborative study of nuclear workers.[168] This is the largest occupational study to date and included a cohort of 407,391 workers with 18,993 deaths and 5.2 million person-years of follow-up. The ERR per Sv for bladder cancer was nonsignificantly negative, estimated at less than 0, with a negative trend with increasing dose (P value of −1.10).

Cancer incidence among medical diagnostic workers in China has been reviewed by Wang et al.[253] who compared 27,011 workers with 25,782 persons in other medical specialties. The cohort included 27,011 medical diagnostic x-ray workers with cumulative doses were 0.55 Sv for those employed before 1970 and 0.08 Sv for the cohort employed after 1970. The RR for cancer of the bladder was significantly elevated with an RR of 2.1 for those employed before 1970 and was nonsignificantly elevated at 1.4 for those employed later. The risk for bladder cancer per unit dose from this study for the 1970–1980 period of beginning employment was an ERR per Sv of 2.0 (95% CI 0.4, 4.3) an EAR of 0.4 (95% CI 0.08, 0.9).

Doody et al. have examined mortality among 143,517 U.S. radiologic technologists during 1926–1990 whose SMR for cancer of the bladder was nonsignificantly reduced at 0.91 (95% CI 0.63, 1.28).[97] Mohan et al. studied cancer and other causes of mortality among 146,022 radiologic technologists in the United States employed from 1940 and later.[99] The SMR for cancer of the bladder in males was significantly reduced at 0.60 (95% CI 0.4, 0.9) and in females it was nonsignificantly reduced at 0.94 (95% CI 0.7, 1.3). Sigurdson et al. studied cancer incidence among 90,305 U.S. radiologic technologists among whom the SIR for bladder cancer was nonsignificantly reduced at 0.93 (95% CI 0.70, 1.17).[101]

Medical Diagnostic Exposure

The risk of bladder cancer has been studied in patients after external exposures in diagnostic radiology. Massachusetts TB patients treated with multiple fluoroscopies have been followed by Davis et al.[364] They reported that for bladder cancer there was an SMR of 0.8 in exposed females and 0.4 in unexposed females. SMRs for exposed and unexposed males were elevated at 1.6 and 1.9, respectively, and this elevation was statistically significant only for the unexposed group. In another study, also of Massachusetts TB patients, the SMR for cancer of the bladder in male controls was elevated at 1.4, and in the exposed males the SMR was 1.2.[105] In the females the SMR for the exposed group was 0.9, and for controls it was 0.6.

Radiation Therapy

Radiation therapy can give quite high doses to specific organs, and patients have been followed after therapy for benign, as well as malignant, conditions. Darby et al. reported on patients who were treated for ankylosing spondylitis in whom cancer of the bladder was nonsignificantly elevated, with an O/E ratio of 1.52.[109] No clear trend of increasing O/E ratio with time was apparent; the highest O/E ratio for bladder cancer was seen in the first 5 years after exposure. A follow-up study by Weiss et al. of 15,577 patients with a mean total body dose of 2.6 Gy found an RR for bladder cancer of 1.08 at 5 to 24.9 years post-treatment and a statistically significant

elevation of 1.81 times greater for more than 25 years postexposure.[266] The estimated ERR per Gy was 0.24 (95% CI 0.09, 0.41) and the EAR was 0.39 (95% CI 0.19, 0.54). Cancer following radiotherapy for peptic ulcer has been studied in over 3700 patients by Griem et al.[112] and later the series was updated by Carr et al.[113] The dose to the abdomen was about 15 Gy and the RR for cancer of the bladder 11 or more years after radiotherapy was nonsignificantly elevated at 1.49 (95% CI 0.50, 4.44). Mattsson et al. studied the incidence of primary malignancies other than breast cancer among women treated with radiation therapy for benign breast disease in whom the RR for bladder cancer was nonsignificantly elevated at 1.64 (95% CI 0.63, 4.31).[114] In women who received radium radiation therapy for benign gynecologic conditions, and in whom the median doses were estimated at 0.21 Gy to the kidney and 6.0 Gy to the bladder, Inskip et al. found that the SMR for bladder cancer was significantly elevated at 2.0, and it increased with time after exposure.[118] The risk factors per unit dose can be derived from this study; the ERR for bladder cancer is 0.20 (95% CI 0.08, 0.35) and the EAR is 0.24 (95% CI 0.01, 0.4).

Studies of second cancers in women treated for cervical carcinoma with radiotherapy show an increase in bladder cancer (Fig. 5-12). One cohort study of women treated for cervical cancer compared 82,616 exposed women with 99,424 unexposed controls from Canada, Denmark, Finland, Norway, Sweden, Yugoslavia, the United Kingdom, and the United States. The study covered 1.28 million person-years at risk, and found a

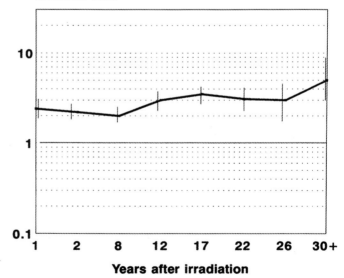

Bladder cancer (cervix series)

Figure 5-12 • RR of bladder cancer by time after treatment for cervical carcinoma with radiation therapy. Error bars indicate 95% CI. (From Boice JD, Jr, et al: Second cancers following radiation treatment for cervical cancer: An international collaboration among cancer registries. J Natl Cancer Inst 1985;74:955–975.)

significant increase in cancer of the bladder. In patients treated for invasive cervical cancer, the O/E ratio for bladder cancer was 2.7 in those treated with radiotherapy and 1.7 in those treated without radiotherapy. In patients who were followed for 10 years or more postexposure, the O/E ratios were 3.5 and 1.2, respectively. In a large case-control study 4188 women who developed second cancers after radiotherapy treatment for cancer of the cervix were compared with 6880 matched controls.[124] The estimated bladder dose was 30 to 60 Gy, and the RR for bladder cancer was significantly elevated at 4.05 (90% CI 1.9, 8.5). The risk factors per unit dose derived from this study are an ERR for bladder cancer of 0.07 (95% CI 0.02, 0.17) and an EAR of 0.12 (95% CI 0.04, 0.3) per 10^4 PYGy. Kleinerman et al. reported on second primary cancer after treatment for cervical cancer in an international registries study.[125] The study evaluated second cancers in 86,193 patients with cervical cancer reported to 13 cancer registries in 5 countries. The O/E ratio for bladder cancer in those treated with radiotherapy was statistically significantly elevated at 3.4 (95% CI 3.1, 3.8) with a mean organ dose of 22 Gy.

In a Japanese study of women also treated for cancer of the cervix, the O/E ratio for bladder cancer was significantly elevated in both groups, with the values being 2.7 and 1.7, respectively; however, some of the increase may have been due to cigarette smoking.[128] A Danish series of 19,470 treated cervical cancer patients was reported by Storm, who found that the O/E for bladder cancer was statistically significantly elevated at 2.9 with radiotherapy but that it was also elevated at 2.5 in those patients who had no radiotherapy.[704] Curtis et al. have studied second cancers following radiotherapy for cancer of the female genital system.[706] For bladder cancer the SIR was statistically significantly elevated at 2.4 (95% CI 1.3, 4.1). Interestingly, in a study of about 700 patients treated for Wilms' tumors with radiotherapy, no increase in bladder cancer was mentioned. Travis et al. have reported on long-term survival and second cancers in over 40,000 testicular cancer patients almost all of whom received infradiaphragmatic radiotherapy.[705] The RR for bladder cancer was significantly increased. Brenner et al. have studied second malignancies in prostate carcinoma patients treated with radiotherapy or surgery and reported a significant increase in bladder cancer risk, with the radiotherapy group having an ERR of 0.77 at times greater than 10 years postexposure compared to the surgery only group.[137]

Internal Exposure

Weapons Testing Fallout

Wiklund et al. have reported that Lapps, who consume reindeer and are presumed to have an increased level of cesium 137, had a nonsignificantly reduced SIR of 0.75 (95% CI 0.24, 1.75) for bladder cancer.[56]

Uranium

Boice et al. studied the cancer mortality in a Texas county with prior uranium mining and milling activities during 1950–2001 and found that the RR for bladder cancer was nonsignificantly reduced at 0.64 (95% CI 0.4, 1.1).[89] Similar results were reported in Pennsylvania and Texas.[90,90a] Studies in uranium miners have not shown a significant increase in bladder cancer. Waxweiler et al. did not report an increase and reported SMRs for bladder cancer of 0.94 (95% CI 0.19, 2.74).[362] A study of uranium enrichment workers by Brown et al. did not find an excess of tumors of the urinary organs and reported an SMR of 0.85 (95% CI 0.31, 1.85).[363] Tirmarche et al. studied the mortality of a cohort of French uranium miners exposed to relatively low radon concentrations and did not find a statistically significant increase in bladder and kidney cancers (as a group).[651] Laurier et al. followed up with the same group and for cancers of the bladder and kidney the SMR was nonsignificantly elevated at 1.1 (95% CI 0.5, 2.0).[186]

Ritz et al. have reported on cancer mortality in uranium processing workers at the Fernald plant in Ohio in whom the SMR for bladder cancer was nonsignificantly increased at 1.15.[192] Dupree-Ellis et al. have reported on mortality in a cohort of 2514 uranium processing workers employed between 1942–1966 at the Mallinkrodt Chemical Works in whom the SMR for bladder cancer was also nonsignificantly increased at 1.16.[193] McGeoghegan et al. examined the mortality and cancer morbidity experience of workers at the Capenhurst uranium enrichment facility during 1946–1995.[242] The cohort included 12,540 workers including 3244 radiation workers with mean doses of 9.85 mSv and for radiation workers the SMR for cancer of the bladder was nonsignificantly elevated at 1.04. McGeoghegan et al. also studied workers at the Springfields uranium production facility during 1946–1995.[243] This included a cohort of 19,454 workers among whom there were 13,960 radiation workers with a mean external dose of 23 mSv and a mean follow-up period of 24.6 years or 479,146 person-years. For radiation workers the SMR for cancer of the bladder was nonsignificantly reduced at 0.92. A meta-analysis of 14 studies, which included 120,000 uranium workers, found a significant decrease with an RR of 0.83 (95% CI 0.71, 0.96) for bladder cancer.[245]

Plutonium

Omar et al. studied the cancer mortality of plutonium workers at the Sellafield plant of British Nuclear Fuels and found that the SMR for bladder cancer was insignificantly elevated at 1.23 for plutonium workers and insignificantly reduced at 0.88 for other radiation workers.[148] Wilkinson et al. studied mortality among plutonium and other workers at a plutonium weapons facility (Rocky Flats in Colorado) in whom the SMR for bladder cancer was 0.93 (90% CI 0.25, 2.4).[286] Wiggs et al. examined mortality through 1990 among white male workers at the Los Alamos National Laboratory, considering both exposures to plutonium and external ionizing radiation.[164] For both types of exposure, the SMR for bladder cancer was statistically significantly reduced at 0.60 (95% CI 0.35, 0.95). The RR for plutonium workers compared to other radiation workers was nonsignificantly elevated. Carpenter et al. examined workers in the United Kingdom who were occupationally exposed to various radionuclides and the SMRs for such workers were all nonsignificantly different from unity.[191] The SMR for bladder cancer was 1.51 for tritium exposures, 0.72 for plutonium exposure, and 0.56 for exposures to other radionuclides.

Chernobyl

The exposures from Chernobyl are the result of both external and internal irradiation. The predominant radionuclides are radioiodines and radiocesiums. The data as of 2000 do not indicate any increase in neoplasms in the general public and for the liquidators, there may be a slight dose-response trend; however, the SMR for all solid cancers is below that of the general population.[157] There are some reports based on a very small series and without any dose estimation or dose-response data published by Romanenko et al.[707] on changes to the uro-epithelium ("Chernobyl cystitis").[708] Review of the topic by the 2005 Chernobyl Forum concluded that these studies have too little statistical power.[69] Rahu et al. have reported on cancer incidence of 5446 male Latvian and Estonian Chernobyl cleanup workers and indicate a nonsignificantly reduced SIR of 0.81 for kidney and bladder cancer as a group.[178]

Iron Miners

Darby et al. reported on radon exposure and cancers other than lung cancer in Swedish iron miners. The cohort included only 1415 miners born between 1880–1919 and 162 observed deaths.[183] The O/E ratio for bladder cancer was nonsignificantly reduced at 0.98 (95% CI 0.32, 2.29).

Thorotrast

Most studies of Thorotrast patients have not reported on bladder cancer but in the Danish series of Andersson et al., however, this category was considered, and among a cohort of 1095 patients a nonsignificantly elevated SIR of 1.4 (95% CI 0.5, 3.1) was reported for bladder cancer.[213] In the German Thorotrast series the risk of bladder cancer was not elevated, with five cases observed in both the patient and control groups.[314] Nyberg reported in the Swedish Thorotrast series the SIR for bladder cancer was insignificantly elevated at 1.2 (95% CI 0.2, 3.5).[222] Travis et al. reported on cancer incidence and mortality after cerebral angiography with radioactive Thorotrast and found a nonsignificant reduction in RR of bladder cancer of 0.8 (95% CI 0.3, 1.9).[219]

Radioiodine

Studies examining tumors after administration of radioiodine have yielded mixed and inconsistent results. The bladder is of interest because there is a physiologic excretion of radioiodine through the urinary tract. Among studies of the potential carcinogenic effects of diagnostic doses of radioiodine administered to perform thyroid scanning, the largest and most recent of these studies included 35,074 patients who were matched with the Swedish cancer registry.[270] In this study no statistically significant increase in cancer of the kidney or bladder was noted, and there was a combined SIR of 1.08 (95% CI 0.95, 1.22).

After treatment for hyperthyroidism, Hoffman et al. indicated an RR for bladder cancer was reduced at 0.9, but again, due to the small number of cases observed, the confidence limits were so wide (95% CI 0.01 to 62.6) as to make the estimated RR of little meaning.[202] In a much larger study Holm et al. reported no excess of bladder cancer and the estimated dose to the bladder was about 0.14 Gy.[271] Ron et al. have reported on cancer mortality among 35,593 hyperthyroid patients.[201] The SMR for bladder cancer was nonsignificantly elevated at 1.08 for those receiving iodine 131, 0.97 for those receiving iodine 131 alone, and 1.3 for those treated with surgery only.

During treatment for thyroid cancer the quantities of radioiodine that are administered are 10 to 20 times higher than for treatment of hyperthyroidism so that one would expect the absorbed doses to be higher by about the same amount. Edmonds et al. reported that in a series of 365 patients, there was a small but significant excess in deaths from cancer of the bladder.[204] In a much larger series, Hall et al. found that the SIR for bladder cancer was nonsignificantly elevated at 1.61 (95% CI 0.44, 4.13).[203]

Radium

There are several reports of subsequent cancers in patients treated with radium 224 for various conditions. Wick et al. studied late effects in ankylosing spondylitis patients treated with radium 224 among whom there were 626 exposed and 725 control patients with a mean follow-up time of 21 years. The mean injected activity was 0.17 MBq/kg and the mean alpha skeletal dose was 0.67 Gy. The O/E ratio for urinary system cancer was 1.16 for those exposed and 0.73 for the controls. Nekolla et al. studied malignancies in patients treated with high doses of radium 224 and found a statistically significant elevation in the rate ratio for bladder cancer at 2.0 (one-sided 95% CI 1.2).[224]

Brachytherapy

In the literature of tumors arising after internal pelvic radiotherapy, case reports are scattered. As an example, Kerr et al. reported on one case of a rhabdomyosarcoma of the urinary bladder occurring 18 years after interstitial radiotherapy for a squamous cell carcinoma.[710] In another case report, Winters et al. reported two cases of bladder cancer arising about 6 years after iodine 125 implants for prostate cancer.[711] The authors postulate that these may have been due to the radiation exposure; however, with the very short latent period and without assessment of other risk factors (e.g., absence of a dose-response relationship), this remains a matter of conjecture.

Summary

The bladder appears to be sensitive to radiogenic tumor induction. Despite this, the most common cause of bladder cancer is cigarette smoking, and a number of other causative factors are known as well. All of these need to be considered in evaluation of any specific case. Most occupational studies are negative, and the positive correlations come primarily from the atomic bomb survivors and patients who received very high bladder doses from radiotherapy.

Most authoritative reports do give risk estimates for bladder cancer. The 1990 ICRP report estimates the probability of fatal bladder cancer after exposure of the general population to be 0.30 $(10^{-2}Sv^{-1})$.[248] The 1990 BEIR V report concluded that radiation can cause cancer of the bladder and, to a lesser extent, cancer of the kidney and suggested use of the atomic bomb survivor risk estimates.[3] The recently released BEIR VII report provides a lifetime risk estimate for bladder cancer of 25 excess deaths for a population of 100,000 persons exposed to 0.1 Gy.

UNSCEAR 2006 also has summarized those epidemiological studies that can be used to derive risk estimates for bladder cancer.[86] These are shown in Table 5-16. It is clear that there is a positive association between radiation and bladder cancer in the atomic bomb survivors and after high-dose radiotherapy, however, most low-dose studies of nuclear workers and medical applications do not show increased risk of bladder cancer (perhaps due to limited statistical power).

OVARIAN CANCER

General

Cancer of the ovary is more common in industrialized nations, with the exception of Japan.[358] Annually, about 24,000 new patients are diagnosed in the United States, and over 13,000 deaths are reported. Most tumors are serous or pseudomucinous cystadenocarcinomas, and most have a relatively poor prognosis. Studies of migrant populations suggest environmental influences may be present.[700] A number of studies also suggest that endocrine function plays a role. Higher rates are seen in women who have a smaller number of pregnancies or are nulliparous. Early and frequent parity may be associated with an over

50% reduction in risk. Breast cancer is also associated with ovarian cancer. Women with breast cancer have twice the expected risk of subsequent ovarian cancer, and conversely, women with ovarian cancer have a three- to fourfold increased risk of breast cancer. Oral contraceptives may reduce the risk of ovarian cancer. There are some unusual genetic associations, including the Peutz-Jeghers syndrome, basal cell nevus syndrome, and gonadal dysgenesis.

External Exposure

Background Radiation and Populations Near Nuclear Installations

In a study of terrestrial radiation in Connecticut, there was a lower mortality from carcinoma of the ovary in the high-background radiation areas than in areas of lower background.[21] There are three papers concerning potential environmental uranium contamination and the possibility of increased risk of ovarian cancer in the public. The papers by Boice et al. indicated a nonsignificant decrease around a uranium mining and milling facility in Texas and a nonsignificant decrease near uranium facilities in Pennsylvania and Colorado.[89,90,90a] A nonsignificant decrease was found by Boice et al. in a study of persons residing near the Hanford site.[91] Lopez-Abente et al. have reported on solid tumor mortality near Spain's four nuclear power plants and four uranium fuel cycle facilities where the RR for ovarian cancer was nonsignificantly elevated at 1.02.[283]

Atomic Bomb Survivors

Incidence and mortality sstudies of the atomic bomb survivors report risks for ovarian cancer.[10,279,359] The 1958–1998 incidence study yields ERR estimates for ovarian cancer of 0.61 (90% CI 0, 0.15) per Gy and an ER of 0.56 (90% CI 0.02, 1.3) cases per $(10^4 PYGy)^{-1}$.[319] There is an estimated excess of 11 cases in the total 245 cases found. There was a statistically significant linear relationship between dose and risk (Fig. 5-13). No effect of age at exposure, time since exposure, or of attained age was found. Risk estimates derived from the 1958–1987 mortality study indicate an ERR at 1 Sv of 1.2 (95% CI 0.2, 2.8) and an EAR of 0.7 (95% CI 0.1 to 1.4) $\times (10^4 PYSv)^{-1}$. In the 2003 update studies of mortality of atomic bomb survivors during 1950–1997, Preston et al. studied a cohort of 86,572 individuals with an average external dose of 0.23 Sv in whom there was a statistically significant excess of ovarian cancer at dose levels of 1 Sv, with an ERR of 0.94 (90% CI 0.07, 2.0).[281]

Occupational Exposure

In contrast to the atomic bomb survivor data, almost all occupational studies have shown either no relation or a nonsignificant relationship between ovarian cancer and occupational radiation exposure. However, some of the

Table 5-16 • Risk Estimates for Cancer Incidence and Mortality from Studies of Radiation Exposure: Cancer of the Urinary Bladder*

Study	Average Excess Relative Risk at 1 Sv	Average Excess Absolute Risk $(10^4 PYSv)^{-1}$
External Low-LET Exposures		
Incidence		
A-bomb Life Span Study[319]		
Males	0.63 (0.17–1.25)	0.47 (<0–1.60)
Females	1.74 (0.71–3.22)	0.52 (0.12–1.13)
Age at exposure		
<20	1.00 (0.16–2.32)	<0 (<0–0.46)
20–40	0.95 (0.23–2.01)	0.69 (<0–1.89)
>40	0.78 (0.14–1.70)	2.28 (0.21–5.01)
Time since exposure		
12–15	<0 (<0–1.06)	<0 (<0–292.76)
15–30	0.98 (0.17–2.20)	0.50 (<0–1.19)
>30	1.00 (0.44–1.74)	1.28 (0.33–2.50)
All	0.92 (0.46–1.50)	0.51 (0.14–1.02)
Cervical cancer case control[6]	0.07 (0.02–0.17)	0.12 (0.04–0.3)
Canada National Dose Registry—males only[153]	1.4 (<0–8.2)	NA
Capenhurst uranium facility[242]	10.33 (<0–57.24)	NA
U.K. Springfields uranium workers[243]	2.68 (< –4.11–14.50)	NA
Mortality		
A-bomb Life Span Study[281]		
Males	1.03 (0.07–2.53)	<0 (<0–313.73)
Females	1.37 (0.15–3.40)	<0 (<0–170.04)
Age at exposure		
<20	<0 (<0–2.28)	<0 (<0–43.45)
20–40	1.52 (<0–4.72)	<0 (<0–176.04)
>40	1.36 (0.34–2.89)	<0 (<0–848.46)
Time since exposure		
12–15	<0 (<0–2.73)	<0 (<0–118.39)
15–30	0.87 (<0–2.87)	<0 (<0–203.71)
>30	1.76 (0.51–3.73)	<0 (<0–334.58)
All	1.17 (0.36–2.30)	<0 (<0–226.53)
Benign gynecological disease[118]	0.20 (0.08–0.35)	0.24 (0.1–0.4)
Metropathia hemorrhagica[116]	0.40 (0.15–0.66)	0.55 (0.2–0.9)
Ankylosing spondylitis[266]	0.24 (–0.09–0.41)	0.39 (0.19–0.54)
Peptic ulcer[113]	2.45 (<0–17.20)	NA
U.S. Los Alamos Laboratory workers[164]	<0	NA
Nuclear industry workers in Japan[150]	<0	NA
Nuclear workers in Canada, United Kingdom, United States[166]	>0	NA
U.K. National Registry for Radiation Workers[146]	–0.33 (–1.28–1.61)	NA
IARC 15-country nuclear workers study[167,168]	<0	NA
Internal High-LET Exposures		
Incidence		
Danish and Swedish Thorotrast patients[219]	0.8 (0.3–1.9)	NA
Mortality		
U.S. Thorotrast patients[219]	∞ (0.2–∞)	NA

*The studies listed are those for which quantitative estimates of risk could be made.
Adapted from United Nations Scientific Committee of the Effects of Atomic Radiation (UNSCEAR): Sources and effects of ionizing radiation: 2006 report to the General Assembly with annexes. New York, United Nations, 2007.

studies are limited by the small number of female radiation workers. Three large studies in the United Kingdom have all been negative. Beral et al. included an analysis of 3115 deaths among 22,552 atomic weapons workers during 1946–1979, comparing exposed and nonexposed workers for cancer of the ovary.[144] They reported a ratio rate of 0.00 (95% CI 0.00, 40.8). A cohort analysis of the U.K. National Registry of Radiation Workers by Kendall et al. included 95,217 workers over 1.2 million person-years at risk and indicated a nonsignificantly elevated SMR of 1.44 for cancer of the ovary.[145] A second analysis in 1999 of 124,743 workers in the U.K. National Registry of Radiation Workers by Muirhead et al. using a lagged analysis reported a nonsignificantly reduced SMR

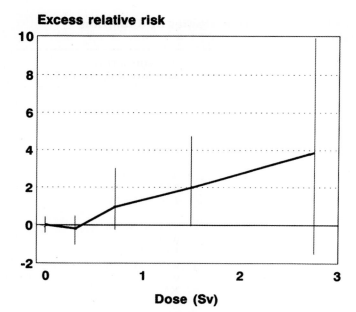

Excess relative risk

Ovarian cancer incidence (A-bomb)

Figure 5-13 • ERR of ovarian cancer in atomic bomb survivors at different dose levels. Bars indicate 95% CI. (From Thompson D, Mabuchi K, Ron E, et al: Cancer incidence in atomic bomb survivors. II: Solid tumors, 1958–1987. RERF Technical Report 5-92, Hiroshima, Japan, Radiation Effects Research Foundation, 1992.)

of 0.86 (95% CI 0.41, 1.58).[146] In a study of workers at the British Sellafield plant, the SMR for ovarian cancer was 0.97 in radiation workers and 0.81 in other workers.[360] A report on the Sellafield plant by Omar et al. indicated a nonsignificant decrease in ovarian cancer among nonplutonium radiation workers with an SMR of 0.60 and incidence was insignificantly increased (based on two cases).[148]

Cardis et al. reported on cancer mortality among nuclear industry workers in three countries in a very large study of 95,673 workers with over 2 million person-years at risk and 15,825 deaths.[166] The trend for ovarian cancer was nonsignificant at 0.49 with a P value of 0.31. Cardis et al. have reported the cancer mortality results from a 15-country collaborative study of nuclear workers.[168] This is the largest occupational study to date and included a cohort of 407,391 workers with 18,993 deaths and 5.2 million person-years of follow-up. The ERR per Sv for ovarian cancer was nonsignificantly negatively estimated at less than 0, with a negative trend with increasing dose (P value of −0.93). Sont et al. also reported on the relationship of cancer incidence and occupational radiation exposure based on the National Dose Registry of Canada and included a cohort of 191,333 persons with an average dose for males of 11.5 mSv and an average dose for the cohort of 6.64 mSv.[153] The SIR for ovarian cancer was nonsignificantly elevated at 1.07. Gilbert et al. have published a number of studies

concerning workers at national laboratories or U.S. federal facilities. In a study of workers at the Hanford National Laboratory during 1945–1986, they reported an SMR of 0.89 for cancer of the female genital organs other than the uterus.[361] The SMR was 0.78 in the radiation-monitored female workers and 1.02 for the unmonitored females.

Cancer incidence among medical diagnostic workers in China was reviewed by Wang et al. in 1988, who compared 27,011 workers with 25,782 persons in other medical specialties.[102] While the risk of cancer overall was elevated by 50%, the RR of 0.95 for ovarian cancer was not elevated. In a 2002 follow-up report, Wang et al. reported the RR for cancer of the ovary was nonsignificantly increased at 1.4.[253] Sigurdson et al. studied cancer incidence in 90,305 U.S. radiologic technologists and found that the SIR for ovarian cancer was nonsignificantly reduced at 0.88 (95% CI 0.71, 1.05).[101]

McGeoghegan et al. have reported on the mortality of 12,540 workers (including 3244 radiation workers) at the Capenhurst uranium enrichment facility during 1946–1995.[242] No case of ovarian cancer was identified in radiation workers. They also studied the cancer mortality experience of 19,454 workers (including 13,960 radiation workers) at the Springfields uranium production facility during 1946–1995.[243] The SMR for ovarian cancer was nonsignificantly reduced for radiation workers at 0.66.

Medical Exposure

Few studies have examined radiation therapy for benign diseases and the subsequent risk of ovarian cancer. Many patients were treated with radiotherapy for ankylosing spondylitis. Darby et al. have extended the follow-up of this group, and cancer of the ovary was not elevated, with a reported O/E of 0.93.[109] Mattsson et al. have reported on cancer incidence among 3090 women who received radiation therapy for benign breast disease and found that the RR for ovarian cancer was nonsignificantly increased at 1.08.[114]

In studies of second cancers in women treated for cervical carcinoma with radiotherapy, there is a consistent decrease in risk of secondary ovarian cancer, even though doses are on the order of 30 Gy. Perhaps the reason for the difference between these studies and the risks derived from the atomic bomb survivors is due to cell killing. In a cohort study of women treated for cervical cancer, 82,616 exposed women were compared with 99,424 unexposed controls. The women were from Canada, Denmark, Finland, Norway, Sweden, Yugoslavia, the United Kingdom, and the United States, and the study covered 1.28 million person-years at risk.[124] There was a significant decrease in cancer of the ovary that was directly exposed in the primary radiotherapy beam. In patients treated for invasive cervical cancer, the O/E ratio for ovarian cancer was 0.7 for those treated with radiotherapy and

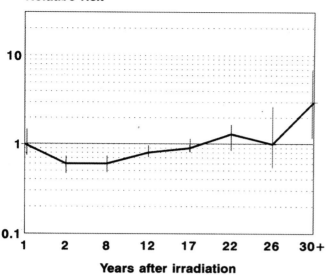

Relative risk

Ovarian cancer (cervix series)

Figure 5-14 ● RR of ovarian cancer by time after treatment for cervical carcinoma with radiation therapy. Error bars indicate 95% CI. (From Boice JD, Jr, et al: Second cancers following radiation treatment for cervical cancer: An international collaboration among cancer registries. J Natl Cancer Inst 1985;74:955–975.)

0.1 for those treated without radiotherapy. In patients who were followed for 10 years or more the O/E ratio was not much different. The RR for ovarian cancer over time is shown in Figure 5-14, and it can be seen that the RR rises above unity for only one of the eight data points. In a large case-control study, 4188 women who developed second cancers after treatment for cancer of the cervix were compared with 6880 matched controls.[126] The RR for cancer of the ovary was not significantly different from unity at 0.45 (90% CI 0.2, 1.0). In a Japanese study of women also treated for cancer of the cervix, the O/E ratio for ovarian cancer was 0.5 in those treated with radiotherapy and 0.7 in those treated without radiotherapy.[128]

Internal Exposure

The studies examining ovarian cancer after administration of radioiodine have yielded negative results. These include studies of the potential carcinogenic effects of diagnostic doses of radioiodine administered to perform thyroid scanning. One of the largest of these studies included 35,074 patients who were matched with the Swedish cancer registry.[270] As a group, there was no increase in cancer of the female genital organs, and the SIR was 0.86 (95% CI 0.78, 0.94). After treatment for hyperthyroidism, Hoffman et al. indicated an RR for ovarian cancer of 2.2 (95% CI 0.3, 24.6).[202] In a much larger study Holm et al. reported that there was no increase in cancer of the female genital organs as a group, and the combined SIR was 1.00 (95% CI 0.85, 1.15).[271] Estimated

doses to female genital organs were reported to average 0.05 Gy. During treatment for thyroid cancer, the quantities of radioiodine administered are in the range of 10 to 20 times higher than for treatment of hyperthyroidism, or in the range of 0.5 to 1.0 Gy to the ovaries. Edmonds et al. reported that in a series of 365 patients, there was no excess of ovarian cancer.[204] But in a much larger series, Hall et al. found that there was an excess risk for female genital organs as a group with an SIR of 2.03 (95% CI 1.2, 3.20).[203] Ron et al. have reported on cancer mortality among 35,593 hyperthyroid patients.[201] The SMR for ovarian cancer was nonsignificantly elevated. The SMR was 1.09 for those receiving any iodine 131 and 1.07 for those receiving iodine alone.

Thorotrast, a contrast medium containing thorium, was used for angiography and, to a much lesser extent, for sinus studies. This material remains in the body and has been associated with a number of tumor types. In a follow-up of Danish Thorotrast patients, Andersson et al. reported an SIR of 2.4 (95% CI 1.0, 5.0) for ovarian cancer.[213] In the German Thorotrast series there was no evidence of an excess of ovarian cancer, with four cases observed in both the patient and control groups.[212] A study by Nekolla et al. of 455 patients treated with radium 224 for TB, ankylosing spondylitis, and a few other diseases indicated that ovarian cancer occurred in four patients and the rate ratio was nonsignificantly elevated.[224] Nyberg et al. reported on cancer incidence after a 40-year follow-up among Swedish patients exposed to radioactive Thorotrast.[222] The SIR for ovarian cancer was nonsignificantly elevated.

A report on the Sellafield plant by Omar et al. indicated a nonsignificant increase in ovarian cancer among plutonium workers with an SMR of 1.58 (based on only one case).[148] Incidence was also nonsignificantly increased based on the same one case. Carpenter et al. examined workers in the United Kingdom who were occupationally exposed to tritium, plutonium, and other radionuclides in whom the SMRs for ovarian cancer in each group were all nonsignificant.[191]

Summary

With the exception of the borderline significant atomic bomb survivor data, not much epidemiologic evidence of radiation induction of ovarian cancer exists. Interpretation of some of the studies is complicated by potential cell killing, and many of the occupational studies do not have many females included. The Chinese x-ray worker study is an exception, and doses were probably at least the same as in many atomic bomb survivors, but no increase in ovarian cancer was identified. The UNSCEAR 1988 Committee, relying predominantly on the Japanese data, derived a risk estimate for cancer of the ovary, using the multiplicative risk model, that was 3.1 (90% CI 0.9 to 6.8) excess lifetime deaths for 1000 persons exposed to 1 Gy of low-LET radiation at high-dose rate.[370] The BEIR V

Table 5-17 • Risk Estimates for Cancer Incidence and Mortality from Studies of Radiation Exposure: Ovary*

Study	Average Excess Relative Risk at 1 Sv	Average Excess Absolute Risk $(10^4 PYSv)^{-1}$
External Low-LET Exposures		
Incidence		
A-bomb Life Span Study[319]		
Age at exposure		
<20	1.16 (0.15–2.86)	0.71 (0.09–1.72)
20–40	<0 (<0–0.71)	<0 (<0–0.71)
>40	1.73 (0.20–4.45)	3.24 (0.45–7.21)
Time since exposure		
12–15	<0 (<0–0.04)	<0 (<0–0.71)
15–30	1.47 (0.37–3.26)	1.04 (0.21–2.3)
>30	0.23 (<0–1.11)	0.54 (<0–1.92)
All	0.61 (0.08–1.35)	0.59 (0.07–1.34)
Cervical cancer case control[126]	0.01 (–0.02–0.14)	0.05 (–0.08–0.6)
Stockholm skin hemangioma[589]	0.62	0.33
Mortality		
A-bomb Life Span Study[281]		
Age at exposure		
<20	1.53 (0.19–4.06)	<0 (<0–185.15)
20–40	0.92 (<0–2.65)	<0 (<0–386.99)
>40	1.33 (<0–4.25)	<0 (<0–717.59)
Time since exposure		
5–15	<0 (<0–9171.6)	<0 (<0–187.74)
15–30	2.65 (0.78–6)	<0 (<0–298.86)
>30	0.88 (<0–2.41)	<0 (<0–513.47)
All	1.18 (0.39–2.31)	<0 (<0–348.4)
^{226}Ra for uterine bleeding[118]	0.41 (–0.69–1.51)	NA
Mortality		
U.K. x-ray for uterine bleeding[116]	0.03 (–0.06–0.15)	0.08 (–0.15–0.41)
U.K. National Registry for Radiation Workers[146]	82.8 (<–1.95–2583)	NA
IARC 15-country nuclear workers study[167,168]	<0	NA
Internal High-LET Exposures		
Incidence		
Danish and Swedish Thorotrast patients[219]	4.3 (1.1–24.3)	NA

*The studies listed are those for which quantitative estimates of risk could be made.
Adapted from United Nations Scientific Committee of the Effects of Atomic Radiation (UNSCEAR): Sources and effects of ionizing radiation: 2006 report to the General Assembly with annexes. New York, United Nations, 2007.

Committee did not derive a separate risk factor.[3] The ICRP 1990 estimated a probability of fatal cancer 10 $(10^{-4}Sv^{-1})$ for exposure of an entire population and of 8 $(10^{-4}Sv^{-1})$ for workers.[248] UNSCEAR 2006 has summarized risk factors that can be obtained from epidemiological studies (Table 5-17) and concluded that although the body of evidence is not strong, the Japanese LSS provides some evidence that ovarian cancer is inducible by ionizing radiation.[86]

UTERINE CERVIX AND CORPUS CANCER

General

Worldwide, cervical cancer is the second most common cancer in women, but in developing countries it is the most frequent cancer.[358] Highest rates occur in Asia, South America, and Africa, while low rates are found in Israel. Endometrial (uterine corpus) cancer is one third as frequent as cervical cancer. Rates of endometrial cancer are generally low in Asia and Africa. In the United States, rates in black women are about one half those of white women. The annual incidence of endometrial cancer in white females is about 15 per 100,000. Cancer of the endometrium is more common in nulliparous women. Tall and obese women are at greater risk probably as a result of increased endogenous estradiol in such women. Obese women have a two- to fivefold increase in risk. Menopause may have a protective influence. Exogenous estrogens are a major risk factor, with increases in cancer associated with use of oral conjugated estrogens administered for replacement therapy and use of sequential oral unopposed estrogen contraceptives. During the 1970s rates in the United States increased due to the use of postmenopausal estrogens. Subsequent incorporation of progesterone in oral contraceptives prevented this problem. The risk of cervical cancer is higher with earlier age at first intercourse and rises with the number of sexual partners throughout life. Thus, there is very likely a sexually transmitted factor (human papilloma virus). Debate as to whether circumcision decreases the risk is inconclusive, although poor penile hygiene appears to increase risk. In most studies there is also an increased risk of cervical cancer with smoking, and smokers have an RR of about 2 compared with nonsmokers. In the United States about 20% to 25% of cervical cancers may be attributable to smoking.[700]

External Exposure

Background Radiation and Populations Near Nuclear Facilities

Two studies have examined the potential relationship between natural background radiation and the risk of cervical cancer. In a large study in China, cervical cancer was significantly more frequent in the high-background area (age-adjusted, site-specific cancer mortality of 2.94 per 10^5 person-years) than in the area with low-background radiation (0.94 per 10^5 person-years).[30] The authors indicated that this finding was difficult to relate to radiation exposure. In contrast, a study of terrestrial radiation in Connecticut showed no correlation of mortality from either endometrial cancer or cervical cancer with terrestrial radiation exposure.[21] There are three papers concerning potential environmental uranium contamination and the possibility of increased risk of cervical and uterine corpus cancers in the public. The papers by Boice et al. indicated a nonsignificant decrease around a uranium mining and milling facility in Texas in uterine corpus cancer and a nonsignificant increase in cervical cancer near a uranium facility in Pennsylvania.[89,90] A significant decrease was found in cervical cancer and a nonsignificant increase in endometrial cancer near a Colorado uranium facility.[90a] A nonsignificant increase in uterine corpus cancer and a nonsignificant decrease in cervical cancer was found by Boice et al. in a study of persons residing near the Hanford National Laboratory.[91]

Atomic Bomb Survivors

The data on the potential relationship between uterine cancer and radiation exposure have been complicated by early reports of the mortality of the atomic bomb survivors. Those reports suggested a relationship, but there was no statistical significance in the relationship. However, neither the 1958–1987 incidence[319] nor the 1958–1998 mortality study[359] of the atomic bomb survivors show any significant increase in cancer of the uterus (Fig. 5-15). The ERR at 1 Gy reported in the incidence study was 0.29 (90% CI −0.14, 0.95) for endometrial cancer and 0.06 (90% CI −0.14, 0.31) for cervical cancer. The

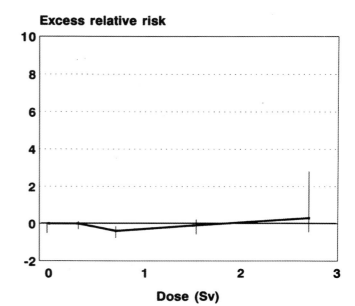

Excess relative risk

Uterine cancer incidence (A-bomb)

Figure 5-15 ● ERR of cancer of the uterus in atomic bomb survivors at different dose levels. Bars indicate 95% CI. (From Thompson D, Mabuchi K, Ron E, et al: Cancer incidence in atomic bomb survivors. II: Solid tumors, 1958–1987. RERF Technical Report 5-92, Hiroshima, Japan, Radiation Effects Research Foundation, 1992.)

estimated excess and total cases for endometrial and cervical cancer were 4 in 184 and 5 in 978, respectively.[319] In the mortality study through 1987, the corresponding values were 0.1 and 0.3 $(10^4 PYSv)^{-1}$. In the 2003 update studies of their mortality during 1950–1997, by Preston et al., the survivors comprised a cohort of 86,572 persons with an average external dose of 0.23 Sv and a nonsignificant excess of uterine cancer at dose levels of 1 Sv with a corresponding ERR of 0.17 (90% CI −0.10, 0.52).[281]

Occupational Exposure

Studies of occupationally exposed workers have not shown an increase in uterine cancer with radiation exposure. Beral et al.[143] indicate a nonsignificantly elevated ratio in the rates of cancer of the uterus in exposed versus nonexposed workers, of 3.10 (90% CI 0.06 to 51.7), and Kendall et al.[145] indicated a nonsignificantly elevated SMR of 1.47 for uterine cancer. A second analysis in 1999 of 124,743 workers in the U.K. National Registry of Radiation Workers by Muirhead et al. using a lagged analysis reported a nonsignificantly increased SMR for uterine cancer of 1.29 (95% CI 0.69, 2.20).[146] In one study of the radiation workers at the Sellafield plant, no cases of uterine cancer were observed.[360] Another report concerning the Sellafield plant by Omar et al. indicated a nonsignificant increase in uterine cancer among nonplutonium radiation workers with an SMR of 1.35 (based on only two cases) and incidence was also nonsignificantly decreased.[148] Habib et al. have reported on cancer incidence among Australian nuclear industry–monitored radiation workers and indicated that no cases of cervical or uterine cance were identified.[152]

Sont et al. reported on cancer incidence and occupational radiation exposure based on the National Dose Registry of Canada in a study that included a cohort of 191,333 persons with an average dose for males of 11.5 mSv and an average dose for the cohort of 6.64 mSv.[153] The SIR for uterine cancer was significantly reduced at 0.71. In the United States, Gilbert's study of the Hanford workers from 1945–1986 yielded an SMR of 0.63 for uterine cancer.[361] Frome reported a mortality study of 106,020 employees in the nuclear industry at Oak Ridge, Tennessee, in whom the SMR for cancers of the cervix and uterus in black and white females was nonsignificant.[160]

Cardis et al. reported on cancer mortality among nuclear industry workers in three countries in a large study of 95,673 workers with over 2 million person-years at risk and 15,825 deaths.[166] The trend for cervical cancer was nonsignificantly decreased at 0.63 with a P value of 0.226. For uterine cancer the trend was significantly increased at 1.17 with a P value of 0.092. Cardis et al. also have reported the cancer mortality results from a 15-country collaborative study of nuclear workers. This is the largest occupational study to date and included a cohort of 407,391 workers with 18,993 deaths and 5.2 million person-years of follow-up.[168] The ERR per Sv for cervical cancer was nonsignificantly negative at −0.11 (90% CI < 0, 131) and for other cancers of the uterus the ERR per Sv was nonsignificantly elevated at 0.16 (90% CI < 0, 94.1).

McGeoghegan et al. have reported on the mortality of 12,540 workers (including 3244 radiation workers) at the Capenhurst uranium enrichment facility during 1946–1995.[242] No case of uterine caner was identified in radiation workers. They also studied cancer mortality experience of 19,454 workers (including 13,960 radiation workers) at the Springfields uranium production facility during 1946–1995 in whom the SMR for uterine cancer was nonsignificantly elevated for radiation workers at 2.25.[243]

The cancer incidence among medical diagnostic radiation workers in China has been reviewed by Wang et al. in a study which included 27,011 such workers with 25,782 persons in other medical specialties.[102] The x-ray workers had a 50% higher risk of developing cancer, RR 1.5, and for cancer of the uterine cervix the RR was 4.6. This increase was not statistically significant, however, because it was based on only three cases observed versus 0.66 expected. Doody et al. reported on mortality among 143,517 U.S. radiologic technologists during 1926–1990.[97] Doses were not evaluated. The SMR for uterine cancer was nonsignificantly reduced at 0.87 (95% CI 0.59, 1.13) and the SMR for cervical cancer was significantly

reduced at 0.27 (95% CI 0.16, 0.39). Sigurdson et al. studied cancer incidence in 90,305 U.S. radiologic technologists and found that the SIR for uterine and cervical cancer considered together was significantly reduced at 0.80 (95% CI 0.69, 0.90).[101] Mohan et al. studied cancer and other causes of mortality among 146,022 radiologic technologists employed from 1940 and later in whom the SMRs for both uterine and cervical cancer were significantly reduced at 0.31 (95% CI 0.2, 0.4).[98,99]

Medical Exposure

The influence of diagnostic medical radiation on the risk of uterine cancer has been studied only in regard to the repeated fluoroscopies of the chest in Massachusetts TB patients. In one study Davis et al. reported that the SMR for cancer of the cervix was significantly elevated only for the unexposed controls with a value of 1.9, and not in the exposed patients.[105] In another report Davis et al. observed that the SMR for cervical cancer was nonsignificantly elevated for exposed females (1.9) as well as for unexposed females (1.8).[364] Eight cases were reported in each group. Darby et al. pointed out that uterine cancer mortality was not increased in patients treated for ankylosing spondylitis, the O/E ratio being 1.02.[109] Follow-up of patients who received intrauterine radium radiotherapy for benign uterine bleeding has been performed by Inskip et al.[118] The study included 4153 women who were studied over 110,000 person-years at risk. No increase in cancer of the uterine cervix was observed, but there was a significant increase in all uterine cancers as a group. The median dose to the uterus was estimated to be 32 Gy. The authors acknowledged that whether the increase was radiation-related was difficult to ascertain, because hormonal abnormalities would predispose to both uterine bleeding and subsequent cancer. The increase was not related to organ dose over the range from 10 to 60 Gy, but in this dose range there are undoubtedly cell-killing effects. Mattsson et al. have reported on cancer incidence among 3090 women who received radiation therapy for benign breast disease in whom the RR for uterine cancer was nonsignificantly elevated at 1.12.[114]

Studies of secondary cancers in women treated for carcinoma of the cervix do not demonstrate an increase in subsequent uterine cancer even though doses are on the order of 150 Gy to portions of the uterus. Some of this may be the result of cell killing. In a cohort study of women treated for cervical cancer, 82,616 exposed women were compared with 99,424 unexposed controls.[124] The women were from Canada, Denmark, Finland, Norway, Sweden, Yugoslavia, the United Kingdom, and the United States and were followed over 1.28 million person-years at risk during which there was a significant decrease in cancer of the uterus. In patients treated for invasive cervical cancer, the O/E ratio for uterine cancer was 0.6 for those treated with radiotherapy and 0.1 for those treated without radiotherapy. In patients

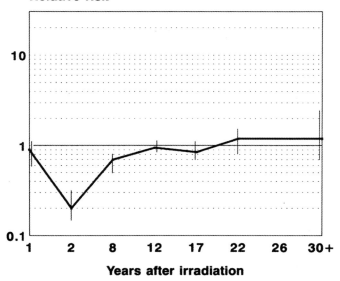

Relative risk

Years after irradiation

Uterine cancer (cervix series)

Figure 5-16 • RR of uterine cancer by time after treatment for cervical carcinoma with radiation therapy. Error bars indicate 95% CI. (From Boice JD, Jr, et al: Second cancers following radiation treatment for cervical cancer: An international collaboration among cancer registries. J Natl Cancer Inst 1985;74:955–975.)

who were followed for 10 years or more, the O/E ratio was not much different. The RR for uterine cancer over time is shown in Figure 5-16, and it can be seen that the RR does not significantly rise above unity for any of the eight data points.

In a large case-control study 4188 women who developed second cancers after treatment for cancer of the cervix were compared with 6880 matched controls.[126] The RR for cancer of the uterus was 1.34 (90% CI 0.8 to 2.3). In a Japanese study of women also treated for cancer of the cervix, the O/E ratio for uterine cancer was significantly reduced, at 0.5 in those treated with radiotherapy.[128] In another study by Ewertz et al., uterine corpus tumors were not increased.[712] In one publication Parkash et al. report, for example, on six cases of uterine papillary serous carcinoma after radiotherapy.[713] However, conclusions derived from such case reports need to be taken in the context of the findings of much larger and scientifically designed studies.

Internal Exposure

The studies examining uterine cancer after administration of radioiodine have generally yielded nonsignificant results. Among studies of the potential carcinogenic effects of diagnostic doses of radioiodine administered to perform thyroid scanning, the largest and most recent included 35,074 patients who were matched with the Swedish cancer registry.[270] In this group there was no increase in cancer of the female genital organs and the

SIR was 0.86 (95% CI 0.78, 0.94). After treatment for hyperthyroidism, Hoffman et al. indicated a nonsignificantly elevated RR of 2.3 (95% CI 0.6, 9.0) for uterine cancer.[202] In a much larger study Holm et al. reported no increase in cancer of the female genital organs as a group, the combined SIR being 1.00 (95% CI 0.85, 1.15).[271] Ron et al. have reported on cancer mortality among 35,593 hyperthyroid patients.[201] The SMR for uterine cancer was significantly reduced at 0.69 (95% CI 0.54, 0.88) for those receiving any iodine 131 and 0.61 (95% CI 0.38, 0.93) for those receiving only iodine.

During treatment for thyroid cancer the quantities of radioiodine administered are 10 to 20 times higher than for treatment of hyperthyroidism so that one would expect the absorbed doses to be higher by about the same amount. Edmonds et al. reported that in a series of 365 patients, there was no excess of uterine cancer.[204] In a much larger series, Hall et al. found an excess risk for female genital organs as a group, with an SIR of 2.03 (95% CI 1.20, 3.20).[203]

Some patients who have received Thorotrast for diagnostic medical purposes (such as angiograms) had a significant residual amount of activity in the abdomen, especially the liver, spleen, and lymph nodes. While these patients have shown a highly increased risk of liver tumors, there has been no consistent increase in uterine cancer. In a Danish Thorotrast series the SIR for cancer of the cervix uteri was 1.2 (95% CI 0.4, 2.6), and for the corpus uteri it was 0.4 (95% CI 0.0, 2.1).[213] A study by Nekolla et al. of 455 patients treated with radium 224 for TB, ankylosing spondylitis, and a few other diseases indicated that uterine cancer occurred in five and the rate ratio was nonsignificantly elevated at 1.9.[224] Nyberg et al. reported on cancer incidence after a 40-year follow-up among Swedish patients exposed to radioactive Thorotrast in whom the SIR for uterine corpus cancer was nonsignificantly elevated.[222]

A report on the Sellafield plant by Omar et al. indicated there were no cases of uterine cancer among plutonium workers.[148] Carpenter et al. examined workers in the United Kingdom who were occupationally exposed to tritium, plutonium, and other radionuclides and the SMRs for uterine cancer in each group were all nonsignificantly different from unity.[191]

Summary

The epidemiologic literature does not support radiation induction of uterine neoplasms. While there are a few anecdotal case reports in the literature, these should not be taken to prove a causal relationship. In fact, the epidemiologic literature, which is vastly stronger, cannot identify a relationship. As a result none of the major scientific consensus groups including BEIR V[3] and ICRP[250] have given risk estimates for uterine neoplasms. UNSCEAR 2006 has summarized those epidemiological studies that provide risk factors for uterine cancer

Table 5-18 • Risk Estimates for Cancer Incidence and Mortality from Studies of Radiation Exposure: Uterine Cancer*

Study	Average Excess Relative Risk at 1 Sv	Average Excess Absolute Risk $(10^4 PYSv)^{-1}$	Study	Average Excess Relative Risk at 1 Sv	Average Excess Absolute Risk $(10^4 PYSv)^{-1}$
External Low-LET Exposures			**External Low-LET Exposures—cont'd**		
Incidence			Mortality—cont'd		
A-bomb Life Span Study[319]			Time since exposure		
Age at exposure			12–15	0.31 (<0–1.23)	<0 (<0–0.26)
<20	0.38 (<0–0.9)	0.75 (<0–2.59)	15–30	<0 (<0–<0)	<0 (<0–0.07)
20–40	<0 (<0–0.33)	0.20 (<0–2.85)	>30	0.52 (0.01–1.24)	<0 (<0–1229.1)
>40	<0 (<0–0.41)	0.09 (<0–4.88)	All	0.09 (<0–0.44)	<0 (<0–0.33)
Time since exposure			Benign gynecological		
12–15	<0 (<0–0.28)	<0 (<0–1.61)	disorders[118]		
15–30	<0 (<0–0.09)	<0 (<0–0.67)	All uterus	0.006	0.14
>30	0.53 (0.17–0.99)	2.86 (0.83–5.31)	Cervix	−0.01	−0.02
All	0.10 (<0–0.32)	0.09 (<0–1.48)	Metropathia[116]		
Cervical cancer[126]			All uterus	0.09	0.24
Age at treatment			Cervix	0.06	0.09
<45	0.0023	NA	Spondylitis[266]		
45–54	0.0048	NA	All uterus	−0.01	−0.02
55–64	0.0008		Cervix	−0.13	−0.18
≥65	0.0000		Other uterus	0.18	0.16
Time since treatment			IARC 15-country nuclear		
1–<5	−0.0045		workers study[167,168]		
5–<10	0.0024		Cervix	−0.11 (<0, 131)	NA
10–<15	−0.0020		Other uterus	0.16 (<0, 94.1)	NA
≥15	0.0307				
Mortality			**Internal High-LET Exposures**		
A-bomb Life Span Study[281]			Incidence		
Age at exposure			Danish and Swedish		
<20	0.42 (<0–1.68)	<0 (<0–333.82)	Thorotrast patients[219]		
20–40	0.17 (<0–0.77)	<0 (<0–1.61)	Uterine cervix	0.6 (0.2–1.8)	NA
>40	<0 (<0–0.51)	<0 (<0–3.53)	Uterine corpus	0.6 (0.2–1.8)	NA

*The studies listed are those for which quantitative estimates of risk could be made.
Adapted from United Nations Scientific Committee of the Effects of Atomic Radiation (UNSCEAR): Sources and effects of ionizing radiation: 2006 report to the General Assembly with annexes. New York, United Nations, 2007.

following radiation exposure (Table 5-18) and concluded that there is no strong ionizing dose response for uterine cancer and that the absence of an association between cervical cancer and radiation is a consistent finding even after very high radiation doses.[86] They also concluded that for cancer of the uterine corpus (endometrial cancer) the evidence is largely negative and that if there is an association with radiation it is confined to very high doses. The 2006 National Academy of Sciences Committee on Radiation Screening and Compensation Programs Report was more definite and concluded that there is no convincing epidemiologic evidence that uterine cancer is induced by ionizing radiation.[257]

PROSTATE CANCER

General

Prostate cancer is the most common cancer in elderly males, and the highest rates in the world are observed in U.S. blacks. Rates in U.S. whites are about one half those in blacks. Many elderly males have nonsymptomatic tumors, and in autopsy series more than 50% of males over the age of 80 have microscopic evidence of this tumor. The causes of the tumor remain generally obscure. At various times sexual activity, vasectomy, dietary fat intake, hormonal factors, and cirrhosis have been implicated as causes but have yet to be confirmed. Radiation does not appear to be a cause of prostate cancer.[358,700]

External Exposure

Background Radiation and Populations Near Nuclear Installations

In a study of the influence of terrestrial radiation in Connecticut on cancer mortality, Walter et al. found that the incidence of prostate cancer was higher in the low-background areas.[21] Increased exposure to natural cosmic radiation occurs to airline crews and there have been a number of studies including information on their

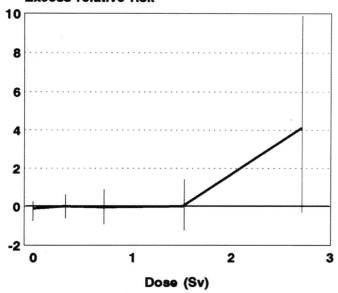

Excess relative risk

Prostate cancer incidence (A-bomb)

Figure 5-17 • ERR of cancer of the prostate in atomic bomb survivors at different dose levels. Bars indicate 95% CI. (From Thompson D, Mabuchi K, Ron E, et al: Cancer incidence in atomic bomb survivors. II: Solid tumors, 1958–1987. RERF Technical Report 5-92, Hiroshima, Japan, Radiation Effects Research Foundation, 1992.)

risks of prostate cancer. Pukkala et al. studied over 10,000 Nordic airline pilots and found a nonsignificant increase in prostate cancer.[39] Band et al. studied 2740 pilots at doses of 6 mSv per year and employed for an average of 20 years, for a total average dose about 120 mSv, and found that they had a significantly increased SIR and a nonsignificantly increased SMR.[40] There are three papers concerning potential environmental uranium contamination and the possibility of increased risk of prostate cancer in the public. The papers by Boice et al. indicated a nonsignificant decrease around a uranium mining and milling facilities in Texas and in Pennsylvania, and a nonsignificant increase near a Colorado facility.[89,90,90a]

Atomic Bomb Survivors

The incidence data for prostate cancer in atomic bomb survivors are shown graphically in Figure 5-17, where it is apparent that there was no excess except for 1 point at 2.5 Sv.[280] In the 1958–1997 update, Preston et al. reported a nonsignificant ERR per Gy of 0.11 (90% CI −0.10, 0.54) and EAR of 0.34 (90% CI −0.64, 1.6) per 10^4PYGy.[319] The estimated excess cases were 4 in a total of 387 cases. In the 1958–1987 LSS mortality study of atomic bomb survivors, the calculated ERR at 1 Sv was 0.3 (95% CI −0.3, 1.6), and the EAR was 0.2 (95% CI −0.2, 0.9) × $(10^4$PYSv$)^{-1}$. In the 2003 update studies by Preston et al. of mortality of atomic bomb survivors

during 1950–1997 it was found that in males there was a nonsignificant excess of prostate cancer at dose levels of 1 Sv amounting to an ERR of 0.21 (90% CI < −0.3, 0.96).[281]

Occupational Exposure

Few occupational studies of external exposure have shown a relationship between radiation and prostate cancer. In the United Kingdom, Darby et al. studied radiation workers in experimental government programs and reported an SMR of 1.88 but an RR for prostate cancer that was significantly low at 0.38 (90% CI 0.17, 0.80) compared with controls.[52] In the latest 2004 review Muirhead et al. studied a cohort of 21,357 test partipants and reported a nonsignificantly increased SMR of 1.15 (95% CI 0.94, 1.39) for prostate cancer in test participants and a nonsignificantly decreased SMR compared to controls.[55] The RR for incidence was nonsignificantly elevated at 1.22 compared to controls.

For other nuclear workers Beral et al., in studying over 39,000 atomic energy workers, did not find an increase and reported an SMR of 1.00 (95% CI 0.67, 1.45) for prostate cancer.[143] In a similar study of atomic weapons workers Beral et al. found the ratio in the rates of exposed versus nonexposed to be 2.23 (95% CI 1.13, 4.40) for prostate cancer.[144] Although this suggested a statistically significant association between accumulated dose and prostate cancer, this excess is not necessarily causally related because as workers accumulate dose they get older, and as they get older the natural incidence of prostate cancer rises. To carry the argument in the other direction, accumulated dose is related to age, but it is not the cause of the age. A study of 95,000 U.K. atomic workers by Kendall et al. found a nonsignificantly elevated SMR of 1.10 for prostate cancer.[145] A second expanded analysis of the same group of 124,743 workers in the U.K. National Registry of Radiation Workers carried out by Muirhead et al. in 1999 using a lagged analysis indicated a nonsignificantly reduced SMR for prostate cancer of 0.98 (95% CI 0.86, 1.13).[146] At Sellafield in the United Kingdom, Smith et al. report a nonsignificantly elevated SMR of 1.20 for prostate cancer.[360] McGeoghegan et al. reported on the mortality and cancer morbidity experience of employees at the Chapelcross plant of British Nuclear Fuels during 1955–1995 who made up a cohort of 2628 workers with median doses of 39 mSv.[149] In radiation workers the SMR for cancer of the prostate was nonsignificant at 1.00. A report on the Sellafield plant by Omar et al. indicated a nonsignificant increase in prostate cancer among non-plutonium radiation workers with an SMR of 1.07 but with an incidence that was nonsignificantly decreased.[148]

Ashmore et al. reported the first analysis of mortality and occupational radiation exposure based on the National Dose Registry of Canada which included a cohort of 206,620 individuals and 5426 deaths.[154] The average exposure for males was 10.6 mSv and their SMR for prostate cancer was nonsignificantly decreased at 0.86 (90% CI 0.70, 1.05). Sont et al. also reported on a study of cancer incidence and occupational radiation exposure based on the National Dose Registry of Canada, which included a cohort of 191,333 persons with an average dose of 11.5 mSv for males in whom the SIR for prostate cancer was significantly reduced at 0.83.[153] In 2004 Zablotska et al. reported on mortality of Canadian nuclear workers and concluded that for prostate cancer there was a nonsignificantly decreased SMR of 0.75 (95% CI 0.49, 1.1).[155]

Artalejo et al. reported on the occupational exposure to ionizing radiation and mortality among 5657 workers of the former Spanish Nuclear Energy Board whose mean exposure was 11.42 mSv.[151] The SMR for prostate cancer was nonsignificantly reduced at 0.73 (95% CI 0.29, 1.51). Iwasaki et al. conducted an analysis of mortality of nuclear industry workers in Japan.[150] The study included 176,000 male workers with 5527 deaths. For average annual doses that were 3.5 mSv before 1982 and 1.2 mSv after 1982, the SMR for prostate cancer was nonsignificantly decreased at 0.95 (95% CI 0.65, 1.34). Habib et al. have reported on cancer incidence among Australian nuclear industry–monitored radiation workers and indicated a nonsignificantly decreased SIR of 0.96 for prostate cancer.[152] Rahu et al. studied the cancer incidence of 5446 male Latvian and Estonian Chernobyl cleanup workers and reported that no cases of prostate cancer were found.[178]

In the United States several occupational studies have reported findings relative to prostate cancer. In a study of Hanford workers from 1945–1986, Gilbert et al. reported an SMR of 0.96 for prostate cancer, with no real difference between radiation-monitored male workers and those who did not work with radiation.[361] In a combined analysis of several federal facilities, Gilbert et al. also reported SMRs for prostate cancer as follows: 1.00 at Hanford, 1.36 (95% CI 0.7 to 2.3) at Oak Ridge, and 0.97 at Rocky Flats.[157] Fry et al. reported a study of mortality and morbidity among 3145 persons occupationally exposed to 50 or more mSv (5000 mrem) in a year, in whom the mean external exposure was 153 mSv, and the SMR for prostate cancer was nonsignificantly elevated.[161]

Cragle et al. indicated that cancer of the prostate in workers at the Savannah River plant was less frequent than expected both in workers paid on an hourly basis and in the combined group of hourly and salaried workers, with SMRs of 0.60 and 0.47, respectively. In a group of salaried workers, the SMR was nonsignificantly elevated at 1.35.[288] In a study of workers at the Mound facility, Wiggs et al. reported that the SMR for prostate cancer was nonsignificantly elevated at 1.86 (95% CI 0.68 to 4.06).[156] Frome reported a mortality study of 106,020 employees in the nuclear industry at Oak Ridge, Tennessee.[160] The SMR for cancer of the prostate in black and white males was nonsignificant. Howe et al.

studied the mortality of U.S. nuclear power industry workers and found them to have a nonsignificantly decreased risk of prostate cancer with an SMR of 0.60 (95% CI 0.33, 1.01).[159]

In a study of 8977 male Canadian atomic energy workers Gribbin et al. reported a nonsignificantly elevated SMR of 1.42 (95% CI 0.71 to 1.94) for prostate cancer.[260] Finally, Wilkinson et al. reported a nonsignificantly elevated SMR of 1.21 (90% CI 0.71 to 2.56) for prostate cancer at the Rocky Flats weapons facility.[286] In a study of Oak Ridge workers Checkoway et al. reported an SMR of 0.92 (95% CI 0.37 to 1.90) for prostate cancer.[284] In yet another study of Oak Ridge workers, Wing et al. found a nonsignificant increase in prostate cancer, with an SMR of 1.12 (95% CI 0.53 to 2.05).[285]

Cardis et al. investigated cancer mortality among nuclear industry workers in three countries in a very large study of 95,673 workers with over 2 million person-years at risk and 15,825 deaths.[166] The trend for prostate cancer was nonsignificantly reduced at −1.68 with a P value of 0.953. Cardis et al. have reported the cancer mortality results from a 15-country collaborative study of nuclear workers.[168] This is the largest occupational study to date and included a cohort of 407,391 workers with 18,993 deaths and 5.2 million person-years of follow-up. The ERR per Sv for prostate cancer was nonsignificantly positive at 0.77 (90% CI < 0, 4.58).

An increase in prostate cancer was reported by Ennow et al. in a study of 4281 Danish radiotherapists employed between 1954–1982.[714] An RR of 6.25 was reported. This finding must be taken in context. In actuality there were only four cases of cancer identified. How four cases of prostate cancer could result in an RR of over 6 is unclear, and the high RR value is suspect. In contrast, a nonsignificant increase in prostate cancer was reported by Smith et al. in British radiologists employed before 1921 (O/E ratio 1.61), and no increase was found in those employed after that time (O/E ratio 0.71).[584] Berrington et al. reported on 100 years of experience among U.K. radiologists in whom they found a nonsignificantly increased SMR for prostate cancer of 2.14 for those employed from 1897–1920 and a nonsignificantly increased SMR of 1.26 for those employed after 1920.[94] Doody et al. studied the mortality among 143,517 U.S. radiologic technologists during 1926–1990 whose doses were not evaluated and they found the SMR for prostate cancer was nonsignificantly reduced at 0.79 (95% CI 0.56, 1.08).[97] Sigurdson et al. investigated the cancer incidence in 90,305 U.S. radiologic technologists in whom they found that the SIR for prostate cancer was nonsignificantly elevated at 1.02 (95% CI 0.89, 1.16).[101] Mohan et al. studied cancer and other causes of mortality among 146,022 radiologic technologists employed from 1940 and later, in whom they found the SMR for prostate cancer nonsignificantly reduced at 0.89 (95% CI 0.7, 1.1).[98,99]

Medical Exposure

A study of Massachusetts TB patients who received many fluoroscopies during the course of treatment did not show a radiation-related increase in prostate cancer. The SMRs for prostate cancer were 1.2 in the exposed males and 1.1 in the unexposed controls.[364] Studies of patients who received radiation therapy for benign conditions have been performed. In one study of 14,554 patients treated for ankylosing spondylitis, for example, cancer of the prostate was not significantly elevated with a reported O/E of 1.16.[109] Carr et al. performed a follow-up study of 3719 patients treated with radiotherapy for peptic ulcer with doses to the abdomen of about 15 Gy, and found that the RR for prostate cancer after radiotherapy in the period 0 to 10 years postexposure was nonsignificantly reduced at 0.29 and in the follow-up period of 11 to 62 years postexposure it was also nonsignificantly reduced at 0.84.[113]

Internal Exposure

In a study of Swedish Lapps who may ingest more cesium 137 than other populations, Wiklund et al. have found a significant decrease of prostate cancer. They report an SIR of 0.30 (95% CI 0.12 to 0.63).[56] Darby et al. studied radon and cancers in Swedish iron miners and found a nonsignificant increase in prostate cancer with an O/E ratio of 1.20 (95% CI 0.81, 1.73).[183] A study of uranium miners by Waxweiler et al. has reported a nonsignificant increase in cancer of the prostate with an SMR of 1.18 (95% CI 0.47 to 2.43).[362] A study of uranium enrichment workers by Brown et al., while not reporting prostate cancer separately, did report a significantly lower than expected SMR for cancers of all male genital organs of 0.16 (95% CI 0.03 to 0.86).[363] Ritz et al. have reported on cancer mortality in uranium processing workers at the Fernald plant in Ohio.[192] The SMR for prostate cancer was nonsignificantly increased at 1.44. Dupree-Ellis et al. have reported on mortality in a cohort of 2514 uranium processing workers employed between 1942–1966 at the Mallinkrodt Chemical Works; their SMR for prostate cancer was nonsignificantly increased at 1.15.[193] McGeoghegan et al., in reporting on the mortality of 12,540 workers (including 3244 radiation workers) at the Capenhurst uranium enrichment facility during 1946–1995, indicated that the SMR for prostate cancer was nonsignificantly reduced in radiation workers at 0.79.[242] They also studied the cancer mortality experience of 19,454 workers (including 13,960 radiation workers) at the Springfields uranium production facility during 1946–1995 and observed that the SMR for prostate cancer was nonsignificantly reduced for radiation workers at 0.89.[243]

Occupational internal contamination from plutonium has not been associated with an increase in prostate cancer. In a 42-year follow-up of the Manhattan Project workers, no cases of prostate cancer were found.[715] In a study of Rocky Flats workers who received a body burden of at least 74 Bq (2 nCi) of plutonium, Wilkinson et al. reported nonsignificantly increased RRs for prostate cancer of 3.74 (90% CI 0.29 to 42.3) and 4.90 (90% CI 0.38 to 55.8), using a biologically implausible 2- and 5-year latent period, and an RR of 10.6 (90% CI 0.76 to 127.15) using a reasonable 10-year latent period.[286] However, these estimates were based on only two observed cases in the exposed group and one in the unexposed group. In a study by Wing et al. workers monitored for internal contamination had an SMR for prostate cancer of 1.12 (95% CI 0.53 to 2.05).[285] A report on the Sellafield plant by Omar et al. indicated a nonsignificant increase in prostate cancer with an SMR of 1.03 in plutonium workers whose incidence of prostate cancer was nonsignificantly decreased.[148] Wiggs et al. found an RR of 1.00 for prostate cancer in a follow-up of Los Alamos plutonium workers.[164] Carpenter et al. examined workers in the United Kingdom who were occupationally exposed to tritium, plutonium, and other radionuclides.[191] The SMRs for prostate cancer in the tritium and plutonium group were nonsignificantly different from unity, although the SMR for the "other radionuclides"–exposed group was significantly elevated with an SMR of 1.53.

The few studies examining prostate cancer after administration of radioiodine have yielded generally negative results. Among studies of the potential carcinogenic effects of diagnostic doses of radioiodine administered to perform thyroid scanning, the largest and most recent included 35,074 patients who were matched with the Swedish cancer registry.[270] No increase in cancer of the male genital organs as a group was observed in the exposed men and their SIR was 0.98 (95% CI 0.84, 1.14).

After treatment for hyperthyroidism, Holm et al. reported no increase in cancer of the male genital organs as a group, and there was a combined SIR of 1.00 (95% CI 0.79, 1.25).[271] During treatment for thyroid cancer the quantities of radioiodine that are administered are 10 to 20 times higher than for treatment of hyperthyroidism. Hall et al. found that there was no excess risk for male genital organs as a group, the SIR being 0.85 (95% CI 0.23, 2.18).[203] Ron et al. have reported on cancer mortality among 35,593 hyperthyroid patients in whom the SMR for prostate cancer was significantly reduced at 0.67 (95% CI 0.47, 0.93) for those receiving any iodine 131 and 0.50 (95% CI 0.24, 0.91) for those receiving only iodine.[201]

Thorotrast, a contrast medium that was used widely for angiography, and to a much lesser extent for sinus studies, remains in the body. It has been associated with leukemia, tumors of the liver, gallbladder, bile ducts, and in cases where the material was directly instilled and remained in place, cancer of the nasal sinuses. In a Danish Thorotrast series the SIR for prostate cancer was not significantly elevated, at 1.5 (95% CI 0.6 to 3.3).[213] In a German series there were 16 cases in the

Thorotrast-injected patients, versus 11 in the control group, which did not represent a statistically significant increase.[211] A study by Nekolla et al. of 455 patients treated with radium 224 for TB, ankylosing spondylitis, and a few other diseases indicated that the frequency of prostate cancer in such patients was nonsignificantly elevated with a rate ratio of 1.2.[224] Nyberg et al. reported on cancer incidence after a 40-year follow-up among Swedish patients exposed to radioactive Thorotrast.[222] The SIR for prostate cancer was nonsignificantly elevated.

Summary

A large number of epidemiological studies have looked for an increased risk of prostate cancer after radiation exposure. At the present time there is no clear evidence that prostate cancer is induced by radiation. Because prostate cancer is very common, and the incidence rates increase rapidly with age, any study that purports to show a dose-related increase should account for this bias factor. The BEIR V Committee does not give a risk estimate for the disease and only indicates that "although the data suggest there may be a weak association between prostate cancer and radiation, the sensitivity of the prostate to the induction of cancer by irradiation appears to be comparatively low."[3] Neither the UNSCEAR 1988,[370] 1994,[369] 2000,[375] and 2006[86] reports, nor the ICRP 1990[248] report has ever provided risk estimates for prostate cancer induction. The UNSCEAR 2006 Committee report has summarized risk estimates for prostate cancer from various epidemiological studies (Table 5-19) and concluded that there is little indication of radiation effects on prostate cancer risks.[86] The 2006 National Academy of Sciences Committee on Radiation Screening and Compensation Programs Report was more definite and concluded that there is no convincing epidemiologic evidence that prostate cancer is a radiogenic disease.[257]

PENIS, TESTES, AND SCROTAL CANCER

General

Cancers of the penis and scrotum are relatively rare. The highest incidence rates are in Brazil, and the lowest are in Israel. Rates are low in populations with a high socioeconomic level, suggesting that hygiene is an important factor. Circumcision appears to be protective. Men with penile cancer have a higher risk of having wives with cervical cancer, which may also suggest a viral etiology. Exposure to polycyclic hydrocarbons, mineral oils, and shale oils is associated with an increase in the frequency of squamous cell carcinoma of the scrotum (particularly in chimney sweeps).[358,700] Cancer of the testes usually occurs in white males under the age of 50. It is very rare in Asians and Africans. Rates in U.S. blacks are about one quarter those in whites. The causes of testicular tumors are largely unknown, but undescended

testes and gonadal dysgenesis and dysfunction appear to be related to increased risk.

External Exposure

Neither the 1958–1998 incidence[279–281,319,716] nor the mortality studies[717] of the atomic bomb survivors has reported an increase in tumors of male genital organs. Virtually none of the very large studies of external occupational exposure have shown a statistically significant risk of penis, testes, or scrotal cancer. The U.K. study by Darby et al. included 22,347 workers exposed to fallout and who worked in experimental government programs.[52] With over 440,000 person-years of observation the RR for testicular cancer was 1.01 (90% CI 0.41 to 2.46). Another U.K. study by Beral et al. included 39,546 atomic energy workers and over 630,000 person-years of observation and reported a nonsignificant elevation of testicular cancer with an SMR of 1.53 (95% CI 0.73, 2.81).[143] In a similar study of atomic weapons workers, they reported that the ratio of the rates for testes cancer between exposed and nonexposed employees was nonsignificantly increased at 4.61 (95% CI 0.02, 1032.2).[144] In a third U.K. study by Kendall et al., which included 95,217 workers and over 1.2 million person-years at risk, a nonstatistically significant decreased SMR for testicular cancer of 0.79 was observed.[145] In 1999, in a second expanded analysis using a lagged analysis of the same group of 124,743 workers in the U.K. National Registry of Radiation Workers, Muirhead et al. found a nonsignificantly reduced SMR for of 0.71 (95% CI 0.26, 1.54).[146] In a study of the Sellafield workers in the United Kingdom, Smith et al. report nonsignificantly elevated SMRs for testicular cancer in both radiation workers and other workers.[360] The values were 1.57 and 1.61, respectively. McGeoghegan et al. reported on the cancer mortality and morbidity experience of employees at the Chapelcross plant of British Nuclear Fuels during 1955–1995.[149] The cohort included 2628 workers with median doses of 39 mSv. In radiation workers, no case of testicular cancer was identified.

Sont et al. reported on the relation between the incidence of cancer and occupational radiation exposure based on the National Dose Registry of Canada, which included a cohort of 191,333 persons with an average dose for males of 11.5 mSv and an average dose for the cohort of 6.64 mSv.[153] The SIR for testicular cancer in this group was nonsignificantly elevated at 1.02. Habib et al. have reported on cancer incidence among Australian nuclear industry–monitored radiation workers and no cases of testicular cancer were identified.[152] Rahu et al. studied the cancer incidence in 5446 male Latvian and Estonian Chernobyl cleanup workers and indicated that they exhibited a nonsignificantly reduced SIR of 0.92 for testicular cancer.[178]

Most of the U.S. occupational studies yield similar findings. Gilbert et al., reporting on Hanford workers

Table 5-19 • Risk Estimates for Cancer Incidence and Mortality from Studies of Radiation Exposure: Prostate Cancer*

Study	Average Excess Relative Risk at 1 Sv	Average Excess Absolute Risk $(10^4 PYSv)^{-1}$
External Low-LET Exposures		
Incidence		
A-bomb Life Span Study[319]		
Age at exposure		
<20	0.12 (<0–1.38)	<0 (<0–0.42)
20–40	0.03 (<0–0.7)	<0 (<0–1.84)
>40	0.11 (<0–0.7)	<0 (<0–2.96)
Time since exposure		
12–15	<0 (<0–1.14)	<0 (<0–325.76)
15–30	<0 (<0–0.31)	<0 (<0–0.38)
>30	0.36 (<0–0.93)	<0 (<0–2207.9)
All	0.12 (<0–0.51)	<0 (<0–0.38)
Canada National Dose Registry[153]	0.1 (<0–3.5)	NA
Capenhurst uranium facility[242]	−1.31 (<−1.31–12.76)	NA
U.K. Springfields uranium workers[243]	0.41 (<−2.90–9.27)	NA
Mortality		
A-bomb Life Span Study[281]		
Age at exposure		
<20	<0 (<0 – >10,000)	<0 (<0–45.63)
20–40	<0 (<0–1.1)	<0 (<0–473.9)
>40	1.01 (0.01–2.78)	<0 (<0–910.84)
Time since exposure		
5–15	<0 (<0–0.38)	<0 (<0–59.26)
15–30	<0 (<0–1.33)	<0 (<0–184.91)
>30	0.69 (<0–0.97)	<0 (<0–623.82)
All	0.4 (<0–1.31)	<0 (<0–298.22)
Ankylosing spondylitis[266]	0.14 (0.02–0.28)	NA
Peptic ulcer[113]	−1.6 (<−1.6–4.5)	NA
Nuclear workers in Canada, United Kingdom, United States[166]	<0	NA
U.K. National Registry for Radiation Workers[146]	0.29 (−1.13–2.95)	NA
Nuclear power industry workers in the U.S.[159]	−2.5 (<−2.51–26.4)	NA
U.S. Oak Ridge workers, 1943–1947[267]	NA	NA
U.S. Oak Ridge X-10 and Y-12[160]	2.06 (<0–24.6)	NA
U.S. Los Alamos Laboratory workers[164]	<0	NA
IARC 15-country nuclear workers study[167,168]	0.77 (<0, 4.58)	NA
Internal High-LET Exposures		
Incidence		
^{224}Ra TB and ankylosing spondylitis patients[224]	∼1.3	NA
Danish and Swedish Thorotrast patients[219]	4.5 (1.6–16.3)	NA
Mortality		
German Thorotrast patients[221]	∼0.9	NA
U.S. Thorotrast patients[219]	0.2 (0–5.1)	NA

*The studies listed are those for which quantitative estimates of risk could be made.
Adapted from United Nations Scientific Committee of the Effects of Atomic Radiation (UNSCEAR): Sources and effects of ionizing radiation: 2006 report to the General Assembly with annexes. New York, United Nations, 2007.

during 1945–1986, found an SMR of 0.82 for cancer of the testes and other male genital organs.[361] The SMR was 0.71 in radiation workers and 1.44 in the nonradiation workers. Very few references to testicular, scrotal, or penile cancer are reported in most epidemiologic studies concerning medical exposure. Frome reported a mortality study of 106,020 employees in the nuclear industry at Oak Ridge, Tennessee, in whom the SMR for cancer of the testes in black and white males was nonsignificantly reduced.[160] Groves et al. conducted a 40-year cancer mortality study of 40,581 Korean War Navy veterans with potential exposure to high-intensity radar which also emit ionizing radiation.[165] The SMR for testicular cancer in such veterans was nonsignificantly decreased at 0.60 (95% CI 0.25, 1.43). Doody et al. reported on mortality among 143,517 U.S. radiologic technologists during 1926–1990.[97] Doses were not evaluated. The SMR for testicular cancer was nonsignificantly reduced at 0.39 (95% CI 0.08, 1.08). Sigurdson et al. studied cancer incidence in 90,305 U.S. radiologic technologists and found that the SIR for testicular cancer was nonsignificantly elevated at 1.32 (95% CI 0.76, 2.13).[101] Mohan et al. studied cancer and other causes of mortality among 146,022 radiologic technologists employed from 1940 and later and reported that the SMR for testicular cancer was nonsignificantly reduced at 0.55 (95% CI 0.2, 1.3).[98,99]

Cardis et al. investigated cancer mortality among nuclear industry workers in three countries in a very large study of 95,673 workers with over 2 million person-years at risk and 15,825 deaths.[166] The trend for testicular cancer in these workers was observed to be nonsignificantly reduced at −0.26 with a P value of 0.604. Cardis et al. have reported the cancer mortality results from a 15-country collaborative study of nuclear workers.[168] This is the largest occupational study to date and included a cohort of 407,391 workers with 18,993 deaths and 5.2 million person-years of follow-up. The ERR per Sv for testicular cancer was nonsignificantly negative, estimated at less than 0, and had a negative trend value with increasing dose (P value of −0.01).

Ritz et al. have reported on cancer mortality in uranium processing workers at the Fernald plant in Ohio. The SMR for testicular cancer was nonsignificantly reduced at 0.67.[192] Dupree-Ellis et al. have reported on mortality in a cohort of 2514 uranium processing workers employed between 1942–1966 at the Mallinkrodt Chemical Works.[193] The SMR for testicular cancer was nonsignificantly reduced at 0.93. McGeoghegan et al. have reported on the mortality of 12,540 workers (including 3244 radiation workers) at the Capenhurst uranium enrichment facility during 1946–1995.[242] No case of testicular cancer was identified in radiation workers at the site. They also studied cancer mortality experience of 19,454 workers (including 13,960 radiation workers) at the Springfields uranium production facility during 1946–1995.[243] The SMR for testicular cancer was nonsignificantly reduced for radiation workers at 0.61. Darby et al. studied cancers in Swedish iron miners and did not identify any case of testicular cancer.[183]

One case report of a penile angiosarcoma that developed 18 years after radiotherapy for a penile ulcer is reported by Prescott et al.[718] There are several case reports in the literature of soft-tissue sarcomas in other body parts after radiotherapy, but they are rare enough that no definite causal relationship or risk factors can be derived.

Internal Exposure

A decrease in mortality from male genital cancers was found in Swedish Lapps who are presumed to have ingested more cesium 137 than the rest of the Swedish population.[56] The SIR was 0.35 (95% CI 0.15, 0.75). In uranium enrichment workers no increase in cancers of the male genital organs was found by Brown et al. who reported an SMR of 0.16 (95% CI 0.01, 0.86).[363] The few studies examining testicular, scrotal, or penile

cancer after administration of radioiodine have yielded negative results. There have been studies of the potential carcinogenic effects of diagnostic doses of radioiodine administered to perform thyroid scanning. In a large study by Holm et al. there was no increase in cancer of the male genital organs as a group, the SIR being 0.98 (95% CI 0.84, 1.14).[270] After treatment for hyperthyroidism, Holm et al. also reported that there was no increase in cancer of the male genital organs as a group, the combined SIR being 1.00 (95% CI 0.79, 1.25).[271] In a series of patients treated with radioiodine for thyroid cancer, Hall et al. reported that there was no excess risk for male genital organs as a group, reporting an SIR of 0.85 (95% CI 0.23, 2.18).[203] In a Danish Thorotrast series the SIR for cancer of male genital sites other than prostate and testes was nonsignificantly elevated.[213]

A report on the Sellafield plant by Omar et al. indicated a nonsignificant excess of testicular cancer in plutonium workers (based on two cases) but no cases of other male genital cancers.[148] Carpenter et al. examined workers in the United Kingdom who were occupationally exposed to tritium, plutonium, and other radionuclides.[191] The SMRs for testicular cancer were significantly elevated in the tritium exposed group at 8.37, but in the plutonium and other radionuclide exposure groups the SMRs were nonsignificantly different from unity.

Summary

The epidemiologic literature shows no causal association between male genital cancer and radiation exposure. The BEIR V[3] and BEIR VII[18] reports, the 1990 ICRP report,[248] and the 2006 UNSCEAR Report[86] do not give risk estimates for cancer of these sites after radiation exposure. The BEIR V Committee stated that "the existing data imply that the human testis is relatively insensitive to the carcinogenic effects of radiation."[3] The 2006 National Academy of Sciences Committee on Radiation Screening and Compensation Programs Report was more definite and concluded that there is no epidemiologic evidence to suggest that testicular cancer is induced by ionizing radiation.[257]

ESOPHAGEAL CANCER
General

Cancer of the esophagus varies widely in frequency throughout the world. Areas of very high rates include the Caspian region of Iran, the southern regions of the Russian Federation, and western and northern China. Between high and low areas, mortality rates vary by as much as a factor of 100. In the United States incidence rates are fourfold higher in blacks than in whites and this tumor is responsible for over 10,000 deaths annually (more than rectal cancer), representing 0.9% of all cancers and 5% of all gastrointestinal cancers. For reasons which are unclear, the incidence of esophageal adenocarcinoma in the United States is increasing at a rate faster than nearly any other cancer. Americans of Chinese ancestry have incidence rates comparable with those of whites; thus, environmental agents seem to be responsible for most of these tumors. In Curaco, where esophageal cancer is the most common malignant tumor of both men and women, the tumor appears to be due to a cocarcinogen present in an herbal tea and certain roots that are chewed. Nitrosamines also may be responsible for this tumor in some areas. Some studies indicate an association between drinking hot beverages (such as tea) with esophageal cancer. Other reported associations are with nitrates and nitrosamines in the diet, chewing of the betel nut, consumption of pickled foods, and nutritional deficiency.

A relation exists between cancer of the esophagus and smoking.[719] In relation to nonsmokers, RRs are 3.4 for smoking 10 to 19 g of tobacco per day and 5.1 for more than 20 g of tobacco per day. Another well-known relation is that of alcohol consumption. There is a clear dose response with this cancer and daily ethanol consumption. Relative risks are 3.8 to 5.6 for consumption of 41 to 80 g per day, 10 to 11 for 81 to 120 g per day, and about 100 for more than 120 g per day.[358] At present alcohol and tobacco are thought to account for 80% to 90% of esophageal cancer in North and South America, as well as in Europe and Japan.[700]

More than 90% of malignant tumors of the esophagus are squamous cell in type. Adenocarcinomas also may arise either as a result of extension from the stomach or from rests of adenomatous tissue. In these cases, chronic gastric reflux and development of a "Barrett's" esophagus increases the risk of adenocarcinomas. Increased risk of esophageal cancer is found in some vitamin deficiency states such as the Plummer-Vinson syndrome. Many epidemiologic studies searching for an association between radiation and esophageal cancer are negative. As we will see, some of the studies have smoking and alcohol consumption as confounding factors.

External Exposure

Background Radiation and Populations Near Nuclear Facilities

In a very large study conducted in areas of high natural background radiation in China, no increase in esophageal cancer was found.[29,30] The age-adjusted mortality from esophageal cancer in the high-background area was 1.40 per 10^5 per person-years and 1.49 per 10^5 per person-years in the control area.

Another paper on the high-background area of China was published in 2000 by Tao et al. and had 1.7 million person-years of study from 1979–1995.[33] The authors did not find a radiation effect for esophageal cancer.

Increased exposure to natural cosmic radiation occurs in airline crews and there have been a number of studies addressing their risk of various cancers including esophageal cancer. Band et al., in a study of 2740 pilots at doses of 6 mSv per year over an average of 20 years for total average dose of about 120 mSv, found a nonsignificantly decreased SIR and a nonsignificantly decreased SMR.[40]

No increase in cancer of digestive organs was found in populations living near nuclear plants in the United States.[78] For all facilities combined, the SMR was 0.97 before start-up in the study areas and 1.02 after start-up. This can be compared with the slightly higher SMRs in the control areas of 1.03 and 1.04, respectively, before and after start-up. There are three papers concerning potential uranium contamination and the possibility of increased risk of esophageal cancer in the public by Boice et al., which indicated a nonsignificant increase around a uranium mining and milling facility in Texas, a significant decrease near a facility in Pennsylvania, and nonsignificant results near a Colorado facility.[89,90,90a] A nonsignificant decrease was found by Boice et al. in a study of persons residing near the Hanford site.[91] Bauer et al. have reported on cancer mortality due to local fallout from Soviet atmospheric nuclear weapons testing at the Semipalatinsk test site in Kazakhstan.[533] Effective doses ranged from 20 mSv to about 4 Sv. The dose-response LRT for esophageal cancer was nonsignificantly increased in males at a P value of 0.0011 but for females it was significant at less than 0.0001. The estimated ERR per Sv for the exposed cohort was nonsignificantly increased at 0.18 (95% CI −0.09, 0.66).

Atomic Bomb Survivors

Major studies of the atomic bomb survivors include an incidence[319] and a mortality study.[8] The incidence studies included 37,270 exposed persons and 42,702 unexposed controls. The group is 55% female and has a follow-up of 53 years. The incidence study has observed 352 cases of esophageal cancer versus 336 expected. The ERR per Gy is 0.52 (90% CI 0.15, 1.0), and the EAR is 0.58 (90% CI 0.18, 1.1) per $(10^4 PYGy)^{-1}$.[319] In the mortality studies through 1987 there are 1,203,100 person-years of observation and 103 deaths from esophageal cancer versus 91 expected. In the 2003 update studies of mortality of atomic bomb survivors during 1950–1997, Preston et al. investigated a cohort of 86,572 persons with an average external dose of 0.23 Sv.[281] In males there was a statistically significant excess of esophageal cancer at dose levels of 1 Sv, with an ERR of 0.61 (90% CI 0.15, 1.2). In females there was a higher statistically significant excess at dose levels of 1 Sv, with an ERR of 1.7 (90% CI 0.46, 3.8). The Japanese data show that esophageal cancer is an extreme example in which RR of mortality changes dramatically with time after exposure or attained age. The mortality data from Japan indicate that ERRs are significantly lower in men than in women. Incidence data do show a nonsignificant effect of age at exposure but no evidence of an effect due to

Excess relative risk

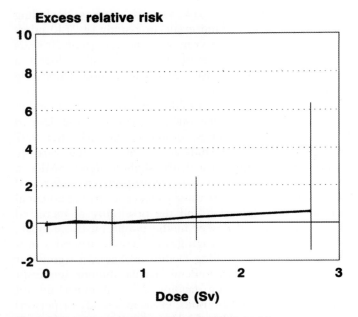

Esophageal cancer incidence (A-bomb)

Figure 5-18 ● ERR of esophageal cancer in atomic bomb survivors at different dose levels. Bars indicate 95% CI. (From Thompson D, Mabuchi K, Ron E, et al: Cancer incidence in atomic bomb survivors. II: Solid tumors, 1958–1987. RERF Technical Report 5-92, Hiroshima, Japan, Radiation Effects Research Foundation, 1992.)

time since exposure or attained age. The incidence data are consistent with a linear-dose response (Fig. 5-18).

Occupational Exposure

A large number of occupational studies are predominantly negative with respect to radiation induction of esophageal cancer. A study of 22,347 U.K. workers exposed to fall-out and other sources has a nonsignificant RR of 1.37 (90% CI 0.78 to 2.41) for esophageal cancer.[52] Two other large occupational studies have been performed in the United Kingdom. A study by Beral et al. included an analysis of 3115 deaths among 22,522 atomic weapon workers during 1946–1979.[144] In this study the ratio of rates for esophageal cancer in exposed as compared to nonexposed employees was 1.03 (95% CI 0.44 to 2.39). A cohort analysis of the U.K. National Registry of Radiation Workers by Kendall et al., which included 95,217 workers over 1.2 million person-years at risk, reported an SMR of 1 for esophageal cancer.[145] A second expanded analysis of the same group in 1999 of 124,743 workers in the U.K. National Registry of Radiation Workers by Muirhead et al. using a lagged analysis reported a nonsignificantly reduced SMR of 0.84 (95% CI 0.69, 1.01).[146] A report on the Sellafield plant by Omar et al. indicated a nonsignificant increase in esophageal cancer among nonplutonium radiation workers with an SMR of 1.10.[148] Incidence was also nonsignificantly increased.

McGeoghegan et al. reported on the mortality and cancer morbidity experience of employees at the Chapel-cross plant of British Nuclear Fuels during 1955–1995.[149] The cohort included 2628 workers with median doses of 39 mSv. In radiation workers the SMR for cancer of the esophagus was nonsignificantly decreased at 0.74. Habib et al. have reported on cancer incidence among Australian nuclear industry–monitored radiation workers and found a nonsignificantly reduced SIR of 0.67 for esophageal cancer.[152] Rahu et al. have reported on cancer incidence of 5446 male Latvian and Estonian Chernobyl cleanup workers for whom they have indicated a nonsignificantly increased SIR of 1.39 for esophageal cancer.[178]

Large occupational studies have been performed in the United States and Canada. Gilbert et al. have reported on workers at the Hanford National Laboratory, in whom they found an SMR of 0.8 for esophageal cancer.[287] Gilbert et al. did report an increased incidence of esoph-ageal cancer in the 1993 updated combined analysis of workers at Hanford, Oak Ridge, and Rocky Flats, but the authors interpreted this as being due to bias or chance fluctuation.[158] Fry et al. reported a study of mor-tality and morbidity among 3145 persons occupationally exposed to 50 or more mSv (5000 mrem) in a year whose mean external exposure was 153 mSv.[161] Their SMR for esophageal cancer was nonsignificantly elevated.

Cragle et al. reporting on workers at the Savannah River plant, indicated that there were no cases of esoph-ageal cancer.[288] Wiggs et al. found an SMR of 0.80 in a follow-up study of Los Alamos workers.[164] At the Mound facility in Ohio the SMR for esophageal cancer was 1.15 (95% CI 0.14 to 4.15),[156] and in one Canadian study of 8977 nuclear workers there was an SMR of 0.80 (95% CI 0.26 to 1.88).[260] Ashmore et al. reported the first analysis of mortality and occupational radiation exposure based on the National Dose Registry of Canada which included a cohort of 206,620 individuals and 5426 deaths. The average exposure for males was 10.6 mSv and their SMR for esophageal cancer was significantly reduced at 0.73 (90% CI 0.53, 0.99).[154] Sont et al. also reported on the relation between cancer incidence and occupational radi-ation exposure based on the National Dose Registry of Canada; their study included a cohort of 191,333 persons with an average dose for males of 11.5 mSv and an average dose for the cohort of 6.64 mSv.[153] The SIR for esophageal cancer in males was significantly reduced at 0.41 and in females it was nonsignificantly elevated at 1.36. In 2004, Zablotska et al. reported on the mortality of Canadian nuclear workers and concluded that for esophageal cancer there was a nonsignificantly decreased SMR of 0.78 (95% CI 0.43, 1.31).[155] Groves et al. con-ducted a 40-year cancer mortality study of 40,581 Korean War Navy veterans with potential exposure to high-intensity radar sources which also emit ionizing radia-tion.[165] The SMR for esophageal cancer in such veterans was nonsignificantly increased at 1.08 (95% CI 0.82, 1.42).

Three somewhat more controversial studies also yielded negative results for an association with occupational exposure and esophageal cancer. Wilkinson et al. found an SMR of 0.94 (90% CI 0.26 to 2.43) for esophageal cancer at the Rocky Flats plant.[286] For Oak Ridge nuclear plant workers Checkoway et al. reported an SMR of 0.89 (95% CI 0.24 to 2.28) using U.S. comparisons and 1.08 (95% CI 0.29 to 2.77) using Tennessee comparisons.[284] Wing et al., reporting on Oak Ridge workers, found an SMR 0.58 (95% CI 0.21 to 1.27) for esophageal cancer.[285] Frome reported a mortality study of 106,020 employees in the nuclear industry at Oak Ridge, Tennessee, in whom the SMR for cancer of the esophagus in black and white males and females was nonsignificantly different from unity.[160] Iwasaki et al. conducted a second analysis of mortality of nuclear industry workers in Japan.[150] The study included 176,000 male workers and 5527 deaths. Average annual doses were 3.5 mSv before 1982 and 1.2 mSv after 1982. For esophageal cancer the SMR was nonsignificantly decreased at 0.84 (95% CI 0.68, 1.02) although there was a positive trend with increasing dose.

Cardis et al. investigated cancer mortality among nuclear industry workers in three countries in a very large study of 95,673 workers with over 2 million person-years at risk and 15,825 deaths, in whom they found that the trend for esophageal cancer was nonsignificantly increased at 0.32 with a P value of 0.365.[166] Cardis et al. also have reported the cancer mortality results from a 15-country collaborative study of nuclear workers.[168] This is the largest occupational study to date and included a cohort of 407,391 workers with 18,993 deaths and 5.2 million person-years of follow-up. The ERR per Sv for esophageal cancer was nonsignificantly negative, estimated at less than 0 with a negative trend with increasing dose (P value of −0.78).

Ritz et al. have reported on cancer mortality in uranium processing workers at the Fernald plant in Ohio.[192] The SMR for esophageal cancer was nonsignificantly increased at 1.20. Dupree-Ellis et al. have reported on mortality in a cohort of 2514 uranium processing workers employed between 1942 and 1966 at the Mallinkrodt Chemical Works.[193] The SMR for esophageal cancer was nonsignificantly increased at 1.35. McGeoghegan et al. have reported on the mortality of 12,540 workers (including 3244 radiation workers) at the Capenhurst uranium enrichment facility during 1946–1995.[242] The SMR for esophageal cancer was nonsignificantly reduced in radiation workers at 0.39. They also studied cancer mortality experience of 19,454 workers (including 13,960 radiation workers) at the Springfields uranium production facility during 1946–1995.[243] The SMR for esophageal cancer was nonsignificantly reduced for radiation workers at 0.77.

Cancer incidence among medical diagnostic workers in China was reported in 1988 by Wang et al. who compared 27,011 workers with 25,782 persons in other medical specialties.[102] The x-ray workers had a 50% higher risk of developing cancer and an excess of esophageal cancer for which the ERR was 2.49, a statistically significant increase. The authors indicated, however, that the risk was not related to dose and was too high for risk factors derived from other radiation studies. They suggested that other factors such as diet and alcohol might have played a role. In a 2002 follow-up report the risk prevailed and Wang et al. reported that for those employed before 1970 with cumulative doses of 551 mSv, the RR was significantly increased at 2.72.[253] For those employed after 1970 with a cumulative mean dose of 82 mSv, the RR was also significantly increased at 2.49.

In a study of British radiologists employed before 1920, Smith et al. reported an O/E mortality ratio of 1.18 that is not statistically significant.[584] For those employed after 1920 the O/E ratio was 0.0. Berrington et al. have analyzed 100 years of experience in U.K. radiologists and reported a nonsignificantly increased SMR for esophageal cancer of 1.25 for those employed from 1897–1920 and a nonsignificantly decreased SMR of 0.35 for those employed after 1920.[94] Doody et al. reported on mortality among 143,517 U.S. radiologic technologists during 1926–1990.[97] Doses were not evaluated. Their SMR for esophageal cancer was nonsignificantly reduced at 0.67 (95% CI 0.43, 1.01). Sigurdson et al. studied the cancer incidence in 90,305 U.S. radiologic technologists and found that the SIR for esophageal cancer was nonsignificantly elevated 1.02 (95% CI 0.59, 1.63).[101] Mohan et al. studied cancer and other causes of mortality among 146,022 radiologic technologists employed from 1940 and later.[98,99] The SMR for esophageal cancer in males was nonsignificantly reduced at 0.67 (95% CI 0.4, 1.0) and for females it was nonsignificantly reduced at 0.95 (95% CI 0.6, 1.5).

Medical Exposure

Esophageal cancer has been studied in patients after external exposures in diagnostic radiology. Massachusetts TB patients treated with multiple fluoroscopies have been followed by Davis et al.[105] They have indicated an SMR of 2.3 for esophageal cancer in exposed females, but this was based on only four cases. The SMR for exposed males was elevated at 2.1, but it was even higher (2.5) for unexposed male controls. In another study also of Massachusetts TB patients, the SMR in exposed and unexposed males was significantly elevated, with SMRs of 4.0 and 4.2, respectively.[364] The authors indicated smoking was the most likely cause of the excess.

Radiation therapy can give quite high doses to specific organs, and patients have been followed after therapy for benign as well as malignant conditions. In patients who were treated for ankylosing spondylitis, the estimated mean dose to the esophagus was over 4 Gy; cancer of the esophagus was significantly elevated, with an O/E of 2.20.[109] Mattsson et al. have reported on cancer incidence among 3090 women who received radiation therapy for benign breast disease. The RR for esophageal cancer was nonsignificantly increased at 2.80 based on only one case.[114] Carr et al. performed a follow-up study of 3719 patients treated with radiotherapy for peptic ulcer with doses to the abdomen of about 15 Gy.[113] No cases of esophageal cancer were found after radiotherapy in the period 0 to 10 years postexposure and in the follow-up period of 11 to 62 years postexposure the RR was nonsignificantly reduced at 0.97. An incidence study of women treated for cervical cancer compared 82,616 exposed women with 99,424 unexposed controls.[124] The women were from Canada, Denmark, Finland, Norway, Sweden, Yugoslavia, the United Kingdom, and the United States; the study covered 1.28 million person-years at risk. Excess risk was found for leukemia and cancers of the esophagus; for the latter, the O/E ratio was 1.5 in those treated with radiotherapy and 1.0 in those with no radiotherapy, but the RR did not vary with time after treatment, and the authors indicated that the excess risk was not likely to be related to the radiation exposure. When patients treated for in situ cervical cancer were followed, the RRs were 1.0 and 0.5, in those with and without radiation, respectively. Curtis et al. evaluated second cancer risk among women with a genital system cancer and found that cancers related to smoking (including esophagus) were notably increased among cervical cancer patients.[706] Travis et al. have reported on long-term survival and second cancers in over 40,000 testicular cancer patients.[705] The RR for esophageal cancer was marginally increased at 1.7 (95% CI 1.0, 2.6).

Internal Exposure

The effects of radiation exposure resulting from internal deposition of radionuclides has also been studied. Such exposures have occurred as a result of occupational settings and medical uses of radionuclides. In a study of persons with internal exposure at Oak Ridge National Laboratory, Wing et al. found no increase of esophageal cancer, reporting an SMR of 0.82 (95% CI 0.69, 0.96).[285] In a study of workers with internal plutonium exposure at the Rocky Flats plant, Wilkinson et al. reported SMRs of 3.26 (90% CI 0.25, 36.81) and 3.68 (90% CI 0.29, 41.56) using biologically implausible 2- and 5-year latent periods.[286] These excesses are not significantly different from unity and, moreover, when a plausible 10-year latent period was used, no cases of esophageal cancer were observed in the exposed group. In a long-term follow-up of the Manhattan Project plutonium workers, no esophageal cancer has been seen.[671] A report on the Sellafield plant by Omar et al. of plutonium workers indicated a nonsignificant increase in esophageal cancer with an

SMR of 1.20.[148] Incidence was also nonsignificantly increased. Carpenter et al. examined workers in the United Kingdom who were occupationally exposed to tritium, plutonium, and other radionuclides.[191] The SMRs for esophageal cancer in each group were all nonsignificant. Gusev et al. found a nonsignificant increase in esophageal cancer among nine villages in heavily contaminated areas around the Semipalatinsk nuclear test site.[720] In the same area Bauer et al. reported a significant increase in esophageal cancer but only in women.[533]

Studies in uranium miners have not shown an increase in cancer of the esophagus; for example, an SMR of 0.72 (95% CI 0.09 to 2.6) has been reported by Waxweiler et al.[362] A 2004 update of French uranium miners by Laurier et al. reported a nonsignificantly reduced SMR of 0.7 for esophageal cancer.[186] Darby et al. studied cancers in Swedish iron miners and found a nonsignificant increase in esophageal cancer with an O/E ratio of 1.36 (95% CI 0.37, 3.47).[183]

There have been studies of the potential carcinogenic effects of diagnostic doses of radioiodine administered to perform thyroid scanning. In the largest and most recent of these studies, which included 35,074 patients who were matched with the Swedish cancer registry, there was no increase in the overall risk of digestive cancer.[270] Esophageal cancer was not mentioned specifically. In patients treated with radioiodine for hyperthyroidism, Hoffman et al. did not report on the esophagus separately but did indicate that for digestive organs, as a group, the RR was 0.8 (95% CI 0.4, 1.7).[202] Similarly, for patients treated for thyroid cancer with radioiodine, the SIR for all digestive organs was 1.23 (95% CI 0.79, 1.84); in nonexposed persons the SIR was 1.17 (95% CI 0.84, 1.67). Ron et al. has more recently reported on cancer mortality among 35,593 hyperthyroid patients. The SMR for esophageal cancer was 1.00 for those receiving any iodine 131 and 1.15 for those receiving only iodine 131.[201]

Thorotrast, a contrast medium that was used widely for angiography and to a much lesser extent for sinus studies, remains in the body and has been associated with some types of tumors. In German Thorotrast patients there have been reports of increased cancer of the esophagus, with seven deaths due to esophageal cancer in the 2334 Thorotrast patients and only one death in 1912 controls. This increased risk may be secondary to smoking, because cancers of the larynx and pancreas were also increased.[211,212] Five deaths were due to larynx cancer in the Thorotrast group and only one in the control group. Additionally, in a Danish Thorotrast series, the SIR was nonsignificantly elevated at 1.1 (95% CI 0.0, 6.2).[213]

SUMMARY

Epidemiologic studies do not show a consistent increase in the risk of esophageal cancer following internal or

Table 5-20 • Risk Estimates for Cancer Incidence and Mortality from Studies of Radiation Exposure: Esophageal Cancer*

Study	Average Excess Relative Risk at 1 Sv	Average Excess Absolute Risk $(10^4 PYSv)^{-1}$
External Low-LET Exposure		
Incidence		
A-bomb Life Span Study[319]		
Males	0.48 (0.09, 1)	<0 (<0, 1112.5)
Females	0.7 (<0, 2.28)	0.02 (<0, 0.45)
Age at exposure		
<20	1.34 (0.44, 2.82)	<0 (<0, 262.07)
20–40	<0 (<0, 0.76)	<0 (<0, 501.33)
>40	0.33 (<0, 1.06)	1.90 (0.46, 3.93)
Time since exposure		
12–15	0.9 (<0, 5.21)	<0 (<0, 282.42)
15–30	0.59 (<0, 1.51)	0.32 (0.04, 0.83)
>30	0.45 (0.03, 1.08)	4.72 (3.64, 5.98)
All	0.51 (0.14, 0.99)	0.19 (<0, 0.53)
Cervical cancer cohort[124]	0.26 (–1.1–1.3)	0.16 (–0.6–1.3)
U.K. Springfields uranium workers[243]	–1.96 (<–2–5.95)	NA
Mortality		
A-bomb Life Span Study[281]		
Males	0.55 (0.09–1.17)	0.25 (0.01–0.82)
Females	1.4 (0.2–3.37)	<0 (<0–151.21)
Age at exposure		
<20	1.38 (0.18–3.6)	<0 (<0–141.53)
20–40	0.59 (<0–1.93)	<0 (<0–353.89)
>40	0.6 (0.05–1.37)	1.95 (0.72–3.6)
Time since exposure		
5–15	1.3 (0.16–3.24)	<0 (<0–<0)
15–30	0.81 (0.09–1.92)	<0 (<0–373.73)
>30	0.4 (<0–1.23)	<0 (<0–493.7)
All	0.69 (0.24–1.28)	<0 (<0–386.68)
Ankylosing spondylitis[266]	0.17 (0.09–0.25)	0.23 (0.1–0.3)
Metropathia hemorrhagica[116]	–0.58 (<–0.2–13.9)	–0.94 (–7–22.5)
Nuclear workers in Canada, United Kingdom, United States[166]	>0	NA
U.K. National Registry for Radiation Workers[146]	–0.095 (<–1.95–4.06)	NA
U.S. Los Alamos Laboratory workers[164]	>0	NA
Nuclear workers in Japan[721]	>0	NA
Nuclear industry workers in Japan[150]	>0	>0
IARC 15-country nuclear workers study[167,168]	<0	
Internal Low-LET Exposure		
Mortality		
Semipalatinsk study[533]	0.18 (–0.09, 0.66)	NA

*The studies listed are those for which quantitative estimates of risk could be made.
Adapted from United Nations Scientific Committee of the Effects of Atomic Radiation (UNSCEAR): Sources and effects of ionizing radiation: 2006 report to the General Assembly with annexes. New York, United Nations, 2007.

external radiation exposure, and a number of the studies have not controlled for the significant bias factors and known esophageal carcinogens such as smoking and alcohol. The UNSCEAR 1988 risk estimate for cancer of the esophagus, using the multiplicative risk model, was 3.4 (90% CI 0.8, 7.2) excess lifetime cancer deaths for 1000 persons exposed to 1 Gy of low-LET radiation at high-dose rate.[370] The BEIR V Committee indicated that the data from the various studies are consistent with those from the atomic bomb survivors, in whom the RR is estimated to approximate 1.58 per Gy (organ dose).[3] This would be an ERR of 0.58. The newer Japanese

data would suggest a risk of about one half of this and with confidence limits that include 0 risk. Thus, the BEIR conclusion should be considered on a historical basis. The ICRP 1990 report, which also does not take into account the newer Japanese data, estimates the lifetime risk of fatal esophageal cancer for exposure of the entire population to be 30 $(10^{-4}Sv^{-1})$.[248] Some studies have been summarized by UNSCEAR 2006 and can be used to derive risk estimates (Table 5-20).[86] UNSCEAR 2006 concluded that there is clearly an association of radiation and esophageal cancer in the Japanese LSS, although since esophageal cancer is relatively infrequent, there is insufficient statistical sensitivity to detect an excess in most occupational low-dose studies. They also indicated that the data are insufficient to characterize the shape of the dose response curve or to establish a dose-rate effectiveness factor.

STOMACH CANCER
General

In 1980 stomach cancer was considered to be the single most common form of cancer in the world, accounting for about 10% to 11% of all new cases.[358] Incidence rates in general have been decreasing over the last decade. Now lung cancer is probably more common. The highest incidence areas are Japan, Korea, and parts of China. In the United States rates are about twice as high in blacks as in whites, and risks are generally higher in males than in females. Rates are about twice as high in persons with low socioeconomic status as in those with high socioeconomic status. Diet probably has an impact on the incidence of stomach cancer, with higher nitrate, nitrosamines, and salt intake associated with higher risk. Close relatives of stomach cancer patients have about a two- to threefold higher risk than controls. Whether this is genetic or environmental is unknown. Persons with blood type A and those who have had gastric surgery also have been shown to be at increased risk in some studies.[700] Ninety-five percent of malignant stomach tumors are adenocarcinomas. The most common sites are the lesser curvature and antral portions of the stomach.

External Exposure

Background Radiation and Populations Near Nuclear Facilities

In a study of terrestrial radiation in Connecticut, no association between background radiation levels and stomach cancer was found.[21] One study of areas of high and low natural background radiation in China has suggested a positive association with stomach cancer.[29] Whether this is due to radiation remains uncertain, because some areas of China have high rates of stomach cancer for other reasons, and this finding is based on only a small difference in the number of cases (53 in the high-background region and 47 in the low-background region). A paper by Sun et al. compared a high-background area and a neighboring control area in Guangdong, China, and covered 1.7 million person-years of study from 1979–1995.[32] Dose rates in the high-background area were 4.3 mSv per year and in the control areas it was about 1.6 mSv per year. The ERR per Sv for stomach cancer compared to the control area was nonsignificantly decreased at −0.27 (95% CI −1.37, 2.69). Another paper in the same area of China was published in 2000 by Tao et al. and covered 1.7 million person-years of study

from 1979–1995.[33] The authors did not find a radiation effect and the RR of stomach cancer was 0.75 (95% CI 0.44, 1.30). Increased natural cosmic radiation occurs to airline crews and there have been a number of studies on their risks of stomach cancer. Pukkala et al., in studying over 10,000 Nordic airline pilots, found a nonsignificant decrease in their frequency of the disease.[39] Band et al. reported a study of 2740 pilots exposed to doses of 6 mSv per year over an average of 20 years for a total average dose about 120 mSv, in whom they found a nonsignificantly decreased SIR and a nonsignificantly decreased SMR for stomach cancer.[40]

Studies on the effects of fallout within the United States from weapons testing at the Nevada test site have been negative in relation to stomach cancer.[456] There was a significant decrease in the fallout area compared with the rest of the United States, with an OR of 0.60 (90% CI 0.43 to 0.84). This is probably the result of lifestyle differences. No increase or consistent trend in stomach cancer rates has been found in the United States in populations living around nuclear installations. Before start-up of facilities, the SMR for stomach cancer when all facilities were combined was 0.92 in the study counties and 1.03 in the control counties. After facility operation the SMRs were 0.96 and 1.03, respectively.[78] There are three papers concerning potential uranium contamination and the possibility of stomach cancer in the public. Boice et al. indicated a nonsignificant increase around a uranium mining and milling facility in Texas and Colorado, and no difference near a facility in Pennsylvania.[89,90,90a] A nonsignificant decrease was found by Boice et al. in a study of persons residing near the Hanford site.[91] Lopez-Abente et al. have reported on solid tumor mortality near Spain's four nuclear power plants and four uranium fuel cycle facilities where the RR for stomach cancer was nonsignificantly different from unity at 1.02.[283] Bauer et al. have reported on cancer mortality due to local fallout from Soviet atmospheric nuclear weapons testing at the Semipalatinsk test site in Kazakhstan.[533] The effective doses to the exposed subjects ranged from 20 mSv to about 4 Sv. The dose-response (LRT) for stomach cancer was nonsignificantly positive at a P value of 0.0146 in males and significantly positive at a value of less than 0.0001 in females. The estimated ERR per Sv for the exposed cohort was 0.95 (95% CI 0.17, 3.49).

Atomic Bomb Survivors

The 1998 incidence study of the atomic bomb survivors has found a statistically significant increase for cancer of the stomach.[319] During 1958–1998, 4730 cancers were observed versus 4579 expected (an excess of 151 cases) for the individuals who received 0.005 Gy or more. The ERR at 1 Gy was 0.34 (90% CI 0.22, 0.47), and the EAR was 9.5 (90% CI 6.1, 14) $\times$ $(10^4 PYSv)^{-1}$. The LSS mortality study data for the period from 1958–1987 also demonstrated a statistically significant increase in cancer of stomach.[8]

Compared with the 1107 expected 1163 (an excess of 56) stomach cancer deaths were observed in 1,203,100 person-years of observation for the 41,000 persons who received 0.01 Sv or more. In this study the ERR at 1 Sv was estimated to be 0.2, and the EAR was 1.9 $(10^4 PYSv)^{-1}$. In the 2003 update studies of mortality of atomic bomb survivors during 1950–1997, Preston et al. had a cohort of 86,572 persons with an average external dose of 0.23 Sv.[281] In males there was a statistically marginally significant excess of stomach cancer at dose levels of 1 Sv, with an ERR of 0.20 (90% CI 0.04, 0.39). In females there was a statistically significant excess at dose levels of 1 Sv, and an ERR of 0.65 (90% CI 0.40, 0.95).

A report of the atomic bomb survivors by Ito et al. has suggested that the frequency of poorly differentiated adenocarcinoma was somewhat higher in the group exposed to more than 0.01 Gy than in a no-exposure group.[722] The atomic bomb survivor incidence data indicate that the ERR for females is higher than that for males. The ERR at 1 Sv is 0.21 for males of all ages and 0.47 for females. The ERR at 1 Sv decreases with increasing age at exposure. For females the values are 2.19 for 0 to 9 years, 1.09 for 10 to 19 years, 0.62 for 20 to 39 years, and 0.15 for 40-plus years of age at exposure. For males corresponding values are −0.26, 0.42, 0.25, and 0.10, respectively. There was no effect of age at exposure or of attained age. A linear dose-response fit the data (Fig. 5-19).[279]

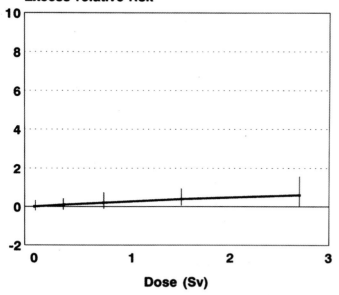

Excess relative risk

Stomach cancer incidence (A-bomb)

Figure 5-19 • ERR of stomach cancer in atomic bomb survivors at different dose levels. Bars indicate 95% CI. (From Thompson D, Mabuchi K, Ron E, et al: Cancer incidence in atomic bomb survivors, II: Solid tumors, 1958–1987. RERF Technical Report 5-92, Hiroshima, Japan, Radiation Effects Research Foundation, 1992.)

Occupational Exposure

Occupational studies have shown either no relation between occupational radiation exposure and the risk of stomach cancer or a nonsignificant increase. Three large studies in the United Kingdom have all been negative. Darby et al. have reported an RR for stomach cancer of 0.78 (90% CI 0.49 to 1.23) in workers exposed to fallout or who worked in experimental government programs.[52] In the latest 2004 review Muirhead et al. studied a cohort of 21,357 test participants and reported a significantly decreased SMR of 0.78 (95% CI 0.63, 0.96) for stomach cancer in test participants and a nonsignificantly increased risk compared to controls.[55] The RR compared to controls for incidence was nonsignificantly elevated at 1.04.

Beral et al. performed an analysis of 3373 deaths among 39,546 nuclear workers during 1946–1979 and reported a significantly low SMR for stomach cancer of 0.70 (95% CI 0.55 to 0.88).[143] In a similar study of 22,522 atomic weapons workers, Beral et al. found a rate ratio of 1.01 (95% CI 0.55 to 1.84) comparing exposed to nonexposed employees.[144] A cohort analysis of the U.K. National Registry of Radiation Workers by Kendall et al. followed 95,217 workers over 1.2 million person-years at risk and indicated an SMR of 0.91.[145] A second analysis in 1999 of 124,743 workers in the U.K. National Registry of Radiation Workers by Muirhead et al. using a lagged analysis reported a significantly reduced SMR for stomach cancer of 0.83 (95% CI 0.73, 0.94).[146] A report on the Sellafield plant by Omar et al. indicated a nonsignificant increase in stomach cancer among nonplutonium radiation workers with an SMR of 1.30. Incidence was nonsignificantly decreased.[148] McGeoghegan et al. reported on the mortality and cancer morbidity experience of employees at the Chapelcross plant of British Nuclear Fuels during 1955–1995.[149] The cohort included 2628 workers with median doses of 39 mSv. In radiation workers the SMR for cancer of the stomach was nonsignificantly decreased at 0.90.

Artalejo et al. reported on mortality among 5657 workers of the former Spanish Nuclear Energy Board whose mean exposure was 11.42 mSv and the SMR for stomach cancer was nonsignificantly decreased at 0.81 (95% CI 0.33, 1.72).[151] Habib et al. have reported on cancer incidence among Australian nuclear industry–monitored radiation workers and indicated an SIR for stomach cancer nonsignificantly different from unity at 0.96.[152] Rahu et al. have reported on cancer incidence of 5446 male Latvian and Estonian Chernobyl cleanup workers and indicate a nonsignificantly decreased SIR of 0.96 for stomach cancer.[178]

In a large Canadian study of 8977 radiation workers Gribbin et al. reported an SMR of 0.61 (95% CI 0.32 to 1.07) for stomach cancer.[260] Ashmore et al. reported the first analysis of mortality and occupational radiation exposure based on the National Dose Registry of Canada which included a cohort of 206,620 individuals and 5426 deaths.[154] The average exposure for males was 10.6 mSv and the SMR for stomach cancer was significantly reduced at 0.54 (90% CI 0.43, 0.68). Sont et al. also reported on incidence and occupational radiation exposure based on the National Dose Registry of Canada, which included a cohort of 191,333 persons with an average dose for males of 11.5 mSv and an average dose for the cohort of 6.64 mSv.[153] The SIR for stomach cancer in males was significantly reduced at 0.41 and in females it was nonsignificantly reduced at 0.75.

Gilbert et al. have published a number of studies concerning workers at national laboratories or federal facilities. In a study of workers at the Hanford National Laboratory during 1945–1986, there was an SMR of 0.77 for stomach cancer.[361] In a combined analysis the SMR for stomach cancer was 0.73 at Hanford, 1.03 at Oak Ridge, and 0.89 at Rocky Flats.[157] Fry et al. reported a study of mortality and morbidity among 3145 persons occupationally exposed to 50 or more mSv (5000 mrem) in a year.[161] The mean external exposure was 153 mSv. The SMR for stomach cancer was nonsignificantly reduced. Howe et al. reported on the mortality of U.S. nuclear power industry workers and found a nonsignificantly decreased risk of stomach cancer with an SMR of 0.81 (95% CI 0.47, 1.32).[159] Cragle et al. studied workers at the Savannah River facility for stomach cancer in whom the O/E ratio was 0 to 0.64.[288] At the Mound facility in Ohio, Wiggs et al. reported an SMR for stomach cancer of 0.56 (95% CI 0.07 to 2.04).[156] In other studies, Wilkinson et al., reporting on the Rocky Flats facility, indicated an SMR of 0.84 (90% CI 0.33 to 1.77).[286] For stomach cancer in workers at the Oak Ridge National Laboratory, Checkoway et al. estimated an SMR of 0.57 (95% CI 0.19 to 1.33) using a U.S. comparison and an SMR of 0.70 (95% CI 0.23 to 1.63) if a Tennessee comparison was used.[284] Wing et al.[285] indicated an SMR of 0.86 (95% CI 0.29 to 1.38) and Frome[160] reported that the SMR in black and white males and females was nonsignificantly reduced in all groups. Wiggs et al. found a significantly reduced SMR for stomach cancer of 0.70 in a follow-up of Los Alamos workers.[164] Iwasaki et al. conducted a second analysis of mortality of nuclear industry workers in Japan.[150] The study included 176,000 male workers with 5527 deaths and average annual doses of 3.5 mSv before 1982 and 1.2 mSv after 1982. For stomach cancer the SMR was significantly decreased at 0.89 (95% CI 0.81, 0.98).

Cardis et al. investigated cancer mortality among nuclear industry workers in three countries in a very large study of 95,673 workers with over 2 million person-years at risk and 15,825 deaths.[166] The trend for stomach cancer was nonsignificantly decreased at −0.21 with a P value of 0.582. Cardis et al. also have reported the cancer mortality results from a 15-country collaborative study of nuclear workers.[168] This is the largest occupational study to date and included a cohort of 407,391 workers with 18,993 deaths and 5.2 million person-years of follow-up. The ERR per Sv for stomach cancer was nonsignificantly positive at 0.49 (90% CI < 0, 3.92).

Ritz et al. have reported on cancer mortality in uranium processing workers at the Fernald plant in Ohio whose SMR for stomach cancer was nonsignificantly increased at 1.34.[192] Dupree-Ellis et al. have reported on mortality in a cohort of 2514 uranium processing workers employed between 1942–1966 at the Mallinkrodt Chemical Works.[193] The SMR for stomach cancer was significantly reduced at 0.38 (95% CI 0.12, 0.89). McGeoghegan et al. have reported on the mortality of 12,540 workers (including 3244 radiation workers) at the Capenhurst uranium enrichment facility during 1946–1995.[242] The SMR for stomach cancer was nonsignificantly reduced in radiation workers at 0.90. They also studied the cancer mortality experience of 19,454 workers (including 13,960 radiation workers) at the Springfields uranium production facility during 1946–1995 and found that the SMR for stomach cancer was nonsignificantly reduced in radiation workers at 0.92.[243] A meta-analysis of 14 studies, which included 120,000 uranium workers, found a significant reduction with RR of 0.76 (95% CI 0.62, 0.89) for stomach cancer.[245]

The cancer incidence among medical diagnostic workers in China was reported by Wang et al. in 1988.[102] Their study compared 27,011 workers with 25,782 persons in other medical specialties. For stomach cancer the RR was 1.26, not significantly different from unity. In a 2002 follow-up report, Wang et al. reported that for those employed before 1970 whose cumulative doses were 551 mSv, the RR for cancer of the stomach was nonsignificantly increased at 1.01.[253] For those employed after 1970 with a cumulative mean dose of 82 mSv, the RR was significantly increased at 1.63.

Aoyama et al. conducted a mortality survey of over 12,000 male Japanese radiological technologists during 1969–1993.[95] The cohort had an average dose of 466 mSv. The SMR for stomach cancer was significantly decreased at 0.65 (95% CI 0.53, 0.79). Smith et al. have reported on British radiologists in whom the O/E ratio was 1.20 and was not statistically significant for those employed before 1920.[584] For those employed after 1920 the O/E for stomach cancer was 0.68. Berrington et al. have reported on 100 years experience in U.K. radiologists in whom they found a nonsignificantly increased SMR for stomach cancer of 1.38 for those employed from 1897–1920 and a nonsignificantly increased SMR of 1.03 for those employed after 1920.[94] Doody et al. reported on mortality among 143,517 U.S. radiologic technologists during 1926–1990 whose doses were not evaluated.[97] The SMR for stomach cancer was significantly reduced at 0.67 (95% CI 0.50, 0.88). Sigurdson et al. studied cancer incidence in 90,305 U.S. radiologic technologists and found that the SIR for stomach cancer was nonsignificantly reduced at 0.85 (95% CI 0.58, 1.20).[101] Mohan et al. studied cancer and other causes of mortality among 146,022 radiologic technologists employed from 1940 and later.[98,99] The SMR for stomach cancer in males was nonsignificantly reduced at 0.84 (95% CI 0.6, 1.1) and for females it was nonsignificantly reduced at 0.81 (95% CI 0.6, 1.1).

Medical Exposure

Davis et al. reported on follow-up of Massachusetts TB patients who were treated using multiple fluoroscopies in whom the SMRs for stomach cancer in females were not significantly elevated.[105] An SMR of 1.5 was found for exposed females versus 1.1 in nonexposed females. The SMR for exposed males was significantly decreased at 0.3 but was higher (1.4) for unexposed male controls. In another report, also of TB patients, Davis et al. found that SMRs for stomach cancer in all exposed patients and female unexposed controls were below unity.[364] The SMR for unexposed males was 1.1, which was not significantly elevated.

A few studies have examined radiation therapy for benign diseases and the subsequent risk of stomach cancer. Mattsson et al. have reported on cancer incidence among 3090 women who received radiation therapy for benign breast disease. The RR for stomach cancer was nonsignificantly increased at 1.82.[114] Griem et al. have reported on 1457 patients treated for peptic ulcer with radiotherapy and 763 nonirradiated patients.[112] In the former, whose estimated stomach dose was 16 to 17 Gy, the estimated excess risk of stomach cancer was 5.5×10^{-4} person $Gy)^{-1}$. Carr et al. performed a follow-up study of the same group with doses to the abdomen of about 15 Gy.[113] Their RR for stomach cancer in the period 0 to 10 years postexposure was nonsignificantly elevated at 1.11 (95% CI 0.28, 4.49) and in the follow-up period of 11 to 62 years postexposure the RR was significantly elevated at 2.60 (95% CI 1.33, 5.09).

In early reports of patients treated with radiotherapy for ankylosing spondylitis, an excess of stomach cancer was reported in the first 9 years after treatment.[108] Darby et al. have extended the follow-up of this group, and cancer of the stomach was not significantly elevated, with a reported O/E of 1.01.[109] Doses to the stomach were variable, but most were thought to be in the range of 0 to 5 Gy. Follow-up of patients who received intra-uterine radium radiotherapy for benign uterine bleeding has been performed by Inskip et al.[118] The study included 4153 women who were followed over 110,000 person-years at risk. They showed no increase in cancer of the stomach. A nonsignificant increase of stomach cancer (ERR at 1 Sv of 1.01, 90% CI < 0 to 2.8) was reported in women treated for metropathia hemorrhagica.[116]

Other studies have followed patients treated for malignancies with radiotherapy to ascertain the subsequent risk of stomach cancer. An incidence study of women treated for cervical cancer compared 82,616 exposed women with 99,424 unexposed controls.[124] Covering 1.28 million person-years at risk, no excess was identified for cancer of the stomach, the O/E ratio being 1.0 in those treated with radiotherapy and 0.9 in those who were treated without radiotherapy. However, in another study by the same group matching 4188 women with second cancers with 6880 controls, excess risk was seen for cancer of the stomach.[126] The dose to the stomach was estimated to be about 2 Gy, and the RR for stomach cancer was 2.08 (90% CI 1.1 to 4.0). In a study of 1507 patients treated for HD, Tucker et al. reported an increase in stomach cancer, with four cases observed.[436] The O/E ratio was 10 (95% CI 2.8, 26.4). Three of the cases occurred 5 to 9 years after therapy, which would represent an implausibly short latent period. Data on patients followed 10 years or more indicated an O/E ratio of 20, but this was the result of only one case being observed and only a fraction of one case being expected (95% CI, 0.3, 112), a statistically nonsignificant difference.

Van Leeuwen et al. have reported on second cancer risk in 1909 testicular cancer patients and found a boarderline increased RR for stomach cancer of 3.7 (95% CI 1.0, 6.8).[723] Similar findings were reported by Travis et al. who examined long-term survival and second cancers in over 40,000 testicular cancer patients almost all of whom received infradiaphragmattic radiotherapy in whom the RR for stomach cancer was significantly increased.[705]

Internal Exposure

Wiklund et al. have reported that Lapps, who consume reindeer meat presumed to contain a high level of cesium 137, have a significantly increased SIR for stomach cancer of 2.25 (95% CI 1.21, 2.77).[56] The authors indicated that an increased risk of stomach cancer is found with high-salt diets, smoked foods, potential presence of aflatoxin in food, and lack of fresh vegetables, all of which are characteristic of the Lapp diet. Similar results were reported by Hassle et al.[724] Few reports have evaluated tumor incidence in relation to occupational exposure with internal deposition of radionuclides. One study of uranium miners found a nonsignificant increase in cancer of the stomach with an SMR of 1.50 (95% CI 0.68 to 2.84).[362] In another study of uranium enrichment workers, the SMR for stomach cancer was 1.69 (95% CI 0.81 to 3.10). However, the cohort with the assumed greatest exposure had the lowest risk of stomach cancer.[363] No case of stomach cancer was observed in the plutonium workers of the Manhattan Project.[671] Wing et al. reported that workers who were monitored for internal contamination at Oak Ridge National Laboratory had an SMR for stomach cancer of 0.79 (95% CI 0.29, 1.72).[285] At the Rocky Flats plant Wilkinson et al. reported that workers with a plutonium body burden of more than 74 Bq (>2 nCi) had nonsignificantly elevated RRs for stomach cancer of

1.84 (90% CI 0.20, 14.4), and 2.18 (90% CI 0.23, 17.1) if biologically implausible latent periods of 2 and 5 years, respectively, were used.[286] When a reasonable 10-year latent period was considered, no stomach cancers were observed in the exposed group. Wiggs et al. found a reduced RR of 0.74 in a follow-up of Los Alamos plutonium workers.[164] A report on the Sellafield plant by Omar et al. indicated a nonsignificant decrease in stomach cancer with an SMR of 0.96 among plutonium workers and a nonsignificant decrease in incidence as well.[148] Carpenter et al. examined workers in the United Kingdom who were occupationally exposed to tritium, plutonium, and other radionuclides.[191] The SMRs for stomach cancer in each group were all nonsignificantly reduced. A 2004 update of French uranium miners by Laurier et al. reported a nonsignificantly increased SMR of 1.1 for stomach cancer.[186] Among villages in heavily contaminated areas around the Semipalatinsk nuclear test site, Bauer et al. reported a significant increase in stomach cancer.[533]

Darby et al. studied radon and cancers in Swedish iron miners and found a significant increase in stomach cancer with an O/E ratio of 1.45 (95% CI 1.04, 1.98).[183] Auvinen et al. did not find an increased risk of stomach cancer due to radon and other radionuclides in drinking water based on a case-cohort study in Finland.[725] A significantly decreased RR of 0.59 for stomach cancer was found by Mifune et al. when studying cancer mortality in the spa area of Japan with a high radon background.[612] Ye et al. also found a decrease for stomach cancer in radon spa areas but it was nonsignificantly different from unity.[726]

Reports concerning the medical applications of radioiodine are of particular interest because of the normal physiologic excretion of radioiodine by the gastric mucosa. The largest and most recent study of patients receiving diagnostic doses of radioiodine included 35,074 patients who were matched with the Swedish cancer registry, in which there was no increase in digestive cancers as a group.[270] In patients treated for hyperthyroidism, who receive larger amounts of radioiodine, two large studies give slightly different results. In a study by Holm et al. patients examined at 10 or more years of follow-up had a slightly increased SIR of 1.33 (95% CI 1.01, 1.71) for stomach cancer.[271] On the other hand, a study by Hoffman et al. indicated that for cancer of the digestive organs as a group, the RR was 0.8 (95% CI 0.4, 1.7).[202] Ron et al. has more recently reported on cancer mortality among 35,593 hyperthyroid patients.[201] The SMR for stomach cancer was not significantly different from unity at 1.05 for those receiving any iodine 131 and was nonsignificantly reduced at 0.97 for those receiving iodine 131 alone.

In patients who receive very large doses of radioiodine for thyroid cancer therapy, a nonsignificant increase was reported by Hall et al.[203] They reported an SIR of 1.75 (95% CI 0.71, 3.61), and in the nonexposed patients the SIR was 0.99 (95% CI 0.36, 2.15). In the radioiodine-treated patients the estimated dose to the stomach was 2.1 Gy. In another study of patients treated for thyroid cancer, Edmonds et al. report a nonsignificantly increased O/E ratio of 1.1 for stomach cancer.[204]

Thorotrast, a contrast medium containing thorium, which was used widely for angiography and to a much lesser extent for sinus studies, remains in the body and has been associated with a number of tumor types. In a study of Danish Thorotrast patients the SIR for stomach cancer was 1.0 (95% CI 0.4 to 2.1).[213] The German series[211,212] report 30 deaths due to stomach cancer in the 2334 Thorotrast patients and 43 stomach cancer deaths in the smaller group of controls. The Japanese Thorotrast studies do not mention an increase of stomach cancer.[215,677] Nyberg et al. reported on cancer incidence after a 40-year follow-up among Swedish patients exposed to radioactive Thorotrast.[222] The SIR for stomach cancer was significantly elevated at 10.5 (95% CI 3.9, 23.0). The Portuguese study mentions that there were eight stomach cancers, but it is not clear if this is over or under the expected number.[216] The BEIR IV Committee did not list stomach cancer as a risk in its combined analysis of the Thorotrast studies.[575] Even though the above large studies have not shown an increase in stomach cancer following Thorotrast injections, there is a case report of at least one cancer occurring in such a patient.[727] This case report is not only in contrast to the other larger studies, but the tumor type was a well-differentiated adenocarcinoma, and the Japanese experience would suggest that poorly differentiated types are more commonly induced by radiation. No increase in stomach cancer has been found in radium dial painters.[229]

A study by Nekolla et al. of 455 patients treated with radium 224 for TB, ankylosing spondylitis, and a few other diseases indicated that the rate ratio for stomach cancer was nonsignificantly elevated at 1.1.[224] Wick and Nekolla also reported on late effects in ankylosing spondylitis patients treated with radium 224.[225] There were 626 exposed and 725 control patients with a mean follow-up time of 21 years. The mean injected activity was 0.17 MBq per kg and mean alpha skeletal dose was 0.67 Gy. The study showed an increase in the O/E ratio of 1.48 for those exposed.

Summary

Risk estimates for stomach cancer can be derived from certain epidemiologic studies. The risk is clearly increased in atomic bomb survivors but not so much in the cervix series, very little in the radioiodine series, and little or not at all in most occupational series. From the atomic bomb survivor data, there appears to be a higher excess RR in females than in males, but this is not seen in all studies.

There also appears to be a decrease in RR with age at exposure of over 30 years.[86]

The UNSCEAR 1988 risk estimate for cancer of the stomach, using the multiplicative risk model, is 12.6 (90% CI 6.6 to 19.9) excess lifetime fatal cancers per 1000 persons exposed to 1 Gy of low-LET radiation at high-dose rate.[370] The BEIR V Committee used a risk model based on the mortality of the atomic bomb survivors, in whom the RR of fatal stomach cancer per Gy was 1.19 (or an ERR of 0.19).[3] This broadly fits risk factors derived from other studies as well. The ICRP 1990 report estimates the lifetime mortality from exposure of an entire population to be 110 ($10^{-4}Sv^{-1}$).[248]

The UNSCEAR 2006 Committee report summarized radiation risk factors for stomach cancer that could be derived from epidemiological studies (Table 5-21).[86] The updated information from the Japanese LSS study and the peptic ulcer radiotherapy study continue to show a positive dose-response relationship. The LSS data indicates that the ERR decreases with increasing age at exposure but the EAR does not. Most nuclear worker studies do not show an excess of stomach cancer but the doses are typically quite low, limiting statistical power.

SMALL INTESTINAL CANCER

General

Cancer of the small intestine is very rare, and even though the small intestine accounts for over 75% to 90% of the surface area of the gastrointestinal tract, only about 5% of GI malignancies occur therein. No definite etiologic factors for the disease have been identified.[700] Most radiation epidemiologic studies do not mention the small intestine, but those that do have not shown evidence of a consistent radiation-related carcinogenic effect. The few studies that have given data are summarized here.

External Exposure

An occupational exposure study in the United Kingdom by Beral et al. included an analysis of 3115 deaths among 22,552 atomic weapons workers during 1951–1982.[143] The rate ratio of exposed to nonexposed employees for small bowel cancers was 0.00 (95% CI 0.00 to 16.3). A report on the Sellafield plant by Omar et al. found no cancers of the small intestine among nonplutonium radiation workers.[148] McGeoghegan et al. reported on the mortality and cancer morbidity experience of employees at the Chapelcross plant of British Nuclear Fuels during 1955–1995.[149] Their study cohort included 2628 workers with median doses of 39 mSv in whom no case of small intestine cancer was identified. Habib et al. have reported on cancer incidence among Australian nuclear industry–monitored radiation workers in whom they found a significantly elevated SIR of 6.12

(95% CI 1.98, 18.99) for cancer of the small intestine (based on only three cases).[152] Rahu et al. reported on the cancer incidence in 5446 male Latvian and Estonian Chernobyl cleanup workers and indicated they had a nonsignificantly elevated SIR of 4.05 for cancer of the small intestine (but this was based on only one case).[178]

Cardis et al. investigated cancer mortality among nuclear industry workers in three countries in a very large study of 95,673 workers with over 2 million person-years at risk and 15,825 deaths.[166] The trend for small bowel cancer was nonsignificantly positive at 0.36 with a P value of 0.360. Cardis et al. have reported the cancer mortality results from a 15-country collaborative study of nuclear workers.[168] This is the largest occupational study to date and included a cohort of 407,391 workers with 18,993 deaths and 5.2 million person-years of follow-up. The ERR per Sv for cancer of the small intestine was nonsignificantly positive at 3.18 (90% CI < 0, 28.3).

McGeoghegan et al. have reported on the mortality of 12,540 workers (including 3244 radiation workers) at the Capenhurst uranium enrichment facility during 1946–1995 and indicated that no case of small intestinal cancer was identified in radiation workers in that cohort.[242] They also studied cancer mortality experience of 19,454 workers (including 13,960 radiation workers) at the Springfields uranium production facility during 1946–1995 and found that the SMR for cancer of the small intestine was nonsignificantly reduced for radiation workers at 0.48.[243]

Sigurdson et al. studied the cancer incidence in 90,305 U.S. radiologic technologists and found that the SIR for cancer of the small intestine was nonsignificantly reduced at 0.42 (95% CI 0.10, 1.12).[101]

Mattsson et al. have reported on cancer incidence among 3090 women who received radiation therapy for benign breast disease.[114] The RR for cancer of the small intestine was nonsignificantly reduced at 0.72. In two studies of women treated with radiotherapy for cancer of the cervix, no radiation-related increase was found. In a case-control study, Boice et al. reported that for cancers of the small bowel the RR was 1.0 (90% CI 0.3 to 2.9), and the estimated dose to the small bowel was 10 to 20 Gy.[126] In the other, a cohort study, the O/E ratio for second cancers in patients given radiotherapy for cervical cancer was significantly elevated at 2.2, but the O/E ratio was even higher (4.3) in the control patients treated without radiotherapy, and, therefore, the increase was undoubtedly not due to radiation exposure.[124]

Internal Exposure

In the medically exposed Danish Thorotrast patient series, the SIR for cancer of the small intestine was 7.4 (95% CI 0.9, 27), but the confidence limits encompassed unity. It should be noted that this ratio was based on only two observed cases. Nyberg et al. reported on cancer incidence after a 40-year follow-up among Swedish patients exposed

Table 5-21 • Risk Estimates for Cancer Incidence and Mortality from Studies of Radiation Exposure: Stomach Cancer*

Study	Average Excess Relative Risk at 1 Sv	Average Excess Absolute Risk $(10^4 PYSv)^{-1}$
External Low-LET Exposures		
Incidence		
A-bomb Life Span Study[319]		
Males	0.26 (0.14–0.42)	2.45 (0.92–4.49)
Females	0.51 (0.33–0.72)	4.36 (2.78–6.15)
Age at exposure		
<20	0.56 (0.32–0.85)	2.74 (1.52–4.19)
20–40	0.39 (0.22–0.59)	6.18 (3.42–9.32)
>40	0.23 (0.07–0.41)	7.99 (2.25–14.59)
Time since exposure		
12–15	0.37 (<0–0.92)	2.4 (0.66–5.21)
15–30	0.31 (0.15–0.5)	2.71 (1.32–4.4)
>30	0.42 (0.27–0.58)	6.75 (4.28–9.48)
All	0.37 (0.26–0.49)	3.61 (2.42–4.96)
Cervical cancer case control[6]	0.54 (0.05–1.5)	NA
Swedish benign breast disease[114]	1.3 (0–4.4)	NA
Stockholm skin hemangioma[589]	<0	<0
U.K. Springfields uranium workers[243]	–1.96 (< –2–9.73)	NA
Mortality		
A-bomb Life Span Study[281]		
Males	0.11 (<0–0.3)	0.32 (<0–1.33)
Females	0.5 (0.27–0.75)	1.46 (0.55–2.56)
Age at exposure		
<20	0.72 (0.29–1.27)	0.51 (<0–1.27)
20–40	0.42 (0.18–0.71)	2.78 (1.06–4.82)
>40	0.12 (<0–0.31)	3.46 (<0–8.03)
Time since exposure		
12–15	0.17 (<0–0.48)	0.17 (<0–1.25)
15–30	0.22 (0.02–0.46)	0.62 (<0–1.76)
>30	0.46 (0.23–0.73)	3.89 (2.19–5.83)
All	0.28 (0.14–0.42)	0.94 (0.31–1.71)
Ankylosing spondylitis[266]	–0.004 (–0.05–0.05)	NA
Yangjiang background radiation[34,35]	–0.27 (–1.37–2.69)	NA
Peptic ulcer[113]	0.2 (0–0.73)	NA
Metropathia hemorrhagica[116]	1.01 (<0.2–2.8)	5.72 (< –2.4–16)
Benign gynecological disease[118]	0.27 (–4.25–4.8)	0.83 (<0–72.7)
Nuclear workers in Canada, United Kingdom, United States[166]	<0	NA
U.K. National Registry for Radiation Workers[146]	–0.032 (–0.95–1.49)	NA
Canadian National Dose Registry[154]	12.5 (<0–33) (males)	NA
Nuclear industry workers in Japan[150]	>0	>0
Nuclear power industry workers in the United States[159]	19.5 (–2.23–141)	NA
Japanese radiological technologists[95]	<0	<0
IARC 15-country nuclear workers study[167,168]	0.49 (<0, 3.92)	
Internal Low-LET Exposures		
Incidence		
Swedish hyperthyroid patients[271]	1.32 (0.04–2.84)	NA
Mortality		
U.S. thyrotoxicosis patients[201]	>0	NA
Semipalatinsk Study[533]	0.95 (0.17, 3.49)	NA
Internal High-LET Exposures		
Incidence		
^{224}Ra ankylosing spondylitis patients[225]	1.56	NA
^{224}Ra ankylosing spondylitis patients[224]	~ 1.2	NA
Danish Thorotrast patients[272]	1.82 (0.61–5.66)	NA
Danish and Swedish Thorotrast patients[219]	2.7 (1.1–7.9)	NA
Mortality		
German Thorotrast patients[212,221]	0.6	NA

*The studies listed are those for which quantitative estimates of risk could be made.
Adapted from United Nations Scientific Committee of the Effects of Atomic Radiation (UNSCEAR): Sources and effects of ionizing radiation: 2006 report to the General Assembly with annexes. New York, United Nations, 2007.

to radioactive Thorotrast.[222] The SIR for small intestinal cancer was significantly elevated at 12.0 (95% CI 2.4, 35.2) but based on only two cases in the exposed group and one case in the control group. A report on Sellafield workers by Omar et al. indicated a nonsignificant increase in plutonium workers of small bowel cancer with an SMR of 2.63 (also based on only two cases).[148] The incidence was also nonsignificantly increased. Carpenter et al. examined workers in the United Kingdom who were occupationally exposed to tritium, plutonium, and other radionuclides.[191] The SMRs for small bowel cancer in each group were all nonsignificantly different from unity. A 2004 update of French uranium miners by Laurier et al. reported a nonsignificantly increased SMR of 1.4 for cancer of the small intestine, colon, and rectum as a group.[186]

Summary

The 1988,[370] 1994,[369] 2000,[375] and 2006[86] UNSCEAR reports and the 1990 ICRP report[248] do not give any risk estimate for cancer of the small bowel following radiation exposure. The BEIR V Committee indicates that "no carcinogenic effects of radiation on the small intestine have been evident in any of the irradiated human populations studied to date."[3] The UNSCEAR 2006 report mentions that the weak epidemiological evidence, in particular the lack of any trend with dose in the cervical case-control study and the lack of expected increase in risk with time in the cervical cancer cohort study, indicates that the small intestine is not susceptible to cancer induction, even at high doses.[86]

COLON CANCER

General

Colon cancer is most common in industrialized countries. Perhaps the highest rate in the world is found in the white male population of Connecticut. Nonhereditary factors appear to play a major role in etiology, because migrants to an area soon have rates approaching that of the local population. A genetic component is also a factor, at least for some cancer-prone families. Colorectal cancer is increased almost 20-fold among persons with long-standing ulcerative colitis. There are a large number of studies relating colorectal cancer to diet. Positive associations have been reported for intake of red meat and diets low in fiber and high in dietary fat. Some studies have reported an increase in risk of colon cancer with either cholelithiasis or cholecystectomy. This may reflect an effect of altered bile acids, but the association remains controversial. For reasons that are unknown, colorectal cancers are shifting from occurring mostly in the rectum to occurring more often in the colon. Tumors of the rectum and colon appear to be etiologically different because colon cancer is more frequent in females, and rectal tumors are more common in males.[358,700,728]

External Exposure

Background Radiation

Two studies have examined the relationship between natural background radiation and the risk of colon cancer. In a large study in China, colon cancer was more frequent in the high-background area (age-adjusted, site-specific cancer mortality of 2.38 per 105 person-years) than in the area with low-background radiation (1.70 per 105 person-years).[29] Tao et al. reported on cancer mortality in the high-background radiation areas of Yangjiang, China, during 1979–1995 where the average annual exposure was 6.4 mSv (including internal exposure).[33] The exposed were divided into low-, medium-, and high-dose groups and compared with a control group. In all of the groups the findings were nonsignificant relative to colon cancer. The RRs were 0.58 (95% CI 0.05 to 6.41), 1.68 (95% CI 0.28 to 10.08), and 1.27 (95% CI 0.18 to 9.03), respectively. No relationship was identified in a study of terrestrial radiation in Connecticut.[21] Increased exposure to natural cosmic radiation occurs to airline crews and there have been a number of studies that include information on the risk of colon cancer. Pukkala et al.,[39] studying over 10,000 Nordic airline pilots, found a nonsignificant decrease in colon cancer and Band et al.[40] in a study of 2740 pilots exposed at doses of 6 mSv per year for an average of 20 years (for a total average dose of about 120 mSv) found a nonsignificantly decreased SIR and a nonsignificantly increased SMR.

Fallout and Populations Near Nuclear Facilities

Studies of fallout within the United States as a result of nuclear weapons testing at the Nevada test site showed a decrease in colon cancer in high fallout areas compared with low fallout areas and a significant decrease compared with the rest of the United States, with an OR of 0.53 (95% CI 0.46 to 0.76).[456] As a group, populations living around United States nuclear plants have not shown an increase in colon and rectal cancer rates.[78] The SMRs for all facilities combined before start-up were 1.00 in the study counties and 1.05 in the control counties. After facility operation, the values were 1.06 and 1.06, respectively. There are three papers concerning potential environmental uranium contamination and the possibility of colon/rectal cancer in the public. Boice et al. indicated a nonsignificant increase around a uranium mining and milling facility in Texas and a significant decreases near uranium facilities in Pennsylvania and Colorado.[89,90,90a] A nonsignificant decrease was found by Boice et al. in a study of persons residing near the Hanford National Laboratory.[91] Lopez-Abente et al. have reported on solid tumor mortality near Spain's four nuclear power plants and four uranium fuel cycle facilities and the RR for colorectal cancer was not significantly different from unity at 1.01.[283]

Atomic Bomb Survivors

In a study of colorectal cancer incidence in the LSS sample of atomic bomb survivors reported by Nakatsuka et al., there was an excess risk of colon cancer, the ERR at 1 Sv being 0.8 (90% CI 0.37, 1.36).[729] Later follow-up by Preston et al. also indicated a statistically significant increase for cancer of the colon.[319] In the 1958–1998 period, 1516 cases were observed compared with 1438 expected (an excess of 78 cases) for the persons who received 0.01 Sv or more and a mean dose of 0.23 Sv. They estimated an ERR at 1 Gy of 0.54 (95% CI 0.30, 0.81) and an EAR of 8.0 (95% CI 4.4, 12) $(10^4 PYSv)^{-1}$. There was a decreasing EAR with increasing time since exposure as well as with increasing attained age. The dose-response relationship was quite linear up to 2 Gy, after which the slope increased.

The LSS mortality study data as of 1985 also demonstrated a statistically significant increase in colon cancer that did not occur until 15 years after exposure.[10] There were 129 deaths from colon cancer versus 117 expected (an excess of 12) during the 1,203,100 person-years of observation for the 41,000 persons who received 0.01 Sv or more. The ERR at 1 Sv was 0.5, and the absolute excess risk of colon cancer deaths was 0.5 $(10^4 PYSv)^{-1}$. Preston et al. reported on mortality of atomic bomb survivors from 1950–1997.[281] In males there was a statistically significant excess of colon cancer at dose levels of 1 Sv, with an ERR of 0.54 (90% CI 0.13, 1.2). In females there was a statistically significant excess at dose levels of 1 Sv, and an ERR of 0.49 (90% CI 0.11, 1.1).

Occupational Exposure

Studies of occupational exposure have not shown a significant radiation-related increase in colon cancer. There are multiple large U.K. studies of occupational exposure of radiation and nuclear workers. Darby et al. have reported an RR for cancer of the large intestine and rectum of 1.12 (95% CI 0.78 to 1.61).[52] Beral et al. indicate a ratio rate of exposed to nonexposed atomic energy authority employees of 0.92 (95% CI 0.46 to 1.85),[143] and an SMR 0.92 (95% CI 0.46 to 1.85) among atomic weapons workers.[144] Kendall et al. indicate an SMR of 1.01 for colon cancer.[145] Muirhead et al. performed a second analysis of the U.K. National Registry for Radiation Workers and studied a cohort of 124,743 workers with mean doses of 30.5 mSv.[146] Both a lagged and unlagged analysis for cancer of the large intestine (colon) gave nonsignificant results with an SMR of 0.95 (95% CI 0.84 to 1.07) and 0.94 (95% CI 0.82 to 1.07), respectively. There was also a nonsignificant negative dose response with an ERR per Sv of −0.71 (90% CI −1.36 to 0.49). Muirhead et al. also studied mortality and incidence of cancer during 1952–1998 in men from the United Kingdom who participated in the United Kingdom's atmospheric nuclear weapons tests and experimental programs whose doses were not estimated.[54] Their incidence rate for cancer of the colon

and rectum and the RR was not significantly different from unity at 1.02 (90% CI 0.90, 1.17).

A report on Sellafield workers by Omar et al. indicated a nonsignificant increase in colon cancer among nonplutonium radiation workers with an SMR of 1.10 and incidence was also nonsignificantly increased.[148] McGeoghegan et al. reported on the mortality and cancer morbidity experience of employees at the Chapelcross plant of British Nuclear Fuels during 1955–1995.[149] The cohort included 2628 workers with median doses of 39 mSv. In radiation workers the SMR for cancer of the colon was nonsignificant and decreased at 0.99.

Artalejo et al. reported on mortality among workers of the former Spanish Nuclear Energy Board with a cohort of 5657 workers and mean exposure of 11.42 mSv.[151] The SMR for colon cancer was nonsignificantly reduced at 0.83 (95% CI 0.33 to 1.72). Habib et al. have reported on cancer incidence among Australian nuclear industry–monitored radiation workers and indicated a nonsignificantly increased SIR of 1.23 for colon cancer.[152] Rahu et al. studied the cancer incidence of 5446 male Latvian and Estonian Chernobyl cleanup workers and indicated an SIR not significantly different from unity at 0.99 for colon and rectal cancer considered together.[178]

There are several Canadian occupational radiation exposure studies. Gribbin reported an SMR for colon cancer of 1.00 (95% CI 0.61 to 1.55).[260] Sont et al. analyzed cancer incidence and occupational radiation exposure based on the National Dose Registry of Canada, which included a cohort of 191,333 persons with an average dose for males of 11.5 mSv and an average dose for the cohort of 6.64 mSv.[153] The SIR was 0.89 (90% CI 0.79 to 0.99). Ashmore et al. analyzed the mortality and occupational radiation exposure based on the National Dose Registry of Canada which included a cohort of 206,620 individuals with 5426 deaths.[154] The average exposure for males was 10.6 mSv and their SMR for colon cancer was significantly reduced at 0.854 (90% CI 0.729 to 0.995).

In the United States, Gilbert's study of the Hanford workers from 1945–1986[361] yielded an SMR of 0.84 for colon cancer, and the combined study[157] indicated the following SMRs for colon cancer: Hanford, 0.95: Oak Ridge, 0.41; and Rocky Flats, 0.46. No increase was seen in a later combined analysis.[158] Howe et al. reported on the mortality of U.S. nuclear power industry workers and found a nonsignificantly decreased risk of colon cancer with an SMR of 0.75 (95% CI 0.53, 1.04).[159] In workers at the Savannah River facility, Cragle et al. indicated an O/E ratio of 2:1.2, which was statistically nonsignificant.[288] At the Mound facility an increase in colon cancer was reported, but the SMR of 1.28 (95% CI 0.55 to 2.52) was not statistically different from unity.[156]

Wilkinson et al. reported an SMR for colon cancer of 0.63 (90% CI 0.29, 1.88) at Rocky Flats.[286] For Oak Ridge worker populations, Checkoway et al. estimated an SMR of 0.63 (95% CI 0.30, 1.16) using U.S. comparisons and 0.79 (95% CI 0.38 to 1.45) using Tennessee statistics as a comparison.[284] Wing et al. report an SMR of 0.89 (95% CI 0.62 to 1.24) for Oak Ridge workers.[285] Frome reported a mortality study of employees in the nuclear industry at Oak Ridge, Tennessee, which covered 106,020 employees with 27,982 deaths and the SMR for cancer of the large intestine (colon) in white males was nonsignificantly reduced at 0.81.[160] Fry et al. conducted a study of mortality and morbidity among persons occupationally exposed to 50 or more mSv (5000 mrem) in a year, which included 3145 subjects with 588 deaths.[161] The mean external exposure was 153 mSv and the SMR for colon cancer was nonsignificantly elevated at 1.42 (95% CI 0.77, 2.38). Wiggs et al. found a significantly reduced SMR of 0.73 for colon cancer in a follow-up study of Los Alamos workers.[164]

Cardis et al. investigated cancer mortality among nuclear industry workers in three countries in a very large study of 95,673 workers with over 2 million person-years at risk and 15,825 deaths.[166] The trend for colon cancer was nonsignificantly negative at −0.83 with a P value of 0.797. Cardis et al. have also reported the cancer mortality results from a 15-country collaborative study of nuclear workers.[168] This is the largest occupational study to date and included a cohort of 407,391 workers with 18,993 deaths and 5.2 million person-years of follow-up. The ERR per Sv for colon cancer was nonsignificantly positive at 0.21 (90% CI < 0, 3.07).

There are a number of studies concerned with medical occupational exposure and the risk of colon cancer. In a study of British radiologists Smith et al. reported an O/E ratio for colon cancer of 1.28, which was not significantly increased for those employed before 1920.[584] For those employed after 1920, the O/E ratio was 0.61. Berrington et al. reported 100 years of experience in British radiologists with regard to mortality from cancer and other causes during 1897–1997.[94] The cohort included 1338 male radiologists whose doses were not quantified. The SMR for cancer of the intestine for all radiologists post-1920 was nonsignificantly reduced at 0.63. Doody et al. reported on mortality among U.S. radiologic technologists during 1926–1990 including 143,517 technologists with 7345 deaths whose doses were not evaluated.[97] The SMR for colon cancer was significantly below that expected at 0.78 (95% CI 0.67, 0.90). Sigurdson et al. studied the cancer incidence in 90,305 U.S. radiologic technologists and found that the SIR for colon cancer was nonsignificantly elevated at 1.06 (95% CI 0.94, 1.17).[101] Mohan et al. studied cancer and other causes of mortality among 146,022 radiologic technologists employed from 1940 on in whom the SMR for colon cancer in males was significantly reduced at 0.75 (95% CI 0.6, 0.9) and in females it was significantly reduced at 0.80 (95% CI 0.7, 0.9).[98,99] The cancer

incidence among medical diagnostic workers in China was reported Wang et al. in 1988.[102] Their study compared 27,011 radiation workers with 25,782 persons in other medical specialties. The x-ray workers had a 50% higher risk of developing cancer (RR 1.5), but for colon cancer the RR was nonsignificantly reduced at 0.93. However in a 2002 follow-up study, also by Wang et al., the RR for cancer of the colon and rectum is nonsignificantly reduced at 0.85 (95% CI about 0.7, 1.05).[253] Aoyama et al. has studied the mortality of Japanese technologists during of 1969–1993.[95] This was a cohort study of over 12,000 male radiological technicians with an average dose of 466 mSv in whom the SMR for colon cancer was nonsignificantly increased at 1.29 (95% CI 0.90, 1.80).

Medical Exposure

Diagnostic medical irradiation as a cause of colon cancer has been studied only in regard to the repeated fluoroscopies of the chest in Massachusetts TB patients. In one study Davis et al. reported that the SMRs for colon cancer were only significantly different from unity for the unexposed male controls, in whom it was significantly elevated.[105] In another study Davis et al. reported that SMRs for colon cancer were nonsignificantly above unity for exposed males and females as well as for unexposed males.[364]

Radiation therapy for benign conditions has not indicated a definite link between colon cancer and radiation, although Darby et al. pointed out that colon cancer mortality was increased by 30% in patients treated for ankylosing spondylitis.[109] Colon cancer has been known to be associated with ankylosing spondylitis without radiation exposure, probably as a result of ulcerative colitis occurring in this condition. Mattsson et al. have reported on cancer incidence among 3090 women who received radiation therapy for benign breast disease.[114] The RR for colon cancer was nonsignificantly elevated at 1.80. Carr et al. studied malignant neoplasms after radiation therapy for peptic ulcer in 3719 patients who received mean doses to part of the colon of 14.8 Sv and lower doses elsewhere in the colon.[113] The RR was nonsignificantly increased at 2.60 (95% CI 0.28, 24) 0 to 10 years after exposure and was nonsignificantly decreased 11 to 62 years after exposure at 0.95 (95% CI 0.54, 1.67). Lundell et al. studied 14,351 subjects who received radiation therapy for skin hemangiomas.[589] The mean dose to the intestine was estimated to range from 1 mSv to 1 Sv with a mean of 30 mSv and the SIR for colon cancer was nonsignificantly increased at 1.02 (95% CI 0.6, 1.8).

Follow-up of patients who received intrauterine radium radiotherapy for benign uterine bleeding was conducted by Inskip et al.[118] The study included 4153 women who were studied over 110,000 person-years at risk, in whom there was no increase in cancer of the colon. A study by Darby et al. indicated a slight excess of colon

Relative risk

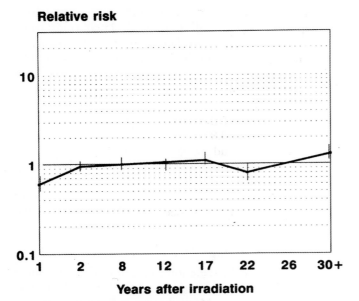

Colon cancer (cervix series)

Figure 5-20 ● RR of colon cancer by time after treatment for cervical carcinoma with radiation therapy. Error bars indicate 95% CI. (From Boice JD, Jr, et al: Second cancers following radiation treatment for cervical cancer: An international collaboration among cancer registries. J Natl Cancer Inst 1985;74:955–975.)

cancer in the same type of patients.[116] A similar study by Ryberg et al. reported there were nonsignificant increases in tumors of the rectum, colon, and nervous system.[297]

Follow-up studies after radiotherapy for cervical cancer do not show a radiation-related increase in colon cancer (Fig. 5-20). An incidence study of women treated for cervical cancer included 82,616 exposed women compared with 99,424 unexposed controls.[124] No excess was identified for cancer of the colon; the O/E ratio was 1.0 in those treated with radiotherapy and 1.1 in those without radiotherapy. Another study that compared 4188 women with second cancers with 6880 controls, reported an RR for colon cancer of 1.02 (90% CI 0.7, 1.6), with an estimated dose to the colon of 24.2 Gy.[126] In a smaller case-control study no excess was found.[127] Brenner et al. have studied second malignancies in prostate carcinoma patients treated with radiotherapy or surgery and reported a nonsignificant increase in colon cancer risk with the radiotherapy group with an ERR of 0.24 at times greater than 10 years postexposure compared to the surgery only group.[137] A large study by Baxter et al. of 30,552 prostate cancer patients who received radiotherapy and 55,263 who had surgery only did not find an increase in cancer in nonirradiated portions of the colon (i.e., other than cecum, sigmoid, and rectum).[730]

In children treated with radiotherapy for cancer, the data are different from those reported for the cervix radiotherapy series. Hawkins et al. have reported childhood cancer survivors to have an increased risk of

second primary tumors in the digestive tract, with an RR of 10 (95% CI 5 to 20).[307] Most of this risk was from five cases of colon cancer observed in over 10,100 patients studied. In a follow-up study of 1507 HD patients, Tucker et al. observed four cases of colon cancer compared with 1.2 expected, for an O/E of 3.5 (95% CI 0.9, 8.8).[436] Travis et al. have reported on long-term survival and second cancers in over 40,000 testicular cancer patients almost all of whom received infradiaphragmatic radiotherapy of about 30 Gy and the RR for colon cancer was significantly increased.[705]

Internal Exposure

Some studies have provided information on the risk of colon cancer following internal exposure. In Swedish Lapps, who eat reindeer meat and are presumed to have increased concentrations of cesium 137, the frequency of colon cancer was significantly lower than expected, with an SMR of 0.25 (95% CI 0.05, 0.74).[56] A study of miners has not revealed an increase in cancer of the intestine or colon, an SMR of 0.69 (95% CI 0.28, 1.41) being reported.[362]

Ritz et al. reported on cancer mortality in uranium processing workers at the Fernald plant in Ohio.[192] The SMR for colon cancer was nonsignificantly increased at 1.05. Dupree-Ellis et al. have reported on mortality in a cohort of 2514 uranium processing workers employed between 1942–1966 at the Mallinkrodt Chemical Works and found the SMR for colon cancer was nonsignificantly increased at 1.11.[193] McGeoghegan et al. reported on the mortality and cancer morbidity experience of workers at the Capenhurst uranium enrichment facility during 1946–1995.[242] The cohort of 12,540 workers included 3244 radiation workers with mean doses of 9.85 mSv. The SMR for colon cancer in radiation workers was nonsignificantly decreased at 0.91 and cancer registrations for colon cancer were also nonsignificantly increased at 1.03. McGeoghegan et al. also studied workers at the Springfields uranium production facility during 1946–1995; the cohort of 19,454 workers included 13,960 radiation workers with a mean external dose of 22.8 mSv.[243] The SMR for cancer of the colon for radiation workers was nonsignificantly reduced at 0.97 and for colon cancer site registrations it was significantly below that expected at 0.73. A meta-analysis of 14 studies, which included 120,000 uranium workers, found a nonsignificant decrease in colorectal cancer with an RR of 0.91 (95% CI 0.78, 1.04).[245] Darby et al. studied radon and cancers in Swedish iron miners and found a nonsignificant decrease in colon cancer with an O/E ratio of 0.88 (95% CI 0.40, 1.67).[183]

Those workers who have been monitored for internal contamination at the Oak Ridge National Laboratory have been studied by Wing et al. who reported an SMR for colon cancer of 0.78 (95% CI 0.40, 1.35).[285] In a study of Rocky Flats workers who had a plutonium body burden of 74 Bq (2 nCi) or more, Wilkinson et al. reported nonsignificant RRs for colon cancer of 0.97 (90% CI 0.07,

10.8) and 1.62 (90% CI 0.11, 18.3), using implausible latent periods of 2 and 5 years.[286] Using a reasonable latent period of 10 years, an RR of 5.70 (90% CI 0.38, 65.2) was found, which was not statistically different from unity because of the very small number of observed cases. No colon cancer has been observed in the 50-year follow-up of the Manhattan Project plutonium workers.[671] Wiggs et al. found an RR of 1.00 in a follow-up of Los Alamos plutonium workers.[164] A report on Sellafield workers by Omar et al. found a nonsignificant increase in colon cancer in plutonium workers with an SMR of 1.02 and incidence was also nonsignificantly increased.[148] Carpenter et al. examined workers in the United Kingdom who were occupationally exposed to tritium, plutonium, and other radionuclides among whom the SMRs for colon cancer in each group were all nonsignificantly reduced.[191] A 2004 update of French uranium miners by Laurier et al. reported a nonsignificantly increased SMR of 1.4 for cancer of the small intestine, colon, and rectum as a group.[186]

The literature generally does not reveal a significant increase in the frequency of colon cancer after internal administration of radioiodine. The largest and most recent of studies of the potential carcinogenic effects of diagnostic doses of radioiodine administered to perform thyroid scanning included 35,074 patients who were matched with the Swedish cancer registry.[270] Colon cancer was not reported separately, but there was no increase in digestive cancers as a group. Patients treated for hyperthyroidism have been followed in several studies. Holm et al.[271] reported a combined SIR for cancers of the colon and rectum of 1.17 (95% CI 0.97, 1.39), while Hoffman et al. reported an RR of 0.8 (95% CI 0.4, 1.7) for digestive organs as a group.[202] Ron et al. have more recently reported on cancer mortality among 35,593 hyperthyroid patients among whom the SMR for colon and rectal cancer considered together was nonsignificantly different from unity.[201] The SMR was 1.11 for those receiving any iodine 131 and 1.15 for those receiving iodine 131 alone. For thyroid cancer patients treated with radioiodine, colon cancer has not been considered alone, but Hall et al. have indicated an SIR for all digestive organs of 1.23 (95% CI 0.79, 1.84) versus an SIR of 1.17 (95% CI 0.84, 1.67) in nonexposed controls.[203] Rubino et al. also studied the risk of colorectal cancer after radioiodine treatment for thyroid cancer.[731] The authors stated that there is an almost significant increased risk of colorectal cancer, however, inspection of the data contained in the paper reveals that the conclusions were based on only 15 cases and the P value for trend with dose was 0.1.

Patients who have received Thorotrast for diagnostic medical purposes such as angiograms have had a significant residual amount of radioactivity in the abdomen, especially the liver, spleen, and lymph nodes.[229] While these patients have shown a highly increased risk of liver tumors, they have shown no consistent increase in the risk of colon cancer. In the Danish Thorotrast series the SIR for colon cancer was 1.3 (95% CI 0.6, 2.5).[213] The German Thorotrast series found less than the expected number of digestive system cancers as a group.[212] There were 10 deaths due to colon cancer in the 2334 Thorotrast patients and 16 colon cancer deaths in the 1912 control persons. No increase in colon cancer was found in the radium dial painters.[229] Nekolla et al. reported on malignancies in a cohort of 899 patients treated with high doses of radium 224 administered intravenously.[224] Colon doses were not estimated and the rate ratio for colon cancer was nonsignificantly decreased at 0.65. Nyberg et al. reported on cancer incidence after a 40-year follow-up among Swedish patients exposed to radioactive Thorotrast among whom the SIR for colon cancer was nonsignificantly elevated at 1.8 (95% CI 0.8, 3.6).[222]

Summary

The UNSCEAR 1988 risk estimate for radiogenic cancer of the colon, using a multiplicative risk model, was 7.9 (90% CI 3.6, 13.4) excess lifetime fatal cancers for 1000 persons exposed to 1 Gy of low-LET radiation at high-dose rate.[370] The BEIR V Committee[3] pointed out that the atomic bomb survivor data did not show an increase in risk for at least 15 years after exposure, following which the ERR was then 0.85 per Gy or 0.8 fatal cases per 10^4PYGy. The ICRP 1990 lifetime fatal risk estimate for a population of all ages exposed to low doses of radiation is 8.5 ($10^{-4}Sv^{-1}$), and for workers it is 6.8 ($10^{-4}Sv^{-1}$).[248]

The 2000 UNSCEAR report indicates data on the Japanese atomic bomb survivors are consistent with a linear-dose response.[375] The effects of gender, age at exposure, and time since exposure on the ERR per Sv are not clear, although the EAR per Sv does increase with increasing time since exposure in the LSS. Changes over time in baseline rates in Japan make it difficult to decide how to transfer risks across populations. Also the lack of precision in low-dose studies of external low-LET radiation and of internal low-LET and high-LET radiation do not allow conclusions to be drawn. Risk factors for colon cancer from epidemiological studies have been summarized by UNSCEAR 2006 (Table 5-22), and it was concluded that there is evidence that colon cancer can be induced by ionizing radiation, compatible with a linear dose-response pattern.[86] The evidence for this comes almost entirely from the Japanese LSS data. The LSS data also suggest that the ERR decreases with increasing age at exposure.

RECTAL CANCER

General

The incidence of rectal cancer is lower than that of cancer of the colon. The geographic incidence is broadly similar.

Table 5-22 • Risk Estimates for Cancer Incidence and Mortality from Studies of Radiation Exposure: Colon Cancer*

Study	Average Excess Relative Risk at 1 Sv	Average Excess Absolute Risk $(10^4 PYSv)^{-1}$
External Low-LET Exposures		
Incidence		
A-bomb Life Span Study[319]		
Males	0.85 (0.52–1.26)	1.41 (0.1–3.07)
Females	0.42 (0.14–0.76)	1.46 (0.69–2.45)
Age at exposure		
<20	0.81 (0.46–1.24)	0.99 (0.31–1.92)
20–40	0.44 (0.14–0.82)	1.78 (0.56–3.46)
>40	0.45 (<0–1.13)	3.11 (0.22–6.54)
Time since exposure		
12–15	2.02 (<0–9.3)	<0 (<0–349.91)
15–30	1.24 (0.51–2.25)	1.14 (0.44–2.09)
>30	0.52 (0.3–0.78)	2.95 (1.32–4.89)
All	0.64 (0.42–0.9)	1.44 (0.76–2.27)
Cervical cancer case control[6]	0 (−0.01–0.02)	0.01 (−0.09–0.18)
Sweden metropathia cohort[297]	5 (−2.2–16)	NA
Stockholm skin hemangioma[589]	0.37	0.11
Canada National Dose Registry[153]	2.6 (<0–7.5)	NA
Capenhurst uranium facility[242]	−1.3 (<−1.3–23.97)	NA
U.K. Springfields uranium workers[243]	11.41 (<−6.27–36.45)	NA
U.K. Chapelcross workers[149]	2.1 (<−2.65–13.92)	NA
Mortality		
A-bomb Life Span Study[281]		
Males	0.53 (0.04–1.2)	<0 (<0–707.28)
Females	0.5 (0.06–1.09)	<0 (<0–623.23)
Age at exposure		
<20	1.13 (0.32–2.34)	<0 (<0–210.88)
20–40	0.23 (<0–0.84)	<0 (<0–966.47)
>40	0.38 (<0–1.12)	<0 (<0–1440.1)
Time since exposure		
12–15	<0 (<0–2.85)	<0 (<0–74.98)
15–30	1.12 (0.27–2.41)	<0 (<0–457.15)
>30	0.3 (<0–0.73)	<0 (<0–1309.2)
All	0.51 (0.17–0.94)	<0 (<0–656.32)
Benign gynecological disease[118]	0.51 (−0.8–5.61)	3.2 (−0.9–7.1)
Metropathia haemorrhagica[116]	0.13 (0.01–0.26)	0.92 (0.1–1.8)
Peptic ulcer[113]	−0.01 (<−0.01–0.07)	NA
U.K. National Registry for Radiation Workers[146]	−0.71 (−1.36–0.49)	NA
Nuclear power industry workers in the United States[159]	−2.28 (<−2.51–10.5)	NA
5 rem study in United States[161]	1.8 (−1–6.1)	2.6 (−1.4–8.6)
Japanese radiological technologists[95]	0.62 (−0.2–1.7)	0.6 (−0.2–1.7)
IARC 15-country nuclear workers study[167,168]	0.21 (<0, 3.07)	
Internal High-LET Exposures		
Incidence		
Danish and Swedish Thorotrast patients[219]	1.5 (0.7–3)	NA
Mortality		
German Thorotrast patients[212,221]	~0.5	NA
U.S. Thorotrast patients[219]	∞ (0.5–∞)	NA

*The studies listed are those for which quantitative estimates of risk could be made.
Adapted from United Nations Scientific Committee of the Effects of Atomic Radiation (UNSCEAR): Sources and effects of ionizing radiation: 2006 report to the General Assembly with annexes. New York, United Nations, 2007.

In contrast, however, rates in immigrants to an area tend to remain similar to those in the country of origin.[358] While many reports group colon and rectal cancers together, in this text we have chosen to discuss them separately, because the two organ sites seem to have different susceptibilities relative to radiation carcinogenesis. In the Japanese atomic bomb survivor incidence data, there is a potentially linear dose-response relationship for colon cancer, but no relationship between radiation dose and rectal cancer.

External Exposure

Background Radiation and Public Near Nuclear Facilities

In a Connecticut study of background terrestrial radiation, Walter et al. found less rectal cancer in the higher radiation areas than in the lower radiation areas.[21] Tao et al. reported on cancer mortality in the high-background radiation areas of Yangjiang, China, during 1979–1995 where the average annual exposure was 6.4 mSv (including internal exposure).[33] The RR for rectal cancer was not significantly different from unity at 1.01 (95% CI 0.20, 5.23).

No increase in colon and rectal cancer was found in a study of populations living around U.S. nuclear facilities.[78] Lopez-Abente et al. have reported on solid tumor mortality near Spain's four nuclear power plants and four uranium fuel cycle facilities where the RR for colorectal cancer was not significantly different from unity at 1.01.[283] Increased exposure to natural cosmic irradiation occurs to airline crews and there have been a number of studies which included information on their rectal cancer rates. Pukkala et al., in studying over 10,000 Nordic airline pilots, found a nonsignificant decrease. Band et al. in a study of 2740 pilots with doses of 6 mSv per year over an average of 20 years (for a total average dose about 120 mSv) found a significantly decreased SIR.[40] Blettner et al. also reviewed additional studies and found variable but nonsignificant results.[41,42]

Atomic Bomb Survivors

In a study specifically of colorectal cancer incidence in the atomic bomb survivor LSS sample reported by Nakatsuka et al. there was no excess risk of rectal cancer.[729] Later follow-up by Preston et al. also did not indicate a significant ERR; at 1 Gy was not significantly elevated at 0.19 (90% CI −0.04, 0.47) and the EAR was 0.56 (90% CI −0.13, 1.4) cases per 10^4PYGy. As of 1998, there were an estimated 14 excess cases out of a total 838 rectal cancer cases.[319] The LSS mortality study data as of 1985 demonstrated a statistically significant increase in colon cancer, but, again, cancer of the rectum was not increased. In the 2003 update studies of mortality of atomic bomb survivors during 1950–1997, Preston et al. analyzed a cohort of 86,572 persons with an average external dose of 0.23 Sv.[281] In males there was a statistically nonsignificant decrease of rectal cancer at dose levels of 1 Sv, with an ERR of −0.25 (90% CI < −0.3, 0.15). In females there was a statistically significant excess at dose levels of 1 Sv, and an ERR of 0.75 (90% CI 0.16, 1.6).

Occupational Exposure

The large occupational exposure studies of atomic workers in the United Kingdom have not shown an increase in rectal cancer; these include the studies of Darby et al.[52] and Beral et al.,[143] who found a nonsignificant ratio rate of rectal cancer in exposed to nonexposed employees of 2.09 in a study of atomic weapons workers (95% CI 0.9 to 4.8). A study by Kendall et al. reported an SMR for rectal cancer of 0.82.[145] A second analysis in 1999 of 124,743 workers in the U.K. National Registry of Radiation Workers by Muirhead et al. using a lagged analysis yielded a significantly reduced SMR for rectal cancer of 0.79 (95% CI 0.66, 0.94).[146] A report on Sellafield workers by Omar et al. indicated a nonsignificant decrease in rectal cancer among nonplutonium radiation workers with an SMR of 0.89 and incidence was also nonsignificantly decreased.[148] McGeoghegan et al. reported on the mortality and cancer morbidity experience of employees at the Chapelcross plant of British Nuclear Fuels during 1955–1995 with a cohort of 2628 workers who had a median dose of 39 mSv.[149] In the radiation workers the SMR for cancer of the rectum was nonsignificantly decreased at 0.84. Habib et al. have reported on the cancer incidence among Australian nuclear industry–monitored radiation workers in whom they found a nonsignificant SIR of 0.98 for rectal cancer.[152] Rahu et al. have reported on cancer incidence in 5446 male Latvian and Estonian Chernobyl cleanup workers and indicate a nonsignificant SIR of 0.99 for their rates of colon and rectal cancer considered together.[178]

One study of Canadian atomic workers has yielded an SMR for rectal cancer of 1.52 (95% CI 0.85 to 2.51). Ashmore et al. reported the first analysis of mortality and occupational radiation exposure based on the National Dose Registry of Canada which included a cohort of 206,620 individuals and 5426 deaths.[154] The average exposure for males was 10.6 mSv. The SMR for rectal cancer was significantly reduced at 0.66 (90% CI 0.50, 0.87). Sont et al. also reported on the relation between cancer incidence and occupational radiation exposure based on the National Dose Registry of Canada, which included a cohort of 191,333 persons with an average dose for males of 11.5 mSv and an average dose for the cohort of 6.64 mSv. The SIR for rectal cancer in males was significantly reduced at 0.71 and in females it was nonsignificantly reduced at 0.79.

None of the large occupational exposure studies in the United States has shown any significant or consistent association between radiation and rectal cancer. The study of Hanford workers from 1945–1986 by Gilbert et al. found an SMR of 0.67 for rectal cancer.[361] The combined study of several federal facilities reported SMRs for cancer of the rectum as follows: Hanford, 0.76; Oak Ridge, 0.16; and Rocky Flats, 0.56.[157] In a follow-up study of the same group no significant increase was found.[158] At the Savannah River plant, Cragle et al. did not identify any cases of rectal cancer.[288] At the Mound facility in Ohio, Wiggs et al. reported an SMR of 0.46 (95% CI 0.01 to 2.54) for rectal cancer.[156] In other studies of workers at U.S. government facilities, the results have also been negative. Wilkinson et al. reported an SMR of 0.53 (90%

CI 0.01 to 1.66) for rectal cancer at Rocky Flats.[286] Checkoway et al. found an SMR of 0.74 (95% CI 0.20 to 1.90) using U.S. comparison data and 1.09 (95% CI 0.30 to 2.79) using Tennessee comparison data.[284] Wing et al. reported a significantly reduced SMR for rectal cancer of 0.42 (95% CI 0.14 to 0.99) for rectal cancer in Oak Ridge National Laboratory workers.[285] Frome reported that the SMR in black and white males and females was nonsignificantly reduced in all categories.[160] Fry et al. reported a study of mortality and morbidity among 3145 persons occupationally exposed to 50 or more mSv (5000 mrem) in a year with a mean external exposure of 153 mSv and their SMR for rectal cancer was nonsignificantly reduced.[161] Wiggs et al. found a significantly reduced SMR of 0.58 for rectal cancer in a follow-up of Los Alamos workers.[164] Iwasaki et al. conducted a second analysis of mortality of nuclear industry workers in Japan.[150] The study included 176,000 male workers and 5527 deaths. Average annual doses were 3.5 mSv before 1982 and 1.2 mSv after 1982. For rectal cancer the SMR was nonsignificantly decreased at 0.87 (95% CI 0.70, 1.06).

Cardis et al. investigated cancer mortality among nuclear industry workers in three countries in a very large study of 95,673 workers with over 2 million person-years at risk and 15,825 deaths.[166] The trend for rectal cancer was nonsignificant at 0.99 with a P value of 0.161. Cardis et al. also have reported the cancer mortality results from a 15-country collaborative study of nuclear workers.[168] This is the largest occupational study to date and included a cohort of 407,391 workers with 18,993 deaths and 5.2 million person-years of follow-up. The ERR per Sv for rectal cancer was nonsignificantly positive at 1.27 (90% CI < 0, 7.62).

Ritz et al. have reported on cancer mortality in uranium processing workers at the Fernald plant in Ohio whose SMR for rectal cancer was nonsignificantly increased at 1.05.[192] Dupree-Ellis et al. have reported on mortality in a cohort of 2514 uranium processing workers employed between 1942–1966 at the Mallinkrodt Chemical Works and the SMR for rectal cancer was nonsignificantly increased at 1.48.[193] McGeoghegan et al. have reported on the mortality of 12,540 workers (including 3244 radiation workers) at the Capenhurst uranium enrichment facility during 1946–1995.[242] The SMR for rectal cancer was nonsignificantly reduced in radiation workers at 0.81. They also studied cancer mortality experience of 19,454 workers (including 13,960 radiation workers) at the Springfields uranium production facility during 1946–1995 in whom the SMR for rectal cancer was nonsignificantly reduced for radiation workers at 0.96.[243]

Cancer incidence among medical diagnostic workers in China has been reviewed by Wang et al. who compared 27,011 workers with 25,782 persons in other medical specialties.[102] While the x-ray workers had a 50%

higher risk of developing cancer of several types, the RR for rectal cancer was nonsignificantly elevated at 1.10. Aoyama et al. conducted a mortality survey of over 12,000 male Japanese radiological technologists during 1969–1993.[95] The cohort had an average dose of 466 mSv. The SMR for rectal cancer was nonsignificantly decreased at 0.95 (95% CI 0.59, 1.43). A study of British radiologists by Smith et al. found an O/E ratio of 0.44 for rectal cancer, which was not statistically different from 1.0 for those radiologists employed before 1920.[584] For those employed after 1920 the O/E ratio was 0.35. Berrington et al. have reported on 100 years experience in U.K. radiologists and reported a nonsignificantly decreased SMR for rectal cancer of 0.34 for those employed from 1897–1920 and a nonsignificantly decreased SMR of 0.83 for those employed after 1920.[94] Doody et al. reported on mortality among 143,517 U.S. radiologic technologists during 1926–1990 but doses were not evaluated.[97] The SMR for rectal cancer was nonsignificantly reduced at 0.78 (95% CI 0.56, 1.06). Sigurdson et al. studied cancer incidence in 90,305 U.S. radiologic technologists and found that the SIR for rectal cancer was significantly reduced at 0.62 (95% CI 0.48, 0.76).[101] Mohan et al. studied cancer and other causes of mortality among 146,022 radiologic technologists employed from 1940 and later and the SMR for rectal cancer in males was nonsignificantly reduced at 0.86 (95% CI 0.6, 1.3) and in females it was also nonsignificantly reduced at 0.85 (95% CI 0.6, 1.2).[98,99]

Medical Exposure

In studying Massachusetts TB patients who received multiple chest fluoroscopies during treatment, Davis et al. found that SMRs for rectal cancer were above unity for both exposed and unexposed persons but were not significantly different from each other.[105] In a second study the results were similar and SMRs for rectal cancer were nonsignificantly above unity for all exposed and unexposed groups except for the male exposed patients, who had a nonsignificantly low SMR of 0.6.[364] There are at least two studies in which patients received radiotherapy for benign conditions, and they were then followed with reference to the occurrence of rectal cancer. In the ankylosing spondylitis series, cancer of the rectum was not significantly elevated, with a reported O/E ratio of 1.07.[109] Follow-up of patients who received intrauterine radium radiotherapy for benign uterine bleeding by Inskip et al. included 4153 women who were studied over 110,000 person-years at risk.[118] An excess of cancer of the rectum was identified, but it did not change with time after irradiation or radiation dose. In addition the risk of rectal cancer was not elevated in the 10-year survivors. The estimated dose to the rectum was 3 Gy. Mattsson et al. have reported on the cancer incidence among 3090 women who received radiation therapy for benign breast disease among whom the RR for rectal

Relative risk

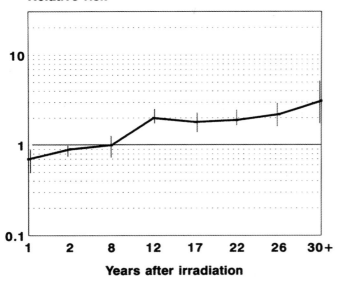

Years after irradiation

Rectal Cancer (cervix series)

Figure 5-21 • RR of rectal cancer by time after treatment for cervical carcinoma with radiation therapy. Error bars indicate 95% CI. (From Boice JD, Jr, et al: Second cancers following radiation treatment for cervical cancer: An international collaboration among cancer registries. J Natl Cancer Inst 1985;74:955–975.)

cancer was nonsignificant at 1.97.[114] No increase in rectal cancer was found by Griem et al. in a study of patients treated with radiotherapy for peptic ulcer.[112] Carr et al. performed a follow-up study of the same group of 3719 patients with doses to the abdomen of about 15 Gy.[113] No cases of rectal cancer were found after radiotherapy in the period 0 to 10 years postexposure and in the follow-up period of 11 to 62 years postexposure the RR was non-significantly reduced at 0.49.

In contrast to the results observed at lower doses, when radiotherapy has included the rectum in the primary beam and the absorbed doses have been in excess of 30 to 60 Gy, there does appear to have been an increased risk of rectal cancer at times more than 10 years after exposure (Fig. 5-21). An incidence study of women treated for cervical cancer that included 82,616 exposed women compared with 99,424 unexposed controls drawn from Canada, Denmark, Finland, Norway, Sweden, Yugoslavia, the United Kingdom, and the United States, covering 1.28 million person-years at risk, excess risk was found for cancer of the rectum, the O/E ratio being 1.3 in those treated with radiotherapy but also 1.3 in those treated without radiotherapy.[124] For women followed more than 10 years, there did appear to be more elevation of the O/E ratio for radiation-treated women (O/E ratio of 1.8) than for those treated in other ways (O/E ratio of 1.3). The ERR after 30 years was 3.1. In a case-control study of women treated for cervical cancer, which matched 4188 women with controls, an excess of rectal cancer was

found, the RR for rectal cancer being 1.83 (90% CI 1.2 to 2.8), with estimated average dose to the rectum of 30 to 60 Gy.[126] In a case-control study the number of persons was smaller, but, again, statistically significant excess risks were found for cancer of the rectum.[127] A Japanese study of cervical cancer patients including 5725 patients treated with radiotherapy alone and 4161 treated with surgery alone found a significant excess for cancer of the rectum, with an O/E ratio of 1.9 in those treated with radiotherapy versus 0.5 in those treated with surgery alone.[128] Brenner et al. have studied second malignancies in prostate carcinoma patients treated with radiotherapy or surgery and reported a significant increase in rectal cancer risk with the radio-therapy group having an ERR of 1.05 at times greater than 10 years postexposure compared to the surgery only group.[137] A large study by Baxter et al. of 30,552 prostate cancer patients who received radiotherapy and 55,263 who had surgery only also showed a significant increase in the hazards ratio for rectal cancer of 1.7 (95% CI 1.4, 2.2) in the irradiated group.[730]

Internal Exposure

No increase in rectal cancer was found in a study of Swedish Lapps, who may have ingested more cesium 137 than other populations; the SMR for rectal cancer was 0.96 (95% CI 0.39, 1.98).[56] There is only a limited amount of data on rectal cancer in relationship to internal occupational radiation exposure. Most studies of internal contamination have either not examined the issue or not reported the data because no excess was found. Studies in uranium miners have not revealed an increase in cancer of the rectum, an SMR of 0.27 (95% CI 0.01, 1.50) being reported.[362] A 2004 update of French uranium miners by Laurier et al. reported a nonsignificant SMR of 1.4 for cancer of the small intestine, colon, and rectum as a group.[186] Darby et al. studied radon and cancers in Swedish iron miners and found a significant increase in rectal cancer with an O/E ratio of 1.94 (95% CI 1.03, 3.31).[183] This finding is of dubious scientific significance given the dosimetry of radon.

Wing et al. found no increase in Oak Ridge workers who were monitored for internal contamination, an SMR of 0.43 (95% CI 0.05, 1.57) being reported for rectal cancer.[285] Wiggs et al. found a nonsignificantly elevated RR in a follow-up of Los Alamos plutonium workers.[164] A report on Sellafield workers by Omar et al. indicated a nonsignificant increase in mortality from rectal cancer among plutonium workers with an SMR of 1.01 and inci-dence was nonsignificantly increased.[148] Carpenter et al. studied workers in the United Kingdom who were occu-pationally exposed to tritium, plutonium, and other radio-nuclides and the SMRs for rectal cancer in each group were all nonsignificantly reduced.[191] One might suppose that the radium dial painters who ingested large quantities of radium might have an increase in rectal cancer; however, no increase was found in this population.[229]

Few, if any, studies have reported results for cancer of the rectum as a specific site following internal exposure as a result of medical procedures. A study of 35,074 patients who received diagnostic doses of radioiodine and were matched with the Swedish cancer registry reported no increase in digestive cancers as a group.[270] In patients treated with radioiodine for hyperthyroidism, Holm et al.[271] reported an SIR for colon and rectum combined of 1.17 (95% CI 0.97, 1.39), and Hoffman et al.[202] reported an RR for cancer of the digestive organs of 0.8 (95% CI 0.4, 1.7). Ron et al. reported on cancer mortality among 35,593 hyperthyroid patients.[201] The SMR for colon and rectal cancers considered as a group was not significantly different from unity. The SMR was 1.11 for those receiving any iodine 131 and 1.15 for those receiving iodine 131 alone.

In patients who received much larger doses of radioiodine during treatment for thyroid cancer, Hall et al. found an SIR for all digestive organs of 1.23 (95% CI 0.79, 1.84) and an SIR in nonexposed controls of 1.17 (95% CI 0.84 to 1.67).[203] In the Danish Thorotrast series no increase in rectal cancer was found, the reported SIR for this tumor being 0.8 (95% CI 0.2, 1.9).[213] Nyberg et al. reported on cancer incidence after a 40-year follow-up among Swedish patients exposed to radioactive Thorotrast.[222] The SIR for rectal cancer was nonsignificantly elevated. A study by Nekolla et al. of 455 patients treated with radium 224 for TB, ankylosing spondylitis, and a few other diseases indicated that rectal cancer occurred in eight and the rate ratio was nonsignificantly reduced at 0.9.[224]

Summary

The epidemiologic data indicate that compared with the colon, the rectum has a relatively low sensitivity to radiation-induced cancer. A statistically significant risk is evident only after extremely high radiation therapy doses. Neither the 1988[370] and 1994 UNSCEAR reports[369] nor the BEIR V Report[3] give a radiation risk estimate for cancer of the rectum. Likewise, ICRP 1990 does not give any risk estimate for rectal cancer associated with radiation exposure.[248] The UNSCEAR 2006 Committee reviewed risk estimates from epidemiological studies.[86] These are shown in Table 5-23 and it can be seen that most studies do not show a statistically significant relationship between rectal cancer and radiation exposure (especially at doses less than 1 Gy) but there is an excess evident at very high rectal doses (tens of Gy).

HEPATOBILIARY SYSTEM CANCER
General

Cancer of the liver is the eighth most common cancer in the world. High-incidence areas are found in sub-Saharan Africa and East and Southeast Asia. In the United States

rates tend to be high in populations of Asian origin and in Eskimos. A close relationship exists between the geographical incidence of hepatocellular carcinoma and the prevalence of persons with chronic hepatitis B or C, and a high dietary intake of aflatoxins. High alcohol intake also has been related to an increased incidence of hepatomas in some, but not all, studies. Nevertheless, when all the cohort studies of issue are combined, it appears that alcoholics have about a 50% increase in risk of liver cancer compared with nonalcoholics.[358,700]

Gallbladder cancer and cancer of the bile duct are quite rare, representing about 1% of all cancers. The frequency of gallbladder cancer is highest in females, particularly among American Indians, Japanese, and Latin Americans. Gallstones are thought to be the cause of 30% of gallbladder cancers in blacks and 50% to 90% in whites and American Indians.

External Exposure

Background Radiation and Populations Near Nuclear Facilities

In the 1980 Chinese high-background study, mortality from liver cancer was higher in the control area than in the high-background area. An additional report in 1990 found nonsignificantly different rates in the two areas (13.92 vs. 12.05 per 10^5 person-years).[29] Tao et al. reported on cancer mortality in the high-background radiation areas of Yangjiang, China, during 1979–1995 where the average annual exposure was 6.4 mSv (including internal exposure) and indicated that the RR for liver cancer was nonsignificantly reduced at 0.75 (95% CI 0.54, 1.05).[33]

No significant increase in the rates of liver cancer was found in populations living around U.S. nuclear facilities.[78] For all facilities combined, the SMRs for liver cancer before facility start-up were 0.94 in the study counties and 1.01 in the control counties. After operation the values were 0.98 and 0.96, respectively. There are three papers concerning potential uranium environmental contamination and the possibility of an increased risk of liver cancer in the public by Boice et al., which indicated a nonsignificant decrease around a uranium mining and milling facility in Texas and nonsignificant increases near facilities in Pennsylvania and Colorado.[89,90,90a] Bauer et al. have reported on cancer mortality due to local fallout from Soviet atmospheric nuclear weapons testing at the Semipalatinsk test site in Kazakhstan.[533] Effective doses there ranged from 20 mSv to about 4 Sv and the dose-response for liver cancer was nonsignificantly reduced at a P value of 0.4448 in males and 0.3632 in females. The estimated ERR per Sv for the exposed cohort was negative at −0.08 (95% CI −0.41, 1.00).

Atomic Bomb Survivors

An 1958–1998 incidence study of atomic bomb survivors by Preston et al. reported on ERR per Gy for liver cancer

Table 5-23 • Risk Estimates for Cancer Incidence and Mortality from Studies of Radiation Exposure: Rectal Cancer*

Study	Average Excess Relative Risk at 1 Sv	Average Excess Absolute Risk $(10^4 PYSv)^{-1}$
External Low-LET Exposures		
Incidence		
A-bomb Life Span Study[319]		
Males	<0 (<0–0.28)	<0 (<0–0.35)
Females	0.46 (0.08–0.97)	0.40 (0.03–1.11)
Age at exposure		
<20	0.16 (<0–0.6)	0.1 (<0–0.58)
20–40	0.12 (<0–0.58)	<0 (<0–1.7)
>40	0.24 (<0–0.97)	0.64 (<0–3.44)
Time since exposure		
12–15	<0 (<0–2.47)	2.44 (1.15–4.47)
15–30	<0 (<0–<0)	<0 (<0–0.12)
>30	0.32 (0.05–0.66)	0.59 (<0–2.02)
All	0.18 (<0–0.46)	0.19 (<0–0.64)
Canada National Dose Registry[153]	13.8 (3.7–33.6)	NA
U.K. Springfields uranium workers[243]	−0.17 (< −3.42–11.95)	NA
Mortality		
A-bomb Life Span Study[281]		
Males	<0 (<0–0.33)	<0 (<0–601.18)
Females	0.95 (0.28–1.86)	<0 (<0–488.26)
Age at exposure		
<20	0.48 (<0–1.82)	<0 (<0–167.7)
20–40	0.2 (<0–1.08)	<0 (<0–590.5)
>40	0.49 (<0–1.37)	1.11 (<0–3.23)
Time since exposure		
12–15	0.38 (<0–2)	<0 (<0–262.78)
15–30	<0 (<0–0.4)	<0 (<0–426.25)
>30	0.68 (0.11–1.47)	<0 (<0–848.25)
All	0.36 (<0–0.88)	<0 (<0–532.76)
U.K. National Registry for Radiation Workers[146]	1.69 (−0.12–5.01)	NA
IARC 15-country nuclear workers study[167,168]	1.27 (<0, 7.62)	NA
Metropathia haemorrhagica[116]	0.04 (−0.09–0.16)	NA
Benign gynaecological disease[118]	0.03 (−0.14–0.19)	NA
Internal High-LET Exposures		
Incidence		
Danish and Swedish Thorotrast patients[219]	1.8 (0.6–5.3)	NA

*The studies listed are those for which quantitative estimates of risk could be made.
Adopted from United Nations Scientific Committee of the Effects of Atomic Radiation (UNSCEAR): Sources and effects of ionizing radiation: 2006 report to the General Assembly with annexes. New York, United Nations, 2007.

of 0.30 (90% CI 0.11, 0.55) and an EAR of 4.3 (90% CI 0.2, 7.2) cases per $10^4 PYGy$.[319] There were an estimated 54 excess cases out of a total 1494 liver cancer cases. The incidence data up to 1997 are shown graphically for both liver and gallbladder in Figures 5-22 and 5-23. There was a statistically significant increase in incidence with dose up to 2 Gy, after which there was a sharp decline. There was no difference in risk between males and females, nor was there any effect of time since exposure or attained age. There was very low risk for those exposed under the age of 10 or over the age of 45. For cancer of the gallbladder, there was no radiation effect, with an ERR per Gy of −0.05 (90% CI <−0.3, 0.3) and an EAR of −0.01 (90% CI <0.01, 0.51) with 549 cases identified versus 551 expected.[319]

In the LSS mortality study of atomic bomb survivors through 1985, 48 deaths were due to liver cancer versus 46 expected during the 1,203,100 person-years of observation.[10] The calculated ERR at 1 Sv was 0.5, which is similar to that in the incidence study. The EAR, at 1.3 $(10^4 PYSv)^{-1}$, is also quite similar. In the 2003 update studies of mortality of atomic bomb survivors during 1950–1997, Preston et al. had a cohort of 86,572 persons with an average external dose of 0.23 Sv.[281] In males there was a statistically significant excess of liver cancer at dose levels of 1 Sv, with an ERR of 0.39 (90% CI 0.11, 0.68). In females there was a statistically significant excess at dose levels of 1 Sv, with an ERR of 0.35 (90% CI 0.07, 0.72). In males there was a statistically significant excess of

Excess relative risk

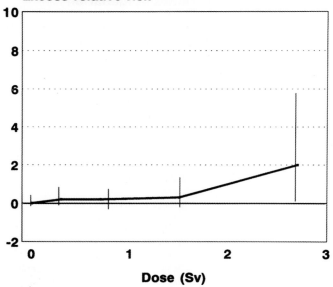

Liver cancer incidence (A-bomb)

Figure 5-22 • ERR of liver cancer in atomic bomb survivors at different dose levels. Bars indicate 95% CI. (From Thompson D, Mabuchi K, Ron E, et al: Cancer incidence in atomic bomb survivors. II: Solid tumors, 1958–1987. RERF Technical Report 5-92, Hiroshima, Japan, Radiation Effects Research Foundation, 1992.)

Excess relative risk

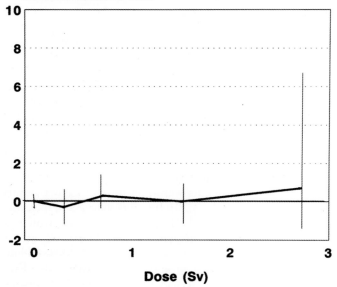

Gallbladder cancer incidence (A-bomb)

Figure 5-23 • ERR of gallbladder cancer in atomic bomb survivors at different dose levels. Bars indicate 95% CI. (From Thompson D, Mabuchi K, Ron E, et al: Cancer incidence in atomic bomb survivors. II: Solid tumors, 1958–1987. RERF Technical Report 5-92, Hiroshima, Japan, Radiation Effects Research Foundation, 1992.)

gallbladder cancer at dose levels of 1 Sv, with an ERR of 0.89 (90% CI 0.22, 1.9). In females there was a nonsignificant excess of gallbladder cancer at dose levels of 1 Sv, with an ERR of 0.16 (90% CI −0.17, 0.67).

Occupational Exposure

Few, if any, occupational studies of external exposure have shown a relationship between radiation and the risk of liver or gallbladder cancers. In the United Kingdom, Darby et al. reported an RR for liver and gallbladder cancer of 1.90 (90% CI 0.76 to 4.95) in radiation workers in experimental government programs.[52] In the latest 2004 review, Muirhead et al. studied a cohort of 21,357 test participants and reported a nonsignificantly decreased SMR of 0.98 (95% CI 0.51, 1.71) for liver cancer in test participants and a nonsignificantly decreased risk compared to controls.[55] The RR compared to controls for incidence was significantly elevated at 1.83. In studying more than 39,000 U.K. nuclear workers, Beral et al. found a ratio rate of exposed to nonexposed employees of 1.37 (95% CI 0.02, 24.1) for liver cancer and a rate of 0.00 (95% CI 0.00 to 4.23) for gallbladder cancer.[143] In another study of atomic weapons workers, Beral et al. reported a rate ratio of 1.37 (95% CI 0.02, 24.1) for liver cancer and 0.00 (95% CI 0.00, 4.23) for gallbladder cancer.[144] A study by Kendall et al. of over 95,000 workers found an SMR of 0.89 for liver cancer.[145] A second expanded analysis in 1999 of 124,743 workers in the U.K. National Registry of Radiation Workers by Muirhead et al. using a lagged analysis reported a nonsignificantly reduced SMR for liver and gallbladder cancers of 0.78 (95% CI 0.56, 1.06).[146] A report on Sellafield workers by Omar et al. indicated a significant decrease in liver and gallbladder cancer among nonplutonium radiation workers with an SMR of 0.20.[148] McGeoghegan et al. reported on the cancer mortality and morbidity experience of employees at the Chapelcross plant of British Nuclear Fuels during 1955–1995.[149] The cohort included 2628 workers with median doses of 39 mSv. In radiation workers the SMR for cancer of the liver was nonsignificantly decreased at 0.42.

Habib et al. have reported on cancer incidence among Australian nuclear industry–monitored radiation workers in whom they found a nonsignificantly increased SIR of 1.19 for liver cancer and no cases of gallbladder cancer.[152] Iwasaki et al. conducted a second analysis of mortality of nuclear industry workers in Japan which included 176,000 male workers with 5527 deaths.[150] Average annual doses were 3.5 mSv before 1982 and 1.2 mSv after 1982. For liver cancer the SMR was nonsignificantly increased at 1.04 (95% CI 0.94, 1.14) and the SMR for biliary cancer was nonsignificantly reduced at 0.96 (95% CI 0.75, 1.21). Artalejo et al. reported on mortality among 5657 workers of the former Spanish Nuclear Energy Board whose mean exposure was 11.42 mSv and whose SMR for liver cancer was nonsignificantly increased at 1.51 (95% CI 0.86, 2.46).[151]

Ashmore et al. reported the first analysis of mortality and occupational radiation exposure based on the National Dose Registry of Canada which included a cohort of 206,620 individuals and 5426 deaths.[154] The average exposure for males was 10.6 mSv and their SMR for liver cancer was nonsignificantly reduced at 0.70 (90% CI 0.0.41, 1.12). The results for gallbladder cancer were also nonsignificantly reduced with an SMR of 0.71 (90% CI 0.37, 1.24). Sont et al. analyzed the relation between the cancer incidence and occupational radiation exposure based on the National Dose Registry of Canada, and reported on a cohort of 191,333 persons with an average dose for males of 11.5 mSv and an average dose for the cohort of 6.64 mSv.[153] The SIR for liver cancer in males was nonsignificantly reduced at 0.92 and in females it was nonsignificantly elevated at 1.33. The SIR for gallbladder cancer in males was nonsignificantly reduced at 0.78 and in females it was nonsignificantly reduced at 0.45.

In the United States a number of occupational studies have reported findings relative to liver cancer. In a study of Hanford workers from 1945–1986, Gilbert et al. reported an SMR of 0.94 for liver cancer.[361] A nonsignificant decrease in liver cancer was reported by Gilbert et al. in a combined analysis of workers at Hanford, Oak Ridge, and Rocky Flats facilities.[158] Fry et al. reported a study of mortality and morbidity among 3145 persons occupationally exposed to 50 or more mSv (5000 mrem) in a year.[161] The mean external exposure was 153 mSv. The SMR for liver cancer was nonsignificantly reduced.

Wiggs et al. found a nonsignificantly reduced SMR of 0.64 for liver and gallbladder cancer in a follow-up of Los Alamos workers.[164] Cragle et al. indicated that no cancers of the liver were identified in workers at the Savannah River plant.[288] Wilkinson et al. reported a nonsignificantly elevated SMR of 1.39 (90% CI 0.28 to 3.59) for liver cancer in plutonium workers.[286] Frome reported a mortality study of 106,020 employees in the nuclear industry at Oak Ridge, Tennessee, in whom the SMR for cancer of the liver in black and white males and females was nonsignificantly different from unity.[160] Studies in miners have revealed no increase in cancer of the liver and biliary tract, with an SMR of 0.71 (95% CI 0.09 to 2.56) being reported by Waxweiler et al.[362]

Cardis et al. investigated cancer mortality among nuclear industry workers in three countries in a very large study of 95,673 workers with over 2 million person-years at risk and 15,825 deaths.[166] The trend for liver cancer was nonsignificant at 0.01 with a P value of 0.495. The trend for biliary cancer was nonsignificantly reduced at −0.86 with a P value of 0.806. Cardis et al. also have reported the cancer mortality results from a 15-country collaborative study of nuclear workers.[168] This is the largest occupational study to date and included

a cohort of 407,391 workers with 18,993 deaths and 5.2 million person-years of follow-up. The ERR per Sv for liver cancer was nonsignificantly positive at 6.47 (90% CI < 0, 27) and the ERR per Sv for biliary tract cancer was nonsignificant and estimated at less than 0 with a negative trend with increasing dose (P value of −0.67).

Ritz et al. have reported on cancer mortality in uranium processing workers at the Fernald plant in Ohio among whom the SMR for liver cancer was nonsignificantly increased at 1.62.[192] Dupree-Ellis et al. have reported on mortality in a cohort of 2514 uranium processing workers employed between 1942 and 1966 at the Mallinkrodt Chemical Works.[193] The SMR for liver cancer was nonsignificantly reduced at 0.42. McGeoghegan et al. have reported on the mortality of 12,540 workers (including 3244 radiation workers) at the Capenhurst uranium enrichment facility during 1946–1995.[242] The SMR for liver cancer was nonsignificantly reduced in radiation workers at 0.60. They also studied cancer mortality experience of 19,454 workers (including 13,960 radiation workers) at the Springfields uranium production facility during 1946–1995.[243] The SMR for liver cancer was nonsignificantly elevated for radiation workers at 1.16. A meta-analysis of 14 studies, which included 120,000 uranium workers, found a nonsignificant decrease in liver cancer with an RR of 0.84 (95% CI 0.62, 1.07).[245]

Among medical diagnostic workers in China, a study in 1988 by Wang et al. compared 27,011 workers with 25,782 persons in other medical specialties and found that the x-ray workers had an excess of liver cancer (ERR 1.40).[102] But, because the excess was not related to time after irradiation or dose, it was considered by the authors to be the result of causes other than radiation. In a 2002 follow-up report, Wang et al. reported that for those employed before 1970 cumulative doses were 551 mSv and the RR for cancer of the liver was significantly increased at 1.39, but for those employed after 1970 with a cumulative mean dose of 82 mSv, the RR was nonsignificantly decreased at 0.85.[253] Aoyama et al. conducted a mortality survey of over 12,000 male Japanese radiological technologists during 1969–1993.[95] Their cohort had an average dose of 466 mSv with an SMR for liver cancer that was nonsignificantly decreased at 0.82 (95% CI 0.63, 1.04). Doody et al. reported on mortality among 143,517 U.S. radiologic technologists during 1926–1990 whose doses were not evaluated.[97] The SMR for liver cancer was nonsignificantly reduced at 0.73 (95% CI 0.51, 1.02). Sigurdson et al. studied the cancer incidence in 90,305 U.S. radiologic technologists and found that the SIR for liver cancer was nonsignificantly reduced at 0.83 (95% CI 0.42, 1.47).[101] Their SIR for gallbladder cancer was also nonsignificantly decreased at 0.67 (95% CI 0.18, 1.72). Mohan et al. studied cancer and other causes of mortality among 146,022 radiologic technologists employed from 1940 and later.[98,99] The SMR for liver cancer in males was nonsignificantly reduced at 0.98

(95% CI 0.6, 1.4) and for females it was nonsignificantly reduced at 0.89 (95% CI 0.7, 1.2).

Medical Exposure

Studies of Massachusetts TB patients who received many fluoroscopies during the course of treatment have not shown a radiation-related increase in liver cancer. In one study the SMRs for liver cancer in all groups were 1.0 or less.[105] In another study by the same authors, SMRs in both male controls and exposed were nonsignificantly elevated, as was the case for exposed female patients.[364] Nonexposed females had a nonsignificantly low SMR of 0.3, based on one case observed. Follow-up studies of patients who received radiation therapy include an investigation of 14,554 patients treated for ankylosing spondylitis in whom cancer of the liver was not significantly elevated, an O/E of 1.10 being reported.[109] This is somewhat surprising in view of the Japanese atomic bomb survivor data and because in the treatment of the spine in the ankylosing spondylitis patients, at least a portion of the liver would have been in the primary radiation beam. Mattsson et al. have reported on cancer incidence among 3090 women who received radiation therapy for benign breast disease and their RR for liver cancer was nonsignificantly reduced at 0.86.[114]

Patients who received radiotherapy for peptic ulcer also would have had a portion of the left lobe of the liver in the primary beam. In spite of this, Griem et al. did not find an increase in liver cancer in such patients.[112] Carr et al. performed a follow-up study of the same group of 3719 patients treated with radiotherapy for peptic ulcer with doses to the abdomen about 15 Gy.[113] No cases of liver cancer were found after radiotherapy in the period 0 to 10 years postexposure and, in the follow-up period of 11 to 62 years postexposure, the RR was nonsignificantly reduced at 0.84.

In a follow-up of patients who received intrauterine radium radiotherapy for benign uterine bleeding, which included 4153 women who were studied over 110,000 person-years at risk by Inskip et al., found no increase in the frequency of liver or gallbladder cancer.[118] Likewise, no increase in liver cancer was found by Darby et al. in patients treated with radiotherapy for uterine bleeeding.[116]

There are some reports of second cancers in patients treated with radiation therapy for malignant diseases. In an incidence study of women treated for cervical cancer, which included 82,616 exposed women compared with 99,424 unexposed controls, excess risk was found for leukemia and cancers of the esophagus, small intestine, rectum, pancreas, and other genital tumors.[124] No excess was identified for cancer of the liver. The O/E ratio for liver cancer was 1.0 in those treated with radiotherapy and 2.3 in those treated without radiotherapy. For cancer of the gallbladder, the O/E ratio was 0.8 for patients treated with radiotherapy and 1.0 for those treated in other ways. In another report of a large cohort study, Boice et al. reported an O/E ratio of 1.0 in patients treated with radiotherapy for invasive cervical cancer and 0.9 in those treated without radiotherapy.[127] A Japanese study of 5275 cervical cancer patients treated with radiotherapy alone and 4161 treated with surgery alone found the O/E ratio in the exposed group to be 0.267 (4 cases observed vs. 15 expected), which was significantly low.[128] It was also lower than expected in the group treated by surgery alone. The results of these three large cervical cancer follow-up series are also surprising, given the risks estimated from atomic bomb survivors and because the dose to the upper abdominal organs in the cervical cancer radiotherapy patients is estimated to be 1 to 3 Gy.

Kovalic et al. have reported on hepatocellular carcinoma as a second neoplasm after successful radiotherapy treatment of children with Wilms' tumors.[732] In the national Wilms' Tumor Study, in which there was follow-up of 2438 patients over 14,381 person-years of observation, four cases of hepatocellular carcinoma were observed after latent periods of 9 to 16 years. The radiation doses were in the range of 35 Gy. Three of the four patients also had chemotherapy, and the effect of this is unknown in relation to risk of these tumors. In larger studies of childhood cancer survivors, other authors have not found a statistically significant increase in liver cancer. Hawkins et al.[307] reported only one case of liver cancer among 10,106 survivors of childhood cancer, and Tucker et al.[436] and Rosenberg et al.[140] did not report an increase in liver cancer after treatment for HD. In these patients some of the liver would have been in the primary radiation therapy beam with the "inverted Y" radiotherapy.

Internal Exposure

In a study of Swedish Lapps, who may ingest more cesium 137 than other populations, Wiklund et al. did not find a significant excess of hepatobiliary cancers.[56] They reported an SMR of 1.32 (95% CI 0.49, 2.88) for the hepatobiliary system and an SMR of 0.45 (95% CI 0.01, 2.53) for liver cancers alone. No increase in hepatobiliary cancer has been found in the radium dial painters.[229] Occupational contamination from internally deposited plutonium was not associated with an increase in liver cancer, in a 50-year follow-up of Manhattan Project workers, with no cases of liver cancer being found.[671] In a study of Rocky Flats workers who accumulated a plutonium body burden of at least 74 Bq (2 nCi), Wilkinson et al. reported RRs for liver cancer of 0.80 (90% CI 0.06, 9.1) and 0.91 (90% CI 0.07, 10.3), using biologically implausible latent periods of 2 and 5 years, respectively, and no cases of liver cancer when a reasonable 10-year latent period was used.[286] A report on Sellafield workers by Omar et al. indicated a significant decrease in liver and gallbladder cancer among plutonium workers with an SMR of 0.19.[148] Carpenter et al. examined workers in the United Kingdom who were occupationally exposed to tritium, plutonium, and other radionuclides.[191] The SMRs for liver and gallbladder cancer in each group were all nonsignificantly different from unity. A 2004 update of French uranium miners by Laurier et al. reported a nonsignificantly increased SMR of 1.3 for cancer of the liver, gallbladder, and pancreas as a group.[186] Darby et al. studied radon and cancers in Swedish iron miners and found a nonsignificant increase in liver and gallbladder cancer with O/E ratios of 1.93 (95% CI 0.83, 3.81) and 1.41 (95% CI 0.29, 4.12), respectively.[183]

Data on liver cancer following administration of radioiodine are scarce. It should not be expected that there would be an increase in risk because radioiodine is neither accumulated nor excreted by the liver. No increase was reported by Holm et al. in the large series of patients who received diagnostic doses.[270] Ron et al. has more recently reported on cancer mortality among 35,593 hyperthyroid patients.[201] The SMR for liver cancer was nonsignificantly reduced at 0.87 for those receiving any iodine 131 and 0.97 for those receiving iodine 131 alone. In patients who received larger doses for radiotherapy, the SIR for liver cancer was nonsignifianctly increased at 1.19 (95% CI 0.62, 2.08),[271] and in the two large series of patients treated for thyroid cancer the occurrence of liver cancer was not mentioned.[203,204]

Thorotrast, a contrast medium containing thorium, was used extensively as a contrast agent for angiography and to a much lesser extent for sinus studies. This medium remains in the body and has been associated with leukemia, tumors of the liver, gallbladder, bile ducts, and, in cases where the material was directly instilled and remained in place, cancer of the nasal sinuses. German Thorotrast patients[211,212] make up the largest study series, involving 5139 Thorotrast-exposed patients and 5151 controls; 347 cases of liver cancer were observed in the exposed group compared with 2 in the control group (RR of about 200). Latent periods ranged from 16 to more than 40 years. The shorter latent periods were typically seen at the higher dose rates and higher total absorbed radiation doses. The alpha dose to the liver in this series was estimated to be in the range of 2 to 15 Gy. In a later follow-up of 2326 German Thorotrast patients and 1890 controls, an excess of primary liver cancer (410 vs. 2 cases) was observed after the 15th year of exposure.[733] Risks after 40 years of exposure were estimated to be 500 per 10^4 person Gy for men and 300 per 10^4 person Gy for women. In a Danish Thorotrast series the SIR for liver cancers was strikingly elevated at 126 (95% CI 100, 157), and for gallbladder cancers the SIR was elevated at 14 (95% CI 8.1, 24). The risk of peritoneal tumors was also elevated, with an SIR of 8.6.[213,217] A more recent follow-up of these patients has been reported by Andersson et al.[734] Among 1003 patients there were 127 liver cancers (45 hepatocellular carcinomas, 41 cholangiocarcinomas, and 33 hemangiosarcomas). The median time from injection to diagnosis was 35 years. The risk estimate was 712 cases per 10,000 persons per Gy. This value is considerably higher than earlier

estimates. Nyberg et al. reported on cancer incidence after a 40-year follow-up among Swedish patients exposed to radioactive Thorotrast.[222] The SIR for liver and gallbladder cancer was significantly elevated at 39.2 (95% CI 30.2, 49.9).

The intial report of the Portuguese Thorotrast series of 2434 patients also revealed striking increases in hemangioendotheliomas, cholangiocarcinomas, and hepatomas. No risk estimates were calculated.[216] There is a 2003 report by dos Santos Silva et al. on the 50-year follow-up of mortality of Portuguese Thorotrast patients.[220] The cohort included 1096 systemically exposed and 240 locally exposed. The SMR for liver cancer in the systemically exposed was significantly increased at 338. The RR of systemically exposed versus locally exposed was significantly increased at 42.4. In Japanese Thorotrast patients between 1945–1990,[215,677] there were 357 persons who were autopsied,[735] among whom there were 240 malignant liver tumors and 4 malignant peritoneal tumors. Dose rates were estimated from autopsy specimens and the resulting mean organ dose rates were as follows: liver, 0.26 Gy per year; spleen, 0.91 Gy per year; and bone marrow, 0.085 Gy per year.

A study by Nekolla et al. of 455 patients treated with radium 224 for TB, ankylosing spondylitis, and a few other diseases indicated that liver cancer occurred in seven patients and was significantly elevated with a rate ratio of 3.0.[224] However, in another study, Wick and Nekolla reported on late effects in ankylosing spondylitis patients treated with radium 224 of whom there were 626 exposed and 725 control patients with a mean follow-up time of 21 years.[225] The mean injected activity was 0.17 MBq per kg and the mean alpha skeletal dose was 0.67 Gy. The study showed a decrease in the O/E ratio for liver cancer among those exposed of 1 to 2.3.

Summary

A number of epidemiologic studies show increases in the risk of liver cancer after radiation exposure. As with most other tumor types, there are negative results from the very large studies of atomic workers. In Japanese atomic bomb survivors the risk reaches statistical significance only at doses near 1 Sv. In the Thorotrast patients the risk is relatively very high. The UNSCEAR 1988 report gave no unified risk estimate for cancer of the hepatobiliary system.[370] The 1990 ICRP report estimated for a population of all ages the lifetime risk of death from liver cancer after exposure to low doses was $15 \times (10^{-4} \text{ Sv}^{-1})$.[248] In the BEIR IV report the lifetime cancer risk from alpha irradiation of the liver was estimated to be about 300 cases per 10^4 person Gy from intravenously administered Thorotrast, and the risk from chronic beta irradiation was estimated to be about 10 times lower.[575]

UNSCEAR 2006 has summarized the radiation risk estimates that can be obtained from epidemiological studies (Table 5-24).[86] They indicate that while an

Table 5-24 • Risk Estimates for Cancer Incidence and Mortality from Studies of Radiation Exposure: Liver Cancer*

Study	Average Excess Relative Risk at 1 Sv	Average Excess Absolute Risk $(10^4 PYSv)^{-1}$
External Low-LET Exposures		
Incidence		
A-bomb Life Span Study[319]		
Males	0.42 (0.18–0.7)	0.29 (<0–1.96)
Females	0.39 (0.09–0.76)	0.52 (0.12–1.14)
Age at exposure		
<20	0.5 (0.21–0.85)	0.48 (0.09–1.08)
20–40	0.21 (<0–0.54)	0.72 (<0–2.02)
>40	0.61 (0.14–1.23)	3.03 (0.02–6.75)
Time since exposure		
12–15	0.54 (<0–2.18)	<0 (<0–0.92)
15–30	0.57 (0.13–1.19)	0.39 (0.02–1.08)
>30	0.37 (0.16–0.61)	1.23 (0.24–2.69)
All	0.41 (0.22–0.63)	0.5 (0.12–1.06)
Cervical cancer cohort[124]	–0.06 (–0.37–0.4)	–0.03 (–0.16–0.2)
Swedish benign breast disease[114]	0.09 (<0–1.4)	NA
U.K. Springfields uranium workers[243]	–1.96 (< –2.08–21.58)	NA
Mortality		
A-bomb Life Span Study[281]		
Males	0.61 (0.33–0.94)	<0 (<0–0.89)
Females	0.36 (0.05–0.74)	<0 (<0–1091.7)
Age at exposure		
<20	0.46 (0.13–0.89)	<0 (<0–0.34)
20–40	0.58 (0.23–1.01)	0.3 (<0–1.58)
>40	0.45 (0.09–0.92)	2 (<0–4.59)
Time since exposure		
12–15	0.24 (<0–0.84)	<0 (<0–0.25)
15–30	0.68 (0.19–1.33)	0.08 (<0–0.91)
>30	0.51 (0.25–0.81)	0.9 (0.01–2.21)
All	0.51 (0.30–0.75)	<0 (<0–0.41)
Ankylosing spondylitis[266]	–0.09 (–0.24–0.2)	NA
Peptic ulcer[113]	–0.03 (< –0.03–0.31)	NA
Benign gynecological disease[118]	–2.18(–3.26–0.3)	NA
Yangjiang background radiation[34, 35]	–0.99 (–1.60–0.1)	NA
Nuclear workers in Canada, United Kingdom, United States[166]	~0	NA
Nuclear workers in Japan[721]	>0	NA
IARC 15-country nuclear workers study[167,168]		
Liver	6.47 (<0, 27)	
Biliary tract	<0	
Internal Low-LET Exposures		
Mortality		
Semipalatinsk Study[533]	–0.08 (–0.41, 1)	NA
Internal High-LET Exposures	**Average Relative Risk**	
Incidence		
Danish Thorotrast patients[272]	194.2 (31–1216)	
Danish and Swedish Thorotrast patients[219]	∞ (44.2–∞)	
Mortality		
German Thorotrast patients[221]	25 Gy^{-1}	
Portuguese Thorotrast patients[736]	5.7	
U.S. Thorotrast patients[219]	22.5 (1.8–464.3)	

*The studies listed are those for which quantitative estimates of risk could be made.
Adapted from United Nations Scientific Committee of the Effects of Atomic Radiation (UNSCEAR): Sources and effects of ionizing radiation: 2006 report to the General Assembly with annexes. New York, United Nations, 2007.

association of liver cancer with radiation has not been demonstrated in medical radiation therapy and worker studies involving external or internal low-LET exposures, the updated Japanese LSS mortality data continue to show a strong dose response. Transfer of these risk factors to other populations is difficult due to high-background liver cancer rates in Japan primarily due to infection with hepatitis C virus. Studies of Thorotrast patients clearly show increased risks of liver cancer which have persisted for 50 years.

PANCREAS CANCER

General

Pancreatic cancer is almost invariably fatal within a year or two, with 5-year survival rates of only about 2%. It is the fourth most common cause of cancer death in both sexes in the United States. Highest incidence rates in the world are in U.S. blacks and in Korean males in Los Angeles. Smoking appears to have a dose-related effect on the risk of pancreatic cancer, with smokers having about a two- to fourfold higher risk than nonsmokers. This risk declines to normal about 10 years after cessation of smoking. At the present time smoking is estimated to be responsible for 20% to 40% of pancreatic cancer in males and 10% to 20% in females.[358,700] No definite causal relation has been found between alcohol or coffee drinking, chronic pancreatitis, diabetes mellitus, or chemical exposures.

The BEIR V report of the National Academy of Sciences has indicated that "excess mortality from the disease has been observed inconsistently in irradiated human populations and has borne no clear relationship to dose or time after irradiation."[3] The possible exceptions to this are the very high doses such as those associated with abdominal radiotherapy. The 2005 BEIR VII report was unable to find enough literature to derive risk estimates for pancreatic cancer.[18] Occasionally there is an attempt to link unusual pancreatic tumors (such as islet cell tumors) and radiation exposure. Such tumors have not been shown to be caused by radiation exposure; however, there is a well-known (and probably genetically based) relationship between pancreatic islet cell tumors and other endocrine neoplasms. If this cell type is encountered, multiple endocrine neoplasia type I should be considered. There are no reports of tumors of this pancreatic cell type being induced by radiation.

External Exposure

Background Radiation and Populations Near Nuclear Facilities

In a study of terrestrial background radiation and cancer incidence in Connecticut, Walter et al. found no

difference in incidence of pancreatic cancer between areas of high and low natural background.[21]

In another population study, Jablon et al. found no evidence of a consistent trend in cancer of the digestive organs in populations living around U.S. nuclear facilities.[78] There are three papers concerning potential environmental uranium contamination and the possibility of increased pancreatic cancer risk among the public. The papers by Boice et al. indicated a nonsignificant increase around uranium mining and milling facilities in Texas and Colorado, and a nonsignificant decrease near a uranium facility in Pennsylvania.[89,90,90a] A nonsignificant decrease in pancreatic cancer was found by Boice et al. in a study of persons residing near the Hanford National Laboratory site.[91]

High Natural Background Radiation Areas

Tao et al. have studied cancer mortality in the high-background radiation in Yangjiang, China, between 1979–1995.[33] The authors compared a high-background area and a neighboring control area in Guangdong, China, with 1.7 million person-years of study. Dose rates in the high-background area were 4.3 mSv per year and in the control areas it was about 1.6 mSv per year. A nonsignificant increased RR for cancer of the pancreas was reported at 3.3 (95% CI 0.48, 26.7). Pukkala et al. studied the incidence of cancer among Nordic airline pilots over five decades and reported a nonstatistically reduced SIR for cancer of the pancreas at 0.92 (95% CI 0.48, 1.61).[39]

Atomic Bomb Survivors

Neither early incidence nor mortality studies of atomic bomb survivors have shown an increase in the frequency of pancreatic cancer (Fig. 5-24). In the 1958-1998 incidence study reported by Preston et al., all resk estimates are nonsignificant with an ERR per Gy of 0.26 (95% CI −0.07, 0.68) and an EAR of 0.46 (95% CI −0.13, 1.5) cases per $(10^4 PYGy)^{-1}$.[319] There were an estimated 11 excess cases out of 512 total cases. The 1990 and 1991 reports on mortality by Shimizu et al. found a nonsignificant reduction in RR for cancer of the pancreas at 0.89 (90% CI < 0, 1.23), an ERR per 10,000 PYGy of −0.10 (90% < 0 to 0.20), and an attributable risk of −3.0% (90% CI < 0, 6.2).[10,717] In a 2003 report Preston et al. reported a total of 86,572 persons in the study with 9335 solid cancer deaths versus 8895 expected for an excess of 440 solid cancer deaths with 48% of the atomic bomb survivor population still alive.[281] There was a negative relationship between radiation dose and cancers of the pancreas. For males the ERR was −0.11 (90% CI < −0.3, 0.44) at 1 Sv and the EAR was −0.15 (90% CI < −0.4, 0.58) per 10,000 PYGy; the attributable risk (%) was −1.9% (90% CI < 6 to 7.5). For females the ERR was −0.01 (90% CI −0.28, 0.45) at 1 Sv and the EAR was −0.01 (90% CI −0.35 to 0.45) per 10,000 PYGy; the attributable risk (%) was −0.2% (90% CI < 5.0, 7.6).

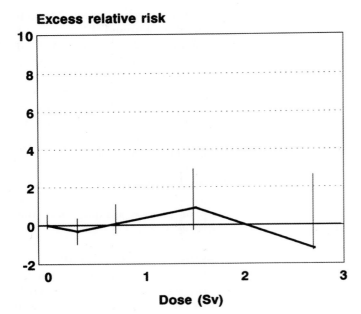

Excess relative risk

Pancreas cancer incidence (A-bomb)

Figure 5-24 • ERR of pancreas cancer in atomic bomb survivors at different dose levels. Bars indicate 95% CI. (From Thompson D, Mabuchi K, Ron E, et al: Cancer incidence in atomic bomb survivors. II: Solid tumors, 1958–1987. RERF Technical Report 5-92, Hiroshima, Japan, Radiation Effects Research Foundation, 1992.)

Occupational Exposure of Nuclear Workers

Virtually none of the very large studies of external radiation occupational exposure have shown a statistically significant risk of pancreatic cancer. Many studies have been performed in the United Kingdom. One U.K. study by Darby et al. included 22,347 workers exposed to fallout and who worked in experimental U.K. government programs.[52] With over 440,000 person-years of observation, the RR for pancreatic cancer was nonsignificantly reduced at 0.87 (90% CI 0.50 to 1.50). Another study by Darby et al. concerned 21,358 servicemen who participated in nuclear weapons tests and the RR was nonsignificantly elevated at 1.11 (95% CI 0.74, 1.68).[701] Muirhead et al. reported the follow-up of mortality and incidence of cancer from 1952–1998 in men from the United Kingdom who participated in the United Kingdom's atmospheric nuclear weapons tests and experimental programs.[54] The SMR for pancreatic cancer was nonsignificantly reduced at 0.82 and the RR was nonsignificantly elevated at 1.08 (90% CI 0.81, 1.42).

A U.K. study by Beral et al. included 39,546 radiation workers and over 630,000 person-years of observation; there was an SMR for pancreatic cancer of 0.93 and a nonsignificant ratio rate between exposed to nonexposed employees of 1.24 (95% CI 0.54, 2.84).[143] In a third U.K. study, by Beral et al. of atomic weapons workers, there was a rate ratio of 1.24 (95% CI 0.54, 2.84).[144] In a fourth

U.K. study by Kendall et al., which included 95,217 workers and over 1.2 million person-years, a significantly decreased SMR of 0.77 for pancreatic cancer was observed.[145] In 1999 Muirhead et al. reported on the second analysis of the National Registry for Radiation Workers, which included a cohort of 124,743 workers with means doses of 30 mSv.[146] Using a lagged analysis, the RR for cancer of the pancreas was nonsignificantly elevated at 1.08 (95% CI 0.81, 1.42). Fraser et al. reported on cancer mortality in over 39,000 radiation monitored employees of the U.K. Atomic Energy Authority during 1946–1986 and the rate ratio for pancreatic cancer was nonsignificantly reduced at 0.65 (95% CI 0.38, 1.12).[702]

Smith et al. examined mortality among over 14,000 workers at the Sellafield plant and reported a nonsignificant reduction in SMR for cancer of the pancreas at 0.92.[360] An additional 1994 Sellafield study by Douglas et al. examined cancer mortality and morbidity among workers.[147] There were 14,282 workers with an average dose of 128 mSv per worker. The SMR for pancreatic cancer remained nonsignificantly reduced and was 0.94. A 1999 report on Sellafield workers by Omar et al. indicated a nonsignificant decrease in pancreatic cancer among nonplutonium radiation workers with an SMR of 0.93 and SIR was also nonsignificantly decreased.[148] McGeoghegan et al. reported on the mortality and cancer morbidity experience of a cohort of 2628 workers with median doses of 39 mSv at the Chapelcross plant of British Nuclear Fuels with a mean follow-up of 24.3 years and 63,967 person-years of study.[149] The SMR for cancer of the pancreas was nonsignificantly elevated at 1.02.

Iwasaki et al. reported a second analysis of mortality of nuclear industry workers in Japan, which included 176,000 male workers with 5527 deaths.[150] Average annual doses were 3.5 mSv before 1982 and 1.2 mSv after 1982. For cancer of the pancreas, the SMR was nonsignificantly reduced at 0.98 (95% CI 0.82, 1.17). Habib et al. have reported on cancer incidence among Australian nuclear industry–monitored radiation workers and indicated a nonsignificantly reduced SIR of 0.42 for pancreatic cancer.[152]

There are multiple studies of Canadian nuclear workers. In a study of atomic energy workers in Canada, Gribbin et al. reported an SMR of 0.88 (95% CI 0.47 to 1.50) for pancreatic cancer.[260] Zablotska et al. performed analysis of mortality among Canadian nuclear power industry workers after chronic low-dose exposure to ionizing radiation.[155] The SMR for pancreatic cancer was significantly reduced at 0.63 (95% CI 0.39 to 0.95). Ashmore et al. reported the first analysis of mortality and occupational radiation exposure based on the National Dose Registry of Canada, which included a cohort of 206,620 individuals with 5426 deaths and among whom the average exposure for males was 11 mSv.[154] The SMR for cancer of the pancreas was significantly reduced at 0.80 (90% CI 0.65 to 0.98). Sont et al. analyzed cancer incidence in a similar group with cohort of 191,333 persons with an average dose for males of 11.5 mSv and an average dose for the cohort of 6.6 mSv.[153] The SIR ratio for cancer of the pancreas in males was significantly reduced at 0.74 (90% CI 0.59 to 0.93) and nonsignificantly reduced in females.

The reports from most of the U.S. occupational nuclear worker studies yield similar negative findings. Gilbert et al. reporting on Hanford workers during 1945–1986 found an SMR of 0.96 for pancreatic cancer.[361] In a combined study of U.S. federal facilities, they reported SMRs for pancreatic cancer as follows: Hanford, 0.89; Oak Ridge, 0.73; and Rocky Flats, 0.71.[157] No increase was reported in a later follow-up paper either.[158] Cragle et al. studied workers at the Savannah River plant and observed two cases of pancreatic cancer versus 0.79 expected, the difference being nonsignificantly different from unity.[288] At the Mound facility in Ohio, Wiggs et al. found an SMR for pancreatic cancer of only 0.25 (95% CI 0.01 to 1.39).[156] Frome et al. conducted a study of 28,008 employees of Oak Ridge World War II nuclear industry workers.[267] The SMR for cancer of the pancreas was nonsignificantly reduced at 0.93. Frome et al. also conducted a mortality study of 106,020 employees in the nuclear industry at Oak Ridge, Tennessee.[160] The SMR for cancer of the pancreas in white males was nonsignificantly reduced at 0.95 and for nonwhite males it was 1.01; for white females the SMR was 0.18 and for nonwhite females it was 0.14.

Fry et al. conducted a study of mortality and morbidity among 3145 persons occupationally exposed to 50 or more mSv in a year.[161] The mean external exposure was 153 mSv. The SMR for cancer of the pancreas in males was nonsignificantly reduced at 0.65 (95% CI 0.18 to 1.69). Howe et al. analyzed the mortality experience of 53,698 U.S. nuclear power industry workers after chronic low-dose exposure to ionizing radiation.[159] There was a significantly reduced SMR for cancer of the pancreas at 0.62 (95% CI 0.37 to 0.98). At the Rocky Flats facility in Colorado, Wilkinson et al. found an SMR of 0.55 (90% CI 0.19 to 1.26).[286] In the studies of Oak Ridge workers, Checkoway et al. reported an SMR of 0.97 (95% CI 0.47 to 1.78) using U.S. comparison data and 0.94 (95% CI 0.45 to 1.73) using Tennessee data for comparison.[284] Wing et al. found an SMR of 1.09 (95% CI 0.44 to 1.81) following external exposure and an SMR of 0.95 after internal exposure.[285] Wiggs et al. found an SMR of 0.89 for pancreatic cancer in a follow-up of Los Alamos workers.[164] In a study of 3564 workers at the Pantex nuclear weapons facility by Acquavella et al. there was only one case of pancreatic cancer and the SMR for cancer of the pancreas was nonsignificantly reduced at 0.26 (95% CI 0.01 to 1.43).[703]

Cardis et al. investigated cancer mortality among nuclear industry workers in three countries in a very large study of 95,673 workers with over 2 million person-years at risk and 15,825 deaths.[166] The trend for pancreatic cancer was nonsignificantly positive at 1.20 with a P value of 0.115. Cardis et al. also have reported the cancer mortality results from a 15-country collaborative study of nuclear workers.[168] This is the largest occupational study to date and included a cohort of 407,391 workers with 18,993 deaths and 5.2 million person-years of follow-up. The ERR per Sv for pancreatic cancer was nonsignificantly positive at 2.10 (90% CI −0.59, 6.77).

In contrast to the vast majority of the occupational worker literature, there is one study by Kauppinen that purports to have found a significant association between pancreatic cancer and occupational exposure.[737] However, this was a questionnaire study of next of kin with only a 50% response rate and was based on only three cases in the supposedly exposed group and four in the control group. The study also had other statistically significant findings which have never been supported in other literature (such as increased incidence of pancreatic cancer due to exposure to mild cold temperature but not severe cold temperatures).

Occupational Exposure of Medical Workers

Smith et al. reported on occupational exposure and follow-up of British radiologists for whom the O/E ratio of 3.23 for pancreatic cancer was significantly increased in those employed before 1920.[584] This was based on six observed cases versus 1.9 expected. For those employed after 1920 the O/E was 0.80. A follow-up by Berrington et al. included 100 years of observation on 2698 British radiologists.[94] Mortality from pancreatic cancer again was statistically significantly elevated, with an SMR of 3.88 in those employed before 1920. It was reduced with an SMR of 0.87 in those employed after 1920. The increase in those employed before 1920 may be simply due to chance, just as those statistically significant decreases reported above would not be attributable to radiation. Therefore, any such finding must be taken in light of the other studies quoted here.

Cancer incidence among medical diagnostic workers in China has been reviewed by Wang et al. who compared 27,011 workers with 25,782 persons in other medical specialties.[738] While the x-ray workers had a 50% higher risk of developing all types of cancer (RR 1.5, 95% CI 1.3, 1.7), the RR for pancreatic cancer was 0.45. The doses of the workers were likely to be on the order or 1 Gy or more because the workers often had depressed white blood cell counts, and when this was noted they were given time off work so that their marrow could recover. In a 2002 follow-up study, Wang et al. reported cumulative doses were 0.55 Sv for those employed before 1970 and 82 mSv for the cohort employed after 1970.[253] The RR for cancer of the pancreas was nonsignificantly reduced with an RR of 0.85.

There have been multiple studies of very large numbers of U.S. radiologic technologists. Burnett et al. have examined cancer mortality in health and science technicians. There was a nonsignificant increase in the PCMR at 1.26 (95% CI 0.78 to 1.92) for cancer of the pancreas.[96] Doody et al. studied mortality among 143,517 U.S. radiologic technologists from 1926–1990.[97] The SMR for cancer of the pancreas was nonsignificantly reduced at 0.83 (95% CI 0.67 to 1.02). Mohan et al. also examined cancer and other causes of mortality among radiologic technologists in the United States in a study of 146,022 radiologic technologists employed from 1940 and later.[99] The SMR for cancer of the pancreas in males was nonsignificantly reduced at 0.99 (95% CI 0.8 to 1.2) and for females it was also nonsignificantly reduced at 0.93 (95% CI 0.8 to 1.1). Sigurdson et al. performed another cancer incidence study among x-ray workers (U.S. Radiologic Technologists Health Study, 1983–1998).[101] The study included 90,305 radiologic technologists and the SIR for pancreatic cancer was nonsignificantly elevated at 1.02 (95% CI 0.76, 1.29).

Medical External Exposure of Patients

Studies that have examined medical diagnostic exposure and the occurrence of pancreatic cancer include a study by Davis et al. of Massachusetts TB patients treated using multiple chest fluoroscopies.[364] The reported SMRs for pancreas cancer were not significantly different from unity or from those of unexposed controls. In another study of the same type of patients SMRs for pancreatic cancer in both male and female exposed and nonexposed groups were again not significantly different from unity.[105]

Early studies reported a significant increase in the frequency of pancreatic cancer after radiation therapy for ankylosing spondylitis.[108] Actually, however, the only statistically significant increase was seen in the first 5 years after treatment, perhaps due to confusion about the symptoms of pancreatic cancer and back pain from ankylosing spondylitis. In a 1987 follow-up by Darby et al. cancer of the pancreas was not significantly elevated, with an O/E of 1.02 being reported.[109] The paper points out that the RR for pancreas and prostate cancers are increased but these diseases are prone to be confused with ankylosing spondylitis as they cause back pain. Other confounding factors mentioned is the known increase in colon cancer in patients with ankylosing spondylitis. Another report of ankylosing spondylitis in 1994 by Weiss et al. included 15,577 patients with a mean total body dose of 2.64 Gy.[266] The paper also contains a dose-response graph for pancreatic and prostate cancer. Statistically significant elevated risks were found, however, the elevated relative risks for pancreatic cancer were felt to be confounded regarding accuracy of diagnosis.

Griem et al. have reported an increase in pancreatic cancer (RR 1.87, 95% CI 1.0, 3.4) among patients treated with radiotherapy for peptic ulcer disease.[112] The dose to the pancreas was about 13 Gy. The authors indicated that the excess may be noncausal and due to smoking or inaccuracies in death certificates. A follow-up study of the same population of 3719 patients was reported by Carr et al.[113] The RR for cancer of the pancreas after radiotherapy was 1.26 in the period 0 to 10 years postexposure and 2.73 (95% CI 1.46, 5.13) in the follow-up period of 11 to 62 years postexposure. The increased relative risk was felt to be inverse with the absorbed dose.

There have been additional reports after other types of radiotherapy for benign disease. Lundell et al. studied risk of solid tumors after irradiation of hemangiomas in infancy.[589] They reported a statistically significant increased ERR per Gy for pancreatic cancer of 25.1 (95% CI 5.5, 57.7), which was based on only nine cases; the authors recognized this was a high value and concluded it may be due to chance especially in view of the doses to the pancreas. Mattsson et al. studied the incidence of primary malignancies other than breast cancer among women treated with radiation therapy for benign breast disease. The RR was nonsignificantly elevated at 1.25 (95% CI 0.56, 2.73).[114] In a study by Inskip et al. of patients who received intrauterine radium radiotherapy for benign uterine bleeding, 4153 women were studied over 110,000 person-years at risk.[118] An excess (SMR of 1.5) of cancer of the pancreas was observed. The authors themselves were puzzled by this finding because the increase appeared a long time after irradiation, and there was little relationship to dose. Doses were also much lower than those incurred from radiotherapy for ankylosing spondylitis and also lower than in the cervical cancer series that did not show a radiation-related increase. The authors did note that none of the cancers in their highest dose group were confirmed histologically, and they mentioned a known association between uterine myomas and pancreatic cancer.

In an incidence study of women treated for cervical cancer, 82,616 exposed women were compared with 99,424 unexposed controls (Fig. 5-25).[124] Excess risk was found for leukemia and cancers of the esophagus, small intestine, rectum, pancreas, and other genital tumors. The O/E ratio of 1.3 for pancreatic cancer was also significantly elevated in those treated with radiotherapy, and it was 0.9 in those with no radiotherapy. However, the RR was high only 0 to 4 years after treatment, so the risk was not likely to be related to the radiation exposure. In another study that matched 4188 women with second cancers with 6880 controls, excess risk was seen for cancers of the bladder, rectum, vagina, cecum, uterus, stomach, NHL, and leukemia.[126] As in the previous study, cancer of the pancreas was increased, but in this study it was not dose related. The RR for cancer of the pancreas was nonsignificantly increased at 1.39 (90% CI 0.7 to 2.7), with an estimated average dose of 1.9 Gy. In a case-control study the number of persons was smaller, but statistically significant

Relative risk

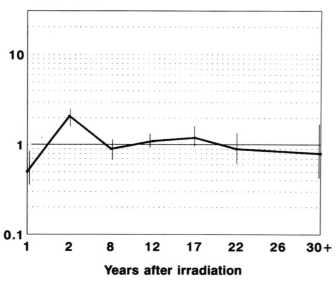

Years after irradiation

Pancreas Cancer (cervix series)

Figure 5-25 • RR of pancreas cancer by time after treatment for cervical carcinoma with radiation therapy. Error bars indicate 95% CI. (From Boice JD, Jr, et al: Second cancers following radiation treatment for cervical cancer: An international collaboration among cancer registries. J Natl Cancer Inst 1985;74:955–975.)

excess risks were found for leukemia and cancers of the stomach, rectum, uterus, bladder, and bone, but no excess was found for cancer of the pancreas.[127] Kleinerman et al. also reported an international registry study and second primary cancer after treatment for cervical cancer.[125] The study evaluated second cancers in 86,193 patients with cervical cancer reported to 13 cancer registries in 5 countries. The pancreatic dose was estimated to average 2 Gy and the O/E ratio for pancreatic cancer was marginally elevated at 1.2 (95% CI 1.0, 2.0), but the O/E ratio was even higher at 1.5 (95% CI 1.1 to 2.0) in patients treated only by surgery. A Japanese study of 5275 cervical cancer patients treated with radiotherapy alone and 4161 treated with surgery alone reported a nonsignificantly elevated O/E ratio of 1.26 for pancreatic cancer in those treated with radiotherapy.[128] In a Danish study of second primary cancers after treatment for cervical cancer Storm found elevated rates of pancreatic cancer at very long post-treatment times in both irradiated and nonirradiated patients and postulated that smoking may be responsible.[704] Birdwell et al. specifically studied gastrointestinal cancer after treatment of HD and reported a four- to fivefold excess of pancreatic cancer after absorbed pancreatic doses of 4.2 to 34 Gy.[739] There are occasional anecdotal case reports after abdominal radiotherapy for testicular tumors that report secondary pancreatic cancer.[740] However, these case reports do not fulfill the criteria for casual relationships or epidemiologic significance. Travis et al. have reported on long-term survival

and second cancers in over 40,000 testicular cancer patients, almost all of whom received infradiaphragmatic radiotherapy to about 27 Gy.[705] The RR for pancreatic cancer was signifcantly increased.

Internal Exposure

Fallout and Other Contamination

No difference in mortality from pancreatic cancer was found in Swedish Lapps, who are presumed to ingest more cesium 137 than the rest of the Swedish population.[741] The SMR for pancreatic cancer was 0.7 (95% CI 0.19, 1.79). Boice et al. have studied cancer mortality in a Texas county with prior uranium mining and milling activities.[89] The SMR for pancreatic cancer was 1.01 (95% CI 0.8, 1.3).

Miners and Nuclear Workers

There is significant literature on the potential relationship between uranium exposure and pancreatic cancer. In uranium miners Waxweiler et al. observed a nonsignificant increase in cancer of the pancreas, an SMR of 1.37 (95% CI 0.63, 2.60) being reported.[362] In uranium enrichment workers no increase in pancreatic cancer was found by Brown et al. who reported an SMR of 0.91 (95% CI 0.39 to 1.51).[363] Tirmarche et al. have studied the mortality of a cohort of French uranium miners.[651] There was no increase in tumors of the liver, gallbladder, and pancreas which were considered together in the analysis. Laurier et al. reported an update on cancer mortality among the French cohort of uranium miners.[186] The reported SMR for liver, gallbladder, and pancreas tumors as a group was nonsignificantly elevated at 1.3 (95% CI 0.8, 2.0). Darby et al. studied radon and cancers in Swedish iron miners and found a nonsignificant decrease in pancreas cancer with an O/E ratio of 0.59 (95% CI 0.24, 1.21).[183]

McGeoghegan et al. have published a report of a cohort of 12,540 workers including 3244 radiation workers at the Capenhurst facility with mean doses of 9.85 mSv, among whom the SMR for cancer of the pancreas was nonsignificantly elevated at 1.18 and the RR was nonsignificantly elevated at 1.2.[242] They also published a report of a cohort of 19,454 workers including 13,960 radiation workers with a mean external dose of 22.8 mSv and a mean follow-up period of 24.6 years, or 479,146 person-years of study at the Springfields uranium production facility.[243] The SMR for pancreatic cancer was less than expected at 0.9 and the RR was nonsignificantly elevated at 1.3. Pinkerton et al. reported on the mortality among a cohort of uranium mill workers in a small study with limited statistical power concerning evaluation of mortality among 1484 men employed in 7 uranium mills in Colorado.[742] The SMR for cancer of the pancreas was 1.08 (95% CI 0.85, 1.35). Ritz also reported on cancer mortality in uranium processing workers and found a nonsignificantly elevated SMR for cancer of the pancreas of 1.17 (95% CI 0.69, 1.85).[447] Dupree-Ellis et al. have reported on mortality in a cohort of 2514 uranium processing workers employed between 1942–1966 at the Mallinkrodt Chemical Works, among whom the SMR for pancreas cancer was nonsignificantly elevated at 1.18.[193]

Plutonium and Radium Workers

There is also some information on the potential relationship between plutonium exposure and pancreatic cancer. In occupational studies Voelz et al. reported no pancreatic cancers in the 50-year follow-up of Manhattan Project plutonium workers.[671] Wing et al. reported an SMR of 0.95 (95% CI 0.44, 1.81) for pancreatic cancer in Oak Ridge workers monitored for internal contamination.[285] Wilkinson et al. did not find any cases of pancreatic cancer in Rocky Flats plutonium workers with a plutonium body burden of more than 74 Bq (2 nCi).[286] Wiggs et al. found nonsignificant reduction in RR (0.72) for pancreatic cancer in a follow-up of Los Alamos plutonium workers.[164]

Omar et al. reported on the cancer mortality and morbidity among plutonium workers at the Sellafield plant of British Nuclear Fuels, among whom there was a nonsignificantly elevated rate ratio of 1.13 with an SMR of 1.04 for plutonium workers and 0.93 for other workers.[148] Carpenter et al. examined cancer mortality in about 17,000 workers in the United Kingdom who were exposed to tritium, plutonium, and other radionuclides.[191] The SMR for pancreatic cancer was nonsignificantly reduced for all at 0.92, 0.68, and 0.48, respectively. No increase in the frequency of pancreatic cancer was found in the radium dial painters.[229]

Medical Internal Exposure of Patients

Most studies of patients who have received radioiodine for diagnostic or cancer therapeutic purposes have not reported results relative to pancreatic cancer. One study by Holm et al. of patients who received radioiodine for treatment of hyperthyroidism indicated an SIR for pancreatic cancer of 1.17 (95% CI 0.82, 1.62).[271] A more recent study of over 35,000 patients treated for hyperthyroidism in the United States was performed by Ron et al. and found a nonsignificantly elevated SMR of 1.10 for those who received iodine 131 and an SMR of 1.05 for those treated surgically.[201]

In a Danish Thorotrast series the SIR for pancreatic cancer was nonsignificantly elevated at 1.9 (95% CI 0.6, 4.3).[213] The German Thorotrast series did report an elevation of pancreatic cancer, with 20 cases in the 2334 followed patients versus 4 in the 1912 controls.[212] The reason for this difference is obscure and may have something to do with smoking or the intensity of follow-up in the two groups, because other nonradiogenic tumors (such as prostate and larynx) also were increased. Nyberg et al. reported on cancer incidence after a 40-year follow-up among Swedish patients exposed to radioactive Thorotrast.[222] The SIR for pancreatic cancer was significantly elevated at 2.9 (95% CI 1.1, 6.4). Travis et al. reported on site-specific cancer incidence and mortality after cerebral angiography with radioactive Thorotrast and found a statistically significant increase in pancreatic cancer with an SIR of 2.4, however, this did not appear to be a function of the dose received.[219] Pancreatic cancer was not increased in the Japanese Thorotrast studies.[735] Nekolla et al. have studied malignancies in patients treated with high doses of radium 224 and they have reported a nonsignificantly increased rate ratio of 1.8 with a lower 95% CI of 0.75.[224]

Summary

The epidemiologic literature does not demonstrate an association between pancreatic cancer and radiation exposure except perhaps at very high doses such as those associated with abdominal radiotherapy. Hence, the UNSCEAR 2000[375] report, the BEIR V[3] and VII[18] reports, and the 1990 ICRP[248] report give no risk estimates for cancer of the pancreas after radiation exposure. The UNSCEAR 2006 report reviewed available literature and risk estimates from studies where they could be estimated (Table 5-25) and concluded that there is little, if any, evidence for associations between pancreatic cancer and radiation exposure whether in relation to external or internal low-LET radiation or internal high-LET radiation.[86]

BONE TUMORS

General

Tumors of bone and cartilage account for about 0.5% of all malignant neoplasms. Bone cancer causes approximately 2000 new cancer cases annually in the United States and approximately 1000 deaths. Malignant bone tumors are divided into several types, with osteosarcoma accounting for 38%; chondroblastic sarcoma, 17%; Ewing's sarcoma, 15%; and all other histologic forms, 30%. There is a male-female sex ratio of 1:3; 5-year survival is approximately 30% for radiation-induced tumors of bone. An overall fatality rate of 75% to 80% is usually seen. Approximately half of bone tumors are present as localized disease, and the other half are equally divided between regional and distant spread.

The various types of tumors are quite age dependent. Osteosarcomas tend to occur in teenagers and in adults who have predisposing Paget's disease. Ewing's sarcoma occurs in childhood and early adult life. Fibrosarcomas mostly occur in middle-aged adults and chondrosarcomas in older adults. There is a relative lack of geographical variation in incidence rates, which argues against a common environmental etiology. There may be some evidence of a familial tendency for osteogenic sarcoma in families with multiple tumors. An increase in bone

Table 5-25 • Risk Estimates for Cancer Incidence and Mortality from Studies of Radiation Exposure: Pancreatic Cancer*

Study	Average Excess Relative Risk at 1 Sv	Average Excess Absolute Risk $(10^4PYSv)^{-1}$
External Low-LET Exposures		
Incidence		
A-bomb Life Span Study[319]		
Males	0.09 (<0–0.63)	<0 (<0–0.36)
Females	0.54 (0–1.26)	0.44 (0.05–1.04)
Age at exposure		
<20	1 (0.01–2.71)	<0 (<0–264.97)
20–40	0.24 (<0–0.94)	0.13 (<0–1.13)
>40	0.07 (<0–0.67)	<0 (<0–1.43)
Time since exposure		
12–15	<0 (<0–<0)	<0 (<0–<0)
15–30	<0 (<0–0.59)	<0 (<0–0.27)
>30	0.62 (0.12–1.28)	1.22 (0.46–2.27)
All	0.29 (<0–0.72)	0.22 (<0–0.63)
Canadian National Dose Register[153]	6.9 (<0–27.1)	NA
Cervical cancer case-control study[6]	0.21 (–0.16–0.89)	NA
Stockholm skin hemangioma[589]	25.1 (5.5–57.7)	1.7
Swedish benign breast disease[114]	–0.37 (<0–0.8)	NA
U.K. Springfields uranium workers[243]	3.6 (< –12.05–34.01)	NA
Mortality		
A-bomb Life Span Study[281]		
Males	0.02 (<0–0.65)	<0 (<0–621.53)
Females	<0 (<0–0.41)	<0 (<0–535.39)
Age at exposure		
<20	0.56 (<0–1.82)	<0 (<0–218.32)
20–40	<0 (<0–0.41)	<0 (<0–745.72)
>40	<0 (<0–0.28)	<0 (<0–1307.5)
Time since exposure		
12–15	<0 (<0–<0)	<0 (<0–153.39)
15–30	<0 (<0–0.78)	<0 (<0–410.14)
>30	<0 (<0–0.51)	<0 (<0–1051.6)
All	<0 (<0–0.33)	0.14 (0.02–0.35)
Canadian National Dose Register[154]		
Males	7.3 (<0–19)	NA
Females	<0 (<0–18.3)	NA
U.K. National Registry for Radiation Workers[146]	<0 (<0–2.31)	NA
Nuclear power industry workers in the United States[159]	–9.38 (< –2.5–89.7)	NA
IARC 15-country nuclear workers study[167,168]	2.1 (<0, –0.59, 6.77)	
Peptic ulcer[113]	0.04 (0–0.08)	NA
Benign gynecological disease[118]	0.14 (–2.76–28.84)	NA
Internal High-LET Exposures		
Incidence		
Danish and Swedish Thorotrast patients[219]	3.8 (1.3–12.3)	NA
Mortality		
U.S. Thorotrast patients[219]	0.9 (0.1–4.4)	NA

*The studies listed are those for which quantitative estimates of risk could be made.
Adapted from United Nations Scientific Committee of the Effects of Atomic Radiation (UNSCEAR): Sources and effects of ionizing radiation: 2006 report to the General Assembly with annexes. New York, United Nations, 2007.

tumors occurs after use of alkylating agents in treatment of childhood cancer. The attributable risk due to radiation is estimated to be less than 10%.[358,700]

Modifying Factors

The absolute radiation risk estimates are somewhat clouded by the fact that many of the population groups exposed to external irradiation received irradiation in body areas where the spontaneous incidence of osteosarcomas is low. For example, the most common site of osteosarcoma is the distal femur (i.e., peripheral skeleton). The patients exposed either for treatment of tinea capitis or for ankylosing spondylitis received the radiation predominantly to the axial skeleton. Individuals who received internal exposures from radium are somewhat difficult to evaluate because the different radioisotopes of radium decay with substantially different rates; thus, the dose is delivered by alpha radiation to different portions of the bone on the basis of the position of the radionuclide in the metabolic cycle of bone. Radium 224 (physical half-life, 3.62 days) yields a relatively high endosteal dose, whereas longer-lived radium 226 decays mainly within the bone volume. An additional problem in deriving risk estimates is the appropriate relative biologic effectiveness (RBE) to be used for alpha particles. In general, the ICRP quality or radiation weighting factor of 20 has been used by most authors. Fractionation is a major modifying factor that has been rather clearly demonstrated in the case of radium 224. Contrary to most other types of irradiation, for radium the effectiveness of a given dose increases as the time of irradiation is protracted. Thus, the absolute risk factors rise if the radium 224 is administered over weeks and years rather than in a single injection. The risk factors appear to be relatively similar for children and adults, as well as for males and females.[743,744]

The latent period for appearance of bone tumors varies widely among the reported studies. With injections of short-lived radium 224, bone sarcomas have been seen as early as 4 years after exposure, with very few being seen after 22 years. Similar appearance times have been identified for therapeutic irradiation, with a mean latent period of 10 years.[745] This is in contrast to continuous irradiation from radium 226, in which bone sarcomas have been seen as long as 52 years after the start of the exposure. The most comprehensive model of bone sarcoma induction for use with alpha radiation, based on human epidemiologic data, has been developed by Marshall and Groer.[746] The model was developed to explain the unusual characteristics of the appearance of the osteosarcoma (i.e., no tumors appeared at or below 9 Gy) in the radium dial painters. The model postulates that two events must be produced in the cell by the alpha radiation to initiate malignant transformation. A number of other sophisticated postulates are also contained in the model, which roughly fits the epidemiologic data in humans. This, however, does not prove the correctness of the postulates; at present, the linear and linear-quadratic dose-response relationships are still considered possible.

External Exposure

Background Radiation and Populations Living Near Nuclear Facilities

One study has examined the potential relationship between background radiation and the risk of skeletal cancer. A large study in China found that osteosarcoma was nonsignificantly less frequent in the high-background area (age-adjusted, site-specific cancer mortality for females of 0.52 per 10^5 person years) than in the area with low-background radiation (0.59 per 10^5 person years).[29] Tao et al. reported on cancer mortality in the high-background radiation areas of Yangjiang, China, during 1979–1995

where the average annual exposure was 6.4 mSv (including internal exposure).[33] The RR for bone cancer was nonsignificantly elevated at 1.33 (95% CI 0.14, 12.8). Jablon et al. have not reported an increase in mortality from bone and joint cancer in populations living around U.S. nuclear facilities as a result of operations.[78] The SMR in study areas was 0.96 before plant operations began and 0.99 after operation. This can be compared with an SMR of 1.01 in the control areas before plant operation and 0.96 afterward. Lopez-Abente et al. have reported on solid tumor mortality near Spain's four nuclear power plants and four uranium fuel cycle facilities indicating that the RR for bone cancer was not significantly different from unity at 0.97.

Increased exposure to natural cosmic radiation occurs in airline crews and there have been a number of studies which include information on their risks of bone or soft-tissue cancers. Pukkala et al., in studying over 10,000 Nordic airline pilots, found no case of bone cancer and nonsignificant decrease of soft-tissue cancers.[39] There was, however, a significant increase in melanoma. Band et al., in a study of 2740 pilots at doses of 6 mSv per year over an average of 20 years for a total average dose about 120 mSv, found a nonsignificantly increased SIR and a nonsignificant increase in SMR for melanoma.[40] This increase in melanoma may be due to sun exposure of the aircrew while at rest stops.

There are three papers concerning potential uranium contamination and the possibility of bone and connective tissue cancers in the public. The papers by Boice et al. indicated a nonsignificant increase in bone cancer and a nonsignificant decrease in connective tissue cancer around a uranium mining and milling facility in Texas and a nonsignificant decrease in bone cancer and a nonsignificant increase in connective tissue cancer near a facility in Pennsylvania.[89,90] Nonsignificant findings were reported for both bone and connective tissue cancer near a Colorado uranium facility.[90a] A nonsignificant decrease in both cancer types was found by Boice et al. in a study of persons residing near the Hanford site.[91]

Fallout

In a study of fallout resulting from nuclear tests in Nevada, Machado et al. reported an OR of 0.48 (90% CI 0.15 to 1.52), comparing the high-fallout areas that occurred in southwestern Utah with the remainder of Utah, and a significantly low OR of 0.31 (90% CI 0.40 to 0.95) when comparison was made with the United States as a whole.[456]

Atomic Bomb Survivors

The incidence and mortality studies of the atomic bomb survivors do report case numbers. The incidence study during 1958–1998 observed 32 cases of bone and connective tissue cancer. The ERR per Gy was slightly increased, but the EAR was not.[319] In the comparable mortality study, there were 1,203,100 person-years of observation and there were 24 deaths versus 19 expected.[10]

Occupational Exposure

A large number of external low-LET exposure occupational studies are negative with respect to radiation induction of bone cancer. Even with large numbers of persons studied, the estimated RRs have wide confidence limits because the number of observed cases is usually small. A study of 22,347 U.K. workers exposed to fallout and other sources reported a nonsignificantly elevated RR of 1.34 for bone cancer (90% CI 0.09 to 31.38).[52] A study by Beral et al. included an analysis of 3373 deaths among 39,546 United Kingdom workers during 1946–1979.[143] The ratio of rates for bone cancer comparing the exposed to nonexposed employees was nonsignificantly elevated at 1.36 (95% CI 0.02 to 43.3). A follow-up study of the same group by Fraser et al. also reported a nonsignificant increase of 2.04 (95% CI 0.69 to 6.09).[702] Another cohort analysis of the U.K. registry of radiation workers by Kendall et al. included 95,217 workers over 1.2 million person-years at risk and reported an insignificantly low SMR of 0.68 for bone cancer.[145] A second analysis in 1999 of 124,743 workers in the U.K. National Registry of Radiation Workers by Muirhead et al. using a lagged analysis reported a nonsignificantly reduced SMR for bone cancer of 0.52 (95% CI 0.14, 1.34).[146]

In a study of 14,327 workers at the Sellafield plant of British Nuclear Fuels, Smith et al. reported an SMR for bone cancer of 0.56 in radiation workers and a higher SMR of 1.22 in other workers.[360] A report on Sellafield workers by Omar et al. indicated a nonsignificant decrease in bone cancer among nonplutonium radiation workers with an SMR of 0.81 and there was a nonsignificant increase in the SMR for connective tissue cancer (based on three cases).[148] McGeoghegan et al. reported on the cancer mortality and morbidity experience of employees at the Chapelcross plant of British Nuclear Fuels during 1955–1995.[149] The cohort included 2628 workers with median doses of 39 mSv. In radiation workers no cases of bone or connective tissue cancer were identified.

Artalejo et al. reported on the mortality among 5657 workers of the former Spanish Nuclear Energy Board with mean exposure of 11.42 mSv.[151] The SMR for bone cancer was significantly elevated at 2.95 (95% CI 1.08, 6.43). Habib et al. have reported on the cancer incidence among Australian nuclear industry–monitored radiation workers and indicated a nonsignificantly elevated SIR of 2.51 for bone cancer and 1.43 for connective tissue cancer.[152] Rahu et al. reported on the cancer incidence of 5446 male Latvian and Estonian Chernobyl cleanup workers and have indicated a nonsignificantly reduced SIR of 0.40 for their rates of bone and connective tissue cancer considered together.[178]

Ashmore et al. reported the first analysis of mortality and occupational radiation exposure based on the National Dose Registry of Canada which included a cohort of 206,620 individuals with 5426 deaths.[154] The average exposure for males was 10.6 mSv and their SMR for bone cancer was significantly decreased at 0.36 (90% CI 0.10, 0.93). Sont et al. also reported on the relation between cancer incidence and occupational radiation exposure based on the National Dose Registry of Canada, which included a cohort of 191,333 persons with an average dose for males of 11.5 mSv and an average dose for the cohort of 6.64 mSv.[153] The SIR for bone cancer in males was nonsignificantly reduced at 0.70 and in females it was nonsignificantly reduced at 0.69.

In one of the large occupational studies in the United States and Canada, Gilbert et al. have reported on workers at Hanford in whom they found an SMR for bone cancer of 0.51 for all workers (0.44 for radiation-monitored male workers and 0.74 for unmonitored male workers).[361] No increase was identified in a later follow-up.[158] Wiggs et al. found a SMR which was not significantly different from unity of 1.04 for bone cancer in a follow-up of Los Alamos radiation workers.[164] Cragle et al. reporting on 9860 white male workers at the Savannah River plant, indicated that there was no significant increase in bone cancer, with only one death from the disease in the entire group.[288] At the Mound facility in Ohio, no deaths from bone cancer were reported.[156] Likewise, Wilkinson et al. did not report any deaths from bone cancer at the Rocky Flats weapons plant.[286]

Cardis et al. investigated cancer mortality among nuclear industry workers in three countries in a very large study of 95,673 workers with over 2 million person-years at risk and 15,825 deaths.[166] The trend for bone cancer was nonsignificantly negative at −1.21 with a P value of 0.887. Cardis et al. also have reported the cancer mortality results from a 15-country collaborative study of nuclear workers.[168] This is the largest occupational study to date and included a cohort of 407,391 workers with 18,993 deaths and 5.2 million person-years of follow-up. The ERR per Sv for bone cancer was nonsignificant and estimated at less than 0, with a negative trend with increasing dose (P value of −0.66).

Cancer rates among medical diagnostic workers in China were reviewed by Wang et al. in 1988 who compared 27,011 workers with 25,782 persons in other medical specialties.[102] The x-ray workers had a 50% higher risk of developing some form of cancer and a significant increase of bone cancer (RR of 9.56). However, this was based on only one case observed in those employed for less than 5 years and three cases observed in those employed for 5 to 9 years. No cases were observed in those employed for 15 years or more, indicating that there was unlikely to be any relationship to radiation. In a 2002 follow-up report, Wang et al. reported the RR for cancer of the bone was nonsignificantly increased at 1.2 for all groups.[253] Mohan et al. studied cancer and other causes of mortality among 146,022 radiologic technologists employed from 1940 and later.[98,99] The SMR for bone cancer in males was nonsignificantly reduced at 0.40 (95% CI 0.1, 1.5) and for females it was nonsignificantly reduced at 0.36 (95% CI 0.1, 1.1).

Diagnostic Medical Exposure

The risk of bone cancer has been studied in patients after external exposures in diagnostic radiology. Massachusetts TB patients treated with multiple fluoroscopies have been followed by Davis et al., who have indicated an SMR of 1.3 in exposed females and 0.0 in unexposed females.[364] The SMR for exposed males was significantly elevated at 4.2 and was 2.0 for unexposed males. In another study also of Massachusetts TB patients,[105] the SMR for bone cancer in male controls was nonsignificantly elevated at 1.6, and in the exposed males the SMR was nonsignificantly elevated at 5.3 (two cases). In the females the SMR for the exposed group was nonsignificantly elevated at 4.8 (two cases), and for controls it was 0.0. Note should be made that the data are based on very few cases.

Radiation Therapy

In treatment of tinea capitis, bone tumors have been reported in at least two studies. UNSCEAR 1977 reviewed these latter studies, and, assuming that the skull forms about 25% of total bone mass in children, derived an absolute lifetime risk factor of three to five cases in 1 million persons for each 10 mGy.[316] Most studies involving external irradiation yield risk estimates that may vary with the skeletal site involved. The BEIR 1980 report indicated that different portions of the skeleton may have different radiosensitivities.[13] Thus, analysis of the British ankylosing spondylitis patients who received approximately 10 Gy to the "spine" shows that of 1400 such patients, only 1 developed bone sarcoma in the spine itself, whereas four developed sarcomatous lesions in the pelvis.[747] Only 1.3 deaths were expected from bone sarcoma versus the 4 that occurred. In this series, the mean dose to the endosteal bone is uncertain; however, it is estimated that the mean dose to the bone marrow was 3.21 Gy. In a more recent follow-up study, Darby et al. reported an O/E ratio of 2.95, which is still based only on the four cases.[109] Secondary neoplasms in 4153 women who received radiation therapy for benign gynecologic conditions have been studied by Inskip et al.[118] In the 109,911 person-years of observation, no cases of bone cancer were identified. No cases of bone cancer were identified by Griem et al. in the follow-up of 1831 patients treated with radiotherapy for peptic ulcer.[112] In 2002, Carr et al. performed a follow-up study of the same group of 3719 patients and no cases of bone cancer were found.[113]

Studies of second cancers in women treated for cervical carcinoma with radiotherapy do not reveal a consistent increase in bone cancer, even though doses to part of the skeleton are on the order of tens of Gy. The estimated RR was 1.23 (90% CI 0.3, 5.6) in a cohort study of women treated for cervical cancer involving 82,616 exposed women compared with 99,424 unexposed controls from Canada, Denmark, Finland, Norway, Sweden, Yugoslavia, the United Kingdom, and the United States.[126] Covering 1.28 million person-years at risk, a nonsignificant increase in cancer of the bone was found. In patients treated for invasive cervical cancer, the O/E ratio was 1.9 for those treated with radiotherapy and 0.0 for those treated without radiotherapy.[124]

In a study by Evans et al. of about 700 patients treated for Wilms' tumors with radiotherapy, subsequent bone cancer was not observed, even though there were 19 patients with benign exostoses or osteochondromas.[547] Osteosarcomas have been reported after radiation therapy for Ewing's tumor, although the series are too small to develop risk estimates.[748] In a study by Hawkins et al. of 10,106 childhood cancer survivors, there was a significant increase (20-fold) in the number of sarcomas.[307] Risk was particularly high (400-fold) in patients with familial retinoblastomas. In fact, in patients with this entity the risk was 200-fold normal even without radiotherapy or chemotherapy. Sagerman et al. have reported that approximately 1.5% of children treated for retinoblastoma will develop radiation-induced malignancies, with about half of these being osteosarcomas.[749] It should be noted, however, that children with heritable retinoblastomas are at increased risk for other tumor types even outside the radiation therapy field.[750]

In a study of patients treated for HD, Tucker et al. reported an O/E ratio of 31 (95% CI 3.5, 111.8) based on two cases versus 0.1 expected.[436] It should be remembered that most patients received both radiotherapy and chemotherapy.[138] Woodard et al. have reported on 16 cases of malignant bone tumors that arose 4 to 31 years after irradiation for HD.[751] The median absorbed dose was 40 Gy, and it was estimated that up to 25% of the skeleton was exposed in the primary beam. The same authors also reported on the survival of 59 patients with postirradiation osteosarcomas and 20 with malignant fibrous histiocytomas. The 5-year, disease-free survival rate for osteosarcomas was 17% compared with a 3-year disease-free survival rate for malignant fibrous histiocytoma of 58%.[752] A similar pattern of subsequent tumors was also reported by Laskin et al.[753] and in children by Newton et al.[754] A postirradiation case of multicentric osteosarcoma has been reported by Tillotson et al.[755] and there are case reports of chondrosarcomas.[756]

Arlen et al. have described 50 cases of radiation-induced osteosarcoma following radiation therapy for various neoplasms.[757] Reported doses ranged from 12 to 240 Gy, and the mean latent period was 9 years. Both osseous and soft-tissue sarcomas have been identified by other authors as well after successful radiation therapy

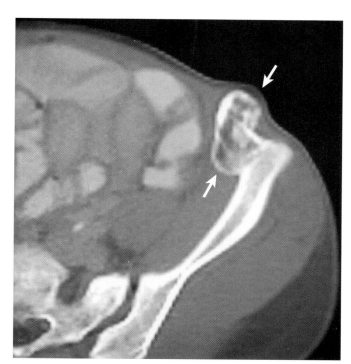

Figure 5-26 • Benign osteochondroma seen on a CT scan arising from the anterior portion of the left iliac crest ten years after pelvic radiotherapy.

for many tumor types, including HD, breast cancer seminoma, and cervical cancer. The doses received covered a wide range, with a median dose of 60 Gy in 6 weeks. The median latent period is between 11 and 15 years.[758,759]

Radiation-induced osteochondromas have been reported in 6% of long-term surviving children who received radiation therapy. It has been postulated that this represents a growth disturbance in the epiphyseal plate rather than a true neoplasm (Fig. 5-26).[760] These benign "tumors" have been noted in the spine, pelvis, scapula, and ribs.[761]

Internal Radiation

For an extensive description of the potential carcinogenic effects of internally deposited radionuclides, the reader is referred to the BEIR IV report of the U.S. National Academy of Sciences.[575] The endosteal dose is important because osteosarcomas appear to arise from the endosteal cells; therefore, the dose to these cells rather than the mean dose to the bone is important. The dose from radium 224, with its short half-life of 3.6 days, is largely delivered while the radium is still on the bone surface. The dose to endosteal cells (bone surface) is between 7 and 9 times that of the bone dose. Radium 226, on the other hand, is distributed throughout the bone before it is completely decayed. Radium 226 has an endosteal dose that is only about two thirds of the mean bone value.[762] It should be noted that the dose delivered from

radium is alpha radiation; thus, depending on the quality or radiation weighting factor used, the appropriate risk estimate for low-LET radiation may be lower than those obtained from the radium studies by a factor of as much as 20.

Diagnostic Internal Exposure

Patients who received Thorotrast (thorium 232 dioxide) for diagnostic purposes have been followed by a number of groups with reference to induction of bone tumors. This is because thorium 232 decays to radium 224. The Danish study by Andersson et al. reported a nonsignificantly increased SIR of 5.0 (95% CI 0.1 to 28) based on only one observed case.[213] This is in contrast to the German series that suggests a probable excess with 4 deaths from bone cancer observed in 2334 patients and only 1 death in the 1912 controls.[211,212] In a Japanese study of 282 patients there was 1 osteosarcoma reported.[215,677] In the initial report of about 2500 Portuguese Thorotrast patients there were five primary bone tumors in the exposed group and none in the control subjects.[216] There is a 2003 report by dos Santos Silva et al. on the 50-year follow-up of mortality of Portuguese Thorotrast patients. The cohort included 1096 systemically exposed and 240 locally exposed. The SMR for bone cancer in the systemically exposed was significantly increased at 12.8. The relative risk of systemically exposed versus locally exposed was significantly increased at 7.6.

Several authors have attempted to calculate risk estimates for Thorotrast based on the assumption that 25 mL of injected Thorotrast gives an average dose rate from translocated radium 224 to the marrow-free skeleton of about 0.01 Gy per year. The BEIR IV Committee's estimated risk is 55 to 120 excess bone sarcomas per 10^4 person Gy average skeletal dose.[575] More recently, Travis et al. have concluded that the association between Thorotrast and bone tumors is not entirely convincing.[763] The only report that has considered bone sarcomas after administration of radioiodine is by Hoffman et al. who reviewed patients treated at the Mayo Clinic for hyperthyroidism.[202] Patients treated with radioiodine compared with those treated with surgery showed a nonsignificant increase in RR (4.3 with 95% CI 0.02 to 854); one bone tumor was found in each of the groups.

Radiation Therapy

Following World War II, a preparation known as Peteostor containing the short-lived radium 224 was administered intravenously for therapy of TB and ankylosing spondylitis.[743,764] Due to the short physical half-life of radium 224 (3.62 days), most of the dose is delivered to the bone surface. The average skeletal dose is estimated to have been about 4 Gy. In the radium 224 patients the risk appears to be minimal at times more than 30 years after exposure. Several studies have been performed regarding these patients, one beginning in 1952 and another in 1971. In the first study, 54 bone sarcomas were identified in 900 patients. The average skeletal dose exceeded 0.9 Gy. The second study examined 1000 patients who received less than 0.9 Gy to the skeleton. Two sarcomas have been identified in these 1000 patients, one occurring at a dose of 0.67 Gy.[13] The risk appears to be higher from a given total dose of radium 224 if the radium is administered over a longer time period rather than in a single injection.[765]

A study by Nekolla et al. of 455 patients treated with radium 224 for TB, ankylosing spondylitis, and a few other diseases indicated that connective tissue tumors occurred in seven and the rate ratio was significantly elevated at 80.[224] Wick and Nekolla also reported on late effects in ankylosing spondylitis patients treated with radium 224, among whom there were 626 exposed and 725 control patients with a mean follow-up time of 21 years.[225] The mean injected activity was 0.17 MBq/kg and the mean alpha skeletal dose was 0.67 Gy. The study showed an increase in the O/E ratio for bone cancer among those exposed of 4 to 1.3.

In a more recent study of 800 patients treated with radium 224 for bone TB and ankylosing spondylitis, Chemelevsky et al. reported 56 bone sarcomas compared with the 0.2 expected.[766] The authors again suggest that protraction of the injections over 15 months results in a higher (double) risk than the same activity injected over 5 months. However, whether this is a real difference or an artifact of the analysis remains unclear. The distribution of appearance times of the bone sarcomas in radium 224 patients is similar to that of leukemia in the atomic bomb survivors, ranging from 3.5 to 25 years, and averaging about 11 years in both juveniles and adults. Additionally, the absence of head sinus carcinomas in this group supports the hypothesis that accumulation of radon 222 in these cavities causes the tumors in radium dial painters exposed to radium 226.[767] The protraction effects suggest that the number of lifetime induced bone sarcomas from radium 224 in people of all ages is 40 cases in 1 million persons for each 10 mGy for a single injection of radium 224, versus 200 cases in 1 million persons for each 10 mGy if the injections are administered weekly over several years. The dose used in this risk estimate refers to the average skeletal dose.

Occupational Exposure

Studies in uranium miners have not shown a significant increase in these cancers. Waxweiler et al. did not observe any of these tumors and reported an SMR of 1.53 (95% CI 0.04 to 8.77).[362] A 2004 update of French uranium miners by Laurier et al. reported a nonsignificantly reduced SMR of 0.7 for bone cancer.[186] Ritz et al. have reported on cancer mortality in uranium processing workers at the Fernald plant in Ohio, among whom no bone cancers were identified.[192] Dupree-Ellis et al. have reported on mortality in a cohort of 2514 uranium processing workers employed between 1942–1966 at the Mallinkrodt Chemical Works.[193] The SMR for bone cancer was nonsignificantly elevated at 1.20 based on one case. McGeoghegan et al. reported on the mortality of 12,540 workers (including 3244 radiation workers) at the Capenhurst uranium enrichment facility during 1946–1995 and no case of bone cancer was identified in radiation workers.[242] They also studied cancer mortality experience of 19,454 workers (including 13,960 radiation workers) at the Springfields uranium production facility during 1946–1995, among whom the SMR for bone cancer was nonsignificantly reduced for radiation workers at 0.67.[243] A meta-analysis of 14 studies, which included 120,000 uranium workers, found a nonsignificant decrease in bone cancer with an RR of 0.93 (95% CI 0.53, 1.33).[245] Darby et al. studied radon cancers in Swedish iron miners and did not identify any case of bone cancer.[183]

A report on the Sellafield plant by Omar et al. indicated that no case of bone cancer was identified among plutonium workers there.[148] Carpenter et al. examined workers in the United Kingdom who were occupationally exposed to tritium, plutonium, and other radionuclides.[191] The SMRs for both bone and connective tissue in each group were all nonsignificantly different from unity. Occupational epidemiologic studies conducted at the U.S. weapons facilities that have plutonium workers have generally not reported on bone cancer in relation to plutonium body burden.[286] There was, however, a report of the follow-up of the Manhattan Project plutonium workers, in whom one fatality in the group due to an osteogenic sarcoma of the sacrum was observed.[671] Whether this was due to chance or to plutonium remains unclear. It should be noted that the sacrum is a very unusual location for spontaneous osteogenic sarcoma in an adult in the absence of predisposing Paget's disease (which this patient did not have).

Radium dial painters internally contaminated with long-living radioisotopes (radium 228, half-life of 5.8 years; radium 226, half-life of 1600 years) number about 2000, and this population has been followed for five decades.[768–770] The radium dial industry began about 1913 in the United States and used mainly young women and girls to apply a paint combining zinc sulfide and radium to dials of clocks, watches, and other instruments (Fig. 5-27). The radium allowed the paint to be luminous. The women often pointed the brushes between their lips and, thus, inadvertently ingested large quantities of radium. This material accumulates in the bone, and autopsies conducted 20 years later revealed that up to 95% of the radium still remained in the body. These data have been reviewed in the BEIR IV report.[575]

Rowland et al. have reported that in the United States there were 3054 radium dial painters employed prior to 1950.[328] As early as 1929 bone sarcomas were identified in these workers. Of all 4059 radium workers in the U.S.

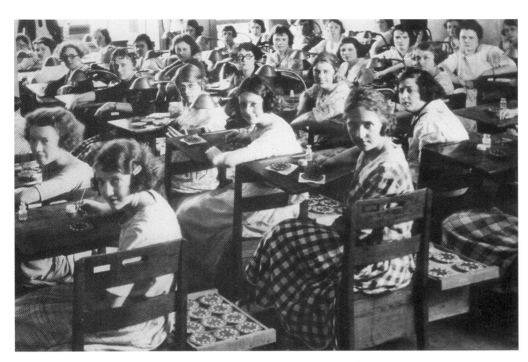

Figure 5-27 • Radium dial painters. Typically these were very young women who pointed their brushes between their lips, and thereby ingested large amounts of radium. (Case courtesy of the Argonne National Laboratory Radium Registry, Argonne, Ill.)

Registry, by 1984 there were 84 in whom bone sarcomas were identified. The minimum latent period was 7 years. In contrast to the risk in radium 224 patients, which appears to become greatly reduced after about 30 years, the risk for the radium dial painters appears to continue for at least 60 years. There is also a U.K. series of 1200 female dial painters reported by Baverstock et al.[771] These women ingested much less radium than their U.S. counterparts, and there was only one death due to bone sarcoma in this group compared to the 0.17 expected. The sarcomas occurred at unusual locations such as the foot, scapula, and pelvis (Figs. 5-28 and 5-29). From the data it appears that radium 228 is about 1.5 times as effective per Gy as radium 226 in producing bone sarcomas. Originally, there was

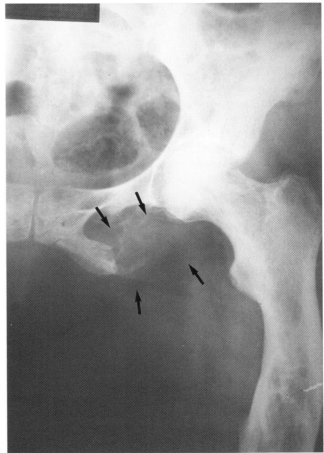

Figure 5-29 • Osteogenic sarcoma with bone destruction of the left ischium of the pelvis in a radium dial painter. (Case courtesy of the Argonne National Laboratory Radium Registry, Argonne, Ill.)

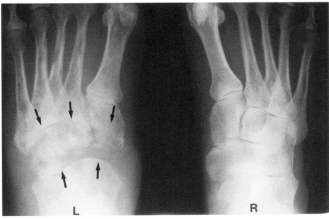

Figure 5-28 • Osteogenic sarcoma with destruction of the left tarsal bones in a radium dial painter. (Case courtesy of the Argonne National Laboratory Radium Registry, Argonne, Ill.)

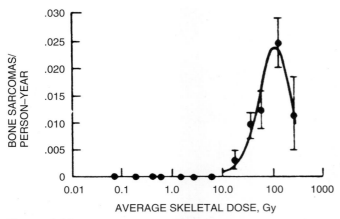

Figure 5-30 • Dose-response relation for bone sarcomas. There is an apparent threshold at about 10 Gy. (From the Committee on the Biological Effects of Ionizing Radiations (BEIR): Health risks of radon and other internally deposited alpha-emitters. BEIR IV. Washington, DC, National Academy Press, 1988.)

thought to be a threshold for induction of these tumors at about 5 to 10 Gy, but later a few cases occurred at doses calculated to be below 5 Gy. Because the time to appearance of these tumors lengthened with the smaller radium burdens, some authors have calculated that mathematically there exists a practical threshold for these tumors at about 0.8 Gy.[229] Whether an actual threshold exists on a mathematical basis remains a matter of debate, but a glance at the dose-response curves for both radium dial painters and Thorotrast patients (Fig. 5-30) certainly suggests a practical threshold. Risk estimation after radium ingestion is very complex and depends on the type of radium ingested. For a more detailed discussion the reader is referred to the BEIR IV report.[575]

Summary

The epidemiologic data show convincing excesses of bone and connective tissue tumors after radiation therapy and after internal contamination with large amounts of alpha-emitting radionuclides. There remains an argument as to whether a practical threshold exists relative to the alpha emitters. There has been no clear excess demonstrated as a result of external occupational exposure or at low activities of internal radionuclides. There is no clear statistically significant excess identified in the atomic bomb survivors. Most authoritative reports give risk estimates for bone cancer although usually not at low doses. The 1988 UNSCEAR Report did not quote a risk factor for bone cancer after external low-dose, low-LET radiation.[370] The 1990 BEIR V Committee concluded that it also was unable to derive a risk estimate at low doses of low-LET radiation but that "the data currently available from the study of the Japanese A-bomb survivors provide no evidence of an excess of bone cancer resulting from low-LET irradiation at levels in the 0 to 4 Gy range."[3]

In persons with internal radium burdens the lifetime risk of bone cancer was judged to be about 2×10^{-2} per person Gy.

The 1990 ICRP report estimates the probability of fatal bone cancer after exposure of the general population to be 5 $(10^{-2}Sv^{-1})$.[248] This ICRP risk estimate is mostly based on data from radium 224 data. Radium 224 actually gives a dose predominantly to the bone surface rather than to the whole bone. In this circumstance the ICRP risk estimate is probably too high.[772] The UNSCEAR 2006 Committee has summarized radiation risk factors regarding bone and connective tissue cancer from epidemiological studies (Table 5-26) and concluded that there is an increased risk of bone sarcomas following low-LET radiation in the range of tens of Gy, and that risk factors cannot be derived at doses below a few Gy.[86] Persons receiving substantial activities of high-LET radiation, in particular, radium 224, 226, and 228, and the plutonium workers at Mayak in Russia have clearly shown exposure-related, increased risk of bone tumors.

SOFT-TISSUE TUMORS

No increase in soft-tissue tumors has been evident at low levels of radiation exposure and most low-level radiation studies either do not report on soft-tissue tumors or group them together with bone cancers. The 1958–1998 incidence data on atomic bomb survivors indicates 149 cases of sarcomas. About half of these were from bone (11), connective tissue (32), and uterus (26). There numbers are too small to derive risk estimates.[319] Cardis et al. have reported the cancer mortality results from a 15-country collaborative study of nuclear workers.[168] This is the largest occupational study to date and included a cohort of 407,391 workers with 18,993 deaths and 5.2 million person-years of follow-up; the ERR per Sv for connective tissue tumors was nonsignificantly positive at 0.32 (90% CI < 0, 11.5).

Many retrospective studies in the literature indicate that a variety of soft-tissue tumors may follow external radiotherapy (Fig. 5-31). The tumors may arise from a variety of tissues including fibrous or neural tissue, fat, muscle, blood vessels, and lymphatic tissue. Radiation probably accounts for less than 5% of all bone and soft-tissue sarcomas.[773] The predominant types appear to be malignant fibrous histiocytomas, fibrosarcoma, neural sheath tumors, and angiosarcoma. In retrospective analyses, Sordillo et al. found that 10% of patients with extraosseous osteosarcoma had prior radiotherapy.[759] Foley et al.[774] and Ducatman et al.[775,776] found that 6% to 11% of patients with malignant peripheral nerve sheath tumors had prior radiotherapy. Radiation-induced synovial sarcomas appear to be rare or nonexistent although there is at least one case report.[777]

Radiation-induced soft-tissue sarcomas typically arise in or near the radiation field and may occur within

Table 5-26 • Risk Estimates for Cancer Incidence and Mortality from Studies of Radiation Exposure: Malignancies of the Bone and Connective Tissue*

Study	Average Excess Relative Risk at 1 Sv	Average Excess Absolute Risk $(10^4 PYSv)^{-1}$
External Low-LET Exposures		
Incidence		
A-bomb Life Span Study[319]		
Males	3.34 (0.9–9.69)	<0 (<0–<0)
Females	<0 (<0–<0)	<0 (<0–9.75)
Age at exposure		
<20	4.33 (0.9–16.11)	<0 (<0–<0)
20–40	3.16 (<0–24.05)	<0 (<0–12.66)
>40	<0 (<0–<0)	<0 (<0–<0)
Time since exposure		
12–30	1.27 (0.07–4.55)	<0 (<0–10.87)
>30	2.28 (0.23–9.32)	<0 (<0–18.77)
All	1.64 (0.4–4.31)	<0 (<0–14.36)
Retinoblastoma patients (bone and soft tissue sarcoma)[781]	0.19 (0.14–0.32)	NA
Childhood radiotherapy (international)[138]	0.06 (0.01–0.2)	NA
Childhood cancer, U.K. (bone)[795]	0.16 (0.07–0.37)	NA
Cervical cancer case control (connective tissue)[6]	−0.05 (−0.11–0.13)	−0.01 (−0.03–0.03)
Cervical cancer case control (bone)[6]	0.02 (−0.03–0.21)	NA
Canada National Dose Registry[153]		
Bone	<0	<0
Connective tissue	<0	<0
Mortality		
A-bomb Life Span Study[281]		
Male	1.24 (0.03–4.47)	<0 (<0–24.4)
Female	<0 (<0–3.15)	<0 (<0–25.43)
Age at exposure		
<20	2.11 (<0–11.62)	<0 (<0–7.21)
20–40	8.26 (0.7–50.09)	<0 (<0–<0)
>40	<0 (<0–0.01)	<0 (<0–35.48)
Time since exposure		
12–30	1.33 (0.05–4.7)	0.08 (0.01–0.26)
>30	<0 (<0–4.2)	<0 (<0–31.08)
All	0.88 (<0–3.03)	<0 (<0–21.23)
Ankylosing spondylitis (bone and connective and soft tissue)[266]	0.44	0.097
Nuclear workers in Canada, United Kingdom, United States (bone)[166]	<0	NA
Nuclear workers in Canada, United Kingdom, United States (connective tissue)[166]	>0	NA
U.S. Oak Ridge workers, 1943–1947 (bone)[267]	NA	NA
U.S. radiologic technologists[796]	<0	<0
Canadian National Dose Registry[154]	−0.9 (−57.5–55.7)	NA
IARC 15-country nuclear workers study[167,168]		
Bone	<0	
Connective tissue	0.32 (<0, 11.5)	
Internal High-LET Exposures		
Incidence		
[224]Ra ankylosing spondylitis patients (bone and connective tissue)[225]	4.3	NA
German thorotrast patients (bone sarcoma)[221]	~3.3	NA
Mortality		
U.S. radium luminizers (bone)[234,556,797,798]	NA	~13
Portuguese Thorotrast patients (bone)[799]	7.08 (1.65–30.3)	NA
U.S. Thorotrast patients[219]	∞ (0.1–∞)	NA

*The studies listed are those for which quantitative estimates of risk could be made.
Adapted from United Nations Scientific Committee of the Effects of Atomic Radiation (UNSCEAR): Sources and effects of ionizing radiation: 2006 report to the General Assembly with annexes. New York, United Nations, 2007.

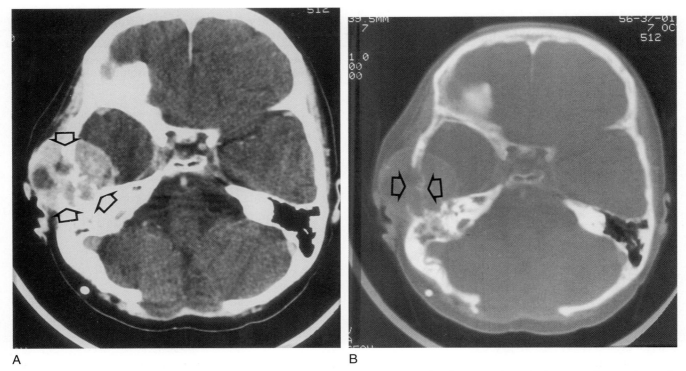

A   B

Figure 5-31 • Sarcoma arising in the right temporal portion of the skull in a 15-yr-old female, 11 yrs after radiotherapy to this area for another tumor. The soft-tissue CT scan (**A**) shows a round, enhancing mass, and the bone windows (**B**) show destruction of the skull.

a few years or decades later. Most reports in the literature lump together osteosarcoma and soft-tissue sarcomas, however, there are some reports on nonosseous soft-tissue sarcomas. The literature also points out that chemotherapy, including dactinomycin[778] and procarbazine,[779] also can increase the risk of soft-tissue sarcomas. Soft-tissue sarcomas are also more common in siblings of childhood cancer patients,[780] and the increased risk of second sarcoma in treated retinoblastoma patients argues for a genetic component for increased sarcoma risk.[781]

Steeves and Bataini have reported that 4 of 1000 patients followed after megavoltage radiation therapy of the head and neck developed second tumors.[782] There were sarcomas (two osteogenic, one fibrosarcoma) and one sarcomatoid epithelioma. In a study of 2311 subjects who were treated during childhood with radiation for enlarged tonsils or adenoids, 32 neural tumors and 54 salivary gland tumors have been reported.[783] Ducatman et al. have reviewed 109 patients with neurofibrosarcoma and indicate that 12 cases arose in previously irradiated areas, but this study was complicated because 7 of the 12 had stigmata of von Recklinghausen's disease.[776]

An increasing number of studies have examined the risk of second bone tumors after radiation therapy for breast and pelvic cancers. Taghian et al. reviewed 6919 patients treated for breast cancer in France between 1954–1983 in whom there were 11 sarcomas, 9 of which were within the irradiated field.[784] These were osteosarcomas, malignant fibrous histiocytomas, and other

soft-tissue sarcomas. The mean latent period was 9.5 years (range 4 to 24). The radiation doses averaged 45 Gy delivered in 18 fractions. The cumulative risk was 0.2% at 10 years. Rubino et al. reported the risk of subsequent bone or soft-tissue sarcoma in a cohort of 6597 breast cancer patients and found 12 cases versus 1.7 expected for an SIR of 7.0 (95% CI 3.7, 11.7).[785]

There are multiple reports of angiosarcomas of the breast occurring after radiotherapy for breast cancer. This was initially thought to be related to chronic lymphedema and (in contrast to data for other sarcomas) some studies show no releation to radiation dose.[786–788] Angiosarcomas have also been reported after pelvic radiation.[789] Ruka et al. found 22 cases of sarcomas among 531 patients irradiated for pelvic tumors over the previous 38 years.[790] The tumors covered a wide range of types including neurofibrosarcomas, fibrosarcomas, hemangiosarcomas, and others. Somewhat similar findings have also been reported by Wiklund et al. in reviewing 33 cases of postirradiation sarcomas.[791] Jacobsen et al. reported an analysis of second primary tumors in 6187 men treated for testicular cancer in the period between 1943–1987.[792] Thirteen sarcomas were found (RR equals 4) and the latent period ranged from 5 to 34 years. Seven of the tumors were within the radiation field, and three were located at the periphery. Brenner et al. have studied second malignancies in prostate carcinoma patients treated with radiotherapy or surgery and reported that within the radiation field there was a significant increase in sarcoma risk with the radiotherapy group having an ERR of 1.45 at times greater than 5 years postexposure compared to the surgery only group.[137] The risk was increased (but nonsignificantly) at times greater than 10 years postexposure. The risk of distant sarcomas was nonsignificantly elevated for both time periods. Schlemmer et al. have reported a case of soft-tissue sarcoma arising in the groin of a Thorotrast patient.[793] Hasson et al. have reported an extraosseous osteosarcoma in the neck of a different Thorotrast patient.[794]

Summary

Radiation is likely to be responsible for less than a few percent of soft tissue sarcomas. However, some types have been reported to be increased, especially in or near a radiation therapy field.

NONMELANOMA SKIN CANCER

General

An excellent review of radiation effects on the skin has been produced by the ICRP and the reader is referred to this for a more detailed discussion.[800] Although skin cancers were the first malignant tumors reported to be induced by radiation (in 1902), and 50 cases were described by 1911, there still are few data available on the frequency and the risks of these tumors. The incidence rates of skin cancer vary substantially among populations. While skin cancer is the most common form of cancer in whites, it is much less common in dark-skinned ethnic groups. As an example, whites in Hawaii have annual rates of 138 per 100,000, while in Hawaiian Asians the rate is only 3.1 per 100,000. There also appears to be a genetic component because there are high rates in those of Irish, Scottish, and Welsh ancestry.

The most common cell type is basal cell carcinoma. Squamous cell carcinomas are about one third to one sixth as common. Both cell types are most common on the head and neck, and somewhat less common on the arms, and much less common on other body parts. In blacks there appears to be a higher risk in areas that have been subjected to previous trauma, burn scars, and chronic ulcers. Skin cancer is not usually included in radiation mortality risk estimates because of the very low mortality associated with this tumor type. The statistics of the incidence of skin carcinomas are somewhat difficult to evaluate because often melanomas are included with basal cell carcinoma and squamous cell carcinoma. In the United States, there are 700,000 cases and 9000 deaths annually from skin carcinomas. If melanomas are excluded, the number of deaths is reduced to about 2000 annually.

The fatality rate for nonmelanoma skin cancers that are radiation-induced appears to be 1% to 3%. The incidence of nonmelanoma skin cancer shows wide geographic variation. High incidence rates have been reported in Tasmania, Australia, British Columbia, Canada, and Texas. Rates in males are about twice those in females. Rates are much higher in whites than in blacks, and the tumors occur mostly in areas of sunlight-exposed skin such as the face, head and neck, and arms. Some chemicals can cause these tumors, including polycyclic hydrocarbons, mineral cutting oils, and arsenic. In non-pigmented races about 90% to 95% of tumors are attributable to sunlight. In blacks most tumors are related to chronic skin trauma.[700] The rate of mortality from squamous cell carcinoma (SCC) is about 1% or less. If metastases are present the 5-year survival is about 50%. The mortality rate from basal cell carcinoma (BCC) is close to 0, and the metastasis rate is about 0.1%. Considering that BCC may be induced by radiation about 10 times as frequently as SCC, the ICRP has chosen a conservative lethality rate of 0.2% for radiation-induced skin cancers.[800]

Modifying Factors

The epidemiologic studies suggest that the effect of ultraviolet irradiation and ionizing radiation may be more than additive. The latent period for induction of skin tumors is extremely wide, with a mean of slightly greater than 20 years. As mentioned in the discussion of genetic effects, patients with xeroderma pigmentosum have a much higher incidence of skin tumors due to faulty repair of DNA following ultraviolet radiation. In general, the skin appears to have a relatively low sensitivity in regard to radiation carcinogenesis. Patients with A-T have cells that are sensitive to ionizing radiation cell-killing effects, but there is no evidence of increased cancer after ionizing radiation exposure. The frequency of A-T in Jewish children of Moroccan ancestry is about five times higher than in most populations, and how much of a role this may play in the findings reported in Israeli children is unknown. Patients with nevoid basal cell carcinoma syndrome (NBCS) develop large numbers of basal cell carcinomas. In contrast to A-T patients, those with NBCS have cells of normal sensitivity in regard to radiation killing effects, but they have a great sensitivity to induction of skin cancers by radiation. After radiation therapy (and sometimes within 1 year), such patients often have basal cell carcinomas developing in and about the radiation field. There is no evidence that patients with either vitiligo or psoriasis have increased sensitivity to radiation induction of skin cancers.

Squamous cell skin cancer rates are high among albino blacks, but there is nothing known about radiation sensitivity of this group. The BEIR 1980 report indicated that the types of tumors found after radiation exposure are more commonly SC and BC carcinomas.[13] There appears to be a significant difference depending on anatomic location, with SCCs predominantly on the hands and BCCs on the head and neck. Basal cell carcinomas appear to dominate at lower dose levels, whereas SCCs occur at much higher dose levels and are usually associated with radiodermatitis or ulceration. Other types of tumors, including fibrosarcomas, melanomas, and sweat gland tumors, have occasionally been reported.[801–803] Because most skin tumors are often relatively innocuous and easily treated, it is possible that most of the studies may suffer from underreporting of the tumors. A final problem in studying the data is that the skin is classed as an organ, and it is very rare that the entire skin of an individual is uniformly irradiated. Thus, allowances must be made for the skin area actually irradiated in the various studies.

External Irradiation

Background Exposure and Populations Near Nuclear Installations

Tao et al. reported on cancer mortality in the high-background radiation areas of Yangjiang, China, during 1979–1995 where the average annual exposure was 6.4 mSv (including internal exposure).[33] The RR for skin cancer there was nonsignificantly elevated at 1.16 (95% CI 0.37, 3.65). There are three papers concerning potential environmental uranium contamination and the possibility of skin cancer in the public. The papers by Boice et al. indicated nonsignificant increases around uranium mining and milling facilities in Texas and Pennsylvania and a nonsignificant decrease near a Colorado uranium facility.[89,90,90a] A nonsignificant increase of skin cancer was reported by Boice et al. in a study of persons residing near the Hanford National Laboratory site.[91]

Fallout and Atomic Bomb Survivors

In 1954 there was unexpected fallout on the Marshall Islands from thermonuclear testing. There was also fallout on a Japanese fishing boat, the *Lucky Dragon*. Many of the 239 Marshall Islanders and the 18 fishermen developed skin erythema, blistering, and subsequent skin depigmentation and atrophy as a result of skin doses from beta- and gamma-emitting radionuclides. The skin doses were in excess of 10 Gy. No increase in skin malignancies have been seen in these populations.[459]

Originally, there was no excess of skin cancer identified in the atomic bomb survivors. This may be because the studies were primarily mortality studies, and mortality from skin cancer is very low. At the end of the last decade there began to appear reports of an increased incidence of skin cancer at Nagasaki (Fig. 5-32).[804–807] The incidence study from Hiroshima and Nagasaki includes 41,000 persons who received 0.01 Sv or more and an average dose of 0.23 Sv. For the period 1958–1998, there were an estimated 40 cases among a total of 330 nonmelanoma skin cancers leading to an ERR per Gy of 0.17 (90% CI 0.003, 0.55) and an EAR of 0.35 (90% CI 0, 1.1) cases per $(10^4 PY\ Gy)^{-1}$.[319] The ERR decreased rapidly with increasing age at exposure. The dose response is consistent with linear, although the best fit is with a spline of increased slope above 1 Gy.[319]

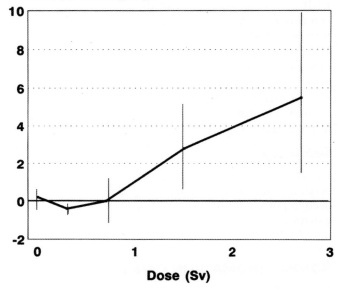

Excess relative risk

Nonmelanoma skin cancer incidence (A-bomb)

Figure 5-32 • ERR of nonmelanoma skin cancer in atomic bomb survivors at different dose levels. Bars indicate 95% CI. (From Thompson D, Mabuchi K, Ron E, et al: Cancer incidence in atomic bomb survivors. II: Solid tumors, 1958–1987. RERF Technical Report 5-92, Hiroshima, Japan, Radiation Effects Research Foundation, 1992.)

Occupational Exposure

Most occupational studies report mortality rather than incidence and, therefore, are somewhat limited with respect to skin cancer. However, a number of occupational studies report on the mortality or incidence of skin cancer. Overall, with the possible exception of the early radiologists and the uranium miners, there has been no consistant increase in skin cancer found. In a study by Darby et al. of U.K. men who participated in nuclear weapons tests, no deaths were reported for nonmelanoma skin cancers.[52] In the latest 2004 review Muirhead et al. have a cohort of 21,357 test partipants and reported a nonsignificantly decreased SMR of 0.51 (95% CI 0.06, 1.82) for nonmelanoma skin cancer in test participants.[55] The RR compared to controls for incidence was nonsignificantly decreased at 0.88. Rahu et al. reported on the cancer incidence of 5446 male Latvian and Estonian Chernobyl cleanup workers and indicated a nonsignificantly reduced SIR of 0.63 for nonmelanoma skin cancer.[178]

For nuclear workers Beral et al. reported a nonsignificantly increased rate ratio of 1.36 (95% CI 0.02 to 43.3) for melanoma and other skin cancers.[143] In another group of atomic energy workers, a follow-up study of the workforce by Fraser et al. reported a rate ratio of 0.50 (95% CI 0.06 to 4.73).[702] Using a 10-year lag, Kendall et al. reported an SMR of 0 for nonmelanoma skin cancers.[145] A second analysis in 1999 of 124,743 workers in the U.K.

National Registry of Radiation Workers by Muirhead et al. using a lagged analysis reported a significantly reduced SMR for nonmelanoma skin cancer of 0.31 (95% CI 0.06, 0.90) but this was based on only three cases.[146]

Ashmore et al. reported the first analysis of mortality and occupational radiation exposure based on the National Dose Registry of Canada which included a cohort of 206,620 individuals and 5426 deaths.[154] The average exposure for males was 10.6 mSv. Gilbert et al. studied the Hanford workers from 1945–1986 and reported a decreased SMR for skin cancer of 0.80.[361] Cragle et al. studied workers at the Savannah River plant and reported SMRs of 0.40 (two cases) in workers paid on an hourly basis and 0.92 (two cases) in salaried workers.[288] Wiggs et al. reported on workers employed between 1947–1979 at the Mound facility in Ohio, among whom the SMR for skin cancer was nonsignificantly elevated at 2.28 (95% CI 0.62 to 5.85), based on four cases.[156] Wilkinson et al. reported on workers employed at the Rocky Flats weapons facility and reported an SMR of 1.02 (90% CL 0.28 to 2.64) based on three cases.[286] Cardis et al. investigated cancer mortality among nuclear industry workers in three countries in a very large study of 95,673 workers with over 2 million person-years at risk and 15,825 deaths.[166] The trend for skin cancer was nonsignificantly reduced at 0.36 with a P value of 0.358.

The occurrence of skin cancer in uranium miners has been raised as a possibility in several reports from Czechoslovakia. In contrast to the subjects of most other literature reported in this section, these miners were predominantly exposed to alpha irradiation, which would not penetrate to the basal layer of the skin. In the reports, cumulative doses to the basal layer of the skin are estimated in the range of 10 to 20 Sv assumedly from beta radiation. It is unlikely, however, that beta dosimetry under mining conditions is accurate. Sevcova et al. initially reported an increase of BCC of the face.[808] In a later follow-up of about 3000 Czech miners, there were 27 skin cancers compared with 4.7 expected. The SMR was reported to be 5.7 (90% CI 4.1 to 7.8). These miners had a special program for surveillance of skin cancers that would be expected to detect more skin cancer than normally appears in national registry statistics. In another report of miners (including coal miners) by Sevcova et al., the O/E ratio for coal and surface miners was below unity, whereas for the uranium miners the O/E ratio was 5.2 (90% CI 2.3 to 10.3).[809] These studies are in contrast to a report by Waxweiler et al. of uranium miners, who found a nonsignificantly increased SMR for skin cancer of 2.16 (95% CI 0.70 to 5.04).[362]

Ritz et al. have reported on cancer mortality in uranium processing workers at the Fernald plant in Ohio.[192] The SMR for skin cancer was nonsignificantly reduced at 0.62. Dupree-Ellis et al. have reported on mortality in a cohort of 2514 uranium processing workers employed between 1942–1966 at the Mallinkrodt Chemical Works.[193] The SMR for skin cancer was nonsignificantly reduced at 0.75. Several Canadian mortality surveillance studies and a niobium workers' study in Norway have not reported an excess of skin cancer deaths.[575]

Matanowski et al. have reported on the experience of U.S. radiologists compared with other medical specialists.[2] An increased risk was found for those employed before 1930 (RR 10.0 with 90% CI 3.5 to 28.3) as well as those employed between 1930–1959 (RR 3.3 with 90% CI 1.5 to 7.5). For the early group the estimated dose to the skin was in the range of 10 Gy. This leads to an estimated ERR of about 0.9 per Gy. Smith et al. found that radiologists employed before 1920 had a significantly increased O/E ratio for deaths from skin cancer of 7.79 (six observed vs. 0.8 expected).[584] For those employed after 1920 the O/E ratio was 1.96 (two observed vs. 1.02 expected). The O/E ratio was 2 to 0.57 for those employed from 1921–1935 and 0 to 0.44 for those employed from 1936–1954, neither of which was significantly increased. Mohan et al. studied cancer and other causes of mortality among 146,022 radiologic technologists employed from 1940 and later.[98,99] The SMR for skin cancer in males was significantly reduced at 0.63 (95% CI 0.4, 0.9) and for females it was also significantly reduced at 0.70 (95% CI 0.5, 0.9). In 1988, Wang et al. studied Chinese radiologic technologists, in whom they found a nonsignificantly increased RR of 1.48 for deaths from skin cancer.[102] The authors estimated that whole-body penetrating doses to many of the workers exceeded 1 Gy. In a 2002 follow-up report, Wang et al. reported for those employed before 1970 whose cumulative doses were 551 mSv the RR for cancer of the skin was significantly increased at 4.31 but for those employed after 1970 with a cumulative mean dose of 82 mSv, the RR was lower and nonsignificantly increased at 2.74.[253]

Diagnostic Medical Exposure

Very few studies have reported the occurrence of skin cancer after diagnostic exposures. Three studies have followed various populations of patients who received multiple fluoroscopic studies of the chest during treatment of TB.[320,322,364] Mean skin doses ranged from 8.5 to 13 Gy, and several skin cancers were identified. The risk factors from these studies were in the range of 0.7 cases annually in 1 million persons exposed for each 0.01 Gy. In a follow-up report, Davis et al. reported SMRs for deaths from skin cancer as follows: 0.8 in exposed females, 2.0 in unexposed females, 0.9 in exposed males, and 1.6 in exposed males.[105] The 1991 ICRP report on skin cancer includes data collected from several studies of patients exposed to multiple fluoroscopies.[810] The collected group contains data from 6285 patients in whom the average cumulative dose was 9.6 Gy; however, the RR was only 1.06, and the absolute excess risk was 0.02 $(10^{-4} PYGy)^{-1}$.

Radiation Therapy

The occurrence of skin tumors in children treated for tinea capitis was examined by both Shore[293] and Modan[295] with rather different results. The study by Shore indicated that there were 24 patients with skin cancer in the exposed group of 2215 children and 2 skin cancers in the control group of 1395 children. No skin cancers were identified in the patients who were black. In the study by Modan, on the other hand, only 1 skin cancer was identified in 10,902 children given scalp irradiation and none in the control series. Both BCCs and SCCs or combinations of these were reported (Fig. 5-33). More recent updates by the same group have reported that the patients who developed cancers reported more radiodermatitis and epilation, suggesting that they may have received higher doses than originally recorded.[811,812] It was also clear that they were more frequent sunbathers, again suggesting that there is a potentiating effect of ultraviolet light.

In a study by Shore the number of skin cancers observed indicated that the absolute risk rose with age.[293] There appeared to be a mean interval of approximately 45 years between the x-ray therapy and skin cancer diagnosis. The differences in the rate of tumor induction reported between these two studies may depend on a number of factors, including ethnic background, fairness of the skin, and the time period over which the populations were observed. Continued study of a New York group of children treated for tinea capitis by Shore et al. reported 83 cases of skin cancer among the 1680 white patients treated by radiotherapy versus 2 expected.[813] All 83 had BCCs, but 4 also had SCC. The estimated scalp doses were in the range of 3.3 to 5.5 Gy. In the control group there were 16 skin cancers compared with 14.3

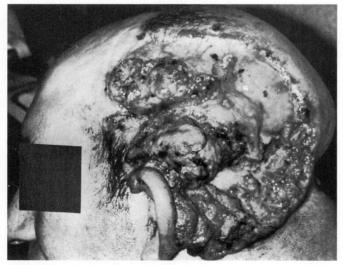

Figure 5-33 • Radiation-induced squamous cell carcinoma invading the scalp and meninges. The tumor was believed to have been induced by childhood treatment for ringworm of the scalp. (From Rubin P and Casarett GW: Clinical Radiation Pathology. Philadelphia, WB Saunders, 1966.)

expected. It was estimated from this study that tumors occurred four times as frequently in areas that received a lot of sunlight as in areas shielded from the sun by hair or clothing. In contrast to the whites, there were no skin cancers found among the 550 irradiated black patients. Two studies have examined patients treated with superficial x-rays for treatment of benign dermatoses.[814] The doses were typically given in fractionated regimens. The results were not clear-cut, because distribution differed between irradiated and control groups. Actual absorbed dose was also uncertain. Lindelof et al. reported increased cancer among 14,140 patients who had received orthovoltage x-ray treatments for various skin disorders.[815] The possible effect of the skin disorders and therapy (such as application of arsenic, tars, and UV light) on subsequent cancer incidence is difficult to determine. Veien et al. reported on 1107 patients who had received radiotherapy for treatment of 3675 warts on their hands or feet.[816] The treatment was a single dose of 30 Gy with low-energy x-rays. Follow-up was from 5 to 22 years, and no skin cancers were observed.

Four other groups were treated with radiation therapy for other reasons, and again the results are diverse. Hempelmann found 9 of 2872 persons irradiated for thymic enlargement to have skin cancer versus 3 among a group of 5055 controls.[420] Skin doses ranged from about 0.4 to 15 Gy, with a mean of 3.3 Gy. The absolute risk was not substantially different between those who received less than 4 Gy and those who received more than 4 Gy. The risk estimates did differ, depending on the number of fractions given in the dose regimen. In a follow-up study Hildreth et al. found a significantly elevated RR of 3.4 after an average skin dose of 3 Gy.[817] In the ankylosing spondylitis patients, on the other hand, Court-Brown and Doll found no excess of skin cancer among the 15,300 patients treated.[106] The cumulative skin dose in the primary beam was estimated to be 10 to 15 Gy. In a follow-up study of the same group by Darby et al. there were five skin cancer deaths compared with 3.8 expected (O/E ratio of 1.36).[109] The difference was not significantly different from unity. The mean dose to the skin of the trunk was estimated to be about 1.8 Gy. In the group of women treated with radiotherapy for postpartum mastitis, no excess of skin cancer was identified. In this latter group, the average skin dose was 2.8 Gy, with an average follow-up of 25 years; 6 cancers were found versus 7.4 expected from normal incidence. In a follow-up study of the same group of mastitis patients, Shore et al. did not find an excess of skin cancer.[521] The O/E ratio was 14 to 10.7 or 1.3, which was not significantly increased. In another study, Van Daal et al. reviewed 257 patients treated between 1932–1963 for benign diseases of the head and neck.[818] Skin doses ranged from 1 to 60 Gy with a median of about 10 Gy. There were 30 skin cancers identified of which 27 were of the basal cell type. A risk factor of 0.9 per $(10^4 PYGy)^{-1}$ was reported. Schneider et al. have reported on 2958 patients treated to the tonsils and nasopharynx with an average cumulative dose of 3.75 Gy.[341] After a mean follow-up period of 35 years for skin cancer, there was an RR of 1.4 (90% CI 1.1 to 1.7). Furst et al. studied 18,030 patients treated for skin hemangioma from 1920–1959 in Sweden.[302] Most were treated at about 6 months of age with either radium 226 sources or orthovoltage x-ray. In these patients 224 cancers were observed, which yielded an RR of 1.18 (95% CI 1.03 to 1.35).

Few studies report on the occurrence of skin cancer after radiotherapy for malignant diseases. Boice et al. reported on a cohort study of women treated previously for cancer of the cervix.[124] In those women treated for invasive cervical cancer with radiotherapy there was an O/E ratio for nonmelanoma skin cancers that was nonsignificantly increased. In a follow-up of Japanese women treated for cancer of the cervix, Arai et al. reported a nonsignificantly elevated O/E ratio for skin cancer of 1.6 (five observed, 3.2 expected).[128] Hay et al. studied 547 men who were irradiated for treatment of testicular tumors in whom 8 skin cancers were observed (all outside the primary treatment field).[597] Because there was no control group with equivalent surveillance, the authors were not sure whether there was a radiation effect or simply bias due to increased surveillance. It should be noted here that there may be a slightly increased subsequent risk of skin cancer in children who have been treated with radiotherapy for retinoblastoma.[819] Whether this is the result of radiation exposure or of a genetic susceptibility is not clear.

Internal Exposure

Only a very limited amount of information relative to internal exposure and the subsequent development of skin cancer is available. In Swedish Lapps, Wiklund et al. reported an SIR of 0.36 for skin cancer and melanoma compared with the Swedish population.[56] No data are reported relative to skin cancer and the internal administration of radioiodine for thyroid scanning or therapy. Wilkinson et al. reported on Rocky Flats plutonium workers who had body burdens of 74 Bq (2 nCi) or more and found no deaths from skin cancer in the exposed group but two deaths in the unexposed group.[286] Carpenter et al. examined workers in the United Kingdom who were occupationally exposed to tritium, plutonium, and other radionuclides.[191] The SMRs for melanoma and skin cancer (treated together) in each group were all nonsignificantly different from unity. In the series of Danish Thorotrast patients, Andersson et al. reported 10 cases of skin cancer for an SIR of 1.2 (95% CI 0.6 to 2.3).[213]

Summary

A number of studies indicate an association between nonmelanoma skin cancer and radiation. The positive studies are predominantly of whites and involve therapeutic doses to areas that are also affected by sunlight. A few genetic conditions confer particular susceptibility. The induced tumors are predominantly basal or squamous cell carcinomas. From a composite of the literature the ICRP suggests that a multiplicative model is most appropriate for nonmelanoma skin cancer and that the RR remains constant throughout life.[810] The absolute risk estimates are 22×10^{-8} per cm^2 per PYGy for UV-exposed skin and 1.3×10^{-8} per cm^2 per PYGy for non-UV-exposed skin. The estimated ERR is 0.61 per Gy for UV-exposed skin and 0.05 per Gy for UV-shielded skin. This yields a similar value of 0.55 for total-body irradiation. The ICRP 1990 report gives an estimate for the probability of fatal skin cancer in the whole population and for workers of $2 \ (10^{-2}Sv^{-1})$.[248]

The UNSCEAR 2006 Committee has summarized radiation risk estimates for nonmelanoma skin cancer that can be derived from the epidemiological literature (Table 5-27) and concluded that there is strong evidence that nonmelanoma skin cancer and specifically BCC is inducible by ionizing radiation with relative risk strongly decreasing with increasing age at exposure.[86] The issue of interaction between exposure to solar UV radiation and ionizing radiation remains unclear. ERRs may be lower on solar exposed sites, whereas EARs may be higher on solar-exposed sites.[249]

MELANOMA

General

Melanomas do not appear to be induced by ionizing radiation, and, therefore, the fatality rate for other forms of skin cancer that are radiation-induced appears to be 1% to 3%.

External Irradiation

Background Exposure and Populations Near Nuclear Installations

There are three papers concerning potential environmental uranium contamination and the possibility of skin cancer/melanoma in the public. The papers by Boice et al. indicated nonsignificant increases around uranium mining and milling facilities in Texas and Pennsylvania and a nonsignificant decrease near a Colorado facility.[89,90,90a]

Fallout and Atomic Bomb Survivors

There was a study by Caldwell et al. of soldiers exposed to fallout during nuclear testing that showed a nonsignificant excess (RR 1.8, 95% CI 0.7 to 3.7).[822] Both the incidence and mortality data from the Japanese atomic bomb survivor LSS yield risk estimates that are nonsignificantly different from unity regardless of sex, time since exposure, or age at exposure.[281,319]

Table 5-27 • Risk Estimates for Cancer Incidence and Mortality from Studies of Radiation Exposure: Nonmelanoma Skin Cancer*

Study	Average Excess Relative Risk at 1 Sv	Average Excess Absolute Risk $(10^4 PYSv)^{-1}$
External Low-LET Exposures		
Incidence		
A-bomb Life Span Study[319]		
Males	1.27 (0.65–2.17)	1.23 (0.65–1.96)
Females	1.37 (0.81–2.12)	1.07 (0.68–1.56)
Age at exposure		
<20	5.69 (3.16–10.27)	<0 (<0–150.01)
20–40	0.9 (0.38–1.66)	0.98 (0.43–1.72)
Time since exposure		
12–15	<0 (<0–1.73)	0.38 (0.04–1.42)
15–30	0.9 (0.2–2.08)	0.42 (0.16–0.84)
>30	1.53 (1–2.24)	2.31 (1.62–3.14)
All	1.33 (0.89–1.88)	1.12 (0.79–1.52)
Childhood Exposure		
Israel tinea capitis[812,820]	0.7 (0.35–1.32)	1.31 (0.94–1.77)
New York tinea capitis (whites)[821]	0.6 (0.3–1.1)	1.9 (0.5–3.3)
Rochester thymic irradiation[817,820]	1.05 (0.5–1.84)	15.9 (7.5–27.9)
Tonsil irradiation[341,820]	0.11 (0.04–0.19)	10.2 (3.3–18.3)
Adult Exposure		
Cervical cancer cohort[124,820]	<0 (<0–0.01)	<0 (<0–0.6)
Massachusetts TB fluoroscopy D6[820]	0.007 (0–0.03)	0.9 (<0–4.5)
New York mastitis[820]	0.12 (<0–0.38)	60 (<0–193.5)
Internal High-LET Exposures		
Incidence		
Danish and Swedish Thorotrast patients[219]	1.3 (0.6–2.8)	NA

*The studies listed are those for which quantitative estimates of risk could be made. Adapted from United Nations Scientific Committee of the Effects of Atomic Radiation (UNSCEAR): Sources and effects of ionizing radiation: 2006 report to the General Assembly with annexes. New York, United Nations, 2007.

Occupational Exposure

In a study by Darby et al. of U.K. men who participated in nuclear weapons tests the SMR for malignant melanoma was 1.05, and for controls it was 0.91, with an RR of 1.25 (90% CI 0.44 to 3.59).[52] In the latest 2004 review Muirhead et al. studied a cohort of 21,357 test participants and reported that the incidence of melanoma compared to controls also was nonsignificantly elevated at 1.09.[55] Rahu et al. have reported on cancer incidence of 5446 male Latvian and Estonian Chernobyl cleanup workers and indicated the SIR for melanoma in such workers that was nonsignificantly elevated at 1.88.[178]

For nuclear workers Beral et al. reported a nonsignificantly increased rate ratio of 1.36 (95% CI 0.02 to 43.3)

for melanoma and other skin cancers.[143] In another group of atomic energy workers, a follow-up study of the workforce by Fraser et al. reported a rate ratio of 0.50 (95% CI 0.06 to 4.73).[702] Using a 10-year lag, Kendall et al. reported an SMR of 1.03 for malignant melanoma.[145] McGeoghegan et al. reported on the mortality and cancer morbidity experience of employees at the Chapelcross plant of British Nuclear Fuels during 1955–1995.[149] The cohort included 2628 workers with median doses of 39 mSv. In radiation workers no case of melanoma was identified. A second analysis in 1999 of 124,743 workers in the U.K. National Registry of Radiation Workers by Muirhead et al. using a lagged analysis reported a nonsignificantly reduced SMR for melanoma of 0.92 (95% CI 0.60, 1.35).[146]

Ashmore et al. reported the first analysis of mortality and occupational radiation exposure based on the National Dose Registry of Canada which included a cohort of 206,620 individuals and 5426 deaths.[154] The average exposure for males was 10.6 mSv. The SMR for melanoma was nonsignificantly reduced at 0.73 (90% CI 0.49, 1.05). Sont et al. also reported on the relationship between cancer incidence and occupational radiation exposure based on the National Dose Registry of Canada, which included a cohort of 191,333 persons with an average dose for males of 11.5 mSv and an average dose for the cohort of 6.64 mSv.[153] The SIR for melanoma in males was significantly elevated at 1.21 and in females it was nonsignificantly elevated at 1.11. Habib et al. have reported on cancer incidence among Australian nuclear industry–monitored radiation workers and indicated a nonsignificantly increased SIR of 1.03 for melanoma.[152] Darby et al. studied radon and cancers in Swedish iron miners and did not identify any cases of melanoma.[183]

A report in 1981 by Austin et al. reported increased melanoma at Lawrence Livermore Laboratory among workers who reported that they had "worked around radioactive materials."[823] A subsequent 1997 analysis by Moore et al. did find an excess compared with regional incidence rates, but it also showed that the cases did not have more radiation exposure than the controls.[824] An additional study of Lawrence Livermore National Laboratory published in 2004 by Whorton et al. reported that the melanoma excess occurred from 1974–1985, but that there was a reduction to community rates during 1986–1997.[825] A study of workers at Los Alamos National Laboratory failed to show an excess of melanoma.[826]

Cardis et al. reported on cancer mortality among nuclear industry workers in three countries.[166] This is a very large study of 95,673 workers and includes over 2 million person-years at risk and 15,825 deaths. For melanoma the trend was nonsignificantly reduced at 0.21 with a P value of 0.416. Cardis et al. also have reported the cancer mortality results from a 15-country collaborative study of nuclear workers.[168] This is the largest occupational study to date and included a cohort of 407,391

Table 5-28 • Risk Estimates for Cancer Incidence and Mortality from Studies of Radiation Exposure: Cutaneous Melanoma*

Study	Average Excess Relative Risk at 1 Sv	Average Excess Absolute Risk $(10^4 PYSv)^{-1}$
External Low-LET Exposures		
Incidence		
A-bomb Life Span Study[319]		
Males	0.01 (<0–2.66)	<0 (<0–6.99)
Females	<0 (<0–0.57)	<0 (<0–1.56)
Age at exposure		
<40	<0 (<0–0.68)	<0 (<0–1.09)
>40	0.07 (<0–2.73)	<0 (<0–<0)
Time since exposure		
12–30	<0 (<0–2.1)	<0 (<0–5.05)
>30	<0 (<0–0.96)	<0 (<0–2.18)
All	<0 (<0–0.74)	<0 (<0–0.03)
Canadian National Dose Register[153]	4.3 (<0–19.6)	NA
Capenhurst uranium facility[242]	–1.3 (< –1.3–10.51)	NA
U.K. Springfields uranium workers[243]	4.38 (–0.21–11.78)	NA
U.K. Chapelcross workers[149]	0.15 (< –2.23–6.43)	NA
Mortality		
A-bomb Life Span Study[281]		
Male	1.91 (<0–15.25)	0.03 (<0–0.13)
Female	<0 (<0–<0)	<0 (<0–5.84)
Age at exposure		
<40	0.66 (<0–4.11)	<0 (<0–1.13)
>40	<0 (<0–0.58)	0.36 (0.14–2.32)
Time since exposure		
12–30	<0 (<0–0.4)	<0 (<0–<0)
>30	0.66 (<0–4.11)	<0 (<0–11.93)
All	0.3 (<0–2.1)	<0 (<0–6.25)
Canadian National Dose Register[154]	44.9 (–67.1–156.8) (males)	NA
Canadian National Dose Register[154]	–0.1 (–1340–1339) (females)	NA
IARC 15-country nuclear workers study[167,168]	0.15 (<0, 131)	
Internal High-LET Exposures		
Incidence		
Danish and Swedish thorotrast patients[219]	0.4 (0.1–2.1)	NA

*The studies listed are those for which quantitative estimates of risk could be made.
Adapted from United Nations Scientific Committee of the Effects of Atomic Radiation (UNSCEAR): Sources and effects of ionizing radiation: 2006 report to the General Assembly with annexes. New York, United Nations, 2007.

workers with 18,993 deaths and 5.2 million person-years of follow-up. The ERR per Sv for melanoma was nonsignificantly positive at 0.15 (90% CI < 0, 5.44) with a negative trend with increasing dose (P value of −0.06).

McGeoghegan et al. have reported on the mortality of 12,540 workers (including 3244 radiation workers) at the Capenhurst uranium enrichment facility during 1946–1995.[242] The SMR for melanoma was nonsignificantly reduced in radiation workers at 0.49. They also studied the cancer mortality experience of 19,454 workers (including 13,960 radiation workers) at the Springfields uranium production facility during 1946–1995.[243] The SMR for melanoma was significantly reduced for radiation workers at 0.19. Carpenter et al. examined workers in the United Kingdom who were occupationally exposed to tritium, plutonium, and other radionuclides.[191] The SMRs for melanoma and skin cancer (treated together) in each group were all nonsignificantly different from unity. Study of the Danish and Swedish Thorotrast patients shows a small ERR per Sv of 0.4 (95% CI 0.1, 2.1).[219]

Few studies report on the occurrence of skin cancer after radiotherapy for malignant diseases. Boice et al. reported on a cohort study of women treated previously for cancer of the cervix.[124] In those women treated for invasive cervical cancer with radiotherapy there was an O/E ratio for melanoma of 0.8; in those who did not get radiotherapy it was 1.0.

Summary

There is little or no consistent scientific evidence that malignant melanomas are induced by radiation. The UNSCEAR 2006 Committee has summarized radiation risk estimates for melanoma that can be derived from the epidemiological literature (Table 5-28).[86] For melanoma, solar UV radiation has the potential to seriously confound the data and one would expect a positive bias in any estimated dose response if solar UV radiation is not taken into account.[249]

REFERENCES

1. Seltser, R. and P.E. Sartwell, The influence of occupational exposure to radiation on the mortality of radiologists and other specialists. Am J Epidemiol, 1965. 81:2–22.
2. Matanowski, G.M., et al., The current mortality rates of radiologists and other physician specialists: Specific causes of death. Am J Epidemiol, 1975. 101:199–210.
3. National Research Council (NRC). Committee on the Biological Effects of Ionizing Radiations (BEIR), Health effects of exposure to low-levels of ionizing radiation. BEIR V. 1990, Washington, DC: National Academy Press.
4. Tanaka, K., M. Takechi, and N. Kamada, Mutation of RAS oncogene in atomic bomb radiation-exposed leukemia. J Radiat Res (Tokyo), 1991. 32(4):378–388.
5. Kamada, N., et al., Cytogenetic and molecular changes in leukemia among atomic bomb survivors. J Radiat Res (Tokyo), 1991. 32(suppl 2):257–265.
6. Boice, J.D., Jr., et al., Radiation dose and leukemia risk in patients treated for cancer of the cervix. J Natl Cancer Inst, 1987. 79(6):1295–1311.
7. Neriishi, K., et al., The observed relationship between the occurrence of acute radiation effects and leukemia mortality among A-bomb survivors. Radiat Res, 1991. 125(2):206–213.
8. Pierce, D.A., et al., Studies of the mortality of atomic bomb survivors. Report 12, Part I: Cancer: 1950–1990. Radiat Res, 1996. 146(1):1–27.
9. Preston, D.L., et al., Effect of recent changes in atomic bomb survivor dosimetry on cancer mortality risk estimates. Radiat Res, 2004. 162(4):377–389.
10. Shimizu, Y., H. Kato, and W.J. Schull, Studies of the mortality of A-bomb survivors. 9. Mortality, 1950–1985: Part II. Cancer mortality based on the recently revised doses (DS86). Radiat Res, 1990. 121(2):120–141.
11. Preston, D., E. Ron, and D. Thompson, Cancer incidence in atomic bomb survivors. Part III. Leukemia, lymphoma and multiple myeloma, 1950—1987. In Cancer Incidence in Atomic Bomb Survivors. 1994, Hiroshima, Japan: Radiation Effects Research Foundation.
12. Preston, D.L., et al., Cancer incidence in atomic bomb survivors. Part III. Leukemia, lymphoma and multiple myeloma, 1950–1987. Radiat Res, 1994. 137(suppl 2):S68–S97.
13. National Research Council (NRC), The effects on populations of exposure to low levels of ionizing radiation. BEIR III. 1980, Washington, DC: National Academy of Sciences, p. xiii.
14. Beebe, G., H. Kato, and C.E. Land, Studies of the mortality of A-bomb survivors: Mortality experience of A-bomb survivors, 1950–1974. 1977, Hiroshima, Japan: Radiation Effects Research Foundation.
15. Ron, E., and B. Modan, Thyroid and other neoplasms following childhood scalp irradiation. In Radiation Carcinogenesis: Epidemiology and Biological Significance, J. Boice and J. Fraumeni, eds. 1984, New York: Raven Press.
16. Ichimaru, M., et al., Incidence of leukemia in A-bomb survivors by dose, years after exposure, age and type of leukemia, 1950–71. 1976, Hiroshima, Japan: Radiation Effects Research Foundation.
17. Moriyama, I. H. Kato, Mortality experience of A-bomb survivors, 1970–1972, 1950–1972. 1973, Hiroshima, Japan: A.B.C. Commission.
18. National Research Council (NRC), Committee on the Biological Effects of Ionizing Radiations (BEIR), Health risks from exposure to low levels of ionizing radiation. BEIR VII, phase 2. 2006, Washington, DC: National Acadamy Press.
19. Tomonaga, M., T. Matsuo, and R. Carter, A-bomb irradiation and leukemia types: An update. RERF Technical Report 9-91, 1991, Hiroshima, Japan: Radiation Effects Research Foundation.
20. Ichimaru, M., et al., Atomic bombings and leukemia. J Radiat Res (Tokyo), 1991. 32(suppl 2):14–19.
21. Walter, S.D., J.W. Meigs, and J.F. Heston, The relationship of cancer incidence to terrestrial radiation and population density in Connecticut, 1935–1974. Am J Epidemiol, 1986. 123(1):1–14.
22. Iwasaki, T., et al., Cancer mortality rates in different geographical distribution by levels of natural radiation dose in Japan. Proceedings of the International Conference on High Levels of Natural Radiation, Ramsar, Iran, 1990. 1991, Vienna: International Atomic Energy Agency (IAEA).
23. Tirmarche, M., et al., Epidemiologic study of regional cancer mortality in France and natural radiation. Radiat Prot Dosim, 1988. 24:479–482.
24. Jacobson, A., P. Plato, and N. Frigerio, The role of natural radiations in human leukemogenesis. Am J Public Health, 1976. 66:31–37.
25. Hickey, R.J., et al., Low-level ionizing radiation and human mortality: Multi-regional epidemiological studies, a preliminary report. Health Phys, 1981. 40(5):625–641.
26. Mason, T.J. and R.W. Miller, Cosmic radiation at high altitudes and U.S. cancer mortality, 1950–1969. Radiat Res, 1974. 60(2):302–306.
27. Weinberg, C.R., K.G. Brown, and D.G. Hoel, Altitude, radiation, and mortality from cancer and heart disease. Radiat Res, 1987. 112(3):381–390.
28. Edling, C., et al., Effects of low-dose radiation—A correlation study. Scand J Work Environ Health, 1982. 8(suppl 1):59–64.
29. High Background Radiation Research Group (HBRRG), Health survey in high background radiation areas in China: HBRRG, China. Science, 1980. 209(4459):877–880.
30. Wei, L.X., et al., Epidemiological investigation of radiological effects in high background radiation areas of Yangjiang, China. J Radiat Res (Tokyo), 1990. 31(1):119–136.
31. Shimizu, M., et al., Correlation between natural radiation exposure and cancer mortality. J Nihon Univ Sch Dent, 1987. 29:314–320.
32. Sun, Q., et al., Excess relative risk of solid cancer mortality after prolonged exposure to naturally occurring high background radiation in Yangjiang, China. J Radiat Res (Tokyo), 2000. 41(suppl):43–52.
33. Tao, Z., et al., Cancer mortality in the high background radiation areas of Yangjiang, China during the period between 1979 and 1995. J Radiat Res (Tokyo), 2000. 41(suppl):31–41.
34. Tao, Z., Y. Cha, and Q. Sun, (Cancer mortality in high background radiation area of Yangjiang, China, 1979–1995). Zhonghua Yi Xue Za Zhi, 1999. 79(7):487–492.
35. Tao, Z., Analysis of data (1987–1995) from investigation of cancer mortality in high background radiation area of Yangjiang China. Chinese Journal of Radiol Med Prot, 1999. 19:75–82.

36. The United Kingdom Childhood Cancer Study of exposure to domestic sources of ionising radiation. Part 2. Gamma radiation. Br J Cancer, 2002. 86(11):1727–1731.

37. Axelson, O., et al., Leukemia in childhood and adolescence and exposure to ionizing radiation in homes built from uranium-containing alum shale concrete. Epidemiology, 2002. 13(2):146–150.

38. Gundestrup, M. and H.H. Storm, Radiation-induced acute myeloid leukaemia and other cancers in commercial jet cockpit crew: A population-based cohort study. Lancet, 1999. 354(9195):2029–2031.

39. Pukkala, E., et al., Incidence of cancer among Nordic airline pilots over five decades: Occupational cohort study. BMJ, 2002. 325(7364):567.

40. Band, P.R., N.D. Le, et al., Cohort study of Air Canada pilots: Mortality, cancer incidence and leukemia risk. Am J Epidemiol, 1995. 143(2):137–143.

41. Blettner, M., B. Grosche, and H. Zeeb, Occupational cancer risk in pilots and flight attendants: current epidemiological knowledge. Radiat Environ Biophys, 1998. 37(2):75–80.

42. Blettner, M. and H. Zeeb, Epidemiological studies among pilots and cabin crew. Radiat Prot Dosimet, 1999. 86:269–273.

43. Langner, I., et al., Cosmic radiation and cancer mortality among airline pilots: Results from a European cohort study (ESCAPE). Radiat Environ Biophys, 2004. 42(4):247–256.

44. Zeeb, H., et al., Mortality from cancer and other causes among airline cabin attendants in Europe: A collaborative cohort study in eight countries. Am J Epidemiol, 2003. 158(1):35–46.

45. Conard, R., Acute myelogenous leukemia following fallout of radiation exposure. JAMA, 1975. 232:1356–1357.

46. de Vathaire, C.C., and B. de Vathaire, Childhood malignancies in French Polynesia during the 1985–1995 period. Trop Med Int Health, 2004. 9(9):1005–1011.

47. Land, C.E., F.W. McKay, and S.G. Machado, Childhood leukemia and fallout from the Nevada nuclear tests. Science, 1984. 223(4632):139–144.

48. Stevens, W., et al., Leukemia in Utah and radioactive fallout from the Nevada test site. A case-control study. JAMA, 1990. 264(5):585–591.

49. Stevens, W., et al., A case-control study of leukemia deaths in Utah (1952–1981) and exposure to radioactive fallout from the Nevada test site: Final report. 1990, Bethesda, Md: National Cancer Institute, National Institutes of Health.

50. Institute of Medicine, The Five Series Study: Mortality of Military Participants in U.S. Nuclear Weapons Tests. 2000, Washington, DC: National Academy Press.

51. Darby, S.C., et al., Trends in childhood leukaemia in the Nordic countries in relation to fallout from atmospheric nuclear weapons testing. BMJ, 1992. 304(6833):1005–1009.

52. Darby, S.C., et al., A summary of mortality and incidence of cancer in men from the United Kingdom who participated in the United Kingdom's atmospheric nuclear weapon tests and experimental programmes. Br Med J (Clin Res Ed), 1988. 296(6618):332–338.

53. Doll, R., et al., Study of U.K. men who had participated in the U.K. nuclear weapons test programme. J Radiol Prot, 1998. 18(3):209–210.

54. Muirhead, C.R., et al., Follow up of mortality and incidence of cancer 1952–98 in men from the U.K. who participated in the U.K.'s atmospheric nuclear weapon tests and experimental programmes. Occup Environ Med, 2003. 60(3):165–172.

55. Muirhead, C.R., et al., Epidemiological studies of U.K. test veterans: II. Mortality and cancer incidence. J Radiol Prot, 2004. 24(3):219–241.

56. Wiklund, K., L.E. Holm, and G. Eklund, Cancer risks in Swedish Lapps who breed reindeer. Am J Epidemiol, 1990. 132(6):1078–1082.

57. United Nations Scientific Committee on the Effects of Atomic Radiation (UNSCEAR), Sources and effects of ionizing radiation: UNSCEAR 2000 report to the General Assembly, with scientific annexes, Vol. 2, Effects. 2000, New York: United Nations.

58. Osechinsky, I. and A. Martirosov. Haematological diseases in the Belarus Republic after the Chernobyl accident. In International Conference on Health Consequences after the Chernobyl Accident. 1995, Geneva: World Health Organization.

59. Gapanovich, V.N., et al., Childhood leukemia in Belarus before and after the Chernobyl accident: Continued follow-up. Radiat Environ Biophys, 2001. 40(4):259–267.

60. Ivanov, V.K., et al., Cancer risks in the Kaluga oblast of the Russian Federation 10 years after the Chernobyl accident. Radiat Environ Biophys, 1997. 36(3):161–167.

61. Ivanov, V.K., et al., (Incidence of post-Chernobyl leukemia and thyroid cancer in children and adolescents in the Briansk region: evaluation of radiation risks). Vopr Onkol, 2003. 49(4):445–449.

62. Bebeshko, V., et al., Leukemias and lymphomas in Ukraine population exposed to chronic low dose irradiation. In Low doses of ionizing radiation: Biological effects and regulatory control. Contributed papers, International conference held in Seville, Spain. 1997, Vienna: International Atomic Energy Agency (IAEA).

63. Prisyazhniuk, A., et al., The time trends of cancer incidence in the most contaminated regions of the Ukraine before and after the Chernobyl accident. Radiat Environ Biophys, 1995. 34(1):3–6.

64. Noshchenko, A.G., et al., Patterns of acute leukaemia occurrence among children in the Chernobyl region. Int J Epidemiol, 2001. 30(1):125–129.

65. Steiner, M., et al., Trends in infant leukaemia in West Germany in relation to in utero exposure due to Chernobyl accident. Radiat Environ Biophys, 1998. 37(2):87–93.

66. Parkin, D.M., et al., Childhood leukaemia in Europe after Chernobyl: 5 year follow-up. Br J Cancer, 1996. 73(8):1006–1012.

67. Parkin, D.M., et al., Childhood leukaemia following the Chernobyl accident: The European Childhood Leukaemia-Lymphoma Incidence Study (ECLIS). Eur J Cancer, 1992. 29A(1):87–95.

68. Noshchenko, A.G., et al., Radiation-induced leukemia risk among those aged 0–20 at the time of the Chernobyl accident: A case-control study in the Ukraine. Int J Cancer, 2002. 99(4):609–618.

69. Chernobyl Forum and World Health Organization, Health effects of the Chernobyl accident and special health care programmes. 2005, Geneva: World Health Organization.

70. Torok, S., et al., Childhood leukaemia incidence in Hungary, 1973–2002. Interpolation model for analysing the possible effects of the Chernobyl accident. Eur J Epidemiol, 2005. 20(11):899–906.

71. Busby, C. and M. Scott, Increases in leukemia in infants in Wales and Scotland following Chernobyl: Evidence for errors in statuatory risk estimates. Energy Environ, 2000. 11(2):127–139.

72. Committee Examining Radiation Risks of Internal Emitters (CERRIE), Report of the Committee Examining Radiation Risks of Internal Emitters, 2004. Available at: (cited Feb. 11, 2007).

73. Cardis, E., et al., Estimates of the cancer burden in Europe from radioactive fallout from the Chernobyl accident. Int J Cancer, 2006. 119(6):1224–1235.

74. Abylkassimova, Z., et al., Nested case-control study of leukemia among a cohort of persons exposed to ionizing radiation from nuclear weapon tests in Kazakhstan (1949–1963). Ann Epidemiol, 2000. 10(7):479.

75. Kosenko, M., M. Degteva, and N. Petrushova, Estimate of the risk of leukemia to residents exposed to radiation as a result of a nuclear accident in the southern Urals. Phys Soc Respon, 1992. 2:187–197.

76. Krestinina, L.Y., et al., Protracted radiation exposure and cancer mortality in the Techa River Cohort. Radiat Res, 2005. 164(5):602–611.

77. Ostroumova, E., et al., Risk analysis of leukaemia incidence among people living along the Techa River: A nested case-control study. J Radiol Prot, 2006. 26(1):17–32.

78. Jablon, S., Z. Hrubec, and J. Boice, Jr., Cancer in Populations Living Near Nuclear Facilities. 1990, Bethesda, Md: National Institutes of Health.

79. McLaughlin, J.R., et al., Childhood leukemia in the vicinity of Canadian nuclear facilities. Cancer Causes Control, 1993. 4(1):51–58.

80. Sofer, T., et al., Geographical and temporal trends of childhood leukemia in relation to the nuclear plant in the Negev, Israel, 1960–1985. Public Health Rev, 1991. 19(1–4):191–198.

81. Committee on Medical Aspects of Radiation in the Environment (COMARE), The incidence of childhood cancer around nuclear installations in Great Britian. Tenth Report, 2005. Available at www.comare.org.uk/documents/COMARE10th Report.pdf.

82. White-Koning, M.L., et al., Incidence of childhood leukaemia in the vicinity of nuclear sites in France, 1990–1998. Br J Cancer, 2004. 91(5):916–922.

83. Laurier, D., et al., Assessment of the risk of radiation-induced leukaemia in the vicinity of nuclear installations: The Nord-Cotentin radio-ecological study. Rev Epidemiol Sante Publique, 2000. 48(suppl 2):S24–S36.

84. Laurier, D., B. Grosche, and P. Hall, Risk of childhood leukaemia in the vicinity of nuclear installations—Findings and recent controversies. Acta Oncol, 2002. 41(1):14–24.

85. Laurier, D. and D. Bard, Epidemiologic studies of leukemia among persons under 25 years of age living near nuclear sites. Epidemiol Rev, 1999. 21(2):188–206.

86. United Nations Scientific Committee of the Effects of Atomic Radiation (UNSCEAR), Sources and effects of ionizing radiation: 2006 report to the General Assembly with annexes. 2007, New York: United Nations.

87. Talbott, E.O., et al., Long-term follow-up of the residents of the Three Mile Island accident area: 1979–1998. Environ Health Perspect, 2003. 111(3):341–348.

88. Yoshimoto, Y., et al., Research on potential radiation risks in areas with nuclear power plants in Japan: Leukemia and malignant lymphoma mortality between 1972 and 1997 in 100 selected municipalities. J Radiat Prot, 2004. 24:343–368.

89. Boice, J.D., Jr., et al., Cancer mortality in a Texas county with prior uranium mining and milling activities, 1950–2001. J Radiol Prot, 2003. 23(3):247–262.

90. Boice, J.D., Jr., et al., Cancer mortality in counties near two former nuclear materials processing facilities in Pennsylvania, 1950–1995. Health Phys, 2003. 85(6):691–700.

90a. Boice, J.D., Jr., M.T. Mumma, and W.J. Blot, Cancer and non-cancer mortality in populations living near uranium and vanadium mining and milling operations in Montrose County, Colorado, 1950–2000. Radiat Res, 2007. 167:711–726.

91. Boice, J.D., Jr., M.T. Mumma, and W.J. Blot, Cancer mortality among populations residing in counties near the Hanford site, 1950–2000. Health Phys, 2006. 90(5):431–445.

92. Bithell, J.F. and G.J. Draper, Uranium-235 and childhood leukemia around Greenham Common airfield. J Radiat Prot, 1999. 19(3):253–259.

93. Grosche, B., et al., Leukaemia in the vicinity of two tritium-releasing nuclear facilities: A comparison of the Kruemmel Site, Germany, and the Savannah River Site, South Carolina, USA. J Radiol Prot, 1999. 19(3):243–252.

94. Berrington, A., et al., 100 years of observation on British radiologists: Mortality from cancer and other causes 1897–1997. Br J Radiol, 2001. 74(882):507–519.

95. Aoyama, T., et al., Mortality survey of Japanese radiological technologists during the period 1969–1993. Radiat Prot and Dosimet, 1998. 77(1/2):123–128.

96. Burnett, C., C. Robinson, and J. Walker, Cancer mortality in health and science technicians. Am J Ind Med, 1999. 36(1):155–158.

97. Doody, M.M., et al., Mortality among United States radiologic technologists, 1926–90. Cancer Causes Control, 1998. 9(1):67–75.

98. Mohan, A., et al., Mortality among radiologic technologists in the United States (1926–1997): 2nd follow up. Ann Epidemiol, 2000. 10(7):480.

99. Mohan, A.K., et al., Cancer and other causes of mortality among radiologic technologists in the United States. Int J Cancer, 2003. 103(2):259–267.

100. Linet, M.S., et al., Incidence of haematopoietic malignancies in US radiologic technologists. Occup Environ Med, 2005. 62(12):861–867.

101. Sigurdson, A.J., et al., Cancer incidence in the US radiologic technologists health study, 1983–1998. Cancer, 2003. 97(12):3080–3089.

102. Wang, J.X., et al., Cancer among medical diagnostic x-ray workers in China. J Natl Cancer Inst, 1988. 80(5):344–350.

103. Wang, J., et al., Leukemia among medical diagnostic X-ray workers in China. Proc Chin Acad Med Sci Peking Union Med Coll, 1990. 5(4):194–199.

104. Boice, J.D., Jr., et al., Diagnostic x-ray procedures and risk of leukemia, lymphoma, and multiple myeloma. JAMA, 1991. 265(10):1290–1294.

105. Davis, F.G., et al., Cancer mortality in a radiation-exposed cohort of Massachusetts tuberculosis patients. Cancer Res, 1989. 49(21):6130–6136.

106. Court Brown, W.M. and R. Doll, Mortality from cancer and other causes after radiotherapy for ankylosing spondylitis. Brit Med J, 1965. 2:1327–1332.

107. Smith, P.G., Leukemia and other cancers following radiation treatment of pelvic disease. Cancer, 1977. 39(suppl 4):S1901–S1905.

108. Smith, P.G. and R. Doll, Mortality among patients with ankylosing spondylitis after a single treatment course with x rays. Br Med J (Clin Res Ed), 1982. 284(6314):449–460.

109. Darby, S.C., et al., Long term mortality after a single treatment course with x-rays in patients treated for ankylosing spondylitis. Br J Cancer, 1987. 55(2):179–190.

110. Weiss, H.A., et al., Leukemia mortality after x-ray treatment for ankylosing spondylitis. Radiat Res, 1995. 142(1):1–11.

111. Lundell, M. and L.E. Holm, Mortality from leukemia after irradiation in infancy for skin hemangioma. Radiat Res, 1996. 145(5):595–601.

112. Griem, M.L., et al., Cancer following radiotherapy for peptic ulcer. J Natl Cancer Inst, 1994. 86(11):842–849.

113. Carr, Z.A., et al., Malignant neoplasms after radiation therapy for peptic ulcer. Radiat Res, 2002. 157(6):668–677.

114. Mattsson, A., et al., Incidence of primary malignancies other than breast cancer among women treated with radiation therapy for benign breast disease. Radiat Res, 1997. 148(2):152–160.

115. Smith, P.G. and R. Doll, Late effects of x irradiation in patients treated for metropathia haemorrhagica. Br J Radiol, 1976. 49(579):224–232.

116. Darby, S.C., et al., Mortality in a cohort of women given x-ray therapy for metropathia haemorrhagica. Int J Cancer, 1994. 56(6):793–801.

117. Inskip, P.D., et al., Leukemia, lymphoma, and multiple myeloma after pelvic radiotherapy for benign disease. Radiat Res, 1993. 135(1):108–124.

118. Inskip, P.D., et al., Cancer mortality following radium treatment for uterine bleeding. Radiat Res, 1990. 123(3):331–344.

119. Brinkley, D. and J.L. Haybittle, The late effects of artificial menopause by X-radiation. Br J Radiol, 1969. 42(499):519–521.

120. Ron, E. and B. Modan, Leukemia, thyroid cancer and CNS tumors following childhood scalp irradiation: Israel tinea study. In Radiation Carcinogenesis: Epidemiology and Biological Significance, J. Boice and J.F. Fraumeni, eds. 1982, New York: Raven Press.

121. Ron, E., B. Modan, and J.D. Boice, Jr., Mortality after radiotherapy for ringworm of the scalp. Am J Epidemiol, 1988. 127(4):713–725.

122. Damber, L., et al., A cohort study with regard to the risk of haematological malignancies in patients treated with x-rays for benign lesions in the locomotor system. I. Epidemiological analyses. Acta Oncol, 1995. 34(6):713–719.

123. Kleinerman, R.A., et al., Second cancers following radiotherapy for cervical cancer. J Natl Cancer Inst, 1982. 69(5):1027–1033.

124. Boice, J.D., Jr., et al., Second cancers following radiation treatment for cervical cancer. An international collaboration among cancer registries. J Natl Cancer Inst, 1985. 74(5):955–975.

125. Kleinerman, R.A., et al., Second primary cancer after treatment for cervical cancer: An international cancer registries study. Cancer, 1995. 76(3):442–452.

126. Boice, J.D., Jr., et al., Radiation dose and second cancer risk in patients treated for cancer of the cervix. Radiat Res, 1988. 116(1):3–55.

127. Boice, J.D., Jr., et al., Radiation dose and breast cancer risk in patients treated for cancer of the cervix. Int J Cancer, 1989. 44(1):7–16.

128. Arai, T., et al., Second cancer after radiation therapy for cancer of the uterine cervix. Cancer, 1991. 67(2):398–405.

129. Curtis, R.E., et al., Relationship of leukemia risk to radiation dose following cancer of the uterine corpus. J Natl Cancer Inst, 1994. 86(17):1315–1324.

130. Boice, J.D., Jr., et al., Cancer in the contralateral breast after radiotherapy for breast cancer. N Engl J Med, 1992. 326(12):781–785.

131. Storm, H.H., et al., Adjuvant radiotherapy and risk of contralateral breast cancer. J Natl Cancer Inst, 1992. 84(16):1245–1250.

132. Curtis, R.E., et al., Risk of leukemia after chemotherapy and radiation treatment for breast cancer. N Engl J Med, 1992. 326(26):1745–1751.

133. Kaplan, H.G., J.A. Malmgren, and M. Atwood, Leukemia incidence following primary breast carcinoma treatment. Cancer, 2004. 101(7):1529–1536.

134. Grunwald, H.W. and F. Rosner, Acute myeloid leukemia following treatment of Hodgkin's disease: A review. Cancer, 1982. 50(4):676–683.

135. Rosner, F., R.W. Carey, and M.H. Zarrabi, Breast cancer and acute leukemia: Report of 24 cases and review of the literature. Am J Hematol, 1978. 4(2):151–172.

136. Zarrabi, M.H. and F. Rosner, Acute myeloblastic leukemia following treatment for non-hematopoietic cancers: Report of 19 cases and review of the literature. Am J Hematol, 1979. 7(4):357–367.

137. Brenner, D.J., et al., Second malignancies in prostate carcinoma patients after radiotherapy compared with surgery. Cancer, 2000. 88(2):398–406.

138. Tucker, M.A., et al., Bone sarcomas linked to radiotherapy and chemotherapy in children. N Engl J Med, 1987. 317(10):588–593.

139. Tucker, M.A., et al., Leukemia after therapy with alkylating agents for childhood cancer. J Natl Cancer Inst, 1987. 78(3):459–464.

140. Rosenberg, S.A. and H.S. Kaplan, The evolution and summary results of the Stanford randomized clinical trials of the management of Hodgkin's disease: 1962–1984. Int J Radiat Oncol Biol Phys, 1985. 11(1):5–22.

141. Hawkins, M.M., et al., Epipodophyllotoxins, alkylating agents, and radiation and risk of secondary leukaemia after childhood cancer. BMJ, 1992. 304(6832):951–958.

142. Kaldor, J.M., et al., Leukemia following Hodgkin's disease. N Engl J Med, 1990. 322(1):7–13.

143. Beral, V., et al., Mortality of employees of the United Kingdom Atomic Energy Authority, 1946–1979. Br Med J (Clin Res Ed), 1985. 291(6493):440–447.

144. Beral, V., et al., Mortality of employees of the Atomic Weapons Establishment, 1951–82. BMJ, 1988. 297(6651):757–770.

145. Kendall, G.M., et al., Mortality and occupational exposure to radiation: First analysis of the National Registry for Radiation Workers. BMJ, 1992. 304(6821):220–225.

146. Muirhead, C.R., et al., Occupational radiation exposure and mortality: Second analysis of the National Registry for Radiation Workers. J Radiol Prot, 1999. 19(1):3–26.

147. Douglas, A.J., R.Z. Omar, and P.G. Smith, Cancer mortality and morbidity among workers at the Sellafield plant of British Nuclear Fuels. Br J Cancer, 1994. 70(6):1232–1243.

148. Omar, R.Z., J.A. Barber, and P.G. Smith, Cancer mortality and morbidity among plutonium workers at the Sellafield plant of British Nuclear Fuels. Br J Cancer, 1999. 79(7–8):1288–1301.

149. McGeoghegan, D. and K. Binks, The mortality and cancer morbidity experience of employees at the Chapelcross plant of British Nuclear Fuels plc, 1955–95. J Radiol Prot, 2001. 21(3):221–250.

150. Iwasaki, T., et al., Second analysis of mortality of nuclear industry workers in Japan, 1986–1997. Radiat Res, 2003. 159(2):228–238.

151. Rodriguez Artalejo, F., et al., Occupational exposure to ionising radiation and mortality among workers of the former Spanish Nuclear Energy Board. Occup Environ Med, 1997. 54(3):202–208.

152. Habib, R., et al., Cancer incidence among Australian nuclear industry workers. J Occup Health, 2006. 48:358–365.

153. Sont, W.N., et al., First analysis of cancer incidence and occupational radiation exposure based on the National Dose Registry of Canada. Am J Epidemiol, 2001. 153(4):309–318.

154. Ashmore, J.P., et al., First analysis of mortality and occupational radiation exposure based on the National Dose Registry of Canada. Am J Epidemiol, 1998. 148(6):564–574.

155. Zablotska, L.B., J.P. Ashmore, and G.R. Howe, Analysis of mortality among Canadian nuclear power industry workers after chronic low-dose exposure to ionizing radiation. Radiat Res, 2004. 161(6):633–641.

156. Wiggs, L.D., et al., Mortality among workers exposed to external ionizing radiation at a nuclear facility in Ohio. J Occup Med, 1991. 33(5):632–637.

157. Gilbert, E.S., et al., Analyses of combined mortality data on workers at the Hanford Site, Oak Ridge National Laboratory, and Rocky Flats Nuclear Weapons Plant. Radiat Res, 1989. 120(1):19–35.

158. Gilbert, E.S., D.L. Cragle, and L.D. Wiggs, Updated analyses of combined mortality data for workers at the Hanford Site, Oak Ridge National Laboratory, and Rocky Flats Weapons Plant. Radiat Res, 1993. 136(3):408–421.

159. Howe, G.R., et al., Analysis of the mortality experience amongst U.S. nuclear power industry workers after chronic low-dose exposure to ionizing radiation. Radiat Res, 2004. 162(5):517–526.

160. Frome, E.L., et al., A mortality study of employees of the nuclear industry in Oak Ridge, Tennessee. Radiat Res, 1997. 148(1):64–80.

161. Fry, S., E.A. Dupree, and A. Sipe, A study of mortality and morbidity among persons occupationally exposed to 50 or more mSv (5000 mrem) in a year. Phase I: Mortality through 1984. Appl Occup Environ Hygiene, 1996. 11(4):334–343.

162. Silver, S.R., et al., Differences in mortality by radiation monitoring status in an expanded cohort of Portsmouth Naval Shipyard workers. J Occup Environ Med, 2004. 46(7):677–690.

163. Yiin, J.H., et al., Risk of lung cancer and leukemia from exposure to ionizing radiation and potential confounders among workers at the Portsmouth Naval Shipyard. Radiat Res, 2005. 163(6):603–613.

164. Wiggs, L.D., et al., Mortality through 1990 among white male workers at the Los Alamos National Laboratory: Considering exposures to plutonium and external ionizing radiation. Health Phys, 1994. 67(6):577–588.

165. Groves, F.D., et al., Cancer in Korean War Navy technicians: Mortality survey after 40 years. Am J Epidemiol, 2002. 155(9):810–818.

166. Cardis, E., et al., Effects of low doses and low dose rates of external ionizing radiation: cancer mortality among nuclear industry workers in three countries. Radiat Res, 1995. 142(2):117–132.

167. Cardis, E., et al., Risk of cancer after low doses of ionising radiation: Retrospective cohort study in 15 countries. BMJ, 2005. 331(7508):77.

168. Cardis, E., et al., The 15-Country Collaborative Study of Cancer Risk among Radiation Workers in the Nuclear Industry: Estimates of radiation-related cancer risks. Rad Res, 2007. 167:396–416.

169. Baisogolov, G.D., et al., Malignant neoformations of the hematopoietic and lymphoid tissues in the personnel of the 1st plant of atomic industry. Vopr Onkol, 1991. 37(5):553–559.

170. Buldakov, L. and A.K. Guskova, Effects of chronic exposure to radiation. J Physician, 1991. 5:34–39.

171. Nikipelov, B., A. Lizlov, and N.A. Koshurnikova, Experience with the first Soviet nuclear installation: Radiation doses and health. Priroda, 1990. 2:28–30.

172. Koshurnikova, N.A., et al., Mortality from malignancies of the hematopoietic and lymphatic tissues among personnel of the first nuclear plant in the USSR. Sci Total Environ, 1994. 142(1–2):19–23.

173. Doshenko, V., Causes of mortality after considerable occupational chronic total gamma irradiation. J Med Radiol, 1991. 8:40.

174. Hohryakov, V.F. and S.A. Romanov, Lung cancer in radiochemical industry workers. Sci Total Environ, 1994. 142(1–2):25–28.

175. Shilnikova, N.S., et al., Cancer mortality risk among workers at the Mayak nuclear complex. Radiat Res, 2003. 159(6):787–798.

176. Ivanov, V., et al., Medical radiological consequences of the Chernobyl catastrophe in Russia. Estimation of radiation risks. 2004, St. Petersburg, Russia: Nauka.

177. Konogorov, A.P., et al., A case-control analysis of leukemia in accident emergency workers of Chernobyl. J Environ Pathol Toxicol Oncol, 2000. 19(1–2):143–151.

178. Rahu, M., et al., Cancer risk among Chernobyl cleanup workers in Estonia and Latvia, 1986–1998. Int J Cancer, 2006. 119(1):162–168.

179. Kaletsch, U., et al., Childhood cancer and residential radon exposure—Results of a population-based case-control study in Lower Saxony (Germany). Radiat Environ Biophys, 1999. 38(3):211–215.

180. Lubin, J.H., et al., Case-control study of childhood acute lymphoblastic leukemia and residential radon exposure. J Natl Cancer Inst, 1998. 90(4):294–300.

181. Law, G.R., et al., Residential radon exposure and adult acute leukaemia. Lancet, 2000. 355(9218):1888.

182. Steinbuch, M., et al., Indoor residential radon exposure and risk of childhood acute myeloid leukaemia. Br J Cancer, 1999. 81(5):900–906.

183. Darby, S.C., E.P. Radford, and E. Whitley, Radon exposure and cancers other than lung cancer in Swedish iron miners. Environ Health Perspect, 1995. 103(suppl 2):45–47.

184. Darby, S.C., et al., Radon and cancers other than lung cancer in underground miners: A collaborative analysis of 11 studies. J Natl Cancer Inst, 1995. 87(5):378–384.

185. Laurier, D., M. Valenty, and M. Tirmarche, Radon exposure and the risk of leukemia: A review of epidemiological studies. Health Phys, 2001. 81(3):272–288.

186. Laurier, D., et al., An update of cancer mortality among the French cohort of uranium miners: extended follow-up and new source of data for causes of death. Eur J Epidemiol, 2004. 19(2):139–146.

187. Tomasek, L., Leukemia among uranium miners—Late effects of exposure to uranium dust? Health Phys, 2004. 86(4):426–427.

188. Laurier, D., et al., Comment on "Studies of radon-exposed miner cohorts using a biologically based model: Comparison of current Czech and French data with historic data from China and Colorado" by W.F. Heidenreich, L. Tomasek, A. Rogel, D. Laurier, M. Tirmarche (2004) Radiat Environ Biophys 43:247–256, and "Radon-induced lung cancer in French and Czech miner cohorts described with a two-mutation cancer model" by M.J.P. Brugmans, S.M. Rispens, H. Bijwaard, D. Laurier, A. Rogel, L. Tomasek, M. Tirmarche (2004) Radiat Environ Biophys 43:153–163. Radiat Environ Biophys, 2005. 44(2):155–156.

189. Eatough, J.P., Radon and leukemia risk in underground miners: Are working level months the most appropriate exposure parameter? Health Phys, 2004. 86(4):425–426; author reply, 427–428.

190. National Research Council (NRC), Committee on the Biological Effects of Ionizing Radiations (BEIR), Health effects of exposure to radon. BEIR VI. 1999, Washington, DC: National Academy Press.

191. Carpenter, L.M., et al., Cancer mortality in relation to monitoring for radionuclide exposure in three U.K. nuclear industry workforces. Br J Cancer, 1998. 78(9):1224–1232.

192. Ritz, B., Radiation exposure and cancer mortality in uranium processing workers. Epidemiology, 1999. 10(5):531–538.

193. Dupree-Ellis, E., et al., External radiation exposure and mortality in a cohort of uranium processing workers. Am J Epidemiol, 2000. 152(1):91–95.

194. Roldan Schilling, V., et al., Acute leukemias after treatment with radioiodine for thyroid cancer. Haematologica, 1998. 83(8):767–768.

195. Shimon, I., A. Kneller, and D. Olchovsky, Chronic myeloid leukaemia following ^{131}I treatment for thyroid carcinoma: A report of two cases and review of the literature. Clin Endocrinol (Oxford), 1995. 43(5):651–654.

196. Goldman, M.B., et al., Radioactive iodine therapy and breast cancer. A follow-up study of hyperthyroid women. Am J Epidemiol, 1988. 127(5):969–980.

197. Hall, P., et al., Leukaemia incidence after iodine-131 exposure. Lancet, 1992. 340(8810):1–4.

198. Holm, L.E., Cancer risks after diagnostic doses of ^{131}I with special reference to thyroid cancer. Cancer Detect Prev, 1991. 15(1):27–30.

199. Dobyns, B.M., et al., Malignant and benign neoplasms of the thyroid in patients treated for hyperthyroidism: A report of the cooperative thyrotoxicosis therapy follow-up study. J Clin Endocrinol, 1974. 38:976–998.

200. Saenger, E.L., G.E. Thoma, and E.A. Tompkins, Incidence of leukemia following treatment of hyperthyroidism: Preliminary report of the Cooperative Thyrotoxicosis Therapy Follow-up Study. JAMA, 1968. 205(12):855–862.

201. Ron, E., et al., Cancer mortality following treatment for adult hyperthyroidism: Cooperative Thyrotoxicosis Therapy Follow-up Study Group. JAMA, 1998. 280(4):347–355.

202. Hoffman, D.A., et al., Mortality in women treated for hyperthyroidism. Am J Epidemiol, 1982. 115(2):243–254.

203. Hall, P., et al., Cancer risks in thyroid cancer patients. Br J Cancer, 1991. 64(1):159–163.

204. Edmonds, C.J. and T. Smith, The long-term hazards of the treatment of thyroid cancer with radioiodine. Br J Radiol, 1986. 59(697):45–51.
205. Brincker, H., H.S. Hansen, and A.P. Andersen, Induction of leukemia by iodine 131 treatment of thyroid carcinoma. Br J Cancer, 1973. 28:232–237.
206. Teppo, L., E. Pukkala, and E. Saxen, Multiple cancer—An epidemiologic exercise in Finland. J Natl Cancer Inst, 1985. 75(2):207–217.
207. Hall, P. and L.E. Holm, Cancer in iodine-131 exposed patients. J Endocrinol Invest, 1995. 18(2):147–149.
208. Rubino, C., et al., Second primary malignancies in thyroid cancer patients. Br J Cancer, 2003. 89(9):1638–1644.
209. Harrison, J.D. and C.R. Muirhead, Quantitative comparisons of cancer induction in humans by internally deposited radionuclides and external radiation. Int J Radiat Biol, 2003. 79(1):1–13.
210. Mole, R.H., The radiobiological significance of the studies with ^{224}Ra and thorotrast. Health Phys, 1978. 35(1):167–174.
211. Van Kaick, G., et al., Report on the German Thorotrast study. Strahlentherapie, 1986. 80(suppl):114–118.
212. Van Kaick, G., H. Wesch, and H. Luhrs, eds. The German Thorotrast study: Report on 20 years of follow-up. In Risks from Radium and Thorotrast, D. Taylor, ed. 1989, London: British Institute of Radiology.
213. Andersson, M. and H.H. Storm, Cancer incidence among Danish Thorotrast-exposed patients. J Natl Cancer Inst, 1992. 84(17):1318–1325.
214. Mori, T., et al., Summary of entire Japanese Thorotrast follow-up study: Updated 1998. Radiat Res, 1999. 152(suppl 6):S84–S87.
215. Mori, T., et al., Present status of the medical study on Thorotrast administered patients in Japan. Strahlentherapie, 1986. 80(suppl):123–134.
216. da Silva Horta, J., et al., Malignancies in Portuguese Thorotrast patients. Health Phys, 1978. 35(1):137–151.
217. Olsen, J.H., M. Andersson, and J.D. Boice, Jr., Thorotrast exposure and cancer risk. Health Phys, 1990. 58(2):222–223.
218. Taylor, D.M., et al, eds., Risks from Radium and Thorotrast. 1989, London: British Institute of Radiology.
219. Travis, L.B., et al., Site-specific cancer incidence and mortality after cerebral angiography with radioactive Thorotrast. Radiat Res, 2003. 160(6):691–706.
220. dos Santos Silva, I., et al., Mortality after radiological investigation with radioactive Thorotrast: A follow-up study of up to fifty years in Portugal. Radiat Res, 2003. 159(4):521–534.
221. van Kaick, G., et al., The German Thorotrast study: Recent results and assessment of risks. Radiat Res, 1999. 152(suppl 6): S64–S71.
222. Nyberg, U., et al., Cancer incidence among Swedish patients exposed to radioactive Thorotrast: A forty-year follow-up survey. Radiat Res, 2002. 157(4):419–425.
223. Spiess, H. and A. Gerspach, Soft-tissue effects following ^{224}Ra injections into humans. Health Phys, 1978. 35(1):61–81.
224. Nekolla, E.A., et al., Malignancies in patients treated with high doses of radium-224. Radiat Res, 1999. 152(suppl 6):S3–S7.
225. Wick, R.R., et al., Late effects in ankylosing spondylitis patients treated with ^{224}Ra. Radiat Res, 1999. 152(suppl 6):S8–S11.
226. Wick, R.R. and W. Gossner, Follow-up study of late effects in ^{224}Ra treated ankylosing spondylitis patients. Health Phys, 1983. 44(suppl 1):187–195.
227. Wick, R., D. Chmelevsky, and W. Gossner, Radium-224: Risk to bone and hematopoietic tissue in ankylosins spondylitis patients. In The Radiobiology of Radium and Thorotrast, W. Gossner, ed. 1986, Munich: Urban and Schwartzenberg.
228. Wick, R., Recent results of the follow-up of radium-224 treated ankylosing spondylitis patients. In Risks from Radium and Thorotrast, D. Taylor, ed. 1989, London: British Institute of Radiology.
229. Mays, C.W., Alpha-particle-induced cancer in humans. Health Phys, 1988. 55(4):637–652.
230. Spiess, H., C.W. Mays, and D. Chmelevsky, Malignancies in patients injected with radium 224: Taylor, D.M., et al. (eds), In Risks from Radium and Thorotrast. 1989, London: British Institute of Radiology.
231. Polednak, A.P., A.F. Stehney, and R.E. Rowland, Mortality among women first employed before 1930 in the U.S. radium dial-painting industry: A group ascertained from employment lists. Am J Epidemiol, 1978. 107(3):179–195.
232. Spiers, F.W., et al., Leukaemia incidence in the U.S. dial workers. Health Phys, 1983. 44(suppl 1):65–72.
233. Rowland, E., Radium in humans: A review of U.S. studies. 1994, Argonne, Ill: Argonne National Laboratories.
234. Stebbings, J.H., Radium and leukemia: Is current dogma valid? Health Phys, 1998. 74(4):486–488.
235. Alderson, M.R., and S.M. Jackson, Long term follow-up wth menorrhagia treated by irradiation. Br J Radiol, 1971. 44:295–298.
236. Dixon, R.J., The late results of radium treatment for benign uterine hemorrhage. Br J Radiol, 1969. 42:583–594.
237. Hutchison, G.B., Leukemia in patients with cancer of the cervix treated with radiation: A report covering the first 5 years of an international study. J Natl. Cancer Inst, 1968. 49:951–982.
238. Kossman, S.E. and M.A. Weiss, Acute myelogenous leukemia after exposure to strontium-89 for the treatment of adenocarcinoma of the prostate. Cancer, 2000. 88(3):620–624.
239. Modan, B. and A.M. Lilienfeld, Polycythemia vera and leukemia—The role of radiation treatment. Medicine, 1965. 44:305–344.
240. Berk, P.D., et al., Increased incidence of acute leukemia in polycythemia-vera-associated with chlorambucil therapy. N Engl J Med, 1981. 304(8):441–447.
241. Mayer, K., et al., Sulfur-35 therapy used for chondrosarcoma and chordoma. In Therapy in Nuclear Medicine, R.P. Spencer, ed. 1978, New York: Grune and Stratton.
242. McGeoghegan, D. and K. Binks, The mortality and cancer morbidity experience of workers at the Capenhurst uranium enrichment facility 1946–95. J Radiol Prot, 2000. 20(4):381–401.
243. McGeoghegan, D. and K. Binks, The mortality and cancer morbidity experience of workers at the Springfields uranium production facility, 1946–95. J Radiol Prot, 2000. 20(2):111–137.
244. Tirmarche, M., H. Baysson, and M. Telle-Lamberton, Uranium exposure and cancer risk: A review of epidemiological studies. Rev Epidemiol Sante Publique, 2004. 52(1):81–90.
245. The Royal Society, The Health Hazards of Depleted Uranium. 2001, London: The Royal Society.
246. Auvinen, A., et al., Uranium and other natural radionuclides in drinking water and risk of leukemia: A case-cohort study in Finland. Cancer Causes Control, 2002. 13(9):825–829.
247. Hempelmann, L.H., C. Lushbaugh, and G.L. Voelz, What happened to the survivors of the early Los Alamos nuclear accidents? In The Medical Basis for Radiation Accident Preparedness. 1980, New York: Elsevier/North Holland.
248. International Commission on Radiological Protection (ICRP), 1990 Recommendations of the ICRP. Ann ICRP, 1991. 21(1–3):1–201.
249. United Nations Scientific Committee on the Effects of Atomic Radiation (UNSCEAR), Sources and effects of 2006 report to the General Assembly, with annexes. 2006, New York: United Nations.
250. International Commission on Radiological Protection (ICRP), 1990 Recommendations of the ICRP. Ann ICRP, 1991. 21(1–3):132.
251. Kossenko, M.M. and M.O. Degteva, Cancer mortality and radiation risk evaluation for the Techa River population. Sci Total Environ, 1994. 142(1–2):73–89.

252. Travis, L.B., et al., Treatment-associated leukemia following testicular cancer. J Natl Cancer Inst, 2000. 92(14):1165–1171.

253. Wang, J.X., et al., Cancer incidence and risk estimation among medical x-ray workers in China, 1950–1995. Health Phys, 2002. 82(4):455–466.

254. Davis, S., et al., Childhood leukaemia in Belarus, Russia, and Ukraine following the Chernobyl power station accident: Results from an international collaborative population-based case-control study. Int J Epidemiol, 2006. 35(2):386–396.

255. Kossenko, M.M., et al., The Techa River Cohort: Study design and follow-up methods. Radiat Res, 2005. 164(5):591–601.

256. United Nations Scientific Committee on the Effects of Atomic Radiation (UNSCEAR), Sources and effects of ionizing radiation: UNSCEAR 2000 report to the General Assembly, with scientific annexes. 2000, New York: United Nations.

257. National Research Council (NRC), Assessment of the scientific information for the radiation exposure screening and education program. 2006, Washington, DC: National Academy Press.

258. Boice, J.D., Jr., Radiation and non-Hodgkin's lymphoma. Cancer Res, 1992. 52(suppl 19):S5489–S5491.

259. Gilbert, E.S., Mortality of workers at the Oak Ridge National Laboratory. Health Phys, 1992. 62(3):260–264.

260. Gribbin, M.A., J.L. Weeks, and G.R. Howe, Cancer mortality (1956–1985) among male employees of Atomic Energy of Canada Limited with respect to occupational exposure to external low-linear-energy-transfer ionizing radiation. Radiat Res, 1993. 133(3):375–380.

261. Bithell, J.F. and A.M. Stewart, Pre-natal irradiation and childhood malignancy: A review of British data from the Oxford Survey. Br J Cancer, 1975. 31(3):271–287.

262. Inskip, P.D., et al., Incidence of childhood cancer in twins. Cancer Causes Control, 1991. 2(5):315–324.

263. Archer, V.E., J.K. Wagoner, and F.E. Lundin, Jr., Cancer mortality among uranium mill workers. J Occup Med, 1973. 15(1):11–14.

264. Andersson, M., B. Carstensen, and J. Visfeldt, Leukemia and other related hematological disorders among Danish patients exposed to Thorotrast. Radiat Res, 1993. 134(2):224–233.

265. Eheman, C.R., et al., Case-control assessment of the association between non-Hodgkin's lymphoma and occupational radiation with doses assessed using a job exposure matrix. Am J Ind Med, 2000. 38(1):19–27.

266. Weiss, H.A., S.C. Darby, and R. Doll, Cancer mortality following X-ray treatment for ankylosing spondylitis. Int J Cancer, 1994. 59(3):327–338.

267. Frome, E.L., D.L. Cragle, and R.W. McLain, Poisson regression analysis of the mortality among a cohort of World War II nuclear industry workers. Radiat Res, 1990. 123(2):138–152.

268. Wick, R., D. Chemelevsky, and W. Gossner, Current status of the followup of radium 224 treated ankylosing spondylitis patients. In Health Effects of Internally Deposited Radionuclides: Emphasis on Radium and Thorium, G. Van Kaick, ed. 1995, Singapore: World Scientific.

269. Wing, S., et al., A case control study of multiple myeloma at four nuclear facilities. Ann Epidemiol, 2000. 10(3):144–153.

270. Holm, L.E., et al., Cancer risk in population examined with diagnostic doses of ^{131}I. J Natl Cancer Inst, 1989. 81(4):302–306.

271. Holm, L.E., et al., Cancer risk after iodine-131 therapy for hyperthyroidism. J Natl Cancer Inst, 1991. 83(15):1072–1077.

272. Andersson, M., B. Carstensen, and H.H. Storm, Mortality and cancer incidence after cerebral arteriography with or without Thorotrast. Radiat Res, 1995. 142(3):305–320.

273. Ichimaru, M., and T. Ichimaru, Aplastic anemia and atypical leukemia in the A-bomb survivors in control in the fixed cohort of Hiroshima and Nagasaki, 1950–1973. 1977, Hiroshima, Japan: Radiation Effects Research Foundation.

274. Lewis, E., Leukemia, multiple myeloma, and aplastic anemia in American radiologists. Science, 1963. 142:1492–1499.

275. Fry, S., Journalistic epidemiology: The case of polycythemia rubra vera. In REAC/TS Newsletter. 1983, Oak Ridge, Tenn: Oak Ridge Association Universities.

276. Heaney, M.L. and D.W. Golde, Myelodysplasia. N Engl J Med, 1999. 340(21):1649–1660.

277. Finch, S.C., Myelodysplasia and radiation. Radiat Res, 2004. 161(5):603–606.

278. Preissig, S.H., et al., Anaplastic astrocytoma following radiation for a glomus jugular tumor. Cancer, 1979. 43(6):2243–2247.

279. Thompson, D., E. Ron, and D. Preston, Cancer incidence in atomic bomb survivors. Part II: Solid tumors, 1958—1987. In Cancer Incidence in Atomic Bomb Survivors. 1994, Hiroshima, Japan: Radiation Effects Research Foundation.

280. Thompson, D., et al., Cancer incidence in atomic bomb survivors, Part II: Solid tumors, 1958–1987. 1992, Hiroshima, Japan: Radiation Effects Research Foundation.

281. Preston, D.L., et al., Studies of mortality of atomic bomb survivors. Report 13: Solid cancer and noncancer disease mortality: 1950–1997. Radiat Res, 2003. 160(4):381–407.

282. Forman, D., et al., Cancer near nuclear installations. Nature, 1987. 329(6139):499–505.

283. Lopez-Abente, G., N. Aragones, and M. Pollan, Solid-tumor mortality in the vicinity of uranium cycle facilities and nuclear power plants in Spain. Environ Health Perspect, 2001. 109(7):721–729.

284. Checkoway, H., et al., Radiation doses and cause-specific mortality among workers at a nuclear materials fabrication plant. Am J Epidemiol, 1988. 127(2):255–266.

285. Wing, S., et al., Mortality among workers at Oak Ridge National Laboratory: Evidence of radiation effects in follow-up through 1984. JAMA, 1991. 265(11):1397–1402.

286. Wilkinson, G.S., et al., Mortality among plutonium and other radiation workers at a plutonium weapons facility. Am J Epidemiol, 1987. 125(2):231–250.

287. Gilbert, E.S., G.R. Petersen, and J.A. Buchanan, Mortality of workers at the Hanford site: 1945–1981. Health Phys, 1989. 56(1):11–25.

288. Cragle, D.L., et al., Mortality among workers at a nuclear fuels production facility. Am J Ind Med, 1988. 14(4):379–401.

289. Carpenter, A.V., et al., CNS cancers and radiation exposure: A case-control study among workers at two nuclear facilities. J Occup Med, 1987. 29(7):601–604.

290. Preston-Martin, S., W. Mack, and B.E. Henderson, Risk factors for gliomas and meningiomas in males in Los Angeles County. Cancer Res, 1989. 49(21):6137–6143.

291. Burch, J.D., et al., An exploratory case-control study of brain tumors in adults. J Natl Cancer Inst, 1987. 78(4):601–609.

292. Longstreth, W.T., Jr., et al., Epidemiology of intracranial meningioma. Cancer, 1993. 72(3):639–648.

293. Shore, R.E., R.E. Albert, and B.S. Pasternack, Follow-up study of patients treated by x-ray epilation for Tinea capitis: Resurvey of post-treatment illness and mortality experience. Arch Environ Health, 1976. 31(1):21–28.

294. Ron, E., et al., Tumors of the brain and nervous system after radiotherapy in childhood. N Engl J Med, 1988. 319(16):1033–1039.

295. Modan, B., et al., Radiation-induced head and neck tumours. Lancet, 1974. 1(7852):277–279.

296. Sandler, D.P., G.W. Comstock, and G.M. Matanoski, Neoplasms following childhood radium irradiation of the nasopharynx. J Natl Cancer Inst, 1982. 68(1):3–8.

297. Ryberg, M., et al., Malignant disease after radiation treatment of benign gynaecological disorders: A study of a cohort of metropathia patients. Acta Oncol, 1990. 29(5):563–567.

298. Colman, M., M. Kirsch, M. Creditor Radiation-induced tumors: I. Symposium. 1978, Vienna: International Atomic Energy Agency.

299. Munk, J., E. Peyser, and J. Grusskiewicz, Radiation-induced intracranial meningiomas. Clin Radiology, 1969. 20:90–94.

300. Brada, M., et al., Risk of second brain tumour after conservative surgery and radiotherapy for pituitary adenoma. BMJ, 1992. 304(6838):1343–1346.

301. Furst, C.J., M. Lundell, and L.E. Holm, Tumors after radiotherapy for skin hemangioma in childhood. A case-control study. Acta Oncol, 1990. 29(5):557–562.

302. Furst, C.J., et al., Cancer incidence after radiotherapy for skin hemangioma: A retrospective cohort study in Sweden. J Natl Cancer Inst, 1988. 80(17):1387–1392.

302a. Neglia, J.P., L.L. Robison, M Storall, et al., New primary neoplasms of the central nervous system in survivors of childhood cancer: A report from the Childhood Cancer Survivor Study. J Natl Cancer Inst, 2006. 98(21):1528–1537.

303. Salvati, M., et al., A report on radiation-induced gliomas. Cancer, 1991. 67(2):392–397.

304. Shapiro, S. and J. Mealey, Jr., Late anaplastic gliomas in children previously treated for acute lymphoblastic leukemia. Pediatr Neurosci, 1989. 15(4):176–180.

305. Edwards, M.K., et al., Gliomas in children following radiation therapy for lymphoblastic leukemia. Acta Radiol Suppl, 1986. 369:651–653.

306. Fontana, M., et al., Late multifocal gliomas in adolescents previously treated for acute lymphoblastic leukemia. Cancer, 1987. 60(7):1510–1518.

307. Hawkins, M.M., G.J. Draper, and J.E. Kingston, Incidence of second primary tumours among childhood cancer survivors. Br J Cancer, 1987. 56(3):339–347.

308. Kingston, J.E., et al., Patterns of multiple primary tumours in patients treated for cancer during childhood. Br J Cancer, 1987. 56(3):331–338.

309. Nygaard, R., et al., Second malignant neoplasms in patients treated for childhood leukemia: A population-based cohort study from the Nordic countries. The Nordic Society of Pediatric Oncology and Hematology (NOPHO). Acta Paediatr Scand, 1991. 80(12):1220–1228.

310. Sridhar, K. and B. Ramamurthi, Intracranial meningioma subsequent to radiation for a pituitary tumor: Case report. Neurosurgery, 1989. 25(4):643–645.

311. Domenicucci, M., et al., Meningioma following high-dose radiation therapy: Case report and review of the literature. Clin Neurol Neurosurg, 1990. 92(4):349–352.

312. Goss, S., The malignant tumor risk from radium body burdens. Health Phys, 1970. 19:731–737.

313. van Kaick, G., et al., Report on the German Thorotrast Study. Strahlentherapie (Sonderb), 1985. 80:114–118.

314. Van Kaick, G., et al., The German Thorotrast study: Report on 20 years follow-up. In Risks from Radium and Thorotrast, D. Taylor, ed. 1988, Bethesda, Md: British Institute of Radiology.

315. MacMahon, B., Prenatal x-ray exposure and childhood cancer. J Natl Cancer Inst, 1962. 28:1173–1191.

316. United Nations Scientific Committee on the Effects of Atomic Radiation (UNSCEAR), Sources and effects of ionizing radiation: Report to the General Assembly with annexes. 1977, New York: United Nations.

317. Jablon, S. and H. Kato, Childhood cancer in relation to prenatal exposure to atomic bomb radiation. Lancet, 1970. 2:1000–1003.

318. Diamond, E.L., H. Schmerier, and A. Lilienfeld, The relationship of intrauterine radiation to subsequent mortality and development of leukemia in children. Am J Epidemiol, 1973. 97:283–313.

319. Preston, D., et al., Solid cancer incidence in atomic bomb survivors: 1958–1998. Radiat Res, 2007. 168(1):1–64.

320. Preston, D.L., et al., Tumors of the nervous system and pituitary gland associated with atomic bomb radiation exposure. J Natl Cancer Inst, 2002. 94(20):1555–1563.

321. Sadetzki, S., et al., Long-term follow-up for brain tumor development after childhood exposure to ionizing radiation for tinea capitis. Radiat Res, 2005. 163(4):424–432.

322. Shore, R.E., et al., Tumors and other diseases following childhood x-ray treatment for ringworm of the scalp (Tinea capitis). Health Phys, 2003. 85(4):404–408.

323. Karlsson, P., et al., Intracranial tumors after exposure to ionizing radiation during infancy: A pooled analysis of two Swedish cohorts of 28,008 infants with skin hemangioma. Radiat Res, 1998. 150(3):357–364.

324. Little, M.P., et al., Risks of brain tumour following treatment for cancer in childhood: Modification by genetic factors, radiotherapy and chemotherapy. Int J Cancer, 1998. 78(3):269–275.

325. Littman, M., I. Kisch, and A. Keane, Radium-induced malignant turmors of the mastoid and paranasal sinuses. Am J Roentgenol, 1978. 131:733–785.

326. Evans, R., The effect of skeletally deposited alpha ray emitters in man. Br J Radiol, 1966. 39:881–895.

327. Rowland, R., and A. Stehney, Radium-induced malignancies. In Argonne National Laboratory Report. 1978, Argonne, Ill: Argonne National Laboratory.

328. Rowland, R., and H. Lucas, Radium-dial workers. In Radiation Carcinogenesis: Epidemiology and Biological Significance, J.D. Boice and J. Fraumeni, eds. 1984, New York: Raven Press.

329. Fabrikant, J., R. Dickson, and B. Fetter, Mechanisms of radiation carcinogenesis at the clinical level. Br J Cancer, 1964. 18:459–477.

330. da Motta, L., Follow-up study of Portuguese patients given thorium dioxide in the paranasal sinuses. In Swarm, N.L.: Distribution, retention and late effects of thorium dioxide. NY Acad Sci, 1987. 145:811–816.

331. Belsky, J., et al., Salivary gland neoplasms following atomic radiation: Additional cases and reanalysis of combined data in a fixed population, 1957–1970. Cancer, 1975. 35:555–559.

332. Belsky, J.L., et al., Salivary gland tumors in atomic bomb survivors, Hiroshima-Nagasaki, 1957 to 1970. JAMA, 1972. 219(7):864–868.

333. Takeichi, N., F. Hirose, and H. Yamamoto, Salivary gland tumors in atomic bomb survivors, Hiroshima, Japan. I. Epidemiologic observations. Cancer, 1976. 38(6):2462–2468.

334. Takeichi, N., et al., Salivary gland tumors in atomic bomb survivors, Hiroshima, Japan. II. Pathologic study and supplementary epidemiologic observations. Cancer, 1983. 52(2):377–385.

335. Wakabayashi, T., et al., Studies of the mortality of A-bomb survivors, report 7. Part III. Incidence of cancer in 1959–1978, based on the tumor registry, Nagasaki. Radiat Res, 1983. 93(1):112–146.

336. Preston-Martin, S., et al., Prior exposure to medical and dental x-rays related to tumors of the parotid gland. J Natl Cancer Inst, 1988. 80(12):943–949.

337. Saenger, E., et al., Neoplasia following therapeutic radiation for benigh conditions in childhood. Radiology, 1960. 74:889–904.

338. Pifer, J.W., et al., Neoplasms in the Ann Arbor series of thymus-irradiated children: A second survey. Am J Roentgenol Radium Ther Nucl Med, 1968. 103(1):13–18.

339. Janower, M.L. and O.S. Miettinen, Neoplasms after childhood irradiation of the thymus gland. JAMA, 1971. 215(5):753–756.

340. Modan, B., E. Ron, and A. Werner, Thyroid cancer following scalp irradiation. Radiology, 1977. 123(3):741–744.

341. Schneider, A.B., et al., Radiation-induced tumors of the head and neck following childhood irradiation. Prospective studies. Medicine (Baltimore), 1985. 64(1):1–15.

342. Kaste, S.C., G. Hedlund, and C.B. Pratt, Malignant parotid tumors in patients previously treated for childhood cancer: Clinical and

imaging findings in eight cases. AJR Am J Roentgenol, 1994. 162(3):655–659.

343. Wiseman, J.C., I.B. Hales, and A. Joasoo, Two cases of lymphoma of the parotid gland following ablative radioiodine therapy for thyroid carcinoma. Clin Endocrinol (Oxford), 1982. 17(1):85–89.

344. Land, C.E., et al., Incidence of salivary gland tumors among atomic bomb survivors, 1950—1987: Evaluation of radiation-related risk. Radiat Res, 1996. 146(1):28–36.

345. Bone, H., Diagnosis of the multiglandular endocrine neoplasias. Clin Chem, 1990. 36:711–718.

346. Duh, Q.Y., et al., Carcinoids associated with multiple endocrine neoplasia syndromes. Am J Surg, 1987. 154(1):142–148.

347. Kaplan, L., et al., Malignant neoplasms and parathyroid adenoma. Cancer, 1971. 28(2):401–407.

348. Takeichi, N., et al., Parathyroid tumors in atomic bomb survivors in Hiroshima: A review. J Radiat Res (Tokyo), 1991. 32(suppl):189–192.

349. Takeichi, N., et al., Parathyroid tumors in atomic bomb survivors in Hiroshima: Epidemiological study from registered cases at Hiroshima Prefecture Tumor Tissue Registry, 1974–1987. Jpn J Cancer Res, 1991. 82(8):875–878.

350. Takeichi, N., H. Ezaki, and K. Dohi, A review of forty-five years study of Hiroshima and Nagasaki atomic bomb survivors. Thyroid cancer: Reports up to date and a review. J Radiat Res (Tokyo), 1991. 32(suppl):S180–S188.

351. Fujiwara, S., A review of forty-five years study of Hiroshima and Nagasaki atomic bomb survivors. Hyperparathyroidism. J Radiat Res (Tokyo), 1991. 32(suppl):S245–S248.

352. Prinz, R., et al., Radiation-associated hyperparathyroidism: A new syndrome? Surgery, 1977. 82:296–302.

353. Russ, J., E. Scanlon, and S. Sener, Parathyroid adenomas following irradiation. Cancer, 1979. 43:1078–1083.

354. Beard, C.M., et al., Therapeutic radiation and hyperparathyroidism: A case-control study in Rochester, Minn. Arch Intern Med, 1989. 149(8):1887–1890.

355. Christmas, T.J., et al., Hyperparathyroidism after neck irradiation. Br J Surg, 1988. 75(9):873–874.

356. Tisell, L.E., et al., Hyperparathyroidism in persons treated with X-rays for tuberculous cervical adenitis. Cancer, 1977. 40(2):846–854.

357. Cohen, J., T.C. Gierlowski, and A.B. Schneider, A prospective study of hyperparathyroidism in individuals exposed to radiation in childhood. JAMA, 1990. 264(5):581–584.

358. International Agency for Research on Cancer (IARC), Cancer: Causes, occurrence and control, L. Tomatis, ed. 1990, Lyon, France: IARC.

359. Ron, E., D. Preston, and D. Thompson, Cancer incidence in atomic bomb survivors. Part IV. Comparison of cancer incidence and mortality. In Cancer Incidence in Atomic Bomb Survivors. 1994, Hiroshima. Japan: Radiation Effects Research Foundation.

360. Smith, P.G. and A.J. Douglas, Mortality of workers at the Sellafield plant of British Nuclear Fuels. Br Med J (Clin Res Ed), 1986. 293(6551):845–854.

361. Gilbert, E.S., et al., Mortality of workers at the Hanford site: 1945–1986. Health Phys, 1993. 64(6):577–590.

362. Waxweiler, R.J., R. Roscoe, and V. Archer, Mortality follow-up through 1977 of the white underground uranium miners cohort examined by the United States Public Health Service. In International conference on radiation hazards in mining: Control, measurement and medical aspects. 1981, Kingsport, Tenn: Kingsport Press.

363. Brown, D. and T. Bloom, Mortality among uranium enrichment workers, National Institute for Occupational Safety and Health, ed. 1987, Washington, DC: Department of Health and Human Services.

364. Davis, F.G., et al., Cancer mortality after multiple fluoroscopic examinations of the chest. J Natl Cancer Inst, 1987. 78(4):645–652.

364a. Hoffman, F.O., A.J. Ruttenber, A.I. Apostoaei, et al., The Hanford Thyroid Disease Study: An alternative view of the findings. Health Phys, 2007. 92(2):99–111.

365. Smith, P.G., R. Doll, and E.P. Radford, Cancer mortality among patients with ankylosing spondylitis not given X-ray therapy. Br J Radiol, 1977. 50(598):728–734.

366. Goolden, A.W. Radiation cancer: A review with special reference to radiation tumors of the pharynx, larynx and thyroid. Br J Radiol, 1957. 30:626–640.

367. Raven, W. and V. Levinson, Radiation cancer of the pharynx. Lancet, 1954. 2:683–684.

368. Yoshizawa, Y., and T. Takeuchi, Search for the lowest irradiation dose from literature on radiation-induced cancer in pharynx and larynx. Nippon Acta Radiologica, 1974. 34:903–909.

369. United Nations Scientific Committee on the Effects of Atomic Radiation (UNSCEAR), Sources and effects of ionizing radiation: UNSCEAR 1994 report to the General Assembly, with scientific annexes. 1994, New York: United Nations.

370. United Nations Scientific Committee on the Effects of Atomic Radiation (UNSCEAR), Sources and effects of ionizing radiation: Report to the General Assembly with annexes. 1988, New York: United Nations.

371. Catelinois, O., et al., Projecting the time trend of thyroid cancers: Its impact on assessment of radiation-induced cancer risks. Health Phys, 2004. 87(6):606–614.

372. Robbins, J., et al., Thyroid cancer: A lethal endocrine neoplasm. Ann Intern Med, 1991. 115(2):133–147.

373. Duffy, B.J. and P.J. Fitzgerald, Cancer of the thyroid in children: A report of 28 cases. J Clin Endocrinol Metab, 1950. 10:1296–1308.

374. National Council on Radiation Protection and Measurements (NCRP), Induction of thyroid cancer by ionizing radiation: Recommendations of the NCRP report no. 80. 1985, Bethesda, Md: NCRP.

375. United Nations Scientific Committee on the Effects of Atomic Radiation (UNSCEAR), Sources and effects of ionizing radiation: UNSCEAR 2000 report to the General Assembly, with scientific annexes, Vol. 2, Effects. 2000, New York: United Nations.

376. Shore, R.E., Issues and epidemiological evidence regarding radiation-induced thyroid cancer. Radiat Res, 1992. 131(1):98–111.

377. Nagataki, S., ed. Radiation and the Thyroid. Proceedings of the 27th annual meeting of the Japanese Nuclear Medicine Society (1987, Nagasaki, Japan). 1989, Amsterdam: Excerpta Medica.

378. WM, M., Reassessment of the Mayo Clinic experience with well-differentiated thyroid carcinoma. 1981, Minneapolis: American Thyroid Association.

379. Silverberg, E., Cancer statistics, 1982. CA Cancer J Clin, 1982. 32(1):15–31.

380. Martinez-Tello, F.J., et al., Occult carcinoma of the thyroid: A systematic autopsy study from Spain of two series performed with two different methods. Cancer, 1993. 71(12):4022–4029.

381. Furmanchuk, A.W., N. Roussak, and C. Ruchti, Occult thyroid carcinomas in the region of Minsk, Belarus: An autopsy study of 215 patients. Histopathology, 1993. 23(4):319–325.

382. Getaz, E.P., K. Shimaoka, and U. Rao, Anaplastic carcinoma of the thyroid following external irradiation. Cancer, 1979. 43(6):2248–2253.

383. Komorowski, R.A., G.A. Hanson, and J.C. Garancis, Anaplastic thyroid carcinoma following low-dose irradiation. Am J Clin Pathol, 1978. 70(2):303–307.

384. Commission, E., Molecular, cellular, biological characterization of childhood thyroid cancer. In Experimental Collaboration Project, E.D. Williams and N.D. Tronko, eds. 1996, Brussels: European Commission.

385. Thomas, G.A., et al., Association between morphological subtype of post-Chernobyl papillary carcinoma and rearrangement of the RET oncogene. In Radiation and Thyroid Cancer. July 1998, St. John's College, Cambridge, U.K. 1999, Singapore: World Scientific.

386. Bounacer, A., et al., High prevalence of activating ret proto-oncogene rearrangements, in thyroid tumors from patients who had received external radiation. Oncogene, 1997. 15(11):1263–1273.

387. Thomas, G.A., et al., High prevalence of RET/PTC rearrangements in Ukrainian and Belarussian post-Chernobyl thyroid papillary carcinomas: A strong correlation between RET/PTC3 and the solid-follicular variant. J Clin Endocrinol Metab, 1999. 84(11):4232–4238.

388. Santoro, M., et al., Gene rearrangement and Chernobyl-related thyroid cancers. Br J Cancer, 2000. 82(2):315–322.

389. Williams, E.D., et al., Thyroid carcinoma after Chernobyl latent period, morphology and aggressiveness. Br J Cancer, 2004. 90(11):2219–2224.

390. Tronko, N.D., et al., Thyroid cancer in children and adolescents of Ukraine having been exposed as a result of the Chernobyl accident (15 years experience). Int J Radiation Medicine, 2002. 4:222–232.

391. Nikiforov, Y.E., et al., Prevalence of mutations of RAS and p53 in benign and malignant thyroid tumors from children exposed to radiation after the Chernobyl nuclear accident. Oncogene, 1996. 13(4):687–693.

392. Suchy, B., et al., Absence of RAS and p53 mutations in thyroid carcinomas of children after Chernobyl in contrast to adult thyroid tumours. Br J Cancer, 1998. 77(6):952–955.

393. Hillebrandt, S., et al., Polymorphisms in the p53 gene in thyroid tumours and blood samples of children from areas in Belarus. Mutat Res, 1997. 381(2):201–207.

394. Beimfohr, C., et al., NTRK1 re-arrangement in papillary thyroid carcinomas of children after the Chernobyl reactor accident. Int J Cancer, 1999. 80(6):842–847.

395. Lima, J., et al., BRAF mutations are not a major event in post-Chernobyl childhood thyroid carcinomas. J Clin Endocrinol Metab, 2004. 89(9):4267–4271.

396. Schneider, A.B., et al., Dose-response relationships for radiation-induced thyroid cancer and thyroid nodules: Evidence for the prolonged effects of radiation on the thyroid. J Clin Endocrinol Metab, 1993. 77(2):362–369.

397. Colman, N., et al., Thyroid cancer associated with radiation exposure: Dose-effect relationships in biological and environments of low-level radiation. 1976, Vienna: International Atomic Energy Agency (IAEA).

398. Raventos, A. and T. Winship, The latent intervals for thyroid cancer following irradiation. Radiology, 1964. 83:501–508.

399. de Vathaire, F., et al., Long-term effects on the thyroid of irradiation for skin angiomas in childhood. Radiat Res, 1993. 133(3):381–386.

400. Lundell, M., T. Hakulinen, and L.E. Holm, Thyroid cancer after radiotherapy for skin hemangioma in infancy. Radiat Res, 1994. 140(3):334–339.

401. Book, S.A., Age-related variation in thyroidal exposure from fission-produced radionuclides. In Developmental Toxicology of Energy Related Products. 1978, Washington, DC: U.S. Nuclear Regulatory Commission, p. 1017.

402. Ron, E., et al., Thyroid cancer after exposure to external radiation: A pooled analysis of seven studies. Radiat Res, 1995. 141(3):259–277.

403. Cardis, E., et al., Risk of thyroid cancer after exposure to 131I in childhood. J Natl Cancer Inst, 2005. 97(10):724–732.

403a. Ronckers, C.M., A.J. Sigurdson, M. Storall, et al., Thyroid cancer in childhood cancer survivors: A detailed evaluation of radiation dose response and its modifiers. Radiat Res, 2006. 166: 618–628.

404. Maxon, H.R., et al., Clinically important radiation-associated thyroid disease: A controlled study. JAMA, 1980. 244(16): 1802–1805.

405. Momani, M.S., et al., Familial concordance of thyroid and other head and neck tumors in an irradiated cohort: Analysis of contributing factors. J Clin Endocrinol Metab, 2004. 89(5):2185–2191.

406. Kolonel, L.N., et al., An epidemiologic study of thyroid cancer in Hawaii. Cancer Causes Control, 1990. 1(3):223–234.

407. Franceschi, S., et al., Diet and epithelial cancer of the thyroid gland. Tumori, 1990. 76(4):331–338.

408. Ron, E. and B. Modan, Thyroid. In Cancer Epidemiology and Prevention, D. Schottenfeld and J.F. Fraumeni, eds. 1982, Philadelphia: W.B. Saunders.

409. Mazzaferri, E.L., Thyroid cancer and Graves' disease. J Clin Endocrinol Metab, 1990. 70(4):826–829.

410. Robbins, J., Thyroid suppression therapy for prevention of thyroid tumors after radiation exposure. In Radiation-associated Thyroid Cancer, L.J. de Groot and L.A. Frohman, eds. 1977, New York: Academic Press.

411. Satran, L., et al., Thyroid neoplasm after high-dose radiotherapy. Am J Pediatr Hematol Oncol, 1983. 5(3):307–309.

412. Blettner, M., et al., Mortality from cancer and other causes among male airline cockpit crew in Europe. Int J Cancer, 2003. 106(6):946–952.

413. Parker, L.N., et al., Thyroid carcinoma after exposure to atomic radiation: A continuing survey of a fixed population, Hiroshima and Nagasaki, 1958–1971. Ann Intern Med, 1974. 80(5):600–604.

414. Wood, J.W., et al., Thyroid carcinoma in atomic bomb survivors Hiroshima and Nagasaki. Am J Epidemiol, 1969. 89(1):4–14.

415. Parker, L., et al., Thyroid carcinoma diagnosed between 13 and 26 years after exposure to atomic radiation: A study of the ABCC-JNIH, Adult Health Study Population, Hiroshima & Nagasaki, 1958–1971. 1973, Hiroshima, Japan: Atomic Bomb Casualty Commission.

416. Thomas, D.B., et al., Ionizing radiation and breast cancer in men (United States). Cancer Causes Control, 1994. 5(1):9–14.

417. Ezaki, H., N. Takeichi, and Y. Yoshimoto, Thyroid cancer: Epidemiological study of thyroid cancer in A-bomb survivors from extended life span study cohort in Hiroshima. J Radiat Res (Tokyo), 1991. 32(suppl):S193–S200.

418. Bowlt, C. and P. Tiplady, Radioiodine in human thyroid glands and incidence of thyroid cancer in Cumbria. BMJ, 1989. 299(6694):301–302.

419. Kaplan, M.M., et al., Thyroid, parathyroid, and salivary gland evaluations in patients exposed to multiple fluoroscopic examinations during tuberculosis therapy: A pilot study. J Clin Endocrinol Metab, 1988. 66(2):376–382.

420. Hempelmann, L.H., et al., Neoplasms in persons treated with x-rays in infancy: Fourth survey in 20 years. J Natl Cancer Inst, 1975. 55(3):519–530.

421. Shore, R.E., et al., Thyroid cancer among persons given x-ray treatment in infancy for an enlarged thymus gland. Am J Epidemiol, 1993. 137(10):1068–1080.

422. Ron, E., et al., Thyroid neoplasia following low-dose radiation in childhood. Radiat Res, 1989. 120(3):516–531.

423. Schneider, A.B., et al., Incidence, prevalence and characteristics of radiation-induced thyroid tumors. Am J Med, 1978. 64(2):243–252.

424. Refetoff, S., et al., Continuing occurrence of thyroid carcinoma after irradiation to the neck in infancy and childhood. N Engl J Med, 1975. 292(4):171–175.

425. Paloyan, E., et al., Total thyroidectomy and parathyroid autotransplantation for radiation-associated thyroid cancer. Surgery, 1976. 80(1):70–76.

426. DeGroot, L. and E. Paloyan, Thyroid carcinoma and radiation: A Chicago endemic. JAMA, 1973. 225(5):487–491.

427. DeGroot, L.J., et al., Retrospective and prospective study of radiation-induced thyroid disease. Am J Med, 1983. 74(5):852–862.

428. Pottern, L.M., et al., Thyroid nodularity after childhood irradiation for lymphoid hyperplasia: A comparison of questionnaire and clinical findings. J Clin Epidemiol, 1990. 43(5):449–460.

429. Kizer, K.W., Nasopharyngeal radium treatment of veterans. Mil Med, 1996. 161(3):A3.

430. Ronckers, C.M., et al., Cancer mortality after nasopharyngeal radium irradiation in the Netherlands: A cohort study. J Natl Cancer Inst, 2001. 93(13):1021–1027.

431. Yeh, H., et al., Cancer incidence after childhood nasopharyngeal radium irradiation: A follow-up study in Washington County, Maryland. Am J Epidemiol, 2001. 153(8):749–756.

432. Hallquist, A., L. Hardell, and P.O. Lofroth, External radiotherapy prior to thyroid cancer: A case-control study. Int J Radiat Oncol Biol Phys, 1993. 27:1085–1089.

433. van Daal, W.A., et al., Thyroid gland carcinoma as a late sequel of irradiation of the neck region. Ned Tijdschr Geneeskd, 1983. 127(1):12–15.

434. De Jong, S.A., et al., Thyroid carcinoma and hyperparathyroidism after radiation therapy for adolescent acne vulgaris. Surgery, 1991. 110(4):691–695.

435. Mike, V., A.T. Meadows, and G.J. D'Angio, Incidence of second malignant neoplasms in children: Results of an international study. Lancet, 1982. 2(8311):1326–1331.

436. Tucker, M.A., et al., Risk of second cancers after treatment for Hodgkin's disease. N Engl J Med, 1988. 318(2):76–81.

437. Kaplan, M.M., et al., Risk factors for thyroid abnormalities after neck irradiation for childhood cancer. Am J Med, 1983. 74(2):272–280.

438. Hancock, S.L., R.S. Cox, and I.R. McDougall, Thyroid diseases after treatment of Hodgkin's disease. N Engl J Med, 1991. 325(9):599–605.

439. Tucker, M.A., et al., Therapeutic radiation at a young age is linked to secondary thyroid cancer. The Late Effects Study Group. Cancer Res, 1991. 51(11):2885–2888.

440. Sankila, R., et al., Risk of subsequent malignant neoplasms among 1,641 Hodgkin's disease patients diagnosed in childhood and adolescence: A population-based cohort study in the five Nordic countries. Association of the Nordic Cancer Registries and the Nordic Society of Pediatric Hematology and Oncology. J Clin Oncol, 1996. 14(5):1442–1446.

441. Curtis, R.E., et al., Solid cancers after bone marrow transplantation. N Engl J Med, 1997. 336(13):897–904.

442. Bhatia, S., et al., Solid cancers after bone marrow transplantation. J Clin Oncol, 2001. 19(2):464–471.

443. Socie, G., et al., New malignant diseases after allogeneic marrow transplantation for childhood acute leukemia. J Clin Oncol, 2000. 18(2):348–357.

444. de Vathaire, F., et al., Thyroid carcinomas after irradiation for a first cancer during childhood. Arch Intern Med, 1999. 159(22):2713–2719.

445. Cohen, A., et al., Secondary thyroid carcinoma after allogeneic bone marrow transplantation during childhood. Bone Marrow Transplant, 2001. 28(12):1125–1128.

446. Damber, L., et al., Thyroid cancer after x-ray treatment of benign disorders of the cervical spine in adults. Acta Oncol, 2002. 41(1):25–28.

447. Ritz, B., Cancer mortality among workers exposed to chemicals during uranium processing. J Occup Environ Med, 1999. 41(7):556–566.

448. Hahn, K., et al., Thyroid cancer after diagnostic administration of iodine-131 in childhood. Radiat Res, 2001. 156(1):61–70.

449. Holm, L.E., G. Eklund, and G. Lundell, Incidence of malignant thyroid tumors in humans after exposure to diagnostic doses of iodine-131. II. Estimation of thyroid gland size, thyroid radiation dose, and predicted versus observed number of malignant thyroid tumors. J Natl Cancer Inst, 1980. 65(6):1221–1224.

450. Holm, L.E., G. Lundell, and G. Walinder, Incidence of malignant thyroid tumors in humans after exposure to diagnostic doses of iodine-131. I. Retrospective cohort study. J Natl Cancer Inst, 1980. 64(5):1055–1059.

451. Holm, L.E., et al., Thyroid cancer after diagnostic doses of iodine-131: A retrospective cohort study. J Natl Cancer Inst, 1988. 80(14):1132–1138.

452. Holm, L.E., et al., Malignant thyroid tumors after iodine-131 therapy: A retrospective cohort study. N Engl J Med, 1980. 303(4):188–191.

453. Safa, A.M., O.P. Schumacher, and A. Rodriguez-Antunez, Long-term follow-up results in children and adolescents treated with radioactive iodine (^{131}I) for hyperthyroidism. N Engl J Med, 1975. 292(4):167–171.

454. Dickman, P.W., et al., Thyroid cancer risk after thyroid examination with 131I: A population-based cohort study in Sweden. Int J Cancer, 2003. 106(4):580–587.

455. Rallison, M.L., et al., Thyroid disease in children: A survey of subjects potentially exposed to fallout radiation. Am J Med, 1974. 56(4):457–463.

456. Machado, S.G., C.E. Land, and F.W. McKay, Cancer mortality and radioactive fallout in southwestern Utah. Am J Epidemiol, 1987. 125(1):44–61.

457. Kerber, R.A., et al., A cohort study of thyroid disease in relation to fallout from nuclear weapons testing. JAMA, 1993. 270(17):2076–2082.

458. Gilbert, E.S., et al., Thyroid cancer rates and ^{131}I doses from Nevada atmospheric nuclear bomb tests. J Natl Cancer Inst, 1998. 90(21):1654–1660.

459. Conard, R., et al., Review of medical findings in a Marshallese population 26 years after accidental exposure to radioactive fallout. 1980, Upton, NY: Brookhaven National Laboratory.

460. Lund, E. and M.R. Galanti, Incidence of thyroid cancer in Scandinavia following fallout from atomic bomb testing: An analysis of birth cohorts. Cancer Causes Control, 1999. 10(3):181–187.

461. McDougall, I., and W. Grieg, Iodine-125 therapy in Grave's disease: Long-term results in 355 patients. Ann Intern Med, 1976. 85:720.

462. Weidinger, P., P.M. Johnson, and S.C. Werner, Five years' experience with iodine-125 therapy of Graves' disease. Lancet, 1974. 2(7872):74–77.

463. Chapman, E., et al., The collection of radioiodine by the human fetal thyroid. J Endocrinol, 1948. 8:717–720.

464. International Atomic Energy Agency (IAEA), The International Chernobyl Project: Technical Report. 1991, Vienna: IAEA.

465. Kazakov, V.S., E.P. Demidchik, and L.N. Astakhova, Thyroid cancer after Chernobyl. Nature, 1992. 359(6390):21.

466. Bertim, M. and J. Lallemand, Increase of cancers of the thyroid gland in children in Byelarus. Annales D'Endocinologie, 1992. 53(5–6):173–177.

467. Prisyazhniuk, A., et al., Cancer in the Ukraine, post-Chernobyl. Lancet, 1991. 338(8778):1334–1335.

468. Tsyb, A.F., et al., Disease indices of thyroid and their dose dependence in children and adolescents affected as a result of the Chernobyl accident. In Nagasaki Symposium on Chernobyl: Update and Future. 1994, Nagasaki: Elsevier Science B.V., Amsterdam.

469. Tronko, N., et al., Thyroid gland in children after the Chernobyl accident (yesterday and today). In Nagasaki Symposium on Chernobyl: Update and Future. 1994, Nagasaki: Elsevier Science B.V., Amsterdam.

470. Shirahige, Y., et al., Childhood thyroid cancer: Comparison of Japan and Belarus. Endocr J, 1998. 45(2):203–209.

471. Tronko, M.D., et al., Thyroid carcinoma in children and adolescents in Ukraine after the Chernobyl nuclear accident: Statistical data and clinicomorphologic characteristics. Cancer, 1999. 86(1):149–156.

472. Ivanov, V.K., et al., Dynamics of thyroid cancer incidence in Russia following the Chernobyl accident. J Radiol Prot, 1999. 19(4):305–318.

473. Jacob, P., et al., Thyroid cancer risk to children calculated. Nature, 1998. 392(6671):31–32.

474. Jacob, P., et al., Childhood exposure due to the Chernobyl accident and thyroid cancer risk in contaminated areas of Belarus and Russia. Br J Cancer, 1999. 80(9):1461–1469.

475. Astakhova, L.N., et al., Chernobyl-related thyroid cancer in children of Belarus: A case-control study. Radiat Res, 1998. 150(3):349–356.

476. Davis, S., et al., Risk of thyroid cancer in the Bryansk oblast of the Russian Federation after the Chernobyl Power Station accident. Radiat Res, 2004. 162(3):241–248.

477. Ron, E., J. Lubin, and A.B. Schneider, Thyroid cancer incidence. Nature, 1992. 360(6400):113.

478. Shakhtarin, V.V., et al., Iodine deficiency, radiation dose, and the risk of thyroid cancer among children and adolescents in the Bryansk region of Russia following the Chernobyl power station accident. Int J Epidemiol, 2003. 32(4):584–591.

479. Heidenreich, W.F., et al., Time trends of thyroid cancer incidence in Belarus after the Chernobyl accident. Radiat Res, 1999. 151(5):617–625.

480. Ivanov, V.K., et al., Thyroid cancer incidence among liquidators of the Chernobyl accident: Absence of dependence of radiation risks on external radiation dose. Radiat Environ Biophys, 2002. 41(3):195–198.

481. Ivanov, V.K., et al., Thyroid cancer incidence among adolescents and adults in the Bryansk region of Russia following the Chernobyl accident. Health Phys, 2003. 84(1):46–60.

482. Kesniiniene, A., et al., Studies of cancer risk among Chernobyl liquidators: Materials and methods. J Radiol Prot, 2002. 22(3A): A137–A141.

483. Trowbridge, F.L., et al., Iodine and goiter in children. Pediatrics, 1975. 56(1):82–90.

484. Rallison, M.L., et al., Thyroid nodularity in children. JAMA, 1975. 233(10):1069–1072.

485. Rojeski, M.T. and H. Gharib, Nodular thyroid disease: Evaluation and management. N Engl J Med, 1985. 313(7):428–436.

486. Vander, J.B., E.A. Gaston, and T.R. Dawber, The significance of nontoxic thyroid nodules: Final report of a 15-year study of the incidence of thyroid malignancy. Ann Intern Med, 1968. 69(3):537–540.

487. Carroll, B.A., Asymptomatic thyroid nodules: Incidental sonographic detection. AJR Am J Roentgenol, 1982. 138(3):499–501.

488. Woestyn, J. and M. Afschrift, Ultrasonic demonstration of small thyroid nodules. Lancet, 1983. 2(8361):1252.

489. Woestyn, J., et al., Demonstration of nodules in the normal thyroid by echography. Br J Radiol, 1985. 58(696):1179–1182.

490. Horlocker, T., J. Hay, and E. James, Prevalence of incidental nodular thyroid disease detected during high-resolution parathyroid ultrasonography. Thyroidology, 1986. 181:1309–1312.

491. Brander, A., et al., Thyroid gland: US screening in a random adult population. Radiology, 1991. 181(3):683–687.

492. Mettler, F.A., Jr., et al., Thyroid nodules in the population living around Chernobyl. JAMA, 1992. 268(5):616–619.

493. Mortensen, J., L. Woolner, and W.P. Bennett, Gross and microscopic findings in clinically normal thyroid glands. J Clin Endocrinol Metab, 1955. 15:1270–1280.

494. Wang, Z.Y., et al., Thyroid nodularity and chromosome aberrations among women in areas of high background radiation in China. J Natl Cancer Inst, 1990. 82(6):478–485.

495. Radford, E., et al., Effects of elevated gamma ray exposures on the prevalence of thyroid abnormalities in a community. Radiat Res, 1983. 93:C8–C12.

496. Nagataki, S., Delayed effects of atomic bomb radiation on the thyroid. In Radiation and the Thyroid. From the 27th Annual Meeting of the Japanese Nuclear Medicine Society, Nagasaki, Japan. 1987, Amsterdam: Excerpta Medica.

497. Nagataki, S., et al., Thyroid diseases among atomic bomb survivors in Nagasaki. JAMA, 1994. 272(5):364–370.

498. Shore, R.E., et al., Benign thyroid adenomas among persons X-irradiated in infancy for enlarged thymus glands. Radiat Res, 1993. 134(2):217–223.

499. Stewart, R.R., et al., Thyroid gland: US in patients with Hodgkin disease treated with radiation therapy in childhood. Radiology, 1989. 172(1):159–163.

500. Hall, P., et al., Thyroid nodularity after diagnostic administration of iodine-131. Radiat Res, 1996. 146(6):673–682.

501. Rosen, I.B., et al., High-dose radiation and the emergence of thyroid nodular disease. Surgery, 1984. 96(6):988–995.

502. Conard, R., ed., Late effects in Marshall Islanders exposed to fall-out 28 years ago. In Radiation Carcinogenesis: Epidemiology and Biological Significance, J. Boice and J.F. Fraumeni, eds. 1984, New York: Raven Press.

503. Robbins, J. and W. Adams. Radiation effects in the Marshall Islands. In Radiation and the Thyroid: 27th Annual Meeting of the Japanese Nuclear Medicine Society, Nagasaki, Japan. 1987, Amsterdam: Excerpta Medica.

504. Hamilton, T.E., G. van Belle, and J.P. LoGerfo, Thyroid neoplasia in Marshall Islanders exposed to nuclear fallout. JAMA, 1987. 258(5):629–635.

504a. Mushkacheva, G., E. Rabinavich, V. Privalov, et al., Thyroid abnormalities associated with protracted childhood exposure to ^{131}I from atmospheric emissions from the Mayak Weapons Facility in Russia. Radiat Res, 2006. 166:715–722.

505. Davis, S., et al., Thyroid neoplasia, autoimmune thyroiditis, and hypothyroidism in persons exposed to iodine 131 from the Hanford nuclear site. JAMA, 2004. 292(21):2600–2613.

506. Kopecky, K.J., et al., Estimation of thyroid radiation doses for the Hanford thyroid disease study: Results and implications for statistical power of the epidemiological analyses. Health Phys, 2004. 87(1):15–32.

507. Kopecky, K.J., et al., Thyroid ultrasound abnormalities in persons exposed during childhood to ^{131}I from the Hanford nuclear site. Thyroid, 2005. 15(6):604–613.

508. Lindberg, S., et al., Cancer incidence after radiotherapy for skin haemangioma during infancy. Acta Oncol, 1995. 34(6):735–740.

509. Jacob, P., et al., Thyroid cancer risk in areas of Ukraine and Belarus affected by the Chernobyl accident. Radiat Res, 2006. 165(1):1–8.

510. Land, C.E., et al., Breast cancer risk from low-dose exposures to ionizing radiation: Results of parallel analysis of three exposed populations of women. J Natl Cancer Inst, 1980. 65(2):353–376.

511. MacMahon, B., Cole, and J. Brown, Etiology of human breast cancer: A review. J Natl Cancer Inst, 1973. 50(1):21–42.

512. Swift, M., et al., Incidence of cancer in 161 families affected by ataxia-telangiectasia. N Engl J Med, 1991. 325(26):1831–1836.

513. Boice, J.D., Jr., and Miller, R.W., Risk of breast cancer in ataxia-telangiectasia. N Engl J Med, 1992. 326(20):1357–1358; author reply, 1360–1361.

514. Land, C.E., Breast cancer in the RERF Life Span Study. RERF Update. 1993, Hiroshima, Japan: Radiation Effects Research Foundation.

515. Land, C.E., et al., Early-onset breast cancer in A-bomb survivors. Lancet, 1993. 342(8865):237.

516. Iknayan, H.F., Carcinoma associated with irradiation of the immature breast. Radiology, 1975. 114(2):431–433.

517. Reimer, R.R., et al., Breast carcinoma following radiotherapy of metastatic Wilm's tumor. Cancer, 1977. 40(4):1450–1452.

518. Boice, J.D., Jr., et al., Frequent chest X-ray fluoroscopy and breast cancer incidence among tuberculosis patients in Massachusetts. Radiat Res, 1991. 125(2):214–222.

519. Miller, A.B., et al., Mortality from breast cancer after irradiation during fluoroscopic examinations in patients being treated for tuberculosis. N Engl J Med, 1989. 321(19):1285–1289.

520. Shimizu, Y., W.J. Schull, and H. Kato, Cancer risk among atomic bomb survivors: The RERF Life Span Study, Radiation Effects Research Foundation. JAMA, 1990. 264(5):601–604.

521. Shore, R.E., et al., Breast cancer among women given X-ray therapy for acute postpartum mastitis. J Natl Cancer Inst, 1986. 77(3):689–696.

522. Shimizu, Y., et al., Mortality of life span study sample. 1988, Hiroshima, Japan: Radiation Effects Research Foundation.

523. Tokunaga, M., et al., Incidence of female breast cancer among atomic bomb survivors, Hiroshima and Nagasaki, 1950–1980. Radiat Res, 1987. 112(2):243–272.

524. Shore, R.E., et al., Breast neoplasms in women treated with x-rays for acute postpartum mastitis. J Natl Cancer Inst, 1977. 59(3):813–822.

525. Baral, E., L.E. Larsson, and B. Mattsson, Breast cancer following irradiation of the breast. Cancer, 1977. 40(6):2905–2910.

526. Hancock, S.L., M.A. Tucker, and R.T. Hoppe, Breast cancer after treatment of Hodgkin's disease. J Natl Cancer Inst, 1993. 85(1):25–31.

527. Preston, D.L., et al., Radiation effects on breast cancer risk: A pooled analysis of eight cohorts. Radiat Res, 2002. 158(2):220–235.

528. Wanebo, C.K., et al., Breast cancer after exposure to the atomic bombings of Hiroshima and Nagasaki. N Engl J Med, 1968. 279(13):667–671.

529. Jablon, S. and H. Kato, Studies of the mortality of A-bomb survivors. Part V. Radiation dose and mortality, 1950–1970. Radiat Res, 1972. 50(3):649–698.

530. Tokunaga, M., et al., Breast cancer in Japanese A-bomb survivors. Lancet, 1982. 2(8304):924.

531. Tokunaga, M., et al., Incidence of female breast cancer among atomic bomb survivors, 1950–1985. Radiat Res, 1994. 138(2):209–223.

532. Tokunaga, M., et al., Proliferative and nonproliferative breast disease in atomic bomb survivors: Results of a histopathologic review of autopsy breast tissue. Cancer, 1993. 72(5):1657–1665.

533. Bauer, S., et al., Radiation exposure due to local fallout from Soviet atmospheric nuclear weapons testing in Kazakhstan: Solid cancer mortality in the Semipalatinsk historical cohort, 1960–1999. Radiat Res, 2005. 164(4 Pt 1):409–419.

534. Hoffman, D.A., et al., Breast cancer in women with scoliosis exposed to multiple diagnostic x rays. J Natl Cancer Inst, 1989. 81(17):1307–1312.

535. Mackenzie, I., Breast cancer following multiple fluoroscopies. Br J Cancer, 1965. 19:1–8.

536. Myrden, J.A. and J.E. Hiltz, Breast cancer following multiple fluoroscopies during artificial pneumothorax treatment of pulmonary tuberculosis. Can Med Assoc J, 1969. 100(22):1032–1034.

537. Myrden, J.A. and J. Quinlan, Breast carcinoma following multiple fluoroscopies with pneumothorax treatment of pulmonary tuberculosis. Ann R Coll Physicians Surg Can, 1974. 7:45.

538. Boice, J.D., Jr., and Monson, R.R., Breast cancer in women after repeated fluoroscopic examinations of the chest. J Natl Cancer Inst, 1977. 59(3):823–832.

539. Boice, J.D., Jr., M. Rosenstein, and E.D. Trout, Estimation of breast doses and breast cancer risk associated with repeated fluoroscopic chest examinations of women with tuberculosis. Radiat Res, 1978. 73:373–390.

540. Hrubec, Z., et al., Breast cancer after multiple chest fluoroscopies: second follow-up of Massachusetts women with tuberculosis. Cancer Res, 1989. 49(1):229–234.

541. Mettler, F.A., Jr., et al., Breast neoplasms in women treated with x rays for acute postpartum mastitis: A pilot study. J Natl Cancer Inst, 1969. 43(4):803–811.

542. Mattsson, A., et al., Radiation-induced breast cancer: Long-term follow-up of radiation therapy for benign breast disease. J Natl Cancer Inst, 1993. 85(20):1679–1685.

543. Hildreth, N.G., R.E. Shore, and L.H. Hempelmann, Risk of breast cancer among women receiving radiation treatment in infancy for thymic enlargement. Lancet, 1983. 2(8344):273.

544. Hildreth, N.G., R.E. Shore, and P.M. Dvoretsky, The risk of breast cancer after irradiation of the thymus in infancy. N Engl J Med, 1989. 321(19):1281–1284.

545. Lowell, D., R. Martineau, and S. Luria, Carcinoma of the male breast following radiation: Report of a case occurring 35 years after radiation therapy of unilateral pre-pubertal gynecomastia. Cancer, 1968. 22:581–586.

546. Orine, S., R. Chambers, and R. Johnson, Post-radiation carcinoma of male breast bilaterally. JAMA, 1967. 201:707.

547. Evans, A.E., et al., Late effects of treatment for Wilms' tumor: A report from the National Wilms' Tumor Study Group. Cancer, 1991. 67(2):331–336.

548. Li, F.P., et al., Breast carcinoma after cancer therapy in childhood. Cancer, 1983. 51(3):521–523.

549. Janjan, N.A. and D.L. Zellmer, Calculated risk of breast cancer following mantle irradiation determined by measured dose. Cancer Detect Prev, 1992. 16(5–6):273–282.

550. Dershaw, D.D., J. Yahalom, and J.A. Petrek, Breast carcinoma in women previously treated for Hodgkin's disease: Mammographic evaluation. Radiology, 1992. 184(2):421–423.

551. Bhatia, S., et al., High risk of subsequent neoplasms continues with extended follow-up of childhood Hodgkin's disease: Report from the Late Effects Study Group. J Clin Oncol, 2003. 21(23):4386–4394.

552. van Leeuwen, F.E., et al., Long-term risk of second malignancy in survivors of Hodgkin's disease treated during adolescence or young adulthood. J Clin Oncol, 2000. 18(3):487–497.

553. van Leeuwen, F.E., et al., Roles of radiation dose, chemotherapy, and hormonal factors in breast cancer following Hodgkin's disease. J Natl Cancer Inst, 2003. 95(13):971–980.

554. Metayer, C., et al., Second cancers among long-term survivors of Hodgkin's disease diagnosed in childhood and adolescence. J Clin Oncol, 2000. 18(12):2435–2443.

555. Baverstock, K.F., D. Papworth, and J. Vennart, Risks of radiation at low dose rates. Lancet, 1981. 1(8217):430–433.

556. Stebbings, J.H., H.F. Lucas, and A.F. Stehney, Mortality from cancers of major sites in female radium dial workers. Am J Ind Med, 1984. 5(6):435–459.

557. Adams, E.E. and A.M. Brues, Breast cancer in female radium dial workers first employed before 1930. J Occup Med, 1980. 22(9):583–587.

558. Wick, R.R. and W. Gossner. Recent results of the follow-up of radium 224 treated ankylosing spondylitis patients. In Risks from Radium and Thorotrast, D. Taylor, ed. 1988. Bethesda, Md: British Institute of Radiology.

559. Mattsson, A., et al., Dose- and time-response for breast cancer risk after radiation therapy for benign breast disease. Br J Cancer, 1995. 72(4):1054–1061.

560. Lundell, M., et al., Breast cancer risk after radiotherapy in infancy: A pooled analysis of two Swedish cohorts of 17,202 infants. Radiat Res, 1999. 151(5):626–632.

561. Travis, L.B., et al., Breast cancer following radiotherapy and chemotherapy among young women with Hodgkin's disease. JAMA, 2003. 290(4):465–475.

562. Morin Doody, M., et al., Breast cancer mortality after diagnostic radiography: Findings from the U.S. Scoliosis Cohort Study. Spine, 2000. 25(16):2052–2063.

563. Howe, G.R. and J. McLaughlin, Breast cancer mortality between 1950 and 1987 after exposure to fractionated moderate-dose-rate ionizing radiation in the Canadian fluoroscopy cohort study and

a comparison with breast cancer mortality in the atomic bomb survivors study. Radiat Res, 1996. 145(6):694–707.

564. Samet, J.M., Epidemiology of Lung Cancer. 1994, New York: Marcel Dekker.

565. Land, C.E., et al., Radiation-associated lung cancer: A comparison of the histology of lung cancers in uranium miners and survivors of the atomic bombings of Hiroshima and Nagasaki. Radiat Res, 1993. 134(2):234–243.

566. Archer, V.E., et al., Latency and the lung cancer epidemic among United States uranium miners. Health Phys, 2004. 87(5):480–489.

567. Tokarskaya, Z.B., et al., Multifactorial analysis of lung cancer dose-response relationships for workers at the Mayak nuclear enterprise. Health Phys, 1997. 73(6):899–905.

568. Tokarskaya, Z.B., et al., The influence of radiation and nonradiation factors on the lung cancer incidence among the workers of the nuclear enterprise Mayak. Health Phys, 1995. 69(3):356–366.

569. Howe, G.R., Lung cancer mortality between 1950 and 1987 after exposure to fractionated moderate-dose-rate ionizing radiation in the Canadian fluoroscopy cohort study and a comparison with lung cancer mortality in the atomic bomb survivors study. Radiat Res, 1995. 142(3):295–304.

570. Vahakangas, K.H., et al., Mutations of p53 and RAS genes in radon-associated lung cancer from uranium miners. Lancet, 1992. 339(8793):576–580.

571. Whittemore, A.S. and A. McMillan, Lung cancer mortality among U.S. uranium miners: A reappraisal. J Natl Cancer Inst, 1983. 71(3):489–499.

572. Lubin, J., J.D. Boice, and C. Edling, Radon and lung cancer risk: A joint analysis of 11 underground miner studies. 1994, Washington, DC: U.S. Department of Health and Human Services.

573. Lubin, J.H., and K. Steindorf, Cigarette use and the estimation of lung cancer attributable to radon in the United States. Radiat Res, 1995. 141(1):79–85.

574. Prentice, R.L., Y. Yoshimoto, and M.W. Mason, Relationship of cigarette smoking and radiation exposure to cancer mortality in Hiroshima and Nagasaki. J Natl Cancer Inst, 1983. 70(4):611–622.

575. National Research Council (NRC), Committee on the Biological Effects of Ionizing Radiations (BEIR), Health risks of radon and other internally deposited alpha-emitters. BEIR IV. 1988, Washington, DC: National Academy Press, xvi. Available at www.netLibrary.com/urlapi.asp?action=summary&v=1&bookid=15940.

576. Travis, L.B., et al., Lung cancer following chemotherapy and radiotherapy for Hodgkin's disease. J Natl Cancer Inst, 2002. 94(3):182–192.

577. Pierce, D.A., G.B. Sharp, and K. Mabuchi, Joint effects of radiation and smoking on lung cancer risk among atomic bomb survivors. Radiat Res, 2003. 159(4):511–520.

578. Tomasek, L., and V. Placek, Radon exposure and lung cancer risk: Czech cohort study. Radiat Res, 1999. 152(Suppl 6):S59–S63.

579. Tomasek, L., Czech miner studies of lung cancer risk from radon. J Radiol Prot, 2002. 22(3A):A107–A112.

580. Steer, A., et al., Accuracy of diagnosis of cancer among autopsy cases: JNIH-ABCC population for Hiroshima and Nagasaki. Gann, 1976. 67(5):625–632.

581. Jagger, J., Natural background radiation and cancer death in Rocky Mountain states and Gulf Coast states. Health Phys, 1998. 75(4):428–430.

582. Archer, V.E., Cancer death rates and background radiation. Health Phys, 1999. 76(6):692–695.

583. Blettner, M., et al., Mortality from cancer and other causes among airline cabin attendants in Germany, 1960–1997. Am J Epidemiol, 2002. 156(6):556–565.

584. Smith, P.G. and R. Doll, Mortality from cancer and all causes among British radiologists. Br J Radiol, 1981. 54(639):187–194.

585. Jablon, S. and R.W. Miller, Army technologists: 29-year follow up for cause of death. Radiology, 1978. 126(3):677–679.

586. Koshurnikova, N.A., et al., Lung cancer risk due to exposure to incorporated plutonium. Radiat Res, 1998. 149(4):366–371.

587. Gilbert, E.S., et al., Lung cancer in Mayak workers. Radiat Res, 2004. 162(5):505–516.

588. Smith, P.G. and R. Doll, Age and time dependent changes in the rates of radiation induced cancers in patients with ankylosing spondylitis following a single course of x-ray treatmemt. In Late Biological Effects of Ionizing Radiation. 1978, Vienna: International Atomic Energy Agency (IAEA).

589. Lundell, M. and L.E. Holm, Risk of solid tumors after irradiation in infancy. Acta Oncol, 1995. 34(6):727–734.

590. Harvey, E.B. and L.A. Brinton, Second cancer following cancer of the breast in Connecticut, 1935–82. Natl Cancer Inst Monogr, 1985. 68:99–112.

591. Schenker, J.G., R. Levinsky, and G. Ohel, Multiple primary malignant neoplasms in breast cancer patients in Israel. Cancer, 1984. 54(1):145–150.

592. Hill, C.A., L.B. North, and B.M. Osborne, Bronchogenic carcinoma in breast carcinoma patients. AJR Am J Roentgenol, 1983. 140(2):259–264.

593. Kurtz, J.M., et al., Contralateral breast cancer and other second malignancies in patients treated by breast-conserving therapy with radiation. Int J Radiat Oncol Biol Phys, 1988. 15(2):277–284.

594. Neugut, A.I., et al., Lung cancer after radiation therapy for breast cancer. Cancer, 1993. 71(10):3054–3057.

595. Inskip, P.D., M. Stovall, and J.T. Flannery, Lung cancer risk and radiation dose among women treated for breast cancer. J Natl Cancer Inst, 1994. 86(13):983–988.

596. Zablotska, L.B. and A.I. Neugut, Lung carcinoma after radiation therapy in women treated with lumpectomy or mastectomy for primary breast carcinoma. Cancer, 2003. 97(6):1404–1411.

597. Hay, J.H., W. Duncan, and G.R. Kerr, Subsequent malignancies in patients irradiated for testicular tumours. Br J Radiol, 1984. 57(679):597–602.

598. van Leeuwen, F.E., et al., Increased risk of lung cancer, non-Hodgkin's lymphoma, and leukemia following Hodgkin's disease. J Clin Oncol, 1989. 7(8):1046–1058.

599. Kaldor, J.M., et al., Lung cancer following Hodgkin's disease: A case-control study. Int J Cancer, 1992. 52(5):677–681.

600. Gilbert, E.S., et al., Lung cancer after treatment for Hodgkin's disease: Focus on radiation effects. Radiat Res, 2003. 159(2):161–173.

601. Anderson, K.A., et al., Malignant pleural mesothelioma following radiotherapy in a 16-year-old boy. Cancer, 1985. 56(2):273–276.

602. Bilbey, J.H., et al., Localized fibrous mesothelioma of pleura following external ionizing radiation therapy. Chest, 1988. 94(6):1291–1292.

603. Kawashima, A., H.I. Libshitz, and J.M. Lukeman, Radiation-induced malignant pleural mesothelioma. Can Assoc Radiol J, 1990. 41(6):384–386.

604. Lerman, Y., et al., Radiation-associated malignant pleural mesothelioma. Thorax, 1991. 46(6):463–464.

605. Catanese, J., et al., Mediastinal osteosarcoma with extension to lungs in a patient treated for Hodgkin's disease. Cancer, 1988. 62(10):2252–2257.

606. National Council on Radiation Protection and Measurements (NCRP), Evaluation of occupational and environmental exposures to radon and radon daughters in the United States: Recommendations of the NCRP report no. 78. 1984, Bethesda, Md: NCRP.

607. Puskin, J.S., An analysis of the uncertainties in estimates of radon-induced lung cancer. Risk Anal, 1992. 12(2):277–285.

608. Stranden, E., Radon in Norwegian dwellings and the feasibility of epidemiological studies. Radiat Environ Biophys, 1986. 25(1):37–42.

609. Stranden, E., Radon 222 in Norwegian dwellings. In Radon and Its Decay Products: Occurrence, Properties and Health Effects. 1987, Washington, DC: American Chemical Society.

610. Forastiere, F., et al., Lung cancer and natural radiation in an Italian province. Sci Total Environ, 1985. 45:519–526.

611. Hofmann, W., R. Katz, and C.X. Zhang, Lung cancer incidence in a Chinese high background area—Epidemiological results and theoretical interpretation. Sci Total Environ, 1985. 45:527–534.

612. Mifune, M., et al., Cancer mortality survey in a spa area (Misasa, Japan) with a high radon background. Jpn J Cancer Res, 1992. 83(1):1–5.

613. Letourneau, E., et al., Lung cancer mortality and indoor radon concentrations in 18 Canadian cities. In Epidemiology Applied to Health Physics, G. S. Wilkinson ed. 1983, Springfield, Va: National Technical Information Service.

614. Haynes, R.M., The distribution of domestic radon concentrations and lung cancer mortality in England. Radiat Prot Dosim, 1988. 25:93–96.

615. Stockwell, H.G., et al., Lung cancer and indoor radon in Florida. Radiat Prot Dosim, 1988. 24:475–477.

616. Stockwell, H.G., et al., Lung cancer in Florida: Risks associated with residence in the central Florida phosphate mining region. Am J Epidemiol, 1988. 128(1):78–84.

617. Vonstille, W.T. and H.L. Sacarello, Radon and cancer. Journal of Environmental and Health, 1990. 53:25–28.

618. Alavanja, M.C., et al., Residential radon exposure and risk of lung cancer in Missouri. Am J Public Health, 1999. 89(7):1042–1048.

619. Bean, J.A., et al., Drinking water and cancer incidence in Iowa. II. Radioactivity in drinking water. Am J Epidemiol, 1982. 116(6):924–932.

620. Hess, C.T., C.V. Weiffenbach, and S.A. Norton, Environmental radon and cancer correlations in Maine. Health Phys, 1983. 45(2):339–348.

621. Fleischer, R.L., A possible association between lung cancer and a geological outcrop. Health Phys, 1986. 50(6):823–827.

622. Archer, V.E., Association of lung cancer mortality with precambrian granite. Arch Environ Health, 1987. 42(2):87–91.

623. Fleischer, R.L., A possible association between lung cancer and phosphate mining and processing. Health Phys, 1981. 41(1):171–175.

624. Cohen, B.L., Experimental test of the linear no-threshold theory of radiation carcinogenesis. In Environmental Radon: Occurrence, Control and Health Hazards, S.K. Majumdar, ed. 1990, Philadelphia: Pennsylvania Academy of Science.

625. Cohen, B.L., Test of the linear-no threshold theory of radiation carcinogenesis for inhaled radon decay products. Health Phys, 1995. 68(2):157–174.

626. Heath, C.W., Jr., et al., Residential radon exposure and lung cancer risk: Commentary on Cohen's county-based study. Health Phys, 2004. 87(6):647–655; discussion 656–658.

627. Alavanja, M.C., et al., Residential radon exposure and lung cancer among nonsmoking women. J Natl Cancer Inst, 1994. 86(24):1829–1837.

628. Schoenberg, J.B., et al., Case-control study of residential radon and lung cancer among New Jersey women. Cancer Res, 1990. 50(20):6520–6524.

629. Simpson, S.G. and G.W. Comstock, Lung cancer and housing characteristics. Arch Environ Health, 1983. 38(4):248–251.

630. Lees, R.E., R. Steele, and J.H. Roberts, A case-control study of lung cancer relative to domestic radon exposure. Int J Epidemiol, 1987. 16(1):7–12.

631. Letourneau, E.G., et al., Case-control study of residential radon and lung cancer in Winnipeg, Manitoba, Canada. Am J Epidemiol, 1994. 140(4):310–322.

632. Blot, W.J., et al., Indoor radon and lung cancer in China. J Natl Cancer Inst, 1990. 82(12):1025–1030.

633. Lubin, J.H., et al., Risk of lung cancer and residential radon in China: Pooled results of two studies. Int J Cancer, 2004. 109(1):132–137.

634. Svensson, C., G. Eklund, and G. Pershagen, Indoor exposure to radon from the ground and bronchial cancer in women. Int Arch Occup Environ Health, 1987. 59(2):123–131.

635. Svensson, C., G. Pershagen, and J. Klominek, Lung cancer in women and type of dwelling in relation to radon exposure. Cancer Res, 1989. 49(7):1861–1865.

636. Pershagen, G., et al., Residential radon exposure and lung cancer in Sweden. N Engl J Med, 1994. 330(3):159–164.

637. Axelson, O., C. Edling, and H. Kling, Lung cancer and residency: A case referent study on the possible impact of exposure to radon and its daughters in dwellings. Scand J Work Environ Health, 1979. 5:10–15.

638. Damber, L.A. and L.G. Larsson, Lung cancer in males and type of dwelling. An epidemiologic pilot study. Acta Oncol, 1987. 26(3):211–215.

639. Axelson, O., et al., Indoor radon exposure and active and passive smoking in relation to occurrence of lung cancer. Scand J Work Environ Health, 1988. 14:71–79.

640. Pershagen, G., et al., Radon in dwelling and cancer. In IMM Report 2/93. 1993, Stockholm: Karolinska Institute.

641. Wichmann, H.E., et al., Increased lung cancer risk due to residential radon in a pooled and extended analysis of studies in Germany. Health Phys, 2005. 88(1):71–79.

642. Darby, S., et al., Radon in homes and risk of lung cancer: Collaborative analysis of individual data from 13 European case-control studies. BMJ, 2005. 330(7485):223.

643. Darby, S., et al., Residential radon and lung cancer—Detailed results of a collaborative analysis of individual data on 7148 persons with lung cancer and 14,208 persons without lung cancer from 13 epidemiologic studies in Europe. Scand J Work Environ Health, 2006. 32(suppl 1):1–83.

644. Krewski, D., et al., Residential radon and risk of lung cancer: A combined analysis of 7 North American case-control studies. Epidemiology, 2005. 16(2):137–145.

645. Krewski, D., et al., A combined analysis of North American case-control studies of residential radon and lung cancer. J Toxicol Environ Health A, 2006. 69(7):533–597.

646. Lubin, J.H., et al., Lung cancer in radon-exposed miners and estimation of risk from indoor exposure. J Natl Cancer Inst, 1995. 87(11):817–827.

647. Chen, J., Estimated risks of radon-induced lung cancer for different exposure profiles based on the new EPA model. Health Phys, 2005. 88(4):323–333.

648. Sevc, J., E. Kunz, and V. Placek, Lung cancer in uranium miners and long-term exposure to radon daughter products. Health Phys, 1976. 30(6):433–437.

649. Horacek, J., V. Placek, and J. Sevc, Histologic types of bronchogenic cancer in relation to different conditions of radiation exposure. Cancer, 1977. 40(2):832–835.

650. Tomasek, L., et al., Patterns of lung cancer mortality among uranium miners in West Bohemia with varying rates of exposure to radon and its progeny. Radiat Res, 1994. 137(2):251–261.

651. Tirmarche, M., et al., Mortality of a cohort of French uranium miners exposed to relatively low radon concentrations. Br J Cancer, 1993. 67(5):1090–1097.

651a. Leuraud, K., S. Billon, D. Bergot, et al., Lung cancer risk associated to exposure to radon and smoking in a case-control stucy of French uranium miners. Helathy Phys, 2007. 92(4):371–378.

652. Xuan, X.Z., et al., A cohort study in southern China of tin miners exposed to radon and radon decay products. Health Phys, 1993. 64(2):120–131.

653. Ham, J.M., Report of the Royal Commission on the health and safety of workers in mines. 1976, Toronto: Ministry of the Attorney General..

654. Archer, V.E., J.K. Wagoner, and F.E. Lundin, Lung cancer among uranium miners in the United States. Health Phys, 1973. 25(4):351–371.

655. Archer, V.E., J.D. Gillam, and J.K. Wagoner, Respiratory disease mortality among uranium miners. Ann N Y Acad Sci, 1976. 271:280–293.

656. Archer, V.E., G. Saccomanno, and J.H. Jones, Frequency of different histologic types of bronchogenic carcinoma as related to radiation exposure. Cancer, 1974. 34(6):2056–2060.

657. Gilliland, F.D., et al., Radon progeny exposure and lung cancer risk among non-smoking uranium miners. Health Phys, 2000. 79(4):365–372.

658. de Villiers, A.J. and J.P. Windish, Lung cancer in the fluorspar community. I. Radiation, dust, and mortality experience. Brit J Ind Med, 1964. 21:94–109.

658a. Villeneuve, P.J., H.I. Morrison, and R. Lane, Radon and lung cancer risk: An extension of the mortality followup of the Newfoundland Fluorspar Cohort. Health Phys, 2007. 92(2):157–169.

659. Morrison, H.I., et al., Cancer mortality among a group of fluorspar miners exposed to radon progeny. Am J Epidemiol, 1988. 128(6):1266–1275.

660. Jogensen, H.S., A study of mortality among miners in Kiruna, 1950–1970. Work Environ Health, 1973. 10:125–133.

661. Snihs, J.O., The approach to radon problems in non-uranium mines in Sweden. In Third International Congress. 1974, Oak Ridge, Tenn: International Radiation Protection Association.

662. Howe, G.R., et al., Lung cancer mortality (1950–80) in relation to radon daughter exposure in a cohort of workers at the Eldorado Port Radium uranium mine: Possible modification of risk by exposure rate. J Natl Cancer Inst, 1987. 79(6):1255–1260.

663. Hornung, R.W. and T.J. Meinhardt, Quantitative risk assessment of lung cancer in U.S. uranium miners. Health Phys, 1987. 52(4):417–430.

664. Samet, J.M., et al., Lung cancer mortality and exposure to radon progeny in a cohort of New Mexico underground uranium miners. Health Phys, 1991. 61(6):745–752.

665. Muller, J., W.C. Wheeler, and J.F. Gentleman, Study of mortality of Ontario miners, 1955–1977. Part I. Report to the Ontario Ministry of Labour. 1983, Ontario: Ontario Worker's Compensation Board and Atomic Energy Control Board of Canada.

666. Howe, G.R., et al., Lung cancer mortality (1950–80) in relation to radon daughter exposure in a cohort of workers at the Eldorado Beaverlodge uranium mine. J Natl Cancer Inst, 1986. 77(2):357–362.

667. Sevc, J., et al., A survey of the Czechoslovak follow-up of lung cancer mortality in uranium miners. Health Phys, 1993. 64(4):355–369.

668. Radford, E.P. and K.G. Renard, Lung cancer in Swedish iron miners exposed to low doses of radon daughters. N Engl J Med, 1984. 310(23):1485–1494.

669. Chambers, D., et al., Reconstruction of the radon daughter exposure of Beaverlodge uranium miners. 1992, Montreal: International Radiation Protection Association.

670. Woodward, A., et al., Radon daughter exposures at the Radium Hill uranium mine and lung cancer rates among former workers, 1952–87. Cancer Causes Control, 1991. 2(4):213–220.

671. Voelz, G.L., J.N. Lawrence, and E.R. Johnson, Fifty years of plutonium exposure to the Manhattan Project plutonium workers: An update. Health Phys, 1997. 73(4):611–619.

672. Wing, S. and D.B. Richardson, Age at exposure to ionising radiation and cancer mortality among Hanford workers: Follow-up through 1994. Occup Environ Med, 2005. 62(7):465–472.

673. Brown, S.C., et al., Lung cancer and internal lung doses among plutonium workers at the Rocky Flats Plant: A case-control study. Am J Epidemiol, 2004. 160(2):163–172.

674. Kreisheimer, M., et al., Lung cancer mortality among male nuclear workers of the Mayak facilities in the former Soviet Union. Radiat Res, 2000. 154(1):3–11.

675. Hall, P., G. Lundell, and L.E. Holm, Mortality in patients treated for hyperthyroidism with iodine-131. Acta Endocrinol (Copenhagen), 1993. 128(3):230–234.

676. Hoffman, D.A., et al., Cancer incidence following treatment of hyperthyroidism. Int J Epidemiol, 1982. 11(3):218–224.

677. Mori, T., et al., Current status of the Japanese followup study of the thorotrast patients and its relationships to the statistical analysis of the autopsy series. In Risks from Radium and Thorotrast, D. Taylor, ed. 1989, London: British Institute of Radiology.

678. Polednak, A.P., A.F. Stehney, and H.F. Lucas, Mortality among male workers at a thorium-processing plant. Health Phys, 1983. 44(suppl 1):S239–S251.

679. van Leeuwen, F.E., et al., Roles of radiotherapy and smoking in lung cancer following Hodgkin's disease. J Natl Cancer Inst, 1995. 87(20):1530–1537.

680. Kreisheimer, M., et al., Lung cancer mortality among nuclear workers of the Mayak facilities in the former Soviet Union: An updated analysis considering smoking as the main confounding factor. Radiat Environ Biophys, 2003. 42(2):129–135.

681. van Kaick, G., et al., Epidemiological results and dosimetric calculations: An update of the German Thorotrast study. In Effects of Internally Deposited Radionuclides: Emphasis on Radium and Thorium, G. van Kaick, ed. 1995, Singapore: World Scientific.

682. Kusiak, R.A., et al., Carcinoma of the lung in Ontario gold miners: Possible aetiological factors. Br J Ind Med, 1991. 48(12):808–817.

683. Morrison, H.I., et al., Radon-progeny exposure and lung cancer risk in a cohort of Newfoundland fluorspar miners. Radiat Res, 1998. 150(1):58–65.

684. Howe, G.R. and R.H. Stager, Risk of lung cancer mortality after exposure to radon decay products in the Beaverlodge cohort based on revised exposure estimates. Radiat Res, 1996. 146(1):37–42.

685. Rogel, A., et al., Lung cancer risk in the French cohort of uranium miners. J Radiol Prot, 2002. 22(3A):A101–A106.

686. Hodgson, J., and R. Jones, Mortality of a cohort of tin miners 1941–1986. Brit J Indust Med, 1990. 47(10):665–676.

687. Wang, Z., et al., Residential radon and lung cancer risk in a high-exposure area of Gansu Province, China. Am J Epidemiol, 2002. 155(6):554–564.

688. Oberaigner, W., et al., Radon und lungenkrebs in bezirk Imst/Osterreich. In Fortschritte in der Umweltmedizin. 2002, Landsberg am Lech: Ecomed Velagsgesellschaft.

689. Tomasek, L., et al., Study of lung cancer and residential radon in the Czech Republic. Cent Eur J Public Health, 2001. 9(3):150–153.

690. Auvinen, A., et al., Indoor radon exposure and risk of lung cancer: A nested case-control study in Finland. J Natl Cancer Inst, 1996. 88(14):966–972.

691. Ruosteenoja, E., et al., Radon and lung cancer in Finland. Health Phys, 1996. 71(2):185–189.

692. Baysson, H., et al., Case-control study on lung cancer and indoor radon in France. Epidemiology, 2004. 15:709–716.

693. Bochicchio, F., et al., Residential radon exposure, diet and lung cancer: A case-control study in a Mediterranean region. Int J Cancer, 2005. 114(6):983–991.

694. Barros-Dios, J.M., et al., Exposure to residential radon and lung cancer in Spain: A population-based case-control study. Am J Epidemiol, 2002. 156(6):548–555.

695. Lagarde, F., et al., Residential radon and lung cancer among never-smokers in Sweden. Epidemiology, 2001. 12(4):396–404.

696. Pershagen, G., et al., Residential radon exposure and lung cancer in Swedish women. Health Phys, 1992. 63(2):179–186.

697. Darby, S., et al., Risk of lung cancer associated with residential radon exposure in south-west England: A case-control study. Br J Cancer, 1998. 78(3):394–408.

698. Field, R.W., et al., Residential radon gas exposure and lung cancer: The Iowa Radon Lung Cancer Study. Am J Epidemiol, 2000. 151(11):1091–1102.

699. Sandler, D.P., et al., Indoor radon and lung cancer risk in Connecticut and Utah. J Toxicol Environ Health A, 2006. 69(7):633–654.

700. Higginson, J., C. Muir, and N. Munoz, Human Cancer: Epidemiology and Environmental Causes. 1992, Cambridge: Cambridge University Press.

701. Darby, S.C., et al., Further follow up of mortality and incidence of cancer in men from the United Kingdom who part icipated in the United Kingdom's atmospheric nuclear weapon tests and experimental programmes. BMJ, 1993. 307(6918):1530–1535.

702. Fraser, P., et al., Cancer mortality and morbidity in employees of the United Kingdom Atomic Energy Authority, 1946–86. Br J Cancer, 1993. 67(3):615–624.

703. Acquavella, J.F., et al., Mortality among workers at the Pantex weapons facility. Health Phys, 1985. 48(6):735–746.

704. Storm, H.H., Second primary cancer after treatment for cervical cancer: Late effects after radiotherapy. Cancer, 1988. 61(4):679–688.

705. Travis, L.B., et al., Second cancers among 40,576 testicular cancer patients: Focus on long-term survivors. J Natl Cancer Inst, 2005. 97(18):1354–1365.

706. Curtis, R.E., et al., Second cancer following cancer of the female genital system in Connecticut, 1935–82. Natl Cancer Inst Monogr, 1985. 68:113–137.

707. Romanenko, A., et al., Pathology and proliferative activity of renal-cell carcinomas (RCCs) and renal oncocytomas in patients with different radiation exposure after the Chernobyl accident in Ukraine. Int J Cancer, 2000. 87(6):880–883.

708. Vozianov, A., V. Bebeshko, and D. Bazyka, eds. Health Effects of the Chernobyl Accident. 2003, Kiev, Ukraine: Academy of Medical Sciences of the Ukraine.

709. Cohen, S. and S. Johansson, Epidemiology and etiology of bladder cancer. Urol Clin North Am, 1992. 19:421–428.

710. Kerr, M., K. Griegor, and D. Tolley, Rhabdomyosarcoma of the adult urinary bladder after radiotherapy for carcinoma. Clin Oncol (R Coll Radiol), 1999. 1(2):115–118.

711. Winters, J.C. and H.A. Fuselier, Jr., Invasive bladder cancer following 125iodine implants. J Urol, 1992. 148(6):1898–1900.

712. Ewertz, M., et al., Endometrial cancer following treatment for breast cancer: A case-control study in Denmark. Br J Cancer, 1984. 50(5):687–692.

713. Parkash, V. and M.L. Carcangiu, Uterine papillary serous carcinoma after radiation therapy for carcinoma of the cervix. Cancer, 1992. 69(2):496–501.

714. Ennow, K., et al., Epidemiological assessment of the cancer risk among the staff in radiotherapy departments in Denmark. In Low Dose Radiation: Biological Basis of Risk Assessment, K. Baverstock and J. Stather, eds. 1989, London: Taylor and Francis.

715. Voelz, G.L. and J.N. Lawrence, A 42-y medical follow-up of Manhattan Project plutonium workers. Health Phys, 1991. 61(2):181–190.

716. Whatley, W.S., J.W. Thompson, and B. Rao, Salivary gland tumors in survivors of childhood cancer. Otolaryngol Head Neck Surg, 2006. 134(3):385–388.

717. Shimizu, Y., H. Kato, and W.J. Schull, Mortality among atomic bomb survivors. J Radiat Res (Tokyo), 1991. 32(suppl):212–230.

718. Prescott, R. and A. Mainwaring, Irradiation-induced penile angiosarcoma. Postgrad Med J, 1990. 66:576–579.

719. Doll, R., Cancers weakly related to smoking. Br Med Bull, 1996. 52(1):35–49.

720. Gusev, B.I., R.I. Rosenson, and Z.N. Abylkassimova, The Semipalatinsk nuclear test site: A first analysis of solid cancer incidence (selected sites) due to test-related radiation. Radiat Environ Biophys, 1998. 37(3):209–214.

721. Epidemiological Study Group of Nuclear Workers (Japan), First analysis of mortality of nucelar workers in Japan 1986–1992. J Health Phys, 1997. 32:173–184.

722. Ito, C., et al., Study of stomach cancer in atomic bomb survivors. Report 1. Histological findings and prognosis. J Radiat Res (Tokyo), 1989. 30(2):164–175.

723. van Leeuwen, F.E., et al., Second cancer risk following testicular cancer: A follow-up study of 1,909 patients. J Clin Oncol, 1993. 11(3):415–424.

724. Hassle, S., et al., Cancer risk in the reindeer-breeding Saami population of Sweden, 1961–1997. Eur J Epidemiol, 2001. 17(10):969–976.

725. Auvinen, A., et al., Radon and other natural radionuclides in drinking water and risk of stomach cancer: A case-cohort study in Finland. Int J Cancer, 2005. 114(1):109–113.

726. Ye, W., et al., Mortality and cancer incidence in Misasa, Japan, a spa area with elevated radon levels. Jpn J Cancer Res, 1998. 89(8):789–796.

727. Hirose, Y., et al., Erythroleukemia and gastric cancer following Thorotrast injection. Jpn J Med, 1991. 30(1):43–46.

728. Potter, J., et al., Colon cancer: A review of the epidemiology. Epidemiol Rev, 1993. 15:449–545.

729. Nakatsuka, H., et al., Colorectal cancer incidence among atomic bomb survivors, 1950–80. J Radiat Res (Tokyo), 1992. 33(4):342–361.

730. Baxter, N.N., et al., Increased risk of rectal cancer after prostate radiation: A population-based study. Gastroenterology, 2005. 128(4):819–824.

731. Rubino, C., et al., Radiation exposure and familial aggregation of cancers as risk factors for colorectal cancer after radioiodine treatment for thyroid carcinoma. Int J Radiat Oncol Biol Phys, 2005. 62(4):1084–1089.

732. Kovalic, J.J., et al., Hepatocellular carcinoma as second malignant neoplasms in successfully treated Wilms' tumor patients. A National Wilms' Tumor Study report. Cancer, 1991. 67(2):342–344.

733. van Kaick, G., et al., Neoplastic diseases induced by chronic alpha-irradiation—Epidemiological, biophysical and clinical results of the German Thorotrast Study. J Radiat Res (Tokyo), 1991. 32(suppl 2):20–33.

734. Andersson, M., et al., Primary liver tumors among Danish patients exposed to Thorotrast. Radiat Res, 1994. 137(2):262–273.

735. Mori, T., and Y. Kato, Epidemiological, pathological and dosimetric status of Japanese Thorotrast patients. J Radiat Res (Tokyo), 1991. 32(suppl 2):34–45.

736. dos Santos Silva, I., F. Malveiro, et al., Mortality from primary liver cancers in the Portuguese Thorotrast cohort study. In Health Effects of Internally Depositied Radionuclides: Emphasis on Radiation and Thorium, G. van Kaick, ed. 1995, Singapore: World Scientific, pp. 229–233.

737. Kauppinen, T., et al., Pancreatic cancer and occupational exposures. Epidemiology, 1995. 6(5):498–502.

738. Wang, J.X., et al., Cancer incidence among medical diagnostic x-ray workers in China, 1950 to 1985. Int J Cancer, 1990. 45(5):889–895.

739. Birdwell, S.H., et al., Gastrointestinal cancer after treatment of Hodgkin's disease. Int J Radiat Oncol Biol Phys, 1997. 37(1):67–73.

740. Rokkas, T., T. Palmer, and G. Sladen, Tumors of the pancreas as a sequel to abdominal irradiation. Postgrad Med J, 1989. 65:493–496.

741. Wiklund, K., L.E. Holm, and G. Eklund, Mortality among Swedish reindeer breeding Lapps in 1961–85. Arctic Med Res, 1991. 50(1):3–7.

742. Pinkerton, L.E., et al., Mortality among a cohort of uranium mill workers: An update. Occup Environ Med, 2004. 61(1):57–64.

743. Spiess, H. and G. Mays, Protraction effect on bone sarcoma induction of radium 224 in children and adults. In Radionuclide Carcinogenesis, C. Sanders, R. Busch, and G. Ballou, eds. 1973, Springfield, Va, United States Army Environmental Command.

744. Spiess, H. and C.W. Mays, Bone cancers induced by ^{224}Ra (Th X) in children and adults. Health Phys, 1970. 19(6):713–729.

745. Kim, J.H., et al., Radiation-induced soft-tissue and bone sarcoma. Radiology, 1978. 129(2):501–508.

746. Marshall, J.H. and P.G. Groer, A theory of the induction of bone cancer by alpha radiation. Radiat Res, 1977. 71(1):149–192.

747. Edgar, M.A. and M.P. Robinson, Post-radiation sarcoma in ankylosing spondylitis: A report of five cases. J Bone Joint Surg Br, 1973. 55(1):183–188.

748. Smith, L.M., R.S. Cox, and S.S. Donaldson, Second cancers in long-term survivors of Ewing's sarcoma. Clin Orthop Relat Res, 1992. (274):275–281.

749. Sagerman, R.H., et al., Radiation induced neoplasia following external beam therapy for children with retinoblastoma. Am J Roentgenol Radium Ther Nucl Med, 1969. 105(3):529–535.

750. Schimke, R.N., J.T. Lowman, and A.B. Cowan, Retinoblastoma and osteogenic sarcoma in siblings. Cancer, 1974. 34(6):2077–2079.

751. Woodard, H.Q., A.G. Huvos, and J. Smith, Radiation-induced malignant tumors of bone in patients with Hodgkin's disease. Health Phys, 1988. 55(4):615–620.

752. Huvos, A.G. and H.Q. Woodard, Postradiation sarcomas of bone. Health Phys, 1988. 55(4):631–636.

753. Laskin, W.B., T.A. Silverman, and F.M. Enzinger, Postradiation soft tissue sarcomas: An analysis of 53 cases. Cancer, 1988. 62(11):2330–2340.

754. Newton, W.A., Jr., et al., Bone sarcomas as second malignant neoplasms following childhood cancer. Cancer, 1991. 67(1):193–201.

755. Tillotson, C., et al., Postradiation multicentric osteosarcoma. Cancer, 1988. 62(1):67–71.

756. Vanel, D., et al., Chondrosarcoma in children subsequent to other malignant tumours in different locations. Skeletal Radiol, 1984. 11(2):96–101.

757. Arlen, M., et al., Radiation-induced sarcoma of bone. Cancer, 1971. 28(5):1087–1099.

758. Kim, J.H., et al., Radiation induced sarcomas of bone following therapeutic radiation. Int J Radiat Oncol Biol Phys, 1983. 9(1):107–110.

759. Sordillo, P.P., et al., Extraosseous osteogenic sarcoma: A review of 48 patients. Cancer, 1983. 51(4):727–734.

760. Jaffe, N., et al., Radiation induced osteochondroma in long-term survivors of childhood cancer. Int J Radiat Oncol Biol Phys, 1983. 9(5):665–670.

761. Neuhauser, E., et al., Radiation effects of roentgen therapy on the growing spine. Radiology, 1952. 59:637–650.

762. Rowland, R., et al., Some dose response relationships for tumor incidence in radium patients. Annual Report, July 1969–June 1970, R.P. Division. 1970, Washington, DC: Center for Human Radiobiology.

763. Travis, L.B., R.L. Kathren, and J.D. Boice, Jr., Cancer risk following exposure to Thorotrast: Overview in relation to a case report. Health Phys, 1992. 63(1):89–97.

764. Mays, C.W., Risk to bone from present radium 224 therapy. In Biological Effects of Radium 224: Benefit and Risk of Therapeutic Applications, W. Muller and H. Ebert, eds. 1978, The Hague: Nijoff Medical Division.

765. Spiess, H. and C.W. Mays, Protraction effects on bone sarcoma induction of ^{224}Ra in children and adults. In Radionuclide Carcinogenesis. 1973, Washington, DC: U.S. Atomic Energy Commission.

766. Chemelevsky, D., et al., The reverse protraction factor in the induction of bone sarcomas in radium 224 patients. Radiat Res, 1990. 124(suppl 10):S69–S79.

767. Mays, C.W. and H. Shiest. Epidemiological studies of German patients injected with radium 224. In Epidemiology Applied to Health Physics. Proceedings of the Sixteenth Mid-year Topical Meeting of the Health Physics Society, Albuquerque, NM. 1983, Springfield, Va: National Technical Information Service Society.

768. Evans, R.D., A. Keane, and M. Shanahan, Radiation effects in man of long-term skeletal alpha irradiation. In Radiobiology of Plutonium, B. Stover and W. Jee, eds. 1972, Salt Lake City, Utah, University of Utah/JW Press.

769. Rowland, R., et al., Tumor incidence in radium patient. 1971, Argonne, Ill: Argonne National Laboratory.

770. Argonne National Laboratory, Data for radium patients. In Center for Human Biology Exposure. 1977, Argonne, Ill: Argonne National Laboratory.

771. Baverstock, K. and D.G. Papworth, The U.K. radium luminiser survey. In Risks from Radium and Thorotrast, D. Taylor, ed. 1989, London: British Institute of London.

772. Puskin, J.S., N.S. Nelson, and C.B. Nelson, Bone cancer risk estimates. Health Phys, 1992. 63(5):579–580.

773. Brady, M.S., J.J. Gaynor, and M.F. Brennan, Radiation-associated sarcoma of bone and soft tissue. Arch Surg, 1992. 127(12):1379–1385.

774. Foley, K.M., et al., Radiation-induced malignant and atypical peripheral nerve sheath tumors. Ann Neurol, 1980. 7(4):311–318.

775. Ducatman, B.S., et al., Malignant peripheral nerve sheath tumors: A clinicopathologic study of 120 cases. Cancer, 1986. 57(10):2006–2021.

776. Ducatman, B.S. and B.W. Scheithauer, Postirradiation neurofibrosarcoma. Cancer, 1983. 51(6):1028–1033.

777. Egger, J.F., et al., Radiation-associated synovial sarcoma: Clinicopathologic and molecular analysis of two cases. Mod Pathol, 2002. 15(9):998–1004.

778. de Vathaire, F., et al., Role of radiotherapy and chemotherapy in the risk of second malignant neoplasms after cancer in childhood. Br J Cancer, 1989. 59(5):792–796.

779. Menu-Branthomme, A., et al., Radiation dose, chemotherapy and risk of soft tissue sarcoma after solid tumours during childhood. Int J Cancer, 2004. 110(1):87–93.

780. Friedman, D.L., et al., Increased risk of cancer among siblings of long-term childhood cancer survivors: A report from the childhood cancer survivor study. Cancer Epidemiol Biomarkers Prev, 2005. 14(8):1922–1927.

781. Wong, F.L., et al., Cancer incidence after retinoblastoma: Radiation dose and sarcoma risk. JAMA, 1997. 278(15):1262–1267.

782. Steeves, R.A. and J.P. Bataini, Neoplasms induced by megavoltage radiation in the head and neck region. Cancer, 1981. 47(7):1770–1774.

783. Shore-Freedman, E., et al., Neurilemomas and salivary gland tumors of the head and neck following childhood irradiation. Cancer, 1983. 51(12):2159–2163.

784. Taghian, A., et al., Long-term risk of sarcoma following radiation treatment for breast cancer. Int J Radiat Oncol Biol Phys, 1991. 21(2):361–367.

785. Rubino, C., et al., Radiation dose and risk of soft tissue and bone sarcoma after breast cancer treatment. Breast Cancer Res Treat, 2005. 89(3):277–288.

786. Billings, S.D., et al., Cutaneous angiosarcoma following breast-conserving surgery and radiation: An analysis of 27 cases. Am J Surg Pathol, 2004. 28(6):781–788.

787. Aydogdu, M. and G. Trams, Angiosarcoma of the breast after conservatively operated breast carcinoma—a sequela of adjuvant radiotherapy?. Geburtshilfe Frauenheilkd, 1996. 56(1):60–62.

788. Karlsson, P., et al., Soft tissue sarcoma after treatment for breast cancer—A Swedish population-based study. Eur J Cancer, 1998. 34(13):2068–2075.

789. Kim, M.K., et al., Secondary angiosarcoma following irradiation—Case report and review of the literature. Radiat Med, 1998. 16(1):55–60.

790. Ruka, W., et al., Induced soft tissue sarcomas following radiation treatment for uterine carcinomas. Eur J Surg Oncol, 1991. 17(6):585–593.

791. Wiklund, T.A., et al., Postirradiation sarcoma: Analysis of a nationwide cancer registry material. Cancer, 1991. 68(3):524–531.

792. Jacobsen, G.K., et al., Increased incidence of sarcoma in patients treated for testicular seminoma. Eur J Cancer, 1993. 29(5):A664–A668.

793. Schlemmer, H.P., et al., Locoregional late effects of paravascular thorotrast deposits: Results of the German Thorotrast study. J Neuroradiol, 2000. 27(4):253–263.

794. Hasson, J., et al., Thorotrast-induced extraskeletal osteosarcoma of the cervical region: Report of a case. Cancer, 1975. 36(5):1827–1833.

795. Hawkins, M.M., et al., Radiotherapy, alkylating agents, and risk of bone cancer after childhood cancer. J Natl Cancer Inst, 1996. 88(5):270–278.

796. Mohan, A.K., et al., Breast cancer mortality among female radiologic technologists in the United States. J Natl Cancer Inst, 2002. 94(12):943–948.

797. Carnes, B.A., P.G. Groer, and T.J. Kotek, Radium dial workers: Issues concerning dose response and modeling. Radiat Res, 1997. 147(6):707–714.

798. Stehney, A.F., Survival times of pre-1950 U.S. women radium dial workers. In Health Effects of Internally Deposited Radionuclides: Emphasis on Radium and Thorium, G. van Kaick, ed. 1995, Singapore: World Scientific, pp. 149–155.

799. dos Santos Silva, I., et al., Mortality in the Portuguese Thorotrast study. Radiat Res, 1999. 152(suppl 6):S88–S92.

800. International Commission on Radiological Protection (ICRP), The biological basis for dose limitation in the skin: A report of a Task Group of Committee 1 of the ICRP. Ann ICRP, 1991. 22(2):1–104.

801. Mole, R.H., Radiation induced tumours—Human experience. Br J Radiol, 1972. 45(536):613.

802. Black, M.M. and E.W. Jones, Dermal cylindroma following x-ray epilation of the scalp. Br J Dermatol, 1971. 85(1):70–72.

803. Traenkl, H., X-ray induced skin cancer in man in biology of cutaneous cancer. U.S. National Cancer Institute Monograph, 1963. 10:423–432.

804. Sadamori, N., et al., Incidence of skin cancer among Nagasaki atomic bomb survivors (preliminary report). J Radiat Res (Tokyo), 1990. 31(3):280–287.

805. Sadamori, N., M. Mine, and M. Hori, Skin cancer among atom bomb survivors. Lancet, 1989. 1(8649):1267.

806. Sadamori, N., M. Otake, and T. Honda, Study of skin cancer incidence in Nagasaki atomic bomb survivors, 1958–1985. 1991, Hiroshima, Japan: Radiation Effects Research Foundation.

807. Sadamori, N., M. Mine, and T. Honda, Incidence of skin cancer among Nagasaki atomic bomb survivors. J Radiat Res (Tokyo), 1991. 32(suppl 2):217–225.

808. Sevcova, M., J. Sevc, and J. Thomas, Alpha irradiation of the skin and the possibility of late effects. Health Phys, 1978. 35(6):803–806.

809. Sevcova, M., et al., Incidence of skin basalioma in miner and non-miner groups: Comparison of epidemiological studies. Ceskoslovenska Dermatol, 1984. 59:1–5.

810. International Commission on Radiological Protection (ICRP), The biological basis for dose limitation in the skin: A report of a Task Group of Committee 1 of the ICRP. Ann ICRP, 1991. 22(2):1–104.

811. Modan, B., et al., Factors affecting the development of skin cancer after scalp irradiation. Radiat Res, 1993. 135(1):125–128.

812. Ron, E., et al., Radiation-induced skin carcinomas of the head and neck. Radiat Res, 1991. 125(3):318–325.

813. Shore, R.E., et al., Skin cancer incidence among children irradiated for ringworm of the scalp. Radiat Res, 1984. 100(1):192–204.

814. Sulzberger, M.B., R.L. Baer, and A. Borota, Do roentgen-ray treatments as given by skin specialists produce cancers or other sequelae? AMA Arch Derm Syphilol, 1952. 65(6):639–655.

815. Lindelof, B. and G. Eklund, Incidence of malignant skin tumors in 14,140 patients after grenz-ray treatment for benign skin disorders. Arch Dermatol, 1986. 122(12):1391–1395.

816. Veien, N.K., et al., Late effects of x-ray treatment of warts. J Dermatol Surg Oncol, 1982. 8(4):275–281.

817. Hildreth, N.G., et al., Risk of extrathyroid tumors following radiation treatment in infancy for thymic enlargement. Radiat Res, 1985. 102(3):378–391.

818. Van Daal, W.A., et al., Radiation-induced head and neck tumours: Is the skin as sensitive as the thyroid gland? Eur J Cancer Clin Oncol, 1983. 19(8):1081–1086.

819. Meadows, A.T., et al., Patterns of second malignant neoplasms in children. Cancer, 1977. 40(suppl 4):1903–1911.

820. Little, M., M. Charles, and J.W. Hopewell, Assessment of skin doses. National Radiation Protection Board, U.K. 1997, Chilton, U.K.: Didcot.

821. Shore, R.E., et al., Skin cancer after x-ray treatment for scalp ringworm. Radiat Res, 2002. 157(4):410–418.

822. Caldwell, G.G., et al., Mortality and cancer frequency among military nuclear test (Smoky) participants, 1957 through 1979. JAMA, 1983. 250(5):620–624.

823. Austin, D.F., et al., Malignant melanoma among employees of Lawrence Livermore National Laboratory. Lancet, 1981. 2(8249):712–716.

824. Moore, D.H., 2nd, et al., Case-control study of malignant melanoma among employees of the Lawrence Livermore National Laboratory. Am J Ind Med, 1997. 32(4):377–391.

825. Donald Whorton, M., et al., Cancer incidence rates among Lawrence Livermore National Laboratory (LLNL) employees: 1974–1997. Am J Ind Med, 2004. 45(1):24–33.

826. Acquavella, J.F., et al., A melanoma case-control study at the Los Alamos National Laboratory. Health Phys, 1983. 45(3):587–592.

827. Rubin, P., and G. Casarett, Clinical Radiation Pathology. 1966, Philadelphia: W.B. Saunders.

6 Deterministic Effects of Radiation

In contrast to the mutagenic and carcinogenic effects of ionizing radiation, which are assumed to increase in frequency as nonthreshold functions of the dose, the deterministic or "nonstochastic" effects of radiation have appreciable thresholds above which they increase in both frequency and severity with further increase in the dose. With the exception of cataracts, cell killing is central to all deterministic effects. Apoptosis, or programmed cell death, varies among tissues; the dividing cells in radiosensitive tissues undergo apoptosis with a much greater frequency than do the postmitotic cells in other tissues (such as fibroblasts).[1]

An example of such a nonstochastic, or deterministic, radiation effect is bone marrow depression. Almost all individuals who receive a whole-body, single dose of radiation in excess of 5 grays (Gy) will experience bone marrow depression. Additionally, although there is some individual variation, virtually no one who receives less than 0.5 Gy in a single, whole-body exposure will demonstrate clinical bone marrow depression. Thus, for practical purposes, deterministic, or nonstochastic, effects have a threshold dose. The deterministic effects observed in an individual depend on the dose received, volume of tissue irradiated, quality or type of radiation, and time over which the dose is received. Deterministic effects observed also depend on the time of observation after irradiation. A given organ is composed of (1) parenchymal cells that have some specific functions for that organ, (2) structural cells that give the organ its form, and (3) vascular tissue that supplies blood to the organ. Each of these three components usually has a different sensitivity to radiation and a different time course of presentation of deterministic radiation effects. Initial effects that are evident clinically may result from dysfunction of the parenchymal cells; however, if the organ survives, late effects may be due to obliterative vascular changes within the organ (Fig. 6-1). The most comprehensive review of nonstochastic effects may be found in the multivolume text by Rubin and Casarett.[2] Other publications, including textbooks on radiation pathology by Fajardo[3] and Scherer et al.[4] and the UNSCEAR reports,[5–7] also have information on late deterministic effects. For complications of specific radiotherapy schemes, the reader is referred to a comprehensive text by Perez.[8] Although effects of radiation on the embryo and fetus (such as induction of malformations) are deterministic effects, they will be discussed separately in Chapter 8.

Radiation oncologists have devised a scoring system for toxicity in an attempt to have uniform reporting of deterministic effects.[9] The LENT (Late Effects Normal Tissue) system uses the acronym SOMA (subjective, objective, management, and analytic). *Subjective* refers to what is generally reported as symptoms by the patient, *objective* refers to findings of a skilled clinician, *management* refers to measures taken to alleviate or reduce toxicity, and *analytic* refers to laboratory and procedural findings. These measures can be combined into a summary score. The system uses grades 1 to 4 for degree of toxicity. Grade 0 is not used as it would indicate no toxicity, and Grade 5 is not used as it indicates a fatal outcome. SOMA toxicity tables related to various organ systems are presented in Appendix 6.

The realization that deterministic radiation effects occurred in the human followed within 1 year of Roentgen's discovery of x-rays in 1896. Until the mid-1940s, it was a relatively common practice to calibrate the output of x-ray tubes by using deterministic radiation effects on humans. This practice, which involved exposing the skin of the leg or arm until erythema was produced, was abandoned when modern radiation protection and accurate calibration of machinery were introduced. Deterministic effects in humans have since been seen in the few high-level radiation accidents and, clinically, in radiation therapy. Since it is rarely possible to sterilize a cancer without having an adverse effect on the normal surrounding tissue, radiotherapists have developed the concept of a tolerance dose (TD). As discussed in Chapter 2, the tolerance dose depends on the level of risk of deterministic effects on normal tissue that the physician is willing to accept to cure a tumor. The TD5 refers to a dose that is expected to result in a 0% to 5% incidence of serious complications or side effects. It is important to realize that the TD can hardly be termed a dose that is tolerable to a healthy individual but rather refers to the dose that is tolerable or acceptable to the patient to cure a cancer. The significance of the "tolerance dose" for this text is that the practice of radiotherapy using the TD has provided a relatively large body of literature on the

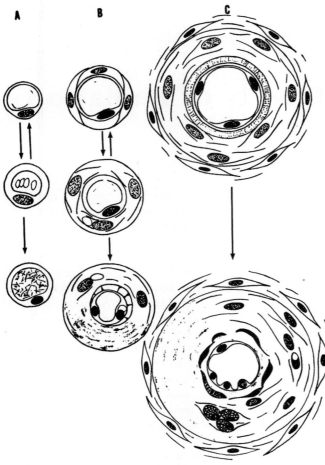

Figure 6-1 • Diagram of radiation injury involving capillary (**A**), arteriole (**B**), and small artery (**C**). Initially the capillary dilates and has increased permeability; later, with narrowing of the lumen and sclerosis of the wall, a thrombus may form causing occlusion of the lumen. Changes in the arteriole are quite similar to those seen in the capillary. With the small artery, less dilatation of the lumen occurs initially, since the wall is more rigid; later progressive damage to the endothelium with narrowing of the lumen occurs. (From Anderson WAD, Kissane JM (eds): Pathology. St. Louis, Mosby, 1977.)

incidence and dose levels required to produce deterministic effects in normal tissue, their time course, and their dependence on quality and temporal distribution of the irradiation.

GENERAL ASPECTS

Radiation effects do not produce pathognomonic, histologic, or morphologic changes that allow a given tissue to be examined and described as having been exposed to ionizing radiation. The tissue can be analyzed for changes that are similar to changes seen following known radiation exposure. If such changes are identified, then radiation can be included in the list of possible etiologies of these changes. Deterministic radiation effects have been classified into a somewhat arbitrary temporal scheme by Rubin

and Casarett.[2] In their scheme, acute effects are those occurring within the first 6 months; subacute, 6 to 12 months; chronic clinical period, 2 through 5 years; and late clinical period, after year 5. Fajardo divides pathologic effects into immediate, acute (days to weeks), and delayed (months to years).[3] Obviously the effects observed are a spectrum of cellular responses occurring over various times, and often these cannot be strictly related to temporal classifications.

Deterministic effects of radiation can be enhanced and suppressed by various modifying agents and conditions. Chemical and physical factors are discussed in Chapter 2, and genetic predisposition causing enhanced radiation damage in Chapter 3. More specific conditions are discussed in Chapter 7 (in the discussion of radiation in combination with other agents). Acute deterministic effects usually result from necrosis of the rapidly proliferative cell lines (particularly those of the intestine, bone marrow, germinal cells, and embryonal tissues); necrosis may be accompanied by transient vascular dilatation at the capillary level. There is rarely a cellular exudate (which might be expected in an inflammatory response), and Fajardo mentions that the suffix *-itis* is usually inappropriate for most acute effects of radiation on tissues such as the skin and heart.[3] Delayed lesions are usually progressive stromal lesions whose full clinical impact comes long after progressive fibrosis can be demonstrated pathologically. Fibrosis is the result of edema followed by fibrinous exudate, fibrin deposition, and collagen formation. The most characteristic delayed radiation lesion is eccentric myointimal proliferation of the small arteries and arterioles. It should be pointed out that the Radiation Effects Research Foundation (RERF) in Hiroshima, Japan, is now using the following categories to classify radiation effects: hereditary, cancer, and noncancer.

SKIN AND MUCOSA

The skin is considered a body organ. It has a surface area of about 2 m^2. The skin serves not only as a barrier against the environment but is also involved in immune function, in control of the body's temperature, and as a medium to provide sensory input. The skin has a series of layers that must be considered to understand potential radiation effects. The outer group of layers is derived from the embryonic ectoderm and makes up the epidermis. The inner layers, which are formed from embryonic mesenchyme, collectively form the dermis. The epidermis is composed of an outer layer of dead cells (stratum corneum). The thickness of this layer, about 20 cells thick, varies markedly in different portions of the body, being thicker on the palms and soles. A middle epidermal layer (stratum granulosum) is about 4 to 5 cells thick and provides a transition between the dead cells and the underlying viable layers (stratum germinativum and stratum spinosum). These two layers determine the majority of

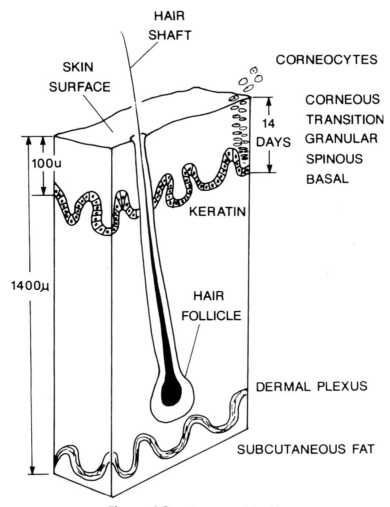

Figure 6-2 • Structure of the skin.

radiation response. There is an underlying, undulating, and proliferating basal cell layer. Cells derived from the basal layer travel toward the surface and eventually die and are sloughed. This process takes about 14 days (Fig. 6-2). The average epidermal layer thickness is 20 to 40 μm on the face and trunk, 40 to 60 μm on the arms and legs, about 85 μm on the backs of the hands, and the greatest thickness on the fingertips is about 150 to 300 μm. Immune functions appear to be a result of Langerhans cells that have migrated from the bone marrow to the skin.

The epidermis is separated from the dermis by a basement membrane. The dermis has two distinct layers: the superficial papillary dermis and the thicker reticular dermis. The dermis is about 1.3 mm in thickness. The superficial layer is composed of collagen bundles and elastic fibers and is the primary layer for thermoregulation and nourishment of the lower layers of the epidermis. The reticular dermis is densely fibrous and is the primary structural layer of the skin. In simplistic terms, the clinical radiation response can be visualized after the skin

structure is understood. Alpha particles are not able to penetrate even the top two or three layers of dead cells in the stratum corneum. Beta radiation can penetrate further and often affects the proliferating cells at the basal layer. More penetrating radiations, such as cobalt 60 photons, may actually be skin sparing because the dose initially increases with depth, sparing the skin and delivering higher doses to deeper tissues.

For appropriate clinical evaluation, it is extremely important to know at least the penetrating ability of the incident radiation, the amount of skin exposed, and the time over which the radiation is delivered. Without this information inappropriate judgments may be made. A vast literature describes the effects of radiation exposure on the skin. As early as 1898, Gassmann described histologic changes of chronic roentgen ulcers.[10] The "radium burn" and radiation dermatitis were described by the early radiation pioneers, including Henri Becquerel and Marie Curie.[11] Comprehensive reports on radiation effects on the skin are recommended to the reader for further reading.[4,12] This portion of the chapter is devoted to skin changes in relatively localized areas. When large areas of skin are exposed there may be the so-called cutaneous radiation syndrome.[13,14] This entity is discussed later in this chapter in the section, "Total-Body Irradiation." The SOMA toxicity table related to skin is presented in Appendix 6.

Low-LET Radiation

Skin erythema, or reddening, occurs if a single dose of 6 to 8 Gy is given, and it is not identified until 1 to 2 days after irradiation. The higher the radiation dose, the more quickly the erythema may be identified. The early erythema is presumably due to release of vasoactive amines. Erythema increases during the first week and usually fades during the second week. It then may return 2 to 3 weeks after the initial insult and last for 20 to 30 days. The second phase of erythema is due to vessel damage; thermographic studies demonstrate increased blood flow during the first 2 to 3 months.[15] This cyclic behavior of the erythema may continue several times. In general, no erythema is expected if radiation doses are below 5 to 6 Gy but if the radiation fields are large and there is an acute dose in excess of 2 Gy, there can be an early erythematous reaction within a few hours. As the dose is fractionated, the threshold for skin erythema rises. If there are 12 daily fractions the dose for erythema of skin rises from about 6 or 8 Gy to about 12 Gy. Acute doses in excess of 8 Gy will produce exudative and erosive changes of the skin. When there are penetrating acute doses in excess of 20 Gy, there is usually a nonhealing ulceration.

The late phase of erythema is probably due to blood vessel damage and is characterized by a blue or mauve discoloration of the skin. This was seen in the Chernobyl patients who received a beta dose at a depth of 1500 μm in the skin of greater than 20 Gy. This was approximately 30% of the dose that was received at a depth of 70 μm. In addition to erythema, edema may be associated with acute exposures. It can appear in a few hours or a few weeks. The higher the dose, the shorter is the period for appearance; there is enough individual variation that dosimetry is imprecise at best. If there is an exudative dermatitis in general, the margins correspond to an acute dose to the basal layer of the epidermis of about 18 Gy. For quite large doses of radiation, there may be additional changes of moist desquamation, formation of bullae, or even a sloughing of the skin. Changes of the skin that have been described in radiation therapy usually involve a course totalling 40 to 50 Gy from an orthovoltage source in 20 to 25 equal fractions over a 4 to 5 week time period. In such circumstances, patients may demonstrate a faint erythema due to capillary dilatation during the first week of treatment. Some epilation is noted at 10 to 14 days. The true erythema usually occurs in the third week of treatment, with the skin becoming red, warm, and edematous.

Moist desquamation begins at the fourth week with oozing of serum. In radiotherapeutic situations, desquamation is usually healed by the time treatment is ended because there is compensatory regeneration in the basal layer of the skin. This regenerative capacity usually exceeds the destructive capacity during conventional radiotherapy. Dry desquamation occurs if irradiation is halted during the third week at the 30 Gy level. In these circumstances, the skin may itch, and scaling and increased pigmentation occur. The erythematous changes and desquamation are almost always confined to the treatment field, although occasionally they may extend beyond it. In addition, a generalized skin reaction may occur, perhaps due to indirect effect of a circulating product resulting from breakdown of tissue as a result of radiation. If doses exceed those discussed, necrosis of the structures underlying the epidermis may occur. Skin ulceration may occur very early with high absorbed doses. These ulcers may heal but ultimately will recur. With more conventional doses such as those used in radiotherapy, painful, slowly healing ulcers may occur and persist for years. The probable cause of these late ulcers is ischemia due to the arteriolar and small artery changes mentioned earlier. With relatively large doses of radiation such as a single dose of 20 to 40 Gy or more, a bullous-type, moist desquamation may occur in 4 weeks. In this situation, small blisters tend to coalesce and rupture.

If the dose is high enough, blisters may be formed from beneath the basal cell layer. At this stage, the clinical lesion may appear very similar to a second- or third-degree thermal burn, but an important differential diagnostic point is that the patient will not remember having been burned. In such circumstances, the bullae may become infected, and there also may be sloughing of the epidermis. A week or two after sloughing of the epidermis, the affected areas may become covered with epidermis, although ulcers tend to recur with later arteriolar obliterative changes. In patients who have developed late radiation ulcers following fractionated radiotherapy with doses of 40 to 120 Gy, there is a reduction in circulation that can be measured by radionuclide techniques. Venous and lymphatic vessel occlusion with swelling of an extremity have also been reported.[16,17]

Some authors have classified skin damage by clinical type.[18] Type I injury has damage limited to the epidermis and dermis without much damage to the subcutaneous tissues. There is an initial erythema, a 3-week latent period, a secondary erythema immediately followed by an exudative epidermatitis, and recovery in 3 to 6 months with or without atrophic changes. Type II injury is a vascular endothelitis, and, at 6 to 8 months postexposure, the acute reactions are renewed with necrosis and ulceration usually requiring surgery. This is the result of damage below the basal layer of the epidermis. In Type III injury there is necrosis within a few weeks of the acute exposure. With radiotherapy, temporary loss of hair

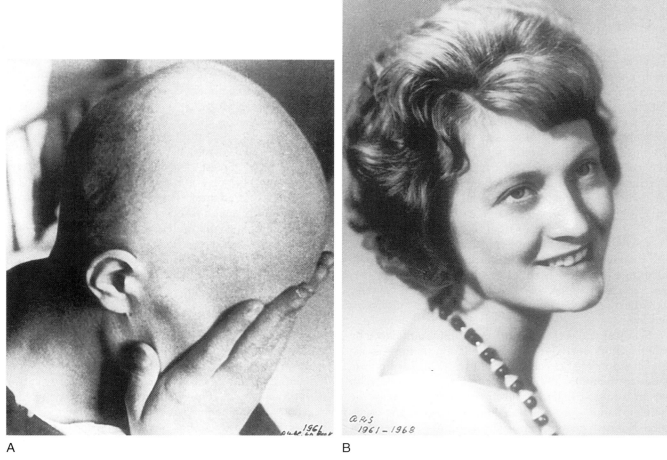

A   B

Figure 6-3 • **A**, Epilation due to radiation following whole-body exposure in a Russian radiation accident in 1961. **B**, Regrowth of hair. Patient seen here is 7 years postexposure.

(epilation) occurs in about 3 weeks with 3 to 5 Gy; hair begins to return during the second month and continues for up to 1 year (Fig. 6-3). Single doses of 7 Gy may cause permanent epilation, with the latent period being less than 3 weeks. Not all body areas have the same radiation epilation sensitivity. The scalp and beard are most sensitive, with chest wall, axillary, abdominal, eyebrow, eyelash, and pubic hair being less sensitive, respectively. Hair follicles of children are more sensitive than those of adults. Hair that has regrown is always finer and slower-growing than the original hair. It may also be of a different color.

Sebaceous glands are of about the same radiosensitivity as hair follicles and are destroyed by an acute dose of 12 to 16 Gy. Sweat glands are somewhat more resistant and may be permanently destroyed by fractionated doses of 30 Gy given over 3 weeks or an acute dose of 25 Gy. In 1947, acneiform changes of the skin following radiation therapy were described. Such changes are seen less often nowadays because of the switch to higher energy therapy sources that reduce the skin dose in relation to the dose at depth. Localized comedones and those of an even more

exaggerated form (known as Favre-Racouchot syndrome) continue to be described.[19,20] Such eruptions usually occur 4 to 6 months after radiotherapy that uses fractionated treatment schemes to total doses of about 60 Gy. These comedones apparently result from degeneration of the connective tissue stroma and plugging of the follicles with keratotic material. Although fingernails are rarely exposed to therapeutic radiation, they can be exposed in accidental or occupational situations, and arrested growth and ridging of the fingernails have been reported. Delayed effects in therapeutic situations may be apparent at 6 months and may progress slowly.

The sequence of pigmentation effects is variable from patient to patient. In some patients, the skin demonstrates gradual hyperpigmentation; however, in blacks, there may be depigmentation of the skin. Increased pigmentation is caused by a radiation-induced increase in enzymatic activity of melanocytes. Depigmentation may occur if the radiation dose has been high enough to destroy the melanocytes. By 1 year, the skin usually demonstrates its final appearance.

Diffuse telangiectasia, suppression of sebaceous gland activity, regrowth of hair, and thin, dry, and semitranslucent skin may result from atrophy. There have been a number of authors that have reported on the individuality and latent period of late skin telangiectasia. Skin telangiectasia often shows progression up to 10 years but is individually variable.[21,22] If moist desquamation occurs during radiotherapy, there is a higher incidence of telangiectasia.[23] With increasing fibrosis, there may be induration of the skin, as well as limitation of motion.[2] The amount of severe fibrosis is greatly influenced by both dose and fractionation. For example, at two fractions per week, severe fibrosis will occur in 20% of persons receiving 36 Gy and 80% of those receiving 43 Gy. For five fractions per week, the corresponding values are 46 Gy and 52 Gy, respectively. The degree of late subcutaneous radiation fibrosis can be assessed using ultrasound[24] and beneficial therapeutic measures include use of pentoxyphilline, tocopherol,[25-27] and interferon gamma.[28] Chronic radiation dermatitis from radioactive gold jewelry has been reported in several patients.[29,30] Such jewelry has either been contaminated with radon or radioactive gold 198.

Skin reaction varies over the body and is influenced by patient factors, including age. In radiation therapy, moist desquamation rarely occurs in children, probably because of the epithelium's ability to recover more rapidly than that in adults. Hyperthyroidism apparently makes the erythema and skin reaction more brisk than usual. Fairer-skinned people demonstrate more skin reaction than do darker-skinned individuals. Those portions of the skin that are moist and subject to friction, such as the axilla, groin, and skin folds, are the most radiosensitive. Sensitive areas appear to be the inner aspect of the neck and antecubital and popliteal spaces, followed in decreasing order by the flexor surface of the extremities, chest, abdomen, face, and back. The extensor surfaces of extremities are somewhat less sensitive. The least-sensitive areas appear to be the nape of the neck, scalp, and the palms and soles. Areas of skin grafting in which the graft is less than 3 months old generally demonstrate greater radiosensitivity than does the normal skin. Interestingly enough, skin grafts older than 1 year normally do not demonstrate much reaction to radiation

Giever et al.[31] and Aristizabel et al.[32] reported enhanced skin reactions with chemotherapy and radiation, particularly for VP16-213 (epipodophyllotoxin) and Adriamycin (doxorubicin hydrochloride), actinomycin D, bleomycin, and methotrexate. The increased skin response is seen not only during the chemotherapy; there can be an increased skin reaction seen up to several months after cessation of actinomycin D. Skin tolerance to radiation depends significantly on the volume of tissue irradiated. As the volume of skin irradiated becomes smaller, the dose required to produce necrosis increases. For example, the skin TD for a circular field of 150 cm^2 is approximately 15 Gy in a single dose, whereas for a circular field of 50 cm^2 the TD is almost 20 Gy.[33,34] For radiotherapy situations the skin tolerance dose is about 50 Gy for a skin area of 100 cm^2, 58 Gy for 16 cm^2, 84 Gy for 4 cm^2, and 392 Gy for 1 cm^2. Occasionally, there are rare atypical skin reactions after radiotherapy that resemble erythema multiforme, pemphigus, hyperkeratosis,[35] lentigo, bullous pemphigoid reactions,[36,37] and other entities. Such reactions can begin in the irradiated area but then become more generalized. Localized radiation-induced scleroderma or exacerbations have been reported after radiotherapy for breast cancer.[38-42] Chemotherapeutic agents may also play a role in the occurrence of such reactions.[43-49] Radiation therapy also can exacerbate existing conditions such as psoriasis.[50] While most of the skin changes described above have occurred as a result of radiotherapy and accidental exposures, these changes (including delayed ulceration) can occur from diagnostic and interventional radiology or cardiology procedures.[51] Temporary epilation has even been reported following CT scans.[52]

Neutron Irradiation

The RBE for single doses of neutrons depends on the neutron energy. The range appears to be between 1.5 and 2.0, and TD for skin erythema of fast neutrons is approximately 2 Gy.[53] Skin reaction with neutrons is much less dependent on the number of fractions given, that is, multiple fractions do not significantly change the total dose required to produce skin changes.

Radiation of the Skin by Radionuclides

The effects on the skin of various radionuclides depend significantly on the half-life and energy spectrum emitted by the radionuclide. In most instances, skin contamination occurs on an accidental basis, with the clinical significance of an accident rarely being a function of the skin dose. Pure alpha-emitting radionuclides pose no skin hazard and predominantly pose an internal contamination hazard. The hazard level of an alpha emitter depends on the chemical nature and solubility of the contaminant, as well as the integrity of the skin as a natural barrier. Gamma-emitting radionuclides (such as cesium 137, cobalt 60, and iridium 192) are often accompanied either by beta emissions or possibly soft x-rays as a result of interaction with a metallic capsule or covering. Industrial radiography sources are the most common cause of problems and can result in a wide spectrum of skin changes (Figs. 6-4 and 6-5). A number of reports and books on the occurrence and treatment of such lesions are available.[13,54-56]

Energetic beta-particle emitters, if left undetected on the skin surface, may ultimately cause erythema, particularly if they are present in high specific-activity amounts. Such accidental situations may be possible in a fission product accident at a commercial nuclear facility.

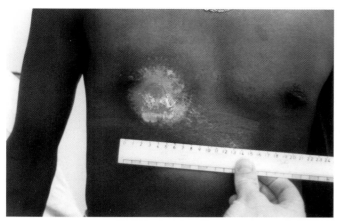

Figure 6-4 • Necrosis of the anterior chest wall in a patient who placed a highly radioactive source next to the chest.

Some beta-emitting radionuclides have been carefully studied (particularly phosphorus 32 and strontium 90), and the following values for beta radiation have been derived: threshold erythema, 5 to 15 Gy; dry desquamation, 17 Gy; and bullous epidermitis, 72 Gy.[57] Additional studies have been published by Krohmer et al.[58]

Skin changes from atomic weapons and discussions of "beta burns" usually arise in many public forums. Beta burns are possible after a nuclear weapon detonation. In early fallout, there are approximately two beta particles for every gamma photon. The maximum range of the beta particles in air (about 6 feet) is much lower than that of the gamma photons. At a planar surface, the beta dose from early fallout beta particles may be about 140 times that of the gamma dose, falling off very quickly with distance. Practical considerations indicate that under actual field conditions, the beta dose is much lower than one would anticipate because (1) clothing is usually worn (particularly shoes), and the human skin has an outer cornified layer composed of dead cells that stop all beta particles with energies of less than 70 keV; (2) most particles of fallout on the skin are expected to have retention times ranging from 2 hours (1000-μm diameter) to 7 hours (50 μm diameter); and (3) most fallout on the ground is not deposited on a perfect planar surface but rather on a very irregular surface. Several reports indicate that at 1 m from a fission product fallout contaminated surface, the beta-gamma ratio is approximately 2 to 3.[59,60]

In a follow-up study of the Japanese fishermen exposed to radioactive fallout in 1954, skin doses were estimated to have been from 1.7 to 6.0 Gy.[61] The equivalent single acute dose is reported to be approximately half: 0.8 to 3 Gy. The external gamma dose from the fallout particles was accompanied by beta radiation fallout, which produced significant skin lesions, including erythema, erosion, occasional necrosis, and skin atrophy. Twenty-three U.S. radar servicemen were also exposed to fallout in the early 1950s. Many experienced discrete

1- to 4-mm round skin lesions that quickly healed. They also experienced ridging of fingernails several months later. It should be noted that discussions of fallout experience in the Marshall Islands and South Pacific may be unique. In the tropical environment, the fission products were attached to calcium oxide from the coral, with the fallout particles sticking to the exposed individuals and clothes. In the continental United States, the situation may be slightly different. In at least one modeling study of fallout, particle size and distribution on the skin significantly affected the calculations.[62] It was concluded that for single particles of less than 500 μm diameter, no particles could cause skin ulceration as long as they were deposited more than 17 minutes after weapon detonation. Regardless of the particle size distribution, in the multiparticle model, skin damage became virtually impossible after a delay time of 10^7 seconds following weapon detonation.

The reactor accident at Chernobyl resulted in a large number of workers having skin contamination with high activities of fresh fission products. These had a beta-gamma ratio of between 10 and 30. Estimated skin doses to a number of patients were in excess of 40 Gy. The energy of the beta particles was sufficient to damage the basal layer of the skin and cause desquamation and a large portal of entry for infection. More than one half of the acute deaths from Chernobyl were a result of the severe skin changes and infection in the face of a depressed bone marrow and immune system (Fig. 6-6). The survivors have skin that is atrophic, telangectatic, keratotic, and has ulcerations, lentigo, and underlying fibrosis.[63]

For many years there has been concern about the effects of skin irradiation by small beta or beta-gamma emitting particles. The reader is referred to a comprehensive NCRP report on the subject.[64] "Hot" particles (also referred to as fleas or specks) are occasionally found in nuclear power plants and commonly contain cobalt 60 or fission products. The cobalt 60 is derived from activation of stable cobalt in the metal of items such as valve seats, while the fission products come from fuel that has escaped through defects in the fuel cladding. The activity of most of the particles is in the range of 400 Bq to 200 kBq. The particles by definition are less than 1 mm in any dimension, yet they can deliver very high doses to small portions of the skin. It is clear that the deterministic effects of radiation in the skin depend markedly on the area irradiated, with much higher doses being tolerated as the field size becomes smaller. A large amount of animal work with small beta-emitting particles has been done, but there is only a limited amount of human data. In one human volunteer experiment, Dean et al. used uranium microspheres and found that 142 Gy produced slight erythema, 400 Gy produced erythema, and 540 Gy produced erythema and a slight possible dry desquamation.[65] The maximum exposure corresponded to

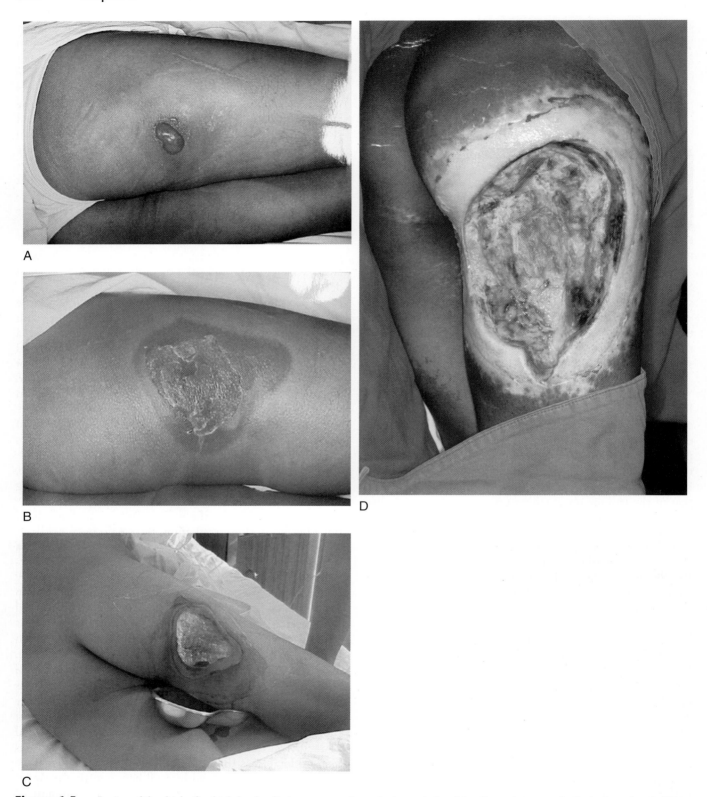

Figure 6-5 ● Lesion of the thigh after high-level radiation exposure from placing an industrial radiography source in the back pocket. **A,** Blister formation, day 4. **B,** Dry and moist desquamation at day 14. **C,** Deep ulceration at day 27. **D,** Massive ulceration down to the bone at 5 months postexposure. Amputation was required.

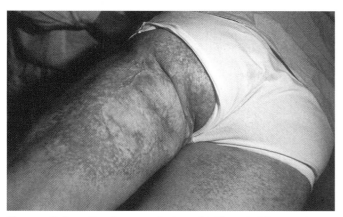

Figure 6-6 • Beta burns on the legs of a Chernobyl fireman 5 years after the accident. The skin is atrophic with underlying fibrosis and surrounding telangiectasia.

10^9 beta particles. No ulceration was found. Two years after the experiment, the exposure sites were not visibly abnormal.

ENDOCRINE GLANDS

The endocrine glands include the pituitary, thyroid, parathyroid, and adrenal glands. In 1908, the adrenals were the first to be studied with regard to deterministic radiation effects by Harvey[66] and later in 1912 by Cottenot.[67] The thyroid was studied in 1923 by Beower and Clark,[68] and the pituitary gland was initially studied only in the 1930s. The historical aspects are well documented by Rubin and Casarett.[2] Most of the endocrine glands are quite radioresistant. The deterministic effects of radiation usually result from degeneration and obliteration of the fine vasculature. Many authors have pointed out the difficulty in assessing deterministic effects of radiation on these glands because their interaction is so complex and they react to many forms of stress and trauma in distant portions of the body. Endocrine abnormalities are relatively common after radiotherapy of the head and neck region. For example, Samaan et al. studied 110 patients who received head and neck irradiation for tumor treatment.[69] The median dose was estimated to be about 50 to 55 Gy. Endocrine deficiencies were found in 91 of the 110 patients and primary pituitary deficiency in 43 patients. Forty of 66 patients receiving neck irradiation with a median dose of 50 Gy showed evidence of primary hypothyroidism. The SOMA toxicity table related to the endocrine system is presented in Appendix 6.

Pituitary Gland

Although there are many different cells in the pituitary gland, the cells of both the anterior and the posterior pituitary all behave as reverting postmitotic cells. The neural elements are more radioresistant than the other portions. A large experience has been gained from radiation therapy of the pituitary for various neoplasms, as well as some nonneoplastic conditions.[70–72] In general, the deterministic effects of high-dose radiation on the pituitary result in hypopituitarism including deficiencies of growth hormone, gonadotropins, thyroid-stimulating hormone, and adrenocorticotropin and require long term endocrine follow-up.[73,74] This is manifested by loss of weight, secondary sexual characteristics, and body hair; dry skin; slow pulse; genital atrophy; and low body temperature. These changes may take 5 to 11 years to occur when the total fractionated dose levels are above 40 Gy. Even very high doses of radiation require several months to cause hypopituitarism. The doses required to produce reduced or absent function are extremely large (usually in excess of 150 Gy). Hypopituitarism has occasionally been reported after external irradiation for nasopharyngeal tumors.[75] This is a very rare complication and, in fact, has only been seen at doses in excess of 90 Gy. When doses in the range of 50 to 85 Gy are examined, subtle disturbances in hormone levels can be identified through radioimmunoassay methods.[75]

The criteria for pituitary hypofunction have been extensively studied, and the fall of urinary gonadotropins during the month subsequent to irradiation appears to be a sensitive indicator. Fuks et al. indicated that cells producing growth hormone may be the most radiosensitive within the pituitary.[72] Acromegaly and Cushing's disease appear to be relatively well controlled by using therapeutic doses of 45 to 55 Gy over 5 weeks. Neuroendocrine effects after cranial radiotherapy in children have been extensively studied. The damage to the hypothalamic-pituitary axis generally results from deterministic effects on the hypothalamus and to a lesser extent on the pituitary. The most sensitive effect is on the production of growth hormone by the anterior pituitary gland, but this is actually secondary to damage of the hypothalamic cells that produce growth hormone–releasing factor.[76] Reduction in growth hormone has been reported with fractionated doses above 18 Gy and with single doses as low as 9 to 10 Gy (as given for total-body radiation in preparation for bone marrow transplant).[77–80] Different tests measure the growth hormone, and depending on the test used, reported results may differ. For example, after 24 Gy of fractionated cranial radiotherapy, there is normal growth hormone response to arginine stimulation but not to insulin.[81] There may be a practical threshold for impairment of growth hormone at about 18 Gy of fractionated cranial radiotherapy.[82] Some authors have suggested that growth hormone deficiency after radiation therapy predicts cardiovascular risk in young adults treated for acute lymphoblastic leukemia.[83]

Even though children treated for leukemia may have biochemical growth hormone deficiency, they still may have normal growth patterns.[84,85] On the other hand, children treated for cranial tumors receive higher fractionated doses of about 30 Gy, and up to 50% of survivors have severe growth retardation.[86] In children treated for brain tumors, about 75% will have growth hormone deficiency, and height below the 10th percentile is seen in about 70%. Reduction in height is more pronounced when irradiation occurs before 8 years of age.[87] When patients receive 50 Gy or more, multiple pituitary hormonal deficiencies usually occur.[88,89]

After a single whole-body exposure of 10 Gy for treatment prior to bone marrow transplantation, severe growth retardation may be seen.[90,91] Reduced growth hormone levels are seen in 42% of such children, but the proportion rises to 87% if they also received additional cranial radiotherapy.[92] Normal growth is usually seen in children who had bone marrow transplantation but did not get prior radiotherapy. In the future, deficiencies in growth hormone may not be such a problem because exogenous growth hormone is becoming available.[93]

Reduction in other pituitary functions can also occur.[94] Reduction in thyroid-stimulating hormone and thyrotropin-releasing hormone levels can occur in children after whole-brain fractionated irradiation of 20 to 30 Gy.[95] Damage to the adrenal or gonadal axis, causing lack of adrenocorticotropic hormone (ACTH), follicle-stimulating hormone (FSH), luteinizing hormone (LH), or LH-releasing hormone (LRH) is more often found in adolescents and adults than children. Quigley et al. showed that 75% of girls treated for acute leukemia with cranial radiotherapy using 24 Gy in 15 fractions over 3 weeks had elevated levels of FSH.[96] Menarche in these girls was early and not delayed, a finding also reported by Noorda et al.[87] Early puberty was also observed by Lieper et al. in 10% of girls treated for acute leukemia.[97] Hamre et al. reported on serum FSH levels and prepubertal development in long-term survivors of acute leukemia.[98] Nine percent of patients who received cranial irradiation had elevated gonadotropins, compared to 49% for craniospinal fields and 93% for those who received craniospinal plus abdominal fields. Constine studied 65 adult patients treated for central nervous system (CNS) malignancies and found abnormalities of hyperprolactinemia, hypothyroidism, and gonadal disturbances in 50% to 80% of patients who received more than 55 Gy.[99] After 40 to 50 Gy of fractionated cranial radiotherapy, the incidence of panhypopituitarism is between 20% and 40%.[100] Littley et al. indicated that 5 years after treatment with fractionated cranial radiotherapy, the incidence of thyroid-stimulating hormone (TSH) deficiency was as follows: 20 Gy, 9%; 35 to 37 Gy, 22%; 40 Gy, 35%; and 42 to 45 Gy, 52%.[101] No pituitary dysfunction was observed in patients who received 12 Gy in six fractions over three days. Sklar et al.[102] and Warner et al.[103] indicated that children with acute lymphatic leukemia (ALL) given cranial radiotherapy are at a significant risk of obesity as young adults.

High-LET Radiation

Much of the recent high-LET experience was reported by Tobias, who used helium ions and proton beams.[71] In using such methods, it has been found that fractionated doses below 200 Gy do not cause necrosis of the pituitary. This may have been a function of the time at which the patients died as a result of their tumors. It is possible that long-term follow-up would have demonstrated necrosis at lower dose levels. Doses in the range of 50 to 110 Gy delivered over 12 days can cause cystic atrophy and, in some cases, fibrosis in the center of the gland.

Radionuclide Irradiation

There is a relatively large experience using yttrium 90, gold 198, strontium 90, and radon seeds for brachytherapy of pituitary lesions. One of the difficulties with use of beta irradiation is that the dosimetry is very difficult to calculate for use in comparison with other forms of therapy. Doses near yttrium 90 therapy spheres have been estimated to be 4000 Gy at 1 mm and 500 Gy at 4 mm.[104] Follow-up studies of patients who received childhood nasopharyngeal radium therapy to treat otitis serosa and who received pituitary doses of about 11 Gy did not demonstrate any significant hormonal deficiencies.[105,106]

Thyroid

There is a very large clinical experience of thyroid irradiation. Human data are available from atomic bomb survivors, fallout studies, accidents, radiotherapy for tumors of the thyroid or the adjacent neck, and radionuclide treatment for hyperthyroidism. The thyroid parenchyma consists of follicles lined by simple epithelium. The follicular cells produce a colloid containing the thyroid hormones. Between the follicles is a very rich network of blood vessels and lymphatics. The epithelial cells are reverting postmitotic cells and are relatively radioresistant. The deterministic changes following large doses of irradiation identified in the thyroid are mediated by the vasculature and may be manifest as inflammatory and edematous changes, followed later by obliteration of the fine vasculature and, ultimately, by radionecrosis or atrophy. The overall relative radiosensitivity of the thyroid is due to the results of vascular damage. Late changes are predominantly concerned with hypothyroidism and various forms of thyroiditis. The SOMA toxicity table related to the thyroid is presented in Appendix 6. Induction of thyroid nodules is covered in detail in Chapter 5.

A large literature has also arisen in the last few years regarding the possible role of radiation in the development of autoimmune (Hashimoto's) thyroiditis. The literature is complicated by the different tests and methodologies used to make the diagnosis, the high prevalence of thyroid abnormalities in the general population, and nonradiation etiologic factors. Autoimmune thyroid disease (AIT) can lead to chronic thyroid inflammation and destruction (Hashimoto's thyroiditis) as well as overactivity (Graves' disease). Hashimoto's thyroiditis is characterized by diffuse involvement of the gland, generalized lymphocytic infiltration, fibrosis, and follicular cell destruction. The process is chronic and progressive and is probably due to the infiltrating T-lymphocytes. The role of thyroid antibodies is less clear but they do serve as markers of thyroid inflammation.

The diagnosis is made by histological examination. The first thyroid antibodies detected were by thyroglobulin (Tg) agglutination but more recently a wide variety of assays for antithyroid peroxidase (ATPO) (also called thyroid antimicrosomal antibodies) have been used. The antibodies are not specific for Hashimoto's thyroiditis as they are found in 70% of patients with Graves' disease and are present in up to 15% of the general population. The incidence of antibodies increases with age. In the Whickham, U.K, longitudinal survey individuals more than 45 years of age, 26% female and 9% male, were antibody positive.[107] The incidence of spontaneous clinical and subclinical hypothyroidism was 7.7% in females, 1.1% in males, and 5.3% overall. In the U.S. NHANES III survey the prevalence of thyroid antibodies for those over 12 years of age was 17% in females, 8.7% in males, and 13% overall.[108] For those 50 to 59 years of age the values were 20.7%, 11%, and 16%, respectively. For the population of 60 years of age the prevalence of thryoid peroxidase (TPO) antibodies was 27%. The incidence of clinical and subclinical hypothyroidism was 4.6% to 6.2% overall. The incidence also varies based on genetic influences and other factors including dietary and concurrent diseases (e.g., diabetes, bowel disease, etc.). The antibodies can reflect a normal autoimmune response and do not necessarily signal the presence of an autoimmune disease.

The definitive diagnosis of autoimmume thyroiditis is made according to current World Health Organization (WHO) standards (2003) based on various combinations of ATPO, antithyroid globulin (ATG), and TSH, in combination with abnormalities detected by ultrasound, palpation, and pathology.[108a] Most of the epidemiologic studies use only a few of these criteria. Autoimmune thyroiditis usually means that a patient has an abnormal thyroid examination and about 90% of these persons will have positive thyroid antibodies in the blood. Radioiodine given therapeutically can rarely induce autoimmune responses in patients with nodular goiters.[109] This certainly is at variance with the fact that very high doses of radioiodine are used for therapy and yet some authors assume that relatively small doses of radioiodine would likely cause autoimmune disease. Nonautoimmune forms of thyroiditis also occur including nonspecific virus-induced subacute thyroiditis, drug-induced thyroiditis (e.g., alpha interferon or amidarone therapy). Increased thyroid antibodies are also seen in about 35% to 40% of patients with thyroid carcinoma.[110]

Low-LET Radiation

AREAS OF HIGH NATURAL BACKGROUND RADIATION

Wang et al. studied large populations living in high background areas of China.[111] While there was an increase in chromosomal abnormalities, there was no evidence of an increase in thyroid nodules, changes in serum levels of thyroid hormones, or elevations in levels of thyroid antibodies as a result of lifetime exposure to increased levels of low-dose-rate gamma radiation.

ATOMIC BOMB SURVIVORS

The atomic bomb survivors were exposed predominantly to external low-LET radiation. Acute effects of external radiation on the thyroid have been identified in autopsies performed on some of the victims at Hiroshima. Liebow examined patients who died 3 to 6 weeks after exposure and identified only a moderate decrease in the follicular size.[112]

In a study of 477 atomic bomb survivors who were in the 1 Gy or greater group and under the age of 20 at exposure, there was no evidence of an increase in clinical or subclinical hypothyroidism when comparison was made to 501 individuals in the 0 Gy group, however, this is in contrast to later studies.[113] In Nagasaki atomic bomb survivors, Nagataki found the prevalence of hypothyroidism in the 0.01 to 0.49 Gy group to be elevated at 4.5% compared with 2.5% in controls.[114,115] These findings are of questionable significance because there was no significant elevation in the 0.5 to 0.99 Gy group. This study based on only 27 cases is sometimes used as evidence for radiation-induced thyroiditis even though the authors state that additional work is needed. The diagnosis of thyroiditis was never actually made in this particular study.

Chikako et al. reported on a study of about 6000 survivors exposed within 1.5 km of hypocenter in whom there was an increase in ATPO in the exposed group compared to the control group, which was not linearly related to dose; the prevalence of ATPO among those with hypothyroidism was significantly lower among the exposed group.[116] Morimoto et al. reported that in individuals less than 20 years of age at the time of the bombing who received 1 Gy or more there was an increase in thyroid cancer and nodules but no statistically significant difference with respect to hypothyroidism or markers of AIT.[117] Fugiwara et al. reported on the prevalence of various types of immune factors but those associated with AIT did not appear to be dose related.[118] An autopsy study by Yoshimoto et al. of about 3800 subjects also did not reveal a statistically significant increase in chronic thyroiditis related to magnitude of radiation dose.[119]

It is noteworthy, nevertheless, that atomic bomb survivors who were under 30 years of age at the time of irradiation have shown a dose-dependent excess of thyroid disease, defined to include nontoxic nodular goiter, diffuse goiter, thyrotoxicosis, chronic lymphocytic thyroiditis, and hypothyroidism.[120] The excess, which became evident within 20 years after irradiation and was not detectable in those exposed at older ages, corresponded to a relative risk of 1.24 at a dose of 1 Gy (P value 0.003). Although many of those affected had multiple diagnoses, the exclusion of persons with thyroid cancer or thyroid adenomas did not modify the risk.

MEDICAL EXTERNAL EXPOSURE

Limited data concerning thyroid function after diagnostic medical exposure are available. Kaplan et al. followed 91 women who received an average of 112 fluoroscopic examinations of the chest during tuberculosis treatment by repeated pneumothorax.[121] No increase in hypothyroidism was seen.

After x-ray therapy of the neck, hyperthyroidism has been reported, but it is quite rare. Reports of the doses needed to cause hypothyroidism from external fractionated irradiation range between 26 and 50 Gy.[122] The individual responses to external radiation of the thyroid may be quite variable; some authors indicate that a normal gland can tolerate doses as high as 60 Gy over 6 weeks without clinical evidence of damage, whereas hypothyroidism occasionally may be seen at doses as low as 10 Gy and may occur in a moderate percentage of long-term survivors of bone marrow transplants who were treated with six whole-body fractions of 2 Gy. Laboratory hypothyroidism may be present in approximately one half of children irradiated for Hodgkin's disease with fractionated doses to the neck of 22 to 44 Gy. Hancock et al. reviewed the records of 1787 patients treated for Hodgkin's disease.[123] The majority of patients received 44 Gy to cervical lymph node areas. Biochemical hypothyroidism was found in 513 patients. Somewhat less than half required medication, and most cases presented 2 to 3 years after therapy, though some still occurred up to 18 years later. The risk for biochemical hypothyroidism was 44% at 20 years after treatment for patients who had received more than 30 Gy and 27% for those in the 7.5 to 30 Gy range. The comparable figures for overt hypothyroidism were 20% and 5%, respectively.

Loeffler et al. specifically followed 437 Hodgkin's disease patients treated with mantle fields to ascertain the rate of Graves' disease.[124] The latter was found in seven patients. The O/E ratio was 5.9 for females and 5.1 for males. In a study of 28 patients given mantle therapy for malignant lymphoma with a thyroid dose of 45 Gy, the incidence of subclinical hypothyroidism was 22%, and no patients had clinical hypothyroidism.[125]

A number of studies have examined hypothyroidism in adults after external radiotherapy. Grande reported

biochemical hypothyroidism in 41% of patients after radiotherapy for head and neck cancer.[126] Similar results were reported by Liening et al.[127] and Tami et al.[128] Reports of hypothyroidism after irradiation of supraclavicular nodes during the course of radiotherapy for breast cancer vary widely. Joensuu[129] reported an incidence of clinical and subclinical hypothyroidism of 21%, while Bruning et al. found a value closer to 80%.[130] Both indicated that the cumulative thyroid dose was 45 to 50 Gy.

Internal Irradiation

NUCLEAR WEAPONS FALLOUT

In 1954, a thermonuclear explosion accidentally deposited large amounts of radioactive iodines in the Marshall Islands. The highest dose was received on the Rongelap atoll. The iodines deposited were a mixture of iodine 131, 132, 133, and 135, and they resulted not only in significant internal contamination, but external contamination and irradiation as well. The deterministic effects identified have included hypothyroidism (both clinical and biochemical). In 4 of 43 subjects biochemical hypothyroidism was demonstrated, and 3 of these subjects were thought to have received a thyroid dose of less than 3.5 Gy. In the course of a 15-year follow-up, 67% of individuals below the age of 10 years developed nodules, as did 15% of the remainder of the population.[131] Thyroid doses in the young age group were felt to range between 10 and 42 Gy, and in the older age group, 30 to 50 Gy. An additional study demonstrated that five Marshallese children who were exposed to the fallout showed some growth retardation, and two young males developed hypothyroidism.[132] In a somewhat later study Robbins et al. indicated that there were 12 cases of subclinical hypothyroidism.[133]

Long-term follow-up of the Marshall Islanders exposed to nuclear weapons fallout and thyroid doses up to 4 Gy by Takahashi et al. did not show an increase in autoimmune hypothyroidism.[134,135] Although there was an early report of an excess of autoimmune thyroiditis reported by Rallison et al.[136] in Nevada and Utah compared to Arizona (assumedly from fallout from weapons testing in Nevada), a subsequent age- and sex-adjusted study by Kerber et al. showed no evidence of a relationship between AIT or other thyroid diseases and individual doses.[137]

The effects of prolonged childhood exposure to[131]I from the Russian Mayak facility showed a nonsignificant decrease in autoimmune thyroiditis with a relative risk (RR) of 0.7 (95% CI 0.4, 1.1) and a nonsignificant decrease in diffuse goiter with an RR of 0.9 (95% CI 0.4, 2.1).[137a]

CHERNOBYL

The Chernobyl accident released very large quantities of radioiodine. Unfortunately, iodine distribution and dosimetry are not precisely known. The International Chernobyl Project did examine the thyroid function of hundreds of persons living in nearby heavily contaminated villages and compared the findings with those of persons living in clean settlements.[138] Five years after the accident there was no evidence of thyroid hypofunction in the general population as a result of the accident. A large number of subsequent studies have been done on children in the fallout regions exposed to radioiodines. The majority of the initial thyroid dose was from iodine 131 (about 80%) and to a lesser extent from shorter-lived radioiodines. The data are complicated by potential effects of iodine deficiency in some areas as well as continuing exposure from cesium 137.

A thorough review of the Chernobyl literature has been conducted by scientists from 22 nations as members of the United Nations Scientific Committee on the Effects of Atomic Radiation (UNSCEAR). Although an increased incidence of thyroid neoplasms has been linked to irradiation from the accident (as discussed in Chapter 5), UNSCEAR 2000 points out, "Even the large screening programme conducted by the Chernobyl Sasakawa Health and Medical Cooperation Project from 1991–1996 involving 160,000 children who were less than 10 years of age at the time of the accident, found no increased risk of hypothyroidism, hyperthyroidism or goiter that could be related to ionizing radiation. Neither was an increase in thyroid antibodies, which is in contradiction to some other minor studies."[7] The Sasakawa study is the largest and best conducted (by far) of the thyroid Chernobyl studies and the only large-scale study of children exposed from Chernobyl. The Sasakawa study reported by Ito et al.[139] and Yamashita et al.[140] included 160,000 children and did not find any increase in thyroid antibodies, hypothyroidism, hyperthyroidism, and cesium 137 contamination. There are quite a number of smaller studies, which typically have less than 200 subjects and are ecological studies based on cesium fallout deposition. These are of questionable value. A study from the Russian oblast of Orelby Kasatkina et al. found significantly higher ATPO and antithymocyte globulin (ATG) levels in the exposed region but for those who had a fine needle aspiration performed the prevalence of autoimmune thyroiditis was the same in the exposed and control areas.[141]

Studies by Vykhovanets et al. covered 1000 children who lived in contaminated areas that were screened but only 53 had blood tests performed and these were compared with 45 children living in other areas.[142] The thyroid dose was derived from unpublished data. Differences were reported as significant but inspection of the actual data indicates that this is probably not so. For example, one reported significant finding was that the level of TSH in the controls was 1.6 ± 1.3 and in the presumably exposed it was 6.1 ± 6.2. There are also data about thyroid echogenicity, which are subjective and apparently obtained with observers' knowledge of where the children were living. Vykhovanets also reported that there was an increase in thyroid autoimmune

disease after Chernobyl in all exposed children in the first decade, but that this effect decreased fourfold and essentially disappeared in the second decade postexposure in persons with dose levels of greater than 0.5 Gy.

Pacini et al. reported on the prevalence of thyroid autoantibodies in children around Chernobyl.[143] The blood samples were drawn 6 to 8 years postexposure and whether these persons will have persistent elevation in antibody levels and whether this truly represents Hashimoto's thyroiditis and might lead to hypothyroidism is unclear. Vermiglio et al. measured the prevalence of ATG and ATPO in 143 children from a contaminated region and compared them with 40 controls.[144] There were statistically significant increases in the exposed group. They also have pointed out the possible effects of iodine deficiency on increasing the incidence of thyroid autoimmunity in Russia.

Increasing availability of nonradioactive iodine to the thyroid gland can precipitate AIT. There are and were programs in the former Soviet Union that supplied iodine tablets (to combat goiter) to school children even before Chernobyl. In addition, there was distribution to the population and use of potassium iodine as a thyroid-blocking agent in the days after the accident. All of these complicate the data. The 2005 Chernobyl project expert summary and review of the literature up to that date has concluded that there is no consistent or conclusive evidence of radiation thyroiditis in the Chernobyl fallout populations.[145] Follow-up of the Chernobyl firemen who suffered from both the acute radiation syndrome, with whole-body doses from 1 to 6 Gy, and inhalation of fission products has not revealed clinical hypothyroidism as of 1993. The incidence of hypothyroidism from smaller doses of iodine 131 is difficult to evaluate.

HANFORD

A recent analysis was conducted relative to releases of radioiodine from the Hanford nuclear facility in Richland, Washington. The study included 3447 subjects who were born between 1940–1946 and were residents near the Hanford plant. The study reported by Davis et al. did not find an increased hypothyroidism or autoimmune thyroiditis related to the releases, dose level, or controls.[146] For hypothyroidism and autoimmune thyroiditis, the slopes of the dose-response curves were negative (−0.006 and −0.026, respectively).

RADIOIODINE THYROID THERAPY

A large experience with radionuclide irradiation of the thyroid gland in humans with iodine 123, 125, and 131 has been documented. Early changes following iodine 131 treatment for benign conditions were described by Freedberg.[147] In these circumstances, patients were given 630 to 5600 MBq of iodine 131 for treatment of angina pectoris and congestive heart failure. Severe necrosis of the thyroid follicles was identified at between 2 and

3 weeks, as well as acute vasculitis, thrombosis, and hemorrhage. One to 3 years later sclerosis of the arteries and fibrous changes, which were most pronounced in the center of the gland, occurred. If doses of radiation are not very large, there may be regeneration of the thyroid parenchyma in a focal and irregular fashion, although the vascular changes continue to occur, with resulting fibrosis.

The dose distributions of iodine 125 and 131 are different within the cellular structure of the thyroid. The dose delivered to the cells from iodine 125 is very localized, with most occurring at the colloid-cell interface. It is estimated that the distribution of dose from iodine 125 will spare approximately 30% of the proliferating cells. Iodine 131, on the other hand, delivers a much more homogeneous dose to the gland and produces diffuse damage, as has been confirmed with electron microscopic studies.[148] Iodine 131 delivers seven times the initial mean dose rate to the thyroid compared with that for an equal activity of iodine 125.[149] Iodine 125 occasionally has been used for therapy of hyperthyroid glands. The differences in dose and homogeneity at the cellular level have not caused a significant difference in clinical results, and the use of iodine 125 for treatment of hyperthyroidism has been abandoned.[150,151]

The use of iodine 131 for the treatment of Graves' disease and toxic multinodular goiters has been studied extensively. One problem is that the natural course of Graves' disease often terminates in hypothyroidism, whether treated with iodine 131 or not. Typical doses administered for such treatments range between 110 and 600 MBq. Some nuclear medicine physicians use the lower doses and try to titrate a patient down to a euthyroid state. This approach often requires several treatments. Another procedure is to use high-dose therapy designed to render the patient hypothyroid with a single dose of radioiodine. Most patients become hypothyroid with administered activities of iodine 131 in the range of 370 to 550 MBq. The actual absorbed dose to the gland is often difficult to calculate in these patients because of uncertainties in the exact size and weight of the gland. Another uncertainty is the biologic half-life of the radioiodine in a hyperthyroid and radiation-damaged gland. It is not unusual for patients receiving such radioactive iodine therapy to be hoarse and to have a sore throat 3 to 10 days after oral administration of the iodine. Occasionally, if there is a large gland that contains a large amount of thyroid hormone, the radiation damage causes the hormone to be released. The patient may experience an acute exacerbation of the hyperthyroidism known as *thyroid storm*. Treatment with propranolol is usually effective in preventing this reaction. In a review of the literature, McDermott indicated that the incidence of thyroid storm is less than 0.5%; however, once present, the fatality rate is high.[152]

Hypothyroidism, when it results from iodine 131 treatment, is usually evident 3 to 4 months after therapy; then the patient must be given replacement thyroid hormone. Transient hypothyroidism following radioiodine therapy for thyrotoxicosis has been described. This may be due to impaired organification of iodide. If iodide trapping becomes diminished, hypothyroidism is likely to be permanent.[153] Becker reviewed the probability in 6000 patients of developing hypothyroidism after surgical and radioiodine treatment for hyperthyroidism.[154] In patients who received 7 to 8 MBq of iodine per gram of gland, there was a 20% probability at 1 year and a 50% probability at 7 years. With 4 MBq/gm, the values were 15% and 30%, respectively. Considering the high uptake of radioiodine in the patient's hyperfunctioning gland, the absorbed dose is usually in excess of 100 Gy and sometimes as high as 400 Gy. That these extremely high doses are necessary with radioiodine indicates that external low-LET radiotherapy appears to be more efficient in producing hypothyroidism on a per-Gy basis. A similar effect was noted in Chapter 5 in the discussion of radiogenic tumors of the thyroid, and it probably results from differences of dose rate and dose distribution. Fajardo reviewed the pathologic findings after internal irradiation of the thyroid.[3] In hyperthyroid patients, large multinucleated cells and breakdown of follicles, with desquamation of the epithelial cells into the lumen, occur within 2 weeks. High-dose iodine 131 for treatment of Graves' disease and toxic nodular goiter can cause transient radiation thyroiditis and increase serum antibody levels but only a few patients show a sustained increase.[155–157]

Factors modifying the response of the thyroid to internal radiation include preexisting disease, particularly hyperthyroidism. Hyperthyroidism results in an increased radiosensitivity, perhaps due to the increased uptake of iodine or to the more active nature of the gland. There also is some evidence that children have more sensitive glands with regard to induction of hypothyroidism than adults.[158] Sex and prior thionamide therapy do not appear to influence the development of subsequent hypothyroidism.[159]

High-LET Radiation

Animal studies indicate that the thyroid is not particularly sensitive to neutron radiation when compared with other tissues. The relative biologic effectiveness (RBE) of monoenergetic 14-MeV neutrons was estimated to be 3.2 when 1 Gy of neutrons was used and 1.8 when 5 Gy of neutrons was given.[160]

Parathyroid Glands

In spite of the extensive experience of neck irradiation for malignancy and treatment of the thyroid for both benign and malignant conditions by radiation, no deterministic clinical effects of radiation on the parathyroid glands have been identified. Both Rubin and Casarett[2] and Fajardo[3] reviewed the literature; the only effect reported has been atrophy of some glands embedded within the thyroid tissue when large doses of radioiodine have been administered. This result indicates the relative resistance of the parathyroid parenchymal cells to radiation and, probably, a moderate vascular resistance as well. Parathyroid changes have been described in animals; however, the parathyroid glands in animals are much closer to the thyroid than in humans, and thus they receive large doses of beta irradiation after iodine 131 administration. There have been reports of hyperfunction of the parathyroids following irradiation of the neck for benign and malignant conditions.[161] The induction of parathyroid adenomas is discussed in Chapter 5. Fujiwara et al. reported increased levels of parathyroid hormone of 6.8% per Gy but the dose response leveled off at about 1 Gy.[162] Calcitonin levels were also increased. The mechanism remains unclear, and there is little, if any, clinical significance since normal individual variation is much greater than the potential radiation effect. There are occasional reports of calcitonin deficiency after radioiodine therapy; however, in most of these cases there has been previous surgery for thyroid carcinoma and the removal of parathyroid glands.[163]

Adrenal Glands

The adrenal glands (usually singly, but sometimes both) can be irradiated in the course of treatment for retroperitoneal or abdominal malignancies. Early studies in the 1920s suggested degeneration of the adrenal cortex; however, this has subsequently been found not to occur. In general, changes in the adrenals are difficult to document because the glands demonstrate a response to stress or trauma whether localized or distant. Soanes et al. examined the clinical response with respect to steroid production and ACTH stimulation in patients undergoing radiotherapy of both adrenal glands.[164,165] Enhancement of the response to administered ACTH occurred, although there was a suggestion that after large doses of radiation, there may be depressed steroidogenesis. Overall, the increase was demonstrated at absorbed fractionated doses greater than 20 Gy; when doses in excess of 35 Gy were given to the adrenals, normal steroidogenesis was demonstrated under nonstress conditions, but response to stress was limited. The relative radioresistance of the adrenals is not surprising because the parenchymal cells of both the adrenal cortex and medulla are reverting postmitotic cells and are, thus, relatively resistant to deterministic effects.

NERVOUS SYSTEM

On a historical basis, the study of radiation-induced changes in the CNS received rather late attention compared to effects on other organ systems. Most authors treat the brain, spinal cord, and peripheral nerves as separate entities since their responses are different; this text will follow the same procedure. It was not until the mid- to late 1930s that damage to the brain was carefully studied. The historical aspects have been well reviewed by Rubin and

Casarett.[2] (The reader is also referred to a superb book on radiation injury to the central nervous system by Gutin et al.[166] as well a review by Schultheiss et al.[167]) Most of the human data comes from radiation therapy of neoplasms, but radiation has been used occasionally for nonmalignant disorders.[168] Scholz reported on the use of whole-brain irradiation in schizophrenia and found that 43 Gy delivered in 3 days resulted in brain damage within 20 months.[169] Bailey et al. reviewed the transient use of cobalt 60 wires to perform lobotomies.[170] Very high doses of radiation delivered on an acute basis may cause what is referred to as the *central nervous system syndrome* or *neurovascular syndrome;* this syndrome will not be included in this section of the text but will be covered later in this chapter in the section, "Total-Body Irradiation." In utero effects are discussed in Chapter 8.

The cells of the mature nervous system include the neurons, the glial cells (including satellite cells and peripheral ganglia), the ependymal lining, and the neuroglia. The sheath about the peripheral nerves is formed from Schwann's cells. The neurons themselves are highly specialized cells that are unable to divide and are, therefore, postmitotic. Various estimates indicate that in normal life 10,000 to 50,000 of these cells are lost each day. Neurons themselves are very resistant to the deterministic effects of radiation. Glial cells, particularly the neuroglial cells, behave as reverting postmitotic cells and divide only under unusual circumstances. Schwann's cells are also reverting postmitotic cells; thus, both of the latter type cells are relatively resistant to radiation injury. The myelin sheath surrounding nerve fibers in the brain and spinal cord (particularly in the white matter of the brain) is also resistant to irradiation. However, radiation therapy may accelerate demyelination in diseases such as multiple sclerosis.[171]

Although the neurons themselves and the neuroglial cells are relatively resistant to radiation-induced death, small doses of radiation can have some effects on their function and may cause stimulation or impulses in the neurons. It is surprising that immediately after doses as low as 0.01 Gy transient abnormalities can be demonstrated on electroencephalography. The changes usually seen are spiking, beginning in the cortical region, with the duration and magnitude depending on dose. These have little, if any clinical importance and the cause of these effects remain unknown. The preceding discussion has referred primarily to the mature system. The developing system, which is actively proliferating in the embryo and in early childhood, is less resistant. Thus, the radioresistance of the nervous system is substantially influenced by the level of maturation. Many of the effects on the nervous system that are manifested, both acutely and at later periods, result from vascular injury, including the diffuse edema identified early and the later necrosis resulting from myointimal proliferation and subsequent fibrosis. There is a basic similarity of the parenchyma of the brain and spinal cord and it appears that the microscopic tissue responses are quite similar. There are no pathognomonic responses of the CNS to radiation, however, selective damage to the gray matter would eliminate radiation as an etiology. The necrosis, malacia, and demyelination of white matter caused by radiation are also seen due to other agents (such as chemotherapy).

Brain

Radiation changes in the brain are of several general types: acute reactions, early delayed reactions, and late delayed reactions. There are several target cell types and pathways by which radiation injury of the CNS may occur. Historically late changes were thought to be secondary to vascular changes but now it appears that the two main target cells are oligodendrocytes as well as endothelial cells. In addition, the vascular changes appear to be preferentially venous (rather than arterial) damage.[167] The SOMA toxicity table related to the brain is presented in Appendix 6.

Low-LET Radiation

Primary brain damage is usually the result of an insult to the glial cells and vascular system, although occasionally an acute demyelinating process is observed.[172] Subacute changes appear to be the result of deterministic effects on proliferating oligodendrocytes and temporary changes in the blood-brain barrier. Abrupt deterioration has been reported in radiotherapy when large fractions (7.5 to 10 Gy) have been used. Excessively large doses or relatively few fractions of large doses (greater than 10 Gy) have caused radiation-induced brain necrosis.[173] A single case of possible radiogenic dementia has been reported.[174]

The tolerance dose of the brain with fractionated radiotherapy over 5 to 6 weeks is thought to be 55 Gy, although small areas of the brain may tolerate doses up to 65 Gy. Postirradiation necrosis has rarely been reported at fractionated doses of less than 60 Gy. Overall, the white matter of the CNS is more susceptible to radionecrosis than is the gray matter or the brain stem. The paraventricular and supraoptic nuclei of the hypothalamus appear to be more radiosensitive than white matter. In the acute clinical period, the response of the brain to irradiation depends on whether the brain was normal initially. The sudden onset of headache, vomiting, and papilledema has often been referred to as "radiation edema," but in most therapeutic circumstances, the clinical presentation has been confused by recent surgery, presence of tumor, and other factors. The actual presence of radiation edema in the usual fractionated radiotherapy scheme appears to be dubious. Elevation of cerebrospinal fluid pressure following fractionated radiotherapy is rare, although single doses in the range of 35 Gy can cause an acute inflammatory reaction with increased capillary permeability and interstitial edema. A single whole-brain dose in the range of 60 Gy is lethal within 2 to 3 days. Demyelinating lesions have been reported within 10 weeks after 55 Gy of fractionated cobalt 60 radiotherapy.[172]

Early delayed reactions appear from a few weeks to a few months after radiation therapy. They are usually self-limited and are easily mistaken for effects of residual tumor or chemotherapy. In children treated for leukemia with methotrexate and radiation, about 60% to 80% will exhibit anorexia, irritability, and a "somnolence syndrome" 2 to 6 months post-therapy, probably due to transient diffuse demyelination. In adults there may be ataxia, nausea, vomiting, dysphagia, dysarthria, and nystagmus. The pathogenesis of this reaction appears to be transient interruption of myelin synthesis perhaps due to abnormalities in capillary permeability. The late delayed reaction has a number of forms, ranging from asymptomatic periventricular white matter changes to decreased mental status, endocrine changes, and even focal necrosis. Seventy percent of cases of focal necrosis present themselves within the first 2 years after radiotherapy although necrosis can occur as early as 3 months.[175] Pathologically, areas of focal necrosis occur preferentially in the white matter and extend to the gray-white matter junction. In late stages there can be clumped chalky calcification. Radiation necrosis occurs with a much higher probability when therapy schemes in 5 weeks exceed 40 Gy in 20 fractions or 60 Gy in 30 fractions, or when fractions exceed 3 Gy.[176,177] With the advent of radiosurgery there are high doses being delivered to small volumes of the brain. Even though the volumes are small, there are still reports of significant radiation reactions.[178] The maximum tolerable dose in children up to the age of 3 is 33% less than that for adults, and Bloom also estimated that for children 3 to 5 years of age, the adult dose has to be reduced by 20%.[179]

Imaging of radiation necrosis with computed tomography (CT) often shows a low-density region with surrounding edema, a variable mass effect, and irregular enhancement after administration of contrast material. Magnetic resonance imaging (MRI) shows areas of decreased signal on T1-weighted images and increased signal on T2 images. Unfortunately, residual tumor has the same imaging characteristics, and it is often not possible to differentiate between these entities with either modality.[180,181] Research using single photon emission computed tomography (SPECT) and positron emission tomography (PET) scanning has been performed, and it appears that using radiotracers (fluorine 18 labeled 2-fluoro-2-deoxyglucose) metabolism can differentiate between these entities. This is because a tumor would have an area of metabolism equal to or greater than that of surrounding brain tissues, while radiation necrosis would have decreased or absent metabolism.[182–185] Dual isotope methods have also been described by Schwartz et al.[186] and others[187] using SPECT. If the area of concern had a high accumulation of thallium 201, there was recurrent tumor rather than necrosis. Recent studies indicate

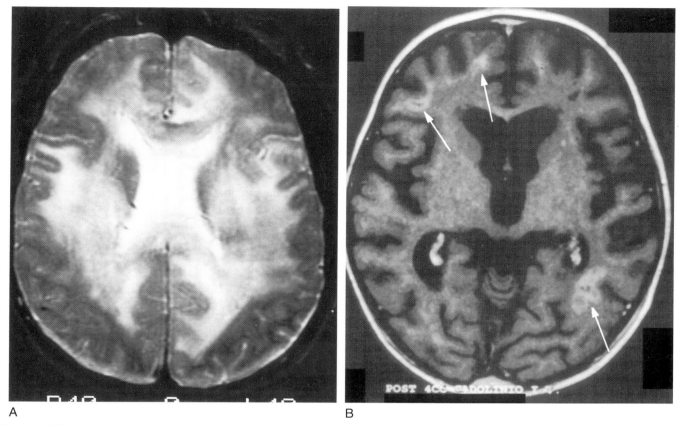

A   B

Figure 6-7 • Imaging changes in the brain after excessive radiation therapy. **A**, Image from a T2-weighted MRI scan shows symmetrical confluent high signal (white) in a periventricular white matter distribution. **B**, Image from a T1-weighted gadolinium-enhanced MRI shows cortical atrophy and mineralizing microangiopathy (*arrows*).

that PET-FDG (fluorodeoxyglucose) in combination with a radiolabeled amino acid analog is also helpful.[188] Histologically, the most characteristic abnormality in delayed radiation necrosis is the exudation of an amorphous, eosinophilic, and structureless substance that can be identified as fibrin. If there is a fibrin exudate along a hypocellular region occurring along the gray-white junction, the picture is almost diagnostic. There are rare reports of delayed brain hemorrhage several years after radiotherapy for pediatric brain tumors.[189]

With the advent of MRI it has become clear that many patients will develop areas of diffusely increased signal in the white matter seen on T2-weighted images (Fig. 6-7A). Reports indicate that 50% to 100% of patients will show these findings after radiotherapy. The changes occur preferentially in the periventricular white matter and may extend out to the gray-white junction. In mild forms the patients appear to have no clinical symptoms, while in patients with extensive MRI changes there is more likely to be more mental impairment such as personality change, confusion, seizure disorders, and learning difficulties.[190,191] Leukoencephalopathy refers to white-matter injury caused by demyelination following treatment with chemotherapeutic agents with or without

associated radiation therapy. It is not seen after radiotherapy alone. The most typical situation is after doses of 20 Gy and with use of methotrexate,[192–194] although it has also been reported after whole-body doses of 10 Gy given prior to bone marrow transplantation.[90] On CT and MRI this entity is indistinguishable from the white matter radiation changes. Cortical gray matter and basal ganglia are not affected. Clinical findings are lethargy, poor school performance, ataxia, spasticity, progressive dementia, and even death.

Another change that is sometimes seen in children treated for leukemia with cranial radiation and methotrexate is mineralizing microangiopathy (Fig. 6-7B).[195] This is seen as calcification in the gray matter, basal ganglia, putamen, and sometimes in the cortex and even the brain stem.[196] There is calcification in small blood vessels that are surrounded by necrotic mineralized necrotic brain tissue. It is not fatal and it is unknown if this produces any specific neurologic signs, although it is often associated with leukoencephalopathy. The entity is seen in about 25% of patients who received intrathecal methotrexate and cranial radiation of 24 Gy and who survive for more than 9 months. Another late change that may be seen in about 50% of patients after cranial radiation therapy is cortical atrophy. This is seen either on CT or MRI as enlarged cortical sulci and enlarged ventricles, usually detectable 1 to 4 years after radiotherapy. This is seen in about one half of patients who have received more than 30 Gy to the brain with fractionated radiotherapy.

Modifying factors influencing radiation effects appear to be preexisting disease, age, anatomic location, arteriosclerosis, and chemotherapy—including systemically administered antimetabolites (methotrexate, 5-fluorouracil), alkylating agents (cisplatinum [BCNU]), plant alkaloids (vincristine), nitrogen mustard, procarbazine, misonidazole, and interleukin-2. In addition to parenchymal changes of the brain due to radiation, there are vascular changes that can be imaged. Koike et al. showed that MRI can visualize radiation-induced telangiectasia in about 20% of children who have received cranial radiotherapy.[197] All doses were 18 to 20 Gy and the abnormalities appeared as early as 3 years but additional lesions still developed 10 years post-therapy. They were seen as small foci of very low signal intensity on T2-weighted images.

The increased sensitivity of the nervous system in children requires radiotherapy treatment schedules to be adjusted according to the age of the patient. Arteriosclerosis may lower tolerance of the brain since the occlusive changes due to radiation may be additive with respect to preexisting arteriosclerotic changes. Sheline[198] and others[193] suggest that chemotherapy may add to the radionecrosis and possibly enhance the level of injury.[198] Both depression and somnolence, probably as a result of a transient encephalopathy, have been reported 6 to 8 weeks after cranial irradiation to dose levels of 24 Gy in 10 to 15 fractions. Such findings have been seen in children and adults treated for acute lymphoblastic leukemia, even with normal cerebrospinal fluid.[199,200] The somnolence is distinct from the more severe neurologic abnormalities produced by intrathecal methotrexate.

Many reports suggest a decline in intelligence quotient (IQ) scores, as well as cognitive dysfunction in children treated with cranial radiation and intrathecal methotrexate for ALL as well as in adults who are treated for primary brain tumors or cranial radiation for small-cell lung cancer.[201] Intellectual decline usually is first noted 4 to 6 months post-therapy and may increase up to 2 to 3 years after which function seems to stabilize. Speculation regarding the etiology of such possible effects includes the theory that cranial irradiation may enhance the intracerebral absorption of the methotrexate (which by itself alone is associated with nervous system dysfunction). The long-term effects of primary radiation therapy for brain tumors in children have been studied by Danoff et al.[202] Tumor doses were 40 to 65 Gy. Performance status was good to excellent in 89% of patients. Mental retardation was found in 17% of patients, and behavioral disorders were found in 39% of the patients, but also in 59% of mothers and 43% of fathers. Mental retardation was greatest in

those less than 3 years of age and in those who had tumors in the region of the thalamus and hypothalamus.

There have been many studies related to the effects of radiation and chemotherapy on cognitive function. These are usually studied by use of achievement tests, aptitude tests, or IQ tests. It is clear that there is a wide range of changes that are seen in survivors of childhood cancers that received cranial radiotherapy. In general the younger the age at irradiation, the greater is the effect. The effects include memory deficits, attention deficit disorders, visual spatial skill impairment, reduction in IQ, and mental retardation. As a result of this, Moore et al. suggested that for some children with brain tumors, treatment without cranial irradiation can minimize morbidity without an increased rate of mortality.[203] Neuropsychologic abnormalities with behavioral disorders and intellectual impairment are seen in up to 50% of children treated for brain tumors with doses of 40 Gy or more in 1.8 to 2.0 Gy daily fractions. The younger the child, the greater is the IQ loss.[94,204,205] The adverse effect may not be evident until 2 to 5 years post-therapy. In general, children who receive 24 Gy of fractionated radiotherapy have a 10- to 15-point loss in IQ.

In children treated for leukemia there does not appear to be neuropsychologic impairment if intrathecal methotrexate is used without radiotherapy. When it is used with radiotherapy the deficit appears to be greater than for radiotherapy alone. A significant reduction in IQ scores occurs when there is 18 Gy of fractionated radiotherapy used with methotrexate.[206–208] Observed declines in IQ appear to be a failure to learn at an appropriate rate rather than loss of previously acquired knowledge.[209] Trautman et al.[210] noted that social class was a much stronger predictor of ultimate IQ than was age at irradiation or radiation dose, while Bleyer et al.[211] indicated that age at irradiation is the most important factor. This stresses the need for controlling of confounding factors in study design. Hyperbaric oxygen therapy has had little, if any, impact on cognitive disorders after brain irradiation.[212] When newer techniques involving highly conformal fractionated partial brain radiotherapy are used, adverse neuropsychological effects are much less common.[213,214] Also, as expected with total-body irradiation in preparation for bone marrow transplantation and doses of 12 to 14 Gy, the incidence of neurobehavioral toxicity is very low.[215] The increasing use of gamma knife radiosurgery (used for treatment of acoustic neuromas, meningiomas, etc.) and other forms of robotic-guided stereotactic irradiation has led to reports of facial and trigeminal neuropathy, headaches, dizziness, and radiation necrosis.[216–219]

Some authors have indicated a correlation between calcification and other abnormalities on CT scans and learning disabilities or seizures, but these conclusions are not confirmed in other studies.[220,221] While the bulk of the literature concerns neuropsychologic effects after childhood cranial radiotherapy, there are a few scattered reports concerning mental impairment in adults. Biologically, there seems much less reason for a radiation effect, and there is always the concern about whether the effects seen are the result of the tumor itself, edema, pre-existing vascular disease, or other factors. Tucker et al. indicated that in adults who received prophylactic CNS radiation for adult leukemia, there were only minimal, subclinical, long-term neuropsychologic changes.[222]

There are a number of published reports of alleged changes in mental function after relatively low doses of radiation. Follow-up studies have been performed and include both Israeli[223] and U.S.[224] children who received about 1 to 2 Gy during treatment of tinea capitus. In the Israel study, males with multiple irradiations had a higher rate of admissions to mental hospitals (34.0 vs. 17.4 per 1000), but this difference was not seen for females. Children irradiated at less than 6 years of age had an RR of mental hospital admissions of 1.7 (95% confidence interval [CI] 1.1 to 2.8), but for older children there was no increased risk. In addition unirradiated siblings had a higher incidence of neurosis and personality disorder. In the U.S. series, there was a 30% excess of psychiatric disorders among the irradiated children; however, a more recent and detailed study by Omran et al. showed only a borderline difference between the two groups.[225] It should be noted that there does not appear to be a good biologic or pathologic basis for effects at these dose levels, and these results are not supported by follow-up studies of children treated for tumors. As with most studies of this type, there is the possibility of recall bias and other potential confounding.

In a controversial paper, Hall et al. concluded that persons treated for cutaneous hemangioma with radiotherapy in infancy had lower cognitive function.[226] This conclusion was based on records of school attendance and cognitive tests of learning ability and logical reasoning (but not IQ tests). The proportion of boys who attended high school decreased with increasing dose from 32% among those not exposed to about 17% in those who received a brain dose of more than 250 mGy. No effect was found with regard to spatial recognition. The mean dose to the brain was 50 mGy. The paper did not take into account potential changes in thyroid function as a function of irradiation and the effect was based on differing levels of brain dose, but there was no external control or comparison group. There also was no difference in results whether the anterior or posterior aspect of the brain received the most radiation. Finally, the magnitude of effects suggested here are considerably higher than that noted at brain doses over 100 times higher given for leukemia treatment. These studies indicated that 24 Gy is associated with about a 10- to 15-point loss of IQ.[207,208]

There are two papers alleging a relationship between radiation and multiple sclerosis. One is simply a case report of a patient who had multiple sclerosis that became worse after radiotherapy.[227] The second paper is unlikely to be valid and is an ecological study in Norway based on latitude, which purports to show an increase in multiple sclerosis varying with latitude and this is assumed to relate to radon exposure.[228] Obviously, the dose from alpha-emitting radon to the brain is orders of magnitude lower than from natural external penetrating background radiation and this hypothesis should not be taken seriously.

Two papers are available concerning population radiation exposure and dementia. A report by Sibley et al. evaluated causes of death among 67,976 female nuclear workers, including those that listed the cause of death as dementia.[229] A positive association was reported but the authors indicate that more research is needed and, of course, there are serious issues about the accuracy of death certificates when the cause of death is listed as dementia. It is also of interest that a study of dementia in the atomic bomb survivors by Yamada et al. did not find any correlation relative to either vascular or Alzheimer's dementia and radiation exposure.[230] There also has been investigation into a possible link of prenatal exposure in the atomic bomb survivors and schizophrenia by Imamura et al. but no relationship was found.[231]

High-LET Radiation

Neutrons, pi-mesons, and heavy nuclei have been the subject of study in the treatment of brain tumors. In general, neutrons produce more injury to normal tissues than might be expected, and the RBE for the brain appears to be about 4 to 5. Increased brain edema following 13 Gy of neutrons over 4 weeks has been reported. Dementia has occurred in some patients with doses of 15.6 Gy over 4 weeks. It has been speculated that the normal brain tissue may be sensitive due to a high hydrogen content. The patient series for the other radiation types are generally small, and injury to normal tissues is difficult to ascertain. For further reading in this area the reader is referred to a chapter on the topic by Laramore.[232]

Internal Exposure

It is clear that high doses of radiation delivered by implanted sealed radioactive sources can give rise to the focal necrotic lesions described earlier.[233,234] These sources can be used alone or in combination with external radiotherapy. Under some circumstances, such as permanent implantation of iodine 125 seeds, the necrosis rate can be as high as 40%.[235]

Spinal Cord

Low-LET Radiation

Deterministic injury of the spinal cord has been reported many times, particularly in cases of radiotherapy of neoplasms that occurred outside the CNS.[167] In general, radiation-induced lesions of the spine have a shorter latent period to their clinical manifestation than do similar brain lesions. The spinal cord often is unable to tolerate the absorbed dose levels necessary to eradicate malignant tumors. In some cases, the original malignancy may be controlled or cured, with the development of the complication of paralysis associated with the level of the irradiation. The so-called radiation myelitis may be either transient or permanent. Myelitis was a clearly identified radiation hazard as early as the 1940s. The diagnosis of radiation myelitis requires that (1) other etiologies must be eliminated, (2) presentation of symptoms should be consistent with radiation myelopathy, and (3) the dose and time of expression must be consistent with spinal cord radiation injury. The SOMA toxicity table related to the spinal cord is presented in Appendix 6.

Acute transient myelitis often appears 2 to 4 months after the termination of radiation therapy. The patient may experience electrical shocklike sensations, tingling, and paresthesias. Often the symptoms are exaggerated by either flexion or extension of the spine (Lhermitte's sign). The pathogenesis appears to be transient demyelination of the ascending sensory neurons. This syndrome usually resolves spontaneously without treatment. Reversal of the transient myelopathy may occur at 2 to 40 weeks.[236,237] In many instances, there is a delayed myelitis. The most radiosensitive portion of the CNS appears to be the upper thoracic segments and the lower lumbar and sacral segments. It had long been thought that the thoracic spinal cord was more sensitive than the cervical cord but this is probably not true. The latent period for delayed myelopathy of the thoracic and cervical spinal cord is about 20 months after radiation therapy, and 75% of cases occur within 30 months. Lumbar myelopathy usually occurs earlier, and the majority of cases appear within 17 months. The signs of radiation myelopathy depend on the level of the lesion in the spinal cord; however, it is irreversible, and there is a high fatality rate. The incidence of delayed myelopathy rises quickly as the radiation therapy scheme exceeds 30 Gy in 10 fractions, 40 Gy in 20 fractions, or 60 Gy in 30 fractions. The patients may experience paralysis, decreased vibration and position sense, spastic quadriplegia, incontinence, and diaphragmatic breathing. Neurologically, the patient may exhibit the Brown-Séquard syndrome due to involvement of the lateral columns of the spinal cord. During this period, the cerebrospinal fluid and pressure are usually normal. If the lower motor neurons are involved, a flaccid paralysis may result. Fajardo points out that the prognosis for delayed radiation myelitis is usually poor, with rarely any evidence of recovery.[3] Survival in cases of cervical and high thoracic myelitis is about 10 months. Death usually results from either pneumonia or urinary tract infection. Clinically, the neurologic level is manifested in anatomic segments lower than the level at which the radiation was given. The acute reversible form of the myelitis may be

due to an abnormality in the synthesis of myelin by the oligodendrogliocytes. Pathologically, the lesions are quite similar to those described in the white matter of the brain with demyelinization and areas of radionecrosis. The delayed form of myelitis has been thought to be due to progressive vascular obliteration and thrombosis, but recently Withers et al. suggested that the death of slowly dividing cells may be the more likely cause.[238] Hyperthermia has been suspected as a contributing factor to acute radiation transverse myelopathy.[239]

The physical factors of the radiation are very important in assessing the risk of myelopathy. If a radiation field is very long, the risk of myelopathy is greater, particularly when adjacent field radiotherapy is performed with overlap in the treatment field. The spinal cord is generally more sensitive than the brain. There is a relationship between the volume of cord irradiated and the tolerance dose. Kramer et al. indicated the maximum acceptable dose to the cervical and lumbar spinal cord to be 50 Gy in 25 fractions over 5 weeks, and to the thoracic cord, 45 Gy delivered over 4.5 to 5 weeks.[173] Other reported tolerance doses range between 35 Gy in 4 weeks and 50 Gy in 5 weeks.[240] If these doses are exceeded, transient radiation myelopathy and, perhaps, paralysis may result. Fitzgerald et al. indicated that 13% of patients who received 40 Gy in an accelerated fractionation scheme and survived 11 months developed progressive myelitis.[241]

Dische et al. examined 754 cases of radiation myelitis that occurred after radiotherapy for lung cancer.[242] They reported that the threshold dose for thoracic radiation myelitis in fractionated radiotherapy was 33.5 Gy. Georgiou et al. reviewed 2410 patients treated with external and internal radiotherapy for carcinomas of the cervix and endometrium.[243] The calculated dose to the lumbosacral plexus was 73 Gy, and only four patients developed lumbosacral plexopathy. The most widely observed dose limit for the spinal cord is 45 Gy in 22 to 25 fractions although there have been reports of myelopathy after 45 Gy when only one field was treated per day. The incidence of myelopathy if the above limits are adhered to is 0.2% or less; however, if the does is 57 to 61 Gy the incidence rises to 5%, and at 68 to 73 Gy the incidence is 50%.[167] Hyperfractionation does not reduce the incidence of myelopathy because there apparently is significantly less repair of radiation damage in the 6-hour intervals than occurs in other tissues. In patients who need to be retreated there appears to be significant recovery of occult radiation damage after about 2 years. Chemotherapy is a very important factor to consider as well since many agents cause myelopathy by themselves or potentiate radiation effects. The agents include methotrexate,[244] cisplatinum, vinblastine, Ara C,[167] and possibly cyclophosphamide.[245]

A few reports on the potential use of magnetic resonance (MR) to help in the diagnosis of radiation myelitis have appeared. The findings are relatively nonspecific: Commonly, no abnormality is seen in the first 3 months; in 3 to 8 months abnormally high signal intensity of T2-weighted images is seen often with contrast enhancement.[246] The high T2 signal and contrast enhancement often resolves in 10 to 24 months. Swelling may or may not be present. This would be difficult to differentiate from residual tumor. Several years after occurrence the MR scans show atrophy of the cord without abnormal signal intensity.[247]

Peripheral Nerves

Low-LET Radiation

Peripheral nerves are among the structures most resistant to radiation damage. Although several researchers have reported peripheral neuropathy, including brachial plexus injury, most of the findings are complicated by other forms of therapy that are in themselves neurotoxic (such as misonidazole).[248] Occasionally, it is also difficult to separate changes due to radiation from those due to surgery, such as scarring around the nerves, as the cause of the neuropathy. Damage to the brachial plexus has been described in individuals who have received doses in the range of 50 Gy in a fractionated course of therapy to the high axillary nodes. A number of articles concern brachial plexus injuries after radiotherapy for breast cancer. Olsen et al. indicated that 5% of patients in a Danish series had disabling plexopathy, and 9% had milder symptoms after administration of 50 Gy in 25 fractions over 5 weeks.[249] Clinical manifestations in cases were parasthesia in 100%, hypasthesia in 74%, weakness in 58%, pain in 47%, and decreased muscle stretch reflexes in 47%. A higher incidence was found in patients also receiving cytotoxic therapy and if fraction sizes were over 2 Gy. A much lower incidence (1.3%) was reported by Pierce et al. with an axillary dose of less than 50 Gy but 5.6% when the dose exceeded 50 Gy.[250] The median time to occurrence was 10.5 months (range 1.5 to 77 months) and 80% of cases completely resolved. The incidence was 0.6% in patients without chemotherapy and 4.5% in patients receiving chemotherapy. There is no evidence that hyperbaric oxygen therapy slows or reverses radiation-induced brachial plexopathy[251] and no other therapies have been forthcoming.[252] There is controversy as to whether electrophysiologic studies are useful in differentiating radiation-induced cases from neoplastic plexopathy. Optic nerve changes are discussed in the following section on the eye.

High-LET Radiation

The RBE of neutrons for the spinal cord and brain may be equal to or higher than that for skin. Few published data concern the RBE of neutrons for the human spinal cord.

Radionuclides

No significant changes on the CNS following administration of unsealed radionuclides have been demonstrated in humans.

EYE AND EAR

Eye

Deterministic effects of radiation on the eye were noted as early as 1897, and by 1908, corneal changes were clearly recognized as deterministic effects. In the 1950s, there was extensive investigation of radiogenic eye damage, particularly concerning cataract formation. The historical aspects are well reviewed by Rubin and Casarett.[2] More recent summary publications are also available.[253–256] Most of the tissues around the eye have the same sensitivity as skin; however, the lens is particularly radiosensitive, with subsequent production of opacities within the lens and cataract formation. The SOMA toxicity table related to the eye is presented in Appendix 6.

The cornea and the sclera are protective portions of the eye. The epithelium of the cornea is composed of a basal layer of vegetative intermitotic cells (as in the skin), as well as squamous cells of other varieties and collagen. The iris is located behind the cornea and in front of the lens, the choroid, and the ciliary bodies. These structures are composed of fibroblasts, smooth muscle, vascular structures, and simple columnar and mesenchymal epithelium. Many of these cells are reverting postmitotic cells. The retina is very complex in formation and has reverting postmitotic cells, as well as fixed postmitotic cells. The lens of the eye is an avascular structure covered by a capsule. The anterior surface of the lens has a layer of epithelial cells that become thicker and denser as they mature and ultimately form the inner mass of the lens. In the anterior portion, the lens epithelium behaves as reverting postmitotic cells. Near the equator of the lens, the epithelial cells divide regularly and thus behave as vegetative intermitotic cells. The accessory glands around the eye (including Moll's glands, sebaceous meibomiam glands, and the lacrimal glands) all contain reverting or fixed postmitotic cells. The ductal epithelium for some of these glands does contain vegetative intermitotic cells. Thus, the excretory ducts, particularly in the meibomiam glands, are relatively sensitive to deterministic effects of radiation, as are the equatorial regions of the optic lens and the basal layer of the cornea. The neurons of the retina probably represent the most radioresistant cells in the eye.

Low-LET Radiation

Because a large portion of the eye, particularly the conjunctiva, is composed of epithelial cells, it reacts as the skin does during the acute clinical period. There may be erythema and, if the dose is high enough, dry or moist desquamation. The eyebrows are quite resistant to epilation, even when it occurs at other sites. Permanent epilation of the eyebrows occurs after a fractionated dose of 30 Gy over 3 weeks. Fractionated doses of 20 Gy cause reddening with vascular prominence, and, as the orthovoltage dose approaches 40 to 50 Gy, a confluent mucositis appears. At this stage, the lacrimal gland has thick secretions, and the eye easily becomes infected. During this period, the patient may experience photophobia. Lacrimal glands are relatively resistant to radiation and most patients tolerate fractionated therapy schemes to total doses of 30 to 40 Gy without severe symptoms of a dry eye. Atrophy of the glands occurs at cumulative fractionated doses in the range of 50 to 60 Gy. The sclera is quite resistant to radiation effects, although damage has been reported in cases of application of beta-emitting plaques where the doses exceeded 20 Gy in a single exposure. The iris of the eye can be affected, and fractionated doses in excess of 70 Gy can produce an acute iritis. The cornea demonstrates very few effects until fractionated doses are in the range of 50 Gy. At that point, a superficial punctate keratitis may develop. Deep keratitis and ulceration of the cornea are quite rare unless very high doses are given over a short time period. Changes in the choroid, lens, retina, and optic nerve are almost never seen in the acute period. The changes seen during the acute clinical period are not pathognomonic of radiation, and an effort must be made to ensure that they are not due to infection. At very high dose levels (which may sometimes result from combining several radiotherapy schemes), if the dose level reaches 100 Gy over the course of a year, a panophthalmitis, which may require enucleation, can develop. At least one report of spontaneous corneal rupture after strontium irradiation for a conjunctival carcinoma has been published. This may have been a complication of the tumor rather than a radiation effect alone.[257]

In the period from 6 months to 2 years (subacute clinical period), telangiectasia may develop in the skin and the conjunctiva. During that time, scarring of the cornea may progress if deep keratitis was present during the acute period. Hemorrhage into the vitreous and retina may occur from telangiectatic changes in the retina. Areas of fluffy exudate may be seen in the retina and the choroid, with associated atrophy.[2]

Radiation retinopathy, as a complication of radiotherapy, was described as early as 1930. It can be produced by external beam radiotherapy at doses as low as 15 Gy but is more common at fractionated doses of 30 to 35 Gy. At total fractionated doses of 70 to 80 Gy, retinopathy will occur in 85% of eyes. Exudates, hemorrhages, microaneurysms, cotton wool spots, telangiectasia, and retinal capillary nonperfusion occur at 4 to 36 months (mean 18 months) after radiotherapy. The earliest changes identified by fluorescein angiography are capillary dilatation, closure, and microaneurysm formation (predominantly on the arterial side). Telangiectatic vessels are a feature of established retinopathy.[258,259] The incidence of retinopathy has been reported to be about 85% after treatment of the orbit with radiotherapy, 45% after treatment of paranasal sinus lesions, and 36% after treatment of nasopharynx lesions.[260] Up to 60% of patients surviving bone marrow transplant therapy after chemotherapy and total-body radiation may develop occlusive microvascular retinopathy.[261] These changes may progress to blindness. Diabetes and chemotherapy, when combined with radiation, seem to have an additive effect in production of retinopathy.[262,263]

Radiation optic neuropathy may temporarily cause decreased vision that may later improve over several months. This entity involves the anterior optic nerve and is characterized acutely by hyperemia and disc swelling. Peripapillary hemorrhages and subretinal fluid may also be present. With external irradiation, the total fractionated mean dose causing this effect is 55 Gy, with a range of 36 to 72 Gy. The mean latent period following radiotherapy is 19 months (5 to 36 months). After treatment of choroidal melanomas with gamma knife radiosurgery using one fraction of 40 to 80 Gy, there is a high incidence of both radiation retinopathy and neovascular glaucoma.[264] Both radiation retinopathy and optic neuropathy appear to be secondary to vascular damage.[262,265,266] Several authors have reported on the magnetic resonance appearance of radiation-induced optic neuropathy.[267–269] In general, there was gadolinium enhancement of the optic nerve with slight swelling even at 6 to 36 months post-radiotherapy with dose levels in the range of 55 to 62 Gy.

Cataracts are the most frequent delayed reaction in the eye. Radiation cataracts are among the few lesions that pathologically are quite characteristic for radiation injury. Radiation cataracts are due to damage to the germinative zone of lens epithelial DNA but there are also likely contributions from deterministic cytoplasmic effects, protein cross-linking, and disruption of ion pumps and membrane channels. Even though the cataract initially appears clinically in the posterior pole, the pathogenesis of the radiation cataract is usually damage to the germinal layer located at the equator of the lens. With the inhibition of mitosis and actively proliferating cells, there is interference with differentiation. The damaged cells migrate toward the posterior pole, where they undergo degeneration. Most senile cataracts begin in the anterior pole of the lens, whereas radiation cataracts begin as a small dot in the posterior pole. Only an ophthalmologist who is very experienced in radiation effects may be able to provide an accurate assessment. Perhaps the best description of radiogenic cataracts in the literature is that of Cogan et al.[270] As the opacity develops in the posterior pole and enlarges to 3 to 4 mm, a central clear area may be identified. Ultimately, the cataract may progress to the anterior pole of the lens, with development of a nonspecific cataract. While posterior cataracts are characteristic of radiation exposure, they are not

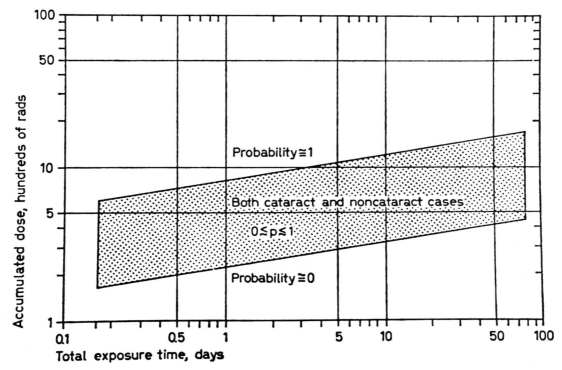

Figure 6-8 • Probability of cataract formation as a function of dose and exposure time. (From Merriam GR, Jr, Szechter A, Focht EF: The effects of ionizing radiations on the eye. (From Merriam GR, Szechter A, Focht EF: The effect of ionizing radiations on the eye. Front Radiat Ther Oncol 1972;6:346–385.)

pathognomonic; in other words, there are other causes that can result in posterior cataracts.

Lens opacities do not always interfere with vision, and thus a clinical cataract requires higher doses. The latent period for production of cataracts from the time of exposure may range from 12 to 35 years, although on the average, it is 2 to 3 years. The higher the absorbed dose, the shorter is the latent period. The incidence of radiation cataracts is dose-, time-, and age-dependent (Fig. 6-8).[271] Single doses of 2 Gy or fractionated doses of 4 Gy can result in the formation of lens opacities.[272] A single dose of 7.5 Gy causes cataract formation in all those exposed. A similar incidence occurs with 14 Gy given over a period of 3 to 12 weeks. In situations in which occupational exposure occurs over a period of years, the threshold for cataract formation appears to be between 6 and 14 Gy.[273,274] The possible threshold reported in other, more recent, studies (discussed later in this chapter) appears to be in the range of 1 Gy or lower.

When radiation-induced cataracts are being considered, other causes of cataracts need to be considered such as drugs (steroids, allopurinol, dilantin, chlorpromazine, tricyclic antidepressants, monoamine oxidase inhibitors, and others), trauma (lasers, UV, microwaves, and penetrating physical injuries), systemic disorders (diabetes, hypocalcemia, riboflavin deficiency), and genetic disorders. Cataracts have been identified in atomic bomb survivors. The term *cataract* often connotes blindness or

at least impaired vision; the vast majority of radiation "cataracts" identified in the atomic bomb survivors were nonprogressive and did not impair vision. There appeared to be a threshold dose below which lenticular opacities were not found.[275,276]

A study of the atomic bomb survivors has indicated that the lenses of children may be more sensitive to the induction of cataracts by ionizing radiation than in adults.[277] Early studies were based on examination of over 2300 individuals. In Hiroshima, the RR for axial opacities and posterior subcapsular changes was 4.8 for individuals exposed to more than 3 Sv while under the age of 15 years. In the age group 15 to 24 years at the time of the bombing, the RR was 2.3 as compared with 1.4 in the age group over 25 years. With regard to posterior subcapsular changes alone, the RR was 2.8 in the 1 to 1.99 Sv group under the age of 15 years and 4.3 in the 2 to 2.99 Sv group. Subsequent reports to elucidate the potential effect of neutron exposure (that was higher at Hiroshima than at Nagasaki) have been published. Unfortunately, the answer is not clear because revisions in the dosimetry (DS86) reduced the estimated neutron component at Hiroshima.[278,279] Minamoto et al. examined the types of cataracts which were present 55 years after exposure in atomic bomb survivors who were exposed before 13 years of age.[280] Positive associations were found for cortical and posterior subcapsular cataract but not for nuclear cataract.

There has been recent discussion as to whether there actually is a threshold dose for cataract formation. Nakashima et al. performed a reanalysis of atomic bomb cataract data to evaluate whether there is a threshold dose for either cortical cataract or posterior subcapsular opacities.[281] Of the 730 persons (aged 55 to 94 years) participating in the study during 2000–2002 (more than 60 years after the bombs), more than half (477) had no lens abnormalities at all. Threshold point estimates were 0.6 and 0.7 Sv, respectively, but there were wide CIs that included 0 Sv as a possibility.

Cucinotta et al. reported on space radiation and cataracts in astronauts.[282] This is of interest since astronauts are exposed to high-energy protons, heavy ions, and secondary particles. Astronauts on Apollo, Skylab, space shuttle, and Mir missions have observed "light flashes" that raise concern for adverse effects on the eye. There is a higher incidence of cataracts in NASA astronauts with lens doses greater than 8 mSv compared to those with lens doses of less than 8 mSv. While many of the cataracts are not clinically significant, occurrence at low doses raises concern over progression over the long term. Increased cataracts in astronauts was also reported by Rasteger et al.[283] Another "low-dose" study is the Beaver Dam Eye Study reported by Klein et al.[284] There were 4926 subjects who had eye examinations and who were questioned about diagnostic x-ray exposure. The only positive finding was for lens opacities and CT scan of the head. The odds ratio (OR) was 1.45 (95% CI 1.08 to 1.95). Doses to the eye from this type of CT scan can be in the range of 10 to 30 mSv.

There have been several studies undertaken regarding cataract formation in the populations exposed to radiation from the Chernobyl accident. Much effort has been focused on the first responders, who suffered acute radiation effects, and the liquidators involved in the extended cleanup and stabilization of the site.[285] Worgul et al. studied 8607 clean-up workers and reported posterior and subcapsular cataracts in 25% of subjects. Dose response was mostly linear, and analysis of various endpoints excluded a threshold greater than 0.7 Gy.[285a] One study investigated the prevalence and the characteristics of lens changes in a pediatric population (5 to 17 years of age) surrounding the Chernobyl area.[286] Of the 1787 subjects (996 exposed, 791 unexposed) in an extensive study, a small (3.6%), but significant, group of exposed children manifested posterior subcapsular (PSC) lens changes consistent with those observed in other exposed individuals, such as the A-bomb survivors. These observations were supported by Fedirko and Khilinska, who found PSC lens changes in a study of 461 children.[287]

There have been a number of other Ukrainian studies of acute radiation sickness (ARS) survivors and liquidators, which reportedly have made estimates of RR by dose and found vascular pathology and deterioration of accommodative capability.[288] Cataract studies also have been conducted at the Medical Radiological Research Center of Russia and at the Republican Research Center of Radiation Medicine and Human Ecology of Belarus.[289] Data from the liquidator studies suggest that exposures to doses on the order of 250 mGy may also be cataractogenic. The Belarusian results to date are mixed: while the liquidators have statistically greater numbers of cataracts than the general population, the evacuees and residents in contaminated areas have statistically fewer cataracts. This unexpected result is being subjected to investigation. There are significant issues with regard to the accuracy of external doses recorded in registries for liquidators. Dosimetry relative to the lens of the eye, and, in particular, for beta radiation, poses significant additional obstacles. In some studies it is not clear whether or how beta radiation may have contributed to the development of cataracts in liquidators. There is some indication that, under certain conditions, the beta contribution to cataract could even exceed that of the gamma component.

Studies of adults who indicate radiation cataracts as a potential complication of radiotherapy as adults have been performed. Sakai et al. reported that 171 patients treated for maxillary carcinoma who survived for 10 years all developed a cataract on the treated side.[290] Studies of children treated for neoplasm relative to the risk of cataracts is hampered, somewhat, by the use of corticosteroids. Many of these patients have received long-term steroids. Posterior subcapsular cataracts were observed by Ogelsby et al. in 42% of patients with rheumatic disease who were treated with long-term steroids.[291] A corticosteroid-induced cataract is similar to that produced by ionizing radiation. Cataract formation was reported by Heyn et al. in 90% of children who were treated for orbital rhabdomyosarcoma.[292] Doses to the lens were calculated from less than 10 Gy to greater than 50 Gy, and the appearance of the cataract ranged from 1 to 4 years after radiotherapy.

The incidence of cataracts in children treated for acute leukemia or other tumors with total-body radiation pre–bone marrow transplant varies widely depending on what literature is examined. Nesbit et al.[293] reported that 2% of survivors of acute leukemia develop posterior subcapsular cataracts, whereas Inati et al.[294] observed a 50% increase in cataract formation in children who were given 24 Gy of fractionated therapy over 2.5 weeks; however, these children also received methotrexate and steroids. The incidence of cataracts following bone marrow transplantation in almost 300 patients has indicated that after 10 Gy of single-dose, whole-body radiation, 80% of children will develop cataracts by 6 years of age compared with 19% given fractionated whole-body radiation of 12 to 15 Gy in 2 to 5 fractions.[295–297] These studies also indicated that about 20% of children treated for aplastic anemia with steroids and given no radiation also developed cataracts. Similar data have been reported by other authors.[298–302] In these cases, the development of cataracts is thought to be of secondary importance since, if and when they occur, they may be surgically corrected. Both steroids[303] and estrogens[304] appear to worsen or accelerate radiation cataracts whereas melatonin (in animal experiments)[305] and heparin[306] have been reported as being potentially beneficial. Other changes have been noted in the eyes of children following radiotherapy, including enophthalmos, stenosis of the lacrimal duct, optic nerve atrophy, and retinopathy. For all these abnormalities, the frequency is very rare below fractionated total doses of 45 Gy.

Hall et al. reported on the incidence of lenticular opacities in patients who were irradiated in infancy for treatment of skin hemagiomas.[307] Lens opacities were found in 37% of those irradiated compared to 20% of controls. Children exposed to a lenticular dose of 1 Gy had a 50% increased risk (OR 1.5, 95% CI 1.10 to 2.05) of developing a posterior subcapsular opacity. Another similar study was reported by Wilde et al., which found an increase in subcapsular puntate opacities and vacuoles occurring at lens doses as low as 0.1 Gy.[308]

Dekaban indicated that in utero radiation, particularly during the first trimester, can result in cataract formation as well as pigmentary degeneration of the retina or microophthalmia.[309] Dekaban's paper includes 26 cases culled from the literature in which the mothers were treated for dysmenorrhea, metrorrhagia, myomata, neoplasms, tuberculous osteomyelitis, and rheumatoid arthritis. Doses ranged from 5.6 Gy to tens of Gy. Two of the 15 cases irradiated during the first trimester were found to have cataracts, and 12 were found to have microophthalmia. No cataracts were identified in children less than 1 year of age who received irradiation to the eye in doses below 13.8 Gy. Bateman indicated that doses in the range of 3 to 5 Gy delivered during the first half of pregnancy are quite damaging to the neurons of the developing retina, although as the neurons mature, they become much more radioresistant.[310] When used in conjunction with radiation therapy, 5-fluorouracil appears to lower the cataractogenic dose. As with other organs that are not rapidly proliferating, the eye ultimately suffers from the radiation damage to the arterioles and capillaries. The radiation causes either reduced lumina or vascular obstruction due to myointimal proliferation.

High-LET Radiation

Neutrons are known to be especially effective in the formation of cataracts. The literature predominantly concerns animals and indicates that the RBE ranges between 4.5 for 1.8 MeV neutrons and 9 for 0.43 MeV neutrons.[311] Cyclotron workers exposed to neutrons were originally thought to have some changes in the lens, although the doses of neutrons were extremely difficult to calculate and the study was a retrospective analysis of only affected persons.[312] In patients undergoing radiotherapy with fast neutrons, no changes were observed with doses of less than 0.8 Gy given as 12 fractions, but there was a minimal permanent loss of vision at doses totalling more than 2.2 Gy.[313]

Radionuclide Irradiation

Those patients who received intravenous radium 224 for treatment of ankylosing spondylitis and tuberculosis have been demonstrated to have an increased incidence of cataract formation.[314] This was particularly apparent since many of the patients were young, and cataract formation was not expected. Cataracts were found in approximately 5% of both juvenile and adult patients; however, the cataract incidence increased significantly with dosage.[315] Cataract formation in these patients occurred at periods of 7 to 26 years after the radium therapy. However, the doses to the lens of the eye have not been estimated; as mentioned with the other effects of radium, it is difficult to evaluate the effect of concurrent disease and drug therapy. The mechanism involved may be due to concentration of radium in the pigmented cells of the iris; such radium biocentration has been observed in rodents and dogs.[316]

Beta radiation induction of cataracts following the application of strontium 90 plaques has been examined.[317] In the past, strontium 90 applicators were used for orbital radiotherapy in the hope that the beta radiation would not cause damage to structures such as the lens. In fact, unique radiation cataracts occur, with the opacities occurring anteriorly in the lens. The average latent period is 2.5 years, and doses causing these changes were similar to those identified for radium applicators. The incidence of lenticular changes ranged from approximately 20% at a dose level of 1.8 to 7.2 Gy, to 42% at 7.2 to 12 Gy, and 73% at doses in excess of 12 Gy to the lens.

There are several reported changes of the eye following iodine 131 therapy. These include nascolacrimal obstruction occurring in about 4% of patients after thyroid cancer therapy and a worsening of exophthalmos after radioiodine therapy for Graves' disease.[318] The latter finding is not radiation related but is a consequence of Graves' disease.[319]

Ear

Even though radiation damage to the middle ear (following radium application) was described as early as 1905, very little work and clinical attention were directed toward this area until the 1950s. There are three excellent historical articles by Berg and Borsanyi.[320-322] Rubin and Casarett also published an excellent review of the historical aspects and clinical and pathologic findings.[2] The external ear consists of the elastic connective tissue, epithelium, and fibroblasts. The middle ear has an epithelial lining in the tympanic cavity. The mucous membrane is squamous and epithelial in nature and is composed of reverting postmitotic cells. The inner ear has many different cells types, but most of the cells are of the reverting postmitotic type. The radiation sensitivity of the external ear, therefore, is similar to that of the skin elsewhere, and the middle and internal ear are relatively radioresistant. Clinical effects that can be identified as results of radiation exposure are primarily due to changes in the fine vasculature, which is moderately radiosensitive.

Low-LET Radiation

Findings related to radiation effects on the ear may be identified very soon after irradiation. They include hearing loss, tinnitus, and earache.[323–326] Tinnitus may occur with localized radiation therapy at levels of 40 Gy. The situation resembles a serous otitis media and is due to hyperemia of the capillaries, increased capillary permeability, and serous exudate. A conductive hearing loss also may be present. Fractionated doses of 40 to 60 Gy will cause acute radiation otitis media in 50% of patients. Often the changes are not clinically evident and may not be found unless they are looked for specifically. From 6 months to a few years after radiotherapy (subacute clinical period), there may be a sudden onset of Meniere's disease.[327] The etiology of these vestibulocerebellar signs is unknown. Usually, the patient recovers within several weeks. In the chronic clinical period, radionecrosis of the auditory ossicles may occur. Previously, exploration was essential to establish the diagnosis and to differentiate the entity from otosclerosis. It is possible at the present time that the diagnosis may be made with high-resolution CT. Necrosis of the ossicles is due to progressive deterioration of the fine vasculature; however, other changes that may occur are atrophy of the spiral ligament, stria vascularis, and basilar membrane. These changes are usually progressive and may not be manifest for 1 to 6 years after radiation therapy. Human data in the chronic period are limited; however, such changes have been described after fractionated therapy of only 40 Gy.[328] The mean fractionated dose causing otologic sequelae is 66 Gy. Quite a few authors have reported on hearing loss to various degrees after radiotherapy.[329] Schot et al. studied patients who were treated with radiotherapy for parotid tumors.[330] Sensorineural hearing loss seldom occurred with cochlear doses of less than 55 Gy but often occurred at doses exceeding 65 Gy.[331] Similar findings after parotid radiotherapy were reported by Singh et al.,[332] Grau et al.,[333] and Wang et al.[334] after irradiation for nasopharyngeal carcinomas. Sensorineural hearing loss is usually more pronounced at high frequencies and has a latent period of 12 months or more.[335] There is some literature suggesting increased ototoxicity with chemotherapy such as cisplatinum.[336] Children may be more sensitive: hearing loss in children following a radiotherapy regimen of 50 Gy in 25 fractions over 5 weeks has been reported.

SALIVARY GLANDS

The salivary glands include the parotid, submaxillary, and sublingual glands. They each have secretions that enter the oral cavity through a duct. Both the parenchymal cells of the gland and the duct cells behave as reverting postmitotic cells and, therefore, are relatively resistant to deterministic effects of radiation. The major exceptions are the relatively large excretory ducts of the parotid, which contain stratified epithelium near the main outlet (similar to that of the oral mucosa, which has vegetative intermitotic cells in the basal layer), and are, therefore, relatively radiosensitive. The pathologic effects of radiation on these glands have been well described by Rubin and Casarett,[2] Fajardo,[3] and Ang et al.[337] Most of the data concerning these structures are derived from radiotherapy experience; however, some human data concerning large single absorbed doses are available. The SOMA toxicity table related to the salivary glands is presented in Appendix 6.

Low-LET Radiation

During the acute clinical period, marked swelling of the salivary glands may follow a large dose of radiation. These changes are predominantly due to increased permeability of the capillaries and may be seen as early as 4 hours. During a fractionated course of radiotherapy, however, there is rarely any swelling seen early, and dryness of the mouth may occur in 3 to 4 weeks. At that time, there is a rise in the serum amylase level, which can be as much as 10 to 20 times preirradiation levels. Other enzymes, including serum glutamic-oxaloacetic transaminase (SGOT), serum glutamic-pyruvic transaminase (SGPT), lactate dehydrogenase (LDH), and alkaline phosphatase, remain normal. As one might expect, urinary excretion of amylase also increases. The effects of single acute doses were studied by Kashima et al.[338] These authors reported results for 33 patients who had received single high doses in the range of 9 to 20 Gy for malignancies in the pharynx. Twenty-four hours after the single dose, surgery was performed, and pathologic study revealed both neutrophilic and eosinophilic infiltration of the interstitial tissues in the serous acinar tissue. Necrotic cell debris was seen in the ducts. The mucous glands showed little change. Such acute changes usually subside within a few days, even if there are to be later changes of xerostomia. There also may be altered taste and diminished appetite.

In the period 1 to 3 months after radiotherapy, the extent of damage varies greatly from case to case.[3] This may be the result of differences in radiotherapy or individual variation. Permanent xerostomia occurs in about 80% of persons receiving fractionated doses of 40 to 60 Gy. There is a large amount of individual variation in salivary flow rates prior to radiotherapy, and in persons with low flow states even 5 to 15 Gy can result in minimal flow. Following most radiotherapy schemes, although there is usually some degree of recovery, dryness of the mouth persists in a large proportion of patients, particularly if the entire salivary gland system has been irradiated. These symptoms may persist into the subacute and chronic clinical periods. Some evidence of residual inflammatory changes can be seen up to 8 months post–radiation therapy with the use of gallium 67 citrate scans.[339] Transient dysfunction of the salivary glands is noted in many patients who have received a single whole-body dose of 10 Gy prior to bone marrow transplantation.[340] Sialograms during the subacute period usually reveal diminished filling of the ducts, but a normal-sized gland. Treatment of the dryness (xerostomia) is symptomatic, consisting of rinsing the mouth with various solutions. If xerostomia persists beyond 1 year, there is very little chance of recovery. As mentioned in the section on bone later in this chapter, this circumstance carries implications for the development of mandibular necrosis and radiation caries.

The rise in serum amylase may be a reasonably useful biochemical and biologic dosimeter in cases of accidental radiation exposure. Kashima et al. indicated that a single dose in the region of 1 to 4 Gy will result in hyperamylasemia of 1000 Somogyi units in 24 to 72 hours.[338] Those patients who receive less than 10 Gy rarely had elevations in excess of 600 Somogyi units. The peak activity may be identified in 9 to 48 hours; these reported enzyme elevations followed treatment of all of the salivary glands. The fractionated doses used in radiotherapy have been well correlated with the subsequent volume of flow of saliva. After dose levels of 10 to 20 Gy the volume of salivary flow is decreased to about 50%. In the range of 50 to 60 Gy of fractionated exposure, volume is reduced to approximately one third. When the total regimen reaches 60 Gy of fractionated exposure the volume of saliva is reduced to approximately 10% 3 months after the cessation of therapy.

High-Let Radiation

At the present time, no substantial literature analyzes the effect of high-LET radiation on the salivary glands.

Radionuclide Irradiation

Following administration of very large doses of iodine 131, a radiation sialitis may be observed. Goolden et al. calculated that after administration of 5.5 to 7.4 GBq of iodine 131, doses to the salivary glands may be as high as 7 to 9 Gy in 12 hours.[341] It is possible that stimulation of these salivary glands (with candy lemon drops) in such instances can accelerate excretion of radionuclide and reduce the symptoms although use in the first 24 hours post–iodine administration may actually increase salivary gland damage.[342] Doses from radioiodine therapy for hyperthyroidism almost never result in significant xerostomia. When higher administered activities of radioiodine are used for treatment of thyroid cancer, the thyroid has been removed and doses to the salivary glands are higher. In these circumstances salivary and lacrimal gland dysfunction (sicca syndrome) can occur.[343] In most cases this is a transient side effect but in some patients it may persist for a long time or appear late. The parotid glands have a greater reduction in function than do the submandibular glands.[344] Amifostine has been shown to have a protective effect with regard to salivary gland damage.[345]

BREAST TISSUE

Effects of radiation on breast tissue following radiation therapy have been well described. In general, breast tissue is quite radioresistant, with the major changes occurring in the skin, although ultimately atrophy of the gland may occur. The changes that occur vary somewhat with the type of radiation used. With orthovoltage radiation sources, the skin reactions are more prominent, whereas with megavoltage radiation and interstitial implants, deep induration is possible. The squamous epithelium of the ducts contains a basal layer of vegetative intermitotic germinal cells that are relatively radiosensitive. The residual portion of the gland behaves as reverting postmitotic cells and is essentially radioresistant. Radiation treatment of the chest wall that includes a prepubertal breast has been reported for benign conditions such as cavernous hemangioma. The result is a small retracted breast unable to respond to hormonal stimulation.[346] Doses to the breast of an infant in excess of 3 Gy may produce later deformity (Fig. 6-9). Furst et al. reviewed the effect of radiation on the breast in 129 women who received about 2.3 Gy to the chest as children for treatment of hemangioma.[347] Breast hypoplasia was reported on the treated side by 57% of the patients and on the contralateral side by 8% of patients. Compared with the stimulated or proliferating breast, the prepubertal breast is relatively radioresistant. With estrogen

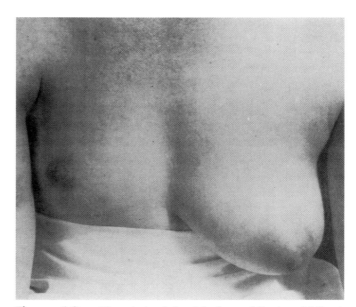

Figure 6-9 • Hypoplasia of the right breast following childhood irradiation for treatment of a cystic hygroma. (From Martin JA: Treatment of cystic hygroma. Texas Med 1954;50:220.)

stimulation, particularly during pregnancy, the radiosensitivity of ductal epithelium increases by 30% to 50%.[348] Failure of lactation after radiotherapy has been reported by several authors.[349,350]

In terms of adverse effects that might be expected following certain doses, Spanos et al. reported late complications in patients who received 60 Gy over 8 weeks, followed by a boost raising the dose to 70 to 110 Gy.[351] In this circumstance, somewhat more than 10% of the patients developed severe fibrosis. Other changes, including induration, atrophy, retraction of the nipple, and telangiectasia, were also identified. Ulceration was seen in less than 20% of the patients. In the prepubertal breast, doses of 15 to 20 Gy delivered over a week will impair development, and higher doses of 30 to 40 Gy will cause permanent fibrosis and atrophy. Robertson et al. reported that in patients with collagen vascular disease, there may be much more severe breast fibrosis after radiotherapy than normally expected.[352] Fajardo described late histopathologic changes, which include dense fibrosis, nonspecific vascular changes, fat necrosis, some atypical fibroblasts, and arterioles with myointimal proliferation.[3] Dysplastic changes and fat necrosis occurring after therapeutic irradiation can easily be confused with true neoplastic changes.[353] The SOMA toxicity table related to the breast is presented in Appendix 6.

RESPIRATORY TRACT

Larynx

There has been a large amount of experience concerning irradiation of the larynx for laryngeal carcinoma. In general, no complications have been identified in radiation therapy schemes in which the dose was less than 2.25 Gy per day for a total dose of 56 to 63 Gy.[354] Edema is seen initially but usually subsides within 7 to 8 weeks following therapy. Occasionally edema persists up to a year, with narrowing that ultimately may require tracheostomy. As a result, aspiration pneumonia may also occur. Pathologically, progressive accumulation of collagen and fibrin in the stroma, with small-vessel telangiectasia and occasional ulceration, may occur. There may be various degrees of atypia of the squamous epithelium. Some of the glands become atrophic, and, as occurs in other tissues, there is myointimal proliferation of the vasculature. One of the peculiarities in radiation therapy of the larynx is the occurrence of chondritis, which may progress to aseptic necrosis.[355,356] Delayed minor reactions include fibrosis of the neck and vocal cords.

Lung

The lung is a relatively radiosensitive organ. An extensive review of the literature on pulmonary responses was published by van den Brenk.[357] Reviews have been written by Davis et al.,[358] Molls,[359] and McDonald et al.[360] (The SOMA toxicity table related to the lung is presented in Appendix 6.) The incidence of complications rises steeply with single doses above 8 Gy.[361] The radiosensitivity of the lung is a limiting factor in total-body radiotherapy for treatment of diffuse metastases and prior to bone marrow transplantation.[362] In single-dose treatment, 8 Gy is the accepted maximum since single doses of 7 to 8 Gy may produce radiation pneumonitis. Massive doses to the thorax have occasionally occurred in accidental criticality situations. At least one person has died within 48 hours after an estimated dose to the thorax of 300 to 500 Gy. The major changes following fractionated pulmonary radiation therapy are radiation pneumonitis, or acute radiation pneumonitis (ARP), and subsequent pulmonary fibrosis. The exact mechanism of radiation pneumonitis is unclear, but it does involve loss of some of the epithelial cells, presence of exudative fluid in the alveolar space, and subsequent thickening of the alveolar walls. In addition to these findings, associations with adult respiratory distress syndrome[363] and bronchiolitis obliterans[364] have been reported.

Some authors have suggested that radiation pneumonitis is the result of a lymphocyte-mediated hypersensitivity reaction, because after unilateral thoracic radiation there was an increase in both lymphocyte lavage and gallium concentration in both lungs.[365] A review of the target cells in radiation pneumopathy by Trott et al. indicated that the target cell population that initiates the pathogenic process in the lung is not known and it may be that no single identifiable target exists.[366] The entire process appears to be the result of complex functional alterations in endothelial cells, pneumocytes, macrophages, and other cells. Several factors have been studied relative to potential predisposition to radiation pneumonitis. High pretreatment plasma levels of interleukin-6[367] and serum KL-6[368] have been associated with increased risk of pneumonitis possibly because cytokine casacades may promote radiation pulmonary injury.[369] The diffusing capacity of carbon monoxide appears to be predictive, but whether other preirradiation lung functions are predictive of those developing severe radiation pneumonitis is debatable.[370-373]

Whether radiation pneumonitis can be reduced in severity by concurrent treatment with corticosteroids is a subject of debate.[374] Because many patients undergoing radiotherapy are also relatively immunosuppressed, some radiation oncologists also administer broad-spectrum antibiotics when a "pneumonitis" is identified. It has been suggested that radiation pneumonitis occurs with equal frequency in those under the age of 70 and those over 70, but that the severity is greater in the older age group.[375]

Low-LET Radiation

Radiation pneumonitis, first described by Grover in 1929, characteristically occurs 3 to 16 weeks after the cessation of radiotherapy. It is characterized by low-grade fever, pleuritic chest pain, dry cough, rales, dyspnea, and fullness in the chest. Later, small amounts of sputum, which can be blood tinged, may be produced. If both lungs are involved, severe respiratory distress, cyanosis, cor pulmonale, and even death from cardiorespiratory failure may occur. The diagnosis is usually made on the basis of radiographic findings of pneumonitis limited to the field of x-ray therapy. Pleural effusions may occur, but they are uncommon.[376,377] Time, dose, and volume aspects are of particular importance in the development of clinical radiation pneumonitis. On the basis of several studies, a clinical threshold of 6 to 7 Gy for single doses has been suggested for the development of acute pneumonitis. A single dose of 10 Gy to both lungs will cause pneumonitis in 84% of patients. This percentage is reduced to about 30% if the single dose is 8 Gy. Five percent of patients who receive a dose of 26.5 Gy in 20 fractions over 4 weeks to both lungs develop pneumonitis. Similarly, 5% of patients receiving a total dose of 20 Gy in 10 fractions over 2 weeks to 1 month develop pneumonitis. As the dose is increased to 30.5 Gy in 20 fractions over 4 weeks to both lungs, 50% of patients will develop pneumonitis, and all patients receiving 30 Gy over 2 weeks in 10 fractions to one lung will develop pneumonitis.

Over the last decade, radiation oncologists have explored dose-volumetric parameters for predicting and avoiding severe radiation pneumonitis. This is expressed as the percentage of the lung that receives a dose of 20 Gy or more (V20), 30 Gy or more (V30), 40 Gy or more (V40), and 50 Gy or more (V50). However, the overall accuracy, sensitivity, specificity, and positive predictive value is only fair.[378] Mean lung dose (MLD) also may be used.[379]

These parameters for fractionated radiotherapy have been studied with regard to grade 2 or greater pneumonitis. With V20 the incidence by dose is as follows: less than 22% volume, 0% incidence of pneumonitis; 22% to 31% volume, 7% incidence; 32 to 40% volume, 13% incidence; and greater than 40% volume, 36% incidence. For total MLD the incidence of grade 2 or greater pneumonitis is 0% at less than 10 Gy, 9% at 11 to 20 Gy, and 24% at 21 to 30 Gy.[380]

The latent period between the development of pneumonitis and radiation therapy is a function of the cellular mitotic index of the cell populations involved. Thus, there is a delay between radiation exposure and expression of injury. Previous or concurrent chemotherapy with agents such as actinomycin D, Adriamycin (doxorubicin hydrochloride), bleomycin, busulfan, dactinomycin, methotrexate, mitomycin C, nitrosoureas, paclitaxel, and tamoxifen predispose patients to the development of radiation pneumonitis.[381–383] "Recall" pneumonitis can occur with radiotherapy after Adriamycin chemotherapy has been discontinued.[384] Abrupt withdrawal of corticosteroids can

unmask subclinical pneumonitis. Clinical radiation pneumonitis is represented pathologically by atypical epithelial cells with congested capillaries and hyaline membrane formation lining the alveolar spaces. In addition, there are mononuclear infiltrates in the alveolar septa. A radiation accident experience in Belarus involved an individual who was exposed in a facility used for sterilization of medical supplies. There was a nonuniform, acute whole-body exposure in the range of 16 Gy. Normally, the patient would have succumbed to a bone marrow syndrome; however, Russian physicians, using their experience from Chernobyl, were able to keep the individual alive until there was marrow regeneration. This was probably the first such individual ever to survive this level of acute exposure. Unfortunately, radiation pneumonitis occurred, and the individual died from pulmonary insufficiency about 90 days postexposure.

The imaging findings associated with radiation pneumonitis have been discussed by many authors.[385–387] The radiologic manifestation of radiation pneumonitis is a hazy alveolar infiltrate corresponding to the shape of the radiation port (Fig. 6-10). As the fibrotic stage progresses, atelectasis, pleural reaction, volume loss, and even calcified plaques may be identified. Radiographic changes of pneumonitis are rare for a dose less than 30 Gy in 3 weeks but are common when the dose exceeds 40 Gy in 4 weeks. Fibrotic changes appear if the dose exceeds 60 Gy delivered over 6 weeks. In general, CT is more sensitive and demonstrates changes earlier than on the standard chest radiographs.[388] Homogeneous or patchy areas of lung "ground glass" opacification and volume loss are the principal findings. The abnormalities are usually, but not always, confined to the radiation fields and are seen in about 80% to 90% of patients within 16 weeks of ending fractionated radiotherapy to the lung, but they may be seen as early as 2 to 4 weeks.[360] At later times fibrosis, traction bronchiectasis, volume loss, mediastinal shifting, pleural thickening, and scarring may be seen.[389] MRI has been used in an attempt to distinguish fibrosis from recurrent tumor, with the idea that radiation fibrosis will not have a high signal on T2-weighted images.[390] This has yet to prove reliable.[358,391,392] Imaging with various nuclear medicine techniques is also possible. Increased uptake of indium 111 penetreotide in early radiation pneumonitis has been reported.[393] PET scans using fluorine 18 FDG have been shown to demonstrate uptake in most irradiated fields for up to 6 months postradiation. There is a fairly large amount of literature on the use of gallium 67 citrate scanning in radiation pneumonitis. While abnormalities are detected when chest radiographs are still normal in many cases, there is activity in both lungs in about 40% of patients only after unilateral lung irradiation.[394,395]

The main permanent change that may occur is pulmonary fibrosis or sclerosis (Fig. 6-11), which may occur in patients who have never clinically manifested

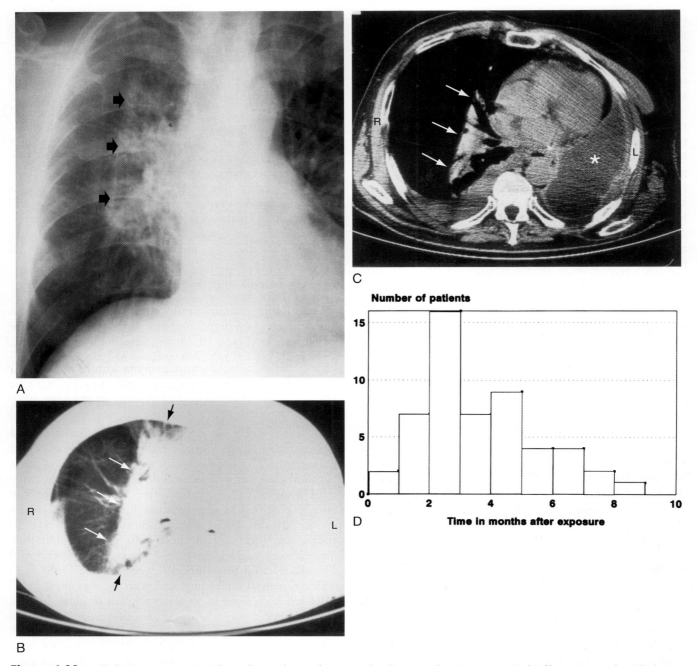

Figure 6-10 ● Radiation pneumonitis. After radiation therapy for a central malignancy, there is a geometrical infiltrate seen in the right lung on the chest radiograph (**A**). Different windows on the same slice of a CT scan (**B** and **C**) show the straight-line infiltrate (*white arrows*). The *black arrows* in image **B** show the direction of the incident radiation. The time course of radiation pneumonitis in 38 patients is shown graphically in part **D**. (From van Dyk J, Keane T, Kan S, et al: Radiation pneumonitis following large single dose irradiation: A re-evaluation based on absolute dose to lung. Int J Radiat Oncol Biol Phys, 1981. 7:461–467.)

acute radiation pneumonitis. If the fibrotic changes are widespread enough, reduction in the pulmonary function of the patient may result. As with most other tissues, the volume irradiated is particularly important in the ability of the patient to tolerate the changes. Irradiation of the total lung may cause reduction in volume and diffusing capacity.[396–398] When smaller volumes of lung are irradiated, diffusing capacity may still be reduced, although patients with previously existing chronic obstructive pulmonary disease (COPD) who receive radiotherapy for lung cancer appear to tolerate the therapy as well as patients without COPD.[399]

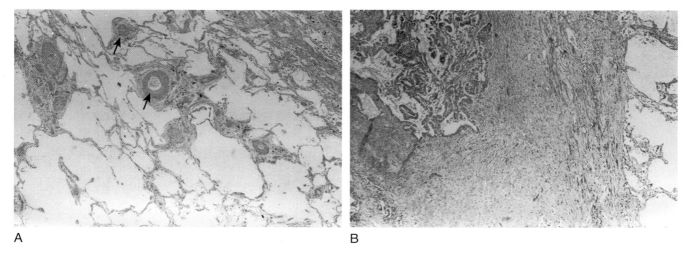

Figure 6-11 • Lung after irradiation for pulmonary metastasis. Sections from autopsy specimen at the edge of the field (**A**) demonstrate arteriolar narrowing and capillary occlusion (*arrows*). Atelectasis is visible in upper right corner. Within the radiation field (**B**) is residual tumor (*upper-left corner*) surrounded by dense fibrosis. (Case courtesy of William Black, MD.)

The pathology of the chronic or late effects includes replacement of the septa by collagen, reduction in the number of functional capillaries, and decreased volume of aerated alveolar space. This may be a function of ischemia because there is myointimal proliferation of the arterioles, and foamy cells in the intima may be seen. The clinical manifestations include reduction in pulmonary function in the irradiated area, with consolidation, volume loss, and susceptibility to infection (particularly fungal infection). A large amount of literature is available concerning radiation pneumonitis and late pulmonary function after radiotherapy of adults. The largest literature probably concerns women who received chest wall irradiation for breast cancer. With tangential fields, lung changes should be in the range of 1% to 2% and with a much lower incidence than was seen with earlier radiotherapy methods, and small and reversible changes in pulmonary function may occur.[400,401] In general, the reliability of radiographic, CT, or nuclear medicine findings for prediction of clinical symptoms or amount of ultimate fibrosis has been poor.[402,403]

There is also a great deal of experience and literature relative to pulmonary reactions after radiotherapy in children. Wohl et al. studied children who are survivors of Wilms' tumors irradiated with a median fractionated lung dose of 20 Gy and at age 2 to 4 years.[404] A number of these patients subsequently had dyspnea and interstitial and pleural thickening. A similar study was performed by Littman et al. in which vital capacity and functional residual capacity were lower in the irradiated group.[405] Both Green et al.[406] and Shaw et al.[407] reported on the follow-up of patients treated for Wilms' tumor. In these patients sometimes the pneumonitis was traced to an infectious etiology, and in those patients receiving whole-lung irradiation there was reduced pulmonary function. A number of studies report on patients who have been followed for Hodgkin's disease. In general, those patients who received mantle field therapy with a dose in the range of 20 to 55 Gy demonstrated restricted lung volume and reduced total lung capacity.[408,409] Tarbell et al. reported on patients treated for Hodgkin's disease with mantle therapy (usually 23 to 43 Gy in 26 fractions); there was about a 3% incidence of radiation pneumonitis, but this rose to about 15% when there was whole-lung radiotherapy.[410] In a group of patients followed for 10 to 20 years by Gustavsson et al., there was right ventricular hypertrophy in 50% of patients, defects on lung perfusion scintigraphy in 80%, and slight to moderate pulmonary fibrosis in 70%.[411] The abnormalities were generally clinically insignificant. Springmeyer et al. examined patients after bone marrow transplantation for assorted conditions.[412] This generally involved whole-body radiation, and analysis of 79 patients demonstrated restrictive ventilatory changes, with a loss of total lung capacity of almost 1 L. Whether prednisone and steroid administration affect the development of the fibrosis remains uncertain; however, the effect, if any, is not significant.

Several drugs often used in conjunction with radiation therapy can produce a higher incidence of pulmonary fibrosis; these include bleomycin sulfate, cyclophosphamide, carmustine (BCNU), and busulfan.[413] Lung nodules have been described after irradiation; whether they represent a nodular form of pneumonitis is uncertain.[414,415] These nodules have been described only in patients receiving concurrent chemotherapy. Inflammatory changes in the bronchi are seen but are generally expressions of superimposed bacterial infections rather than true radiation changes. As will be discussed later in the section,

"Heart and Vessels," mediastinal irradiation can lead to occlusion and narrowing of pulmonary arteries or to fibrosis with resultant pulmonary hypertension.[416]

High-LET Radiation

Significant human data have not been reported for the RBE of neutrons in humans. Pi-meson treatment of pulmonary metastases in doses of 3980 pion rad in 23 fractions over 4 weeks can produce pneumonitis. There are some data on the normal tissue reactions following high-energy neutron beam therapy, and Cohen et al. indicated that 20 Gy in 12 fractions over 4 weeks represents a practical tolerance limit for most sites.[417]

Radionuclide Irradiation

Although extensive research has focused on inhalation of radionuclides by animals, there is very limited and confusing information with regard to humans. Predicting results of significant internal contamination via inhalation is difficult because the distribution of radionuclide deposition depends initially on size of the particles inhaled and ultimately on the solubility of the compound both in the lungs and in the lymph nodes. The major human database concerning radionuclide inhalation comes from uranium miners who inhale dust, radon, and radon daughter products.

Pulmonary fibrosis is difficult to evaluate in uranium miners because they usually have accompanying silicosis and emphysema. A fivefold excess mortality from nonmalignant respiratory diseases (other than tuberculosis) has been found in the Colorado plateau miners.[418] Excess deaths were from silicosis, emphysema, and fibrosis. There was a suggestion in these miners that radon daughter exposure reduced ventilatory function and contributed to the development of emphysema. Even though exposure of animals to high levels of radon daughters leads to interstitial changes and emphysema,[419] most researchers feel that the human epidemiologic studies have been unable to separate the possible effects of radon exposure from those of the other occupational exposures.[420]

There is some experience with inhalation of plutonium in 26 Manhattan Project workers at Los Alamos National Laboratory. An extensive medical follow-up of these workers over 50 years has been performed; no clinically significant deterministic pulmonary changes have been reported (see Chapter 9). A study of interstitial changes on chest x-rays of 326 plutonium workers at the Rocky Flats plant with lung doses from 0 to 28 Sv revealed a 5.3-fold greater risk of abnormal chest x-ray when lung doses were 10 Sv or greater.[421] Extensive study was performed by Okladnikova et al. on the workers of the Russian Mayak facility and 66 cases of plutonium pulmonary fibrosis have been reported.[422] Alpha lung doses ranged from 1.4 to 40 Gy and external gamma doses ranged from 2.1 to 2.9 Gy. In the mild cases the latency period was 17 years and in severe cases it was 7 years.

One patient who ostensibly developed pulmonary fibrosis as a result of Thorotrast (thorium 232 oxide) administration was reported by De Vuyst et al.[423] Whether this case was due to Thorotrast or to idiopathic pulmonary fibrosis is unknown. The proportion of Thorotrast that is deposited in the lungs is typically only 0.7%, which would deliver an estimated average dose to the main pulmonary bronchi of about 0.13 Gy per year.[424] There has been discussion as to whether pulmonary fibrosis can be the result of occupational inhalation of lanthanides. A pulmonary syndrome is induced by stable rare earths that is not the result of radioactivity.[425] Radiation pneumonitis due to lung shunting has been reported as a potential complication after intraarterial treatment with yttrium 90 microspheres for hepatic tumors.[426] Pulmonary fibrosis is a very rare complication of radioiodine therapy. Edmonds et al. reported long-term effects of radioiodine treatment for thyroid cancer including one patient who developed pulmonary fibrosis; however, the patient also had diffuse pulmonary metastases making it difficult to determine the cause of the fibrosis.[427]

HEART AND VESSELS

Low-LET Radiation

The historical annotations concerning radiation effects on the cardiovascular system have been reviewed by Rubin and Casarett.[2] Throughout the literature, particularly the early literature, the heart and great vessels were considered to be radioresistant organs. One of the major reasons for this belief was that it was not technically possible to limit radiation therapy to the mediastinal structures without irradiating large portions of the lung that were much more radiosensitive. With appropriate technical advances, it has been possible to localize the radiation more accurately, and deterministic effects of radiation have now been recognized in the cardiac structures themselves.[428,429] Late effects of radiotherapy on the cardiovascular system include cardiomyopathy, coronary artery disease, pericardial effusions, and constrictive pericarditis.[430] The SOMA toxicity table related to the heart is presented in Appendix 6. Issues concerning premature death or increased mortality due to cardiovascular disease are covered in the section "Radiation-Induced Life Shortening" later in this chapter. Likewise, the cardiovascular syndrome associated with acute radiation sickness is covered later in the section, "Total-Body Radiation."

The myocardium is composed of striated muscle fibers with essentially no regenerative ability. They are classified as fixed postmitotic cells and are thus very resistant to deterministic effects of radiation. The myocardium itself appears capable of withstanding fractionated radiotherapy doses as high as 100 Gy without obvious clinical or microscopic changes being identified. In one case of accidental exposure to an iridium 192 radiography source, there was localized myocardial damage. In that case, the absorbed dose to the myocardium was not calculated; however, the dose was high enough so that there was necrosis of the overlying skin, soft tissue, and rib.[431]

There appears to be a great deal of confusion concerning whether radiation can produce myocarditis. The diagnosis of myocarditis prior to 1987 was not well defined; however, after this point in time criteria have been proposed.[432] By definition, the diagnosis of myocarditis can be made only if myocyte necrosis or degeneration or both are associated with an inflammatory infiltrate adjacent to the myocytes. Most authors who discuss myocarditis indicate that ionizing radiation is not a cause, however, there are several textbooks on the heart, as well as infectious disease, that list ionizing radiation in a differential diagnosis of noninfectious myocarditis.[433] Careful inspection of the references that they quote, however, indicates that myocarditis is not mentioned in the original references. Some confusion arises because many of the early references such as those by Stewart and Fajardo mention pancarditis.[434,435] Review of the original articles indicates that this has been used to mean fibrosis of the myocardium and pericardium, rather than myocarditis. With extremely acute doses of radiation (in excess of 30 Gy), edema may be present in the myocardium along with cellular infiltrates due to the leakage from the vasculature. This has been reported only in one or two accidental situations in which the individual died from other causes within a few days, and the case occurred long before there was an agreed pathologic definition of myocarditis.[436]

The issue of myocarditis may come up in patients receiving fractionated radiotherapy. In these cases, viral causes should be considered, as well as hypersensitivity myocarditis related to drugs. Some drugs that can cause myocarditis include methyldopa, amphotericin, doxorubicin, cyclophosphamide, barbiturates, and lithium, as well as a number of antihypertensive drugs, sulfonamides, theophylline, and antibiotics (penicillin, streptomycin, tetracycline).[437,438] Adriamycin combined with radiation increases the risk of cardiotoxicity. Adriamycin alone is known to damage myocardial myocytes, although it seldom damages the capillaries. The reverse is usually true in radiation injury of the myocardium. Radiation changes in the myocardium are probably more correctly called radiation cardiomyopathy. The interval between radiation and development of these changes usually exceeds 10 years. The specific pathologic changes seen are similar to idiopathic cardiomyopathy, with a variable amount of interstitial fibrosis and myocardial cell hypertrophy. Ultrastructurally, however, there is a difference, with the thickening of the basement membranes in the myocardial cells and the capillaries to several times their normal thickness. While this is not totally specific, a marked degree of basement membrane thickening should suggest radiation-induced cardiomyopathy. Overall, data suggests that 40 Gy

of fractionated dose is considered a threshold for clinical cardiomyopathy in both adults and children. Several commonly used drugs including the anthracyclines (doxorubicin and daunomycin) induce cardiomyopathy by themselves but also are enhanced in terms of toxicity with mediastinal irradiation.[439–442]

Radiation-induced heart disease (RIHD) was described by Stewart et al.[443,444] The majority of radiation-induced cardiac abnormalities have been demonstrated in patients who have received mediastinal irradiation for Hodgkin's disease. The changes most commonly involve the pericardium rather than the heart muscle (myocardium). The changes seen in the pericardium include pericardial effusion, fibrosis, and possibly subsequent constrictive pericarditis. Pericardial or myocardial disease was observed in 6% to 7% of patients who have received a mean fractionated total dose of 42.8 Gy in a radiation therapeutic scheme to a large volume of the heart. Administration of 40 Gy in 16 fractions over 4 weeks has been reported to result in pericarditis in about 5% of patients.[445,446] Patients being treated for Hodgkin's disease demonstrate a high incidence of complications when the total dose exceeds 60 Gy. The acute form of presentation includes pleuritic chest pain, pericardial friction rub, and fever. Pericardial effusion may cause tamponade in some cases.

It has been noted that a large number of asymptomatic young patients treated for Hodgkin's disease with mediastinal irradiation have pericardial effusions, decreased left ventricular reserve, and decreased size of the left ventricular cavity, and diastolic dysfunction.[447,448] Long-term clinical follow-up of these patients may show progression of the subclinical injury to a symptomatic stage.[449] In another study, careful evaluation demonstrated occult or overt cardiac disease in 96% of patients treated with radiotherapy for Hodgkin's disease. The most common finding was constrictive pericarditis.[450] Cardiac complications of radiotherapy can be complicated by the use of anthracyclines. While radiation can affect many portions of the heart, anthracycline damage is usually limited to the myocardium.[451,452]

Carmel and Kaplan reported that pericarditis occurred in 7% of patients who were treated for Hodgkin's disease who had total doses of less than 6 Gy and that this rose to 12% at 6 to 15 Gy, 19% at 15 to 30 Gy, and 50% of those who received more than 30 Gy.[453] Thickening of the pericardium at autopsy was reported by Brosius et al. in slightly less than one half of the patients who had received mediastinal radiotherapy.[454] A higher incidence (70%) was reported by Veinot et al.[455] The dose to the surface of the heart ranged from 30 to 88 Gy in a fractionated scheme. Coronary artery narrowing was also identified. Similar findings were reported by Makinen et al.[456] and Kadota et al.[408] Cosset et al. reported on 499 patients treated for Hodgkin's disease with mediastinal irradiation and indicated that at 10 years, there was a 9.5% incidence of pericarditis and a 3.9% incidence of myocardial infarction.[457] The incidence of pericarditis was significantly higher with total doses of 41 Gy or more. The same group reported that nuclear medicine examination of myocardial perfusion performed 3 to 11 years after mediastinal irradiation for Hodgkin's disease was abnormal in about 70% of asymptomatic patients treated.[458] Fraction size has an influence, and Cosset et al. reported that use of three fractions of 3.3 Gy per week resulted in 9% pericarditis compared with 0% when four fractions of 2.5 Gy per week were used.[459]

There are only a few studies of cardiac function performed where patients who have not had concomitant cytotoxic therapy were examined soon after radiotherapy. Savage et al. performed a study on patients who had their entire cardiac volume irradiated and compared them with those who had at least some portion of their heart shielded.[460] The patients were all irradiated for Hodgkin's disease and examined 2.5 to 21 years after treatment. Those who had their entire heart irradiated had ejection fractions of approximately 55% compared with 63% in those who were partially shielded. Thus, the left ventricular ejection fraction and left ventricular peak filling rates were slightly low but were still within the normal range. Glanzmann et al. reported on long-term follow-up of 352 Hodgkin's patients treated between 1964–1992.[461] Doses to the heart were generally between 30 and 42 Gy; the RR for myocardial infarction was 4.2. Constine et al. reported that when the heart is shielded and modern radiotherapy techniques are used for treatment of Hodgkin's disease, cardiac complication is mild.[462] Swerdlow et al. followed a cohort of 7033 Hodgkin's disease patients; the SMR from myocardial infarction was 9.5 (95% CI 3.5, 20.6) for patients treated with doxorubicin, vinblastine, and dacarbazine regimen, and 14.8 (95% CI 4.8 to 34.5) for patients with supradiaphragmatic radiotherapy and vincristine without anthracylines.[462a] Jakacki et al. pointed out that when thoracic spinal irradiation is given to children, there can be asymmetrical cardiac abnormalities as the heart grows.[463]

In addition to radiotherapy for Hodgkin's disease, the incidence of cardiac and coronary complication have been reported after therapy for breast cancer, total-body irradiation, and benign peptic ulcer. In the 1970s when women were treated for cancer of the left breast, the heart often received substantial doses but modern techniques with tangential fields and electron boost have substantially reduced cardiac complications.[464] In a study by Ikaheimo et al., 24 women treated for breast cancer with echocardiography before and up to 6 months after radiotherapy were examined.[465] There was a slight transient depression of left ventricular function, which was symptomless and normalized within 3 months. They also reported a slight decrease in ventricular size. The etiology that affects this is unclear. The doses received by these patients were 30 to 35 Gy.

Vallis et al. followed more than 2100 patients treated with radiotherapy for early breast cancer between 1982–1988 and found no evidence of excess coronary artery disease associated with left-sided breast cancer.[466] Darby et al. reported, in a prospective study of about 300,000 women treated for early left-sided breast cancer treated from 1973–1982, that their cardiovascular mortality ratio was 1.2 to 1.6, compared to women with a cancer of the right breast treated with radiotherapy.[467] For women treated for cancer of the left breast from 1993–2001 no excess cardiovascular mortality was demonstrated. Similar findings were recently reported by Patt et al.[468] and Giordano et al.[469] Leung et al. reported on long-term complications after total-body radiation treatment for childhood leukemia and found cardiac abnormalities in only 8%.[470] Carr et al. reported a higher than expected frequency of coronary heart disease after irradiation for benign peptic ulcer in patients who received volume-weighted cardiac doses from 1.6 to 3.9 Gy, but in about 5% of patients the heart was in the radiation port and received 7.6 to 18.4 Gy.[471]

Over the last decade, there has been a great deal of interest in using beta or iridium 192 gamma brachytherapy sources to inhibit restenosis of coronary arteries after angioplasty dilatation and stent placement. The brachytherapy has appeared to slow restenosis to some extent by inhibiting neointimal formation[472–474] although late occlusion has still been a problem.[475] Intracoronary brachytherapy is now less common as chemical coated stents are being more commonly used.

Late changes of fibrosis can be seen not only in the pericardium and endocardium but also in the valves. In a study by Perrault et al., 41 patients were examined between 8 and 22 years postradiotherapy for Hodgkin's disease or seminoma, 70% of whom revealed pericardial thickening and 28% mitral or aortic thickening.[476] Most valvular changes occured 10 or more years after exposure.[477] Heidenreich et al. pointed out that valvular disease increased with time after irradiation and that in asymptomatic patients treated for Hodgkin's disease who received mean doses of 43 Gy, mild or greater aortic regurgitation occurred in 60% of patients, compared to 4% of controls, and disease of the other valves is significantly less common.[478]

There are reports of changes in the electrocardiogram in patients being treated for breast carcinoma. The clinical significance of these "radiation-induced" electrocardiographic changes is not completely understood, but they do not appear to be caused by myocardial damage per se. Positional changes or preexisting coronary disease has been implicated in most reports. Occasionally, a high-degree atrioventricular block and acute myocardial infarction have been reported to occur with the pericardial fibrosis.[479–481] There are several case reports in the literature regarding complete atrioventricular block. It is assumed that this is due to postirradiation fibrosis of the atrioventricular node, although there are usually other associated changes, including coronary artery disease.[482] These have all been reported in patients who have received radiation therapy in excess of 40 Gy.[483–486] All of the cases occurred between 10 and 20 years postradiotherapy. Given the large number of patients receiving radiotherapy to the mediastinum, this appears to be a very rare complication. Various other ECG changes, such as Q-T prolongation, ventricular premature complexes, and so on, have been reported in survivors of childhood cancer treated with radiotherapy and anthracyclines.[487] There has been interest in whether radiation therapy can affect cardiac pacemakers. There are occasional isolated case reports of pacemaker failure occurring weeks after radiation therapy.[488,489] However, a test run of multiple types of pacing devices has not shown this to be a real problem, up to 60 Gy.[490]

The fine blood vessels and the connective tissue cells of the heart are only moderately resistant. Following irradiation, both the epicardium and pericardium may demonstrate dense fibrosis, but this always appears to be most prominent in the pericardium. The epicardium may be covered by a thick film of fibrin indistinguishable grossly from fibrinous pericarditis. In the late stages, the myocardium can show diffuse fibrosis, with bands of dense collagen. The exact mechanism of the pericardial fibrosis is uncertain, although ischemia undoubtedly plays a large role. Brosius et al. performed both clinical and autopsy studies on 16 patients who had received more than 35 Gy in fractionated radiotherapy to the heart 5 to 144 months before death.[454] The patients were between 15 and 33 years old. Essentially all of the patients had thickened pericardium, and eight had some interstitial myocardial fibrosis. Epicardial coronary artery narrowing was seen in nearly half of the patients who were studied, compared with only 10% of the control subjects. Damage to individual myocardial cells was not detected in any patient by histologic study. The authors themselves point out that the high incidence of changes here may be because a number of study patients were irradiated with techniques now considered unacceptable by most modern radiotherapists.

Damage to large blood vessels has been reported, although it is much less common than capillary and arteriolar damage. Many case reports of damage to large blood vessels concern patients who have atherosclerotic degenerative changes.[491,492] Thus, the causal relationship with radiation has been impossible to prove. Fajardo indicated that spontaneous rupture of large vessels is often blamed on radiation.[429] He reviewed more than 90 such cases (most of which were fatal) and concluded that in no more than 5 of the 90 cases did radiation appear to be the cause. One case that did appear to be radiation-related involved adult unilateral occlusion of a pulmonary artery.[493] Many studies in animals have concerned the relationship of radiation with the induction or acceleration of atherosclerosis. There are a number of articles in the literature indicating narrowed or occluded coronary arteries years after radiotherapy.[494–501]

There are a large number of recent reports regarding higher than expected incidence of atherosclerosis and/or stenosis in major arteries.[501] Most of the literature concerns wall thickening and stenosis of carotid arteries probably because of the large number of head and neck cancers treated with radiotherapy.[502,503] The long-term incidence of significant carotid stenosis after this type of therapy ranges from 30% to 60%.[504] The reported changes involve the carotid artery[505–508] and brachial artery,[509,510] as well as the aorta[511] and pelvic vessels.[512] Most patients have received fractionated radiotherapy in the range of 40 to 70 Gy. In at least one study of carotid disease by Moritz et al., 30% of patients who received fractionated radiotherapy of 50 Gy had moderate or severe carotid lesions compared with 6% of control patients.[513] In another study by Goodman et al., patients treated for seminoma with unilateral pelvic irradiation with 25 to 26 Gy were followed for an average of 9 years.[514] Only 3 of 19 developed vascular abnormalities, and in 2 patients they were bilateral, indicating that radiation was not likely to be the cause. In the third patient the abnormalities were subclinical. In these reports arterial lesions tended to develop about 3 to 10 years after radiotherapy. Lesions have been reported as occurring as early as 1 month; however, this does not make sense on a radiobiologic basis and almost certainly represents a preexisting lesion. Many patients being treated for tumors with radiotherapy are older and have preexisting cardiovascular disease, and this represents a major bias factor in the case reports. Very few controlled studies are available. In most papers, smoking, as well as the radiation, was thought to play a significant role in the development of atheromatous lesions. Examination of small arteries, arterioles, and capillaries is needed since changes in these structures are undoubtedly responsible for most delayed radiation injury.[429,515–517] Most veins are relatively resistant to radiation, although phlebosclerosis is occasionally seen and rarely there can be thrombosis of the main hepatic vein.[518]

Injury to capillaries has been demonstrated after a single dose to the skin as low as 4 Gy. Smooth-muscle cells and elastic tissues present in large arteries are quite radioresistant. Endothelial cells appear to be the most radiosensitive portions of the entire vascular system. Because capillaries consist only of endothelial cells and are of small diameter, the degenerative changes become apparent earlier in small vessels than in larger vessels. Initially, radiation, even at low doses, causes an increase in capillary permeability, separation of the cell junctions, necrosis or loss of endothelial cells, and damage to the basement membrane. Endothelial renewal and the myointimal proliferation that occur can be concentric but more often are eccentric, causing narrowing or occlusion of the lumen. Interestingly enough, most pure radiation vasculopathies lack leukocytic exudate. In some instances, *foam cells* (lipid-filled macrophages) are identified and are considered by some authors to be pathognomonic.[429] It should be noted that all capillaries are not equally radiosensitive; for example, pulmonary capillaries are more sensitive than myocardial capillaries.[519] Overall, it appears that radiation injury to the microvasculature is the most important factor in delayed nonstochastic effects of radiation, particularly in those tissues that have parenchymal cells that are of the slow or nonrenewal type. There is at least one report by Sasaki et al. of the atomic bomb survivors in which a small but statistically significant increase in systolic and diastolic blood pressure was associated with radiation.[520] The cause of this is uncertain, however, such findings have not been reported in other much more highly exposed groups. There is a report of increased mortality from circulatory diseases in atomic bomb survivors. This is discussed in the section on radiation-induced life shortening near the end of this chapter.

High-LET and Radionuclide Radiation

There are few human data available in regard to cardiac tolerance for high-LET and radionuclide radiation. The question regarding high-LET radiation usually arises when cardiac abnormalities are identified in persons who have inhaled either uranium or plutonium. Even though these are alpha-emitting radionuclides, the radionuclides deposited in the lung contribute little, if any, dose to the heart. For insoluble forms (class Y) of plutonium and uranium, the cardiac dose is approximately one ten-thousandth of the calculated lung dose. Neither uranium nor plutonium concentrate to any significant extent in the heart.

Internal Irradiation

While there are a large number of radionuclide studies performed regarding the heart for diagnostic purposes, the absorbed doses are orders of magnitude lower than those shown to produce identifiable effects from external irradiation. To have deterministic effects on the heart or major vessels, this would require implantation of therapeutic level sources. A single case of intracranial vasculopathy in a patient who had deterministic implantation of gold 198 colloid into the brain was interpreted to be a radiation-induced vasculopathy.[521]

There is one report of mediastinal hemorrhage after treatment of hyperthyroidism with radioactive iodine.[522] Another report appears 4 years later describing a similar event 8 weeks after treatment.[523] Review of the papers indicates that the same authors are reporting the same case twice in different journals 4 years apart. Thousands of persons treated for this disease each year using radioactive iodine do not have such complications, and whether this one case is causally related to radiation is questionable. Hall et al. reported on causes of mortality in 10,552 Swedish hyperthyroid patients treated with iodine 131.[524] The SMR for cardiovascular diseases was significantly elevated at 1.65 (95% CI 1.59 to 1.71), but this was apparently due to the hyperthyroidism rather than to radiation exposure.

GASTROINTESTINAL TRACT

Effects of a given absorbed dose of radiation on the gastrointestinal tract depend significantly on which portion of the tract is irradiated. Radiation sensitivity varies markedly between the midportion and the ends: the esophagus and rectum are relatively radiation-resistant, and the midportions, including the stomach and small intestine, are more sensitive. The reader is referred to a chapter on the subject in a book by Trott and Herrmann[525] and a review article by Coia et al.[526]

With single acute doses of 5 to 15 Gy to the abdominal region, there is rather rapid development of a *gastrointestinal syndrome*. With fractionation of the radiation dose, the gastrointestinal tract can tolerate much higher absorbed doses. In conventional radiotherapy, doses of up to 40 Gy are tolerated; however, patients receiving 45 to 54 Gy have about a 25% risk of stomach ulcer formation, with occasional perforation of the ulcers.[527,528] Imaging features of radiation induced changes in the abdomen have been published by Capps et al.[529]

Oral Cavity and Pharynx

Low-LET Radiation

The epithelial lining of the mouth and pharynx are somewhat more sensitive than the skin because the renewal rate of their cells is higher. A large amount of attention has focused on the combined effects of radiation and chemotherapy. Methotrexate and 5-fluorouracil can produce severe mucositis and esophagitis when used in combination with radiation. The standard descriptions of adverse effects from radiation therapy assume either orthovoltage radiation with 2 Gy five times a week for a total of 50 Gy in 5 weeks, or irradiation with cobalt 60 with a daily dose of 2 Gy and a weekly dose of 12 Gy to a total level of 60 Gy in five weeks. Because there is increased sensitivity of the mucosa compared to skin, changes of radiomucositis will be noted before radiation dermatitis. In the acute period, the mechanisms of injury are quite similar but vary in time of expression. At 10 to 12 Gy, some alteration in taste response is noted.[530] Radiation therapy affects taste deterministically but also by changing the sense of smell. It appears that there are learned aversions developed to foods consumed in proximity with the nausea and vomiting associated with either chemotherapy or radiation therapy. These aversions are typically transient, lasting only a few weeks.[531–534] It appears that radiotherapy affects salty and bitter tastes most, whereas chemotherapy seems to affect sweet and sour tastes. Most patients (more than 75%) receiving fractionated radiotherapy schemes totaling 60 to 70 Gy have impairment in taste for several years.[535]

At the end of the second week of radiotherapy and dose levels of 20 to 24 Gy, dysphasia, soreness, and pain, as well as dryness of the mouth occur, and taste is deteriorated further. There is definite erythema, and patchy mucositis of the palate may be noted. At 30 to 36 Gy, the saliva is thick, and mucositis is identified in the region of the tonsils and the posterior pharynx. At levels of 50 to 60 Gy, mucositis develops into a pseudomembrane involving all tissues including the tongue. Clearing of these changes begins in approximately 2 weeks and is completed within 2 months. The volume of the mucosa irradiated influences the reaction. Higher doses are much better tolerated in small areas than in large areas. Improvement of mucositis and protective effects during radiotherapy have been reported for amifostine,[536-538] sucralfate,[539,540] oral glutamine,[541] and most recently recombinant human keratinocyte growth factor.[542]

In the chronic period, delayed effects include progressive fibrosis of the submucosa, telangiectasia, and interstitial fibrosis of the mucous glands. Areas adjacent to the mucosa, such as Waldeyer's tonsillar ring, demonstrate marked radiosensitivity of the lymphocytes; however, repopulation occurs quite promptly. The skeletal muscle of the tongue is quite radiation-resistant, with changes rarely seen below total fractionated doses of 100 to 500 Gy. Chronic ulcers may occur in the mucosa, in a fashion similar to that for the skin, as the result of arterial intimal fibrosis. Such radiation ulcers are usually flat, with very little associated inflammation. They commonly occur along the lateral border of the tongue, floor of the mouth, and other areas where there is friction or microtrauma. Irradiation of the salivary glands causes the saliva to have an acidic pH, causing the rapid development of dental caries.[543] Thus, oral hygiene is particularly important in patients undergoing courses of radiotherapy; even so, secondary infections of the mucosa (such as thrush) are relatively common. Caries seem to be related to the oral lactobacillus count. Both caries and osteoradionecrosis can be reduced or prevented by application of fluoride. There has been a lot of recent interest in use of dental enamel as a biologic dosimeter. Through the use of electron spin resonance, a measure of dose can be determined.[544-546]

Neutron Radiation

Hussey et al. attempted to obtain an RBE for 50-MeV neutrons by using mucosal reactions in patients.[547] Their best estimate was that in relation to cobalt 60 therapy, the neutron RBE is 2.8.

Esophagus

Low-LET Radiation

The squamous epithelium of the esophagus has approximately the same turnover rate as oral mucosa and, thus, has about the same radiosensitivity. In spite of this, the esophagus is extremely resistant to radiation when compared with the remainder of the gastrointestinal tract. Esophagitis, dysphasia, and later stricture following radiotherapy was reported by Seaman and Ackerman.[548] Early

changes are primarily due to mucosal damage while late damage is primarily related to changes in the muscle wall although mucosal changes may be present. The SOMA toxicity table related to the esophagus is presented in Appendix 6.

The appearance of mucositis in the esophagus is very similar to its appearance in the oropharynx. Symptoms include mild to moderate substernal burning and difficulty in swallowing, beginning at the second or third week after the initiation of radiotherapy, that are sometimes accompanied by sharp chest pain and can be noted at absorbed dose levels as low as 20 Gy. Doses of 20 to 30 Gy over 2 weeks lead to clinical symptoms of esophagitis; however, they are transient. The esophagus can tolerate fractionated doses up to 60 Gy. Lepke et al. identified 40 patients with functional or morphologic abnormalities after radiotherapy.[549] These changes included abnormal motility, mucosal edema, strictures, ulcerations, pseudodiverticula, and fistulae.[550-554] Esophageal motility could be impaired as early as 1 week after radiotherapy, but more generally this finding occurred at 4 to 12 weeks. Improvement of radiation esophagitis and healing of ulceration during therapy has been reported with an oral solution of granulocyte macrophage-colony stimulating factor (rhGM-CSF).

Strictures have been reported to develop 4 to 8 months after completion of radiotherapy at doses from 30 Gy in 2 weeks to 65 Gy in 6.5 weeks. Strictures occurred after 6 to 8 months in some patients who had received 45 Gy over a period of 4 weeks. Higher doses shortened the interval to occurrence, with strictures developing as early as 3 to 4 months. The same study also demonstrated that patients receiving combination chemotherapy and radiotherapy were more likely to have esophageal injury, an observation that has been made by other authors, as well.[555] A study of head and neck cancer patients who received radiotherapy found that strictures were very uncommon when less than 60 Gy was received, and most patients who develop strictures have received more than 60 Gy.[556] Strictures may occur at lower doses in very young patients. Esophagitis can be increased in patients treated with Adriamycin, cisplatinum, 5-fluorouracil, actinomycin D, bleomycin, and methotrexate. Effects by these drugs on late radiation toxicity is unclear. Isolated case reports of esophageal-aortic fistula and tracheoesophageal fistula have also been reported in the literature.[557] The tolerance dose (TD 50/5) has been estimated to be 72 Gy when one third of the esophagus is irradiated, 70 Gy when two thirds is irradiated, and 68 Gy when the entire esophagus is irradiated.[526] With traditional therapy protocols involving higher doses, stricture, perforation, and obstruction may occur (Fig. 6-12). With high-dose conformal radiotherapy, doses in the range of 78 Gy commonly cause late toxicity but it is usually not severe.[558]

Three months after the usual course of radiation therapy, epithelial regeneration appears to be complete. The epithelium often is thicker than normal but may

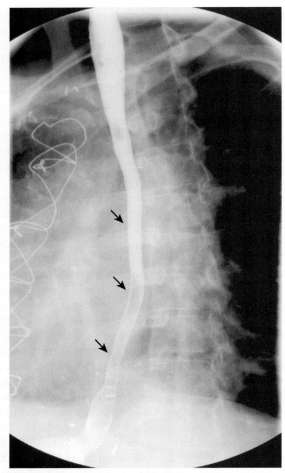

Figure 6-12 • Long smooth radiation stricture of the esophagus after radiation therapy of the mediastinum for Hodgkin's disease. Note also median sternotomy wires from coronary artery bypass graft surgery possibly due to radiation-induced coronary artery disease.

show occasional areas of atrophy. As with the skin, small-vessel telangiectasia, fibrosis of the muscularis and submucosa, and intimal fibrosis of the arterioles occur.

Stomach

Low-LET Radiation

The earliest changes due to radiation identified in the stomach were reported in 1912 by Regaud, who noted atrophy of the glands of the fundic portion of the stomach. In the 1940s, following high-dose gastric irradiation, other deterministic effects of radiation on the stomach became apparent. In a series of 256 patients treated for testicular tumors with retroperitoneal node irradiation, 35 proved to have gastric ulceration.[559] Ironically, not only can radiation cause ulcers, but historically radiation therapy was also used for treatment of peptic ulcer. Fractionated courses of radiation therapy up to an absorbed dose of 20 Gy are well tolerated and suppress gastric acidity; thus, the rationale for its use in benign peptic ulceration. The reduction in gastric acidity appears

before reduction in pepsin levels and indeed before morphologic changes can be demonstrated. This hypoacidity may last for as little as 6 months or up to many years. Doses of 15 Gy given over 10 days have been reported to decrease gastric acidity to 30% of pretreatment levels at 11 months and to 58% of pretreatment levels at 30 months.[560] Doses of 16 Gy given in 10 daily fractions to the stomach cause necrosis of glandular epithelium and loss of chief and parietal cell granules within 6 days after the completion of treatment. By 16 weeks after such a course of therapy, the mucosa histologically returns to normal.[429]

Fractionated treatments of the upper abdomen of up to 50 Gy produce nausea and vomiting. In this regard it should be noted that whole-body doses as low as 1 Gy may produce the same symptoms (see the section later in this chapter, "Total-Body Irradiation"). Radiation ulcers in the stomach are usually single, from 0.5 to 2 cm in diameter and antral in location.[528] They have been reported after fractionated doses to the stomach ranging from 48 to 64 Gy. Patients who develop radiation ulcers usually experience epigastric pain 5 to 6 months after the beginning of therapy. The incidence of ulceration following fractionated radiotherapy is about 6% at 40 to 50 Gy and 17% at 50 to 60 Gy. The tolerance dose of the esophagus, stomach, and intestine is less than that of the mouth because such an ulcer may cause lethal perforation, whereas in the mouth an ulcer is more of a nuisance. Perforation has been reported in 6% of cases with doses about 40 to 50 Gy, 10% at 50 to 60 Gy, and almost 40% at fractionated doses above 60 Gy.[526] Perforation of the stomach is much more common in cases in which the tumor involves the stomach per se.

Additional delayed effects include impairment of gastric motility, dyspepsia, and development of chronic atrophic gastritis, usually as a result of fibrosis of the mucosa. Gastritis occurring 1 to 12 months postradiotherapy may occur as a result mucosal atrophy, fibrosis of submucosal tissue, and spasm or stenosis of the antrum. Late ulceration typically arises at 5 to 6 months postradiotherapy and is indistinguishable from an ordinary ulcer. Dyspepsia occurring 6 months to 4 years postradiotherapy also has been reported. Stenotic reactions are possible but unusual. CT scanning may demonstrate nonspecific gastric wall thickening with stranding of perigastric fat. An unusual entity of massive hyalinization of the gastric submucosa and muscularis following chemotherapy and x-ray therapy has been reported. Its exact pathogenesis and significance remain unknown.[561] The SOMA toxicity table related to the stomach is presented in Appendix 6.

Small Intestine

Low-LET Radiation

The reader is referred to a comprehensive study of the small bowel and large intestine published by

Becciolini[562] and a review article by Coia et al.[526] The small bowel demonstrates mucosal reactions in radiotherapy schemes in which 30 to 40 Gy are given over 4 weeks. Higher doses may cause obstruction and other complications. Prior surgery, with formation of adhesions, reduces the tolerance of the bowel to radiotherapy. The small intestine is quite sensitive to radiation injury because of the rapidly proliferating cells of the mucosal epithelium in the crypts of Lieberkühn. These columnar cells, which divide approximately once every 24 hours, push the more mature cells up the villi to the intestinal lumen, where they mature to their final state when they reach the tips of the villi. The epithelium of the crypt is replaced in fewer than 7 days, making this the most rapidly proliferating tissue and one of the most radiosensitive tissues in the body. The relatively high sensitivity of the mucosal lining compared with underlying vascular and stromal components means that acute changes are of the most clinical significance and that late changes due to arteriolar narrowing rarely occur. Radiosensitivity of the small intestine in radiation therapy is clearly affected by the intestine's ability to move. Because the terminal ileum, the duodenum, and the most proximal portion of the jejunum are relatively fixed, these areas are the most frequently involved in complications of radiation injury. Because the small intestine was relatively inaccessible until the advent of endoscopy, there exists little in the way of human observations. A single case of accidental exposure has, however, been reported.[563] Within 7 days after single doses in excess of 15 Gy, superficial erosion, pyknosis, and sloughing of the epithelium into the lumen occur. At somewhat lower doses, mucosal regeneration begins by 7 days. In therapeutic situations, within 12 to 24 hours after daily doses of 1.5 to 3 Gy, cell necrosis in the walls of the crypts can be identified. There is progressive loss of cells, as well as atrophy of the villi.

During the period of mucosal sloughing, patients experience nausea, vomiting, cramping, pain, diarrhea, fluid and electrolyte imbalance, and sepsis. Hypoproteinemia due to protein leakage through the damaged mucosal cells may occur. The pathophysiology of radiation enteritis is poorly understood, and increased prostaglandin levels have been implicated; however, Lifshitz et al. examined patients receiving radiotherapy and found no increase in prostaglandin levels.[564] Other investigators have concluded that lactose malabsorption is a factor in the nausea, diarrhea, and vomiting experienced by patients undergoing pelvic radiotherapy.[565] Henriksson et al. pointed out that sucralfate (an aluminum hydroxide complex of sulfated sucrose) can protect against radiation-induced diarrhea and bowel discomfort in patients receiving bowel radiotherapy.[566] In acute and subacute radiation enteritis barium studies of the small intestine may show nodular filling defects or "thumbprinting" similar to intestinal ischemia.[529]

The gastrointestinal syndrome that may occur after a large, single, acute absorbed dose usually results in death. It has been described to be a combination of fluid-electrolyte derangement and sepsis. Whether the gastrointestinal syndrome truly exists in humans remains a matter of debate (see the section later in this chapter, "Total-Body Irradiation"). A gastrointestinal radiographic contrast examination of the patient during the acute clinical period generally demonstrates rapid transit time of barium from the stomach to the colon. Hypermotility is demonstrated in just under one half of the patients receiving radiation therapy to the small bowel. Lentz et al. reported that after whole-abdomen radiation therapy in the range of 29 to 51 Gy for gynecologic malignancies, a transient chylous ascites developed in about 3% of patients.[567] Concurrent use of Adriamycin or actinomycin D enhances radiation toxicity of the intestine.

Late radiation injury may take years to become apparent; however, in many patients the injury becomes apparent about 8 to 12 months postradiotherapy. During the chronic period, delayed effects are generally manifested as intermittent abdominal pain or obstruction. The diagnosis is difficult to make without the history of radiation exposure. Additional symptoms include occasional bleeding, diarrhea, cramping, abdominal bloating, nausea, vomiting, and laboratory findings of hypoproteinemia and malabsorption. Patients may show an increase in intraluminal bile-labeled salt content due to impaired reabsorption and bacterial overgrowth, prompting use of cholestyramine for patients with severe diarrhea. Perkins et al. published a radiologic-pathologic correlative study of nine patients with radiation injury of the small bowel.[568] In general, barium studies demonstrate a lack of distensibility of a bowel segment without sharp margins and the persistence of edematous-appearing mucosa with a "saw-toothed" appearance. There also may be separation of bowel loops due to fibrosis, focal areas of narrowing and long segment strictures, as well as fistulas.[529]

Donaldson et al. reviewed the late complications in children after whole-abdominal radiation therapy for Wilms' tumor, teratoma, or lymphoma.[569] Of 14 long-term survivors, 5 developed severe radiation injury, with small-bowel obstruction, within 2 months of therapy completion. The average age at treatment was 6 years, and the treatment was 31 Gy in 7 to 20 fractions over 11 to 39 days. Coia and Hanks reviewed the complications in 1026 patients treated with large-field infradiaphragmatic radiation therapy for Hodgkin's disease and seminoma.[570] The most frequent complications were gastrointestinal injury, such as peptic ulceration, hemorrhage, chronic diarrhea, and intestinal obstruction. The bowel complications occurred in 1% of patients at doses of less than 35 Gy and 3% for doses equal to or greater than 35 Gy. Major bowel complications increase rapidly when large portions of the bowel receive fractionated doses above 50 to 55 Gy. Histologically, during the subacute and chronic period, the villae of the mucosa are often blunt and thickened, and the mucosal cells are often flattened. The lamina propria may be normal or may demonstrate severe fibrosis. Telangiectasia may occasionally occur, as well. Overall, collagen deposition throughout the submucosa is demonstrated most consistently. The arterioles, as in other tissues, show endothelial proliferation and intimal fibrosis.

Colon, Sigmoid, and Rectum

The mucosal cells of the colon have a somewhat longer turnover time (4 to 8 days) than those of the small intestine. There are also fewer epithelial cells at risk for a given surface area, and some of the cells remain in prolonged interphase. Thus, the epithelial portions of most of the colon have somewhat less radiosensitivity than the small intestine and about the same radiosensitivity as the esophagus. The blood vessels and underlying muscle have radiosensitivity similar to that of the remainder of the gastrointestinal tract. The SOMA toxicity table related to the colon and rectum is presented in Appendix 6.

Low-LET Radiation

The pathologic basis of radiation-induced changes in the colon and rectum is similar to that already discussed for the small intestine. Acute changes are easily demonstrated during a course of radiation therapy in which the total dose exceeds 30 to 40 Gy. These changes include hyperemic mucosa and abnormalities in mucus production. Pathologically, the peritoneal surfaces are roughened, with variable amounts of fibrin or fibrous plaques, and shallow mucosal ulcers may be present. When superficial ulcers appear, the changes are usually relatively well healed within a month. Treatment usually consists of low-residue diets and symptomatic management of diarrhea.[571] On barium imaging studies, acute radiation colitis demonstrates mucosal irregularity, nodular mucosa, and cobblestone or sawtooth patterns. With MR imaging, the earliest change is increased signal intensity in the submucosa on T2 images.[529]

Six to 12 months after radiation therapy, the patient may exhibit painless rectal bleeding. In mild stages, the rectal changes consist of mucosal thickening and exudate; however, ultimately there may be progression to ulceration, rectal strictures, or fistulas. The mucous membrane is usually granular, and the ulcers may be either solitary or multiple, usually 1 to 4 cm in diameter, and are located in a transverse direction. The appearance on barium enema in these circumstances may be confused with that of a recurrent tumor. The best method for determining radiation proctitis is by endoscopy. Gehrig et al. indicated that after fractionated radiotherapy, the incidence of proctitis 1 to 6 years later is 0% at 40 Gy, 20% at 60 Gy, and 50% at 90 Gy.[572] The most characteristic findings described by other authors are arteriolar narrowing, telangiectasia (Fig. 6-13), and diminished distensibility.[573,574]

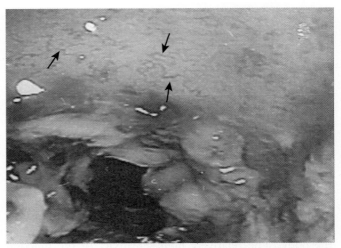

Figure 6-13 • Telangiectasia of the rectum causing bleeding after excessive radiotherapy.

Some relief of radiation proctosigmoiditis can be achieved through the use of rectal steroids[575] or sucralfate.[576] Other therapies that have been used are deterministic application or installation of 4% formalin,[577,578] vitamins E and C,[579] and coagulation argon or laser.[580] Occurrence of fistulas, perforation, and small-bowel or colon injury can lead to mortalities in the range of 25%.[581,582]

Chronic changes consist of shortening and fibrosis of the colon, with occasional areas of tapered stenosis ulcers and fistulas. At this stage, the mucosa may be normal or atrophic. Occasionally mucosal glands are present deep in the muscle, probably as a result of healing ulcers.[583] The strictures generally result from extensive submucosal fibrosis (Fig. 6-14). The radiologic diagnosis may be suggested by an hourglass-type deformity on barium enema or a "lead-pipe" appearance such as is seen with long-standing ulcerative colitis. Treatment of these stenotic areas usually

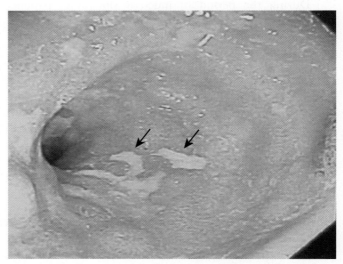

Figure 6-14 • Rectal ulceration and stricture after excessive radiotherapy.

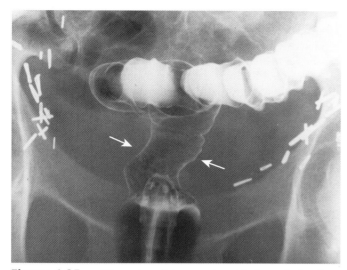

Figure 6-15 • Narrowing of the rectosigmoid after radiation therapy to the pelvis. (Case courtesy of William Black, MD.)

is symptomatic. Dilation is sometimes used, although occasionally surgical intervention is necessary. The pathology of the late changes is a result of progressive endarteritis and subsequent fibrosis (Figs. 6-15 and 6-16).[584] In general, the fixed position of the rectosigmoid portion of the colon causes it to be relatively susceptible to radiation injury when compared to the transverse colon.

The rectum is relatively resistant to radiation, although loss of the epithelium occurs on a transient basis with doses of 30 to 40 Gy. Chau reported the incidence of bowel

complications in supervoltage pelvic irradiation to a total dose of 60 Gy to be between 1% and 3%.[585] As can be expected, the incidence of acute changes increases dramatically with an increase in the volume of tissue irradiated. Daily doses to the entire abdomen in excess of 1 Gy are usually poorly tolerated. In terms of the importance of biologic factors, increasing age, black race, and previous surgery are thought to be associated with a greater number of complications. The anatomic vascular distribution may be of some importance, although it has been demonstrated that intestinal ulcerations do not always occur at the area of maximal irradiation or least vascularity but appear to result more often from combined injury, mechanical trauma, and bacterial action.

Neutron Radiation

Few data are available concerning the RBE of neutrons for the gastrointestinal tract of humans. Data from mice would indicate that the RBE of neutrons with regard to the gastrointestinal tract is higher than for other organ systems.[586,587]

Radionuclide Irradiation

Research findings on the irradiation of the gastrointestinal tract by radionuclides are quite limited. Beta-emitting radionuclides administered as colloids in the peritoneal cavity have been used for many years for treatment of serosal implantation of malignant disease. Doses in the neighborhood of 50 to 70 Gy to the omentum and peritoneal serosal surfaces result in mild radiation

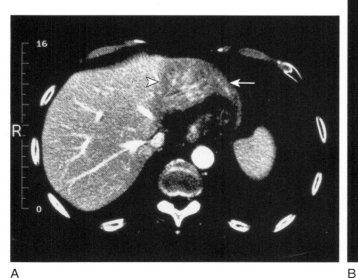

A

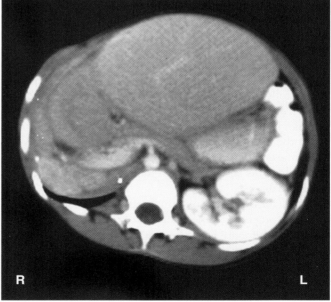

B

Figure 6-16 • Imaging changes seen on CT scan after abdominal radiotherapy. **A,** Low density seen in the lateral aspect of the right lobe of the liver (*arrows*) several months after radiotherapy. **B,** Asymmetry with small volume of the right side of the abdomen 6 years after radiotherapy of the right flank for Wilm's tumor treatment. The left lobe of the liver shows marked compensatory hypertrophy.

sickness, with leukopenia.[54] Long-term gastrointestinal complications, including adhesions and fragility of the bowel, have been found.[588] The experience with radium applications and bowel complications was extensively reviewed by Rubin and Casarett.[2]

LIVER AND BILIARY SYSTEM

Low-LET Radiation

Radiation-induced changes in hepatic cells were described as early as 1924 by Case and Warthin.[589] Although the liver was considered to be generally radioresistant compared to other upper abdominal viscera, it was clear by the mid-1950s that fractionated doses in excess of 40 to 50 Gy resulted in hepatic necrosis. In the mid-1960s, more attention was directed to irradiation of the liver, particularly in terms of radiotherapy schemes. Clinical signs of hepatic injury induced by radiation include an increase in abdominal girth, hepatomegaly, ascites, jaundice, elevated serum alkaline phosphatase, and, occasionally, a clinical picture resembling the Budd-Chiari syndrome.[590–592] Profound thrombocytopenia, particularly in children, has also been reported.[593]

Radiation changes in the liver are primarily due to damage to the fine vasculature and connective tissue. The hepatic cells are relatively resistant to the deterministic effects of radiation. Both the hepatic cells and ductal epithelial cells are long-lived and behave as reverting postmitotic cells. They do not divide regularly; however, following removal or destruction of a large portion of the liver, there is a marked capacity for regeneration. This induced division of hepatic cells and ductal epithelial cells probably causes regenerating areas to be more radiosensitive than normal liver. The most critical portion of the liver appears to be the small central vein in each lobule, and the few pathologic studies that have been done appear to indicate that the most characteristic change following irradiation of the liver is nonspecific venous occlusive damage. Few additional data are available because the adjacent bowel is more sensitive and is the limiting factor when whole-body or whole-abdominal irradiation is used. In addition, radiotherapy of the liver is usually not effective in treatment of metastatic disease.

The liver is able to tolerate fractionated doses of 40 to 50 Gy in 4 weeks to a small portion of the organ.[591,594–596] In children there are liver abnormalities noted after radiotherapy to the liver of 12 to 30 Gy. Chou et al. reported that about 75% of children receiving 7 to 12 Gy total-body irradiation prior to bone marrow transplant developed acute liver dysfunction and about 25% showed signs of hepatic veno-occlusive disease.[597] Thomas et al. reported hepatic fibrosis in 3 of 26 long-term survivors of Wilms' tumors who had received at least 30 Gy in 1.5 to 2 Gy fractions.[598,599]

A number of other complications after radiotherapy ranging from thrombocytopenia to death have also been reported. Effects of conventionally fractionated radiation can be identified at levels of 30 Gy as nonfunctional areas on radionuclide liver scans. On 3-phase CT scanning of the liver in acute radiation injury there is low attenuation of irradiated parenchyma although if there is an underlying fatty infiltration of the liver the parenchyma may be hyperattenuating. Later radiation injury often shows heterogeneous and variable enhancement of veno-occlusive disease and delayed clearance of contrast material.[529,600]

Above dose levels of 30 to 35 Gy delivered in 28 days, the incidence of clinical liver disease varies between 4% and 32%.[601] Feigen et al. indicated that when moving-strip radiotherapy is used to treat the liver, a dose of 2.5 Gy in 10 fractions is near the maximum tolerable dose.[602] It should be noted that after resection of the liver, the remaining regenerating liver is more radiosensitive. As with other organs, the dose fractionation scheme is extremely important in determining tolerance. Fajardo et al. reported that two total abdominal doses of 5 Gy each are sufficient to cause severe hepatic injury.[603] In the acute clinical period, symptoms may occur 2 to 6 weeks after completion of a radiation therapy course in which the liver was included in the radiation port. The clinical manifestations are those described earlier and occasionally are termed *radiation hepatitis*. Radiation-induced liver disease (radiation hepatitis) was reviewed by Lawrence et al.[604] There is often development of anicteric ascites 2 weeks to 4 months after irradiation. Other findings include markedly increased alkaline phosphatase, moderate hepatomegaly, mild right upper quadrant pain, moderately increased aspartate aminotransferase (AST), and mildly increased bilirubin. There is often 10% to 20% mortality. If jaundice is present this is usually the result of combined modality treatment of liver disease.[604]

Pathologic changes typically identified may include severe sinusoidal congestion, hyperemia, hemorrhage, atrophy of the central hepatic cells with dilation of the central vein, and progressive atrophy of the liver cell plates. Treatment consists of bed rest, high-protein-high-calorie diet, diuretics, possibly steroids, and symptomatic treatment of ascites. Spironolactone and steroids have been used in some cases. During this period, the radionuclide sulfur colloid liver-spleen scan often demonstrates depressed or absent activity of the reticuloendothelial cells (Fig. 6-17). This function may return in a few months after fractionated doses up to 23 Gy. There are several reports of other imaging modalities that have been used in cases of hepatic injury. Yankelevitz et al. indicated that on using MRI, there was an increase in signal on T2-weighted scans at 4 weeks after 36 Gy of abdominal radiotherapy.[605] The appearance returned to normal after 60 days post-therapy. Garra et al. reported that there is higher

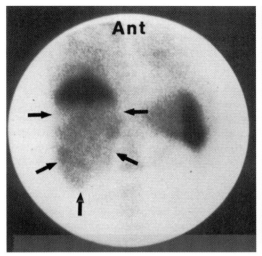 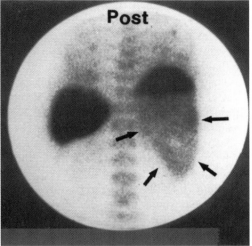

Figure 6-17 • Radiation defect identified on radionuclide liver spleen scan. Only superior aspect of the liver functions normally. Entire lower aspect (*arrows*) is relatively hypofunctional as a result of a recent course of radiotherapy. (Case courtesy of M.J. Guiberteau, MD.)

attenuation in irradiated liver using ultrasound imaging.[606] This is to be expected with fibrotic changes. The SOMA toxicity table related to the liver is presented in Appendix 6.

Hepatic veno-occlusive lesions may occur early but are more characteristic at 3 to 6 months. Many of the small central lobular or sublobular veins develop a fibrous net that ultimately becomes dense and coalesces. Ultimately, narrowing of the lumen, sinusoidal congestion, and liver cell atrophy occur. If enough liver is included in the radiotherapy treatment field, there may be gradual reduction in liver size due to atrophy with recurrent ascites, jaundice, and liver failure. Wharton et al. reported that 11 out of 14 patients treated with whole-abdominal irradiation to doses of 23 to 30 Gy in 8 fractions over 12 days died as a result of the radiation injury.[607] In adults, veno-occlusive disease has been observed after single doses of 10 Gy or fractionated doses of 18 to 30 Gy. A 20% to 25% incidence of veno-occlusive disease has been seen after a single acute dose of 10 Gy followed by bone marrow transplantation.[608,609]

Beyond 6 months, pathologic examination of the liver reveals markedly less congestion, but there is atrophy due to loss of hepatic cells, with a decreased distance between the central veins and the portal spaces. The veno-occlusive disease identified in the liver after radiation therapy is unique and has been compared to similar conditions caused by various alkaloids, urethane, arsphenamine, and long-term oral contraceptives.[610] Antineoplastic drugs, particularly busulfan, dimethylbusulfan, cytarabine, and thioguanine, may also produce this picture alone or in combination with radiation therapy.[603] Hepatic sensitivity is increased when radiation is used in combination with chemotherapeutic agents such as Adriamycin, actinomycin D, 5-fluorouracil, chlorambucil, and vincristine sulfate.[611–613] In fact, a case of fatal radiation hepatitis with

concomitant use of radiation and vincristine was reported by Hansen.[614]

The result of single massive doses of 3 to 100 Gy of x-ray to the liver of rabbits was described by Ariel.[615] Single doses of 3 Gy caused only mild intercellular edema, with the changes completely gone by day 7. At single doses of 30 Gy, dilatation of vessels, hemorrhage, and edema appeared within 12 hours. The edema was greatest at 2 days, but some remained at 7 days. Dose levels of 300 Gy caused immediate edema, compression of the hepatic cells, and, within 2 days, some necrosis. The intrahepatic biliary system is also composed of reverting postmitotic cells. Few human data are available, although the animal data indicate that after radiation exposure, very little alteration is identified in the biliary epithelium. Columnar epithelial cells that line the gallbladder and the extrahepatic ducts are long-lived reverting postmitotic cells relatively resistant to radiation.

High-LET Radiation

Experience with high-LET radiation is extremely limited; however, at least one case of a primary liver tumor was irradiated with the negative pi-meson beam at the Los Alamos National Laboratory. No clinically evident adverse results were identified in doses up to 29 pion Gy in 24 fractions delivered over 3 weeks.

Radionuclide Irradiation

There is a moderate amount of information available concerning effects of internal radionuclide irradiation of the liver in humans. Data stem from three sources: (1) hepatic irradiation for radiotherapeutic purposes, (2) therapeutic intravenous injection of radium, and (3) Thorotrast given for radiographic contrast studies. The patients given Thorotrast administration for angiography are historically the most interesting. These patients have a high incidence of unusual malignancies (see Chapter 5); however, they also have a high incidence of nonmalignant liver disease.[616,617] The changes are predominantly those of cirrhosis or fibrosis. Estimates of the exact radiation dose are difficult, but those that have been made are in the range of 5 to 15 Gy. Some of these changes occurred after periods of 20 to 40 years after administration of the Thorotrast. Injection of radium 224 for ankylosing spondylitis and tuberculosis has resulted in changes in the bone and cartilage. Cirrhosis has been reported in some of these patients, particularly males, but it is not known whether it was secondary to radiation or to alcohol. Therapeutic radionuclide irradiation of the liver has been performed in at least two different circumstances. The first used phosphorus 32 phosphate colloid for patients with metastatic colon cancer. Injection of 550 MBq in the hepatic arterial system resulted in doses estimated at 50 Gy. Temporary radiation hepatitis occurred in at least one patient. Arterial injection of yttrium 90 resin microspheres and 5-fluorouracil has also been used for treatment of hepatic metastases. Injection of 3700 MBq gives an estimated dose of 100 Gy of beta radiation to the liver.[618] In 25 such patients followed for approximately 2 years, no significant abnormalities had been reported.[619]

Marn et al. described the appearance of the liver on CT scan after administration of intraarterial yttrium 90 microspheres for therapy of metastatic disease.[620] Low-attenuation, irregular areas were best seen 8 weeks after therapy and were partially or completely reversible at 16 to 24 weeks. There was little or no change in liver function when these areas were identified. Similar conclusions were reached by Gray et al. who performed liver biopsies 7 to 9 months after the same treatment.[621]

PANCREAS

Low-LET Radiation

The pancreas is composed of both endocrine and exocrine cells. After irradiation, the islet cells show significantly more change than do acinous cells. The radiotherapeutic literature concerning deterministic effects is quite limited because the pancreas is relatively radioresistant compared with the surrounding, more sensitive structures such as the liver and small bowel. Only occasionally have radiation therapy projects allowed depth dose curves that could effectively treat the pancreas without substantially injuring the surrounding structures. These have included the radiotherapy projects at Lawrence Laboratory at Berkeley and the now-discontinued project at Los Alamos National Laboratory facility. Unfortunately, no pathologic studies have been forthcoming from the latter project. Woodruff et al. studied patients from the Lawrence-Berkeley project and demonstrated radiation injury in normal pancreatic parenchyma. Apparently, these changes were fibrosis replacing the exocrine parenchyma and, to a lesser extent, the islets. Pancreatic fibrosis has also been described in several patients who have received high-dose abdominal radiation for testicular tumors.[622,623] The only other report of human experience in the literature is that of Case and Warthin in 1924, a case report of a patient who died 10 weeks after heavy doses of radiation to the epigastrium.[589] Atrophy of acinous cells, as well as necrosis and lymphocytic infiltration of the ductal epithelium, occurred. Most of the pathologic studies have been complicated by autolysis, infection, and tumor involvement of the pancreas at the time of autopsy. Exact dose-response relationships for the pancreas have been difficult to calculate because in the older literature the absorbed dose is difficult to ascertain. Of the limited animal data, the scant amount available has been mostly related to study of pancreatic islets of rats,[624] and several studies in dogs.[625,626]

Overall, the deterministic effects of radiation on the pancreas are substantially less severe than those on the surrounding, more radiosensitive structures such as the liver and small intestine. With some effort, it is possible to achieve dose levels at which an exocrine secretion of the pancreas decreases, with some associated fibrosis. Becciolini et al. analyzed duodenal juice after 50 Gy in 25 fractions and did not find any significant changes or decrease in either trypsin or amylase.[562] Their conclusion was that the pancreas did not contribute to malabsorption in irradiated patients. Steglich et al. studied 27 patients and reported increases in serum lipase activity after pancreatic irradiation, but this also occurred to a lesser degree after pelvic irradiation.[627] There has been one report of pancreatic insufficiency 23 years after abdominal radiotherapy for seminoma, but given the frequency of radiotherapy to this area and the lack of findings from other studies, the insufficiency was probably due to causes other than radiotherapy.[628] Chronic pancreatitis has been reported in a few patients treated for Hodgkin's disease with doses between 36 and 40.5 Gy.[629] Generally, however, this appears to be a rare complication.

URINARY SYSTEM

Kidney

The kidney is a relatively radiosensitive organ when compared with the other intra-abdominal organs and tissues. Its radiosensitivity was demonstrated by both experimental and clinical data in the late 1920s. However, as Rubin and Casarett have pointed out, these data were neglected for the next several decades, only to be rediscovered after many tragic experiences during the 1950s.[2] The kidney consists of three major cell groups of interest, those forming (1) the glomerulus, (2) the renal tubules, and (3) the vascular supply system. The vascular system is particularly important because about one fifth of the body's blood passes through the kidneys each minute. The arterioles supply a rich network about the glomeruli and the renal tubules. The epithelia of the tubules and the glomerular capsule are long-lived, composed of reverting postmitotic cells that rarely divide. The nephrons themselves are unable to regenerate and are constantly being reduced in number with age and injury; however, if an injury is focal, the remaining nephrons may hypertrophy. For another review, the reader is referred to a chapter in a book by Stewart and Williams.[630] The SOMA toxicity tables related to the kidney, ureter, and bladder are presented in Appendix 6.

Low-LET Radiation

From the time of completion of a standard course of radiation therapy up to about 6 months, renal function is usually relatively normal. Occasionally, at dose levels about 4.5 Gy, there may be a diminution of renal plasma levels; when fractionated doses exceed 20 to 24 Gy, a fall in the glomerular filtration rate (GFR) may occur. Measurements of tubular function (such as those that might be obtained with Hippuran) are highly variable in humans, and most other tests, such as blood urea nitrogen (BUN), are usually normal during radiotherapy. There are only fragmentary human data regarding acute changes after single large doses, but animal studies do not follow the same time course as fractionated doses in humans.[631] Pathologically, the acute changes that may be identified are hyperemia, increased capillary permeability with interstitial edema, and degenerative changes in the endothelial cells of the fine vasculature. The occlusive changes that follow are usually in the interlobular arteries and afferent arterioles. In the period 6 to 12 months after treatment (the subacute clinical period), the clinical manifestations of acute radiation nephritis become apparent.

The term *acute radiation nephritis* is a poor choice since the condition is neither acute nor a nephritis; pathologically, it is actually a nephrosclerosis.[429] The patients demonstrate anemia, edema, hypertension, proteinuria, uremia, oliguria, and, in some cases, anuria. The hypertension, which may be malignant, is responsible for most deaths occurring before 12 months. Other clinical complaints include the development of peritoneal and pleural effusions, headaches, nausea and vomiting, and, occasionally, photophobia. Following radiotherapy, the development of these signs is often confused with recurrent tumor or the development of distant metastases. Laboratory studies in patients with acute radiation nephritis demonstrate albuminuria and a low specific gravity. A normochromic, normocytic anemia with a normal platelet count often occurs. The BUN is elevated (usually to about 80 mg/dL). Hematuria is rarely seen and is usually microscopic.

The tolerance dose for the adult kidney appears to be approximately 23 Gy in 5 weeks to the parenchyma of both kidneys. Doses of 28 Gy to both kidneys in 5 weeks carry a high risk of severe radiation nephritis.[632]

In children, serious lesions can develop at lower doses, usually when 20 Gy is exceeded. Reduced creatinine clearance was reported by Mitus et al. in 18% of 108 children who had nephrectomy for malignant disease and received less than 12 Gy to the remaining kidney, and in 33% of those who received 12 to 24 Gy.[633] Radiation nephropathy has also been reported in children receiving bone marrow transplantation therapy.[634,635] After 12 to 14 Gy in 6 to 8 fractions over 3 to 4 days, there was hematuria and elevated creatinine. This is probably the result of both radiation and chemotherapy since long-term studies revealed abnormalities in less than 10% of patients receiving only 12 Gy in 6 fractions of total-body radiation.[636] Obviously if only one kidney is irradiated, there is substantially less clinical effect. Radiation of only one kidney did not cause radiation nephropathy in any of 13 patients receiving between 25 Gy in 6 weeks and 49 Gy in 5 weeks.[637]

Anderson et al. published a report of radiation nephritis demonstrated by CT.[638] In the acute phase there can be delayed excretion of contrast or a persistent nephrogram. In the chronic period the affected kidney is small and contracted. A number of radionuclide studies have been performed to assess both glomerular filtration and tubular secretion after radiotherapy. Dewit et al. reported that no changes were seen after bilateral whole-kidney irradiation of 17 to 18 Gy in 3.5 weeks; however, 40 Gy in 5.5 weeks resulted in a reduction of both parameters by 30% to 40% 3 to 5 years postradiotherapy.[639] When a radionuclide bone scan is performed after radiation therapy of the kidney, there may be increased uptake of the radiotracer by the kidneys. This may occur between 6 months and 2 years after the radiotherapy.[640,641] Whether this is due to microscopic deposition of calcium or perhaps to chemotherapy, which has been reported to also increase uptake of radiotracer, is unknown.

Willet et al. studied the long-term radiation effects on renal function in 86 patients who were treated with fractionated doses of at least 26 Gy during treatment for other tumors.[642] Only one patient developed clinically significant sequelae. For patients who had only 50% of a kidney irradiated, the mean decrease in creatinine clearance was 10%, and for those receiving whole unilateral renal irradiation the decrease was 24%. All changes in creatinine clearance were manifest within 1 year and did not progress. Other authors have reported similar findings.[643]

Some authors have reported cases in which malignant hypertension requiring nephrectomy was needed,[644] while most other authors find a slight increase that can usually be treated medically.[645] Preexisting hypertension may be made worse by renal radiotherapy. There are a few reports of hypertension occurring in children. Koskimies reported three children who developed hypertension more than 10 years after receiving more than 36 Gy to the tumor area.[646]

There have been many reports of both children and adults dying of renal failure and hypertension following therapeutic radiation.[647–649] Pathologic examination in these cases demonstrates the subacute changes of intimal necrosis, subendothelial fibrinous thickening, fibrinoid thrombosis, atrophy of tubules, and replacement with collagen. Myointimal proliferation with intimal "foamy cells" may be seen in some instances. Pathologic examination in established, radiation-induced renal failure often shows total sclerosis of the glomeruli as well. Treatment of acute radiation nephritis usually involves transfusions, bed rest, low-protein diet, and restriction of fluid and salt intake. Steroids have occasionally been tried; however, some researchers think that they may actually be harmful rather than helpful. Development of generalized edema, a BUN in excess of 100 mg/dL, or increasing hypertension is a grave prognostic indicator.[2,429]

Chronic radiation "nephritis" develops during the chronic clinical period (usually 1 to 5 years after radiation), with a mean time of 2 to 3 years. The clinical course involves the slow evolution of anemia, hypertension, and impairment of renal function. In general, the kidneys are small, as measured either by ultrasound or on intravenous pyelograms. It is possible that nuclear medicine studies using any number of radiopharmaceuticals would demonstrate a decrease in renal blood flow. The changes are irreversible and progressive; the treatment is usually symptomatic. Both benign and malignant hypertension may occur in patients after quite long intervals, even without clinical renal impairment.[650,651] The presence and degree of hypertension, as well as the time course, depend on the amount of renal tissue irradiated and the absorbed dose. The pathology of the chronic clinical period is an extension of that process seen in the subacute clinical period and involves progressive nephrosclerosis, degeneration of the fine vasculature with myointimal proliferation, occlusion, sclerosis of the glomeruli, atrophy of tubules, and, finally, interstitial fibrosis. Fajardo discussed the possible interaction of chemotherapy with radiation therapy.[429] Many of the changes induced by radiation can be seen with cancer chemotherapy, including thickening of the basement membrane, glomerular sclerosis, tubular loss, and stromal fibrosis. The nephrotoxic agents include nitrosoureas, methotrexate, cisplatinum, and Adriamycin. In children in whom actinomycin D is used with radiotherapy, a normal creatinine clearance and glomerular filtration rate are seen when the fractionated radiotherapy does not exceed 15 Gy; however, there is progressive renal insufficiency after doses of 20 Gy or more.[652]

Yamada et al. reported on noncancer diseases in the atomic bomb survivors and indicated an increased incidence of renal and ureteral stones.[653] They do point out that this is a new finding needing additional follow-up. Calculi are unlikely to be related to radiation in this population as the radiation dose is orders of magnitude smaller than for radiotherapy patients in whom no such increase is reported.

Ureter and Bladder

The bladder is relatively more radioresistant than the kidneys, with the most resistant portion of the genitourinary system being the ureters. Changes in the ureters and bladder were identified as early as 1930 by Schmitz, who reported the first case of ureteral stricture.[654] Other historical aspects have been well discussed and described by Rubin and Casarett.[2] Bladder injury, as well as distal ureteral problems, became apparent with the wide clinical experience gained through treatment of cervical carcinoma and other pelvic malignancies, particularly with radium therapy. The epithelium of the bladder and ureters is composed of proliferating vegetative intermitotic cells in the deep layer of the epithelium. These germinal cells are analogous to the same cells in the epidermis. Thus, the effects described for skin and mucosa are generally applicable to the mucosa of the urinary bladder.

Low-LET Radiation

Acute cystitis may occur 4 to 6 weeks after a course of radiotherapy. Symptoms include dysuria, nocturia, and frequency. Hyperemia and edema of the mucosa may be seen. At high doses, partial desquamation occurs. In severe cystitis with accompanying infection, ureteritis and transient hydroureter may be identified. The treatment of radiation cystitis is similar to that of cystitis due to other causes. In a series of 527 patients studied after therapy for cervical cancer, Montana et al. indicated that the risk of cystitis was 3% for those with a bladder dose of less than 50 Gy and 12% for those receiving fractionated doses in the range of 80 Gy or more to the bladder.[655] In the subacute clinical period (6 months to 2 years after therapy), painless hematuria may be a sign of trigonal ulcer. Cystoscopically, there is telangiectasia of the vessels in the region of the trigone; if obliteration of the smaller arterioles occurs as well, ulceration and fistula formation may result.

The bladder can usually tolerate 55 to 60 Gy in 20 fractions over 4 weeks.[656] Higher doses may be delivered with radium implants, and the changes observed include erythema, fibrosis, ulceration, and fistula formation. Severe radiation-induced hemorrhagic cystitis following radiotherapy is a relatively rare event.[657] If the distal ureters are involved, strictures and hydronephrosis may result. Goodman and Dalton indicated that pelvic inflammatory disease, urinary tract infection, and surgical manipulation increase the likelihood of ureteral stenosis.[658] In general, doses exceeding 50 to 60 Gy over a 5-week therapeutic regimen or 20 to 25 Gy in a single application carry a relatively high risk of late radiation reactions. With radium application for cervical carcinoma, the dose to the bladder is usually in the range of 50 to 60 Gy and rarely above 70 Gy.[659]

Parliament et al. reported that about 3% (10 of 328) of patients treated with curative intent for cervical carcinoma developed obstructive uropathy.[660] Eight cases were unilateral, and the median time to obstruction was 26 months. Of course, recurrent cervical carcinoma is a much more common cause of obstruction. Behr et al. reported a higher incidence (12%) of hydronephrosis and a very high incidence of incontinence probably due to fibrotic changes of the bladder and urethra.[661] In males treated for prostatic carcinoma, the incidence of incontinence is sometimes reported to be as high as 18% after radiotherapy,[662] while other authors suggest that it is mostly related to surgery.[663] A very large study by Lawton et al. reported on 1020 patients followed for at least 7 years after external beam radiotherapy for prostate cancer.[664] Only a total dose greater than 70 Gy was found to have a significant impact in the incidence of urinary complications. The total incidence of complications was cystitis, 2.6%; hematuria, 3.1%; urethral stricture, 4.6%; and bladder contracture, 0.7%. One case report presented retroperitoneal fibrosis causing ureteral obstruction 13 years after 30 Gy of external beam radiotherapy for stage I testicular carcinoma. That there are quite a number of causes of retroperitoneal fibrosis and there are not more reports after radiotherapy suggest that the fibrosis may not be radiation-related.[665]

In the chronic stages, the bladder may become contracted, thick, and indurated. There may be multiple areas of ulceration, edema, and telangiectasia. Collagen may replace muscular tissue, and breakdown of the bladder wall may occur. There also is submucosal fibrosis which is equally prominent in early and late stages.[666] Patients with bladder cancer who have had cystectomy and a urinary diversion to an ileal loop have a high risk of complication following radiotherapy doses of 55 Gy in 20 fractions over 4 weeks.[667]

High-LET Radiation

Only a limited amount of human experience with high-LET radiation exists; however, reports of the use of fast neutrons to control tumors of the bladder suggest an RBE not significantly different from the RBE of photons.[668]

Radionuclide Irradiation

Renal insufficiency has been reported in patients who have received radium 224, occurring in up to 13% of 222 patients who were given radium injections for treatment of ankylosing spondylitis or tuberculosis.[314] It is uncertain how much renal damage was due to the radium. The complicating factors of renal tuberculosis and drug therapy are unknown. Uranium can cause renal damage as a result of its chemical toxicity, however, workers in uranium plants have not demonstrated an excess mortality due to noncancer renal diseases.[669,670] This is discussed in detail in Chapter 9. Pinney et al. reported an excess of a number of genitourinary diseases in community residents living near the Fernald uranium plant in Ohio.[671] These

findings are suspect in terms of being radiation related. For example, the highest increase was in kidney stones, which are not known to be related to radiation even in radiotherapy patients.

In the last decade, there have been marked changes in radiotherapeutic techniques for treatment of prostate cancer. These include conformal radiotherapy as well as brachytherapy with prostatic iodine 125 or palladium 103 seed implants. After brachytherapy the incidence of dysuria is about 50% and peaks about 1 month after implantation but may not completely resolve for several years.[672] Urethral strictures occur in about 5% of patients with a median time to development of about 2 years,[673] urinary incontinence occurs in about 7% of patients, and erectile dysfunction in about 8% to 50%.[674–676]

REPRODUCTIVE ORGANS

A vast amount of information on the male and female genital tracts has been accumulated as a result of radiotherapy for pelvic malignancies. Few pelvic malignancies are not treated with radiation; the radiation used is not only external but often interstitial or intercavitary as well. That high doses of radiation can be given to the pelvis indicates that most reproductive organs themselves are not particularly sensitive to radiation necrosis even though they may demonstrate other changes. One very interesting difference between irradiation of the male and female is that in the female, radiation may not only cause reduction or obliteration of gamete production but also a decrease in the production of hormones. This, of course, may result in artificial menopause with secondary effects. In the male, there are few, if any, changes in hormone production. Most of the human data were derived from localized radiation, although whole-body radiation has been reported to cause temporary sterility. A review of some of the effects on reproductive organs was published by Lushbaugh and Ricks,[677] as well as Ladner.[678]

It should be pointed out that alterations in gonadal function as a result of radiotherapy can occur by a number of mechanisms. In children cranial irradiation can cause gonadotrophin deficiency or premature puberty,[679] and the reader is referred to the earlier section in this chapter, "Brain," for more details. Deterministic or scattered radiation to the ovary or testes can cause effects, and finally chemotherapeutic agents, such as alkylating agents, can be toxic to the ovaries but more so to the testes.[680,681] The SOMA toxicity tables related to the reproductive organs are presented in Appendix 6.

Ovary

Low-LET Radiation

The ovarian follicles contain the ova. The number of ovarian follicles appears to be maximal at birth or shortly thereafter. The follicles contain oocytes derived from the *oogonia*, vegetative differentiating intermitotic cells that are relatively sensitive to radiation. The oocytes, on the other hand, although somewhat variable according to their stage or position, are more resistant to radiation effects than are the oogonia. The lethal dose (LD_{50}) for human oocytes has been estimated to be less than 2 Gy.[682] A similar pattern occurs in the male, with the spermatogonia more radiosensitive than spermatocytes. With the exception of granulosa cells, the cells in the ovary (the connective tissue, cells of the theca, corpora lutea, and interstitial cells) are relatively resistant to radiation and behave as reverting postmitotic cells.

The ovary is very radiosensitive and demonstrates temporary or reduced sterility with 1.5 to 6.5 Gy in a single dose and with 1.5 to 12 Gy in fractionated doses.[683–686] Permanent sterility results from single doses of 3.2 to 10 Gy or higher fractionated doses.[677,683,684,687–690] The sensitivity of the ovary is greater in older women. This latter finding and the discovery that the ovary appears more resistant than the bone marrow in humans are different from the results expected on the basis of animal data alone. Between 1920–1940, 1.5 to 2.25 Gy in three doses over 3 weeks was administered for the purpose of increasing fertility. There was no evidence of an increase in malformations in subsequently conceived children.[677,691] More recently, Horning et al. examined the reproductive potential of females treated with radiotherapy for Hodgkin's disease.[692] The study reviewed 12 women treated for Hodgkin's disease who subsequently became pregnant, identifying no birth defects after radiotherapy or chemotherapy.

During the acute clinical period, the granulosa cells in the follicle are affected most by radiation. These cells are vegetative intermitotic cells and are, therefore, relatively radiosensitive. Changes in these cells are identified before radiation changes appear in the oocyte. Following radiation exposure of the ovary, there is a fertile period before temporary radiation sterility. This temporary fertile period occurs as a result of the final maturation process of follicles that are late in the stage of development. The temporary sterility that follows is due to radiation damage to those follicles in the intermediate stage of development that have a large amount of granulosa cell proliferation. In the subacute clinical period, there may be complete recovery of the ovaries with a sufficiently small dose. In the chronic, or late clinical period, resumption of growth and development of the ovarian follicles may not occur for a year or two, and the number of follicles present in the ovary is reduced. With large doses that cause permanent sterility, atrophy and degeneration occur, not only in the follicles but also in the interstitial gland cells and corpora lutea. Liebow et al. examined the ovaries in a young girl who died of radiation injury at Hiroshima; the ovaries were found to be totally devoid of follicles.[112] Fajardo points out

that the myointimal proliferation and subsequent obliteration of the lumen of the ovarian arteries and arterioles is more marked than is seen in other areas in the female reproductive tract.[3]

Ovarian irradiation interferes with formation and elimination of estriol and significantly reduces the urinary excretion of total estrogen. Excretion of estrone and estradiol-17 is also reduced but less than estriol. Radiation doses given for reduction of circulating hormone levels in some cancer patients usually ranged from 5.5 to 6.5 Gy.[693] In at least one study whose purpose was to eradicate hormonal function, the patients received 16 Gy.[1] Induction of menopause by radiation requires smaller doses in older females: 90% of women over the age of 40 may be sterilized by a dose of 1.5 Gy whereas only 50% of a group of females under 40 are affected when the dose exceeds 5 Gy.[687] Recovery of ovarian function occasionally follows irradiation with doses presumed to cause sterility. At least one patient, who was reported to have received 6.4 Gy, became pregnant 2 years after irradiation and delivered a normal child.[694]

Stillman et al. reported that 68% of girls treated for childhood cancer and who had both ovaries within the treatment field will demonstrate ovarian failure at a mean ovarian dose of 32 Gy.[695] Ortin et al. reviewed data on 92 girls treated for Hodgkin's disease and followed for a median time of 9 years.[696] None of the girls who underwent pelvic irradiation without prior oophoropexy maintained ovarian function. Ovarian injury was related both to the number of cycles of chemotherapy as well as radiation dose. Wallace et al. pointed out that whole-abdominal radiotherapy to doses of 30 Gy results in ovarian failure in most patients.[697,698] They have also estimated that the LD_{50} for the human oocyte does not exceed 4 Gy. In many girls who receive whole-body radiation either as a single whole-body dose of 10 Gy, or 12 Gy in six fractions over 3 days, there will be ovarian failure, which is occasionally transient.[298] In the patients who receive a single dose of 10 Gy the majority will have abnormal gonadotropin levels and delayed onset of puberty. With the fractionated regimes, one half will have normal puberty and gonadotropin levels. For survivors who retain normal ovarian function after cancer therapy, there is an increased risk of premature menopause.[699]

Uterus

The relative radioresistance of the uterus compared to other structures has been demonstrated by its ability to withstand being used as a cavity for placement of radium during radiotherapy. Rubin and Casarett have termed the radiation tolerance of the uterus "amazing."[2] It is not known what doses are required to cause sterility on the basis of uterine irradiation because most of the therapeutic methods employed have also involved ovarian ablation. Doll and Smith reported a study of 1068 women who were treated for metropathia hemorrhagica.[700] At dose levels ranging from 6.25 to 10.5 Gy, 97% had induced menopause. It has also been reported in other studies that doses of 1.5 to 2.25 Gy in three doses over 3 weeks decreased menstrual periods in 75% of patients; however, over one half became pregnant later.[691] Critchley et al. indicated that female long-term survivors treated as children with total-body radiation and marrow transplantation are at risk for impaired uterine growth and blood flow and that despite estrogen replacement the uterus is often reduced to 40% of normal adult size.[701] Similar findings were reported by Larsen et al.[702]

Applications of radium in the region of the uterine cervix can result in doses to the cervix of 100 to 200 Gy. Hamberger et al. analyzed the dose schedules causing severe complications for treatment of carcinoma of the cervix.[703] Standard radiotherapy doses for endometrial carcinoma used in a preoperative fashion ranged between 45 and 60 Gy over 4 to 7 weeks. Pathologic study of the uterus is difficult after radiotherapy because coexistent tumors cause difficulties in interpretation. In the region of the endometrium, acute necrosis of the glands is identified with hemorrhage and fibrinous exudates. Approximately 6 weeks after radiotherapy, atrophy, which may occasionally be severe, as well as atypia in the cells, occurs. Fajardo indicated that lipid-containing histiocytes have been described in the endometrium and that ulceration is common, probably as a result of endometrial "burns" due to the contact of the endometrium with the radium sources.[3] These often heal and are replaced by scar tissue and fibrosis with telangiectasia of the blood vessels in the area. The myometrium does not appear to develop significant fibrosis or atrophy. Changes in arterioles occur, but such changes are often seen in the outer third of the uterine wall (without a radiation exposure history) as patients increase in age. Fajardo suggests that the finding of foamy histiocytes in the endothelial cells with myointimal proliferation should raise the suspicion of radiation treatment.[3]

The cervix has received special attention because of the frequent use of radium therapy for cervical carcinoma. On removal of a radium applicator, edema and exudate often result, lasting for up to 3 weeks. Atrophy becomes apparent 6 weeks later, with cervical ulceration being relatively common and healing as described earlier. Actual necrosis of the cervix may occur within 1 year of therapy; however, in most instances it is due to recurrent tumor. Scarring of the cervix with atrophic epithelium and dysplasia of the epithelium often occurs years after the therapy. The dysplasia identified is quite common; whether it represents an in situ carcinoma or a benign situation is uncertain. The actual dose to the cervix is difficult to ascertain because such treatments are usually measured in terms of milligram hours of radium, and in recent years, cesium 137 and iridium 192 have been used. As a rule of thumb, a milligram-hour (mghr) of radium is equal to 79 mGy.

Vagina

Low-LET Radiation

The vaginal mucosa reacts in a fashion very similar to that of mucous membrane in other portions of the body, such as the pharynx, including initial stages of moist desquamation, confluent mucositis, and occasional ulceration. Details of cytologic changes in the vaginal epithelium have been carefully described by Graham.[704]

The relative sensitivity of the vaginal lining compared with the endometrium is in large part due to the endometrium being composed of reverting postmitotic cells that are relatively radioresistant, whereas the squamous epithelial lining in the vagina represents proliferating vegetative intermitotic cells that are relatively radiosensitive. Descriptions of the external genitalia in females after irradiation are difficult to find; however, the tolerance to radiation is low compared with that of most skin, probably because of the effects of moisture and friction. Fractionated doses of 30 to 50 Gy are capable of eliciting significant desquamative reaction. Vaginal necrosis has been reported in three patients after radiotherapy. All had preexisting cardiovascular disease and received 70 to 90 Gy to large portions of the vagina.[705]

Testes

Low-LET Radiation

The radiosensitivity of the testes was identified as early as 1906. In general, the human data related to testicular effects come from accidental exposure because the testes are not often irradiated for therapeutic reasons. The testis itself is a very complicated structure containing seminiferous tubules with a complex epithelium composed of Sertoli cells (supporting and nutrient cells) and spermatogenic cells. There are numerous interstitial cells, including the Leydig cells, which produce testosterone. Sperm production begins with type A spermatogonia, which reproduce and give rise to type B spermatogonia. Following several divisions, the type B spermatogonia form primary spermatocytes that move toward the center of the seminiferous tubules. As the primary spermatocyte reaches the lumen, it undergoes division and meiosis so that by the time it becomes a secondary spermatocyte, it has a haploid number of chromosomes. Each secondary spermatocyte then divides to form a spermatid and, finally, mature sperm. The time from stem cell to mature sperm has been estimated to be approximately 60 days. Because type A spermatogonia are vegetative intermitotic cells, they are highly radiosensitive, whereas type B spermatogonia, which are differentiating intermitotic cells, are somewhat less radiosensitive. Some type A spermatogonia have relatively long intermitotic periods; therefore, not all type A spermatogonia are of the same radiosensitivity. The Sertoli and Leydig cells, which are reverting postmitotic cells, are reasonably radioresistant. Following doses as small as 80 mGy, a reduction in the number of spermatogonia occurs. At these low doses, the more resistant and more differentiated cells in the line may continue normal maturation. A reduction in the sperm count may not be evident until 30 to 60 days have passed. The ultimate degree and duration of depletion of the sperm depend on the magnitude of the dose received.

The term *sterility* following radiation is often loosely applied; it may represent complete sterility, temporary subfertility, or fertility with a reduced number of sperm being produced. A number of discussions concern testicular irradiation from accidental exposures.[112,677,706,707] The range of effects reported and the doses are distressingly variable. Heller indicated that doses as low as 0.15 Gy may cause oligospermia and temporary sterility.[708] There are suggestions that a single dose in humans in the range of 5 to 6 Gy may cause permanent sterility. Investigation of human volunteers indicates that 25 fractions of 0.15 to 0.20 Gy daily may cause a decrease in the sperm count.[2] It is of interest that in the few patients treated with radiotherapy to one testicle or to the inguinal nodes to dose levels of 0.6 to 2.5 Gy, a significant percentage (34 of 74 patients) were subsequently able to father children.[709]

Lushbaugh and Casarett have reviewed the literature, finding no case reports of malformed infants from parents who had received prior radiotherapy.[710] Some of these effects may be due to the fact that radiation-damaged spermatogonia are self-destructive. Glucksmann indicated that 5 to 6 Gy in a single dose causes permanent sterility, whereas a single dose of 2.5 Gy causes temporary sterility for 12 months.[684] Hasterlik reported three patients with accidental exposures and average whole-body doses between 0.12 and 1.9 Sv, in whom the sperm count was normal at 10 days, greatly reduced at 7 to 12 months, and normal at 20 months.[515] Overall, Rubin and Casarett estimated that 5 to 6 Gy in a single dose will cause permanent sterility in most men; however, in some cases, that dose has been exceeded without causing sterility. They also indicated that a dose of 2.5 Gy certainly may cause sterility for about 12 months.[2] UNSCEAR 1982 reviewed available literature and reported the following results: (1) temporary sterility of the testes is reported to occur with single doses ranging from 1.5 to 4 Gy and with fractionated doses of 0.1 to 2 Gy, and (2) permanent sterility occurs with single doses ranging from 5 to 9.5 Gy and with fractionated doses of 2 to 6 Gy.[711] Sterility may be temporary for a matter of years before returning fertility. Five individuals who received doses of 2.3 to 3.7 Gy in the Oak Ridge criticality accident were aspermic for 4 months and hypospermic for 21 months; at least one demonstrated "sterility" for several years and subsequently had a normal offspring.[712] Gottlober et al. reported that about 50% of survivors of the acute radiation syndrome at Chernobyl had increased FSH levels indicating impaired fertility.[63]

In the first hours to days after a single dose of 12 Gy, there is necrosis of the germinal cells, and the spermatogonia are distorted and, in many cases, unidentifiable. Necrotic cells are deposited in the lumen of the convoluted tubules; with extremely large absorbed radiation doses, there may be cytoplasmic swelling or vacuolization of the spermatocytes and spermatids.[429] Thickening of the basement membrane and loss of Sertoli cells occur. Regeneration of the spermatogonia may begin as early as 2 to 8 weeks, whereas regeneration of spermatozoa may take months to years. Studies of atomic bomb casualties who had either the hematopoietic or gastrointestinal syndrome found total depletion of the sperm cells.[713]

Both radiation therapy and chemotherapy (particularly alkylating agents) can result in germ cell depletion, oligo or azoospermia, and testicular atrophy. Some authors indicate that Leydig cells are relatively resistant to deterministic effects of radiation at doses as high as 12 Gy, but Kinsella[714] and Howell[715] indicated that with radiation therapy, doses as low as 0.2 Gy of scatter radiation can result in transient elevations in serum FSH levels. At doses over 2 Gy there is Leydig cell dysfunction as evidenced by elevations in LH. Similar results were reported by Hansen et al. in 51 patients treated for testicular cancer and in whom the median dose to the nonremoved testicle was 1.7 Gy.[716] Irradiation at younger ages produces more damage than in adults.[717]

Ortin et al. reviewed data on 148 boys treated for Hodgkin's disease and followed for a median time of 9 years.[696] Sexual maturation was achieved in all boys without the need for androgen replacement. Of eight boys who were treated with radiation alone, three who received a 40 to 45 Gy pelvic dose were able to father children. Three others who received 30 to 44 Gy of pelvic radiation were oligospermic. This was contrasted with an 83% incidence of absolute azoospermia in boys treated with chemotherapy and no pelvic radiation. Shatford et al. found that long-term follow-up of 13 male children treated for Hodgkin's disease with chemotherapy or abdominal radiotherapy showed normal testosterone levels and secondary sexual characteristics but 11 of the 13 remained azoospermic.[718] Huyghe et al. reported on 451 patients treated for testicular tumors in whom fertility decreased from 91% before treatment to 67% after treatment with radiotherapy having more effect than chemotherapy.[719] A general review of gonadal toxicity from cancer treatment was published by Goldman and Johnson.[720] Patients who have received bone marrow transplantation have been studied by Sanders[91] and Deeg[90] who reported that gonadal failure occurred in almost all boys who were postpubertal at the time of irradiation, and that in those irradiated prior to puberty about one half had elevated FSH or LH levels.

High-LET Radiation

RBE data on the reproductive organs have been derived essentially from animals. These results indicate that with high-energy neutrons, the RBE ranges from 2.5 to 3.2; at lower energies (1 MeV), values for the RBE range from 4.1 to 5.5.[721,722]

Radionuclide Irradiation

Irradiation of the testes by radionuclides may result from internal or external exposure. In the case of energetic beta radiation, the sperm cells may be irradiated by external radionuclides.[723,724] Although there may be internal deposition of radionuclides such as cesium, few human data are available. Extensive research data concern the effect of radionuclide administration on the ovaries and testes in mice, but no significant information is available concerning the human.[725–731] There is one report concerning the testicular function in 25 males after radioiodine therapy for thyroid carcinoma.[732] At 3 and 6 months post-therapy all patients showed an elevated FSH and decreased inhibin B levels indicating impaired spermatogenesis and a compensated insuffiency of Leydig cell function. At 18 months, all values of gonadal function had returned to normal. There has been recent surge in treatment of prostate cancer with implantation of brachytherapy seeds. In spite of the high local doses there are reports of the patients fathering children after this type of therapy.[733]

Prostate and Seminal Vesicles

Low-LET Radiation

The prostate and seminal vesicles are quite radioresistant. There is a vast literature derived from radiotherapy of carcinoma of the rectum, prostate, and bladder. On a historical basis, there are several reports of treating benign prostatic hypertrophy with doses in the range of 10 to 20 Gy.[734] A 30% improvement in the symptomatology of those patients was reported. Current treatment schemes for pelvic carcinoma with external radiation therapy call for fractionated doses totaling 60 to 70 Gy; this regimen is usually followed without evidence of adverse effects. Very high doses are occasionally achieved through radioactive implants. Ureteral stricture is a rare complication, but fistula formation has been reported. Fajardo indicated that within weeks of a typical course of external radiotherapy, acute inflammation of the prostate is very uncommon.[3] Within months to years, the parenchyma is reduced in volume, with marked atrophy. Vascular changes may be severe, with myointimal proliferation and foamy cells in the endothelium in a large percentage of cases. In the region of the seminal vesicles, the perivesicular tissue is replaced by dense collagen. Chan et al. used MRI to study 38 patients treated for prostatic or pelvic tumors.[735] The pattern of signal seen in the prostate was variable, but the most common pattern was a diffuse low-signal intensity on T2-weighted images. Tumor usually has an increased signal.

Penis, Urethra, and Scrotum

In general, the penis, urethra, and scrotum appear able to tolerate fractionated radiotherapy of 60 to 65 Gy over 6 to 8 weeks. Treatment for tumors has been performed not only by external radiotherapy but by application of isotope molds using cobalt 60 and iridium 192.[736] Dose schedules of 20 Gy in 2 days, or 50 Gy over 8 days, produced severe reactions with late ulceration, probably due to myointimal obliteration. There have been exposures due to industrial radiography sources that have necessitated surgical resection or amputation.[737] Radiotherapy doses in excess of 65 Gy are associated with penile complications including necrosis and urethral stenosis.[738]

Radiation therapy of the prostate with high doses can cause fibrosis and subsequent urinary incontinence.[739] Potency and the ability to maintain a full erection can be reduced after radiotherapy for prostate cancer, but this is most pronounced in men who were only borderline sexually active to begin with[740] or had psychogenic problems.[741] Mittal studied penile blood flow both before and after prostatic radiotherapy, as well as in individuals who became impotent 2 to 5 months post-therapy.[742] There was no measured change in blood flow.

In the last decade, there have been marked changes in radiotherapeutic techniques for treatment of prostate cancer. These include conformal radiotherapy as well as brachytherapy with prostatic iodine 125 or palladium 103 seed implants. After brachytherapy the incidence of dysuria is about 50% and peaks about 1 month after implantation but may not completely resolve for several years.[672] Urethral strictures occur in about 5% of patients with a median time to development of about 2 years,[673] urinary incontinence occurs in about 7% of patients, and erectile dysfunction in about 8% to 50%.[674–676] Some authors suggest that with brachytherapy if the dose to 50% of the bulb of the penis is maintained at 50 Gy or less, post-treatment potency is maximized.[743]

BONE, CARTILAGE, AND MUSCLE

Low-LET Radiation

Most information about radiation effects on bone and cartilage are derived from experience using radiotherapy.[744] In young children, age 0 to 6 years, 10 Gy produces mild osseous changes, whereas 10 to 20 Gy in fractionated radiotherapy doses produces severe changes (asymmetrical bone growth).[745–751] In general, the higher the dose and the younger the child, the more deformity results. Although animal data indicate that irradiation of bone causes a reduction in the number of blood vessels, it is not thought to be the primary cause of reduction in growth.[752,753]

Otake et al. studied growth retardation as a potential radiation effect following in utero exposure of atomic bomb survivors.[754] Overall, the effect, if any, was small. In the first trimester, all parameters were negative with regard to uterine dose. A positive dose response was seen in the second trimester, but this was small and close to the control level. In the third trimester there was no significant dose effect. Similar results have been reported by Nakashima et al.[755]

There is a relatively large experience with radiation effects on the bone following radiotherapy of children. After treatment for Wilms' tumor, there are growth disturbances and osteochondrosis, and if the radiation is applied assymetrically to the spine, there can be resultant scoliosis.[598,756–759] The most sensitive time appears to be when the children are less than 6 years of age at irradiation or during their adolescent growth spurt. About 10% of children treated with orthovoltage radiation and fractionated radiotherapy doses of greater than 30 to 35 Gy for Wilms' tumor develop scoliosis greater than 20 degrees and require intervention. Few if any changes are seen at fractionated doses of less than 20 Gy. With modern megavoltage techniques, treatment of up to 40 Gy can be performed without significant scoliosis.[760]

In addition to spinal deformity, hypoplasia of other bones has been reported by a number of authors. Leg length discrepancy was also reported by Robertson et al.[761] and by Paulino et al.[762] after treatment of childhood extremity sarcomas. Hypoplasia of various facial bones has been reported after radiotherapy in childhood, including the jaw, orbit, or hemiface.[292,763] Hypoplasia of the ilium also has been reported after radiotherapy of the pelvis.[764,765]

There is an interesting study by Gilsanz et al., who studied reduced bone density in leukemia survivors and concluded that this only occurred in those children who had cranial irradiation and that osteoporosis was not due to the disease or to chemotherapy.[766] In children, radiotherapeutic fractionated doses in excess of 25 Gy to the ends of long bones have been shown occasionally to cause slipped capital epiphyses. Slippage is rare with fractionated doses of less than 25 Gy.[767,768] Risk in children irradiated under the age of 4 is about 47%, and about 5% in older children.[769] This effect apparently results from an arrest in chondrogenesis and vascular changes. Chemotherapy may play a minor role because many patients have received doxorubicin, which has been shown to arrest chondrogenesis temporarily.[768–771] Radiation changes in the epiphyseal region causing disturbances in growth may also be responsible for development of osteochondromas (see the section on bone tumorigenesis in Chapter 5). In addition to slippage of the femoral epiphysis, there also can be aseptic necrosis in some patients. Usually these are children who have received doses in excess of 30 to 40 Gy and chemotherapy.[772]

Adult bone is much more resistant to the effects of radiation, with effects generally attributable to decreased blood flow. Actual necrosis of the bone is quite rare, and fractionated therapeutic doses up to 65 Gy given in 6 to 8 weeks normally do not cause it. Because bone is extremely dense, the absorbed radiation dose in bone varies markedly, depending on the energy of the incident radiation. Thus, it is extremely difficult to identify the precise bone dose necessary to produce necrosis since dose levels reported in the literature may be inaccurate.[771]

The changes demonstrated in adult bone usually include decreased ability to resist infection and increased susceptibility to fractures, with poor subsequent healing. One of the bones that most commonly experiences postradiation complications is the mandible, where it is often extremely difficult to differentiate between actual bone necrosis due to radiation and osteomyelitis.[773,774] Treatment of tumor next to bone and poor dental status are important contributing factors in osteonecrosis of the mandible. Murray et al. examined the incidence of radiation necrosis of the mandible (Fig. 6-18).[775,776] The overall incidence was 19% in their series. Heavy smokers and chronic alcoholics are at high risk for mandibular necrosis due to poor oral hygiene. With newer techniques osteoradionecrosis of the jaw is seen in about 2% to 3% of patients treated for head and neck tumors.[777] Osteonecrosis of the maxillary sinuses has been reported to be as high as 25% after radiation therapy.[778]

The incidence or spontaneous rib fractures after postmastectomy irradiation was reported by Overgaard.[779] High doses per fraction resulted in a 19% incidence of late bone damage compared with 6% in the standard dose fraction. Radiation-induced fractures of the pelvis were identified using radionuclide bone scans in about 30% of women treated for uterine cancer with an average dose of 46 Gy fractionated radiotherapy. Fractures were often symmetric and 84% of patients had pain.[780] Blomlie et al. tried using MRI to evaluate radiation-induced insufficiency fractures of the sacrum.[781] This modality is expensive, and the results can be confusing because the fractures have associated edema and can be confused with metastatic disease. In contrast, it is interesting to note that fractures of the femoral neck occur in less than one tenth of 1% of patients treated for carcinoma of the uterine cervix. In growing cartilage and bone, a single dose of 6 Gy has been demonstrated to cause a reduction in mitotic activity of proliferating chondroblasts. The most radiosensitive cells of the skeleton appear to be the intermitotic chondroblasts. After radiation, distortion of the chondroblast columns and interference with normal growth mechanisms occur.[429] At high absorbed doses, osteoblasts may also be killed. If the bone marrow and underlying blood vessels are unable to recover, both bone and cartilage resorption are impaired. In animals, maximal damage is seen with single doses in the region

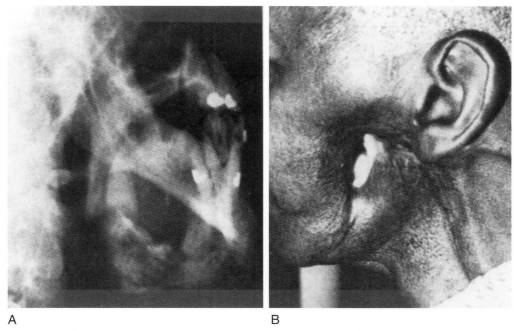

A   B

Figure 6-18 • Radiation necrosis of mandible. **A,** X-ray demonstrates complete necrosis, which occurred 2 years after a calculated dose of 60 Gy of cobalt 60 radiotherapy over 6 weeks. **B,** There also was fistula formation. (From Moss WT, Brand WN, Battifora H: Radiation Oncology, 5th ed. St. Louis, Mosby, 1979.)

of 30 Gy, causing complete cessation of growth. At lower absorbed doses, the changes identified on a radiograph may appear similar to early epiphyseal closure; however, if the blood supply decreases, the bones become sclerotic. Various therapies have been used to treat radiation osteonecrosis with varying degress of success. These include hyperbaric oxygen therapy,[782] pentoxyphilline, tocopherol, and clodronate.[783]

Radiographic and MR imaging findings of radiation effects on bone were described by Mitchell et al.[784] and more recently by Williams et al.[785] Mandibular osteoradionecrosis usually includes ill-defined cortical destruction without sequestration of bone fragments. Most other bones demonstrate osteopenia, disorganization, insufficiency fractures, and trabecular coarsening. CT scanning can show the changes in more detail. MRI is of less value, usually showing increased T1 signal in the medullary space where hematopoietic tissue has been replaced with fat.

Although radiation changes can occasionally be identified in adult teeth (after vascular disruption of the pulp), the developing tooth is more sensitive. Doses of less than 10 Gy will cause arrest of a tooth bud. There have been reports of abnormalities in children's teeth after radiotherapy. These changes include tooth agenesis, arrested root development, enamel dysplasia, and crown abnormalities. Dental abnormalities may occur in up to 82% of children who survive maxillofacial radiotherapy.[786,787] Radiation-induced and natural caries have the same pattern of decay with widespread areas of porosity of enamel and loss of enamel. Radiation damage to dentition following radiotherapy is a significant clinical issue.[543,788]

With mature bone, the deterministic effects of radiation are not apparent for some time. Some of the earliest changes following radiotherapy are areas of decreased radioactivity on radionuclide bone scans (Fig. 6-19). Such areas do not appear with a total fractionated dose of less than 20 Gy but do appear in 60% of regions receiving more than 45 Gy. These changes appear 4 to 6 months after radiotherapy and may persist for up to 19 months.[789] With high doses, pathologically there is an absence of osteoblasts and osteocytes, with subsequent arteriolar intimal thickening. The bone is then subject to necrosis and fracture with minimal trauma. The skeletal changes radiographically evident were best described by Bragg et al., but the doses required to cause such changes are rarely reported.[790] The bone becomes demineralized and has an abnormal coarse trabecular pattern. The process often resembles Paget's disease; however, the appearance of fractures, lack of bone expansion, localized nature, and clinical history generally exclude this diagnosis (Fig. 6-20). It is sometimes difficult to exclude metastases and infection as causes of the radiographic changes identified.

Cartilage, like adult bone, is fairly radioresistant. Doses of 60 to 70 Gy in a prolonged radiotherapy treatment scheme can be tolerated by cartilage.[791,792] Unless

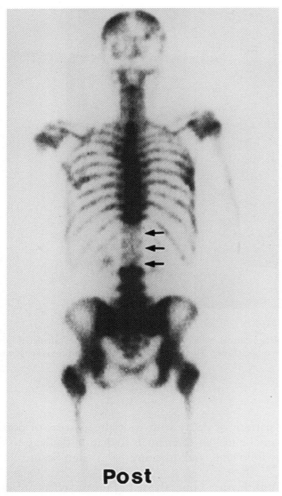

Figure 6-19 • Decreased activity of the lower thoracic and upper lumbar spine seen on radionuclide bone scan 5 months following radiotherapy.

there is stress to the cartilage, clinical manifestations of deterministic radiation effects are rare with the exception of delayed necrosis of the larynx. This is usually manifested by 1 year posttreatment by dysphagia, odynophagia, respiratory obstruction, hoarseness, and recurrent aspiration.[793] There is a case report of localized chondrocalcinosis following radiotherapy.[794]

Deterministic effects of radiation on muscle are distinctly unusual. Acute radionecrosis of skeletal muscle requires absorbed doses in excess of 500 Gy.[795] At lower fractionated doses, from 22 to 54 Gy, atrophy of fibers can be identified (Fig. 6-21). Finally, ischemia due to arterial narrowing may result in fibrosis.[796] The ultimate clinical result of muscle irradiation probably depends not only on the absorbed dose but on the length of the muscle segment irradiated. If the muscle is short and is entirely included in the irradiated field, the resultant detriment may be substantially greater than if only a portion of a long muscle is

irradiated. Heterotopic calcification of soft tissue has been reported as a late radiation effect although it is usually seen in combination with other late effects such as tissue ulceration, fibrosis, nerve damage, or bone necrosis.[797]

Neutron or High-LET Radiation

At the present time, there are few reports on the effects of neutron or high-LET radiation on bone and cartilage. There is one report of normal tissue reactions and complications (including bone necrosis) following high-energy neutron beam therapy that indicates that tissue tolerance is 20 Gy (in 12 fractions over 4 weeks) for all sites. Neutron therapy used for rectum-sparing prostate cancer therapy has been shown to result in soft-tissue injury in surrounding muscle.[798] There is some animal evidence, but extrapolation to humans is, at best, difficult.[799–802]

Radionuclide Irradiation

Human data concerning effects of radionuclides on bone are derived predominantly from three sources: persons occupationally exposed to radium with subsequent internal contamination, patients receiving therapeutic administration of radium, and individuals having intra-articular administration of radionuclides for treatment of arthritis. Radionuclides that concentrate in bone are referred to as volume seekers or surface seekers. The *volume seekers* ultimately are included in the matrix of the bone, although originally they may deposit on the surface. Examples of such volume-seeking radionuclides include isotopes of calcium, strontium, radium 226, and the alkaline earth elements. Plutonium, radium 224, and thorium accumulate on the periosteum and endosteal surfaces and are, therefore, considered *surface seekers*.

In the early 1900s, watch dial figures were painted with luminous compounds containing radium. It was a relatively common practice to point the brush between the lips to make the point finer, causing ingestion and internal contamination with large amounts of radium salts. Records for this group have been kept at the Human Radiobiology section of the Argonne National Laboratory in Chicago.[803] The radioisotopes of radium predominantly involved were radium 226 and 228.[804–806] Actual radiographic bone changes include small destructive areas in flat bones, particularly the skull,[807] fractures of long bones; coarsening of the trabecular pattern; bone infarcts; and aseptic necrosis (Fig. 6-22).[806–809] These changes were only seen when systemic intake exceeding 148 kBq resulted in estimated bone doses in excess of 7 to 8 Sv. A subsequent reanalysis indicates that necrosis was observable in femurs at approximately 0.8 Gy skeletal dose.[810] The radium dial painters had a very high incidence of primary bone tumors (osteosarcoma) and tumors of the cranial sinuses. This topic is more fully discussed in Chapter 5.

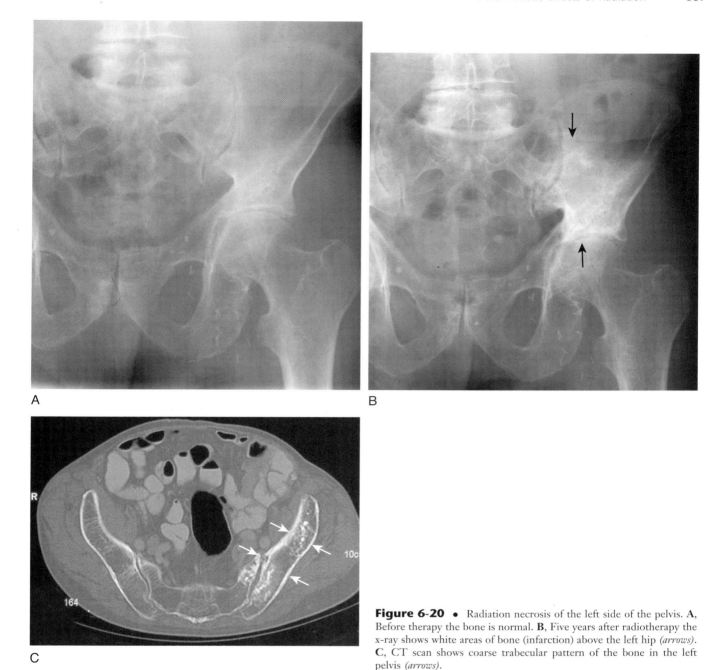

Figure 6-20 • Radiation necrosis of the left side of the pelvis. **A,** Before therapy the bone is normal. **B,** Five years after radiotherapy the x-ray shows white areas of bone (infarction) above the left hip *(arrows)*. **C,** CT scan shows coarse trabecular pattern of the bone in the left pelvis *(arrows)*.

Radium 224 has been and is still used in Germany for treatment of ankylosing spondylitis. It decays rapidly, and, therefore, its dose is delivered predominantly to the endosteal and periosteal surface of the bone. The longer half-life of radium 226 causes the major dose to be to the bone volume. In children injected with radium 224, growth retardation has been demonstrated in 12% to 70% of the cases. The percentage of children demonstrating growth retardation is a function of the age at injection, with the younger children demonstrating the more pronounced changes.[811]

Radionuclides used in intra-articular radiotherapy have included gold 198 colloid, yttrium 90 silicate citrate, phosphorus 32 chromic phosphate, rhenium 186 sulfide, and erbium 169 citrate.[812–816] The main purpose of these injections has been to irradiate the synovial tissue and to sterilize it without causing necrosis of the cartilage. Estimated doses to the synovium of the knee joint using yttrium 90 have been estimated to be approximately 60 to 80 Gy.[816,817] Two cases of joint rupture have been reported, presumably secondary to radiation necrosis of the adjacent cartilage.[818]

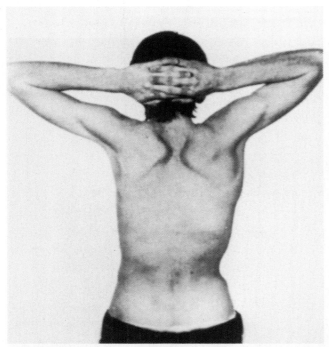

Figure 6-21 • Atrophy of left flank musculature due to radiation therapy for childhood Wilms' tumor. (From Moss WT, Brand WN, Battifora H: Radiation Oncology, 5th ed. St. Louis, Mosby, 1979.)

HEMATOPOIETIC AND LYMPHATIC SYSTEMS

Hematopoietic System

Changes in the hematopoietic system were identified as early as 1904 by Heineke, and as early as 1906 it was known that myelopoiesis was more radiosensitive than erythropoiesis. In 1913, Shouse et al. demonstrated that aplasia of the bone marrow in animals was a cause of death following total-body irradiation.[819] Lethal accidental exposures in humans and the subsequent blood and bone marrow changes were described in 1952 by Hempelmann.[820] The hematopoietic system is one of the most radiosensitive tissues in the body, and the response to radiation is a classic study in the disturbance of the kinetics of various cellular lines (Fig. 6-23).[821,822] Doses of radiation as small as 0.5 to 1 Gy in a single exposure produce obvious responses.

The pathologic aspect of the radiation effects has been extensively discussed both by Rubin and Casarett[2] and by Fajardo.[429] The reader is also referred to a chapter by Nothdurft[823] and to Annex G of the 1988 UNSCEAR Report.[824] The clinical responses of an individual depend markedly on the amount of tissue irradiated. Radiation of a large portion of the bone marrow results in the hematopoietic form of the acute radiation syndrome (discussed later in the chapter in the section, "Acute Radiation Syndromes"). The changes discussed in the text immediately following are applicable to either localized radiation or generalized radiation exposure. A major difference in marrow response between localized and generalized radiation is that in cases in which the bone marrow is irradiated locally, subsequent regeneration may occur more quickly. The kinetics of human hematopoiesis that form the basis of the responses of the cell lines have been well discussed by Cronkite.[825] Erythrocytes, reticulocytes, granulocytes, mature megakaryocytes, and platelets are fixed postmitotic cells. The reticular cells, macrophages, monocytes, plasma cells, and fibroblasts are reverting postmitotic cells. Both categories are relatively resistant to the deterministic effects of radiation. Somewhat more sensitive are the differentiating intermitotic cells, including erythroblasts, myeloblasts, and megakaryoblasts. These cells both divide and differentiate and are moderately radiosensitive. Cells that are relatively sensitive to radiation are vegetative intermitotic cells, such as large- and medium-sized lymphocytes and hemocytoblasts. More recent and detailed descriptions of the hierarchy of the cells in the hematopoietic system by other authors indicate that most cell lines begin with a pluripotent stem cell. From this there are two distinct pathways, one to lymphopoiesis and the other to monocytes, neutrophils, erythrocytes, platelets, and eosinophils. A number of growth factors or cytokines control cell development along different lineages. For example, in the production of neutrophils, cytokines IL-1, IL-3, and IL-6 are effective in the development of multipotent progenitor cells from the stem cells. IL-3 and GM-CSF are used to develop granulocyte/macrophage progenitor cells, and GM-CSF and G-CSF are used in the final development of neutrophils. As we will see later, there have been attempts to stimulate various cell lines after radiation injury using a number of these cytokines.

The kinetic pattern of postradiation events in hematopoietic tissue has been described by a large number of authors but most recently by Fliedner.[826] The time-related pattern of changes identified is a function of the time required for each cell type to complete its development from the stem cell. Due to the short life span of neutrophils (7 to 17 hours) and of platelets (about 10 days), there is rather rapid development of granulocytopenia and thrombocytopenia after radiation-induced injury of a major proportion of the hemopoietic system. The one important exception to this scheme of radiosensitivity is the small lymphocyte. Although it appears to be a nondividing cell and should be relatively resistant to radiation, it is actually very sensitive. It undergoes intermitotic cell death with a D_0 of 0.2 to 0.3 Gy.[827] It is possible that not all the small lymphocytes are radiosensitive and that there may be some very sensitive subpopulations. Lymphocytic depletion may be seen within hours of irradiation, whereas platelets and granulocytes are depleted over days, and depletion of red cells (erythrocytes) occurs over weeks. Late changes of aplastic anemia that are reported in the literature can occur as a result of vascular compromise and fibrosis. Under these circumstances

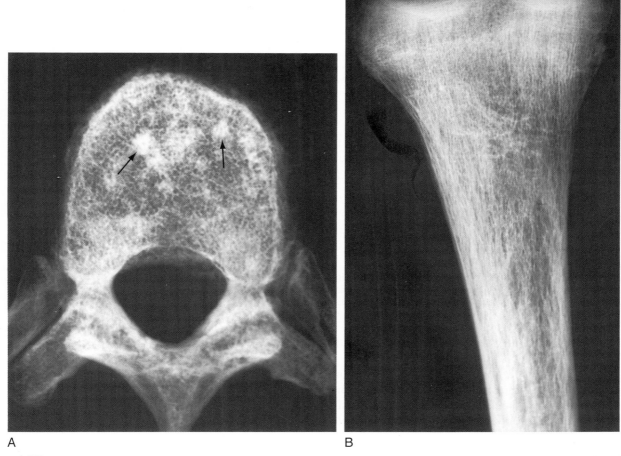

A   B

Figure 6-22 • Radium osteitis. Specimen radiograph of a vertebral body (**A**) and proximal tibia (**B**) from a radium dial painter. The trabecular pattern is coarse and there are small areas of sclerosis (**A**) (*arrows*) probably due to bone infarcts. (Cases courtesy of Argonne National Laboratory Radium Registry.)

all cell lines are equally affected. Such changes are not seen with acute marrow doses of less than 10 to 20 Gy in a relatively acute regimen. Marrow depression usually does not occur with chronic exposure unless doses exceed 0.4 Sv per year.

Low-LET Radiation

Several studies of atomic bomb survivors concerning the potential long-term effects of radiation exposure on granulocyte behavior have been performed. Hollingsworth et al. studied blood bactericidal activity for *E. coli* and found no relationship with radiation exposure.[828] Sasagawa et al. also studied the phagocytic and bactericidal activities of leukocytes in whole blood of Hiroshima and Nagasaki survivors with particular reference to *Staphylococcus aureus*.[829] No effect of radiation exposure was identified. Neutrophil phagocytosis was studied by Barreras et al. in 10 heavily exposed subjects and 10 matched controls.[830] No difference was found. Finch has mentioned the work of Pinkston et al. who examined

random migration and chemotaxis of granulocytes, and again no radiation effects were observed.[831] Finch also pointed out that there was no relationship of either aplastic anemia or polycythemia vera with radiation dose in the atomic bomb survivors. Granulocyte reserves were also measured before and after exercise in a study by Belsky et al.[832] There was no relation to the postexercise increase in circulating granulocytes. Wong et al. evaluated the long-term effects of radiation on hemoglobin levels in atomic bomb survivors over a 40-year period from 1958–1998.[833] Compared to the unexposed survivors, the mean hemoglobin levels for those exposed to a bone marrow dose of 1 Gy were significantly reduced by 0.10 g/dL or 0.67% at 40 years of age, and by 0.24 g/dL or 1.8% at 80 years of age. The etiology of this statistically significant (but clinically insignificant) reduction is unclear.

The International Chernobyl Project studied a large number of hematologic parameters in the populations living in contaminated settlements around the Chernobyl plant.[138] Parameters studied included

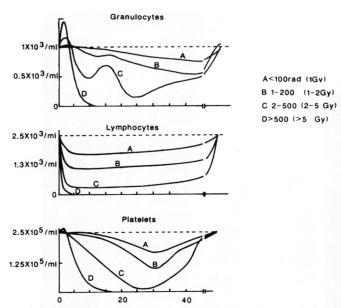

Figure 6-23 • Schematic picture of average time course for various cells in the blood after acute whole-body radiation. (From United Nations Scientific Committee on the Effects of Atomic Radiation [UNSCEAR]: Sources and effects of ionizing radiation: Report to the General Assembly, Vienna, 1988.)

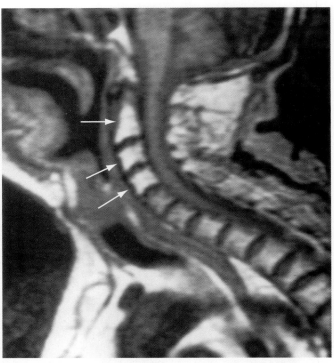

Figure 6-24 • Fatty change in the marrow after radiation therapy. A lateral magnetic resonance scan (T1-weighted) of the cervical spine shows a high signal (*arrows*) in the vertebral bodies of C2–4 after radiation therapy for an oropharyngeal tumor. The normal marrow appearance is seen in the lower vertebral bodies.

hematocrit, hemoglobin, mean corpuscular volume and hemoglobin, total leukocyte and lymphocyte count, differential count, and platelet count. No statistically significant difference was found between persons in contaminated and control villages despite claims to the contrary in the popular press.

The acute changes in bone marrow have been studied in patients receiving fractionated radiotherapy. In a typical fractionated radiotherapy treatment regimen (in which the treatment scheme is normally 2 Gy daily with five fractions weekly), the following changes have been identified. At levels of 4 Gy, there is a moderate decrease in nucleated cells with a marked decrease in the precursors of the red cells and granulocytes. When absorbed doses of 10 Gy are reached, there is a total absence of the undifferentiated and differentiating cellular forms, including all "blast" cells. The marrow often is hemorrhagic. By the end of the 5-week course of 50 Gy, extreme hypoplasia of the marrow and difficulty finding anything but a few plasma cells and lymphocytes result. The typical change identified in the peripheral blood is a fall in the lymphocyte count, with a maximal depression at 10 to 15 days. The count tends to stay depressed until the end of the therapeutic treatment, and recovery occurs 3 to 6 months later. At late stages after localized radiotherapy, there is replacement of the injured marrow by fat and to a lesser extent fibrosis.

There have been a number of reports on the use of MRI in imaging bone marrow changes after radiotherapy.[834,835] In general, the marrow develops an increased

or bright signal on T1-weighted images, which is due to the fatty replacement (Fig. 6-24). Areas of increased signal may either be homogeneous or inhomogeneous. These changes are typically seen weeks to months after the completion of radiotherapy schemes, and there has not been a report of MRI use in accidental situations. It is unlikely that the changes that can been seen occur early enough to be of prognostic value in the acute period.

If either the pelvis or thoracic bone marrow is irradiated in a radiotherapy treatment scheme, it is not unusual for the lymphocyte count to fall to approximately 40% of its original value. The neutrophil count is maximally depressed after 15 to 20 days, again usually to approximately 40% of the pretreatment values. The eosinophil count may change, depending on the site of irradiation. Pelvic irradiation tends to elevate the eosinophil count, whereas treatment of the upper abdomen and thorax may cause a decrease in the eosinophil count. There has been some experience in radiotherapy with half-body irradiation. This was usually given to either the upper or lower half of the body, and initially bone marrow tolerance was expected to be the limiting factor. About 60% of the active marrow is located in the upper half of the body. It was found that single doses of 8 to 10 Gy delivered at a rate of 2 Gy per minute to the upper

Table 6-1 • Chance of Survival Without Medical Treatment After Whole-Body Irradiation

Dose (Gy)	Survival
< 1	Virtually certain
1–2	Probable
2–4.5	Possible
5–6	Virtually impossible

half of the body were well tolerated. There was moderate depression in blood cell counts, but these returned to normal in about 3 to 8 weeks.[836,837] Recovery is faster after lower-body irradiation than upper body because there is less active marrow irradiated. In a patient who is not anemic or treated with chemotherapy prior to localized radiotherapy, the red cell count and platelet (thrombocyte) count are usually not depressed significantly. Major changes may be identified if there is some abnormality in the marrow reserve in other portions of the body. For example, if a patient has extensive marrow infiltration by tumor in portions of the body outside the radiotherapy field, the additional radiation changes on the bone marrow within the field may have effects greater than expected. Regeneration of marrow occurs in many patients after localized radiotherapy. There have been many studies of this subject, and it appears that when the fractionated radiotherapy scheme does not exceed 30 Gy, there is a good chance of marrow regeneration. Some authors report that once dose levels of 40 Gy of localized radiotherapy are exceeded, regeneration in that area is much less likely.[838–840]

When large portions of the bone marrow or the total body are irradiated, the findings are quite different. For acute whole-body irradiation of humans in the dose range of 1 to 6 Gy, clinically important effects result from damage to the bone marrow. This is often referred to as the *hematopoietic syndrome*. Table 6-1 shows the chance of survival of individuals exposed to whole-body irradiation who do not receive medical treatment.

With current medical measures, whole-body doses as high as 12 Gy in 6 fractions of 2 Gy have been used for bone marrow ablation prior to bone marrow transplantation. In the "survival probable" category of patients receiving acute total-body exposures of 1 to 2 Gy, the lymphocyte counts show a marked initial drop, with the minimal values being reached at 2 to 3 days. The exact amount varies from patient to patient; however, the absolute lymphocyte count is usually in the range of 1000 cells/mm^3. This depression persists for several weeks. Granulocytes show a decrease over the first 8 days but do not drop below 2000/mm^3. The minimal value often does not occur for approximately 6 weeks. Recovery takes several months. The platelet count does not change appreciably for 2 to 3 weeks; it may fall into the range

of 50,000/mm^3; however, there is rarely evidence of hemorrhage.

Hematologic changes in the "survival possible" category in which the absorbed dose to the whole body is 2 to 4.5 Gy are as follows. The peripheral lymphocytes undergo a profound and rapid drop, reaching a minimum in approximately 3 days and staying at that level for approximately 5 weeks. The lymphocyte count may be in the range of 500 to 1000 cells/mm^3; however, they do not completely disappear. The course of the granulocytes or leukocytes is much more variable; in many individuals, granulocytes rise in the first 2 to 4 days after exposure. Following this, a decline, which may be interrupted by another increase in leukocytes, occurs for about 8 to 10 days. This rise is termed *an abortive rise*, because it does not persist and is followed by further decline, with minimal levels occurring at approximately 1 month postexposure. The decline is rarely to levels of less than 2000 cells/mm^3. Platelets undergo a rather steady decline from the time of exposure to approximately day 26 but then may return to normal values in about 7 weeks after exposure. The values at the nadir are often below 50,000/mm^3.

In patients receiving more than 5 Gy acute whole-body dose, the marrow rarely recovers, and untreated patients usually die from infection or hemorrhage (Fig. 6-25). In such circumstances, the lymphocytes drop to very low values within hours of exposure. Values below 500 lymphocytes/mm^3 at 24 hours postexposure constitute a very grave prognosis. These minimal values are maintained from the end of day 1 until the patient either dies or has a marrow transplantation. Granulocytes may show the initial transient rise, although again this is a very variable phenomenon. In any case, by day 5 or 6, the granulocytes are usually reduced to levels below 400 cells/mm^3. Platelets demonstrate a gradual decline to minimal levels at 6 to 8 days after exposure; normally, they are reduced to levels below 50,000 cells/mm^3, and bleeding becomes a problem.

There is a large experience in radiotherapy with administration of high-dose, total-body irradiation followed by bone marrow transplantation.[841–843] This has usually been done for treatment of refractory acute leukemias, although it has found application in treatment of multiple myeloma, neuroblastoma, and oat cell carcinoma. The total radiation doses are usually in the range of 7.5 to 15 Gy and are designed to eliminate diseased active bone marrow.

Treatment of bone marrow depression due to accidental external exposure is usually complicated by other injuries such as trauma, burns, or nonpenetrating radiation injuries such as beta burns. In addition to analysis of blood elements, Russian physicians have pointed out that following acute whole-body exposure, other signs that a patient will have irreversible myelodepression were vomiting within the first half hour, diarrhea within 1 to 2 hours, and swelling of the parotid glands in the first

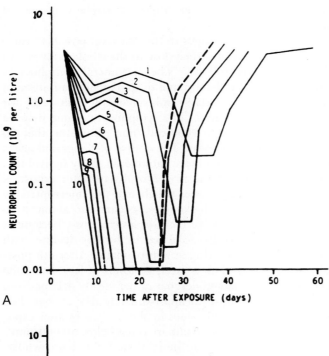

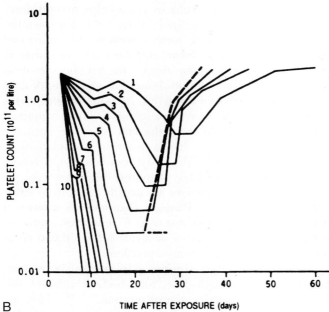

Figure 6-25 • Schematic picture of average time course for neutrophils (**A**) and platelets (**B**) after acute relatively uniform whole-body gamma radiation. The numbers on the lines refers to dose in Gy. The *dotted lines* indicate that recovery may not occur as indicated in all patients. (From United Nations Scientific Committee on the Effects of Atomic Radiation [UNSCEAR]: Sources and effects of ionizing radiation. Report to the General Assembly, Vienna, 1988.)

24 to 36 hours. A number of attempts at bone marrow transplantation have been made with the most experience occurring as a result of the Chernobyl accident. Of the 13 persons who received bone marrow transplants after the Chernobyl accident, only 2 survived, and both

recovered with their native marrow, suggesting that they did not need the transplants.[824] The general conclusion of Russian physicians was that bone marrow transplant, in these circumstances, was not a satisfactory form of treatment and that antibiotics, supportive fluid and electrolyte therapy, antiviral and antifungal therapy, and, possibly, marrow-stimulating agents were better. The typical experimental stimulating agents being used are the cytokines interleukin-3 (IL-3) and GM-CSF. Other experimental cytokines which appear to be useful include G-CSF, IL-6, and PIXY321, which is a genetically engineered fusion protein of recombinant human GM-CSF and IL-3.[844] In the several years after the Chernobyl accident, follow-up studies of the survivors of the acute radiation syndrome have demonstrated normal values of circulating granulocytes, erythrocytes, platelets, and lymphocytes, although the response to stress is slightly suboptimal when compared with normal persons. From a number of accidents it has become clear that when whole-body doses exceed about 10 Gy and when the victim is medically supported with subsequent bone marrow regeneration, fatality still occurs from multiorgan failure.[54,845] There is experience related to the tolerance of bone marrow in accidental situations where there has been chronic exposure. Fliedner et al. indicated that there appears to be a threshold of approximately 10 mSv per day above which hematopoietic effects occur and failure may occur.[846]

Some authors have reported on the occurrence of polycythemia vera after radiation exposure. This was discussed in Chapter 5. Since there are less than 10 cases reported in the literature, there is no dose-response relationship, and no increases have been found in major studies, this entity is not felt to be radiation related. Idiopathic thrombocytic purpura is also not a late finding of radiation exposure. Aplastic anemia finding may occur after very high marrow doses, but it is basically a vascular compromise and should affect all cell lines.

High-LET Radiation

The RBE for neutrons and their effect on the hematopoietic system have been studied by several researchers.[721,847,848] The RBE appears to be low and is probably between 1.0 and 2.0.

Internal Irradiation

There is information on the effects of internal irradiation on the hematopoietic system from several sources. The most important from a historical viewpoint is the group of radium dial painters mentioned in Chapter 5 (in the sections on bone cancer and tumors of the mastoid and paranasal sinuses) and in the section on bone cartilage and muscle in this chapter. These female painters were employed between 1915 and 1930 in the United States and became internally contaminated via the oral route with radium 226 and radium 228. In those patients who received very high skeletal doses, an asymptomatic but statistically significant reduction in the hematocrit was identified, and most received doses in excess of 10 Gy.[849] Sharpe reported no clinically significant reductions of any peripheral cellular elements in long-term follow-up of the New Jersey radium dial painters.[805] Dose rates to the marrow from radium 226 have been calculated to be 16 mGy annually for a burden of 37 kBq.[850]

The other sources of data in humans predominantly are patients receiving therapeutic administrations of radionuclides. Very large amounts of radioiodine are administered to treat patients with metastatic thyroid carcinoma. Often the limiting consideration is the dose to the bone marrow.[851,852] This effect is usually not severe until there have been four or more treatments, and total activity administered is in excess of 18 GBq. The effect on the bone marrow usually can be assessed with peripheral blood counts. There has been a recent resurgence of interest in treatment of widespread bone metastases with unsealed radionuclides, particularly strontium 89. An unwarranted side effect is marrow depression. For this radiopharmaceutical, the estimated marrow dose is 0.01 Gy/MBq.[853] Laing et al. examined the depression of platelets at different levels of administered activity and found the following percentage depression: at 0.7 MBq/kg, 19%; 1.5 MBq/kg, 24%; and 3.0 MBq/kg, 45%.[854] In general, there is no major bone marrow toxicity in terms of either platelets or leukocytes at administered activity levels of less than 3.0 MBq/kg unless there has been prior radiotherapy or chemotherapy. There have been recent advances in nuclear medicine monoclonal immunotherapy for lymphoma patients. Often the bone marrow dose is the limiting factor in treatment and trace compounds are used to produce images and estimate the bone marrow dose prior to actual therapy.[855]

Phosphorus 32 has been used to treat patients with primary polycythemia; generally, multiple administrations are given until the polycythemia is reduced to acceptable levels. The absorbed dose to the bone marrow in such treatment was calculated by Spiers et al. to be in the range of 0.24 Gy for a 37-MBq-injected dose.[856] Typically, this is administered with the specific aim of myelosuppression. The typical intravenously administered activity is 85 MBq/m^2 (not to exceed 185 MBq), and this delivers a marrow dose of about 1 Gy.[857] Some authors have reported on the use of sulfur 35 in treatment of chondrosarcomas or chordomas. This treatment is usually limited by marrow damage. When administered activities are in the range of 370 to 1780 MBq/kg of body weight, significant marrow depression can occur.[858] Use of iron 52 to aid in myeloablation prior to bone marrow transplantation was reported by Jacquy et al.[859] Median administered activity was 22.2 GBq and the estimated marrow dose was 6.25 Gy.

In one accident a patient in Wisconsin received a lethal amount of colloidal gold 198 while being treated for serosal metastatic carcinoma of the ovary by instillation of the colloidal radioactive gold into the peritoneal cavity. Through an error, the activity administered was in millicuries rather than microcuries. The patient subsequently died from hematologic complications. Had the patient survived, hepatic failure undoubtedly would have also occurred. Other reports of bone marrow depression resulting from radiogold and radiosulfur are present in the literature.[860,861]

Ingestion of cesium 137 in an accident in Goiania, Brazil, caused radiation doses in 14 persons that were large enough to result in severe bone marrow depression. Four of the 14 died as a result of infection and hemorrhage.[862] Eight of these persons received granulocyte-macrophage stimulating factor in an uncontrolled manner.[863] Whether there was any benefit remains a matter of speculation.

Lymphatic System

The lymphatic system includes lymph nodes, the spleen, tonsils, thymus, and, although not usually mentioned, the lymphoid tissue in the gastrointestinal tract. A moderate amount of information concerning the effects of radiation on the lymphatic system, mostly derived from patients who received total lymphoid irradiation for Hodgkin's disease, is available. Irradiation of the body in this manner has an extensive effect not only on the lymphatic tissue but also on the immune system.

Low-LET Radiation

The radiotherapy generally delivered for Hodgkin's disease gives absorbed doses in the range of 40 to 70 Gy over 4 to 8 weeks. Fajardo indicated that several patterns in lymph nodes follow radiotherapy.[864] The most common pattern is that of lymphocyte depletion in the cortical portion of the lymph node involving the follicle and the parafollicular cortex. Initially, there may be rather pronounced destruction of the lymphocytes in the lymphatic tissue; however, by the time most biopsies are taken, repopulation has undoubtedly occurred to some extent from other portions of the lymphatic system. Occasionally, a pattern of atrophy of the lymphatic tissue and replacement by fat cells appears. Another possible result is replacement of the parenchyma by fibrous tissue, either as a single focus or in a multifocal fashion. There is a moderate amount of disagreement among pathologists concerning the dose required to produce such changes in lymph nodes. Some claim that therapeutic doses in the range of 50 to 60 Gy cause changes in all lymph nodes; others are often unable to tell whether lymph nodes have been irradiated.[865]

Lymphatic vessels can withstand high doses of radiation. Lymphangiography has been used to estimate lymph flow in patients after radiotherapy, and it appears that if total fractionated doses exceed 20 Gy, reduction in size and number of lymphatic vessels may result. Even when patients develop late skin ulcers after radiotherapy, the changes in the lymphatic vessels are not marked, although some collateral lymphatic circulation may develop.[866] It appears that large single doses in the range of 40 Gy have little effect in terms of reduction of lymph flow and that fractionated doses in the range of 75 Gy given over 60 days in humans do not change lymph flow significantly. The acute effects of radiation on the spleen have been described by Liebow et al.[112] In autopsy studies performed on those who died at Hiroshima between the third and sixth weeks, the spleens contained large cells with atypical nuclei, prominent plasma cells, eosinophils, and frequent hemorrhages. It appears that in these victims (who generally were dying from hematopoietic repression), lymphopoietic regeneration had already begun to occur. Late effects of radiation on the spleen following fractionated splenic radiotherapy for Hodgkin's disease include atrophy with a thick capsule and fibrous trabeculae.[867] As occurs in most organs in the chronic phase of radiation injury, the most reliable change of radiation exposure is proliferation of the intimal lining of the arterioles. Coleman et al. described a decrease in splenic size and activity on radionuclide liver-spleen scans following splenic irradiation for Hodgkin's disease.[868]

High-LET Radiation and Radionuclides

The only data on effects of splenic irradiation are from the Thorotrast patients who received thorium dioxide intravenously as a contrast agent. The splenic dose is difficult to estimate; however, the dose was usually high enough to cause splenic atrophy and fibrosis (Fig. 6-26).[869] When

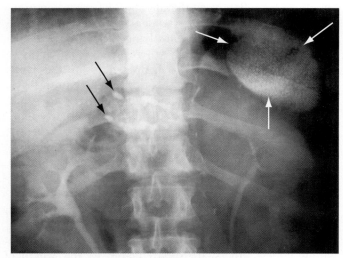

Figure 6-26 ● Intravenous pyelogram in patient who received a Thorotrast (thorium dioxide) injection 35 years earlier. Spleen (*white arrows*) retains thorium and is shrunken and atrophic from the radiation exposure. Some Thorotrast is visible within the several lymph nodes (*black arrows*).

the spleen reaches this stage, associated absence of reticuloendothelial activity is demonstrated on radionuclide liver-spleen scan.

IMMUNE RESPONSE

The immune system is complex and is composed of cells and tissues that protect against infections and cancer. The immune system is comprised of central lymphoid organs (bone marrow and thymus) and peripheral lymphoid tissues including lymph nodes, the spleen, mucosa-associated lymphoid tissue (MALT), and the skin. Many of the aspects of the immune system discussed here have been demonstrated in animal models, and specific human data, where available, have been included. The immune response is primarily mediated by two cell types: the lymphocyte and the macrophage. The exact role of the macrophage in the immune response is not well understood, but it may be regulatory in nature. It appears that the macrophage takes antigen and puts it into a form that is recognizable by the lymphocyte. The major and best understood cell type involved in the immune process is the lymphocyte. Lymphocytes have the following immune functions: (1) recognition of the foreign substance (antigen), (2) induction and regulation of the immune response, (3) causing the response to be very specific, and (4) responsibility for immunologic memory.

Extensive reviews of the subject of ionizing radiation on the immune response of the animal have been published by Anderson.[870,871] Earlier monographs are also available.[872,873] The earlier data and their interpretation are somewhat limited because the cell types involved have subpopulations whose role in the immune response was not well understood. For accurate interpretation of experimental immunologic data, particular attention must be devoted to the subpopulations of the lymphocytes, and their differential radiosensitivity. Radiation effects on the immune system of humans have been confounded by localized exposures, presence of malignancy in radiotherapy situations, and the well-recognized normal decrease in immunocompetence associated with aging.[874,875] For a comprehensive discussion of radiation effect on the immune system, the reader is referred to a chapter by Grosse-Wilde and Schaefer,[876] a review by Hoppe,[877] and a recent extensive review in the UNSCEAR 2006 report.[5] Issues related to autoimmune thyroid disease are discussed earlier in this chapter in the section on deterministic effects on the thyroid gland.

In humans, the immune stem cells appear to arise in the embryonic yolk sac during the second and third weeks of gestation. The cells migrate to the developing liver at approximately the sixth week; thus, the liver is important early in fetal life. The bone marrow becomes important to the immune response only at a later time, although the liver has the potential capacity, if necessary, to produce hematopoietic cells again. Lymphocytes with demonstrable immunoglobulin production are evident in the liver at approximately 9 weeks of gestation. The thymus is the first lymphoid organ to develop, and small lymphocytes are present by the eighth to ninth week of gestation. Later they appear to migrate to the spleen, lymph nodes, and bone marrow. Cytokines are important for maturation and differentiation of not only granulocytes, erythrocytes, and platelets, but lymphocytes as well. Under the influence of interleukins IL-1 and IL-3, some of the pluripotent stem cells in the marrow become committed to the lymphatic lineage. Some of these will enter the thymus to become T-cells with their subtypes (T-helper, T-suppressor, and cytotoxic cells). Others will remain in the bone marrow as B-lymphocytes and will also populate the spleen and lymph nodes.

Cell Types and Function

Lymphocytes can be divided into two major subcategories on the basis of function: *thymus-derived* (T) and *bone marrow*, or *bursa* (B) cells. The two classes do not work completely independently, and there is major cooperation between T- and B-cells. It is also important to realize that there are different types of immune responses and that different cell types may participate in varying degrees. The immune response can be divided into two broad categories: cellular and humoral. *Cellular immunity*, mediated by the T-cells, is important in rejection of incompatible grafts, graft-versus-host disease, and delayed hypersensitivity responses. The *humoral response* is that of antibody synthesis; B-cells are primarily responsible for this type of immunity. The T-cells responsible for cellular immunity appear to have stem cells originating in the bone marrow that migrate via systemic circulation to the thymus, where they mature. As they mature, the surface of the cell changes and they acquire the ability to distinguish foreign molecules.

The B-cells also undergo a maturational cycle. The site at which this maturation takes place is unknown, although it may occur in the bone marrow. Most commonly, the T-cells "help" the B-cells in the humoral response often through the production of cytokines. Cytokines are small proteins that communicate and orchestrate the attack on infections or altered cells. T-cells have several regulatory subpopulations referred to as *helper* and *suppressor* T-cells. An example of the interaction of cell types has been noted in the maturation process of B-cells; with the T-cells, B-cells differentiate into plasma cells, which are then able to secrete antibodies and specific immunoglobulins. The interaction between the two cell types caused confusion in the past, because an abnormality in the function of one cell type may be reflected in the function of another. Once the T- and B-lymphocytes become mature, they migrate to peripheral lymphoid organs, where they are involved in immune responses. The organs to which they migrate are the lymph nodes, the spleen, and lymphoid tissue in the gastrointestinal tract. The T- and B-cells are present in different numbers and in different areas of lymphoid tissue. The thymus and bone marrow are classified as central lymphatic tissue, whereas the spleen, lymph nodes, and gastrointestinal tissues are peripheral lymphoid tissues. The normal thymus contains no lymphoid follicles or B-cells. The lymph nodes, on the other hand, are somewhat different; their cortex contains primary follicles as well as more loosely arranged secondary follicles, or germinal centers. Between the germinal centers are bands, or paracortical, areas, which are thymic-dependent (T-dependent), and the primary follicles and germinal centers contain B-dependent cells. There is substantial circulation of lymphocytes, particularly of T-cells. Through a moderate degree of selectivity, cells that are removed from a particular organ tend to return to that organ when reintroduced into the circulation. This concept of cell "traffic" is important, especially when one considers recovery from radiation injury.[870] The immune competent cells (including B- and T-cells, macrophages, thymocytes, monocytes, natural killer [NK] cells, leukocytes, and erythrocytes) produce antigens, which have been referred to as clusters of differentiation (CD) that are numbered in the order in which they were identified.

Radiation Effects on Lymphocytes

Early experiments demonstrated the marked radiosensitivity of small lymphocytes. Doses as low as 20 to 40 mGy were reported by Stefani to cause significant alterations in motility and morphology of human lymphocytes irradiated and maintained in vitro.[878] One of the most unusual aspects of the response of some lymphocytes to radiation is the timing of cell death. Most cells exposed to moderate levels of radiation do not die until after the first or second cell division following the radiation insult. Small lymphocytes, on the other hand, have been shown to be very susceptible to interphase death without having to enter into mitosis. As with other cell types, the presence of oxygen enhances the radiation sensitivity of lymphocytes. An oxygen enhancement ratio of approximately 2.7 has been documented in animal systems.[879]

With radiation doses in the range of the mean whole-body LD_{50}, changes in the small lymphocytes are so rapid that they can be found within 1 hour.[880] Within 3 days, lymphoid tissues subjected to such doses of radiation may be almost completely devoid of lymphocytes. Assuming that dose administration is not protracted, depletion of lymphocytes in various tissues is dose-dependent up to nearly the lethal range. Apparently some lymphocytes, which are antigen-activated and localized in the gastrointestinal tract, are much more resistant to the effects of ionizing radiation than are nonactivated small lymphocytes. Plasma cells are highly radiation-resistant and can continue to secrete antibody at doses in excess of tens of Gys. There is a misconception perpetuated in many medical texts that radiation exposure is a cause of lymphocytosis. A review of the literature and articles actually quoted usually reveals an error in interpretation or misquoting. In a few very early papers, there is mention of a relative lymphocytosis, but the authors point out that the normal percentage of lymphocytes in peripheral blood was not known in the mid-1940s. Some authors suggest that there may be a lymphocytosis as a precursor of leukemia; however, review of the leukemia cases that occurred in the atomic bomb survivors show that this is not the case.[881] Donati and Gantner[882] indicated that there can be leukocytosis, erythrocytosis, lymphocytosis, and granulocytosis as a result of radiation exposure, however, virtually none of these claims are supported by the literature they reference, and the data were obtained from x-ray workers who presented to clinic with unrelated infections.[883,884]

Miale's textbook on laboratory medicine indicates that overexposure to ionizing radiation causes "reactive" lymphocytes to be found in the peripheral blood.[885] In a review of the literature quoted, the term *refractive* is used and refers to an atypical binucleated lymphocyte.[886] It should be noted that binucleated lymphocytes have been seen more commonly in smokers. Miale also indicated that chronic exposure to radiation can lead to a relative lymphocytosis with leukopenia. Cronkite et al. also mention lymphocytosis and leukocytosis as a result of repeated small radiation exposures.[887] This information was based on other articles or on German literature. Cronkite indicated that he considered this information to be incorrect in light of later experience. In spite of the experience of the last several decades, errors originating from the very old literature regarding lymphocytosis continue to persist in what should be authorative documents.[888]

Depression and Regeneration of Immune Response

Regeneration of lymphatic tissues following irradiation usually follows a certain pattern. The cortical lymphocytes reappear first, followed by germinal center formation. If there has been local irradiation of only certain lymph nodes or of the spleen, regeneration is more rapid than if there has been whole-body exposure, probably because of the circulation of nonirradiated cells repopulating the irradiated tissues.[870]

Depression of the immune response after radiation is primarily due to the radiosensitivity of most small lymphocytes. The major consequence of the immune suppression is increased susceptibility to infection, although an increase in the induction rate of neoplasms is also possible. When the radiation dose is delivered at a reduced dose rate, the radiation is much less effective in producing immune depression. This effect may be due to the repair of radiation damage that is possible during either extended or fractionated exposures.[889] Dose rates of 10 to 40 mGy/minute were much less effective in producing immune depression in rats than 300 to 600 mGy/minute for the same cumulative dose. Overall, evidence indicates that B-lymphocytes show more acute and rapid advancement of radiation injury than do T-lymphocytes. In the B-lymphocytes, redistribution of nuclear chromatin occurs at doses of 0.5 to 1.0 Gy, whereas T-cells require approximately 20 Gy for the same effect. Following irradiation of spleen and lymph nodes, B-cell-dependent areas are depleted more extensively than T-cell-dependent areas. The general observation that B-lymphocytes are more radiosensitive than T-lymphocytes may be due to interphase death, but this does not take into account B-cell heterogeneity. Restoration of the immune response is generally inversely proportional to the dose received, although in mice an intact thymus is required to restore the T-cell response. After low-dose exposures, regeneration may occur via the proliferation of the local, less radiosensitive cells.[890] Following larger doses, regeneration is more probably performed by repopulation from exogenous stem cells rather than proliferation of resistant small lymphocytes. With the larger doses, repopulation is delayed by 9 to 14 days, probably as a result of the maturation that the stem cell must undergo either in the thymus or in the bone marrow. An extensive discussion of the radiosensitivity of the subtypes of the T- and B-cells is given by Anderson et al.[870]

After total lymphoid irradiation there is a significant reduction in the absolute number of T-cells.[891] The results concerning the radiosensitivity of CD4+ T-helper cells and CD8+ T-suppressor cells are controversial.[892] After total lymphoid irradiation the CD4 subset is diminished; one might conclude that T-helper cells are more radiosensitive than suppressor cells. There are subsets of T-helper cells that are either IL-2 or IL-4 secreting. Of these, the IL-4 subset appears more radiosensitive.[893]

Functional Responses of the Immune System

Immunosupression is a consequence of whole-body irradiation at medium to high doses. Localized radiotherapy can also result in systemic suppression. In contrast, many studies have shown that very low doses of ionizing radiation may result in immunostimulatory effects particularly at short times after irradiation. The UNSCEAR 2006 report indicated that because of these divergent effects, ionizing radiation is probably better considered as an "immunomodulatory" rather than an "immunosuppressive" agent.[5] A theory of *hormesis* has been proposed by some scientists. This concept is more fully explored in Chapter 12. The dose of radiation employed, timing with respect to exposure, antigenic challenge, and the types of cells involved are particularly important in observing an effect of augmentation of the immune response. This phenomenon was described as early as 1950 by Taliaferro.[894] In most instances, the augmentation of the immune response was greatest when irradiation was given shortly after administration of an immune challenging substance.[895] It is felt that this augmentation may be due to a radiation-induced injury of a subpopulation of suppressor T-cells responsible for regulation of the response. Similar results also have been obtained with low doses of radiation administered shortly before tumor transplantation. Normally, augmentation occurs at fairly low doses; however, Hellstrom and Hellstrom have described an antitumor response at doses as high as 4 Gy.[896]

As mentioned earlier, the antigen response is humoral and is the function of the B-cells. Because the B-cell is particularly radiosensitive compared with the other lymphocytes, it might be expected that antigen localization and retention may be easily inhibited by radiation. In fact, doses of 4.5 Gy inhibit this response. Although the inductive phase of the antigen response is very radiosensitive, plasma cells and preformed antibodies demonstrate no significant depression after doses as high as 8 Gy. Both in vitro and in vivo responses demonstrate the radiosensitivity of the immune response, which causes antibody production to have a D_{37} value of 0.55 to 0.85 Gy.[870] Both the delayed hypersensitivity response and the graft-versus-host response are more radioresistant than generation of the antibody response, probably because of the relative radioresistance of the T-cell.

Immune Function After Total- and Partial-Body Irradiation

OCCUPATIONAL EXPOSURE

There are a number of studies of the immune status in occupationally exposed groups. Rees et al. did not find significant changes in the immune profiles of 325 male workers occupationally exposed to low-LET radiation at the British Nuclear Fuels Sellafield plant.[897] The cumulative exposures were greater than 200 mSv in a period from 19 to 45 years in one group and less than 27 mSv in a period of 15 to 32 years in the other. No statistically significant differences were found in total counts of circulating T- and B-lymphocytes, CD4+ and CD8+ T-cell subsets, CD4+/CD8+ ratio, or in CD3+/MHC-DR+ ratios. This study took account of possible confounding factors including age, gender, and cigarette smoking and the sample size was large enough for substantiating the conclusion that occupational exposure to low doses does not affect immune profiles of workers.[5] Similar negative findings were reported by Tuschl et al. for employees working at the research reactor of the Austrian Research Center.[898] The authors also reported on 10 nuclear power plant workers exposed to 0.8 to 1.4 mSv as well as tritium inhalation in a 4-week period.[899] The CD4+/CD8+ ratio was increased and there was an increase in absolute numbers of CD4+ T-cells. The authors postulated this was due to potentiation of the immune response.

RADIOTHERAPY

Chaskes et al. examined patients therapeutically exposed to total-body gamma irradiation at dose levels of 1 to 3.5 Gy.[900] The dose rates ranged from 15 mGy/minute to 15 mGy/hour. Reductions in immunoglobulin-A (IgA), immunoglobulin-M (IgM), and immunoglobulin-G (IgG) were reported. Immunoglobulin levels returned to close to normal 7 weeks after total-body irradiation. The order of decreasing sensitivity to irradiation is IgA, IgM, and IgG. The suppression of IgG and IgM was greater when the dose was given at 15 mGy/hour than at 15 mGy/minute.

Because the thymus is involved with the maturation phase of T-lymphocytes, irradiation of the thymus might be expected to lead to profound effects. Irradiation of the thymus demonstrates extremely marked radiosensitivity of the thymic lymphocytes.[901] Morphologic and possibly functional alterations in the thymus of animals result from exposure to doses as small as 50 mGy. Sensitivity of these lymphocytes may be due to the sensitivity of the cell to radiation injury, or it may be secondary to the sensitivity induced by one rapid cellular division. The reticulum cell component of the thymus is much more radioresistant, with no significant changes after a dose of 50 Gy. Data on exposure of the human thymus come from persons accidentally exposed, as well as those undergoing radiation therapy. Findings confirm the marked early radiosensitivity of the lymphocytes within the human thymus.[902] Multiple late effects, including development of thyroid nodules and tumors, have been reported to result from therapeutic irradiation of the thymus. This carcinogenic effect is discussed in Chapter 5. In addition to the risk of developing tumors, children who have received thymic irradiation also have an increased frequency of many uncommon diseases with immunologic overtones such as sarcoid, thyroiditis, and collagen diseases.[903] Immunologic evaluation of the children has revealed a persistent depression of T-cells among the irradiated group.

Total lymphoid radiotherapy for rheumatoid arthritis appears to affect in vitro lymphocyte function with decreased response of peripheral lymphocytes to the mitogens PHA, ConA, and PWM. There is also a decrease in response to allogenic cells in a mixed lymphocyte culture.[904] A selective decrease in T-helper cell antibody response to diphtheria or tetanus toxin is also seen.[905] In spite of clinical remission after such therapy, there has been no change demonstrated after radiation in serum rheumatoid factor titer, antinuclear antibodies, or immunoglobulin-E (IgE) levels.[906] It should be noted that data regarding radiation effects derived from patients with autoimmune diseases should not be broadly applied. Peripheral blood lymphocytes from such patients have been found to be more radiosensitive by a factor of 4 when compared with those from healthy patients. This apparently is associated with a deficiency in DNA repair.[891,907,908]

A decline in T-helper cells has been reported after total lymphoid irradiation for treatment of rheumatoid arthritis.[909] Radiotherapy has been used in hopes of improving the survival of renal transplants. Local irradiation of the allograft has had no beneficial effects.[910,911] Total lymphoid irradiation was not considered beneficial.[912] Cossu et al. reported that lymphocytes in patients with systemic lupus erythematosus are more radiosensitive when the disease is in an active phase compared to patients in the remissive phase.[913] Higher morbidity associated with radiation therapy has been reported in HIV-1+ patients although the mechanism for this is unclear.[914]

While there is an extensive literature on second cancers following radiotherapy, papers concerning changes in immune parameters after radiotherapy are scarce and the actual impact of these changes on health has not been well established.[5] T-cell depression following chest wall irradiation or carcinoma of the breast has been noted.[915] In these cases, the thymus was exposed to doses estimated to be between 20 and 24 Gy. In 1962, Berger et al. reported that after local radiotherapy to the breast, the frequency of cytotoxic T-lymphocyte precursor cells can be reduced by about 25%, although values subsequently return to normal.[916] In addition, immunoglobulin secretion can be reduced.[917] Nakayama et al. studied immune status in patients treated with radiotherapy for lung cancer.[918] The percentage and absolute number of CD4+, CD45RA+ cells and CD56+ (naive T cells), and CD16+ (NK cells) decreased. The percentage of activated CD4+ T-cells and activated CD8+ T-cells increased but not significantly. Similar findings after thoracic irradiation were reported by Ishida et al.[919] Van Mook et al. reported on 24 B-cell chronic lymphocytic leukemia patients who had received splenic irradiation with up to 10 Gy to the spleen in 1 Gy fractions.[920] Six weeks later there was a decrease in absolute lymphocyte count and CD4+ and CD8+ cells but no change in the CD4+/CD8+ ratio. There also was no change in immunoglobulin levels.

Many studies have confirmed decreased immunocompetence following localized radiotherapy for a variety of other tumors.[921–923] Blomgren et al. studied the lymphocyte count and serum immunoglobulin level in children irradiated for treatment of either Wilms' tumor or non-Hodgkin's lymphoma.[924] Tumor doses were from 7 to 32 Gy, and all children received chemotherapy. With the exception of a slightly decreased serum level of IgE in patients treated for lymphoma, there was no difference from healthy controls in immunoglobulin levels, lymphocyte count, or frequency of rosette-forming cells. Because there is some persistent lymphopenia in adults treated for breast cancer, it was supposed here that children who have an intact thymus can recover more rapidly than adults who normally have an atrophied thymus. Posner et al. reported a long-term decrease of total CD4+ cells after treatment with mediastinal radiotherapy for Hodgkin's disease.[925]

Watanabe et al. expanded on this work and pointed out that the long-term decrease was actually due to a decrease in CD4+ and CD8+ naive T-cells and that these effects lasted up to 30 years.[926] In contrast, CD4+ and CD8+ memory T-cell subsets returned to normal or above normal by 5 years postradiotherapy. After whole-body radiotherapy for non-Hodgkin's lymphoma, Safwat et al. recently reported a significant decrease in lymphocytes and an increase in the percentage of CD4+ T-cells and a consequent significant increase in the CD4+/CD8+ ratio due to a higher radiosensitivity of CD8+ T-cell subset after whole-body radiation.[927] Blood samples were collected 24 hours after the end of treatment (1.6 Gy). These results are different from those reported earlier by Clave et al. in which all major T-cell subsets appeared equally radiosensitive while NK cells were relatively radioresistant.[928]

Blomgren et al. studied immune parameters in patients treated with iodine 131 for Graves' hyperthyroidism.[929] The cellular composition and immunologic reactivities of the lymphocytes were abnormal before treatment because this is an autoimmune disease. After iodine administration there was a slight lymphopenia, and the ratio of CD4+ and CD8+ T-lymphocytes, which was increased before treatment, increased further. No other immunologic parameters studied, such as secretion of other Ig classes, mitogenic responses of lymphocytes, and distribution of other lymphocyte subsets, changed to any detectable extent. Wasserman et al. studied changes in blood lymphocyte populations after treatment of patients with iodine 131 for nodular goiter and after treatment with phosphorus 32 for treatment of polycythemia vera.[930] The iodine treatments ranged from 300 to 500 MBq, and there was an increased proportion of helper/inducer T-cells. There was also a decreased ability of the lymphocytes to secrete immunoglobulins, particularly IgM after stimulation with pokeweed antigen. After administration of 150 to 305 MBq of phosphorus 32, there was again decreased secretion of Ig.

ATOMIC BOMB SURVIVORS

There has been extensive study of the immune system in atomic bomb survivors. Ohkita reported that several months after exposure hematolymphoid function of many survivors had almost completely recovered.[931] Immune function has continued to be studied in the atomic bomb survivors since the presence of peripheral chromosomal aberrations and an increase in cancer incidence have been demonstrated. The proportion of T-cells in the peripheral lymphocytes of the heavily exposed survivors was not affected by age or radiation dose. Lymphocyte function, however, was demonstrated to be affected in terms of response to mitogen.[932] Whether this effect is at all responsible for the increase in malignant tumors in the population is not known. The possibility of increased susceptibility to infection has been studied by Kato, who found no correlation between the level of antibody to Epstein-Barr (EB) virus and radiation dose.[933] It does appear that the children who received heavy in utero exposures did have at least a temporary decrease in antibody-producing competence. A study of the titers of anti-EB virus antibodies in the sera of 372 atomic bomb survivors was reported by Akiyama et al.[934] The proportion of persons with high titers was significantly elevated among the exposed survivors; however, the results suggest that reactivation of EB virus in the latent stage occurs more frequently in the survivors, even though this may not be related to radiation dose. Akiyama et al. studied the number of T- and B-cells as well as the phytohemagglutinin (PHA) responsiveness of T-cells in 1047 individuals.[932] The results were nonsignificant but suggested a decrease in T-cells and their PHA responsiveness with dose, and the number of B-cells tended to increase with dose. Akiyama et al.[935] and Bloom et al.[936] also have studied NK cell activity, circulating immune complex, and interferon production in 1300 survivors. None of these were affected by radiation exposure. A third study by Akiyama et al. of the responsiveness of lymphocytes to allogenic antigens in mixed lymphocyte culture showed a significant decrease in responsiveness with increasing dose.[937]

Studies by Yamada et al. showed that differentiation of B-lymphocytes in immune globulin–producing cells and the function of suppressor T-lymphocytes was depressed in the exposed group but not at a statistically significant level.[938] More detailed studies were carried out by Fugiwara et al. using monoclonal antibodies.[939] Total lymphocytes were monitored using Leu-1+ and showed no change with either radiation exposure or age. Use of Leu-2a showed a decrease in cytotoxic suppressor activity related to age but not to radiation. Use of the Leu-3a antibody that detected helper and inducer cells showed a decrease related to age but not to radiation, and finally use of HLA-DR++ antibody that detects monocytes and B-cells again showed a decrease with age but not with radiation. Another study that used monoclonal antibodies by Kusunoki et al. examined mononuclear cells in 1328 atomic bomb survivors.[940] With age some subpopulations of T-cell lymphocytes and B-cells tended to decrease. There was a suggestion that radiation may have accelerated aging of the T-cell–related immune system, but this was not seen for Leu-7 or CD-16 cells, which increased with age and had no relation to radiation exposure. Kusunoki et al. also studied EB antibodies and precursors.[941] They did not find any significant effect of the atomic bomb radiation although their study sample was made up of only 68 persons. Bloom et al. studied multiple immune parameters in Hiroshima.[936] None of the immunologic variables was related to radiation exposure. Finch et al. mentioned work by Pinkston conducted in both Hiroshima and Nagasaki on release of migration inhibition factor from stimulated T-cells and indicated that no

radiation effect was found.[831] More recent studies by Fujiwara et al. studied potential radiation effects on auto-antibodies and immunoglobulins p73 among 2069 atomic bomb survivors.[118] While there was an increase in rheumatoid factor titer and prevalence with radiation, there was no effect on antinuclear antibody, antithyroglobulin antibody, or anti-thyroid-microsomal antibody. There was an increase in IgA level with radiation exposure but no effect on IgG or IgE. The increase in rheumatoid factor is curious because there is no evidence of an increase in clinically evident rheumatoid arthritis among atomic bomb survivors.[942] Shifts towards an inflammatory profile have been reported in the atomic bomb survivors. Neriishi et al. demonstrated a positive association between radiation dose and erythrocyte sedimentation rate, total leukocyte counts, alpha-1 and alpha-2 globulin, and sialic acid.[943] Hayashi et al. found increased levels of C-reactive protein (CRP) and IL-6.[944] This was significantly related to radiation dose with an increase of 30% per Gy for CRP and 10% per Gy for IL-6. Hayashi et al. also later reported a dose-dependent increase in total immunoglobulin levels with IgA and IgM increasing but not IgG or IgE.[945]

In summary, for the atomic bomb survivors, short-term effects of radiation on the immune system were due to dose-dependent bone marrow depletion due to cell death. Late effects have been primarily functional and quantitative abnormalities of T- and B-cells in survivors exposed to high doses (>1 Gy). In contrast to acquired immunity, no significant dose effects have been found regarding innate immunity particularly with regard to function and number of NK cells.

ACCIDENTAL EXPOSURE

Several studies on humans have examined immunoglobulin levels following accidental total-body irradiation. One study of Marshall Islanders included only 13 exposed persons and 46 unexposed controls. Minimal reductions in IgA and IgG were reported.[946] The small numbers of patients examined and difficulty in dose estimates made assessing the importance of these minimal findings difficult. Chang et al. analyzed the immune status in residents of a building constructed with cobalt 60–contaminated steel rods and reported that the mean percentages of CD4+ T-lymphocytes, MHR-DR+ lymphocytes, and the CD4+/CD8+ ratio were lower than in a reference population.[947] UNSCEAR 2006 commented that these findings should be taken with caution given the wide range of cumulative doses and protraction of doses.[948]

There have been many recent claims regarding depression of the immune system in populations living in contaminated villages around the Chernobyl nuclear plant. This is usually discussed in terms of an increased number of visits to hospitals for colds and other illnesses. In the International Chernobyl Project conducted in 1990, no objective evidence of an increase in infections as evidenced by leukocyte count or any abnormality in lymphocyte count was found.[138] The official data relative to specific infections (such as measles, hepatitis, etc.) did not show any relation to the accident. Of course, data relative to hospital and physician visits are often due to concern relative to radiation effects rather than a true increase in disease. The UNSCEAR 2000 report pointed out that: (1) the levels of radiation that Chernobyl populations were exposed to had not been shown to affect the immune system in prior non-Chernobyl studies and (2) the findings of Chernobyl studies were not consistent with the known mechanisms and temporal effects of radiation on the immune system.[7] It also concluded that immunological effects in the general population could not be associated with Chernobyl and, when observed, were likely due to other causes.

Chernobyl studies on the function and number of lymphocyte subsets have yielded conflicting results. There was a report indicating a decrease in lymphocytes in recovery workers, however, this lasted only about a year.[949] Helicopter pilots who received higher doses did not show this effect nor did Chelyabinsk recovery workers.[950,951] Studies on children were also conflicting. Children evacuated from Pripyat also did not have significant differences in immunological parameters from control groups.[952] Children examined 2 years after the accident from Mogilev and Gomel did not show abnormalities in levels of T-lymphocytes, but showed a minor increase in B-lymphocytes.[953]

Additional studies on emergency and cleanup workers have focused on levels and function of T-cells and NK cells. Early studies reported a decrease in T-cell counts and immunoglobulins.[954–956] At 1 to 5 years postexposure there was variable recovery of cellular and humoral immunity. There were also variable responses of B-cell counts. Thirteen years postexposure, none of the patients had developed classic autoimmune disease.

The results of more recent studies in cleanup workers have been controversial and, again, the results differ between studies. Many of the studies have reported an initial decrease in CD3+ and CD4+ cells. Later reports showed an increase in these counts and a late decrease in CD8+ counts. Yarilin et al. reported a decrease in CD3+ cells in groups exposed to 0.1 to 0.5 Gy and another group exposed to 0.5 to 9 Gy; however, there was a decrease in CD8+ cells only in the lower dose group and a decrease in CD8+ cells only in the higher dose group.[957] In other studies of workers in the 30 km zone, Titova et al.[958] reported a decrease in both CD4+ and CD8+ cells and Kurjane et al.[959] reported that doses between 0.01 to 0.5 Gy reduced CD3+, CD4+, and CD8+ T-cells. Kuzmenok et al. did not find any changes in the levels these cell populations 11 to 14 years after the accident.[960] The same study reported a possible increase in response of CD25+ cells to the cytokine interleukin-2, which was not proportional to dose. Kurjane et al.

reported a decrease in NK cells, however, these findings are in contrast to studies of the atomic bomb survivors suggesting radioresistance.[959] In addition, confounding factors exist. Some authors have reported a toxic effect of lead (which was dumped on the reactor) on CD4+ and CD16+ cells.[961] Also, elevated blood levels of lead, zinc, and iron were found in Latvian and other cleanup workers.[959, 961] Chumak et al. reported an accumulation of polyunsaturated fatty acids in peripheral mononuclear cells and esterified fatty acids in cleanup workers 11 to 14 years after exposure, as well as an increase in CD4+ cells and a decrease in CD8+ cells in heavily irradiated workers (also inconsistent with studies of the atomic bomb survivors).[954] Another study of 730 emergency and 1212 recovery workers also reported decreases in CD3+ and CD4+ counts, but unexplained substantial, although smaller, decreases for the control groups.[962]

The immune status of children around Chernobyl has also been studied. Titov et al. reported a variety of findings including a decrease in B-cells and IgM, but only for 30 to 45 days after the accident.[963] A decrease in IgG was reported for 90 days, which later returned to normal and then increased. A study of 1118 children performed 5 years after the accident reported decreased CD3+ and CD4+ levels in children living in contaminated territories compared with children of the same age living in "clean" villages.[952] This is in contrast to the study that showed lower levels of CD3+ and CD4+ cells in children with doses greater than 1 mSv with respiratory disease, compared to control children in uncontaminated areas.[964] However, no decrease was seen in healthy children living in the contaminated zone. Koike et al. reported that children in Gomel had abnormalities in NK cell activity but this was not correlated with the level of ^{137}Cs contamination.[965] Koike et al. also mentioned that children with goiter in contaminated areas had increased serum levels of IgG, IgM, IgE, and a depressed level of NK cell activity. These latter finding are in conflict with the data from the atomic bomb survivors. An in vitro study of lymphocytes by Padovani et al. suggested that there may be an adaptive response with increased radioresistance after a preceding challenge dose of 1.5 Gy.[966]

The consensus of the 2005 Chernobyl Forum was that reported immunological effects of radiation exposure from the Chernobyl accident appear to be related mostly to changes in the numbers or function of peripheral lymphocytes and serum immunoglobulin levels.[145] These effects have been detectable up to the present time. Some of these effects may be due to confounding factors other than direct radiation, such as stress, chronic infections, diet, and chemicals. As a result, it is difficult to interpret the results. Immune effects would normally be expected to be significant in those workers who suffered from the acute radiation syndrome. Studies of children have shown varying results over time and between studies.

The conclusion of the 2005 Chernobyl Forum was that while effects on levels of immune cells and function have been reported in a number of studies, there is significant variation in the results of different Chernobyl studies and some results are at variance with data from the atomic bomb survivors.[145] The possible role of confounding factors, such as heavy metals and the effect of radioiodine on the thyroid, also complicates the issue. To date, at doses of less than several tens of mSv, no clinical effects have been clearly related to abnormal immune function. The UNSCEAR 2006 report stated that while a broad spectrum of immune abnormalities has been reported among Chernobyl victims, it has not been possible to interpret these results, since it has been unclear whether all possible confounding factors have been taken into account.[5]

Summary

The immune system is one of the most complex systems in the body. It protects against infection and cancer. The two major forms of immunity are innate and acquired. Innate immunity provides a rapid defense while acquired immunity develops only after a pathogen and antigens have entered the body. The UNSCEAR 2006 report points out that ionizing radiation is better considered an immunomodulatory agent than an immunosuppressive agent. While high-dose irradiation can lead to immunosuppression, the effects of doses less than 200 mGy or less than 100 mGy/hour remain controversial and the literature is often contradictory. At low doses the primary effects appear to be related to the function and number of T- and B-cell lymphocyte subsets, however, resultant clinically significant effects are difficult to find.

TOTAL-BODY IRRADIATION

There are many circumstances in which humans have been exposed to total-body radiation (Fig. 6-27). These, of course, include the survivors of Hiroshima and Nagasaki, as well as a multitude of accidental exposures. The latter have been well summarized by Fry et al.,[61] Gusev et al.,[54] Ricks et al.,[967] and UNSCEAR.[824] Worldwide there have been about 100 documented fatalities due to radiation accidents since 1946. Most of the data on acute exposures to the whole body come from external irradiation, although at least one fatality was due to internal contamination following a misadministration of gold 198, and several others as a result of internal and external exposure from cesium.[55] There has been one murder attributed to administration of polonium 210.

Although the terms *total-body radiation* and *whole-body radiation* carry the connotation of a homogeneous uniform dose, this is rarely the circumstance. In almost all situations, the dose is delivered in a fashion that irradiates one part of the body substantially more than another. Perhaps the

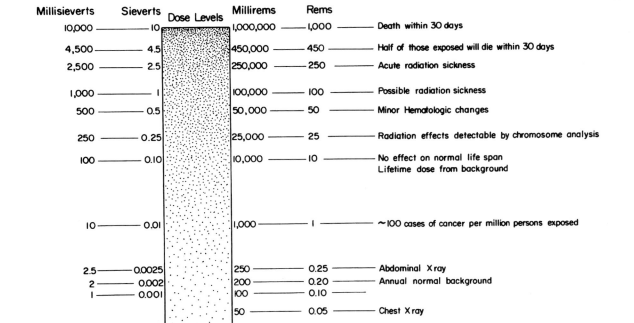

Figure 6-27 • Relative spectrum of sources and effects of various levels of whole-body doses.

closest approach to uniform exposure results from those circumstances in which total-body irradiation is used for therapeutic purposes prior to bone marrow transplantation. In these cases, the patient is irradiated from front and back.

The total-body absorbed dose required to cause death is generally characterized by a median LD_{50}. This abbreviation refers to a dose required to kill 50% of the persons irradiated, and it assumes no medical intervention. It is usually necessary to establish a temporal relationship with regard to the mortality, which usually is referred to as the $LD_{50/30}$ or the $LD_{50/60}$. These are doses that, if given, might be expected to result in death in one half of the individuals within 30 days and 60 days, respectively. The $LD_{50/60}$ in humans is estimated to be 3.5 to 4 Gy, air or surface dose.

A number of more recent estimations of the lethal dose from whole-body radiation have been reported. Most of these have been derived from analyses of the atomic bomb survivor data. Contributing to uncertainties in atomic bomb data is not only the dosimetry but other nonradiation factors such as trauma, nutritional status, and a devastating typhoon on September 17, 1945.[968] The reported doses usually refer to bone marrow dose and $LD_{50/60}$. Estimates by Rotblat[969] using older dosimetry suggested that the $LD_{50/60}$ distance was 892 m from the hypocenter and a dose of 1.5 Gy, but more recent computations of dose (using DS86) at the same distance by Fujita et al.[970] estimated a dose of 2.44 Gy. Work done by Young and the U.S. Defense Nuclear Agency reviewing these and other data concludes that if the deaths of the persons seriously injured on the first day are excluded, the dose is 3.2 Gy, and, if they are not excluded, the dose would be 2.64 Gy.[971] In a study of 7593 persons (1095 of whom died in the first 60 days), Kamada et al. made estimates based on a small sample of girls and with DS86 dosimetry found a relatively high dose of about 4 Gy.[972] The authors suggest that the young female may be more resistant to whole-body exposure. Fujita et al. using DS86 dosimetry for each individual estimated the $LD_{50/60}$ to be in the range of 2.7 to 3.1 Gy when first-day deaths are excluded.[970] Levin et al. made estimates based on occupants of reinforced concrete structures in Nagasaki.[973] Median lethal bone marrow dose estimates were 2.9 Gy using a logarithmic dose scale and 3.4 Gy using a linear dose scale. Thus, most of the data from Japan yield $LD_{50/60}$ bone marrow dose estimates of about 3 Gy. Obviously, the lethal dose of radiation depends on the dose rate, uniformity, and penetration of the radiation, as well as the status of the irradiated individual. A review of the literature concerning the LD_{50} was presented in the 1988 UNSCEAR report.[824]

From the data derived from the Chernobyl accident, it appears that for healthy males who receive medical treatment the $LD_{50/60}$ is at least 4 Gy. Of 21 patients in the 4 to 6 Gy group, 7 survived. For ill cancer patients who are treated with conservative support medications and blood cell infusions, it appears to be about 3.0 to 3.5 Gy marrow dose, but a dose of 2 Gy could kill 30% to 40% of very ill patients. With pretreatment and an appropriate bone marrow match and successful transplantation, a large number of children have survived whole-body acute doses in the range of 9 to 14 Gy.[824]

Shielding portions of the active marrow will have a major effect on survival in acute exposure situations. In men it appears that shielding of 10% of the active marrow will enable nearly all to survive when the body receives a dose close to the $LD_{50/60}$. Active marrow in adults is found in approximate percentages at various sites as follows: skull, 7%; upper limbs, 4%; ribs, 19%; sternum, 3%; cervical vertebrae, 4%; thoracic, 10%; lumbar, 11%; pelvis, 30%; and lower limbs, 11%. For purposes of convenience, some rather arbitrary delineations of the temporal sequence of events identified clinically after whole-body radiation exposure have been made. These are (1) a prodromal period, (2) a latent period, (3) a period of illness, and (4) a period of recovery or demise. The *prodromal period* may occur 1 to 6 hours after the radiation exposure and is a period of transitory symptoms. The time of onset, type, and number of symptoms depend on the radiation dose (Table 6-2).

Some of the symptoms, particularly nausea and vomiting, are difficult to evaluate from a clinical viewpoint, because they may be psychogenic in origin, and care should be taken in using these symptoms exclusively, rather than good dosimetric information, history, and so on. Estimates of the onset, duration, and incidence of symptoms are derived from radiation therapy patients and accident victims. The Japanese data are difficult to use because of the uncertainties in dosimetry. Unfortunately, some authors report the absorbed dose as the skin dose, some do not specify the site, and still others use the midline tissue dose (MTD). In general, to derive MTD if one knows the value in air, tissue attenuation in the average person may be corrected for by using a factor of 0.66. Thus, a dose in air of 10 Gy is equivalent to an MTD of about 6.6 Gy for the average adult. The dose rates at which prodromal symptoms occur are in the range of 0.05/minute and higher. The dose rate also may have an effect on the symptoms manifested; for example, gastrointestinal effects appear to increase as the dose rate increases, but the data from humans concerning dose rate are very limited.

Prodromal symptoms occur with increasing frequency at higher absorbed doses. Anorexia may be seen in 5% of people at doses as low as 0.4 Gy and occurs in 95% of people at approximately 2.75 Gy. The dose-response curve for nausea is somewhat higher, with 5% of people experiencing this symptom at approximately 0.45 Gy and 95% experiencing it at 4.5 Gy. Vomiting occurs at slightly higher levels: 5% experience it at approximately 0.6 Gy, and about 95% at 7 Gy. These doses given are MTD.

Table 6-2 • Symptoms Following Acute Whole-Body Irradiation

Dose Range	Symptom	Percentage	Time Post-exposure
0.5–1.0 Gy	Anorexia	15–50	3–18 hr
	Nausea	5–30	3–20 hr
	Vomiting	15–20	4–16 hr
1–2 Gy	Anorexia	50–90	1–48 hr
	Nausea	30–70	4–30 hr
	Vomiting	20–50	6–24 hr
	Fatigue	25–60	3–72 hr
	Weakness	25–50	3–48 hr
	Bleeding (mild)	10	1–5 wk
	Fever	10–50	2 days–5 wk
	Infection	10–50	1–5 wk
	Death	< 5	5–6 wk
2–3.5 Gy	Anorexia	90–100	1–48 hr
	Nausea	70–90	1–48 hr
	Vomiting	50–80	3–24 hr
	Diarrhea	10	4–8 hr
	Fatigue (moderate)	60–90	2 hr–6 wk
	Weakness (moderate)	50–80	2 hr–6 wk
	Bleeding	10–50	1–5 wk
	Fever	10–80	1–5 wk
	Infection	10–80	2–5 wk
	Ulceration	30	3–5 wk
	Death	5–50	4–6 wk
3.5–5.5 Gy	Anorexia	100	1–72 hr
	Nausea	90–100	1–72 hr
	Vomiting	80–100	3–24 hr
	Diarrhea	10	3–8 hr
	Fatigue	90–100	1 hr–6 wk
	Weakness	90–100	1 hr–6 wk
	Headache	50	4–24 hr
	Bleeding	50–100	6 days–6 wk
	Fever and infection	80–100	6 days–6 wk
	Death	50–99	3.5–6 wk
5.5–7.5 Gy	Anorexia	100	1–72 hr
	Nausea	100	1–72 hr
	Vomiting	100	1–48 hr
	Diarrhea	10	4–6 hr
	Fatigue and weakness (severe)	100	1 hr–2 wk
	Dizziness and disorientation	100	4–48 hr
	Headache	80	4–30 hr
	Bleeding, fever, infection, hypotension	100	10–14 days
	Death	100	2–3 wk

Courtesy of James Conklin, MD.

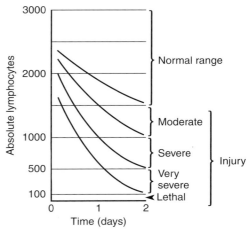

Figure 6-28 • Effect of whole-body irradiation on absolute lymphocyte count, a useful early biologic dosimeter, particularly in cases of accidental exposure. (From Andrews G, et al: Personnel Dosimetry for Radiation Accidents. Vienna, International Atomic Energy Agency, 1965).

damaged gastrointestinal mucosa releasing 5-hydroxytryptamine (5-HT3) with subsequent activation of 5-HT3 receptors. Treatment with 5-HT3 receptor antagonists appears to be quite effective at hemibody single doses up to 8 Gy. The drugs that have been used are granisetron, tropisetron, and ondansetron. Whether the 5-HT3 receptors are responsible for postradiation antegrade and retrograde giant migrating bowel contractions of the small bowel and colon is not known. With respect to evaluation of accidental exposures, the duration and onset of some of the symptoms and peripheral lymphocyte changes may be useful (Fig. 6-28).

As acute dose levels exceed those listed, symptoms merely move forward in time. At dose ranges between 7.5 and 10.5 Gy MTD, death occurs in 100% of individuals at 7 to 15 days. As the MTD is raised to 10 to 20 Gy, death occurs in 100% of patients at 2 to 12 days; with higher MTDs, in excess of 20 Gy, death occurs in 100% of individuals between 2 and 5 days. Although the LD_{50} skin dose estimate of approximately 3.5 to 4 Gy corresponds to an MTD of 1.98 to 2.64 Gy, this estimate represents a situation without good medical care. It is probable that with appropriate medical treatment, the LD_{50} skin dose may be in the range of 6 Gy, or an MTD of 3.96 Gy.

Acute Radiation Syndromes and Sickness

The acronym ARS has been used variably in the literature. Early literature referred to acute radiation *syndromes* while more recent literature has used the term to mean acute radiation *sickness*. The term "syndrome" refers to the predominant underlying tissue that results in death at various absorbed doses. Unfortunately, at high doses there are many tissues damaged and there is interaction

A number of authors have examined the effectiveness of various drugs in preventing or treating radiation-induced nausea and vomiting after high-dose whole-body, lower hemibody, or abdominal radiotherapy.[540,974–980] It appears that much of the nausea and vomiting is due to the of many physiological and pathological mechanisms. For our purposes here, ARS will refer to *acute radiation sickness*.

Depending on the dose levels, major manifestations of acute radiation sickness include signs of hematopoietic depression with concurrent infection and hemorrhage (hematopoietic syndrome). The intestinal, toxemia, and cerebral syndromes occur after large doses with signs of diarrhea, water loss, fever, arterial blood pressure drop, and functional and structural changes of the brain. Occasionally, with very high acute doses to the head or trunk, there may be loss of consciousness, which is sometimes referred to as transient incapacitation (or CNS) syndrome. The concept of a cutaneous radiation syndrome was later introduced to describe the complex pathological changes and interactions resulting from acute radiation exposure of the skin.

There are several phases in the development of ARS. These include initial reaction, latent period, disease manifestation, and late outcomes. The severity and time sequence of each of these phases is broadly dependent on the dose and dose rate. The situation can be quite complex since in many accidental situations in which patients develop ARS, there is relatively nonuniform distribution of the spatial distribution of dose in the body, and as a result most patients combine variants of ARS.

There are a number of national registries that accumulate data on ARS patients. These exist in Brazil, China, France, Russia, and the United States. In addition, there are international registries maintained by the International Atomic Energy Agency (IAEA). To date, these registries indicate that there have been about 400 ARS patients as a result of radiation accidents. Obviously, this number excludes persons who died at Hiroshima and Nagasaki. Historically, approximately 20% of all patients with ARS have fatal outcomes.

There are a number of criteria that have been used for acute radiation *sickness*. At this time, the most useful subdivisions of ARS appear to be in three grades of severity with the fourth grade of severity that covers all other forms with an inevitable fatal outcome. With these, it is possible to determine the necessary recommendations, both in terms of diagnosis and for therapy. ARS has several forms but all manifest themselves within the first 30 days following exposure and are related to the magnitude of the absorbed dose. Although these are listed in order of increasing absorbed dose, there is considerable clinical overlap of the four forms. The IAEA (1998) produced useful summary tables on the methods for early diagnosis of radiation injuries as well as the acute, latent, and critical phases of ARS (Tables 6-3 to 6-5).[981] Even with such classifications, there are essential difficulties in determining the diagnosis and prognosis as well as the outcome, particularly if the situation involves a very uneven distribution of dose or very high doses specifically to the skin, lung, intestine, or hematopoietic tissue.

Table 6-3 • Prodromal Phase of Acute Radiation Sickness (ARS)

Symptoms and Medical Response	DEGREE OF ARS AND APPROXIMATE DOSE OF ACUTE WBE (Gy)				
	Mild (1–2 Gy)	Moderate (2–4 Gy)	Severe (4–6 Gy)	Very Severe (6–8 Gy)	Lethal* (>8 Gy)
Vomiting					
Onset	2 hr after exposure or later	1–2 hr after exposure	Earlier than 1 hr after exposure	Earlier than 30 min after exposure	Earlier than 10 min after exposure
% of incidence	10–50	70–90	100	100	100
Diarrhea	None	None	Mild	Heavy	Heavy
Onset	—	—	3–8 hr	1–3 hr	Within min or 1 hr
% of incidence	—	—	<10	>10	Almost 100
Headache	Slight	Mild	Moderate	Severe	Severe
Onset	—	—	4–24 hr	3–4 hr	1–2 hr
% of incidence	—	—	50	80	80–90
Consciousness	Unaffected	Unaffected	Unaffected	May be altered	Unconsciousness (may last sec/min)
Onset	—	—	—	—	Sec/min
% of incidence	—	—	—	—	100 (at >50 Gy)
Body temperature	Normal	Increased	Fever	High fever	High fever
Onset	—	1–3 hr	1–2 h	<1 hr	<1 hr
% of incidence	—	10–80	80–100	100	100
Medical Response	Outpatient observation	Observation in general hospital, treatment in specialized hospital if needed	Treatment in specialized hospital	Treatment in specialized hospital	Palliative treatment (symptomatic only)

*With appropriate supportive therapy individuals may survive for 6–12 months with whole-body doses as high as 12 Gy.
WBE, whole-body exposure.
Adapted from International Atomic Energy Agency (IAEA), Diagnosis and treatment of radiation injuries: Safety report series, No. 2. Vienna, IAEA, 1998.

Table 6-4 • Latent Phase of Acute Radiation Sickness (ARS)

	DEGREE OF ARS AND APPROXIMATE DOSE OF ACUTE WBE (Gy)				
	Mild (1–2 Gy)	Moderate (2–4 Gy)	Severe (4–6 Gy)	Very Severe (6–8 Gy)	Lethal (> 8 Gy)
Lymphocytes (G/L) (days 3–6)	0.8–1.5	0.5–0.8	0.3–0.5	0.1–0.3	0.0–0.1
Granulocytes (G/L)	>2.0	1.5–2.0	1.0–1.5	≤ 0.5	≤ 0.1
Diarrhea	None	None	Rare	Appears on days 6–9	Appears on days 4–5
Epilation	None	Moderate, beginning on day 15 or later	Moderate, beginning on day 11–21	Complete earlier than day 11	Complete earlier than day 10
Latency period (days)	21–35	18–28	8–18	7 or less	None
Medical response	Hospitalization not necessary	Hospitalization recommended	Hospitalization necessary	Hospitalization urgently necessary	Symptomatic treatment only

G/L, giga/liter; WBE; whole-body exposure.
Adapted from International Atomic Energy Agency (IAEA), Diagnosis and treatment of radiation injuries: Safety report series, No. 2. Vienna, IAEA, 1998.

Comparatively exact assessment of the severity, grade, and prognosis of damage can be reached for patients who are exposed to relatively uniform radiation (the difference of doses accumulated in body parts is less than threefold). The most confident outcome assessment under these circumstances can be drawn for hematopoietic damage. All other situations of clinical syndromes with predominant damage (or shielding) of separate body segments (head, trunk, extremities, pelvis) or organs (lungs or intestine) have to be analyzed on a case-by-case basis from the viewpoint of the clinical signs and damage identified in these organs and structures.

The acute radiation *syndrome* is generally divided into four subgroups: (1) neurovascular syndrome, (2) gastrointestinal syndrome, (3) hematopoietic syndrome, and (4) cutaneous syndrome. These syndromes are classified by degree of severity in Table 6-6. Acute neurological changes generally occur only when the whole-body irradiation dose exceeds 50 Gy. The survival time is usually less than 48 hours. An excellent description of these syndromes was published by Bond et al.[821] and Hempelmann.[982] In general, symptoms are identified almost immediately and consist of disorientation, apathy, ataxia, prostration, and often tremor and convulsions. The seizures may result from minimal external stimuli. The cause of death is believed to be a function of several causes, including vascular damage, meningitis, myelitis, and encephalitis. Fluid infiltrates into the meninges, brain, and choroid plexus, causing marked edema. The resulting pressure may cause pressure on critical

Table 6-5 • Findings of Critical Phase of Acute Radiation Sickness (ARS) Following Whole-Body Exposure (WBE)

	DEGREE OF ARS AND APPROXIMATE DOSE OF ACUTE WBE (Gy)*				
	Mild (1–2 Gy)	Moderate (2–4 Gy)	Severe (4–6 Gy)	Very Severe (6–8 Gy)	Lethal (>8 Gy)
Onset of symptoms (days)	>30	18–28	8–18	<7	<3
Lymphocytes (G/L)	0.8–1.5	0.5–0.8	0.3–0.5	0.1–0.3	0.0–0.1
Platelets (G/L)	60–100	30–60	25–35	15–25	<20
	10–25%	25–40%	40–80%	60–80%	80–100%[†]
Clinical manifestations	Fatigue, weakness	Fever, infections, bleeding, weakness, epilation	High fever, infections, bleeding, epilation	High fever, diarrhea, vomiting, dizziness and disorientation, hypotension	High fever, diarrhea, unconsciousness
Lethality (%)	0	0–50 Onset 6–8 wk	20–70 Onset 4–8 wk	50–100 Onset 1–2 wk	100 1–2 wk
Medical response	Prophylactic	Special prophylactic treatment from days 14–20; isolation from days 10–20	Special prophylactic treatment from days 7–10; isolation from the beginning	Special treatment from the first day; isolation from the beginning	Symptomatic only

*1 Gy = 100 rads.
[†]In very severe cases, with a dose >50 Gy, death precedes cytopenia.
Adapted from International Atomic Energy Agency (IAEA), Diagnosis and treatment of radiation injuries: Safety report series, No. 2. Vienna, IAEA, 1998.

Table 6-6 • Degrees of Various Types of Acute Radiaton Syndromes

Observation	Degree 1	Degree 2	Degree 3	Degree 4
Hematopoietic Syndrome 24–48 h				
Lymphocytes (10^9 cells/L)	>1.5	1.0–1.5	0.5–1.0	<0.5
Granulocytes (10^9 cells/L)	>2	4–6	6–10	>10
Platelets (10^9 cells/L)	>100	50–100	50–100	50–100
3–7 days				
Lymphocytes (10^9 cells/L)	>1.0	0.5–1.0	0.1–0.5	<0.1
Granulocytes (10^9 cells/L)	>2	>2	>5	>5
Platelets (10^9 cells/L)	>100	50–100	20–50	<20
Gastrointestinal Syndrome				
Diarrhea frequency	2–3/day	4–6/day	7–9/day	>10
Stool consistency	Bulky	Loose	Very loose	Watery
Blood in stool	Occult	Intermittent	Persistent	Gross
Abdominal cramps/pain	Minimal	Tolerable	Intense	Unbearable
Vomiting	See neurovascular syndrome	—	—	—
Nausea	See neurovascular syndrome	—	—	—
Neurovascular Syndrome				
Nausea	Mild	Tolerable	Intense	Unbearable
Vomiting	1/day	2–5/day	6–10/day	>10/day
Anorexia	Able to eat and drink	Decreased intake	No significant intake	Parenteral nutrition
Fatigue	Normal	Normal	Needs some assistance	Prevents daily activity
Headache	Mild	Mild	Intense	Intense
Temperature (°C)	<38	38–40	>40 less than 24 hr	>40 for more than 24 hr
Heart rate	>100	>100	>100	>100
Blood pressure	>100/70	<100/70 unstable	<90/60 transient	<80/? hypotensive
Neurological	None	Mild	Significant interference with normal activity	Life threatening, possible loss of consciousness
Cutaneous Syndrome				
Erythema (hours–30 days)	Minimal transient	Moderate <10 cm² or <10% body surface area	Marked 10–40% body surface area	Severe >40% body surface area
Altered sensation/itching (hours–days)	Pruritis	Slight or intermittent pain	Moderate persistent pain	Severe persistent pain
Edema (5 days–8 wk)	Present asymptomatic	Symptomatic	Secondary dysfunction	Total dysfunction
Blistering (5 days–8 wk)	Absent or rare	Rare with hemorrhage	Bullae with sterile fluid	Bullae with hemorrhage
Desquamation (5 days–8 wk)	Absent	Patchy dry	Patchy moist	Confluent moist
Ulcer/necrosis (5 days–8 wk)	Epidermal only	Dermal	Subcutaneous	Deep tissue involvement
Hair loss (2–8 wk)	Thinning	Patchy easily visible	Complete reversible	Complete irreversible
Onycholysis (2–8 wk)	Absent	Partial	Partial	Complete

From U.S. Department of Health and Human Services. Accessed Oct. 10, 2007 at www.remm.nlm.gov/ars.htm.

structures. Although these changes can be identified in animals, they have rarely been seen in humans, and some of the deaths in this category may actually result from cardiovascular shock.[706] There has been little pathologic examination of human tissue in these circumstances; however, in animals, the brain is grossly congested, with infiltration of granulocytes into the brain tissue. Perivascular hemorrhage and edema, as well as increased vascular permeability, has been identified.[429,983,984] Some investigators suggest that in the same dose range, there is a syndrome of cardiovascular shock. In humans, a rapid drop in blood pressure has been identified in some accidental situations (usually in which there has been nonuniform exposure, with the greater part being to the upper torso).

When acute absorbed skin doses in the range of 7 to 50 Gy are received, the gastrointestinal syndrome (group IV) may occur. In most circumstances, after the prodromal period, a latent period of approximately 1 to 4 days during which the patient is asymptomatic occurs. The clinical progress of the syndrome is a manifestation of the radiosensitivity and failure of both the gastrointestinal syndrome and the bone marrow. The symptoms include lethargy, diarrhea, dehydration, and sepsis. The earliest pathologic changes can be identified as degenerative abnormalities in the small-bowel epithelium. If the absorbed skin dose does not exceed approximately 12 Gy, regeneration of the bowel epithelium is possible. With higher doses, initial loss of the intestinal stem cells at the base of the mucosal crypts occurs, with subsequent denudation of the mucosa. As the intestinal vascular barrier is broken, there is marked fluid and electrolyte loss into the intestinal lumen and sepsis caused by the bacteria in the intestine that now have access to the bloodstream. Sepsis, of course, is aggravated by the decrease in granulocytes that normally would be available to combat it. Fluid loss is exacerbated by a failure of reabsorption of fluid in the colon.

Many researchers have indicated that the presence of bile in the intestine is one of the main factors in causation of radiation-induced diarrhea. In animal systems cannulation or ligation of the bile duct will prevent the diarrhea. Normally bile salts are reabsorbed in the distal ileum; when reabsorption does not take place, an inordinately large amount of bile salts gains access to the colon. The abnormalities in secretion of fluid into the bowel and reabsorption may cause a large loss of electrolytes, particularly sodium and, to a lesser extent, potassium. Infection plays a role as early as 24 hours. Not only is the white blood cell count reduced, but other mechanisms normally operable to combat infection such as lymphoid elements (Peyer's patches) are depleted. Antibiotics have been demonstrated to reduce the bacteremia, although their effect on the ultimate mortality rate is questionable. Other investigators indicate that treatment with antibiotics may increase the mean survival time.

In general, there are very limited human data on the gastrointestinal syndrome, and almost all available findings are derived from animal data. Death resulting from these changes usually occurs at 3 to 14 days postexposure. In the absorbed skin dose range of 2 to 7 Gy, the hematopoietic syndrome may be encountered. After the prodromal period, the duration of the asymptomatic latent period is 1 to 3 weeks. The signs and symptoms result from radiation damage to the bone marrow, lymphatic organs, and immune response. In this syndrome, rapid reduction in the lymphocytes (Table 6-7) and a somewhat more delayed reduction of leukocytes, platelets, and red cells occur. The granulocytopenia leads to infection, and the thrombocytopenia leads to hemorrhage. Mean survival is usually 2 to 6 weeks, with the nadir of the various blood elements occurring approximately 30 days after exposure. Death usually results from hemorrhage and infection. Transfusions and antibiotics are usually indicated. There

Table 6-7 • Change of Lymphocyte Counts (G/L) in Initial Days of Acute Radiation Sickness (ARS) Depending on Dose of Acute Whole-Body Exposure

Degree of ARS	Dose (Gy)	Lymphocyte Counts (G/L)* After 6 Days Since First Exposure
Preclinical phase	0.1–1.0	1.5–2.5
Mild	1.0–2.0	0.7–1.5
Moderate	2.0–4.0	0.5–0.8
Severe	4.0–6.0	0.3–0.5
Very severe	6.0–8.0	0.1–0.3
Lethal	>8.0	0.0–0.05

*Expressed as 10^9 cells/L.
Adapted from International Atomic Energy Agency (IAEA), Diagnosis and treatment of radiation injuries: Safety report series, No. 2. Vienna, IAEA, 1998.

may be additional signs of impaired gastrointestinal function and fluid imbalance from the radiation received by the bowel. The histologic changes and peripheral blood count variations were discussed earlier in the chapter, in the section on hematopoietic tissue.

There has been an additional more recently described "syndrome" related to extensive irradiation of the skin. The cutaneous syndrome is important because of the interaction of the immune and barrier functions of the skin which, when compromised, cause a synergistic effect with the injury to other systems resulting in markedly increased mortality.[13,14,985]

Chernobyl

It is instructive to review the Chernobyl accident since that single accident includes about one third of all cases of ARS in the world's literature. There are several publications that have described the acute health effects of the Chernobyl accident in detail.[54,824,986] The possible diagnosis of ARS was initially considered for 237 persons. One hundred fifteen patients from this group were transported to the Radiation Medicine Department of the Institute of Biophysics (Moscow). Within several days, the acute radiation syndrome was verified in 104 of these persons. Thirty additional patients were also verified to have acute radiation syndrome when considered retrospectively, for a total of 134. The doses and outcomes of these patients are shown in Table 6-8.

All expected major clinical symptoms of ARS and their combinations were observed in personnel involved in the accident who had total-body gamma exposures of more than 1 Gy. The gastrointestinal syndrome was observed in 15 patients and radiation pneumonitis was detected in eight patients. Combinations of these syndromes with severe widespread beta dermatitis occurred

Table 6-8 • Doses, Number, and Outcome of 134 Chernobyl Patients with Acute Radiation Sickness (ARS)

Degree of ARS	Dose Range (Gy)	Number of Patients	Number of Short-Term Deaths	Number of Survivors
Mild (I)	0.8–2.1	41	0 (0%)	41
Moderate (II)	2.2–4.1	50	1 (2%)	49
Severe (III)	4.2–6.4	22	7 (32%)	15
Very severe (IV)	6.5–16	21	20 (95%)	1
Total	0.8–16	134	28	106

in 19 patients (Table 6-9). Skin doses exceeded bone marrow doses by a factor of 10 to 30 in some patients and in these patients some had estimated skin doses in the range of 400 to 500 Gy. This local radiation damage to the skin resulted in significant aggravation of existing pulmonary and hepatic or renal abnormalities. Beta burns were the primary cause of death in a number of patients and significantly increased the severity of ARS. When skin injury exceeded 50% of the body surface area, this was a major contributing cause to morbidity and mortality.

In the early period (14 to 23 days postexposure) 15 patients died of skin or intestinal complications and 2 patients died of pneumonitis. In the period 24 to 48 days after exposure, there were six deaths from skin or lung injury and two from secondary infections following bone marrow transplantation. A patient who had severe ARS developed acute diffuse interstitial pneumonia with rapid development of hypoxemia, incompatible with life. Bacterial and fungal pneumonia was not confirmed at autopsy, and it appeared that there was acute radiation pneumonitis with possible cytomegalovirus being present. Two deaths at relatively late periods (days 86 to 96) were related to infectious complications of local radiation injury of the skin and renal insufficiency. One female patient died at 112 days from brain hemorrhage. Underlying bone marrow failure was the major contributor to all the deaths during the first 2 months.

Three deaths were believed to occur unnecessarily as a result of inappropriate bone marrow transplantation. Bone marrow transplantation in patients with doses below 9 Gy only worsened the ARS therapy results due to the development of side effects. (It is now clear that the percentage of radiation accident victims who can get a definite benefit from such transplantation is very small.) Recovery of myelopoiesis and survival is possible following whole-body exposures of 6 to 8 Gy, and this was found after rejection of haploidentical transplant (three cases) as well as in patients who were not transplanted due to absence of an appropriate donor (four cases). There were no fatalities in the ARS grade II (2 to 4 Gy doses), excluding the one female patient who died from brain hemorrhage in the late term. For those patients with ARS grades III–IV, the fatal outcomes in this group resulted primarily from acute severe cutaneous injuries from lung damage and from a combination of skin and intestinal damage combined with a bone marrow depression. Within 14 years after the accident, 14 additional ARS survivors of grade I–III died from other various causes.

RADIATION-INDUCED LIFE SHORTENING

Radiation-induced life shortening in rats was described as early as 1944. The experimental literature through 1960 indicated that irradiated animals appeared to age more rapidly than control groups. In the early 1960s, Casarett suggested that aging resulted from endothelial damage of the arterioles and fibrotic changes in the interstitial cells.[987] Only in the mid-1970s did the concept of radiation-induced life shortening and premature aging come under serious criticism by Walburg[988] and Storer.[989] These investigators indicated that life-shortening effects identified after radiation could best be explained by an increase in neoplastic diseases.

Table 6-9 • Relationship of ARS Degree and Percentage Skin Burns and Dose in Chernobyl Patients

Number of Patients	ARS Severity Grade	PERCENTAGE OF SKIN SURFACE RADIATION BURN			Approximate Absorbed Skin Dose (Gy)
		50%–100%	10%–50%	1%–10%	
31	I	0	1	2	8–12
43	II	1	9	2	12–20
21	III	3	15	3	20–25
20	IV	9	10	1	>20

The animal data on radiation-induced life shortening have been well summarized by UNSCEAR.[711] In general, the data refer to low-dose radiation; it is clear that at high doses (with cell killing) the effects of radiation may indeed shorten life through very specific causes. Although scattered reports in the literature have suggested that low doses of radiation, either alone or combined with suboptimal ambient temperatures, may actually lengthen the lifespan of animals, these reports have not been replicated consistently. It is possible that in some animals an increased resistance results from stress, possibly mediated through hormonal or immune factors. The preponderance of the animal evidence, however, clearly indicates that after low- and high-LET radiation (in low and medium dose ranges) shortening of the lifespan may result primarily from an acceleration or increased incidence of neoplastic conditions.

The human epidemiologic data concerning lifespan shortening are based on atomic bomb survivors, patients exposed to radiotherapy, and occupationally exposed persons. The epidemiologic studies have many associated limitations, which have been described at length in Chapter 4. Specifically, these problems include small sample size, lack of an adequate control group, inaccuracy of records, and differences in assessment of the absorbed dose and its temporal distribution.

Atomic Bomb Survivors and Persons Exposed to Fallout

Conard examined Marshall Islanders, who were exposed to fallout, for various signs of aging; however, the irradiated group consisted of only 334 persons, too small a group for statistically reliable results.[990] Examination of the survivors from Hiroshima and Nagasaki for signs of life shortening has been conducted serially by various authors.[991–996] Autopsy correlations of aging, particularly the soluble-insoluble collagen ratio, have also been examined.[997] Overall, the collagen ratio in heavily exposed individuals was not significantly different from that of individuals who were not exposed.

Shimizu et al. reported on noncancer mortality in the atomic bomb survivors.[998] Data from the Life Span Study (LSS) during 1950–1985 suggest an excess risk of noncancer mortality among survivors exposed at young ages in the high-dose range. The risks identified are very small and are much less than for cancer, and there was a suggestion of dose response for circulatory disease. For all subjects the excess relative risk (ERR) at 2 Gy was 0.06 (RR of 1.06). Using clinical data from the Adult Health Study of atomic bomb survivors during 1958–1986, Wong et al. also observed an increased RR of myocardial infarction during later years (1968–1986) in heavily exposed (0.2 Gy) survivors who were under age 40 at the time of exposure, but no significant increase in those irradiated at older ages.[120] There was also an increase in the specific categories of thyroid disease, cirrhosis of the liver, and uterine myomata.

The RR at 1 Gy (100 rad) with 95% CI was as follows: hypertension, 1.02 (0.98 to 1.06); ischemic heart disease, 1.04 (0.96 to 1.13); myocardial infarction, 1.15 (0.83 to 1.62); hypertensive heart disease, 0.99 (0.94 to 1.06); aneurysm, 0.97 (0.83 to 1.33); stroke, 0.97 (0.86 to 1.14); thyroid disease, 1.30 (1.16 to 1.47); cataract, 1.03 (0.97 to 1.10); gastric ulcer, 1.02 (0.92 to 1.16); duodenal ulcer, 0.89 (0.80 to 1.05); cirrhosis, 1.14 (1.04 to 1.27); uterine myoma, 1.46 (1.27 to 1.70); prostatic hyperplasia, 1.01 (0.88 to 1.22); dementia, 1.11 (0.94 to 1.64); and Parkinson's disease, 1.44 (0.94 to 2.57). The increase in cirrhosis was probably of an infective (rather than radiation) nature, and more study is underway to determine if hepatitis antigens were present in these cases.

On further follow-up to 1997, the risks of mortality from diseases other than cancer remained elevated by about 14% per Sv, with significant increases for heart disease, stroke, digestive diseases, and respiratory diseases, but with no evidence of radiation effects at doses below 0.5 Sv.[999] The prevalence of aortic atherosclerosis, as diagnosed radiographically, was also elevated,[1000] along with the plasma levels of CRP and IL-6,[944] the latter increases being noteworthy in view of the fact that low-level inflammatory responses are widely accepted as a risk factor for the diseases in question. The median loss of life expectancy from cancer and other diseases in members of the LSS cohort, analyzed through 1995, was estimated to approximate 2.6 years in those exposed to doses of 1.0 Gy or more and 2 months in those exposed to doses between 0.005 and 1.0 Gy.[1001]

Radiotherapy Patients

Radiotherapy data are useful because the dose and field of exposure are relatively well defined. Limitations of such studies are that the exposure is not whole-body exposure and the patient is usually being irradiated for a malignant disease. Treatment of malignant diseases is rarely limited to radiotherapy; thus, complicating factors, such as chemotherapy, often confound the data. Usually, the radiotherapy studies have examined either patients with specific neoplasms in which there is a fair survival or individuals in whom radiotherapy was given for benign conditions. Court-Brown and Doll examined patients treated with radiotherapy for ankylosing spondylitis between the years 1935–1954.[1002] Over 14,000 persons were included in this sample. In this and a later study, mortality in the group of treated patients was greater than for members of the general population.[1003] There was a substantial excess of deaths from causes other than cancer; however, they appeared to be associated with the ankylosing spondylitis. Such causes of death included lesions of the aortic valve, regional enteritis, amyloid degeneration, nephritis, effect of drugs, and proneness to accidents. There was, in addition, a clear increase in deaths from leukemia and cancer in the heavily irradiated sites, which was attributed to radiation exposure.

Another study in which radiation therapy was used for treatment of benign conditions was for presumed thymic enlargement. Hempelmann et al. compared 3000 irradiated children with 5000 nonirradiated siblings.[1004] Although thyroid tumors increased, there was no evidence of a nonspecific increase in mortality. This result is not surprising because the radiation field involved only the neck and upper thorax; however, it does indicate that if there were substantial effects on the immune system from thymic irradiation, they apparently were not significant enough to result in increased infections or other conditions that would affect mortality.

Conversely, in patients surviving 10 or more years after radiotherapy for peptic ulcer, the risk of coronary heart disease (adjusted for confounders) increased significantly with the cardiac dose, ranging from 1.0 for the lowest cardiac dose category (mean volume-weighted dose of 1.6 Gy, with mean in-field dose of 7.6 Gy) to 1.51 for the highest cardiac dose category (mean volume-weighted dose of 3.9 Gy, with mean in-field dose of 18.4 Gy).[471] Compatible but inconclusive data on mortality from cardiovascular disease have been reported from other studies of patients treated with radiation for various benign conditions, including abnormal uterine bleeding[690,1005–1008] and other gynecological disorders.[1009] Also, as noted in an earlier section of this chapter, adverse effects of radiation on the heart and blood vessels have been observed to increase the risk of cardiovascular disease in patients surviving radiotherapy for Hodgkin's disease,[444,1010–1013] as well as in those treated for cancers of the breast[1014,1015] and testicular seminoma.[1016,1017]

Occupational Exposure

Data with respect to life shortening from radiogenic causes other than cancer have been studied for three major occupational groups: radiologists, x-ray technologists, and radium dial painters. It was reported in the late 1940s that radiologists demonstrated an increased rate of leukemia.[1018] In 1948, Dublin and Speigelman indicated that the death rate from leukemia was higher in radiologists than in any other recorded medical specialty.[1019] This finding was confirmed by Warren, who also indicated that although the mortality rate for physicians was about the same as for the general adult population, radiologists died on the average 5.2 years earlier than nonexposed physicians.[1020] In addition, medical specialists (other than radiologists) exposed to radiation had a shorter lifespan than nonexposed physicians. This appeared to be from many causes of death, including neoplasms, degenerative changes, and infections. This finding of nonspecific life shortening prompted a reexamination of the data by Seltser and Sartwell.[1021] They found that the age distribution of the group of radiologists used by Warren was different from that of the other groups and that average age at death was a misleading parameter.

Another study by Seltser and Sartwell on U.S. radiologists was reported in 1965.[1022] In that study, the mortality experience of several medical specialty societies was analyzed, with over 30,000 physicians being included. The individuals were assigned to groups by suspected radiation exposure, including high exposure (radiologists), intermediate exposure (internists), and low exposure (ophthalmologists and otorhinolaryngologists). In fact, radiologists had a median age at death 5 years earlier than that of the low-exposure group. This life shortening could not be attributed to leukemia but was associated with many causes of death. Newer data on radiologists were subsequently reported by Warren in 1966.[1023] He indicated that the mean age at death of radiologists rose constantly in the periods studied: 55.8 years in the years 1934–1939, 59.3 years in the period 1940–1949, 64.5 years from 1950–1959, and 70.1 years from 1960. British radiologists have also been studied.[1024] Included in this study were 1377 radiologists who practiced between the years 1897–1956. It was assumed that exposure prior to 1921 was high and that after that date radiation protection measures reduced exposure. There was no evidence of nonspecific life shortening, although cancer mortality was increased in those entering practice before 1921. An extension of this study over the next 20 years was published in 1981.[1025] The overall noncancer death rate among radiologists was lower than in two of the three comparison groups and thus again did not demonstrate any evidence of nonspecific life shortening. The British data have been criticized with respect to statistical adequacy and the uncertainties in dosimetry.[1022] The UNSCEAR Committee in its 1982 report concluded that the data from the early radiologists did demonstrate a real increase in leukemia and skin cancer and that if a nonspecific lifespan-shortening effect was present in the early radiologists, it has disappeared in recent years.[711]

Studies concerning radiology technicians have been reported from Japan[1026,1027] and the United States for men trained as radiographers during World War II.[1028] In the Japanese studies, the number of deaths identified was lower than expected, perhaps because of underreporting or some other problem with the survey. No evidence of nonspecific life shortening was identified. In the study of the World War II U.S. radiographers, no information on lifespan shortening was reported. In general, the data on the technologists is much more limited than that on the radiologists and is, therefore, statistically less significant.

Mortality in the radium dial painters in the United States was reported by Polednak.[1029] As discussed in Chapter 5 (in the section on bone cancer), these women were exposed to radium 226 and 228. The population studied was exposed between 1915–1929 and included 634 persons. The initial study demonstrated a significant increase in osteosarcomas and tumors of the paranasal sinuses. A later study by Stehney was extended and concluded that once the radium tumor deaths were removed, the survival of the exposed group was indistinguishable from that of a control group of the same age.[1030] Workers in 15 nuclear power utilities in the United States followed for the 18 years between 1979–1997 showed a strongly positive and statistically significant association between radiation dose and mortality from heart disease, with an ERR of 8.78 per Sv.[1031] Positive but statistically nonsignificant associations for mortality from leukemia (excluding chronic lymphocytic leukemia) and all solid cancers combined were also observed, with ERRs per Sv of 5.67 and 0.506, respectively.

For whole-body irradiation at low-dose levels and partial-body exposure even at moderate dose levels, it is difficult to find any cause of lifespan shortening other than induction of neoplasms. Certainly, when high doses are delivered to large portions of the body (causing subsequent hematologic derangement, alteration of the immune response, and cell killing), lifespan shortening results from deterministic effects of radiation on particular cell lines.

UNSCEAR 2006 concluded that while the LSS data involving acute exposure have indicated an association between ionizing radiation and cardiovascular disease, this is not entirely clear from other Japanese studies such as the Adult Health Study (AHS).[5] Other studies of chronic or fractionated exposure have not indicated an association between cardiovascular disease and exposure. Even the LSS data are not sufficient to either determine appropriate risk models for a potential association with cardiovascular disease or to derive risk coefficients. At present, the scientific evidence is not sufficient to conclude that there is a causal relationship between ionizing radiation and cardiovascular disease at doses of less than 0.5 to 1.0 Sv.

Due to the high incidence of cardiovascular disease in nonexposed populations, the multifactorial nature and diversity of cardiovascular disease entities, as well the need to eliminate large confounding factors, it is unlikely that epidemiological studies will be able to add significant understanding to the potential and nature of any possible causal relationship. Answers regarding low-dose exposure and cardiovascular disease will likely only come from radiobiological and mechanistic studies. If an increase in cardiovascular disease is found in a population exposed to doses of less than 0.5 to 1.0 Sv, the chance that radiation is the cause is extremely low and other etiologies should be explored.

BIOCHEMICAL INDICATORS OF RADIATION INJURY

For many years, scientists have examined the possibility of using biochemical indicators to assess the level of radiation injury in humans. It had been hoped that these methods might provide useful biologic dosimetry as the early hematologic changes had. An ideal biochemical indicator would be one that was dose-dependent over a wide range and that would give some indication of when the radiation exposure actually occurred. In addition, one would like the ideal biochemical test to be able to be performed rapidly, ideally from a sample (such as blood or urine) easily obtained from the patient. Radiation-induced biochemical effects are of two general classes. The first class includes effects of degradation due to radiation injury, and the second includes changes induced by the functional response of the body to the radiation injury. Overall, although some biochemical changes have been identified, they have not proved to be particularly useful as a biologic dosimeter because very few of them have good dose-response relationships, and most have substantial individual variation from patient to patient. The areas that have been studied will be briefly reviewed here; for more information, including animal data, the reader is referred to the proceedings of a symposium organized by the IAEA.[1032]

Metabolites of nucleic acids increase after radiation exposure in animals. The mechanism of breakdown of DNA is unclear; however, its viscosity is known to decrease with increasing dose. In rats, the blood plasma and urinary excretion of deoxycytidine, deoxyuridine, and uridine increase with radiation exposure up to levels of 2 to 4 Gy. Goldberg indicated that radiation therapy for gynecologic malignancies leads to increased urinary output of ribonuclease (RNase) in each mL of urine and each mg of creatinine during the last week of therapy.[1033] The therapy regimen quoted was a 60-week course of administration of 50 to 85 Gy. It was concluded that changes in urine RNase activity were specifically related to radiation. The mechanism presumably involved is release of this enzyme from nonmalignant cells or from regressing tumor. Unfortunately, the dose-response relationship was not examined in these patients. Excretion of pyrimidines (particularly deoxycytidine) has been studied in animals; unfortunately, excretion of deoxycytidine by humans is rather low, and the normal range of excretion is very large and is affected by age. Another substance, beta-aminoisobutyric acid (BAIBA), a metabolic derivative of thymidine, has been measured in the urine of humans and animals. An increase in the level of BAIBA has appeared in the urine of patients after both therapeutic and accidental exposures.[1034,1035] Normal excretion of BAIBA does not exceed 20 mg per day. In the patients exposed accidentally at Oak Ridge, Lockport, and Los Alamos, significantly elevated excretion levels of BAIBA were identified. All of these patients had received in excess of 1 Gy of acute whole-body radiation, and BAIBA rose to levels of 20 to 50 mg per day. Unfortunately, the dose-response curve is erratic. It is known that normal BAIBA excretion varies substantially among individuals and is controlled to a high degree by genetic determinants. Smith and Langlands indicated that in a group of males who received 1.5 Gy of 4-MeV x-rays to the abdomen, only a small increase in excretion was identified, although individual variation was extensive.[1036] They concluded that without preirradiation control data, the test is not particularly useful. In addition to breakdown products derived from nucleic acids, increased excretion of products resulting from the protein breakdown has been observed. Changes in the activity of proteolytic enzymes have been studied only in animals; however, urinary excretion of amino acids has been studied in humans. Enhanced levels of excretion of cysteic acid, valine, leucine, hydroxyproline, phenylalanine, arginine, aspartic acid, proline, threonine, and tryptophan have occasionally been reported after accidental exposure.[820,1034,1037,1038]

Increased excretion of creatine following irradiation was reported as early as 1923. Gerber et al. reported that although the creatine-creatinine ratio in rats was linear with dose, the same phenomenon did not occur in humans.[1035] After radiation accidents, the creatine-creatinine ratio increased in many patients, although the dose-response correlation is very poor. Excretion of taurine following radiation exposure has been examined. Taurine is a metabolic product of cysteine. In animals, the urinary excretion of taurine rises very rapidly up to absorbed doses of approximately 2 to 3 Gy, plateauing at higher doses. Taurine excretion has been examined after accidental radiation exposure and after radiation therapy.[1034] An increased level of taurine can be identified, although the reason for the increase is uncertain. Interestingly enough, in animals, several days after the acute radiation exposure, taurine excretion levels actually decrease to below the normal value. Desai et al. reported that intensive cytotoxic chemotherapy or radiation therapy leads to a reduction in plasma taurine concentration.[1039] Taurine is a nonessential amino acid and is the most abundant free amino acid in the intracellular space. The mechanism of this decrease was not clear because the precursor amino acids methionine and cystine were not reduced. Urinary excretion of 5-hydroxyindoleacetic acid (5-HIAA) increases in rats with radiation doses up to approximately 8 Gy. Some researchers report that after local irradiation the 5-HIAA urinary level also rises in humans.[1040] Abnormalities in tryptophan metabolism were studied by Streffer, who concluded that changes in tryptophan are extremely dependent on age, sex, and many other factors.[1041] Serum marker KL-6 antigen has been used as an indicator of disease activity in patients with interstitial pneumonia. Hamada et al. studied serum KL-6 levels in a patient with radiation pneumonia and reported that it was more sensitive to lung damage than was lactate dehydrogenase and procollagen type III N-terminal peptide or CRP.[1042] Porciani et al. studied radiotherapy patients and reported significant

reductions in the polyamines spermidine and spermine both in the urine and red blood cells following treatment.[1043]

Hofmann et al. examined increased serum amylase in 41 patients after whole-body as well as head and neck irradiation.[1044] There was a dose-independent serum amylase increase if the salivary glands were within the radiation field. Differentiation of pancreatic amylase from salivary amylase indicated that after whole-body irradiation, there was either only a small or no increase in pancreatic amylase. Dubray et al. found a significant increase in serum salivary amylase if the dose exceeded 0.5 Gy, and a 2.5-fold increase was seen in 91% of patients when the dose exceeded 2 Gy to the salivary glands.[1045] Becciolini et al. proposed the use of salivary gland amylase and tissue polypeptide antigen (TPA) as a potential biochemical dosimeter for space flights.[1046]

In summary, searches for biochemical indicators of radiation injury for use as a biologic dosimeter have been rather disappointing. Although many excreted metabolites show linear dose-responses in animals, the reaction in humans is much more variable and usually only occurs at high absorbed doses. In addition, the effects of radiation quality, dose rate, and partial- versus total-body irradiation are unknown for most of these biochemical changes. The major use of these biochemical indicators at the present time is that when urinary excretion of these compounds is significantly elevated (greater than 1 Gy) high absorbed doses of radiation exposure cannot be excluded. In such circumstances, hematologic data, as well as clinical signs and symptoms, should be more useful.

FATIGUE

Whether fatigue is a deterministic effect of radiation, a psychologic manifestation of stress, or a result of associated disease is often a matter of debate. At present the answer is not entirely clear; however, at this point the symptom is clearly multidimensional in nature and multifactorial in origin. A short summary of the literature will be presented here. Fatigue is difficult to define, but in everyday use the word is related to a feeling of tiredness. There have been many diseases that have been reported to have fatigue as a symptom including multiple sclerosis, systemic lupus erythematosus, myocardial infarction, chronic fatigue syndrome, and even simpler entities such as anemia. Fatigue is also considered to be a symptom of depression.

Much of the literature related to fatigue and radiation exposure comes from cancer patients who have had radiotherapy. Up to 70% to 80% of cancer patients report fatigue during radiotherapy or chemotherapy.[1047] This may persist for several years after the treatment has ended but it gradually declines over time.[1048] The mechanisms that have been proposed for the fatigue include malnutrition, accumulation of toxic end products from cell breakdown, anemia, infections, pain causing lack of sleep, concurrent drugs, and immobilization resulting in lack of conditioning. Both chemotherapy and radiotherapy have been associated with reported fatigue. Between 75% and 100% of patients report fatigue during chemotherapy.[1049,1050] During radiotherapy the following frequencies have been reported of patients with fatigue: 93% chest irradiation, 68% head and neck, and 65% to 72% abdomen and pelvis.[1051,1052] If scales of fatigue are used, there appears to be an increase in mean score as radiotherapy progresses.[1053] While it might be supposed that these effects are the result of toxic breakdown products in the body, there has been no literature to relate the fatigue to any particular metabolite or measurable substance. There is, however, evidence that psychotherapy given to patients undergoing radiotherapy results in a modest reduction of reported symptoms.[1054]

Persons who have been in radiation accidents also have reported long-term fatigue. Over one half of the persons who survived the acute radiation syndrome as a result of the Chernobyl accident reports fatigue of various degrees even 20 years later. It may be that the large amount of cell killing and cell repair had a lasting effect; however, even persons with little or no exposure often report fatigue. The International Chernobyl Project examined the frequency of fatigue in persons living in both contaminated and clean villages. The average total dose received by a person living in the contaminated villages for 5 years was about 0.07 Gy. This is a level that is so low that no cell killing or toxic metabolites would be expected. In spite of this, 81% of persons in noncontaminated control villages reported fatigue compared with 89% in contaminated settlements. This extremely high frequency indicates the difficulty of performing such studies and the very large impact of psychologic factors.

REFERENCES

1. Fry, R.J., Deterministic effects. Health Phys, 2001. 80(4):338–343.
2. Rubin, P. and G. Casarett, Clinical Radiation Pathology. 1966, Philadelphia, Saunders.
3. Fajardo, L., Pathology of Radiation Injury. 1982, New York, Masson.
4. Scherer, E., C. Streffer, and K. Trott, Radiopathology of Organs and Tissues, E. Scherer, C. Streffer, and K. Trott, eds. 1991, Berlin, Springer-Verlag.
5. United Nations Scientific Committee on the Effects of Atomic Radiations (UNSCEAR), Sources and effects of ionizing radiation: 2006 report to the General Assembly with annexes. 2006, New York, United Nations.
6. United Nations Scientific Committee on the Effects of Atomic Radiation (UNSCEAR), Sources and effects of ionizing radiation: 1993 report to the General Assembly, with scientific annexes. 1993, New York, United Nations.
7. United Nations Scientific Committee on the Effects of Atomic Radiation (UNSCEAR), Sources and effects of ionizing radiation: 2000 report to the General Assembly, with scientific annexes. 2000, New York, United Nations.
8. Perez, C., Principles and Practice of Radiation Oncology, 4th ed. 2003, Philadelphia, J.B. Lippincott.
9. Rubin, P., et al., RTOG late effects working group. Overview: Late effects of normal tissues (LENT) scoring system. Int J Radiat Oncol Biol Phys, 1995. 31(5):1041–1042.
10. Gassmann, A., Zur histologie der Rontgenulcera. Forschr Geb Rontgenstrahlen, 1898. 2:199–207.
11. Dewing, S., Modern Radiology in Historical Prospectives. 1960, Springfield, Ill, Charles C. Thomas.
12. International Commission on Radiological Protection (ICRP), The biological basis for dose limitation in the skin: A report of a Task Group of Committee 1 of the International Commission on Radiological Protection. Ann ICRP, 1991. 22(2):1–104.
13. Gottlober, P., G. Krahn, and R.U. Peter, Cutaneous radiation syndrome: Clinical features, diagnosis and therapy. Hautarzt, 2000. 51(8):567–574.
14. Peter, R.U., Cutaneous radiation syndrome in multi-organ failure. Br J Radiol Suppl, 2005. 27:180–184.
15. White, R.L., et al., Thermographic changes following preoperative radiotherapy in head and neck cancer. Radiology, 1975. 117(2): 469–471.
16. Bardychev, M. and A. Zyb, Regional blood circulation in late radiation ulcers of the skin. Med Radiol, 1973. 19:2:47–54.
17. Bardychev, M., T. Oliper, and L. Guseva, Clinics and treatment of radiation fibrosis with disorders of regional haemo- and lympho-circulation of the extremeties and secondary neuritis. Med Radiol, 1978. 23(8):34–40.
18. Gongora, R. and H. Magdelenat, Accidental acute local irradiations in France and their pathology. In Proceedings of a Workshop. 1985, Sacaly, France: Br J Radiol, 1986. 19:12–15.
19. Aversa, A.J. and R. Nagy, Localized comedones following radiation therapy. Cutis, 1983. 31(3):296–303.
20. Friedman, S.J. and W.P. Su, Favre-Racouchot syndrome associated with radiation therapy. Cutis, 1983. 31(3):306–310.
21. Turesson, I. and H.D. Thames, Repair capacity and kinetics of human skin during fractionated radiotherapy: Erythema, desquamation, and telangiectasia after 3 and 5 year's follow-up. Radiother Oncol, 1989. 15(2):169–188.
22. Turesson, I., Individual variation and dose dependency in the progression rate of skin telangiectasia. Int J Radiat Oncol Biol Phys, 1990. 19(6):1569–1574.
23. Bentzen, S.M. and M. Overgaard, Relationship between early and late normal-tissue injury after postmastectomy radiotherapy. Radiother Oncol, 1991. 20(3):159–165.
24. Gottlober, P., et al., Sonographic determination of cutaneous and subcutaneous fibrosis after accidental exposure to ionising radiation in the course of the Chernobyl nuclear power plant accident. Ultrasound Med Biol, 1997. 23(1):9–13.
25. Delanian, S., S. Balla-Mekias, and J.L. Lefaix, Striking regression of chronic radiotherapy damage in a clinical trial of combined pentoxifylline and tocopherol. J Clin Oncol, 1999. 17(10):3283–3290.
26. Delanian, S. and J.L. Lefaix, Reversibility of radiation-induced fibroatrophy. Rev Med Interne, 2002. 23(2):164–174.
27. Georges, C., J.L. Lefaix, and S. Delanian, Case report: Resolution of symptomatic epidural fibrosis following treatment with

combined pentoxifylline-tocopherol. Br J Radiol, 2004. 77(922):885–887.

28. Gottlober, P., et al., Interferon-gamma in 5 patients with cutaneous radiation syndrome after radiation therapy. Int J Radiat Oncol Biol Phys, 2001. 50(1):159–166.

29. Simon, N. and J.H. Harley, Skin reactions from gold jewelry contaminated with radon deposit. JAMA, 1967. 200:254–255.

30. Luria, L.W., H. Berman, and S. Satchidanand, Chronic radiation dermatitis from radioactive gold jewelry. N Y State J Med, 1983. 83(5):741–743.

31. Giever, R., et al., Enhanced radiation reaction following combination chemotherapy for small cell carcinoma of the lung. Radiat Oncol Biol Phys, 1982. 8:921–923.

32. Aristizabel, N., et al., Adriamycin-irradiation cutaneous complications. Int J Radiat Oncol Biol Phys, 1977. 2:325–331.

33. Patterson, R., The Treatment of Malignant Disease by Radium and X-Rays. 1956, London, Edward Arnold Press.

34. Von Essen, C.F., Roentgen therapy of skin and lip carcinoma: Factors influencing success and failure. AJR, 1960. 83:556–570.

35. Pujol, R.M., et al., Postirradiation multiple minute digitate porokeratosis. J Cutan Med Surg, 2001. 5(2):126–130.

36. Peter, R.U., et al., Radiation lentigo: A distinct cutaneous lesion after accidental radiation exposure. Arch Dermatol, 1997. 133(2):209–211.

37. Thoma-Greber, E., et al., Bullous skin reactions after soft roentgen radiotherapy of HIV-associated Kaposi sarcomas. Hautarzt, 1997. 48(5):339–342.

38. Auclair, C., et al., Clastogenic inosine nucleotide as components of the chromosome breakage factor in scleroderma patients. Arch Biochem Biophys, 1990. 278(1):238–244.

39. Bleasel, N.R., et al., Radiation-induced localized scleroderma in breast cancer patients. Australas J Dermatol, 1999. 40(2):99–102.

40. Davis, D.A., et al., Localized scleroderma in breast cancer patients treated with supervoltage external beam radiation: Radiation port scleroderma. J Am Acad Dermatol, 1996. 35(6):923–927.

41. Haustein, U.F., Exacerbation of progressive scleroderma following roentgen therapy. Hautarzt, 1990. 41(8):448–450.

42. Phan, C., et al., Matched-control retrospective study of the acute and late complications in patients with collagen vascular diseases treated with radiation therapy. Cancer J, 2003. 9(6):461–466.

43. Fleischer, A.B., Jr., et al., Skin reactions to radiotherapy—A spectrum resembling erythema multiforme: Case report and review of the literature. Cutis, 1992. 49(1):35–39.

44. Pandya, A.G., A.H. Kettler, and S. Bruce, Radiation-induced erythema multiforme: An unusual presentation with elastic tissue phagocytosis. Int J Dermatol, 1989. 28(9):600–602.

45. Girolomoni, G., E. Mazzone, and G. Zambruno, Pemphigus vulgaris following cobalt therapy for bronchial carcinoma. Dermatologica, 1989. 178(1):37–38.

46. Winkelmann, R.K., et al., Pseudosclerodermatous panniculitis after irradiation: An unusual complication of megavoltage treatment of breast carcinoma. Mayo Clin Proc, 1993. 68(2):122–127.

47. Ross, E.V., Ichthyosiform scaling secondary to megavoltage radiotherapy. Cutis, 1991. 48(1):59–60.

48. Maor, M.H., Dermatophytosis confined to irradiated skin: A case report. Int J Radiat Oncol Biol Phys, 1988. 14(4):825–826.

49. Low, G.J. and J.H. Keeling, Ionizing radiation-induced pemphigus: Case presentations and literature review. Arch Dermatol, 1990. 126(10):1319–1323.

50. Schreiber, G.J. and R. Muller-Runkel, Exacerbation of psoriasis after megavoltage irradiation: The Koebner phenomenon. Cancer, 1991. 67(3):588–589.

51. Vlietstra, R.E., et al., Radiation burns as a severe complication of fluoroscopically guided cardiological interventions. J Interv Cardiol, 2004. 17(3):131–142.

52. Imanishi, Y., et al., Radiation-induced temporary hair loss as a radiation damage only occurring in patients who had the combination of MDCT and DSA. Eur Radiol, 2005. 15(1):41–46.

53. Field, S.B., R.L. Morgan, and R. Morrison, The response of human skin to irradiation with x-rays or fast neutrons. Int J Radiat Oncol Biol Phys, 1976. 1(5-6):481–486.

54. Gusev, I.A., A.K. Guskova, and F.A. Mettler, Medical Management of Radiation Accidents, 2nd ed. 2001, Boca Raton, Fla, CRC Press.

55. International Atomic Energy Agency (IAEA), Dosimetry and medical aspects of the radiological accident in Goiania. 1998, Vienna, IAEA.

56. Oliveira, A.R., et al., Localized lesions induced by ^{137}Cs during the Goiania accident. Health Phys, 1991. 60(1):25–29.

57. Low-Beer, B., External use of radioactive phosphorus: Erythema studies. Radiology, 1946. 47:213–222.

58. Krohmer, J., Physical measurements on various beta ray applicators. AJR, 1951. 66(5):791–796.

59. Goulding, F. and G. Cowper, Hazard due to beta radiation from fission products deposited on the ground after an atomic explosion. 1953, Chalk River Nuclear Laboratory Report, Ontario.

60. Brennan, J., Beta-gamma skin hazard in the post-shot contaminated area, in Military Effects Test, Program of Operation. 1953, Upshot-Knothole.

61. Hübner, K.F., S.A. Fry, and Radiation Emergency Assistance Center/Training Site (REAC/TS), The medical basis for radiation accident preparedness: Proceedings of the REAC/TS International Conference: The medical basis for radiation accident preparedness, October 18–20, 1979, Oak Ridge, Tennessee, U.S. 1980, New York, Elsevier/North Holland.

62. Mikhail, S., Beta radiation doses from fallout particles deposited on the skin, E.S. Associates, eds. 1971, Burlingame, Calif: U.S. Army.

63. Gottlober, P., et al., The outcome of local radiation injuries: 14 years of follow-up after the Chernobyl accident. Radiat Res, 2001. 155(3):409–416.

64. National Council on Radiation Protection and Measurements (NCRP) and U.S. Nuclear Regulatory Commission, Limit for exposure to "hot particles" on the skin: Recommendations of the NCRP. NCRP report no. 106. 1989, Bethesda, Md, The Council, p.vi.

65. Dean, P.N., J. Langham, and L.M. Holland, Skin response to a point source of fissioned uranium-235 carbide. Health Phys, 1970. 19(1):3–7.

66. Harvey, W., On the pathological effects of roentgen rays in animal tissues. Pathol Bacteriol, 1908. 12:549.

67. Cottenot, P., A. Mulon, and A. Zimmerman, Action des rayons X sur la corticale surrenale. Society Biol, 1912. 63:717.

68. Beower, J. and J. Clark, Resistance of the thyroid gland to the action of radium rays: The results of experimental implantation of radium needles in the thyroid of dogs. AJR, 1923. 10:632.

69. Samaan, N.A., et al., Hypothalamic, pituitary and thyroid dysfunction after radiotherapy to the head and neck. Int J Radiat Oncol Biol Phys, 1982. 8(11):1857–1867.

70. Sommers, S., Effects of ionizing radiation upon endocrine glands. In Pathology of Irradiation, C. Berdjis, ed. 1971, Baltimore, Williams and Wilkins.

71. Tobias, C., Pituitary radiation. In Radiation, Physics and Biology: Recent Advances in the Diagnosis and Treatment of Pituitary Tumors, J. Linfoot, ed. 1976, New York, Raven Press.

72. Fuks, Z., et al., Long-term effects on external radiation on the pituitary and thyroid glands. Cancer, 1976. 37(suppl 2):1152–1161.

73. Sklar, C. and L. Constine, Chronic neuroendocrinological sequelae of radiation therapy. Int J Radiat Oncology Biol Phys, 1995. 31(5):1113–1121.

74. Rose, S.R., et al., ACTH deficiency in childhood cancer survivors. Pediatr Blood Cancer, 2005. 45(6):808–813.

75. Samaan, N.A., et al., Hypopituitarism after external irradiation for nasopharyngeal cancer. In Recent Advances in Diagnosis and

Treatment of Pituitary Tumors, J. Linfoot, ed. 1979, New York, Raven Press.

76. Shalet, S.M., Growth and hormonal status of children treated for brain tumours. Childs Brain, 1982. 9(3-4):284–293.

77. Schmiegelow, M., et al., Growth hormone response to a growth hormone-releasing hormone stimulation test in a population-based study following cranial irradiation of childhood brain tumors. Horm Res, 2000. 54(2):53–59.

78. Schmiegelow, M., et al., Cranial radiotherapy of childhood brain tumours: Growth hormone deficiency and its relation to the biological effective dose of irradiation in a large population based study. Clin Endocrinol (Oxford), 2000. 53(2):191–197.

79. Schmiegelow, M., et al., Gonadal status in male survivors following childhood brain tumors. J Clin Endocrinol Metab, 2001. 86(6):2446–2452.

80. Schmiegelow, M., et al., Dosimetry and growth hormone deficiency following cranial irradiation of childhood brain tumors. Med Pediatr Oncol, 1999. 33(6):564–571.

81. Dickinson, W.P., et al., Differential effects of cranial radiation on growth hormone response to arginine and insulin infusion. J Pediatr, 1978. 92(5):754–757.

82. Rappaport, R. and R. Brauner, Growth and endocrine disorders secondary to cranial irradiation. Pediatr Res, 1989. 25(6):561–567.

83. Link, K., et al., Growth hormone deficiency predicts cardiovascular risk in young adults treated for acute lymphoblastic leukemia in childhood. J Clin Endocrinol Metab, 2004. 89(10): 5003–5012.

84. Moell, C., et al., Suppressed spontaneous secretion of growth hormone in girls after treatment for acute lymphoblastic leukaemia. Arch Dis Child, 1989. 64(2):252–258.

85. Shalet, S.M., The effects of cancer treatment on growth and sexual development. Clin Oncol (R Coll Radiol), 1985. 4:223–238.

86. Lannering, B. and K. Albertsson-Wikland, Growth hormone release in children after cranial irradiation. Horm Res, 1987. 27(1):13–22.

87. Noorda, E.M., et al., Adult height and age at menarche in childhood cancer survivors. Eur J Cancer, 2001. 37(5):605–612.

88. Herber, S.M., et al., Growth of long term survivors of childhood malignancy. Acta Paediatr Scand, 1985. 74(3):438–441.

89. Bajorunas, D.R., et al., Endocrine sequelae of antineoplastic therapy in childhood head and neck malignancies. J Clin Endocrinol Metab, 1980. 50(2):329–335.

90. Deeg, H.J., R. Storb, and E.D. Thomas, Bone marrow transplantation: A review of delayed complications. Br J Haematol, 1984. 57(2):185–208.

91. Sanders, J.E., et al., Growth and development following marrow transplantation for leukemia. Blood, 1986. 68(5):1129–1135.

92. Sanders, J.E., Late effects in children receiving total body irradiation for bone marrow transplantation. Radiother Oncol, 1990. 18(suppl 1):82–87.

93. Livesey, E.A., et al., Endocrine disorders following treatment of childhood brain tumours. Br J Cancer, 1990. 61(4):622–625.

94. Duffner, P.K., et al., The long-term effects of cranial irradiation on the central nervous system. Cancer, 1985. 56(suppl 7):1841–1846.

95. Andler, W., K. Roosen, and H. Clar, Endocrinological investigations in 68 children with brain tumors. In Tumours of the Central Nervous System in Infancy and Childhood, D. Voth, P. Gutjahr, and C. Langmaid, eds. 1982, Berlin, Springer-Verlag.

96. Quigley, C., et al., Normal or early development of puberty despite gonadal damage in children treated for acute lymphoblastic leukemia. N Engl J Med, 1989. 321(3):143–151.

97. Lieper, A., et al., Precocious and premature puberty associated with treatment of acute lymphoblastic leukemia. Arch Dis Child, 1987. 62:1107–1112.

98. Hamre, M.R., et al., Gonadal function in survivors of childhood acute lymphoblastic leukemia: Abstract. Proc Am Soc Clin Oncol, 1985. 4:166.

99. Constine, L.S., et al., Hyperprolactinemia and hypothyroidism following cytotoxic therapy for central nervous system malignancies. J Clin Oncol, 1987. 5(11):1841–1851.

100. Eastman, R.C., P. Gorden, and J. Roth, Conventional supervoltage irradiation is an effective treatment for acromegaly. J Clin Endocrinol Metab, 1979. 48(6):931–940.

101. Littley, M.D., et al., Radiation-induced hypopituitarism is dose-dependent. Clin Endocrinol (Oxford), 1989. 31(3):363–373.

102. Sklar, C.A., et al., Changes in body mass index and prevalence of overweight in survivors of childhood acute lymphoblastic leukemia: Role of cranial irradiation. Med Pediatr Oncol, 2000. 35(2):91–95.

103. Warner, J.T., et al., Body composition of long-term survivors of acute lymphoblastic leukaemia. Med Pediatr Oncol, 2002. 38(3):165–172.

104. Notter, G., A technique for destruction of the hypophysis using yttrium 90 spheres. Acta Radiol, 1959. 184(suppl):1–128.

105. Ronckers, C.M., et al., Late health effects of childhood nasopharyngeal radium irradiation: Nonmelanoma skin cancers, benign tumors, and hormonal disorders. Pediatr Res, 2002. 52(6):850–858.

106. Ronckers, C.M., et al., No convincing evidence for a causal relationship between childhood nasopharyngeal radium irradiation and head-neck tumors or hormone-related disorders later in life: A retrospective cohort study. Ned Tijdschr Geneeskd, 2004. 148(36):1775–1780.

107. Vanderpump, M.P., et al., The incidence of thyroid disorders in the community: A twenty-year follow-up of the Whickham Survey. Clin Endocrinol (Oxford), 1995. 43(1):55–68.

108. Hollowell, J.G., et al., Serum TSH, T(4), and thyroid antibodies in the United States population (1988 to 1994): National Health and Nutrition Examination Survey (NHANES III). J Clin Endocrinol Metab, 2002. 87(2):489–499.

108a. World Health Organization (WHO), Principles and menthods for assessing autoimmunity associated with exposure to chemicals. Envirn Health Crit, no 236. 2003, Geneva, WHO.

109. DeGroot, L. and J. Jameson, eds. In *Endocrinology*, 4th ed., vol. 2. 2001, Philadelphia, W.B. Saunders.

110. Spencer, C.A., et al., Serum thyroglobulin autoantibodies: Prevalence, influence on serum thyroglobulin measurement, and prognostic significance in patients with differentiated thyroid carcinoma. J Clin Endocrinol Metab, 1998. 83(4):1121–1127.

111. Wang, Z.Y., et al., Thyroid nodularity and chromosome aberrations among women in areas of high background radiation in China. J Natl Cancer Inst, 1990. 82(6):478–485.

112. Liebow, A., S. Warran, and E. DeCoursey, Pathology of atomic bomb casualties. Am J Pathol, 1947. 25:853–1028.

113. Morimoto, I., et al., Serum TSH, thyroglobulin and thyroid disorders in atomic bomb survivors exposed in youth: A study 30 years after exposure. 1985, Hiroshima, Japan, Radiation Effects Research Foundation.

114. Nagataki, S., ed. Radiation and the Thyroid: Proceedings of the 27th Annual Meeting of the Japanese Nuclear Medicine Society (1987, Nagasaki, Japan). 1989, Amsterdam, Excerpta Medica.

115. Nagataki, S., et al., Thyroid diseases among atomic bomb survivors in Nagasaki. JAMA, 1994. 272(5):364–370.

116. Chikako, I., et al., Study on the effect of atomic bomb radiation on thyroid function. Hiroshima J Med Sci, 1987. 36:13–24.

117. Morimoto, I., et al., Serum TSH, thyroglobulin, and thyroidal disorders in atomic bomb survivors exposed in youth: 30-year follow-up study. J Nucl Med, 1987. 28(7):1115–1122.

118. Fujiwara, S., et al., Autoantibodies and immunoglobulins among atomic bomb survivors. Radiat Res, 1994. 137(1):89–95.

119. Yoshimoto, Y., et al., Prevalence rate of thyroid diseases among autopsy cases of the atomic bomb survivors in Hiroshima, 1951–1985. Radiat Res, 1995. 141(3):278–286.

120. Wong, F.L., et al., Noncancer disease incidence in the atomic bomb survivors: 1958–1986. Radiat Res, 1993. 135(3):418–430.

121. Kaplan, M.M., et al., Thyroid, parathyroid, and salivary gland evaluations in patients exposed to multiple fluoroscopic examinations during tuberculosis therapy: A pilot study. J Clin Endocrinol Metab, 1988. 66(2):376–382.

122. Markson, J.L. and G.E. Flatman, Myxoedema after deep x-ray therapy to the neck. Br Med J, 1965. 5444:1228–1230.

123. Hancock, S.L., R.S. Cox, and I.R. McDougall, Thyroid diseases after treatment of Hodgkin's disease. N Engl J Med, 1991. 325(9):599–605.

124. Loeffler, J.S., et al., The development of Graves' disease following radiation therapy in Hodgkin's disease. Int J Radiat Oncol Biol Phys, 1988. 14(1):175–178.

125. Feyerabend, T., et al., Incidence of hypothyroidism after irradiation of the neck with special reference to lymphoma patients: A retrospective and prospective analysis. Acta Oncol, 1990. 29(5):597–602.

126. Grande, C., Hypothyroidism following radiotherapy for head and neck cancer: Multivariate analysis of risk factors. Radiother Oncol, 1992. 25(1):31–36.

127. Liening, D.A., et al., Hypothyroidism following radiotherapy for head and neck cancer. Otolaryngol Head Neck Surg, 1990. 103(1):10–13.

128. Tami, T.A., et al., Thyroid dysfunction after radiation therapy in head and neck cancer patients. Am J Otolaryngol, 1992. 13(6):357–362.

129. Joensuu, H. and J. Viikari, Thyroid function after postoperative radiation therapy in patients with breast cancer. Acta Radiol Oncol, 1986. 25(3):167–170.

130. Bruning, P., et al., Primary hypothyroidism in breast cancer patients with irradiated supraclavicular lymph nodes. Br J Cancer, 1985. 51(5):659–663.

131. Larsen, P. and R. Conard, Thyroid hypofunction appearing as a delayed manifestation of accidental exposure to radioactive fallout in a Marshallese population. 1978, Upton, NY, Brookhaven National Laboratories.

132. Sutow, W. and R. Conard, The effects of fallout radiation on Marshallese children. In Radiation Biology of the Fetal and Juvenile Mammal, R. Sikov and D.D. Mahlum, eds. 1969, Washington, DC, U.S. Atomic Energy Commission.

133. Robbins, J. and W. Adams. Radiation effects in the Marshall Islands. In Radiation and the Thyroid: 27th Annual Meeting of the Japanese Nuclear Medicine Society (1987, Nagasaki, Japan). 1987, Amsterdam, Excerpta Medica.

134. Takahashi, T., et al., Thyroid Disease in the Marshall Islands: Findings from 10 years of Study. 2001, Sendai, Japan, Tohoku University Press.

135. Takahashi, T., et al., A progress report of the Marshall Islands nationwide thyroid study: An international cooperative scientific study. Tohoku J Exp Med, 1999. 187(4):363–375.

136. Rallison, M.L., et al., Natural history of thyroid abnormalities: Prevalence, incidence, and regression of thyroid diseases in adolescents and young adults. Am J Med, 1991. 91(4): 363–370.

137. Kerber, R.A., et al., A cohort study of thyroid disease in relation to fallout from nuclear weapons testing. JAMA, 1993. 270(17):2076–2082.

137a. Muschkacheva, G., E. Rabinovich, V. Privalov, et al., Thyroid abnormalities associated with protracted childhood exposure to ^{131}I from atmospheric emissions from the Mayak weapons facility in Russia. Radiat Res, 2006. 166:715–722.

138. International Atomic Energy Agency (IAEA), The International Chernobyl Project: Technical Report. 1991, Vienna, IAEA.

139. Ito, M., et al., Childhood thyroid diseases around Chernobyl evaluated by ultrasound examination and fine needle aspiration cytology. Thyroid, 1995. 5(5):365–368.

140. Yamashita, S. and Y. Shabita. Chernobyl: A decade later. In Proceedings of the 5th Chernobyl Sasakawa Medical Cooperation Symposium 1996, Kiev, October 14–15. 1996, Amsterdam, Elsevier.

141. Kasatkina, E.P., et al., Effects of low level radiation from the Chernobyl accident in a population with iodine deficiency. Eur J Pediatr, 1997. 156(12):916–920.

142. Vykhovanets, E.V., et al., ^{131}I dose-dependent thyroid autoimmune disorders in children living around Chernobyl. Clin Immunol Immunopathol, 1997. 84(3):251–259.

143. Pacini, F., et al., Prevalence of thyroid autoantibodies in children and adolescents from Belarus exposed to the Chernobyl radioactive fallout. Lancet, 1998. 352(9130):763–766.

144. Vermiglio, F., et al., Post-Chernobyl increased prevalence of humoral thyroid autoimmunity in children and adolescents from a moderately iodine-deficient area in Russia. Thyroid, 1999. 9(8):781–786.

145. Chernobyl Forum and World Health Organization, Health effects of the Chernobyl accident and special health care programmes. 2005, Geneva, World Health Organization.

146. Davis, S., et al., Thyroid neoplasia, autoimmune thyroiditis, and hypothyroidism in persons exposed to iodine 131 from the Hanford nuclear site. JAMA, 2004. 292(21):2600–2613.

147. Freedberg, A., G. Kurland, and H. Blumgart, The pathologic effects of iodine 131 on the normal thyroid gland of man. Endocrinol Metab Clin North Am, 1952. 12:1315–1348.

148. Lewitus, Z. and J. Rechnic, Electron-microscopic and isotopic evidence for a difference between the radiobiological effects of iodine 13 and iodine 125. In Radioaktive Isotope in Klinik und Forschung, Band II, R. Hofer, ed. 1975, Vienna, Urban and Schwarzenberg.

149. Snyder, W., et al., Absorbed dose per unit cumulated activity for selected radionuclides and organs. In Medical Internal Radiation Dose Committee. 1975, New York, Society of Nuclear Medicine.

150. Berger, M., Distribution of absorbed dose around point sources of electrons and beta particles in water and other media. J Nucl Med, 1971. 12(suppl):5–23.

151. Siemsen, J.K., et al., Early results of ^{125}I therapy of thyrotoxic Graves' disease. J Nucl Med, 1974. 15(4):257–260.

152. McDermott, M.T., et al., Radioiodine-induced thyroid storm: Case report and literature review. Am J Med, 1983. 75(2):353–359.

153. Connell, J.M., et al., Transient hypothyroidism following radioiodine therapy for thyrotoxicosis. Br J Radiol, 1983. 56(665):309–313.

154. Becker, D.V., Comparison of treatments for hyperthyroidism. In Radiation and the Thyroid: Proceedings of the 27th Annual Meeting of the Japanese Nuclear Medicine Society (1987, Nagasaki, Japan), S. Nagataki, ed. 1989, Amsterdam, Excerpta Medica.

155. McGregor, A.M., et al., Effects of radioiodine in thyrotropin binding inhibiting immunoglobulins in Graves' disease. Clin Endocrinol (Oxford), 1979. 11:437–444.

156. Nygaard, B., et al., Thyrotropin receptor antibodies and Graves' disease, a side-effect of ^{131}I treatment in patients with nontoxic goiter. J Clin Endocrinol Metab, 1997. 82(9):2926–2930.

157. Wallaschofski, H., et al., Induction of TSH-receptor antibodies in patients with toxic multinodular goitre by radioiodine treatment. Horm Metab Res, 2002. 34(1):36–39.

158. Werner, S., H.B. Hamilton, and M. Nemeth, Therapeutic effects from repeated diagnostic doses of iodine 131 in adults and juvenile hypothyroidism. J Clin Endocrinol, 1952. 12:1349.

159. Cunnien, A.J., et al., Radioiodine-induced hypothyroidism in Graves' disease: Factors associated. J Nucl Med, 1982. 23(11):978–983.

160. Malone, J.F., et al., The response of rat thyroid, a highly differentiated tissue, to single and multiple doses of gamma or fast neutron irradiation. Br J Radiol, 1974. 47(561):608–615.

161. Pisell, L., et al., Hyperparathyroidism and radiation therapy. Ann Int Med, 1978. 89:216–217.

162. Fujiwara, S., et al., Levels of parathyroid hormone and calcitonin in serum among atomic bomb survivors. Radiat Res, 1994. 137(1):96–103.

163. Body, J.J., N. Demeester-Mirkine, and J. Corvilain, Calcitonin deficiency after radioactive iodine treatment. Ann Intern Med, 1988. 109(7):590–591.

164. Soanes, W.A., R. Cox, and J. Maher, The effects of roentgen irradiation on the adrenal cortical function in man. AJR, 1961. 85:133–144.

165. Soanes, W.A. and C.C. Dodson, The adrenal response to irradiation on patients with testicular tumors. J Urol, 1954. 72(4):705–711.

166. Gutin, P., S. Leibel, and G.E. Sheline, eds., Radiation Injury to the Nervous System. 1991, New York, Raven Press.

167. Schultheiss, T.E., et al., Radiation response of the central nervous system. Int J Radiat Oncol Biol Phys, 1995. 31(5):1093–1112.

168. Gilbert, H. and A. Kagan, eds., Radiation Damage to the Nervous System. 1980, New York, Raven Press.

169. Scholz, W. and Y. Hsii, Late damage from roentgen irradiation of the human brain. Arch Neurol Psychiat, 1938. 40:928.

170. Bailey, O.T., J. Woodward, and T. Putnam, Tissue reactions of the human frontal white mater to gamma cobalt 60 radiation. In Response of the Central Nervous System to Ionizing Radiation, T. Haley and R. Snider, eds. 1964, Boston, Little, Brown.

171. Peterson, K., et al., Effect of brain irradiation on demyelinating lesions. Neurology, 1993. 43(10):2105–2112.

172. Rider, W., Radiation damage to the brain: A new syndrome. J Can Assoc Radiol, 1963. 14:67–69.

173. Kramer, S., M. Southard, and C. Mansfield, Radiation effects and tolerance of the central nervous system. Front Radiat Ther Oncol, 1972. 6:332–345.

174. Wachowski, T. and H. Chenault, Degenerative effects of large doses of roentgen rays on the human brain. Radiology, 1945. 45:227–246.

175. Safdari, H., et al., Radiation necrosis of the brain: Time of onset and incidence related to total dose and fractionation of radiation. Neuroradiology, 1985. 27(1):44–47.

176. Lee, A.W., et al., Clinical diagnosis of late temporal lobe necrosis following radiation therapy for nasopharyngeal carcinoma. Cancer, 1988. 61(8):1535–1542.

177. Marks, L.B. and D.P. Spencer, The influence of volume on the tolerance of the brain to radiosurgery. J Neurosurg, 1991. 75(2):177–180.

178. Tolly, T.L., et al., Early CT findings after interstitial radiation therapy for primary malignant brain tumors. AJNR Am J Neuroradiol, 1988. 9(6):1177–1180.

179. Bloom, H.J., Intracranial tumors: Response and resistance to therapeutic endeavors, 1970–1980. Int J Radiat Oncol Biol Phys, 1982. 8(7):1083–1113.

180. Valk, P.E., et al., PET of malignant cerebral tumors after interstitial brachytherapy: Demonstration of metabolic activity and correlation with clinical outcome. J Neurosurg, 1988. 69(6):830–838.

181. Tran, T.A., et al., Radiologic-pathologic conferences of the University of Texas M.D. Anderson Cancer Center: Delayed cerebral radiation necrosis. AJR Am J Roentgenol, 2003. 180(1):70.

182. Di Chiro, G., et al., Cerebral necrosis after radiotherapy and/or intraarterial chemotherapy for brain tumors: PET and neuropathologic studies. AJR Am J Roentgenol, 1988. 150(1):189–197.

183. Thiel, A., et al., Enhanced accuracy in differential diagnosis of radiation necrosis by positron emission tomography-magnetic resonance imaging coregistration: Technical case report. Neurosurgery, 2000. 46(1):232–234.

184. Ricci, P.E., Differentiating recurrent tumor from radiation necrosis: Time for re-evaluation of positron emission tomography? AJNR Am J Neuroradiol, 1998. 19(3):407–413.

185. Langleben, D.D. and G.M. Segall, PET in differentiation of recurrent brain tumor from radiation injury. J Nucl Med, 2000. 41(11):1861–1867.

186. Schwartz, R.B., et al., Radiation necrosis vs. high-grade recurrent glioma: Differentiation by using dual-isotope SPECT with 201TI and 99mTc-HMPAO. AJNR Am J Neuroradiol, 1991. 12(6):1187–1192.

187. Stokkel, M., et al., Differentiation between recurrent brain tumour and post-radiation necrosis: The value of 201Tl SPET versus 18F-FDG PET using a dual-headed coincidence camera—A pilot study. Nucl Med Commun, 1999. 20(5):411–417.

188. Hustinx, R., et al., PET imaging for differentiating recurrent brain tumor from radiation necrosis. Radiol Clin North Am, 2005. 43(1):35–47.

189. Allen, J.C., et al., Brain and spinal cord hemorrhage in long-term survivors of malignant pediatric brain tumors: A possible late effect of therapy. Neurology, 1991. 41(1):148–150.

190. Curran, W.J., et al., Magnetic resonance imaging of cranial radiation lesions. Int J Radiat Oncol Biol Phys, 1987. 13(7):1093–1098.

191. Tsuruda, J.S., et al., Radiation effects on cerebral white matter: MR evaluation. AJR Am J Roentgenol, 1987. 149(1):165–171.

192. Kay, H.E., et al., Encephalopathy in acute leukaemia associated with methotrexate therapy. Arch Dis Child, 1972. 47(253):344–354.

193. Rubinstein, L.J., et al., Disseminated necrotizing leukoencephalopathy: A complication of treated central nervous system leukemia and lymphoma. Cancer, 1975. 35(2):291–305.

194. Peylan-Ramu, N., et al., Computer assisted tomography in methotrexate encephalopathy. J Comput Assist Tomogr, 1977. 1(2):216–221.

195. Bleyer, W.A. and T. Griffin, White matter necrosis, mineralizing microangiopathy and intellectual abilities in survivors of childhood leukemia. In Radiation Damage to the Central Nervous System: A Delayed Therapeutic Hazard, H. Gilbert and A. Kagan, eds. 1980, New York, Raven Press.

196. Price, D.B., G.C. Hotson, and J.P. Loh, Pontine calcification following radiotherapy: CT demonstration. J Comput Assist Tomogr, 1988. 12(1):45–46.

197. Koike, S., et al., Asymptomatic radiation-induced telangiectasia in children after cranial irradiation: Frequency, latency, and dose relation. Radiology, 2004. 230(1):93–99.

198. Sheline, G.E., W.M. Wara, and V. Smith, Therapeutic irradiation and brain injury. Int J Radiat Oncol Biol Phys, 1980. 6(9):1215–1228.

199. Freeman, J.E., P.G. Johnston, and J.M. Voke, Somnolence after prophylactic cranial irradiation in children with acute lymphoblastic leukaemia. Br Med J, 1973. 4(5891):523–525.

200. Proctor, S.J., J. Kernaham, and P. Taylor, Depression as component of post-cranial irradiation somnolence syndrome. Lancet, 1981. 1(8231):1215–1216.

201. Meadows, A.T., et al., Declines in IQ scores and cognitive dysfunctions in children with acute lymphocytic leukaemia treated with cranial irradiation. Lancet, 1981. 2(8254):1015–1018.

202. Danoff, B.F., et al., Assessment of the long-term effects of primary radiation therapy for brain tumors in children. Cancer, 1982. 49(8):1580–1586.

203. Moore, B.D., III, J.L. Ater, and D.R. Copeland, Improved neuropsychological outcome in children with brain tumors diagnosed during infancy and treated without cranial irradiation. J Child Neurol, 1992. 7(3):281–290.

204. Duffner, P.K., M.E. Cohen, and P. Thomas, Late effects of treatment on the intelligence of children with posterior fossa tumors. Cancer, 1983. 51(2):233–237.

205. Kun, L.E., R.K. Mulhern, and J.J. Crisco, Quality of life in children treated for brain tumors. Intellectual, emotional, and academic function. J Neurosurg, 1983. 58(1):1–6.

206. Longeway, K., et al., Treatment of meningeal relapse in childhood acute lymphoblastic leukemia. II. A prospective study of intellectual loss specific to CNS relapse and therapy. Am J Pediatr Hematol Oncol, 1990. 12(1):45–50.

207. Tamaroff, M., et al., Immediate and long-term posttherapy neuropsychologic performance in children with acute lymphoblastic leukemia treated without central nervous system radiation. J Pediatr, 1982. 101(4):524–529.

208. Ochs, J., et al., Comparison of neuropsychologic functioning and clinical indicators of neurotoxicity in long-term survivors of childhood leukemia given cranial radiation or parenteral methotrexate: A prospective study. J Clin Oncol, 1991. 9(1):145–151.

209. Mulhern, R.K., et al., Late neurocognitive sequelae in survivors of brain tumours in childhood. Lancet Oncol, 2004. 5(7):399–408.

210. Trautman, P.D., et al., Prediction of intellectual deficits in children with acute lymphoblastic leukemia. J Dev Behav Pediatr, 1988. 9(3):122–128.

211. Bleyer, W.A., et al., Influence of age, sex, and concurrent intrathecal methotrexate therapy on intellectual function after cranial irradiation during childhood: A report from the Children's Cancer Study Group. Pediatr Hematol Oncol, 1990. 7(4):329–338.

212. Hulshof, M.C., et al., Hyperbaric oxygen therapy for cognitive disorders after irradiation of the brain. Strahlenther Onkol, 2002. 178(4):192–198.

213. Torres, I.J., et al., A longitudinal neuropsychological study of partial brain radiation in adults with brain tumors. Neurology, 2003. 60(7):1113–1118.

214. Steinvorth, S., et al., Cognitive function in patients with cerebral arteriovenous malformations after radiosurgery: Prospective long-term follow-up. Int J Radiat Oncol Biol Phys, 2002. 54(5):1430–1437.

215. Peper, M., et al., Neurobehavioral toxicity of total body irradiation: A follow-up in long-term survivors. Int J Radiat Oncol Biol Phys, 2000. 46(2):303–311.

216. Sato, K., et al., Radiation necrosis and brain edema association with CyberKnife treatment. Acta Neurochir Suppl, 2003. 86:513–517.

217. Noren, G., Long-term complications following gamma knife radiosurgery of vestibular schwannomas. Stereotact Funct Neurosurg, 1998. 70(suppl 1):65–73.

218. Vermeulen, S., et al., Stereotactic radiosurgery toxicity in the treatment of intracanalicular acoustic neuromas: The Seattle Northwest gamma knife experience. Stereotact Funct Neurosurg, 1998. 70(suppl 1):80–87.

219. Morita, A., et al., Risk of injury to cranial nerves after gamma knife radiosurgery for skull base meningiomas: Experience in 88 patients. J Neurosurg, 1999. 90(1):42–49.

220. Brouwers, P. and D. Poplack, Memory and learning sequelae in long-term survivors of acute lymphoblastic leukemia: Association with attention deficits. Am J Pediatr Hematol Oncol, 1990. 12(2):174–181.

221. Chessells, J.M., et al., Neurotoxicity in lymphoblastic leukaemia: Comparison of oral and intramuscular methotrexate and two doses of radiation. Arch Dis Child, 1990. 65(4):416–422.

222. Tucker, J., et al., Minimal neuropsychological sequelae following prophylactic treatment of the central nervous system in adult leukaemia and lymphoma. Br J Cancer, 1989. 60(5):775–780.

223. Ron, E., et al., Mental function following scalp irradiation during childhood. Am J Epidemiol, 1982. 116(1):149–160.

224. Shore, R.E., R.E. Albert, and B.S. Pasternack, Follow-up study of patients treated by x-ray epilation for tinea capitis: Resurvey of post-treatment illness and mortality experience. Arch Environ Health, 1976. 31(1):21–28.

225. Omran, A.R., et al., Follow-up study of patients treated by x-ray epilation for tinea capitis: Psychiatric and psychometric evaluation. Am J Public Health, 1978. 68(6):561–567.

226. Hall, P., et al., Effect of low doses of ionising radiation in infancy on cognitive function in adulthood: Swedish population based cohort study. BMJ, 2004. 328(7430):19.

227. Murphy, C.B., et al., Clinical exacerbation of multiple sclerosis following radiotherapy. Arch Neurol, 2003. 60(2):273–275.

228. Bolviken, B., et al., Radon: A possible risk factor in multiple sclerosis. Neuroepidemiology, 2003. 22(1):87–94.

229. Sibley, R.F., et al., Nested case-control study of external ionizing radiation dose and mortality from dementia within a pooled cohort of female nuclear weapons workers. Am J Ind Med, 2003. 44(4):351–358.

230. Yamada, M., et al., Prevalence and risks of dementia in the Japanese population: RERF's adult health study Hiroshima subjects. Radiation Effects Research Foundation. J Am Geriatr Soc, 1999. 47(2):189–195.

231. Imamura, Y., et al., Lifetime prevalence of schizophrenia among individuals prenatally exposed to atomic bomb radiation in Nagasaki City. Acta Psychiatr Scand, 1999. 100(5):344–349.

232. Laramore, G., Injury to the central nervous system after high-LET radiation. In Radiation Injury to the Nervous System, P. Gutin, S. Leibel, and G.E. Sheline, eds. 1991, New York, Raven Press.

233. Leibel, S., P. Gutin, and R. Davis, Factors affecting radiation injury after interstitial brachytherapy for brain tumors. In Radiation Injury to the Nervous System, P. Gutin, S. Leibel, and G.E. Sheline, eds. 1991, New York, Raven Press.

234. Bampoe, J., et al., Brain necrosis after permanent low-activity iodine-125 implants: Case report and review of toxicity from focal radiation. Brain Tumor Pathol, 2000. 17(3):139–145.

235. Wowra, B., H.P. Schmitt, and V. Sturm, Incidence of late radiation necrosis with transient mass effect after interstitial low dose rate radiotherapy for cerebral gliomas. Acta Neurochir (Wien), 1989. 99(3–4):104–108.

236. Lewanski, C.R., J.A. Sinclair, and J.S. Stewart, Lhermitte's sign following head and neck radiotherapy. Clin Oncol (R Coll Radiol), 2000. 12(2):98–103.

237. Fein, D.A., et al., Lhermitte's sign: Incidence and treatment variables influencing risk after irradiation of the cervical spinal cord. Int J Radiat Oncol Biol Phys, 1993. 27(5):1029–1033.

238. Withers, H., et al., Normal tissue radioresistance in clinical radiotherapy. In Biological Basis and Clinical Implications of Tumor Radioresistance. Proceedings of the Second Rome International Symposium, G.H. Fletcher, C. Nervi, and H. Withers, eds. 1980, Paris, Masson et Cie.

239. Douglas, M.A., L.C. Parks, and J. Bebin, Sudden myelopathy secondary to therapeutic total-body hyperthermia after spinal-cord irradiation. N Engl J Med, 1981. 304(10):583–585.

240. Phillips, T.L. and F. Buschke, Radiation tolerance of the thoracic spinal cord. Am J Roentgenol Radium Ther Nucl Med, 1969. 105(3):659–664.

241. Fitzgerald, R.H., Jr., R.D. Marks, Jr., and K.M. Wallace, Chronic radiation myelitis. Radiology, 1982. 144(3):609–612.

242. Dische, S., M.F. Warburton, and M.I. Saunders, Radiation myelitis and survival in the radiotherapy of lung cancer. Int J Radiat Oncol Biol Phys, 1988. 15(1):75–81.

243. Georgiou, A., P.W. Grigsby, and C.A. Perez, Radiation induced lumbosacral plexopathy in gynecologic tumors: Clinical findings and dosimetric analysis. Int J Radiat Oncol Biol Phys, 1993. 26(3):479–482.

244. Antunes, N.L., et al., Radiation myelitis in a 5-year-old girl. J Child Neurol, 2002. 17(3):217–219.

245. Schwartz, D.L., et al., Radiation myelitis following allogeneic stem cell transplantation and consolidation radiotherapy for non-Hodgkin's lymphoma. Bone Marrow Transplant, 2000. 26(12):1355–1359.

246. Alfonso, E.R., et al., Radiation myelopathy in over-irradiated patients: MR imaging findings. Eur Radiol, 1997. 7(3):400–404.

247. Wang, P.Y., W.C. Shen, and J.S. Jan, MR imaging in radiation myelopathy. AJNR Am J Neuroradiol, 1992. 13(4):1049–1055; discussion, 1056–1058.

248. Kinsella, T., R. Weischselbaum, and G.E. Sheline, Radiation injury of cranial and peripheral nerves. In Radiation Damage to the Nervous System, H. Gilbert and A. Kagan, eds. 1980, New York, Raven Press.

249. Olsen, N.K., et al., Radiation-induced brachial plexopathy: Neurological follow-up in 161 recurrence-free breast cancer patients. Int J Radiat Oncol Biol Phys, 1993. 26(1):43–49.

250. Pierce, S.M., et al., Long-term radiation complications following conservative surgery (CS) and radiation therapy (RT) in patients with early stage breast cancer. Int J Radiat Oncol Biol Phys, 1992. 23(5):915–923.

251. Pritchard, J., et al., Double-blind randomized phase II study of hyperbaric oxygen in patients with radiation-induced brachial plexopathy. Radiother Oncol, 2001. 58(3):279–286.

252. Schierle, C. and J. Winograd, Radiation-induced brachial plexopathy: Review. Complication without a cure. J Reconstructive Microsurgery, 2004. 20(2):149–152.

253. Brady, L.W., et al., Complications from radiation therapy to the eye. Front Radiat Ther Oncol, 1989. 23:238–250; discussion, 251–254.

254. Alberti, W., Effects of radiation on the eye and ocular adnexa. In Radiopathology of Organs and Tissuies, E. Scherer, C. Streffer, and K. Trott, eds. 1991, Berlin, Springer-Verlag.

255. Gordon, K.B., D.H. Char, and R.H. Sagerman, Late effects of radiation on the eye and ocular adnexa. Int J Radiat Oncol Biol Phys, 1995. 31(5):1123–1139.

256. Parsons, J.T., et al., Response of the normal eye to high dose radiotherapy. Oncology (Williston Park), 1996. 10(6):837–847; discussion, 847–848, 851–852.

257. Phillip, W., et al., Spontaneous corneal rupture after strontium irradiation of a conjunctival squamous cell carcinoma. Ophthalmologica, 1987. 195(3):113–118.

258. Amoaku, W.M. and D.B. Archer, Fluorescein angiographic features, natural course and treatment of radiation retinopathy. Eye, 1990. 4 (Pt 5):657–667.

259. Archer, D.B., W.M. Amoaku, and T.A. Gardiner, Radiation retinopathy—Clinical, histopathological, ultrastructural and experimental correlations. Eye, 1991. 5 (Pt 2):239–251.

260. Amoaku, W.M. and D.B. Archer, Cephalic radiation and retinal vasculopathy. Eye, 1990. 4 (Pt 1):195–203.

261. Lopez, P.F., et al., Bone marrow transplant retinopathy. Am J Ophthalmol, 1991. 112(6):635–646.

262. Brown, G.C., et al., Radiation retinopathy. Ophthalmology, 1982. 89(12):1494–1501.

263. Thompson, G.M., C.S. Migdal, and R.J. Whittle, Radiation retinopathy following treatment of posterior nasal space carcinoma. Br J Ophthalmol, 1983. 67(9):609–614.

264. Haas, A., et al., Incidence of radiation retinopathy after high-dosage single-fraction gamma knife radiosurgery for choroidal melanoma. Ophthalmology, 2002. 109(5):909–913.

265. Parsons, J.T., et al., The effects of irradiation on the eye and optic nerve. Int J Radiat Oncol Biol Phys, 1983. 9(5):609–622.

266. Nakissa, N., et al., Ocular and orbital complications following radiation therapy of paranasal sinus malignancies and review of literature. Cancer, 1983. 51(6):980–986.

267. Young, W.C., et al., Radiation-induced optic neuropathy: Correlation of MR imaging and radiation dosimetry. Radiology, 1992. 185(3):904–907.

268. Hudgins, P.A., et al., Radiation-induced optic neuropathy: Characteristic appearances on gadolinium-enhanced MR. AJNR Am J Neuroradiol, 1992. 13(1):235–238.

269. Guy, J., et al., Radiation-induced optic neuropathy: A magnetic resonance imaging study. J Neurosurg, 1991. 74(3):426–432.

270. Cogan, C., D. Donaldson, and A. Reese, Clinical and pathological characteristics of radiation cataract. Arch Ophthalmol, 1952. 47:55.

271. Merriam, G.R. and E.F. Focht, A clinical study of radiation cataracts and the relationship dose. AJR, 1957. 77:759–785.

272. Merriam, G.R., A. Szechter, and E.F. Focht, The effects of ionizing radiations on the eye. Front Radiat Ther Oncol, 1972. 6:346–385.

273. Charles, M.W. and P. Lindop, Skin and eye irradiation: Examples of some limitations of international recommendations in radiological protection: Application of the dose limitation system for radiation protection. 1979, Vienna, IAEA.

274. Bendel, I., W. Schuttmann, and B. Arndt, Cataract of the lens as a late effect of ionizing radiation in occupationally exposed persons. In Late Biological Effects of Ionizing Radiation. 1978, Vienna, IAEA.

275. Schull, W.J., Late radiation responses in man: Current evaluation from results from Hiroshima and Nagasaki. Adv Space Res, 1983. 3(8):231–239.

276. Otake, M. and W.J. Schull, The relationship of gamma and neutron radiation to posterior lenticular opacities among atomic bomb survivors in Hiroshima and Nagasaki. Radiat Res, 1982. 92(3):574–595.

277. Choshi, K., et al., Ophthalmologic changes related to radiation exposure and age in adult health study sample, Hiroshima and Nagasaki. Radiat Res, 1983. 96(3):560–579.

278. Otake, M. and W.J. Schull, Radiation-related posterior lenticular opacities in Hiroshima and Nagasaki atomic bomb survivors based on the DS86 dosimetry system. Radiat Res, 1990. 121(1):3–13.

279. Otake, M. and W.J. Schull, A review of forty-five years study of Hiroshima and Nagasaki atomic bomb survivors. Radiation cataract. J Radiat Res (Tokyo), 1991. 32(suppl):283–293.

280. Minamoto, A., et al., Cataract in atomic bomb survivors. Int J Radiat Biol, 2004. 80(5):339–345.

281. Nakashima, E., K. Neriishi, and A. Minamoto, A reanalysis of atomic-bomb cataract data, 2000–2002: A threshold analysis. Health Phys, 2006. 90(2):154–160.

282. Cucinotta, F.A., et al., Space radiation and cataracts in astronauts. Radiat Res, 2001. 156(5 Pt 1):460–466.

283. Rastegar, N., P. Eckart, and M. Mertz, Radiation-induced cataract in astronauts and cosmonauts. Graefes Arch Clin Exp Ophthalmol, 2002. 240(7):543–547.

284. Klein, B.E., et al., Diagnostic x-ray exposure and lens opacities: The Beaver Dam Eye Study. Am J Public Health, 1993. 83(4):588–590.

285. Junk, A.K., et al., Long-term radiation damage to the skin and eye after combined beta- and gamma-radiation exposure during the reactor accident in Chernobyl. Klin Monatsbl Augenheilkd, 1999. 215(6):355–360.

285a. Worgul, B.V., Y.I. Kundiyev, N.M. Sergiyenko, et al., Cataracts among Chernobyl clean-up workers: Implications regarding permissible eye exposures. Radiat Res, 2007. 167:233–243.

286. Day, R., M.B. Gorin, and A.W. Eller, Prevalence of lens changes in Ukrainian children residing around Chernobyl. Health Phys, 1995. 68(5):632–642.

287. Fedirko, P. and V. Khilinska, The state of the lens in children residing in the zone of radioactive contamination: Analysis of results of a long-term observation. Oftalmol Zh, 1998. 2:155–158.

288. Fedirko, P., Chernobyl catastrophe and the eye: Some results of a prolonged clinical-epidemiological investigation. Oftalmol Zh, 1999. 2:69–73.

289. Ivanov, V., et al., Medical Radiological Consequences of the Chernobyl Catastrophe in Russia. Estimation of Radiation Risks. 2004, St. Petersburg, Russia, Nauka.

290. Sakai, S., et al., A study of the late effects of radiotherapy and operation on patients with maxillary cancer: A survey

more than 10 years after initial treatment. Cancer, 1988. 62(10):2114–2117.

291. Oglesby, R., et al., Cataracts in patients with rheumatic diseases treated with corticosteroids. Further Observations. Arch Ophthalmol, 1961. 66:41–46.

292. Heyn, R., et al., Late effects of therapy in orbital rhabdomyosarcoma in children: A report from the Intergroup Rhabdomyosarcoma Study. Cancer, 1986. 57(9):1738–1743.

293. Nesbit, M.E., et al., Evaluation of long-term survivors of childhood acute lymphoblastic leukemia (ALL). Proc Am Assn Cancer Res, 1982. 23:107.

294. Inati, A., et al., Efficacy and morbidity of central nervous system "prophylaxis" in childhood acute lymphoblastic leukemia: Eight years' experience with cranial irradiation and intrathecal methotrexate. Blood, 1983. 61(2):297–303.

295. Deeg, H.J., et al., Cataracts after total body irradiation and marrow transplantation: A sparing effect of dose fractionation. Int J Radiat Oncol Biol Phys, 1984. 10(7):957–964.

296. Tichelli, A., et al., Cataract formation after bone marrow transplantation. Ann Intern Med, 1993. 119(12):1175–1180.

297. Hamon, M.D., et al., Incidence of cataracts after single fraction total body irradiation: The role of steroids and graft versus host disease. Bone Marrow Transplant, 1993. 12(3):233–236.

298. Barrett, A., J. Nicholls, and B. Gibson, Late effects of total body irradiation. Radiother Oncol, 1987. 9(2):131–135.

299. Appelbaum, F.R. and E.D. Thomas, Treatment of acute leukemia in adults with chemoradiotherapy and bone marrow transplantation. Cancer, 1985. 55(suppl 9):2202–2209.

300. Aristei, C., et al., Cataracts in patients receiving stem cell transplantation after conditioning with total body irradiation. Bone Marrow Transplant, 2002. 29(6):503–507.

301. Frisk, P., et al., Cataract in children after autologous bone marrow transplantation: A common, but curable complication. Lakartidningen, 2002. 99(13):1444–1447.

302. Flandin, I., et al., Impact of TBI on late effects in children treated by megatherapy for stage IV neuroblastoma: A study of the French Society of Pediatric Oncology. Int J Radiat Oncol Biol Phys, 2006. 64(5):1424–1431.

303. van Kempen-Harteveld, M.L., et al., Cataract after total body irradiation and bone marrow transplantation: Degree of visual impairment. Int J Radiat Oncol Biol Phys, 2002. 52(5):1375–1380.

304. Dynlacht, J.R., et al., Effect of estrogen on radiation-induced cataractogenesis. Radiat Res, 2006. 165(1):9–15.

305. Karslioglu, I., et al., Radioprotective effects of melatonin on radiation-induced cataract. J Radiat Res (Tokyo), 2005. 46(2):277–282.

306. Belkacemi, Y., et al., Cataractogenesis after total body irradiation. Int J Radiat Oncol Biol Phys, 1996. 35(1):53–60.

307. Hall, P., et al., Lenticular opacities in individuals exposed to ionizing radiation in infancy. Radiat Res, 1999. 152(2):190–195.

308. Wilde, G. and J. Sjostrand, A clinical study of radiation cataract formation in adult life following gamma irradiation of the lens in early childhood. Br J Ophthalmol, 1997. 81(4):261–266.

309. Dekaban, A.S., Abnormalities in children exposed to x-radiation during various stages of gestation: Tentative timetable of radiation injury to the human fetus, part I. J Nucl Med, 1968. 9(9):471–477.

310. Bateman, J.L., Ion irradiation. In Pathology of Irradiation, C. Berjis, ed. 1971, Baltimore, Williams and Wilkins.

311. Merriam, G.R., Jr., et al., The dependence of RBE on the energy of fast neutrons. IV. Induction of lens opacities in mice. Radiat Res, 1965. 25:123–138.

312. Abelson, P. and P. Kruger, Cyclotron-induced radiation cataracts. Science, 1949. 110:655–657.

313. Roth, J., et al., Effects of fast neutrons on the eye. Br J Ophthalmol, 1976. 60(4):236–244.

314. Spiess, H. and A. Gerspach, Soft-tissue effects following ^{224}Ra injections into humans. Health Phys, 1978. 35(1):61–81.

315. Stefani, F.H., H. Speiss, and C.W. Mays, Cataracts in patients injected with a solution of radium 224, colloidal platinum and the red dye eosin (Peteosthor). In Risks from Radium and Thorotrast. 1988, Bethesda, Md, British Institute of Radiology.

316. Taylor, G.N., et al., Radium-induced eye melanomas in dogs. Radiat Res, 1972. 51(2):361–373.

317. Thomas, C.I., J.P. Storaasli, and H.L. Friedell, Lenticular changes associated with beta radiation of the eye and their significance. Radiology, 1962. 79:588–597.

318. Burns, J.A., et al., Nasolacrimal obstruction secondary to I(131) therapy. Ophthal Plast Reconstr Surg, 2004. 20(2):126–129.

319. Bartalena, L., et al., Relation between therapy for hyperthyroidism and the course of Graves' ophthalmopathy. N Engl J Med, 1998. 338(2):73–78.

320. Berg, N. and M. Lindgren, Dose factors and morphology of delayed radiation lesions of the internal and middle ear in rabbits. Acta Radiol, 1961. 56:305–319.

321. Borsanyi, S., The effects of radiation therapy on the ear with particular reference to radiation otitis media. South Med J, 1952. 55:740–743.

322. Borsanyi, S. and C. Blanchard, Ionizing radiation and the ear. JAMA, 1962. 181:958–961.

323. Leach, W., Irradiation of the ear. J Laryngol Otol, 1965. 79:870–880.

324. Dias, A., Effects on the hearing of patients treated by irradiation in the head and neck area. J Laryngol Otol, 1966. 80(3):276–287.

325. Moretti, J.A., Sensori-neural hearing loss following radiotherapy to the nasopharynx. Laryngoscope, 1976. 86(4):598–602.

326. Coplin, J., et al., Hearing loss after therapy with radiation. Am Dis Child, 1981. 135:1066–1067.

327. Gabriele, P., et al., Vestibular apparatus disorders after external radiation therapy for head and neck cancers. Radiother Oncol, 1992. 25(1):25–30.

328. Gyorkey, J. and F.J. Pollock, Radiation necrosis of the ossicles. Arch Otolaryngol, 1960. 71:793–796.

329. Talmi, Y.P., Y. Finkelstein, and Y. Zohar, Postirradiation hearing loss. Audiology, 1989. 28(3):121–126.

330. Schot, L.J., et al., Late effects of radiotherapy on hearing. Eur Arch Otorhinolaryngol, 1992. 249(6):305–308.

331. Honore, H.B., et al., Sensori-neural hearing loss after radiotherapy for nasopharyngeal carcinoma: Individualized risk estimation. Radiother Oncol, 2002. 65(1):9–16.

332. Singh, I.P. and N.J. Slevin, Late audiovestibular consequences of radical radiotherapy to the parotid. Clin Oncol (R Coll Radiol), 1991. 3(4):217–219.

333. Grau, C., et al., Sensori-neural hearing loss in patients treated with irradiation for nasopharyngeal carcinoma. Int J Radiat Oncol Biol Phys, 1991. 21(3):723–728.

334. Wang, L.F., et al., A long-term study on hearing status in patients with nasopharyngeal carcinoma after radiotherapy. Otol Neurotol, 2004. 25(2):168–173.

335. Raaijmakers, E. and A.M. Engelen, Is sensorineural hearing loss a possible side effect of nasopharyngeal and parotid irradiation? A systematic review of the literature. Radiother Oncol, 2002. 65(1):1–7.

336. Walker, D.A., et al., Enhanced cis-platinum ototoxicity in children with brain tumours who have received simultaneous or prior cranial irradiation. Med Pediatr Oncol, 1989. 17(1):48–52.

337. Ang, K.K., L.C. Stephens, and T.E. Schultheiss, Oral Cavity and salivary glands. In Radiopathology of Organs and Tissues, E. Scherer, C. Streffer, and K. Trott, eds. 1991, Berlin, Springer-Verlag.

338. Kashima, H., W. Kirkham, and J. Andrews, Post-irradiation sialadenitis: A study of clinical features, histopathologic changes and seum enzyme variation following irradiation of human salivary glands. AJR, 1965. 94:271–291.

339. Oates, E., P. Touliopoulos, and D.E. Wazer, Demonstration of unilateral sialadenitis on postradiotherapy gallium-67-citrate imaging. J Nucl Med, 1993. 34(6):953–954.

340. Deeg, H.J., Acute and delayed toxicities of total body irradiation. Seattle Marrow Transplant Team. Int J Radiat Oncol Biol Phys, 1983. 9(12):1933–1939.

341. Goolden, A., J. Mallard, and H. Farran, Radiation sialitis following radiation therapy. Br J Radiol, 1957. 30:210–212.

342. Nakada, K., et al., Does lemon candy decrease salivary gland damage after radioiodine therapy for thyroid cancer? J Nucl Med, 2005. 46(2):261–266.

343. Solans, R., et al., Salivary and lacrimal gland dysfunction (sicca syndrome) after radioiodine therapy. J Nucl Med, 2001. 42(5):738–743.

344. Esfahani, A.F., et al., Semi-quantitative assessment of salivary gland function in patients with differentiated thyroid carcinoma after radioiodine-131 treatment. Hell J Nucl Med, 2004. 7(3):206–209.

345. Capizzi, R.L. and W. Oster, Chemoprotective and radioprotective effects of amifostine: An update of clinical trials. Int J Hematol, 2000. 72(4):425–435.

346. Underwood, G. and L. Gaul, Disfiguring sequelae from radium therapy: Results of a birthmark adjacent to the breast tissue in a female infant. Arch Dermatol Syph, 1948. 57:918–919.

347. Furst, C.J., et al., Breast hypoplasia following irradiation of the female breast in infancy and early childhood. Acta Oncol, 1989. 28(4):519–523.

348. Turner, C. and E. Gomez, Radiosensitivity of cells of the mammary gland. AJR Am J Roentgenol, 1936. 36:79–93.

349. Rostom, A.Y. and S. O'Cathail, Failure of lactation following radiotherapy for breast cancer (letter). Lancet, 1986. 18:163–164.

350. Findlay, P.A., et al., Lactation after breast radiation. Int J Radiat Oncol Biol Phys, 1988. 15(2):511–512.

351. Spanos, W.J., Jr., E.D. Montague, and G.H. Fletcher, Late complications of radiation only for advanced breast cancer. Int J Radiat Oncol Biol Phys, 1980. 6(11):1473–1476.

352. Robertson, J.M., et al., Breast conservation therapy. Severe breast fibrosis after radiation therapy in patients with collagen vascular disease. Cancer, 1991. 68(3):502–508.

353. Clarke, D., et al., Fat necrosis of the breast simulating recurrent carcinoma after primary radiotherapy in the management of early stage breast carcinoma. Cancer, 1983. 52(3):442–445.

354. Mendenhall, W.M., J.T. Parsons, A.A. Mancuso, et al., Larynx. In Principles and Practice of Radiation Oncology, C.A. Perez and L.W. Brady, eds. 2nd ed. 1992, Philadelphia, Lippincott.

355. Alexander, F.W., Micropathology of radiation reaction in the larynx. Ann Otol Rhinol Laryngol, 1963. 72:831–841.

356. Keene, M., et al., Histopathological study of radionecrosis in laryngeal carcinoma. Laryngoscope, 1982. 92(2):173–180.

357. van den Brenk, H., Radiation effects on the pulmonary system. In Pathology of Irradiation, C.C. Berdjis, ed. 1971, Baltimore, Williams and Wilkins.

358. Davis, S.D., D.F. Yankelevitz, and C.I. Henschke, Radiation effects on the lung: Clinical features, pathology, and imaging findings. AJR Am J Roentgenol, 1992. 159(6):1157–1164.

359. Molls, M. and D. van Beunibgen, Radiation injury of the lung. In Radiopathology of Organs and Tissues, E. Scherer, C. Streffer, and K. Trott, eds. 1991, Berlin, Springer-Verlag.

360. McDonald, S., et al., Injury to the lung from cancer therapy: Clinical syndromes, measurable endpoints and potential scoring systems. Int J Radiat Oncol Biol Phys, 1995. 31(5):1187–1203.

361. Phillips, T.L. and L. Margolis, eds., Radiation pathology and the clinical response of lung and oesophagus. In Frontiers of Radiation Therapy and Oncology, vol. 6, J. Vaeth, ed. 1972, Basil: S. Karger.

362. Fowler, J.F. and E.L. Travis, The radiation pneumonitis syndrome in half-body radiation therapy. Int J Radiat Oncol Biol Phys, 1978. 4(11–12):1111–1113.

363. Byhardt, R.W., R. Abrams, and U. Almagro, The association of adult respiratory distress syndrome (ARDS) with thoracic irradiation (RT). Int J Radiat Oncol Biol Phys, 1988. 15(6):1441–1446.

364. Kaufman, J. and R. Komorowski, Bronchiolitis obliterans: A new clinical-pathologic complication of irradiation pneumonitis. Chest, 1990. 97(5):1243–1244.

365. Roberts, C.M., et al., Radiation pneumonitis: A possible lymphocyte-mediated hypersensitivity reaction. Ann Intern Med, 1993. 118(9):696–700.

366. Trott, K.R., T. Herrmann, and M. Kasper, Target cells in radiation pneumopathy. Int J Radiat Oncol Biol Phys, 2004. 58(2):463–469.

367. Chen, Y., et al., Circulating IL-6 as a predictor of radiation pneumonitis. Int J Radiat Oncol Biol Phys, 2001. 49(3):641–648.

368. Hara, R., et al., Serum levels of KL-6 for predicting the occurrence of radiation pneumonitis after stereotactic radiotherapy for lung tumors. Chest, 2004. 125(1):340–344.

369. Fujita, J., et al., The role of anti-epithelial cell antibodies in the pathogenesis of bilateral radiation pneumonitis caused by unilateral thoracic irradiation. Respir Med, 2000. 94(9):875–880.

370. Gopal, R., et al., Effects of radiotherapy and chemotherapy on lung function in patients with non-small-cell lung cancer. Int J Radiat Oncol Biol Phys, 2003. 56(1):114–120.

371. Fujino, M., et al., Characteristics of patients who developed radiation pneumonitis requiring steroid therapy after stereotactic irradiation for lung tumors. Cancer J, 2006. 12(1):41–46.

372. Mehta, V., Radiation pneumonitis and pulmonary fibrosis in non-small-cell lung cancer: Pulmonary function, prediction, and prevention. Int J Radiat Oncol Biol Phys, 2005. 63(1):5–24.

373. Robnett, T.J., et al., Factors predicting severe radiation pneumonitis in patients receiving definitive chemoradiation for lung cancer. Int J Radiat Oncol Biol Phys, 2000. 48(1):89–94.

374. Moss, W., F. Haddy, and S.K. Sweany, Some factors altering the severity of radiation pneumonitis: Variation with cortisone, heparin and antibodies. Radiology, 1960. 75:50.

375. Koga, K., et al., Age factor relevant to the development of radiation pneumonitis in radiotherapy of lung cancer. Int J Radiat Oncol Biol Phys, 1988. 14(2):367–371.

376. Jennings, F. and A. Arden, Development of radiation pneumonitis: Time dose factors. Arch Pathol, 1962. 74:351.

377. Libshitz, H.I. and M.E. Southard, Complications of radiation therapy: Thorax. Semin Roentgenol, 1974. 9:41.

378. Rodrigues, G., et al., Prediction of radiation pneumonitis by dose-volume histogram parameters in lung cancer—A systematic review. Radiother Oncol, 2004. 71(2):127–138.

379. Kim, T.H., et al., Dose-volumetric parameters for predicting severe radiation pneumonitis after three-dimensional conformal radiation therapy for lung cancer. Radiology, 2005. 235(1):208–215.

380. Graham, M.V., et al., Clinical dose-volume histogram analysis for pneumonitis after 3D treatment for non-small cell lung cancer (NSCLC). Int J Radiat Oncol Biol Phys, 1999. 45(2):323–329.

381. Cohen, I.J., et al., Dactinomycin potentiation of radiation pneumonitis: A forgotten interaction. Pediatr Hematol Oncol, 1991. 8(2):187–192.

382. Brice, P., et al., Cardiopulmonary toxicity after three courses of ABVD and mediastinal irradiation in favorable Hodgkin's disease. Ann Oncol, 1991. 2(suppl 2):73–76.

383. Allen, A.M., et al., Body mass index predicts the incidence of radiation pneumonitis in breast cancer patients. Cancer J, 2005. 11(5):390–398.

384. Ma, L.D., et al., "Recall" pneumonitis: Adriamycin potentiation of radiation pneumonitis in two children. Radiology, 1993. 187(2):465–467.

385. Pagani, J.J. and H.I. Libshitz, CT manifestations of radiation-induced change in chest tissue. J Comput Assist Tomogr, 1982. 6(2):243–248.

386. Ikezoe, J., et al., CT appearance of acute radiation-induced injury in the lung. AJR Am J Roentgenol, 1988. 150(4):765–770.

387. Bluemke, D.A., et al., Complications of radiation therapy: CT evaluation. Radiographics, 1991. 11(4):581–600.

388. Park, K.J., et al., Radiation-induced lung disease and the impact of radiation methods on imaging features. Radiographics, 2000. 20(1):83–98.

389. Choi, Y.W., et al., Effects of radiation therapy on the lung: Radiologic appearances and differential diagnosis. Radiographics, 2004. 24(4):985–997; discussion, 998.

390. Glazer, H.S., et al., Radiation fibrosis: Differentiation from recurrent tumor by MR imaging. Radiology, 1985. 156(3):721–726.

391. Bajrovic, A., et al., Is there a life-long risk of brachial plexopathy after radiotherapy of supraclavicular lymph nodes in breast cancer patients? Radiother Oncol, 2004. 71(3):297–301.

392. Hoeller, U., et al., Radiation-induced plexopathy and fibrosis: Is magnetic resonance imaging the adequate diagnostic tool? Strahlenther Onkol, 2004. 180(10):650–654.

393. Valdes Olmos, R.A., et al., Radiation pneumonitis imaged with indium-111-pentetreotide. J Nucl Med, 1996. 37(4):584–588.

394. Kataoka, M., et al., Ga-67 citrate scintigraphy for the early detection of radiation pneumonitis. Clin Nucl Med, 1992. 17(1):27–31.

395. Kataoka, M., et al., Diffuse gallium-67 uptake in radiation pneumonitis. Clin Nucl Med, 1990. 15(10):707–711.

396. Teates, C.D., The effects of unilateral thoracic irradiation on pulmonary blood flow. Am J Roentgenol Radium Ther Nucl Med, 1968. 102(4):875–882.

397. Miller, R.W., et al., Pulmonary function abnormalities in long-term survivors of childhood cancer. Med Pediatr Oncol, 1986. 14(4):202–207.

398. Mefferd, J.M., S.S. Donaldson, and M.P. Link, Pediatric Hodgkin's disease: Pulmonary, cardiac, and thyroid function following combined modality therapy. Int J Radiat Oncol Biol Phys, 1989. 16(3):679–685.

399. Boushy, S.F., A.H. Helgason, and L.B. North, The effect of radiation on the lung and bronchial tree. Am J Roentgenol Radium Ther Nucl Med, 1970. 108(2):284–292.

400. Lingos, T.I., et al., Radiation pneumonitis in breast cancer patients treated with conservative surgery and radiation therapy. Int J Radiat Oncol Biol Phys, 1991. 21(2):355–360.

401. Lund, M.B., et al., The effect on pulmonary function of tangential field technique in radiotherapy for carcinoma of the breast. Br J Radiol, 1991. 64(762):520–523.

402. Rotstein, S., I. Lax, and G. Svane, Influence of radiation therapy on the lung-tissue in breast cancer patients: CT-assessed density changes and associated symptoms. Int J Radiat Oncol Biol Phys, 1990. 18(1):173–180.

403. Groth, S., et al., The effect of thoracic irradiation for cancer of the breast on ventilation, perfusion and pulmonary permeability: A one-year follow-up. Acta Oncol, 1989. 28(5):671–678.

404. Wohl, M.E., et al., Effects of therapeutic irradiation delivered in early childhood upon subsequent lung function. Pediatrics, 1975. 55(4):507–516.

405. Littman, P., et al., Pulmonary function in survivors of Wilm's tumor: Patterns of impairment. Cancer, 1976. 37(6):2773–2776.

406. Green, D.M., et al., Diffuse interstitial pneumonitis after pulmonary irradiation for metastatic Wilms' tumor: A report from the National Wilms' Tumor Study. Cancer, 1989. 63(3):450–453.

407. Shaw, N.J., et al., Pulmonary function in survivors of Wilms' tumor. Pediatr Hematol Oncol, 1991. 8(2):131–137.

408. Kadota, R.P., et al., Cardiopulmonary function in survivors of childhood Hodgkin's lymphoma: A pilot study (abstract). Proc Soc Clin Oncol, 1986. 5:198.

409. do Pico, G.A., et al., Pulmonary reaction to upper mantle radiation therapy for Hodgkin's disease. Chest, 1979. 75(6):688–692.

410. Tarbell, N.J., L. Thompson, and P. Mauch, Thoracic irradiation in Hodgkin's disease: Disease control and long-term complications. Int J Radiat Oncol Biol Phys, 1990. 18(2):275–281.

411. Gustavsson, A., et al., Long-term effects on pulmonary function of mantle radiotherapy in patients with Hodgkin's disease. Ann Oncol, 1992. 3(6):455–461.

412. Springmeyer, S.C., et al., Pulmonary function changes in long term survivors of allogenic marrow transplantation. In Recent Advances in Bone Marrow Transplantation, R.P. Gale, ed. 1983, New York, Alan R. Liss.

413. Einhorn, L., et al., Enhanced pulmonary toxicity with bleomycin and radiotherapy in oat cell lung cancer. Cancer, 1976. 37(5):2414–2416.

414. Taberman, A., Multiple foci of atypical epithelial hyperplasia (tumourlets) in irradiated human lungs. Br J Radiol, 1973. 46:464–466.

415. Cohen, M.D., et al., Lung nodules after whole lung radiation. Am J Pediatr Hematol Oncol, 1983. 5(3):283–286.

416. Butler, P., et al., Pulmonary hypertension after lung irradiation in infancy. Br Med J (Clin Res Ed), 1981. 283(6303):1365.

417. Cohen, L., et al., Normal tissue reactions and complications following high-energy neutron beam therapy. I. Crude response rates. Int J Radiat Oncol Biol Phys, 1989. 16(1):73–78.

418. Waxweiler, R.J., R. Roscoe, and V. Archer, Mortality follow-up through 1977 of the white underground uranium miners cohort examined by the United States Public Health Service. In International Conference on Radiation Hazards in Mining: Control, Measurement and Medical Aspects, Golden, Colorado. 1981, Kingsport, Tenn, Kingsport Press.

419. Cross, F.T., et al., Development of lesions in Syrian golden hamsters following exposure to radon daughters and uranium ore dust. Health Phys, 1981. 41(1):135–153.

420. Samet, J.M., et al., Prevalence survey of respiratory abnormalities in New Mexico uranium miners. Health Phys, 1984. 46(2):361–370.

421. Newman, L.S., M.M. Mroz, and A.J. Ruttenber, Lung fibrosis in plutonium workers. Radiat Res, 2005. 164(2):123–131.

422. Okladnikova, N.D., et al., Occupational diseases from radiation exposure at the first nuclear plant in the USSR. Sci Total Environ, 1994. 142(1-2):9–17.

423. De Vuyst, P., et al., Lung fibrosis induced by Thorotrast. Thorax, 1990. 45(11):899–901.

424. National Research Council (NRC). Committee on the Biological Effects of Ionizing Radiations (BEIR), Health risks of radon and other internally deposited alpha-emitters. BEIR IV. 1988, Washington, DC, National Academy Press.

425. Haley, P.J., Pulmonary toxicity of stable and radioactive lanthanides. Health Phys, 1991. 61(6):809–820.

426. Leung, T.W., et al., Radiation pneumonitis after selective internal radiation treatment with intraarterial 90 yttrium-microspheres for inoperable hepatic tumors. Int J Radiat Oncol Biol Phys, 1995. 33(4):919–924.

427. Edmonds, C.J. and T. Smith, The long-term hazards of the treatment of thyroid cancer with radioiodine. Br J Radiol, 1986. 59(697):45–51.

428. Cohn, K.E., et al., Heart disease following radiation. Medicine (Baltimore), 1967. 46(3):281–298.

429. Fajardo, L., M. Berthrong, and R. Anderson, Radiation Pathology. 2001, New York, Oxford University Press.

430. Schultz-Hector, S., Heart. In Radiopathology of Organs and Tissues, E. Scherer and C. Streffer, eds. 1991, Berlin, Springer-Verlag.

431. Lister, G.D. and T. Gibson, Destruction of the chest wall and damage to the heart by x-irradiation from an industrial source. Br J Plast Surg, 1973. 26(4):328–335.

432. Aretz, H.T., Myocarditis: The Dallas criteria. Hum Pathol, 1987. 18(6):619–624.

433. Weinstein, C. and J.J. Fenoglio, Myocarditis. Hum Pathol, 1987. 18(6):613–618.

434. Fajardo, L.F. and J.R. Stewart, Pathogenesis of radiation-induced myocardial fibrosis. Lab Invest, 1973. 29(2):244–257.

435. Stewart, J.R. and L.F. Fajardo, Radiation-induced heart disease: An update. Prog Cardiovasc Dis, 1984. 27(3):173–194.

436. Karas, J.S., JR, Fatal radiation syndrome from an accidental nuclear excursion. N Engl J Med, 1963. 272:756–761.

437. Fenoglio, J.J., Jr., H.A. McAllister, Jr., and F.G. Mullick, Drug related myocarditis. I. Hypersensitivity myocarditis. Hum Pathol, 1981. 12(10):900–907.

438. Taliercio, C.P., B.A. Olney, and J.T. Lie, Myocarditis related to drug hypersensitivity. Mayo Clin Proc, 1985. 60(7):463–468.

439. Pinkel, D., et al., Doxorubicin cardiomyopathy in children with left-sided Wilms tumor. Med Pediatr Oncol, 1982. 10(5):483–488.

440. Gilladoga, A.C., et al., The cardiotoxicity of adriamycin and daunomycin in children. Cancer, 1976. 37(suppl 2):1070–1078.

441. Billingham, M.E., et al., Anthracycline cardiomyopathy monitored by morphologic changes. Cancer Treat Rep, 1978. 62(6):865–872.

442. Prout, M.N., et al., Adriamycin cardiotoxicity in children: Case reports, literature review, and risk factors. Cancer, 1977. 39(1):62–65.

443. Stewart, J. and L. Fajardo, Radiation-induced heart disease. Radiat Ther Oncol, 1972. 6:274–288.

444. Stewart, J.R., et al., Radiation-induced heart disease: A study of twenty-five patients. Radiology, 1967. 89:302–310.

445. Fajardo, L.F., Radiation-induced coronary artery disease. Chest, 1977. 71(5):563–564.

446. Stewart, J.R. and L.F. Fajardo, Dose response in human and experimental radiation-induced heart disease: Application of the nominal standard dose (NSD) concept. Radiology, 1971. 99(2):403–408.

447. Gottdiener, J.S., et al., Late cardiac effects of therapeutic mediastinal irradiation. Assessment by echocardiography and radionuclide angiography. N Engl J Med, 1983. 308(10):569–572.

448. Heidenreich, P.A., et al., Diastolic dysfunction after mediastinal irradiation. Am Heart J, 2005. 150(5):977–982.

449. Adams, M.J., et al., Cardiovascular status in long-term survivors of Hodgkin's disease treated with chest radiotherapy. J Clin Oncol, 2004. 22(15):3139–3148.

450. Applefeld, M.M. and P.H. Wiernik, Cardiac disease after radiation therapy for Hodgkin's disease: Analysis of 48 patients. Am J Cardiol, 1983. 51(10):1679–1681.

451. Berry, G.J. and M. Jorden, Pathology of radiation and anthracycline cardiotoxicity. Pediatr Blood Cancer, 2005. 44(7):630–637.

452. Adams, M.J. and S.E. Lipshultz, Pathophysiology of anthracycline- and radiation-associated cardiomyopathies: Implications for screening and prevention. Pediatr Blood Cancer, 2005. 44(7): 600–606.

453. Carmel, R.J. and H.S. Kaplan, Mantle irradiation in Hodgkin's disease. An analysis of technique, tumor eradication, and complications. Cancer, 1976. 37(6):2813–2825.

454. Brosius, F.C., 3rd, B.F. Waller, and W.C. Roberts, Radiation heart disease: Analysis of 16 young (aged 15 to 33 years) necropsy patients who received over 3,500 rads to the heart. Am J Med, 1981. 70(3):519–530.

455. Veinot, J.P. and W.D. Edwards, Pathology of radiation-induced heart disease: A surgical and autopsy study of 27 cases. Hum Pathol, 1996. 27(8):766–773.

456. Makinen, L., et al., Long-term cardiac sequelae after treatment of malignant tumors with radiotherapy or cytostatics in childhood. Cancer, 1990. 65(9):1913–1917.

457. Cosset, J.M., et al., Pericarditis and myocardial infarctions after Hodgkin's disease therapy. Int J Radiat Oncol Biol Phys, 1991. 21(2):447–449.

458. Maunoury, C., et al., Myocardial perfusion damage after mediastinal irradiation for Hodgkin's disease: A thallium-201 single photon emission tomography study. Eur J Nucl Med, 1992. 19(10):871–873.

459. Cosset, J.M., et al., Late toxicity of radiotherapy in Hodgkin's disease: The role of fraction size. Acta Oncol, 1988. 27(2):123–129.

460. Savage, D.E., et al., Radiation effects on left ventricular function and myocardial perfusion in long term survivors of Hodgkin's disease. Int J Radiat Oncol Biol Phys, 1990. 19(3):721–727.

461. Glanzmann, C., et al., Cardiac risk after mediastinal irradiation for Hodgkin's disease. Radiother Oncol, 1998. 46(1):51–62.

462. Constine, L.S., et al., Cardiac function, perfusion, and morbidity in irradiated long-term survivors of Hodgkin's disease. Int J Radiat Oncol Biol Phys, 1997. 39(4):897–906.

462a. Swerdlow, A.J., C.D. Higgins, P. Smith, et al., Myocardial infarction mortality risk after treatment for Hodgkin's disease: A collaborative British cohort study. J Natl Cancer Inst, 2007. 99:206–214.

463. Jakacki, R.I., et al., Cardiac dysfunction following spinal irradiation during childhood. J Clin Oncol, 1993. 11(6):1033–1038.

464. Gagliardi, G., et al., Prediction of excess risk of long-term cardiac mortality after radiotherapy of stage I breast cancer. Radiother Oncol, 1998. 46(1):63–71.

465. Ikaheimo, M.J., et al., Early cardiac changes related to radiation therapy. Am J Cardiol, 1985. 56(15):943–946.

466. Vallis, K.A., et al., Assessment of coronary heart disease morbidity and mortality after radiation therapy for early breast cancer. J Clin Oncol, 2002. 20(4):1036–1042.

467. Darby, S.C., et al., Long-term mortality from heart disease and lung cancer after radiotherapy for early breast cancer: Prospective cohort study of about 300,000 women in US SEER cancer registries. Lancet Oncol, 2005. 6(8):557–565.

468. Patt, D.A., et al., Cardiac morbidity of adjuvant radiotherapy for breast cancer. J Clin Oncol, 2005. 23(30):7475–7482.

469. Giordano, S.H., et al., Risk of cardiac death after adjuvant radiotherapy for breast cancer. J Natl Cancer Inst, 2005. 97(6):419–424.

470. Leung, W., et al., Late effects of treatment in survivors of childhood acute myeloid leukemia. J Clin Oncol, 2000. 18(18):3273–3279.

471. Carr, Z.A., et al., Coronary heart disease after radiotherapy for peptic ulcer disease. Int J Radiat Oncol Biol Phys, 2005. 61(3):842–850.

472. Mintz, G.S., et al., Effect of intracoronary gamma-radiation therapy on in-stent restenosis: An intravascular ultrasound analysis from the gamma-1 study. Circulation, 2000. 102(24):2915–2918.

473. Waksman, R., et al., Intracoronary gamma-radiation therapy after angioplasty inhibits recurrence in patients with in-stent restenosis. Circulation, 2000. 101(18):2165–2171.

474. Waksman, R., et al., Five-year follow-up after intracoronary gamma radiation therapy for in-stent restenosis. Circulation, 2004. 109(3):340–344.

475. Costa, M.A., et al., Late coronary occlusion after intracoronary brachytherapy. Circulation, 1999. 100(8):789–792.

476. Perrault, D.J., et al., Echocardiographic abnormalities following cardiac radiation. J Clin Oncol, 1985. 3(4):546–551.

477. Carlson, R.G., et al., Radiation-associated valvular disease. Chest, 1991. 99(3):538–545.

478. Heidenreich, P.A., et al., Asymptomatic cardiac disease following mediastinal irradiation. J Am Coll Cardiol, 2003. 42(4):743–749.

479. Yahalom, J., Y. Hasin, and Z. Fuks, Acute myocardial infarction with normal coronary arteriogram after mantle field radiation therapy for Hodgkin's disease. Cancer, 1983. 52(4):637–641.

480. Prentice, R.T., Myocardial infarction following radiation. Lancet, 1965. 10:388.

481. Hamilton, D.V. and P.I. Reed, Myocardial infarction following radiotherapy for Hodgkin's disease. Br J Clin Pract, 1978. 32(6):181.

482. Orzan, F., et al., Associated cardiac lesions in patients with radiation-induced complete heart block. Int J Cardiol, 1993. 39(2):151–156.

483. Nakao, T., et al., Complete atrioventricular block following radiation therapy for malignant thymoma. Jpn J Med, 1990. 29(1):104–110.

484. Tzivoni, D., et al., Complete heart block following therapeutic irradiation of the left side of the chest. Chest, 1977. 71(2):231–234.

485. Slama, M.S., et al., Complete atrioventricular block following mediastinal irradiation: A report of six cases. Pacing Clin Electrophysiol, 1991. 14(7):1112–1118.

486. Strender, L., J. Lindahl, and L. Larsson, Incidence of heart disease and functional significance of changes in the elcectrocardiogram ten years after radiotherapy for breast cancer. Cancer, 1986. 57:929–934.

487. Larsen, R.L., et al., Electrocardiographic changes and arrhythmias after cancer therapy in children and young adults. Am J Cardiol, 1992. 70(1):73–77.

488. Brooks, C. and M. Mutter, Pacemaker failure associated with therapeutic radiation. Am J Emerg Med, 1988. 6(6):591–593.

489. Lee, R.W., et al., Runaway atrioventricular sequential pacemaker after radiation therapy. Am J Med, 1986. 81(5):883–886.

490. Salmi, J., et al., The influence of electromagnetic interference and ionizing radiation on cardiac pacemakers. Strahlenther Onkol, 1990. 166(2):153–156.

491. Brant-Zawadzki, M., et al., Radiation-induced large intracranial vessel occlusive vasculopathy. AJR Am J Roentgenol, 1980. 134(1):51–55.

492. Painter, M.J., A.M. Chutorian, and S.K. Hilal, Cerebrovasculopathy following irradiation in childhood. Neurology, 1975. 25(2):189–194.

493. Hekali, P., et al., Occlusion of the right pulmonary artery: A rare, late complication of radiation therapy. Ann Clin Res, 1982. 14(1):7–10.

494. Maunory, C., et al., Myocardial perfusion damage after mediastinal irradiation for Hodgkin's disease: A thallium 201 single photon emission tomographic study. Eur J Nucl Med, 1992. 19:871–873.

495. van Son, J.A., L. Noyez, and W.N. van Asten, Use of internal mammary artery in myocardial revascularization after mediastinal irradiation. J Thorac Cardiovasc Surg, 1992. 104(6):1539–1544.

496. Sande, L.M., J. Casariego, and A.R. Llorian, Percutaneous transluminal coronary angioplasty for coronary stenosis following radiotherapy. Int J Cardiol, 1988. 20(1):129–132.

497. McEniery, P.T., et al., Clinical and angiographic features of coronary artery disease after chest irradiation. Am J Cardiol, 1987. 60(13):1020–1024.

498. Joensuu, H., Acute myocardial infarction after heart irradiation in young patients with Hodgkin's disease. Chest, 1989. 95(2):388–390.

499. Gustavsson, A., et al., Late cardiac effects after mantle radiotherapy in patients with Hodgkin's disease. Ann Oncol, 1990. 1(5):355–363.

500. Corn, B.W., B.J. Trock, and R.L. Goodman, Irradiation-related ischemic heart disease. J Clin Oncol, 1990. 8(4):741–750.

501. Fajardo, L.F. and M. Berthrong, Vascular lesions following radiation. Pathol Annu, 1988. 23 Pt 1:297–330.

502. Steele, S.R., et al., Focused high-risk population screening for carotid arterial stenosis after radiation therapy for head and neck cancer. Am J Surg, 2004. 187(5):594–598.

503. Martin, J.D., et al., Carotid artery stenosis in asymptomatic patients who have received unilateral head-and-neck irradiation. Int J Radiat Oncol Biol Phys, 2005. 63(4):1197–1205.

504. Abayomi, O., Neck irradiation, carotid injury and its consequences. Oral Oncol, 2004. 40(9):872–878.

505. Atkinson, J.L., et al., Radiation-associated atheromatous disease of the cervical carotid artery: Report of seven cases and review of the literature. Neurosurgery, 1989. 24(2):171–178.

506. Call, G.K., et al., Carotid thrombosis following neck irradiation. Int J Radiat Oncol Biol Phys, 1990. 18(3):635–640.

507. McGuirt, W.F., et al., Irradiation-induced atherosclerosis: A factor in therapeutic planning. Ann Otol Rhinol Laryngol, 1992. 101(3):222–228.

508. Phillips, G.R., III, et al., Late complications of revascularization for radiation-induced arterial disease. J Vasc Surg, 1992. 16(6):921–924; discussion, 924–925.

509. Atabek, U., et al., Upper extremity occlusive arterial disease after radiotherapy for breast cancer. J Surg Oncol, 1992. 49(3):205–207.

510. Hashmonai, M., et al., Subclavian artery occlusion after radiotherapy for carcinoma of the breast. Cancer, 1988. 61(10):2015–2018.

511. Piedbois, P., et al., Arterial occlusive disease after radiotherapy: A report of fourteen cases. Radiother Oncol, 1990. 17(2):133–140.

512. Pettersson, F. and J. Swedenborg, Atherosclerotic occlusive disease after radiation for pelvic malignancies. Acta Chir Scand, 1990. 156(5):367–371.

513. Moritz, M.W., R.F. Higgins, and J.R. Jacobs, Duplex imaging and incidence of carotid radiation injury after high-dose radiotherapy for tumors of the head and neck. Arch Surg, 1990. 125(9):1181–1183.

514. Goodman, M.J., S.G. Lalka, and S. Reddy, Static and dynamic vascular impact of large artery irradiation. Int J Radiat Oncol Biol Phys, 1993. 26(2):305–310.

515. Dunjic, A., The influence of radiation on blood vessels and circulation. XI. Blood flow and permeability after whole body irradiation. Curr Top Radiat Res Q, 1974. 10(1):170–184.

516. Reinhold, H.S. and G.H. Buisman, Repair of radiation damage to capillary endothelium. Br J Radiol, 1975. 48(573):727–731.

517. Hopewell, J.W., et al., Microvasculature and radiation damage. Recent Results Cancer Res, 1993. 130:1–16.

518. Rahmouni, A., et al., Unusual complication of liver irradiation: Acute thrombosis of a main hepatic vein: CT and MR imaging features. Radiat Med, 1992. 10(4):163–166.

519. Fajardo, L.F. and J.R. Stewart, Experimental radiation-induced heart disease. I. Light microscopic studies. Am J Pathol, 1970. 59(2):299–316.

520. Sasaki, H., et al., The effects of aging and radiation exposure on blood pressure levels of atomic bomb survivors. J Clin Epidemiol, 2002. 55(10):974–981.

521. Nishizawa, S., et al., Post-irradiation vasculopathy of intracranial major arteries in children—Report of two cases. Neurol Med Chir (Tokyo), 1991. 31(6):336–341.

522. Prenger, K.B., et al., Massive mediastinal hemorrhage following treatment of hyperthyroidism with radioactive iodine. Thorac Cardiovasc Surg, 1984. 32(2):122–123.

523. Piers, D.A., et al., Mediastinal hemorrhage after treatment of thyrotoxicosis using radioiodine. Clin Nucl Med, 1988. 13(8):574–576.

524. Hall, P., G. Lundell, and L.E. Holm, Mortality in patients treated for hyperthyroidism with iodine-131. Acta Endocrinol (Copenhagen), 1993. 128(3):230–234.

525. Trott, K. and T. Herrmann, Radiation effects on abdominal organs. In Radiopathology of Organs and Tissues, E. Scherer, C. Streffer, and K. Trott, eds. 1991, Berlin, Springer-Verlag.

526. Coia, L.R., R.J. Myerson, and J.E. Tepper, Late effects of radiation therapy on the gastrointestinal tract. Int J Radiat Oncol Biol Phys, 1995. 31(5):1213–1236.

527. Amory, N. and I. Brick, Irradiation damage of the intestines following 1000 kV roentgen therapy: Evaluation of tolerance dose. Radiology, 1951. 56:49–57.

528. Hamilton, F., Gastric ulcer following irradiation. Arch Surg, 1947. 55:394–399.

529. Capps, G.W., et al., Imaging features of radiation-induced changes in the abdomen. Radiographics, 1997. 17(6):1455–1473.

530. Mossman, K.L., Gustatory tissue response during photon and neutron radiotherapy. Radiat Res, 1982. 91:265–274.

531. Bartoshuk, L.M., Chemosensory alterations and cancer therapies. NCI Monogr, 1990. (9):179–184.

532. Mattes, R.D., et al., A descriptive study of learned food aversions in radiotherapy patients. Physiol Behav, 1991. 50(6):1103–1109.

533. Mattes, R.D., et al., Clinical implications of learned food aversions in patients with cancer treated with chemotherapy or radiation therapy. Cancer, 1992. 70(1):192–200.

534. Schwartz, L.K., et al., Taste intensity performance in patients irradiated to the head and neck. Physiol Behav, 1993. 53(4):671–677.

535. Korcok, M., Taste loss persists after head/neck irradiation. JAMA, 1982. 247(4):422.

536. Antonadou, D., et al., Prophylactic use of amifostine to prevent radiochemotherapy-induced mucositis and xerostomia in head-and-neck cancer. Int J Radiat Oncol Biol Phys, 2002. 52(3):739–747.

537. Kouvaris, J., et al., Cytoprotective effect of amifostine in radiation-induced acute mucositis—A retrospective analysis. Onkologie, 2002. 25(4):364–369.

538. Sasse, A.D., et al., Amifostine reduces side effects and improves complete response rate during radiotherapy: Results of a meta-analysis. Int J Radiat Oncol Biol Phys, 2006. 64(3):784–791.

539. Franzen, L., et al., Effects of sucralfate on mucositis during and following radiotherapy of malignancies in the head and neck region: A double-blind placebo-controlled study. Acta Oncol, 1995. 34(2):219–223.

540. Henriksson, R., et al., Sucralfate: Prophylaxis of mucosal damage during cancer therapy. Scand J Gastroenterol Suppl, 1995. 210:45–47.

541. Huang, E.Y., et al., Oral glutamine to alleviate radiation-induced oral mucositis: A pilot randomized trial. Int J Radiat Oncol Biol Phys, 2000. 46(3):535–539.

542. Hofmeister, C.C. and P.J. Stiff, Mucosal protection by cytokines. Curr Hematol Rep, 2005. 4(6):446–453.

543. Kielbassa, A.M., et al., Radiation-related damage to dentition. Lancet Oncol, 2006. 7(4):326–335.

544. Doi, Y., et al., 13C enriched carbonate apatites studied by ESR: Comparison with human tooth enamel apatites. Calcif Tissue Int, 1981. 33(1):81–82.

545. Pass, B. and J.E. Aldrich, Dental enamel as an in vivo radiation dosimeter. Med Phys, 1985. 12(3):305–307.

546. Aldrich, J.E. and B. Pass, Determining radiation exposure from nuclear accidents and atomic tests using dental enamel. Health Phys, 1988. 54(4):469–471.

547. Hussey, D.H., et al., 50-MEVd leads to Be neutrons: A comparison of normal tissue tolerance in animals with clinical observations in patients. Int J Radiat Oncol Biol Phys, 1982. 8(12):2083–2088.

548. Seaman, W.B. and L.V. Ackerman, The effect of radiation on the esophagus: A clinical and histologic study of the effects produced by the betatron. Radiology, 1957. 68(4):534–541.

549. Lepke, R.A. and H.I. Libshitz, Radiation-induced injury of the esophagus. Radiology, 1983. 148(2):375–378.

550. Hishikawa, Y., et al., Esophageal pseudodiverticulum following high-dose-rate intracavitary irradiation for esophageal cancer. Radiat Med, 1988. 6(6):267–271.

551. Yang, Z.Y., Y.H. Hu, and X.Z. Gu, Non-cancerous ulcer in the esophagus after radiotherapy for esophageal carcinoma—A report of 27 patients. Radiother Oncol, 1990. 19(2):121–129.

552. Kaplinsky, C., et al., Esophageal obstruction 14 years after treatment for Hodgkin's disease. Cancer, 1991. 68(4):903–905.

553. Silvain, C., et al., Treatment and long-term outcome of chronic radiation esophagitis after radiation therapy for head and neck tumors: A report of 13 cases. Dig Dis Sci, 1993. 38(5):927–931.

554. Ellenhorn, J.D., et al., Treatment-related esophageal stricture in pediatric patients with cancer. Cancer, 1993. 71(12):4084–4090.

555. Boal, D.K., P.E. Newburger, and R.L. Teele, Esophagitis induced by combined radiation and adriamycin. AJR Am J Roentgenol, 1979. 132(4):567–570.

556. Laurell, G., et al., Stricture of the proximal esophagus in head and neck carcinoma patients after radiotherapy. Cancer, 2003. 97(7):1693–1700.

557. Fajardo, L.F. and A. Lee, Rupture of major vessels after radiation. Cancer, 1975. 36(3):904–913.

558. Maguire, P.D., et al., Clinical and dosimetric predictors of radiation-induced esophageal toxicity. Int J Radiat Oncol Biol Phys, 1999. 45(1):97–103.

559. Bowers, L. and A.W. Lee, Surgery in radiation injury of the stomach. Surgery, 1947. 22:20–38.

560. Findlay, J.M., et al., Role of gastric irradiation in management of peptic ulceration and oesophagitis. Br Med J, 1974. 3(5934):769–771.

561. Smith, J.C. and R.P. Bolande, Radiation and drug-induced hyalinization of the stomach. Arch Pathol, 1965. 79:310–316.

562. Becciolini, A., Relative radiosensitivities of the small and large intestine. In Advances in Radiation Biology, vol 12. 1987, New York: Academic Press.

563. Drier, J. and T. Browning, Morphologic response of the mucosa of the human small intestine to x-ray exposure. J Clin Invest, 1966. 5:194–204.

564. Lifshitz, S., et al., Plasma prostaglandin levels in radiation-induced enteritis. Int J Radiat Oncol Biol Phys, 1982. 8(2):275–277.

565. Weiss, R.G. and J.A. Stryker, 14C-lactose breath tests during pelvic radiotherapy: The effect of the amount of small bowel irradiated. Radiology, 1982. 142(2):507–510.

566. Henriksson, R., L. Franzen, and B. Littbrand, Effects of sucralfate on acute and late bowel discomfort following radiotherapy of pelvic cancer. J Clin Oncol, 1992. 10(6):969–975.

567. Lentz, S.S., M.F. Schray, and T.O. Wilson, Chylous ascites after whole-abdomen irradiation for gynecologic malignancy. Int J Radiat Oncol Biol Phys, 1990. 19(2):435–438.

568. Perkins, D.E. and H.J. Spjut, Intestinal stenosis following radiation therapy. Am J Roentgenol Radium Ther Nucl Med, 1962. 88:953–966.

569. Donaldson, S.S., et al., Radiation enteritis in children: A retrospective review, clinicopathologic correlation, and dietary management. Cancer, 1975. 35(4):1167–1178.

570. Coia, L.R. and G.E. Hanks, Complications from large field intermediate dose infradiaphragmatic radiation: An analysis of the patterns of care outcome studies for Hodgkin's disease and seminoma. Int J Radiat Oncol Biol Phys, 1988. 15(1):29–35.

571. Gelfand, M.D., et al., Acute irradiation proctitis in man: Development of eosinophilic crypt abscesses. Gastroenterology, 1968. 54(3):401–411.

572. Gehrig, J., et al., Radiation proctocolitis following gynecologic radiotherapy: An endoscopic study. Schweiz Med Wochenschr, 1987. 117(36):1326–1332.

573. den Hartog Jager, F.C., et al., The endoscopic spectrum of late radiation damage of the rectosigmoid colon. Endoscopy, 1985. 17(6):214–216.

574. Haboubi, N.Y., P.F. Schofield, and P.L. Rowland, The light and electron microscopic features of early and late phase radiation-induced proctitis. Am J Gastroenterol, 1988. 83(10):1140–1144.

575. Sanguineti, G., et al., Sucralfate versus mesalazine versus hydrocortisone in the prevention of acute radiation proctitis during conformal radiotherapy for prostate carcinoma: A randomized study. Strahlenther Onkol, 2003. 179(7):464–470.

576. Kochhar, R., et al., Radiation-induced proctosigmoiditis: Prospective, randomized, double-blind controlled trial of oral sulfasalazine plus rectal steroids versus rectal sucralfate. Dig Dis Sci, 1991. 36(1):103–107.

577. Venkatesh, K.S. and P. Ramanujam, Endoscopic therapy for radiation proctitis-induced hemorrhage in patients with prostatic carcinoma using argon plasma coagulator application. Surg Endosc, 2002. 16(4):707–710.

578. Luna-Perez, P. and S.E. Rodriguez-Ramirez, Formalin instillation for refractory radiation-induced hemorrhagic proctitis. J Surg Oncol, 2002. 80(1):41–44.

579. Kennedy, M., et al., Successful and sustained treatment of chronic radiation proctitis with antioxidant vitamins E and C. Am J Gastroenterol, 2001. 96(4):1080–1084.

580. Taylor, J.G., J.A. Disario, and D.J. Bjorkman, KTP laser therapy for bleeding from chronic radiation proctopathy. Gastrointest Endosc, 2000. 52(3):353–357.

581. Fischer, L., et al., Late progress of radiation-induced proctitis. Acta Chir Scand, 1990. 156(11–12):801–805.

582. Harling, H. and I. Balslev, Long-term prognosis of patients with severe radiation enteritis. Am J Surg, 1988. 155(3):517–519.

583. Black, W.C., et al., Quantitation of the late effects of x-radiation on the large intestine. Cancer, 1980. 45(3):444–451.

584. Wood, I., M. Walston, and G. Kurrle, Irradiation injury to the gastrointestinal tract: Clinical features, management and pathogenesis. Aust Ann Med, 1963. 12:143–152.

585. Chau, P., et al., Complications in high dose pelvis irradiation in female pelvic cancer. Am J Roentgenol, 1962. 87:22–40.

586. Hornsey, S. and S.B. Field, The RBE of cyclotron neutrons for effects on normal tissues. Eur J Cancer, 1974. 10(4):231–234.

587. Phillips, T.L., et al., Comparison of RBE values of 15 MeV neutrons for damage to an experimental tumour and some normal tissues. Eur J Cancer, 1974. 10(5):287–292.

588. Hazra, T. and R. Howells, Uses of beta emitters for intracavitary therapy. In Therapy in Nuclear Medicine, R. Spencer, ed. 1978, New York, Grune and Stratton.

589. Case, J. and A. Warthin, The occurrence of hepatic lesions in patients treated by intensive deep roentgen radiation. AJR, 1924. 12:27.

590. Ogata, K., et al., Hepatic injury following irradiation—A morphologic study. Tokushima J Exp Med, 1963. 43:240–251.

591. Ingold, J.A., et al., Radiation hepatitis. Am J Roentgenol Radium Ther Nucl Med, 1965. 93:200–208.

592. Reed, G.B., Jr. and A.J. Cox, Jr., The human liver after radiation injury: A form of veno-occlusive disease. Am J Pathol, 1966. 48(4):597–611.

593. Tefft, M., et al., Irradiation of the liver in children: Review of experience in the acute and chronic phases, and in the intact normal and partially resected. Am J Roentgenol Radium Ther Nucl Med, 1970. 108(2):365–385.

594. Kurohara, S.S., et al., Response and recovery of liver to radiation as demonstrated by photoscans. Radiology, 1967. 89(1):129–135.

595. Kraut, J., M.A. Bagshaw, and E. Glatstein, Hepatic effects of irradiation. In Frontiers of Radiation Therapy and Oncology, vol. 6. J. Vaeth, ed. 1972, Baltimore, University Park Press.

596. Johnson, P.M., F.M. Grossman, and H.L. Atkins, Radiation induced hepatic injury: Its detection by scintillation scanning. Am J Roentgenol Radium Ther Nucl Med, 1967. 99(2):453–462.

597. Chou, R.H., et al., Toxicities of total-body irradiation for pediatric bone marrow transplantation. Int J Radiat Oncol Biol Phys, 1996. 34(4):843–851.

598. Thomas, P.R., et al., Late effects of treatment for Wilms' tumor. Int J Radiat Oncol Biol Phys, 1983. 9(5):651–657.

599. Thomas, P., et al., Radiation associated toxicities in the Second National Wilm's Tumor Study. Int J Radiat Oncol Biol Phys, 1984. 10(suppl 2):88.

600. Willemart, S., et al., Acute radiation-induced hepatic injury: Evaluation by triphasic contrast enhanced helical CT. Br J Radiol, 2000. 73(869):544–546.

601. Schultz, H., et al., Nephroblastoma. Results and complications of treatment. Acta Radiol Oncol Radiat Phys Biol, 1979. 18(5):449–459.

602. Feigen, M., et al., Radiation hepatitis following moving strip radiotherapy. Int J Radiat Oncol Biol Phys, 1983. 9(3):397–400.

603. Fajardo, L.F. and T.V. Colby, Pathogenesis of veno-occlusive liver disease after radiation. Arch Pathol Lab Med, 1980. 104(11):584–588.

604. Lawrence, T.S., et al., Hepatic toxicity resulting from cancer treatment. Int J Radiat Oncol Biol Phys, 1995. 31(5):1237–1248.

605. Yankelevitz, D.F., et al., MR appearance of radiation hepatitis. Clin Imaging, 1992. 16(2):89–92.

606. Garra, B.S., et al., The ultrasound appearance of radiation-induced hepatic injury. Correlation with computed tomography and magnetic resonance imaging. J Ultrasound Med, 1988. 7(11):605–609.

607. Wharton, J.T., et al., Radiation hepatitis induced by abdominal irradiation with the cobalt 60 moving strip technique. Am J Roentgenol Radium Ther Nucl Med, 1973. 117(1):73–80.

608. McDonald, G.B., et al., Veno-occlusive disease of the liver after bone marrow transplantation: Diagnosis, incidence, and predisposing factors. Hepatology, 1984. 4(1):116–122.

609. Trott, K.R. and T. Herrmann, Radiation injury to abdominal organs. Br J Radiol Suppl, 1988. 22:30–32.

610. Bras, G., B. Jelliffe, and K. Stewart, Veno-occlusive of liver with non-portal type cirrhosis occurring in Jamaica. Arch Pathol, 1954. 57:285–300.

611. Tefft, M., A. Mitus, and N. Jaffe, Irradiation of the liver in children: Acute effects enhanced by concomitant chemotherapeutic administration? Am J Roentgenol Radium Ther Nucl Med, 1971. 111(1):165–173.

612. Johnson, F.L. and F.M. Balis, Hepatopathy following irradiation and chemotherapy for Wilms' tumor. Am J Pediatr Hematol Oncol, 1982. 4(2):217–221.

613. Phillips, T.L., Tissue toxicity of radiation-drug interactions. In Radiation-Drug Interactions in the Treatment of Cancer, G. Sokol and R. Maikel, eds. 1980, New York, John Wiley and Sons.

614. Hansen, M., et al., Fatal hepatitis following irradiation and vincristine. Acta Med Scand, 1982. 212:171–174.

615. Ariel, I., Effect of single massive doses of roentgen radiation upon the liver: Experimental study. Radiology, 1951. 57:561–575.

616. da Silva Horta, J., et al., Malignancies in Portuguese Thorotrast patients. Health Phys, 1978. 35(1):137–151.

617. Kato, Y., T. Mori, and T. Kumatori, Thorotrast dosimetric study in Japan. Environ Res, 1979. 18(1):32–36.

618. Grady, E., Adjuvant therapy for colon cancer by internal irradiation to the liver. In Therapy in Nuclear Medicine, R. Spencer, ed. 1978, New York, Grune and Stratton.

619. Ariel, I., Treatment of metastatic cancer to the liver from primary colon and rectal cancer by the intraarterial administration of chemotherapy and radioactive isotopes. In Therapy in Nuclear Medicine, R. Spencer, ed. 1978, New York, Grune and Stratton.

620. Marn, C.S., et al., Hepatic parenchymal changes after intraarterial Y-90 therapy: CT findings. Radiology, 1993. 187(1):125–128.

621. Gray, B.N., et al., Tolerance of the liver to the effects of yttrium-90 radiation. Int J Radiat Oncol Biol Phys, 1990. 18(3):619–623.

622. Brick, I., Effects of million volt radiation on the gastrointestinal tract. Arch Intern Med, 1955. 96:26–31.

623. Case records of the Massachusetts General Hospital. Weekly clinicopathological exercises. Case 31-1970. N Engl J Med, 1970. 283(4):191–201.

624. Spalding, J.F. and C. Lushbaugh, Radiopathology of islets of Langerhans in rats. Fed Proc, 1955. 14:420.

625. Volk, B.W., K.F. Wellmann, and A. Lewitan, The effect of irradiation on the fine structure and enzymes of the dog pancreas. I. Short-term studies. Am J Pathol, 1966. 48(5):721–753.

626. Pieroni, P.L., et al., Effect of irradiation on the canine exocrine pancreas. Ann Surg, 1976. 184(5):610–614.

627. Steglich, R., Untersuchen der serumlpasen als indicator einer radiogenen pankreasaffektion, M. Diuss, ed. 1987, Dresden, Med Akad.

628. Dookeran, K.A., M.M. Thompson, and W.H. Allum, Pancreatic insufficiency secondary to abdominal radiotherapy. Eur J Surg Oncol, 1993. 19(1):95–96.

629. Levy, P., et al., Abdominal radiotherapy is a cause for chronic pancreatitis. Gastroenterology, 1993. 105(3):905–909.

630. Stewart, F. and M. Williams, The urinary tract. In Radiopathology of Organs and Tissues, E. Scherer, C. Streffer, and K. Trott, eds. 1991, Berlin, Springer-Verlag.

631. Maier, J.G. and G.W. Casarett, Pathophysiologic aspects of radiation nephritis in dogs. UR Rep, 1963. 86(Jun 24):1–176.

632. Luxton, R.W. and P.B. Kunkler, Radiation nephritis. Acta Radiol Ther Phys Biol, 1964. 66:169–178.

633. Mitus, A., M. Tefft, and F. Fellers, Long-term followup of renal function in 108 children who underwent nephretomy for malignant disease. Pediatrics, 1969. 44:912–921.

634. Tarbell, N.J., et al., Renal insufficiency after total body irradiation for pediatric bone marrow transplantation. Radiother Oncol, 1990. 18(suppl 1):139–142.

635. Van Why, S.K., et al., Renal insufficiency after bone marrow transplantation in children. Bone Marrow Transplant, 1991. 7(5):383–388.

636. Borg, M., et al., Renal toxicity after total body irradiation. Int J Radiat Oncol Biol Phys, 2002. 54(4):1165–1173.

637. Kim, T.H., C.R. Freeman, and J.H. Webster, The significance of unilateral radiation nephropathy. Int J Radiat Oncol Biol Phys, 1980. 6(11):1567–1571.

638. Anderson, B., et al., Demonstration of radiation nephritis by computed tomography. Comput Radiol, 1982. 6:187–191.

639. Dewit, L., et al., Radiation injury in the human kidney: A prospective analysis using specific scintigraphic and biochemical endpoints. Int J Radiat Oncol Biol Phys, 1990. 19(4):977–983.

640. Titelbaum, D.S., et al., Renal uptake of technetium-99m methylene diphosphonate following therapeutic radiation for vertebral metastases. J Nucl Med, 1989. 30(6):1113–1116.

641. Flanagan, F.L. and F. Dehdashti, Case report: Acute segmental radiation nephritis on bone scintigraphy. Br J Radiol, 1996. 69(828):1175–1177.

642. Willett, C.G., et al., Renal complications secondary to radiation treatment of upper abdominal malignancies. Int J Radiat Oncol Biol Phys, 1986. 12(9):1601–1604.

643. Kim, T.H., P.J. Somerville, and C.R. Freeman, Unilateral radiation nephropathy—The long-term significance. Int J Radiat Oncol Biol Phys, 1984. 10(11):2053–2059.

644. Bloomfield, D.K., D.H. Schneider, and V. Vertes, Renin and angiotensin II studies in malignant hypertension after x-irradiation for seminoma. Ann Intern Med, 1968. 68(1):146–151.

645. Birkhead, B.M., et al., Assessment of renal function following irradiation of the intact spleen for Hodgkin's disease. Radiology, 1979. 130(2):473–475.

646. Koskimies, O., Arterial hypertension developing 10 years after radiotherapy for Wilms's tumour. Br Med J (Clin Res Ed), 1982. 285(6347):996–998.

647. Zuelzer, W.W., H.D. Palmer, and W.A. Newton, Jr., Unusual glomerulonephritis in young children probably radiation nephritis. Am J Pathol, 1950. 26(6):1019–1039.

648. Russell, H., Renal sclerosis, post-radiation nephritis following irradiation of the upper abdomen. Edinb Med J, 1953. 60:474–483.

649. Schreiver, B. and R. Greendyke, Radiation nephritis: Report of a fatal case. Am J Med, 1959. 26:146–151.

650. Luxton, R.W., Radiation nephritis. Q J Med, 1953. 22:215–242.

651. Maier, J.G., Effects of radiation on kidney, bladder, and prostate. Front Radiat Ther Oncol, 1972. 6:196–227.

652. Jaffe, N., et al., Childhood urologic cancer therapy related sequelae and their impact on management. Cancer, 1980. 45(suppl 7):1815–1822.

653. Yamada, M., et al., Noncancer disease incidence in atomic bomb survivors, 1958–1998. Radiat Res, 2004. 161(6):622–632.

654. Schmitz, H., Compolications of the urinary tract due to carcinoma of the cervix or radiation treatment. AJR, 1930. 24:47.

655. Montana, G.S. and W.C. Fowler, Carcinoma of the cervix: Analysis of bladder and rectal radiation dose and complications. Int J Radiat Oncol Biol Phys, 1989. 16(1):95–100.

656. Morrison, R. and T. Deeley, The treatment of carcinoma of the bladder by supervoltage x-rays. Br J Radiol, 1965. 38:449–458.

657. Crew, J.P., C.R. Jephcott, and J.M. Reynard, Radiation-induced haemorrhagic cystitis. Eur Urol, 2001. 40(2):111–123.

658. Goodman, M. and J.R. Dalton, Ureteral strictures following radiotherapy: Incidence, etiology and treatment guidelines. J Urol, 1982. 128(1):21–24.

659. Leisener, H. and O. Kjellgren, Radium reactions in the bladder. Acta Obstet Gynecol Scand, 1959. 38:544–550.

660. Parliament, M., et al., Obstructive ureteropathy following radiation therapy for carcinoma of the cervix. Gynecol Oncol, 1989. 33(2):237–240.

661. Behr, J., M. Winkler, and F. Willgeroth, Functional changes in the lower urinary tract after irradiation of cervix carcinoma. Strahlenther Onkol, 1990. 166(2):135–139.

662. Vanuytsel, L., et al., Radiotherapy in multiple fractions per day for prostatic carcinoma: Late complications. Int J Radiat Oncol Biol Phys, 1986. 12(9):1589–1595.

663. Green, N., D. Treible, and H. Wallack, Prostate cancer: Post-irradiation incontinence. J Urol, 1990. 144(2 Pt 1):307–309.

664. Lawton, C.A., et al., Long-term treatment sequelae following external beam irradiation for adenocarcinoma of the prostate: Analysis of RTOG studies 7506 and 7706. Int J Radiat Oncol Biol Phys, 1991. 21(4):935–939.

665. Moul, J.W., Retroperitoneal fibrosis following radiotherapy for stage I testicular seminoma. J Urol, 1992. 147(1):124–126.

666. Suresh, U.R., et al., Radiation disease of the urinary tract: Histological features of 18 cases. J Clin Pathol, 1993. 46(3):228–231.

667. Fowler, J.W., A.J. Hart, and W. Duncan, The effects of radiotherapy on the integrity of the ureteroileal segment following cystectomy. Br J Urol, 1982. 54(2):126–129.

668. Batterman, J.J., Results of d-T neutron irradiation on advanced tumors of the bladder and rectum. Int J Radiat Oncol Biol Phys, 1982. 8:2159–2164.

669. McGeoghegan, D. and K. Binks, The mortality and cancer morbidity experience of workers at the Capenhurst uranium enrichment facility 1946–1995. J Radiol Prot, 2000. 20(4):381–401.

670. McGeoghegan, D. and K. Binks, The mortality and cancer morbidity experience of workers at the Springfields uranium production facility, 1946–1995. J Radiol Prot, 2000. 20(2):111–137.

671. Pinney, S.M., et al., Health effects in community residents near a uranium plant at Fernald, Ohio, USA. Int J Occup Med Environ Health, 2003. 16(2):139–153.

672. Merrick, G.S., et al., Dysuria after permanent prostate brachytherapy. Int J Radiat Oncol Biol Phys, 2003. 55(4):979–1085.

673. Merrick, G.S., et al., Risk factors for the development of prostate brachytherapy related urethral strictures. J Urol, 2006. 175(4):1376–80; discussion, 1381.

674. Benoit, R.M., M.J. Naslund, and J.K. Cohen, Complications after prostate brachytherapy in the Medicare population. Urology, 2000. 55(1):91–96.

675. Incrocci, L., A.K. Slob, and P.C. Levendag, Sexual (dys)function after radiotherapy for prostate cancer: A review. Int J Radiat Oncol Biol Phys, 2002. 52(3):681–693.

676. Robinson, J.W., S. Moritz, and T. Fung, Meta-analysis of rates of erectile function after treatment of localized prostate carcinoma. Int J Radiat Oncol Biol Phys, 2002. 54(4):1063–1068.

677. Lushbaugh, C. and R. Ricks, Some cytokinetic and histopathological considerations of male and female gonadal tissues. Front Radiat Ther Oncol, 1972. 6:228–248.

678. Ladner, H., Reproductive organs. In Radiopathology of Organs and Tissues, E. Scherer, C. Streffer, and K. Trott, eds. 1991, Berlin, Springer-Verlag.

679. Livesey, E.A. and C.G. Brook, Gonadal dysfunction after treatment of intracranial tumours. Arch Dis Child, 1988. 63(5):495–500.

680. Clayton, P.E., et al., Ovarian function following chemotherapy for childhood brain tumours. Med Pediatr Oncol, 1989. 17(2):92–96.

681. Byrne, J., et al., Effects of treatment on fertility in long-term survivors of childhood or adolescent cancer. N Engl J Med, 1987. 317(21):1315–1321.

682. Wallace, W.H., A.B. Thomson, and T.W. Kelsey, The radiosensitivity of the human oocyte. Hum Reprod, 2003. 18(1):117–121.

683. Patterson, R., The Treatment of Malignant Disease by Radiotherapy. 1963, Baltimore, Williams and Wilkins.

684. Glucksman, A., The effects of radiation on reproductive organs. Br J Radiol, 1947. 1:101–109.

685. Thomas, P., et al., Reproductive and endocrine function in patients with Hodgkin's disease: Effects of oophoropexy and irradiation. Br J Cancer, 1976. 33:225–231.

686. Ray, G., et al., Oophoropexy: A means of preserving ovarian function following pelvic megavoltage radiotherapy for Hodgkin's disease. Radiology, 1970. 96:175–180.

687. Peck, W., et al., Castration of the female by irradiation. Radiology, 1940. 34:176–186.

688. Lacassagne, A., et al., The action of ionizing radiation of the mammalian ovary. In The Ovary. 1962, New York, Academic Press.

689. Rubin, P. and G.W. Casarett, eds., A direction for clinical radiation pathology. In Frontiers in Radiation Therapy and Oncology, vol. 6, J. Vaeth, ed. 1972, Basil, Karger.

690. Smith, P.G. and R. Doll, Late effects of x-irradiation in patients treated for metropathia haemorrhagica. Br J Radiol, 1976. 49(579):224–232.

691. Kaplan, I., Genetic effects in children and grandchildren of women treated for infertility and sterility by roentgen therapy: A report of the study of 33 years. Radiology, 1959. 72:518–521.

692. Horning, S.J., et al., Female reproductive potential after treatment for Hodgkin's disease. N Engl J Med, 1981. 304(23):1377–1382.

693. Diczfaluswy, E., et al., Estrogen excretion in breast cancer patients before and after ovarian irradiation and oophorectomy. J Clin Endocrinol, 1959. 19:1230–1244.

694. Jacox, W., Recovery following human ovarian irradiation. Radiology, 1939. 32:528.

695. Stillman, R.J., et al., Ovarian failure in long-term survivors of childhood malignancy. Am J Obstet Gynecol, 1981. 139(1):62–66.

696. Ortin, T.T., C.A. Shostak, and S.S. Donaldson, Gonadal status and reproductive function following treatment for Hodgkin's disease in childhood: The Stanford experience. Int J Radiat Oncol Biol Phys, 1990. 19(4):873–880.

697. Wallace, W.H., et al., Ovarian failure following abdominal irradiation in childhood: Natural history and prognosis. Clin Oncol (R Coll Radiol), 1989. 1(2):75–79.

698. Wallace, W.H., et al., Ovarian failure following abdominal irradiation in childhood: The radiosensitivity of the human oocyte. Br J Radiol, 1989. 62(743):995–998.

699. Sklar, C., Maintenance of ovarian functin and risk of premature menopause related to cancer treatment. J Nat Cancer Inst Monograph, 2005. 34:25–27.

700. Doll, R. and P.G. Smith, The long-term effects of x irradiation in patients treated for metropathia haemorrhagica. Br J Radiol, 1968. 41(485):362–368.

701. Critchley, H.O., L.E. Bath, and W.H. Wallace, Radiation damage to the uterus—Review of the effects of treatment of childhood cancer. Hum Fertil (Cambridge), 2002. 5(2):61–66.

702. Larsen, E.C., et al., Radiotherapy at a young age reduces uterine volume of childhood cancer survivors. Acta Obstet Gynecol Scand, 2004. 83(1):96–102.

703. Hamberger, A.D., et al., Analysis of the severe complications of irradiation of carcinoma of the cervix: Whole pelvis irradiation and intracavitary radium. Int J Radiat Oncol Biol Phys, 1983. 9(3):367–371.

704. Graham, R., The effect of radiation on vaginal cells on cervical carcinoma—The prognostic significance. Surg Gynecol Obstet, 1947. 84:166–173.

705. Rhomberg, W. and H. Eiter, Radiation-induced vaginal necrosis. Strahlenther Onkol, 1988. 164(9):527–530.

706. Fanger, H. and C.C. Lushbaugh, Radiation death from cardiovascular shock following a criticality accident: Report of a second death from a newly defined human radiation death syndrome. Arch Pathol, 1967. 83(5):446–460.

707. Oakes, W.R. and C.C. Lushbaugh, Course of testicular injury following accidental exposure to nuclear radiations: Report of a case. Radiology, 1952. 59(5):737–743.

708. Heller, C., Radiobiological factors in manned space flights. In Report of the Space Radiation Study Panel of the Life Sciences Committee, W. Langham, ed. 1967, Washington, DC, National Academy of Sciences.

709. Smithers, D.W., D.M. Wallace, and D.E. Austin, Fertility after unilateral orchidectomy and radiotherapy for patients with malignant tumours of the testis. Br Med J, 1973. 4(5884):77–79.

710. Lushbaugh, C.C. and G.W. Casarett, The effects of gonadal irradiation in clinical radiation therapy: A review. Cancer, 1976. 37(suppl 2):1111–1125.

711. United Nations Scientific Committee on the Effects of Atomic Radiation (UNSCEAR), Ionizing radiation: Sources and effects. In UNSCEAR report to the General Assembly, in annex K: Radiation-induced life shortening. 1982, New York, United Nations, p. v.

712. Andrews, G., et al., Report of 21-year medical follow-up of survivors of the Oak Ridge Y-12 accident. In The Medical Basis of Radiation Accident Preparedness. 1980, New York, Elsevier/North Holland.

713. Liebow, A., Encounter with disaster—A medical diary of Hiroshima, 1945. Yale J Biol Med, 1965. 38:61–239.

714. Kinsella, T.J., Effects of radiation therapy and chemotherapy on testicular function. Prog Clin Biol Res, 1989. 302:157–171; discussion, 172–177.

715. Howell, S., Spermatogenesis after cancer treatment: Damage and recovery. J Nat Cancer Inst Monograph, 2005. 34:12–17.

716. Hansen, P.V., et al., Long-term recovery of spermatogenesis after radiotherapy in patients with testicular cancer. Radiother Oncol, 1990. 18(2):117–125.

717. Shalet, S.M., et al., Vulnerability of the human Leydig cell to radiation damage is dependent upon age. J Endocrinol, 1989. 120(1):161–165.

718. Shafford, E.A., et al., Testicular function following the treatment of Hodgkin's disease in childhood. Br J Cancer, 1993. 68(6):1199–1204.

719. Huyghe, E., et al., Fertility after testicular cancer treatments: Results of a large multicenter study. Cancer, 2004. 100(4):732–737.

720. Goldman, S. and F.L. Johnson, Effects of chemotherapy and irradiation on the gonads. Endocrinol Metab Clin North Am, 1993. 22(3):617–629.

721. Geraci, J.P., et al., Cyclotron fast neutron RBE for various normal tissues. Radiology, 1975. 115(2):459–463.

722. de Ruiter-Bootsma, A.L., M.F. Kramer, and D.G. de Rooij, Response of stem cells in the mouse testis to fission neutrons of

1 MeV mean energy and 300 kV x rays: Methodology, dose-response studies, relative biological effectiveness. Radiat Res, 1976. 67(1):56–68.

723. Casey, R., M.A. Jewett, and R.A. Facey, Effective depth of spermatogonia in man. I. Measurement of scrotal thickness. Phys Med Biol, 1982. 27(11):1349–1356.

724. Facey, R.A., Effective depth of spermatogonia in man. II. Calculations for external high-energy beta rays. Phys Med Biol, 1982. 27(11):1357–1365.

725. Srivastava, P.N. and S.R. Chadha, The effect of radiophosphorus on the development of gonads in mice. Strahlentherapie, 1970. 139(6):738–743.

726. Samuels, L.D., Effects of polonium-210 on mouse ovaries. Int J Radiat Biol Relat Stud Phys Chem Med, 1966. 11(2):117–130.

727. Ronnback, C., B. Henricson, and A. Nilsson, Effect of different doses of ^{90}Sr on the ovaries of the foetal mouse. Acta Radiol Suppl, 1971. 310:200–209.

728. Ronnback, C. and A. Nilsson, Influence of oestrogen on the excretion of strontium-90 and -85 in mice. Acta Radiol Ther Phys Biol, 1975. 14(5):485–496.

729. Beaumont, H.M., The radiosensitivity of germ-cells at various stages of ovarian development. Int J Radiat Biol, 1962. 4:581–590.

730. Dobson, R.L., How toxic is tritium? Relevance of high-dose results and gamma-ray data to evaluating low-level, chronic exposure. Environ Health Perspect, 1978. 22:145–147.

731. Lathrop, K., I. Gloria, and P. Harper, Response of mouse foetus to radiation fro Na 99m-TcO4: Biological and environmental effects of low-level radiation, vol 2. 1975, Vienna: IAEA.

732. Wichers, M., et al., Testicular function after radioiodine therapy for thyroid carcinoma. Eur J Nucl Med, 2000. 27(5):503–507.

733. International Commission on Radiological Protection (ICRP), Radiation safety aspects of brachytherapy for prostate cancer using permanently implanted sources: A report of ICRP Pub. 98. Ann ICRP, 2005. 35(3):iii–vi, 3–50.

734. Barringer, B., et al., Roentgen treatment of benign hypertrophy of the prostatic gland. Am J Roentgenol, 1934. 31:350–357.

735. Chan, T. and H. Kressel, Prostate and seminal vesicles after irradiation: MR appearance. J Magn Reson Imag, 1991. 1:503–511.

736. Haile, K. and L. Delclos, The place of radiation therapy in the treatment of carcinoma of the distal end of the penis. Cancer, 1980. 45(suppl 7):1980–1984.

737. Collins, V. and M. Gaulden, A case of child abuse by radiation exposure. In Medical Basis for Radiation Accident Preparedness, K. Hubner and S. Fry, eds. 1980, New York, Elsevier/North Holland.

738. Suchaud, J., et al., Brachytherapy of cancer of the penis: Analysis of 53 cases. J Urol (Paris), 1989. 95(95):27–31.

739. Kaufman, J.J., R.B. Smith, and S. Raz, Radiation therapy in carcinoma of the prostate: A contributing cause of urinary incontinence. J Urol, 1984. 132(5):998–999.

740. Banker, F.L., The preservation of potency after external beam irradiation for prostate cancer. Int J Radiat Oncol Biol Phys, 1988. 15(1):219–220.

741. van Heeringen, C., A. De Schryver, and E. Verbeek, Sexual function disorders after local radiotherapy for carcinoma of the prostate. Radiother Oncol, 1988. 13:47–52.

742. Mittal, B., A study of penile circulation before and after radiation in patients with prostrate cancer and its effect on impotence. Int J Radiat Oncol Biol Phys, 1985. 11:1121–1125.

743. Merrick, G., et al., A comparison of radiation dose to the bulb of the penis in men with and without prostate brachytherapy-induced erectile dysfunction. Int J Radiat Oncol Biol Phys, 2001. 50(3): 597–604.

744. Engleman, M.A., G. Woloschak, and W. Small, Jr., Radiation-induced skeletal injury. Cancer Treat Res, 2006. 128:155–169.

745. Desjardins, A., Osteogenic tumor: Growth injury of bone and muscular atrophy following therapeutic irradiation. Radiology, 1930. 14:296.

746. Stevens, R., Retardation of bone growth following roentgen irradiation of an extensive nevocarcinoma of the skin of an infant four months of age. Radiology, 1935. 25:538–546.

747. Spangler, D., The effect of x-ray therapy for closure of the epiphysis: Preliminary report. Radiology, 1941. 37:310–315.

748. Neuhauser, E., et al., Irradiation effects of roentgen therapy on the growing spine. Radiology, 1951. 9:637–650.

749. Probert, J.C. and B.R. Parker, The effects of radiation therapy on bone growth. Radiology, 1975. 114(1):155–162.

750. Gauwerky, F., On radiation injury of growing bone. I. Stud Med, 1960. 113:325–350.

751. Rausch, L. and E. Ander, Investigations of the relationship between local and general radiation sensitivity. Strahlentherapie [Sonderb], 1966. 62:198–205.

752. Kember, N.F. and J. Coggins, Changes in the vascular supply to rat growth cartilage during radiation injury and repair. Int J Radiat Biol, 1967. 12:143–151.

753. McLean, F. and A. Budy, Radiation, Isotopes and Bone. 1964, New York, Academic Press.

754. Otake, M., et al., A longitudinal study of growth and development of stature among prenatally exposed atomic bomb survivors. Radiat Res, 1993. 134(1):94–101.

755. Nakashima, E., Relationship of five anthropometric measurements at age 18 to radiation dose among atomic bomb survivors exposed in utero. Radiat Res, 1994. 138(1):121–126.

756. Scheibel-Jost, P., et al., Spinal growth after irradiation for Wilms' tumour. Int Orthop, 1991. 15(4):387–391.

757. Makipernaa, A., et al., Spinal deformity induced by radiotherapy for solid tumours in childhood: A long-term follow up study. Eur J Pediatr, 1993. 152(3):197–200.

758. Goldwein, J.W. and J. Meadows, Influence of radiation on growth in pediatric patients. Clin Plast Surg, 1993. 20:455–464.

759. Paulino, A.C., et al., Late effects in children treated with radiation therapy for Wilms' tumor. Int J Radiat Oncol Biol Phys, 2000. 46(5):1239–1246.

760. Rate, W.R., et al., Late orthopedic effects in children with Wilms' tumor treated with abdominal irradiation. Med Pediatr Oncol, 1991. 19(4):265–268.

761. Robertson, W.W., Jr., et al., Leg length discrepancy following irradiation for childhood tumors. J Pediatr Orthop, 1991. 11(3):284–287.

762. Paulino, A.C., Late effects of radiotherapy for pediatric extremity sarcomas. Int J Radiat Oncol Biol Phys, 2004. 60(1):265–274.

763. Larson, D.L., et al., Long-term effects of radiotherapy in childhood and adolescence. Am J Surg, 1990. 160(4):348–351.

764. Smith, R., J.K. Davidson, and G.E. Flatman, Skeletal effects of orthovoltage and megavoltage therapy following treatment of nephroblastoma. Clin Radiol, 1982. 33(6):601–613.

765. Heaston, D.K., H.I. Libshitz, and R.C. Chan, Skeletal effects of megavoltage irradiation in survivors of Wilms' tumor. AJR Am J Roentgenol, 1979. 133(3):389–395.

766. Gilsanz, V., et al., Osteoporosis after cranial irradiation for acute lymphoblastic leukemia. J Pediatr, 1990. 117(2 Pt 1): 238–244.

767. Barrett, I.R., Slipped capital femoral epiphysis following radiotherapy. J Pediatr Orthop, 1985. 5(3):268–273.

768. Walker, S.J., et al., Slipped capital femoral epiphysis following radiation and chemotherapy. Clin Orthop Relat Res, 1981(159):186–193.

769. Silverman, C.L., et al., Slipped femoral capital epiphyses in irradiated children: Dose, volume and age relationships. Int J Radiat Oncol Biol Phys, 1981. 7(10):1357–1363.

770. Edeiken, B.S., H.I. Libshitz, and M.A. Cohen, Slipped proximal humeral epiphysis: A complication of radiotherapy to the shoulder in children. Skeletal Radiol, 1982. 9(2):123–125.

771. Parker, R., Tolerance of mature bone and cartilage in clinical radiation therapy. In Frontiers of Radiation Therapy and Oncology, vol. 6, J. Vaeth, ed. 1972, Basel, Karger.

772. Prindull, G., et al., Aseptic osteonecrosis in children treated for acute lymphoblastic leukemia and aplastic anemia. Eur J Pediatr, 1982. 139(1):48–51.

773. Seldin, H., Radio-osteomyelitis of the jaw. J Oral Surg, 1955. 13:112–119.

774. Regen, E. and W. Wilkins, On rate of healing of fractures and phosphatase activity of callus of adult bone. J Bone Joint Surg Am, 1936. 18:69–79.

775. Murray, C.G., et al., Radiation necrosis of the mandible: A 10-year study. I. Factors influencing the onset of necrosis. Int J Radiat Oncol Biol Phys, 1980. 6(5):543–548.

776. Murray, C.G., et al., Radiation necrosis of the mandible: A 10-year study. II. Dental factors: Onset, duration and management of necrosis. Int J Radiat Oncol Biol Phys, 1980. 6(5):549–553.

777. Schratter-Sehn, A.U., et al., Incidence of osteoradionecrosis after combined radiotherapy-chemotherapy of head and neck tumors. Strahlenther Onkol, 1991. 167(3):165–168.

778. Parker, R.G. and H.C. Berry, Late effects of therapeutic irradiation on the skeleton and bone marrow. Cancer, 1976. 37(suppl 2):1162–1171.

779. Overgaard, M., Spontaneous radiation-induced rib fractures in breast cancer patients treated with postmastectomy irradiation: A clinical radiobiological analysis of the influence of fraction size and dose-response relationships on late bone damage. Acta Oncol, 1988. 27(2):117–122.

780. Abe, H., et al., Radiation-induced insufficiency fractures of the pelvis: Evaluation with 99mTc-methylene diphosphonate scintigraphy. AJR Am J Roentgenol, 1992. 158(3):599–602.

781. Blomlie, V., et al., Radiation-induced insufficiency fractures of the sacrum: Evaluation with MR imaging. Radiology, 1993. 188(1):241–244.

782. David, L.A., et al., Hyperbaric oxygen therapy and mandibular osteoradionecrosis: A retrospective study and analysis of treatment outcomes. J Can Dent Assoc, 2001. 67(7):384.

783. Delanian, S. and J.L. Lefaix, Complete healing of severe osteoradionecrosis with treatment combining pentoxifylline, tocopherol and clodronate. Br J Radiol, 2002. 75(893):467–469.

784. Mitchell, M.J. and P.M. Logan, Radiation-induced changes in bone. Radiographics, 1998. 18(5):1125–1136; quiz, 1242–1243.

785. Williams, H.J. and A.M. Davies, The effect of x-rays on bone: A pictorial review. Eur Radiol, 2006. 16(3):619–633.

786. Sonis, A.L., et al., Dentofacial development in long-term survivors of acute lymphoblastic leukemia. A comparison of three treatment modalities. Cancer, 1990. 66(12):2645–2652.

787. Jaffe, N., et al., Dental and maxillofacial abnormalities in long-term survivors of childhood cancer: Effects of treatment with chemotherapy and radiation to the head and neck. Pediatrics, 1984. 73(6):816–823.

788. Sciubba, J.J. and D. Goldenberg, Oral complications of radiotherapy. Lancet Oncol, 2006. 7(2):175–183.

789. Hattner, R.S., J. Hartmeyer, and W.M. Wara, Characterization of radiation-induced photopenic abnormalities on bone scans. Radiology, 1982. 145(1):161–163.

790. Bragg, D.G., et al., The clinical and radiographic aspects of radiation osteitis. Radiology, 1970. 97(1):103–111.

791. Baclesse, F., Clinical experience with ultrafractionated roentgen therapy. In Progress in Radiation Therapy. 1958, New York, Grune and Stratton.

792. Fletcher, G.H. and R. Klein, Dose-time-volume relationship in squamous cell carcinoma of the larynx. Radiology, 1964. 82:1032–1041.

793. Fitzgerald, P.J. and R.J. Koch, Delayed radionecrosis of the larynx. Am J Otolaryngol, 1999. 20(4):245–249.

794. Collis, C.H., P.A. Dieppe, and J.A. Bullimore, Radiation-induced chondrocalcinosis of the knee articular cartilage. Clin Radiol, 1988. 39(4):450–451.

795. Gerstner, B., R. Lewis, and E. Rickey, Early effects of high intensity x-irradiation of skeletal muscle. J Gen Physiol, 1954. 37:445–459.

796. Zeman, W. and M. Solomon, Effects of radiation on striated muscle. In Pathology of Irradiation, C. Berdjis, ed. 1971, Baltimore, Willliams and Wilkins.

797. Carl, U.M. and K.A. Hartmann, Heterotopic calcification as a late radiation effect: Report of 15 cases. Br J Radiol, 2002. 75(893):460–463.

798. Soulen, R.L., et al., Musculoskeletal complications of neutron therapy for prostate cancer. Radiat Oncol Invest, 1997. 5(2):81–91.

799. Kember, N.F., Radiobiolical investigations with fast neutrons using the cartilage clone system. Br J Radiol, 1969. 42(500):595–597.

800. Dixon, B., The effect of radiation on the growth of vertebrae in the tails of rats. II. Split doses of x-rays and the effect of oxygen. Int J Radiat Biol Relat Stud Phys Chem Med, 1969. 15(3):215–226.

801. Dixon, B., The effect of radiation on the growth of vertebrae in the tails of rats. 3. The response to cyclotron neutrons. Int J Radiat Biol Relat Stud Phys Chem Med, 1969. 15(6):541–548.

802. Kember, N.F., Cell survival and radiation damage in growth cartilage. Br J Radiol, 1967. 40(475):496–505.

803. Rowland, R., et al., Some dose response relationships for tumor incidence in radium patients. In Annual Report, July 1969–June 1970, R.P. Division, ed. 1970, Washington, DC, Center for Human Radiobiology.

804. Aub, J.C., et al., The late effects of internally deposited radioactive materials in man. Medicine, 1952. 31(3):221–329.

805. Sharpe, W.D., Chronic radium intoxication: Clinical and autopsy findings in long-term New Jersey survivors. Environ Res, 1974. 8(3):243–383.

806. Evans, R., The effect of skeletally deposited alpha ray emitters in man. Br J Radiol, 1966. 39:881–895.

807. Looney, W., et al., A clincial investigation of the chronic effects of radium salt administered therapeutically. Am J Roentgenol Radium Ther Nucl Med, 1955. 73:1006–1037.

808. Hasterlik, R.J., A.J. Finkel, and C.E. Miller, The cancer hazards of industrial and accidental exposure to radioactive isotopes. Ann N Y Acad Sci, 1964. 114:832–837.

809. Spiers, F., J. Whitwell, and P. Dorley, Dose in bone marrow cavities from radium 26. In The Effects of Radiation on the Skeleton. 1973, Oxford, Clarendon Press.

810. Stebbings, J.H., Dose-response analyses of osteonecrosis in New Jersey radium workers point to roles for other alpha emitters. Health Phys, 1998. 74(5):602–607.

811. Spiess, H., ^{224}Ra-induced tumours in children and adults. In Delayed Effects of Bone-Seeking Radionuclides, C.W. Mays, et al., eds. 1969, Salt Lake City, University of Utah Press.

812. Ansell, B., et al., Evaluation of intra-articular colloidal gold 198 Au in the treatment of persistent knee effusions. Ann Rheum Dis, 1963. 22:435–439.

813. Makin, M., G.C. Robin, and J.A. Stein, Radio-active gold in the treatment of persistent synovial effusion. Isr Med J, 1963. 22:107–111.

814. Topp, J.R. and E.G. Cross, The treatment of persistent knee effusions with intra-articular radioactive gold: Preliminary report. Can Med Assoc J, 1970. 102(7):709–714.

815. Rosenthal, L., Use of radiocolloids for intra-articulaar therapy for synovitis. In Therapy in Nuclear Medicine, R. Spencer, ed. 1978, New York, Grune and Stratton.

816. Stevenson, A., et al., Cytogenetic and scanning study of patients receiving intra-articular injections of gold 198 and yttriuim 90. Ann Rheum Dis, 1973. 32:112–123.

817. Bowring, C.S. and D.H. Keeling, Absorbed radiation dose in radiation synovectomy. Br J Radiol, 1978. 51(610):836–837.

818. Davis, P. and M.I. Jayson, Acute knee joint rupture after yttrium 90 injection. Ann Rheum Dis, 1975. 34(1):62–63.

819. Shouse, S., S. Warren, and G. Whipple, Aplasia of marrow and fatal intoxication in dogs produced by roentgen irradiation of all bones. J Exp Med, 1913. 53:421.

820. Hempelmann, L.H., H. Lisco, and J. Hoffman, The acute radiation syndrome: A study of 9 cases and a review of the problem. Ann Intern Med, 1952. 36:279.

821. Bond, V.P., T.M. Fliedner, and J. Archambeau, Mammalian Radiation Lethality. 1965, New York, Academic Press.

822. International Atomic Energy Agency (IAEA), Effects of ionizing radiation on the hematopoietic tissue. 1967, Vienna, IAEA.

823. Nothdurft, W., Bone marrow. In Radiopathology of Organs and Tissues, E. Scherer, C. Streffer, and K. Trott, eds. 1991, Berlin, Springer-Verlag.

824. United Nations Scientific Committee on the Effects of Atomic Radiation (UNSCEAR), Sources and effects of ionizing radiation: Report to the General Assembly with annexes. 1988, New York, United Nations.

825. Cronkite, E., Kinetics of human hematopoiesis. In Effects of Ionizing Radiation on the Hematopoietic Tissue. 1967, Vienna, IAEA.

826. Fliedner, T.M., W. Nothdurft, and K.H. Steinbach, Blood cell changes after radiation exposure as an indicator for hemopoietic stem cell function. Bone Marrow Transplant, 1988. 3(2):77–84.

827. Tubiana, M., Clinical treatments of leukemia by splenic irradiation. In Cell Survival After Low Doses of Radiation: Theoretical and Clinical Implications, P. Alper, ed. 1975, London, John Wiley and Sons.

828. Hollingsworth, J. and H.B. Hamilton, Blood bactericidal activity. Report of the Atomic Bomb Casualty (ABC) Commission, ed. 1960, Hiroshima, Japan, ABC Commision.

829. Sasagawa, S., et al., Whole blood phagocytic and bacteriociday activities of atomic bomb survivors. 1989, Hiroshima, Japan, Radiation Effects Research Foundation.

830. Barreras, R. and S. Finch, Peripheral leukocyte phagocytosis and respiratory response to certain macromolecular substances in the ABCC-JNIH Adult Health Study. 1974, Hiroshima, Japan, Atomic Bomb Casualty Commission.

831. Finch, S. and C. Finch, Summary of studies at ABCC-RERF concerning late hematologic effects of atomic bomb exposure in Hiroshima and Nagasaki. 1988, Hiroshima, Japan, Radiation Effects Research Foundation.

832. Belsky, J.L., et al., Leukocyte response to exercise in atomic bomb survivors. Radiat Res, 1972. 50(3):699–707.

833. Wong, F.L., et al., Effects of radiation on the longitudinal trends of hemoglobin levels in the Japanese atomic bomb survivors. Radiat Res, 2005. 164(6):820–827.

834. Kauczor, H.U., et al., Bone marrow changes following radiotherapy. Results of MR tomography. Radiologe, 1992. 32(10):516–522.

835. Stevens, S.K., S.G. Moore, and I.D. Kaplan, Early and late bone-marrow changes after irradiation: MR evaluation. AJR Am J Roentgenol, 1990. 154(4):745–750.

836. Fitzpatrick, P.J. and W.D. Rider, Half body radiotherapy. Int J Radiat Oncol Biol Phys, 1976. 1(3-4):197–207.

837. Salazar, O.M., et al., Single-dose half-body irradiation for palliation of multiple bone metastases from solid tumors: Final Radiation Therapy Oncology Group report. Cancer, 1986. 58(1):29–36.

838. Sykes, M.P., et al., The effects of varying dosages of irradiation upon sternal-marrow regeneration. Radiology, 1964. 83:1084–1088.

839. Sacks, E.L., et al., Bone marrow regeneration following large field radiation: Influence of volume, age, dose, and time. Cancer, 1978. 42(3):1057–1065.

840. Rubin, P., et al., Bone marrow regeneration and extension after extended field irradiation in Hodgkin's disease. Cancer, 1973. 32(3):699–711.

841. Gale, R.P. and R.E. Champlin, Bone marrow transplantation in acute leukaemia. Clin Haematol, 1986. 15(3):851–872.

842. Thomas, E.D., Long-term results of marrow transplantation for leukemia. Bone Marrow Transplant, 1986. 1(suppl):175–176.

843. Barrett, A.J., Bone marrow transplantation. Cancer Treat Rev, 1987. 14(3–4):203–213.

844. MacVittie, T.J., A.M. Farese, and W. Jackson, III, Defining the full therapeutic potential of recombinant growth factors in the post radiation-accident environment: The effect of supportive care plus administration of G-CSF. Health Phys, 2005. 89(5): 546–555.

845. Nagayama, H., et al., Transient hematopoietic stem cell rescue using umbilical cord blood for a lethally irradiated nuclear accident victim. Bone Marrow Transplant, 2002. 29(3):197–204.

846. Fliedner, T.M., et al., Hematopoietic cell renewal as the limiting factor in low-level radiation exposure: Diagnostic implications and therapeutic options. Mil Med, 2002. 167(suppl 2):46–48.

847. Field, S.B., The relative biological effectiveness of fast neutrons for mammalian tissues. Radiology, 1969. 93(4):915–920.

848. Broerse, J.J. and G.W. Barendsen, Relative biological effectiveness of fast neutrons for effects on normal tissues. Curr Top Radiat Res Q, 1973. 8(4):305–350.

849. Polednak, A.P., Long-term effects of radium exposure in female dial workers: Hematocrit and blood pressure. Environ Res, 1977. 13(2):237–249.

850. Marshall, J.H. and S. Hoegerman, Estimation of alpha particle dose from radium 226 to blood. 1974, Argonne, Ill, Argonne National Laboratory.

851. Benua, R., et al., The relaton if radioiodine dosimetry to results and complications in treatment of metastatic thyroid cancer. Am J Roentgenol, 1962. 87:171–182.

852. Keldsen, N., B.T. Mortensen, and H.S. Hansen, Haematological effects from radioiodine treatment of thyroid carcinoma. Acta Oncol, 1990. 29(8):1035–1039.

853. Breen, S.L., J.E. Powe, and A.T. Porter, Dose estimation in strontium-89 radiotherapy of metastatic prostatic carcinoma. J Nucl Med, 1992. 33(7):1316–1323.

854. Laing, A.H., et al., Strontium-89 chloride for pain palliation in prostatic skeletal malignancy. Br J Radiol, 1991. 64(765):816–822.

855. Mettler, F. and M. Guiberteau, Essentials of Nuclear Medicine Imaging, 5th ed. 2006, Philadelphia, W.B. Saunders.

856. Spiers, F.W., A.H. Beddoe, and S.D. King, The absorbed dose to bone marrow in the treatment of polycythaemia by 32P. Br J Radiol, 1976. 49(578):133–140.

857. Chauduri, T., The role of phosphorus 32 in polycythemia vera and leukemia. In Therapy in Nuclear Medicine, R.P. Spencer, ed. 1978, New York, Grune and Stratton.

858. Mayer, K., et al., Sulfur-35 therapy used for chondrosarcoma and chordoma. In Therapy in Nuclear Medicine, R.P. Spencer, ed. 1978, New York, Grune and Stratton.

859. Jacquy, C., et al., Additional myeloablation with 52Fe before bone marrow transplantation. Bone Marrow Transplant, 1997. 19(3):191–196.

860. Rubin, P. and S.H. Levitt, The response of disseminated reticulum cell sarcoma to the intravenous injection of colloidal radioactive gold. J Nucl Med, 1964. 5:581–594.

861. Andrews, J.R., et al., The effects of one curie of sulfur 35 administered intravenously as sulfate to a man with advanced chondrosarcoma. Am J Roentgenol Radium Ther Nucl Med, 1960. 83: 123–134.

862. Brandao-Mello, C.E., et al., Clinical and hematological aspects of 137Cs: The Goiania radiation accident. Health Phys, 1991. 60(1):31–39.

863. Butturini, A., et al., Use of recombinant granulocyte-macrophage colony stimulating factor in the Brazil radiation accident. Lancet, 1988. 2(8609):471–475.

864. Fajardo, L.F. and M. Berthrong, Radiation injury in surgical pathology. I. Am J Surg Pathol, 1978. 2(2):159–199.

865. Lenzi, M. and G. Bassani, The effect of radiation on the lymph and on the lymph vessels. Radiology, 1963. 80:814–817.

866. Kuhm, E., Z. Molnar, and K. Bohm, Late effects of radiotherapy on the lymph system examined by lymphography. In Late Biological Effects of Ionizing Radiation, vol. 1. 1978, Vienna: IAEA.

867. Dailey, M.O., C.N. Coleman, and L.F. Fajardo, Splenic injury caused by therapeutic irradiation. Am J Surg Pathol, 1981. 5(4):325–331.

868. Coleman, C.N., et al., Functional hyposplenia after splenic irradiation for Hodgkin's disease. Ann Intern Med, 1982. 96(1):44–47.

869. van Kaick, G., et al., Malignancies in German Thorotrast patients and estimated tissue dose. Health Phys, 1978. 35(1):127–136.

870. Anderson, R.E. and N.L. Warner, Ionizing radiation and the immune response. Adv Immunol, 1976. 24:215–335.

871. Anderson, R.E. and J.C. Standefer, Radiation injury in the immune system. In Cytotoxic Insult to Tissues, Effects on Cell Linings, C. Potten and J.H. Hendry, eds. 1983, Edinburgh, Churchill Livingstone.

872. Talliaferro, W., L. Talliaferro, and B. Jaroslow, Radiation and Immune Mechanisms. 1964, New York, Academic Press.

873. Micklen, H. and J. Loutit, Tissue Grafting and Radiation. 1966, New York, Academic Press.

874. Waldorf, D.S., R.F. Willkens, and J.L. Decker, Impaired delayed hypersensitivity in an aging population: Association with antinuclear reactivity and rheumatoid factor. JAMA, 1968. 203(10):831–834.

875. Girard, J.P., et al., Cell-mediated immunity in an ageing population. Clin Exp Immunol, 1977. 27(1):85–91.

876. Grosse-Wilde, H. and U. Schafer, Lymphatic system. In Radiopathology of Organs and Tissues, E. Scherer, C. Streffer, and K. Trott, eds. 1991, Berlin, Springer-Verlag.

877. Hoppe, R.T., Effects of irradiation on the human immune system. Front Radiat Ther Oncol, 1989. 23:140–149.

878. Stefani, S. and R. Schrek, Cytotoxic effect of 2 and 5 roentgens on human lymphocytes irradiated in vitro. Radiat Res, 1964. 22:126–129.

879. Vos, O., Radiation sensitivity and post-irradiation repair of mouse lymphatic cells in vivo and in vitro: A study with the parent to F1 hydrid graft-versus-host reaction. Int J Radiat Biol Relat Stud Phys Chem Med, 1967. 13(4):317–333.

880. Cronkite, E., et al., Interaction of radiation and host immune defense mechanisms in malignancy. In Brookhaven National Lab, V.P. Bond, ed. 1974, Upton, NY, Associated Universities, U.S. Atomic Energy Commission.

881. Moloney, W.C. and R.D. Lange, Leukemia in atomic bomb survivors. II. Observations on early phases of leukemia. Blood, 1954. 9(7):663–685.

882. Donati, R. and G. Gantner, Hermatological aspects of radiation exposure. In Blood Disorders Due to Drugs and Other Agents, R. Girdwood, ed. 1973, Amsterdam, Excerpta Medica.

883. Helde, M. and T. Wahlberg, On inconsistencies between radio-hematologic observations. Acta Radiol, 1954. 42:75–80.

884. Helde, M., The connection between Roentgen ray risks for workers and changes in their blood pictures. Acta Radiol, 1946. 27:308–315.

885. Miale, J., Laboratory Medicine Hematology. 1982, St. Louis, Mosby.

886. Dickie, A. and L.H. Hempelmann, Morphologic changes in the lymphocytes of persons exposed to ionizing radiation. J Lab Clin Med, 1947. 32:1045–1059.

887. Cronkite, E., V.P. Bond, and R.A. Conard, The hematology of ionizing radiation. In Atomic Medicine, 4th ed., C. Behrens and E. King, eds. 1964, Baltimore, Williams and Wilkins.

888. Permeggiani, L., In Encyclopedia of Occupational Health and Safety, 3rd ed., T. Hague, ed. 1983, Geneva: International Labour Organization.

889. Courtenay, V.D., Studies on the protective effect of allogeneic marrow grafts in the rat following whole-body irradiation at different dose-rates. Br J Radiol, 1963. 36:440–447.

890. Anderson, R.E. and W.L. Williams, Radiosensitivity of T and B lymphocytes. V. Effects of whole-body irradiation on numbers of recirculating T cells and sensitization to primary skin grafts in mice. Am J Pathol, 1977. 89(2):367–378.

891. Harris, G., et al., Radiosensitivity of peripheral blood lymphocytes in autoimmune disease. Int J Radiat Biol Relat Stud Phys Chem Med, 1985. 47(6):689–699.

892. Anderson, R.E., J.C. Standefer, and S. Tokuda, The structural and functional assessment of cytotoxic injury of the immune system with particular reference to the effects of ionizing radiation and cyclophosphamide. Br J Cancer Suppl, 1986. 7:140–160.

893. Amagai, T., et al., Dysfunction of irradiated thymus for the development of helper T cells. J Immunol, 1987. 139(2):358–364.

894. Talliaferro, W. and I. Talliaferro, Effect of irradiation on hemolysis decline. J Infect Dis, 1950. 87:201.

895. Anderson, R.E., I. Lefkovits, and G.M. Troup, Radiation-induced augmentation of the immune response. Contemp Top Immunobiol, 1980. 11:245–274.

896. Hellstrom, I. and K.E. Hellstrom, Lymphocyte mediated cytotoxicity to tumor antigens. Johns Hopkins Med J Suppl, 1974. 3:37–50.

897. Rees, G.S., et al., Occupational exposure to ionizing radiation has no effect on T- and B-cell total counts or percentages of helper, cytotoxic and activated T-cell subsets in the peripheral circulation of male radiation workers. Int J Radiat Biol, 2004. 80(7):493–498.

898. Tuschl, H., R. Kovac, and A. Wottawa, T-lymphocyte subsets in occupationally exposed persons. Int J Radiat Biol, 1990. 58(4):651–659.

899. Tuschl, H., F. Steger, and R. Kovac, Occupational exposure and its effect on some immune parameters. Health Phys, 1995. 68(1):59–66.

900. Chaskes, S., G.C. Kingdon, and E. Balish, Serum immunoglobulin levels in humans exposed to therapeutic total-body gamma irradiation. Radiat Res, 1975. 62(1):144–145.

901. Anderson, R.E., et al., Radiosensitivity of T and B lymphocytes. IV. Effect of whole body irradiation upon various lymphoid tissues and numbers of recirculating lymphocytes. J Immunol, 1977. 118(4):1191–1200.

902. Andrews, G.A., Criticality accidents in Vinca, Yugoslavia, and Oak Ridge, Tennessee: Comparison of radiation injuries and results of therapy. JAMA, 1962. 179:191–197.

903. Hempelmann, L.H. and J. Grossman, The association of illnesses with abnormal immunologic features with irradiation of the thymic gland in infancy: A preliminary report. Radiat Res, 1974. 58(1):122–127.

904. Weigensberg, M., et al., Suppression of cell-mediated immune responses after total lymphoid irradiation (TLI). I. Characterization of suppressor cells of the mixed lymphocyte reaction. J Immunol, 1984. 132(2):971–978.

905. Tanay, A. and S. Strober, Opposite effects of total lymphoid irradiation on T cell-dependent and T cell-independent antibody responses. J Immunol, 1984. 132(2):979–984.

906. Terr, A.I., R.B. Moss, and S. Strober, Effect of total lymphoid irradiation on IgE antibody responses in rheumatoid arthritis and systemic lupus erythematosus. J Allergy Clin Immunol, 1987. 80(6):798–802.

907. Bhusate, L.L., et al., Increased DNA strand breaks in mononuclear cells from patients with rheumatoid arthritis. Ann Rheum Dis, 1992. 51(1):8–12.

908. McCurdy, D., et al., Delayed repair of DNA damage by ionizing radiation in cells from patients with juvenile systemic lupus erythematosus and rheumatoid arthritis. Radiat Res, 1997. 147(1):48–54.

909. Helfgott, S.M., Total lymphoid irradiation. Rheum Dis Clin North Am, 1989. 15(3):577–582.

910. Pilepich, M.V., et al., Renal graft irradiation in acute rejection. Transplantation, 1983. 35(3):208–211.

911. Hamburger, J., et al., Renal homotransplantation in man after radiation of the recipient: Experience with six patients since 1959. Am J Med, 1962. 32:854–871.

912. Waer, M., et al., Comparison of the immunosuppressive effect of fractionated total lymphoid irradiation (TLI) vs. conventional immunosuppression (CI) in renal cadaveric allotransplantation. J Immunol, 1984. 132(2):1041–1048.

913. Cossu, F., et al., Radiosensitivity of lymphocyte subpopulations in subjects with systemic lupus erythematosis: A in-vitro preliminary study. Minerva Med, 1991. 82(5):239–249.

914. Smith, K.J., et al., Increased cutaneous toxicity to ionizing radiation in HIV-positive patients: Military Medical Consortium for the Advancement of Retroviral Research (MMCARR). Int J Dermatol, 1997. 36(10):779–782.

915. Stjernsward, J., et al., Lymphopenia and change in distribution of human B and T lymphocytes in peripheral blood induced by irradiation for mammary carcinoma. Lancet, 1972. 1(7765):1352–1356.

916. Berger, M., et al., Influence of local radiotherapy of breast cancer patients on the frequency of cytotoxic T lymphocyte precursor cells. Immunobiology, 1990. 180(2–3):261–271.

917. Rotstein, S., et al., Long-term effects on the immune system following local irradiation for breast cancer: Pokeweed mitogen induced immunoglobulin secretion by blood lymphocytes and serum immunoglobulin levels. Eur J Surg Oncol, 1985. 11(2):137–141.

918. Nakayama, Y., et al., Varied effects of thoracic irradiation on peripheral lymphocyte subsets in lung cancer patients. Intern Med, 1995. 34(10):959–965.

919. Ishida, S., Changes in clinical and immunological status after post-thymectomized irradiation for invasive thymoma with myasthenia gravis. Rinsho Shinkeigaku, 1996. 36(5):629–632 (in Japanese).

920. van Mook, W.N., M.M. Fickers, and T.A. Verschueren, Clinical and immunological evaluation of primary splenic irradiation in chronic lymphocytic leukemia: A study of 24 cases. Ann Hematol, 2001. 80(4):216–223.

921. Cosimi, A.B., et al., Cellular immune competence of breast cancer patients receiving radiotherapy. Arch Surg, 1973. 107(4):531–535.

922. Braeman, J., A. Birch, and T.J. Deeley, Depression of in vitro lymphocyte reactivity after radical radiotherapy. Ann Clin Res, 1974. 6(6):338–340.

923. Check, J.H., et al., Effect of radiation therapy on mumps-delayed type hypersensitivity reaction in lymphoma and carcinoma patients. Cancer, 1973. 32(3):580–584.

924. Blomgren, H., et al., Studies on the lymphatic system in longterm survivors treated for Wilms' tumour or non-Hodgkin's lymphoma during childhood. Clin Oncol, 1980. 6(1):3–13.

925. Posner, M.R., et al., Circulating lymphocyte populations in Hodgkin's disease after mantle and paraaortic irradiation. Blood, 1983. 61(4):705–708.

926. Watanabe, N., et al., Long-term depletion of naive T cells in patients treated for Hodgkin's disease. Blood, 1997. 90(9):3662–3672.

927. Safwat, A., et al., The potential palliative role and possible immune modulatory effects of low-dose total body irradiation in relapsed or chemo-resistant non-Hodgkin's lymphoma. Radiother Oncol, 2003. 69(1):33–36.

928. Clave, E., et al., Multicolor flow cytometry analysis of blood cell subsets in patients given total body irradiation before bone marrow transplantation. Int J Radiat Oncol Biol Phys, 1995. 33(4):881–886.

929. Blomgren, H., et al., Blood lymphocyte population following ^{131}I treatment for hyperthyroidism. Acta Endocrinol (Copenhagen), 1991. 124(2):152–158.

930. Wasserman, J., et al., Changes of the blood lymphocyte subpopulations and their functions following ^{131}I treatment for nodular goitre and ^{32}P treatment for polycythemia vera. Int J Radiat Biol Relat Stud Phys Chem Med, 1988. 53(1):159–167.

931. Ohkita, T., A review of thirty years of Hiroshima and Nagasaki atomic bomb survivors. II. Biological effects: A. Acute effects. J Radiat Res, 1975. 16:49–66.

932. Akiyama, M., et al., Peripheral lymphocyte response to PHA and T cell population among atomic bomb survivors. Radiat Res, 1983. 93(3):572–580.

933. Kato, H., et al., Cross-sectional and prospective study on the relationship of EB virus infection and selected risk factors in the ABCC-JNIH Adult Heath Study Sample, Hiroshima and Nagasaki, ABC Commission, ed. 1972, Hiroshima, Japan, Atomic Bomb Casualty Commission.

934. Akiyama, M., et al., Study of the titers of anti-Epstein-Barr virus antibodies in the sera of atomic bomb survivors. Radiat Res, 1993. 133(3):297–302.

935. Akiyama, M., et al., Immunological responses of atomic bomb survivors, RERF, ed. 1988, Hiroshima, Japan, Radiation Effects Research Foundation.

936. Bloom, E.T., et al., Immunological responses of aging Japanese A-bomb survivors. Radiat Res, 1988. 116(2):343–355.

937. Akiyama, M., et al., Age and dose related alteration of in vitro mixed lymphocyte culture response of blood lymphocytes from A-bomb survivors. Radiat Res, 1989. 117(1):26–34.

938. Yamada, Y., et al., Effects of atomic bomb radiation on the differentiation of human peripheral blood B lymphocytes and the function of concanavalin A-induced supressor lymphocytes, ABC Commission, ed. 1984, Hiroshima, Japan, Atomic Bomb Casualty Commission.

939. Fujiwara, S., et al., Analysis of peripheral blood lymphocytes of atomic bomb survivors using monoclonal antibodies. J Radiat Res (Tokyo), 1986. 27(3):255–266.

940. Kusunoki, Y., et al., Age-related alteration in the composition of immunocompetent blood cells in atomic bomb survivors. Int J Radiat Biol Relat Stud Phys Chem Med, 1988. 53(1):189–198.

941. Kusunoki, Y., et al., Immune responses to Epstein-Barr virus in atomic bomb survivors: Study of precursor frequency of cytotoxic lymphocytes and titer levels of anti-Epstein-Barr virus-related antibodies. Radiat Res, 1994. 138(1):127–132.

942. Kato, H., et al., Rheumatoid arthritis and gout in Hiroshima and Nagasaki, Japan: A prevalence and incidence study. J Chronic Dis, 1971. 23(9):659–679.

943. Neriishi, K., E. Nakashima, and R.R. Delongchamp, Persistent subclinical inflammation among A-bomb survivors. Int J Radiat Biol, 2001. 77(4):475–482.

944. Hayashi, T., et al., Radiation dose-dependent increases in inflammatory response markers in A-bomb survivors. Int J Radiat Biol, 2003. 79(2):129–136.

945. Hayashi, T., et al., Long-term effects of radiation dose on inflammatory markers in atomic bomb survivors. Am J Med, 2005. 118(1):83–86.

946. Conard, R.A., et al., Immunohematological studies of Marshall Islanders sixteen years after fallout radiation exposure. J Gerontol, 1971. 26(1):28–36.

947. Chang, W., et al., Chronic low dose gamma radiation exposure and the alteration of the distribution of lymphocyte subpopulations in

residents in radioactive buildings. Int J Radiat Biol, 1999. 75(10):1231–1239.

948. Amundson, S.A., et al., Fluorescent cDNA microarray hybridization reveals complexity and heterogeneity of cellular genotoxic stress responses. Oncogene, 1999. 18(24):3666–3672.

949. Kosianov, A. and Z. Morozov, Characteristic of immunological state of liquidators of industrial accident with radiation components. Proceedings of the Whole Union Conference on Human Immunology and Radiation. 1991, Gomel, Belarus.

950. Ushakov, I., B. Davydov, and S. Soldatov, A Man in the Sky of Chernobyl: A Man and a Radiation Accident. 1994, Rostov-on-Don, Russia, Rostov University Publishing.

951. Akleev, A. and M. Kosenko, Quantitative functional and cytogenetic character of lymphocytes and some indices of immunological status of persons participating in the recovery operation works in Chernobyl. J Haematol Transfusiol, 1991. 36:24–26.

952. Bebeshko, V., et al., Immuno-biology and psychosocial aspects of the health of children after Chernobyl. Disaster Prehospital Disaster Med, 1996. 11:104–107.

953. Galizkaya, N. and et al., Evaluation of the immune system. Zdravookhr, Beloruss (in Russian), 1990. 6:33–35.

954. Chumak, A., et al., Monohydroxylated fatty acid content in peripheral blood mononuclear cells and immune status of people at long times after the Chernobyl accident. Radiat Res, 2001. 156(5 Pt 1):476–487.

955. Bebeshko, V., et al., Acute and remote immunohematological effects after the Chernobyl accident. Environ Sci Pollution Res, 2003. 1(special issue):85–94.

956. Vozianov, A., V. Bebeshko, and D. Bazyka, eds., Health Effects of the Chernobyl Accident. 2003, Kiev, Ukraine, Academy of Medical Sciences of the Ukraine.

957. Yarilin, A.A., et al., Late T cell deficiency in victims of the Chernobyl radiation accident: Possible mechanisms of induction. Int J Radiat Biol, 1993. 63(4):519–528.

958. Titova, L., et al., A comparative evaluation of the content of T-lymphocyte populations alpha 1-thymosin and autoantibodies to epithelial thymic cells in the personnel in the 30-km control zone of the accident at the Chernobyl Atomic Power Electric Station. Radiats Biol Radioecol, 1996. 36(4):601–609.

959. Kurjane, N., et al., Analysis of the immune status in Latvian Chernobyl clean-up workers with nononcological thyroid diseases. Scand J Immunol, 2001. 54(5):528–533.

960. Kuzmenok, O., et al., Late effects of the Chernobyl radiation accident on T cell-mediated immunity in cleanup workers. Radiat Res, 2003. 159(1):109–116.

961. Gridley, D.S., M.J. Pecaut, and G.A. Nelson, Total-body irradiation with high-LET particles: Acute and chronic effects on the immune system. Am J Physiol Regul Integr Comp Physiol, 2002. 282(3):677–688.

962. Bazyka, D., A. Chumak, and N. Byelyaeva, Immune cells in Chernobyl radiation workers exposed to low dose irradiation. Int J Low Radiation, 2003. 1:63–75.

963. Titov, L.P., et al., Effects of radiation on the production of immunoglobulins in children subsequent to the Chernobyl disaster. Allergy Proc, 1995. 16(4):185–193.

964. Chernyshov, V.P., et al., Analysis of blood lymphocyte subsets in children living on territory that received high amounts of fallout from Chernobyl accident. Clin Immunol Immunopathol, 1997. 84(2):122–128.

965. Koike, K., et al., Frequent natural killer cell abnormality in children in an area highly contaminated by the Chernobyl accident. Int J Hematol, 1995. 61(3):139–145.

966. Padovani, L., et al., Do human lymphocytes exposed to the fallout of the Chernobyl accident exhibit an adaptive response? 1. Challenge with ionizing radiation. Mutat Res, 1995. 332(1–2):33–38.

967. Ricks, R.C., S.A. Fry, and Radiation Emergency Assistance Center/Training Site (REAC/TS), The medical basis for radiation accident preparedness. II. Clinical experience and follow-up since 1979: Proceedings of the Second International REAC/TS Conference: The medical basis for radiation accident preparedness, October 20–22, 1988. 1990, New York, Elsevier, p. xli.

968. Fujita, S., H. Kato, and W.J. Schull, The LD$_{50}$ associated with exposure to the atomic bombing of Hiroshima and Nagasaki. J Radiat Res (Tokyo), 1991. 32(suppl):154–161.

969. Rotblat, J., Acute radiation mortality in a nuclear war, NAS, ed. 1986, Washington, DC, National Academy Press.

970. Fujita, S., H. Kato, and W.J. Schull, The LD$_{50}$ associated with exposure to the atomic bombing of Hiroshima. J Radiat Res (Tokyo), 1989. 30(4):359–381.

971. Young, R., Human mortality from uniform low-LET radiation. In NATO RSG V on LD$_{50}$. 1987, Gosport, UK, NATO.

972. Kamada, N., et al., Acute and late effects of A-bomb radiation studied in a group of young girls with a defined condition at the time of bombing. J Radiat Res (Tokyo), 1989. 30(3):218–225.

973. Levin, S.G., R.W. Young, and R.L. Stohler, Estimation of median human lethal radiation dose computed from data on occupants of reinforced concrete structures in Nagasaki, Japan. Health Phys, 1992. 63(5):522–531.

974. Priestman, T.J., J.T. Roberts, and B.K. Upadhyaya, A prospective randomized double-blind trial comparing ondansetron versus prochlorperazine for the prevention of nausea and vomiting in patients undergoing fractionated radiotherapy. Clin Oncol (R Coll Radiol), 1993. 5(6):358–363.

975. Priestman, T.J., et al., Results of a randomized, double-blind comparative study of ondansetron and metoclopramide in the prevention of nausea and vomiting following high-dose upper abdominal irradiation. Clin Oncol (R Coll Radiol), 1990. 2(2):71–75.

976. Priestman, T.J., Controlling the toxicity of palliative radiotherapy: The role of 5-HT3 antagonists. Can J Oncol, 1996. 6(suppl 1):17–22.

977. Priestman, S.G., T.J. Priestman, and P.A. Canney, A double-blind randomised cross-over comparison of nabilone and metoclopramide in the control of radiation-induced nausea. Clin Radiol, 1987. 38(5):543–544.

978. Henriksson, R., et al., The effect of ondansetron on radiation-induced emesis and diarrhoea. Acta Oncol, 1992. 31(7):767–769.

979. Henriksson, R., L. Franzen, and B. Littbrand, Prevention and therapy of radiation-induced bowel discomfort. Scand J Gastroenterol Suppl, 1992. 191:7–11.

980. Henriksson, R., L. Franzen, and B. Littbrand, Does sucralfate reduce radiation-induced diarrhea? Acta Oncol, 1987. 26(1):76–77.

981. International Atomic Energy Agency (IAEA), Diagnosis and treatment of radiation injuries, in Safety Report Series 2. 1998: Vienna, IAEA.

982. Hempelmann, L.H., Example of the acute radiation syndrome in man. N Engl J Med, 1952. 246(20):776–782.

983. Adams, M.J., et al., Radiation-associated cardiovascular disease: Manifestations and management. Semin Radiat Oncol, 2003. 13(3):346–356.

984. Fajardo, L.F. and J.R. Stewart, Cardiovascular radiation syndrome. N Engl J Med, 1970. 283(7):374.

985. Barabanova, A., Acute radiation syndrome with cutaneous syndrome. In Medical Basis for Radiation Accident Preparedness: The Clinical Care of Victims, R. Ricks, M.E. Berger, and F.M. Ohara, Jr., eds. 2002, New York, Parthenon.

986. Mettler, F., A. Guskova, and I. Gusev, Acute health effects and radiation syndromes resulting from the Chernobyl accident. Health Phys, 2007, in press.

987. Casarett, G.W., Concept in criteria of radiologic aging. In Cellular Basis and Etiology of Late Somatic Effects of Ionizing Radiation, J. Harris, ed. 1963, London, Academic Press.

988. Walburg, H., Radiation-induced life shortening and premature aging. Adv Radiat Biol, 1975. 7:145–179.

989. Storer, J.B., Radiation carcinogenesis. In Cancer, F. Becker, ed. 1975, New York, Plenum.

990. Conard, R.A., Effects of ionizing radiation on aging and life shortening in human populations. Front Radiat Ther Oncol, 1972. 6:486–498.

991. Beebe, G.W., H. Kato, and C.E. Land, Studies of the mortality of A-bomb survivors. 4. Mortality and radiation dose, 1950–1966. Radiat Res, 1971. 48(3):613–649.

992. Jablon, S. and H. Kato, Studies of the mortality of A-bomb survivors. 5. Radiation dose and mortality, 1950–1970. Radiat Res, 1972. 50(3):649–698.

993. Anderson, R.E., Longevity in radiated human populations, with particular reference to the atomic bomb survivors. Am J Med, 1973. 55(5):643–656.

994. Beebe, G.W., C. Land, and H. Kato, The hypothesis of radiation accelerated aging and the mortality of Japanese atomic bomb victims. In Late Effects of Ionizing Radiation. 1978, Vienna, IAEA.

995. Kato, H., et al., Mortality from causes other than cancer, 1950–1978: Life Span Study Report 9. 1981, Hiroshima, Japan, Radiation Effects Research Foundation.

996. Kato, H., et al., Studies of the mortality of A-bomb survivors: Report 7, Mortality, 1950–1978. II. Mortality from causes other than cancer and mortality in early entrants. Radiat Res, 1982. 91(2):243–264.

997. Anderson, R.E., T. Yamamoto, and T. Thorslund, Aging in Hiroshima and Nagasaki atomic bomb survivors: Soluble-insoluble collagen ratio. J Gerontol, 1974. 29(2):153–156.

998. Shimizu, Y., H. Kato, and W.J. Schull, Non-cancer mortality in the Life Span Study, 1950–1985. In RERF Update Summer. 1991, Hiroshima, Japan, Radiation Effects Research Foundation.

999. Preston, D.L., et al., Studies of mortality of atomic bomb survivors. Report 13. Solid cancer and noncancer disease mortality: 1950–1997. Radiat Res, 2003. 160(4):381–407.

1000. Yamada, M., et al., Prevalence of atherosclerosis in relation to atomic bomb radiation exposure: An RERF Adult Health Study. Int J Radiat Biol, 2005. 81:821–826.

1001. Cologne, J.B. and D.L. Preston, Longevity of atomic-bomb survivors. Lancet, 2000. 356(9226):303–307.

1002. Court Brown, W.M. and R. Doll, Mortality from cancer and other causes after radiotherapy for ankylosing spondylitis. Brit Med J, 1965. 2:1327–1332.

1003. Smith, P.G. and R. Doll, Mortality among patients with ankylosing spondylitis after a single treatment course with x-rays. Br Med J (Clin Res Ed), 1982. 284(6314):449–460.

1004. Hempelmann, L.H., et al., Neoplasms in persons treated with x-rays in infancy: Fourth survey in 20 years. J Natl Cancer Inst, 1975. 55(3):519–530.

1005. Alderson, M.R. and S.M. Jackson, Long-term follow-up with menorrhagia treated by irradiation. Br J Radiol, 1971. 44:295–298.

1006. Inskip, P.D., et al., Leukemia, lymphoma, and multiple myeloma after pelvic radiotherapy for benign disease. Radiat Res, 1993. 135(1):108–124.

1007. Ryberg, M., B. Nilsson, and F. Pettersson, Cardiovascular death after radiotherapy for benign bleeding disorders. The Radiumhemmet metropathia cohort 1912–1977. J Intern Med, 1990. 227(2):95–99.

1008. Darby, S.C., et al., Mortality in a cohort of women given x-ray therapy for metropathia haemorrhagica. Int J Cancer, 1994. 56(6):793–801.

1009. Brinkley, D. and J.L. Haybittle, The late effects of artificial menopause by x-radiation. Br J Radiol, 1969. 42(499):519–521.

1010. Stewart, J.R. and L.F. Fajardo, Radiation-induced heart disease: Clinical and experimental aspects. Radiol Clin North Am, 1971. 9(3):511–531.

1011. Fajardo, L.F. and J.R. Stewart, Radiation and the coronary arteries: Friend or foe? Int J Radiat Oncol Biol Phys, 1996. 36(4):971–972.

1012. Hancock, S.L., S.S. Donaldson, and R.T. Hoppe, Cardiac disease following treatment of Hodgkin's disease in children and adolescents. J Clin Oncol, 1993. 11(7):1208–1215.

1013. Hudson, M.M., et al., Increased mortality after successful treatment for Hodgkin's disease. J Clin Oncol, 1998. 16(11):3592–3600.

1014. Darby, S., et al., Mortality from cardiovascular disease more than 10 years after radiotherapy for breast cancer: Nationwide cohort study of 90,000 Swedish women. BMJ, 2003. 326(7383):256–257.

1015. Early Breast Cancer Trialists' Collaborative Group, Effects of radiotherapy and of differences in the extent of surgery for early breast cancer on local recurrence and 15-year survival: An overview of the randomized trials. Lancet, 2005. 366:2087–2106.

1016. Lederman, G.S., et al., Cardiac disease after mediastinal irradiation for seminoma. Cancer, 1987. 60(4):772–776.

1017. Huddart, R.A., et al., Cardiovascular disease as a long-term complication of treatment for testicular cancer. J Clin Oncol, 2003. 21(8):1513–1523.

1018. March, H., Leukemia in radiologists. Radiology, 1944. 43:275–278.

1019. Dublin, L. and M. Speigelman, Mortality of medical specialists. JAMA, 1948. 137:1519–1524.

1020. Warren, S., Longevity and causes of death from irradiation in physicians. J Am Med Assoc, 1956. 162(5):464–468.

1021. Seltser, R. and P.E. Sartwell, Ionizing radiation and longevity of physicians. J Am Med Assoc, 1958. 166(6):585–587.

1022. Seltser, R. and P.E. Sartwell, The influence of occupational exposure to radiation on the mortality of radiologists and other specialists. Am J Epidemiol, 1965. 81:2–22.

1023. Warren, S. and O. Lombard, New data on the effects of ionizing radiation on radiologists. Arch Environ Health, 1966. 13:415–421.

1024. Court Brown, W.M. and R. Doll, Expectation of life and mortality from cancer among British radiologists. Br Med J, 1958. 34(5090):181–187.

1025. Smith, P.G. and R. Doll, Mortality from cancer and all causes among British radiologists. Br J Radiol, 1981. 54(639):187–194.

1026. Kitabatake, T., K. Komiyama, and K. Hosoe, Survey on death rate and causes of death in x-ray technicians. Nippon Igaku Hoshasen Gakkai Zasshi, 1965. 25(3):213–223.

1027. Kitabatake, T., T. Watanabe, and M. Nakamura, Mortality and cause of death in Japanese radiological technicians, 1966 to 1972 (author's translation). Nippon Igaku Hoshasen Gakkai Zasshi, 1974. 34(6):440–443.

1028. Miller, R.W. and S. Jablon, A search for late radiation effects among men who served as x-ray technologists in the U.S. Army during World War II. Radiology, 1970. 96(2):269–274.

1029. Polednak, A.P., A.F. Stehney, and R.E. Rowland, Mortality among women first employed before 1930 in the U.S. radium dial-painting industry: A group ascertained from employment lists. Am J Epidemiol, 1978. 107(3):179–195.

1030. Stehney, A.F., Survival times of pre-1950 U.S. women radium dial workers. In Health Effects of Internally Deposited Radionuclides: Emphasis on Radium and Thorium, G. van Kaick, ed. 1995, Singapore, World Scientific, pp. 149–155.

1031. Howe, G.R., et al., Analysis of the mortality experience amongst U.S. nuclear power industry workers after chronic low-dose exposure to ionizing radiation. Radiat Res, 2004. 162(5):517–526.

1032. International Atomic Energy Agency (IAEA), Biochemical indicators of radiation injury in man. 1971, Vienna, IAEA.

1033. Goldberg, D. Alkaline ribonuclease activity in response to therapeutic radiation in the human female. In Biochemical Indicators of Radiation Injury in Man. 1971, Vienna, IAEA.

1034. Andrews, G.A., et al., Accidental radiation excursion at the Oak Ridge Y-12 plant—IV: Preliminary report on clinical and laboratory effects in the irradiated employees. Health Phys, 1959. 2:134–138.

1035. Gerber, G., et al., Urinary excretion of several metabolites in persons accidentally exposed to ionizing radiation. Radiat Res, 1961. 15:314–318.

1036. Smith, H. and A. Langlands, The urinary excretion of beta-aminoisobutyric acid after exposure to radiation. In Biochemical Indicators of Radiation Injury in Man. 1971, Vienna, IAEA.

1037. Ganis, F.M., M.W. Hendrickson, and J.W. Howland, Amino acid excretion in human patients accidentally exposed to large doses of partial-body ionizing radiation (the Lockport Incident). Radiat Res, 1965. 24:278–291.

1038. Jammet, H., et al., Etude de six cas de irradiation totale aique accidentalle Rev Franc Etud Clin. Biol, 1959. 4:210.

1039. Desai, T.K., et al., Taurine deficiency after intensive chemotherapy and/or radiation. Am J Clin Nutr, 1992. 55(3):708–711.

1040. Smith, H. and A.O. Langlands, Alterations in tryptophan metabolism in man after irradiation. Int J Radiat Biol Relat Stud Phys Chem Med, 1966. 11(5):487–494.

1041. Streffer, C., Biochemical post-irradiation changes and radiation indicators. In Biochemical Indicators of Radiation Injury in Man. 1971, Vienna, IAEA.

1042. Hamada, H., et al., Monitoring of serum KL-6 antigen in a patient with radiation pneumonia. Chest, 1992. 101:858–860.

1043. Porciani, S., et al., Polyamines as biochemical indicators of radiation injury. Phys Med, 2001. 17(suppl 1):187–188.

1044. Hofmann, R., et al., Increased serum amylase in patients after radiotherapy as a probable bioindicator of radiation exposure. Strahlenther Onkol, 1990. 166:688–695.

1045. Dubray, B., et al., Post-irradiation hyperamylasemia as a biological dosimeter. Radiother Oncol, 1992. 24:21–26.

1046. Becciolini, A., et al., Serum amylase and tissue polypeptide antigen as biochemical indicators of salivary gland injury during iodine-131 therapy. Eur J Nucl Med, 1994. 21(10):1121–1125.

1047. Smets, E., et al., Fatigue in cancer patients. Br J Cancer, 1993. 68:220–224.

1048. Schwartz, A.L., et al., Fatigue patterns observed in patients receiving chemotherapy and radiotherapy. Cancer Invest, 2000. 18(1):11–19.

1049. Nail, L. and K. King, Fatigue. Semin Oncol Nurs, 1987. 3:257–262.

1050. Love, R.R., et al., Side effects and emotional distress during cancer chemotherapy. Cancer, 1989. 63:604–612.

1051. King, K., et al., Patient's description of the experience of receiving radiation therapy. Oncol Nurs Forum, 1985. 12:55–61.

1052. Ans, J., et al., Assessment of malaise in cancer patients treated with radiotherapy. Cancer Nurs, 1985. 8:306–313.

1053. Greenberg, D., J. Sawicka, and S. Eisenthal, Fatigue syndrome due to localized radiation. J Pain Symp Manage, 1992. 7:38–45.

1054. Forester, B., D. Kornfeld, and J. Fleiss, Psychotherapy during radiotherapy: Effects on emotional and physical distress. Am J. Psychiatry, 1985. 141:22–27.

Effects of Radiation in Combination with Other Agents

As the knowledge of radiation effects has expanded, interactions between radiation and other agents have become apparent. For the most part, attention has been directed to situations in which the combination of radiation with such agents has enhanced the effect of radiation. As mentioned in Chapter 1, some agents are useful as radioprotective agents, but they are limited in number and are rarely considered in clinical and legal situations. Radiosensitizers are of more clinical importance. This chapter will discuss some effects of low-level radiation in combination with other agents; however, for the most part, the interactive effects that have been identified occur at high radiation levels. Typical examples are the combination of radiation therapy and chemotherapy, which increases the incidence of complications, or the effect of radiation therapy on the management of wound healing and other trauma. Information concerning interactive effects is limited and scattered, much is anecdotal, and most experiments in this field have not been optimally designed. An excellent review of the theoretical mathematics and limited data in this field was published by the United Nations Scientific Committee on Effects of Atomic Radiation (UNSCEAR) in its 1982 report and is summarized here.[1] Some additional information on mechanistic models and approaches to evaluation of risk is presented in the National Council on Radiation Protection and Measurements (NCRP) report on comparative carcinogenicity of ionizing radiation and chemicals[2] and in Annex H of the UNSCEAR 2000 report.[3]

NOMENCLATURE

In a discussion of combined effects, the first priority is to define terms. This is somewhat difficult because there are at least two classes of combined effects. In the first situation, ionizing radiation and the other agent may both produce a particular effect. In the second circumstance, ionizing radiation may produce a given effect that is then modified in degree or nature by some agent that is in itself inactive. In the first circumstance, in which radiation and another agent both produce an effect, terms describe a variety of results. *Additivity* refers to a situation in which the effect is the sum of each of the effects expected from the offending agents. *Synergism* describes situations in which the action of radiation and the other agent produces an effect greater than the sum of effects produced by the agents separately. *Antagonism* describes a situation in which combined action is less than would be expected from the sum of each agent acting alone (Fig. 7-1).

In the second circumstance, where the action of radiation is affected by an agent that by itself has no effect, different terminology is normally used. When the secondary agent increases the effect of radiation, the term *sensitization* is used, whereas when the resulting action is less than would be expected from the radiation alone, the action is termed *protection* (Fig. 7-2).

Obviously, these categorizations are somewhat simplistic because certain agents may have various effects at different dose levels. An additional problem in examining combined actions is the question of magnitude of exposure and temporal sequence. In the case of radiation, exposure and absorbed dose are reasonably well defined. However, with other agents, such as temperature, chemotherapy, and even cigarette smoking, exposure is difficult to define (particularly in terms of the concentration of the agent). The length of the exposure to such agents is rarely well quantified. In addition to the complexity caused because some agents, such as tobacco smoke, are really not a single agent but a multitude of initiators, promoters, cocarcinogens, and carcinogens, the effects of radiation in combination with other agents is made more difficult by the interaction that may occur between nonradiation agents. For example, tobacco smoking is causally related to esophageal cancer, as is alcohol. Several studies have indicated that the combined effects of tobacco and alcohol are multiplicative.[4] The relative risk (RR) for a nonsmoker-nondrinker is 1.0, which rises to 5.1 with consumption of 20 g or more of tobacco per day. Drinking more than 80 g of alcohol per day raises the risk to 18, but drinking and smoking this amount raises the RR to 44. Whether there are additional interactive mechanisms with other factors such as Barrett's esophagus

ADDITIVITY

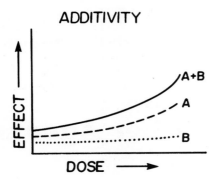

SYNERGISM

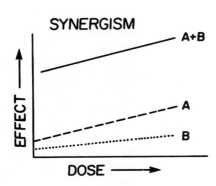

ANTAGONISM

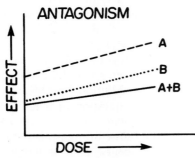

Figure 7-1 • Possibilities of interaction when two agents may both produce a particular effect. *Additivity* is the sum of the two effects; in *synergism*, when *A* combines with *B*, the effect is much greater than would be expected for either one alone. In *antagonism*, addition of agents *A* and *B* causes an effect less than that which would be expected.

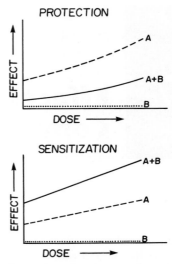

Figure 7-2 • Interaction of two agents when one, *B*, produces no effect when applied by itself but has some effect when applied in combination with *A*. In the circumstance of *protection*, combining *B* with *A* produces less of an effect than would be expected from *A* alone. In *sensitization*, combining *B* with *A* results in a much greater effect than for *A* applied alone.

remains largely unknown. Fortunately, in the case of esophageal carcinoma, the risk from radiation exposure is very low or negligible. Finally, it should be noted that different end points may be used in evaluation of interactions. Some studies report on the interaction between chemotherapy and radiation in terms of subsequent tumor induction. Other studies with the same chemical and radiation administered at high doses may report on deterministic effects due to cell killing. There is no inherent biological reason why the interaction should be the same for both end points, because the underlying mechanisms are likely to be different. For this reason, when an interaction is reported and quoted later in the literature, it is important to be specific relative to the etiologic agent, the end point studied, dose levels, and timing of exposures.

PHYSICAL AGENTS

Temperature

The relationships of high and low temperatures to the effect of ionizing radiation have been carefully studied. Presently, the application of high temperatures is the subject of intense research in the treatment of cancer. The concept of hyperthermia in combination with radiation has been studied since the 1960s.[5,6] Application of heat in the range of 40°C kills mammalian cells. The most likely action at the present time seems to be damage of the plasma membranes. In cell cultures, application of heat increases cell sensitivity to radiation. There appears to be a delay in rejoining of the strand breaks in the DNA and inhibition of DNA synthesis. The action of heat and radiation appears to be synergistic, although timing is very important. Maximal synergistic effect between radiation and heat (in terms of cell killing) is identified when the two agents are given simultaneously.[7] At the present time, very few temperature-dependent effects have been observed in humans, except in radiation therapy. Even this experience is limited because total-body hyperthermia usually requires general anesthesia. It is hoped that localized hyperthermia, through the use of therapeutic ultrasound, in combination with radiation therapy may provide more information. Hot working environments and accidental situations (such as the fire at Chernobyl) do not increase radiation effects, because body temperature remains normal. The relationship of low temperature to radiation effects has been studied in many animal systems.[8,9] The results are difficult to interpret; however, overall treatment with low temperature appears to reduce the life span of the animal. Currently, there is no reported evidence of interaction between radiation and low ambient temperature in humans.

Magnetic Fields, Ultrasound, and Electromagnetic Radiation

Most of the cell culture experiments performed to examine interaction of magnetic fields and radiation effects have produced essentially negative results.[10–12] The effects of ultrasound in combination with radiation on genetic material was studied by Harkanyi et al., who demonstrated that even at power levels as high as 1 watt/cm^2, no chromosomal aberrations in bone marrow could be identified.[13] Data concerning interaction of radiation and electromagnetic fields generally suffer from lack of quantifying parameters in the experimental work. Results of animal experiments using lethality as an end point have shown conflicting results: Some researchers report antagonistic action, although others report an additive action.[14] Few results for humans are available, except some scattered reports in the Russian literature that suggest that exposure to electromagnetic fields and ionizing radiation causes "functional disturbances" of the nervous system, changes in the sedimentation rate of erythrocytes, and dysmenorrhea.[1] The studies are difficult to evaluate because of the diffuse nature of the end points, variability between exposed groups, and lack of individual dosimetry and control groups. Controversy concerning the possible induction of cancer by either electric or magnetic fields has been the subject of a large number of both conferences and summary documents,[15–17] which indicate that the epidemiology is weak, little is known about potential mechanisms, there is lack of appropriate control groups in many studies, and at this time conclusions may be premature.[18–20] In a review of the literature, there is no evidence at this time of an interaction between radiation and either magnetic or electric fields.

Ultraviolet Light

There is extensive literature concerning the interaction of ultraviolet (UV) light and ionizing radiation. With mammalian cells in tissue culture, damage produced by irradiation with x-rays appears to be partially additive with UV damage.[21] With regard to the effect of UV light and x-rays (using chromosome aberrations in human lymphocytes as an end point), Holmberg et al. found the interaction to be synergistic.[22] UV light alone gave a very small yield of dicentrics, whereas combination of UV light with x-rays doubled the yield of dicentrics seen with x-rays alone; however, when stimulated lymphocytes entering

G_1 stage in the cell cycle were used, no synergism was observed.[23] Several animal experiments have examined the effect on skin tumor induction. At least in rats, UV irradiation predominantly produces a keratoacanthoma, whereas epidermal tumors generally followed electron irradiation. There does not appear to be an interaction between irradiation and UV in induction of tumors in rats.[24]

The effect of ultraviolet exposure on the risk of radiation-induced skin cancer is extensively discussed in the section on skin cancer in Chapter 5. In general, there is a two- to fivefold increase in risk in those portions of skin that are subsequently exposed to UV light (such as the face, neck, and hands).[25,26]

Combinations of Ionizing Radiation

Various combinations of therapeutic irradiation, including combinations of gamma or x-rays with heavy ions and fast neutrons and electrons, have been investigated in hopes of finding a more efficacious regimen for cancer treatment. The overall discussion of these radiotherapeutic applications, which is beyond the scope of this text, appears in several sources.[27–29] Zaider and Rossi have published a theoretical description of the interaction of high and low-LET radiation.[30] Although some experiments suggest synergism, the majority of data appear to fit the definition of additivity better.

Inhalation

Inhalation of various noxious agents has been the subject of intense interest, particularly since the experience with asbestos in shipyard workers and radon exposure of uranium miners. Radon may be adsorbed to dust particles that may subsequently be deposited into the respiratory system. The uranium miner studies are somewhat limited because some of the uranium miners have worked as hard rock miners and thus have a background of silicosis. Most lung changes in uranium miners are thought to be due to silicosis. The reader is referred to Chapters 5, 6, and 9 for a more detailed discussion. The only quantitative data regarding inhalation of noxious agents and radiation are from animal research. Combination of polonium 210 with quartz dust leads to more pronounced lung fibrosis than does either agent alone.[31] Many animal experiments have used plutonium and crysotile asbestos fibers. The animal data indicate that the tumor yield in animals receiving both asbestos and plutonium is less than that in the plutonium group alone.[32] The UNSCEAR 1982 report[1] indicated that if asbestos is given by intrapleural injection followed by exposure to radon 222, a synergistic effect in terms of tumor induction results.

Trauma

Radiation in combination with trauma has been of particular interest for accidental exposure, evaluation of the effects of nuclear weapon detonation, and management of patients who have had or are expected to have surgery and radiation therapy for the treatment of malignant neoplasms. An excellent review of the expected effects under many of these circumstances was published by Conklin et al.[33]

The prognosis of acute radiation syndromes is substantially influenced by the presence of combined injuries. At Hiroshima and Nagasaki, when radiation levels were sufficient to cause hematopoietic depression, lack of appropriate granulation tissue formation, poor healing of wounds, and hemorrhage occurred. It has been suggested that prodromal symptoms, sometimes used as biologic dosimeters, may be unreliable when conventional trauma is associated with the radiation injury. A wound that occurs even several days before high-dose irradiation demonstrates a prolonged healing time. An open wound markedly increases the chance of infection, and after whole-body radiation to moderate and high dose levels, mortality increases substantially. To prevent these complications, many investigators recommend that wounds occurring with large radiation exposures be treated and closed as quickly as possible.[33] It is interesting that in some animal systems if a wound is inflicted before irradiation, there is an increase in survival time compared to radiation alone. This may be a function of increased myelopoiesis when the trauma occurs before the radiation.[34]

Analysis of wound healing in radiation therapy has been the subject of many studies. The results encountered are markedly dependent on the fractionation scheme. Montague indicated that radiation therapy given after mastectomy to a dose of 40 grays (Gy) and delivered over 4 weeks at five fractions a week results in delayed wound healing in 6% of patients.[35] When the fractionation scheme is changed so that the weekly dose is given in three fractions rather than five, delayed wound healing occurs in 15% of patients. Similarly, wound infections occurred in 2% of patients who received five fractions weekly, but when the same dose was given in three fractions, the incidence of wound infections increased to 17%. Moderate wound sloughing occurred in 3% of the five-fraction-a-week group but increased to 13.5% when the same dose was given in three fractions. The action of radiation in combination with burns has also been extensively studied. The usual cause of death following burns is fluid and electrolyte imbalance frequently combined with sepsis. Combination of radiation injury and burn increases both the morbidity and mortality of the patient. The combined action, at least in simplistic terms, appears to be synergistic. Messerschmidt et al. indicated that whole-body radiation exposure of mice to 5.1 Gy was associated with a 10% mortality.[36] A second- or third-degree burn produced by a hot metal stamp was associated with a 30% mortality. When the animals received a burn after whole-body irradiation, mortality increased to 90%. It should, however, be noted that mortality did not increase if the burn occurred within 1 hour before the irradiation; this

finding conflicts with those of other researchers, who have indicated an increased mortality when the burns occurred prior to radiation.[37] A major cause of mortality among the Chernobyl firemen was the combination of whole-body radiation and extensive beta burns. The large areas of denuded skin served as a portal of entry for bacteria. Substantial absorbed doses of radiation delay the healing of bone fractures; although the early phases of healing do not appear to be significantly delayed, doses in the range of 7 to 8 Gy cause a fracture to take approximately twice as long to heal. In general, traumatic injuries associated with high-dose radiation injuries substantially increase the morbidity and mortality of the individual. The mechanisms involved are complex. If the radiation is delivered locally (as in radiation therapy), delayed healing and wound infection may result from direct action on the vascular structures and rapidly dividing cells. When the radiation is more generalized, the results identified usually, in part, manifest a depression of the hematopoietic and immune systems resulting in an increased susceptibility to sepsis and fluid and electrolyte imbalance.

CHEMICAL AGENTS

The vast number of known chemical carcinogens, cocarcinogens, and promoters has generated a literature well beyond the scope of the present text. Some of the animal data, which were reviewed and presented in the 1982 report of UNSCEAR, indicate that oxygen has a substantial radiosensitizing effect on tissue as long as the oxygen is present at the time the radiation is administered.[1] A high-calcium and high-fluorine diet may be beneficial when compared with diets relatively deficient in these minerals. After Chernobyl, many persons living in contaminated areas took dietary supplements of selenium in the hope of some protective effect. There is no epidemiological evidence to support this idea and, in fact, increased levels of selenium can be neurotoxic. Because nitro-oxides are rather common air pollutants, these compounds are of particular interest. It appears that when they are administered in combination with alpha irradiation, the incidence of lung cancer in mammals may increase.[1]

Many organic compounds are recognized as radiosensitizers. Some of these compounds modify the primary chemical processes involved in radiation injury. The first class of such compounds includes electron affinic agents and iodine compounds, which act by changing the concentration of radiation-induced free radicals. This class includes compounds containing carbonyl ($C=O$), aldehyde ($-CHO$), nitro ($-NO_2$), and cyano ($CN-$) groups, iodide, iodoacetic acid, iodoproprionic acid, methyliodide, iodobenzoic acid, and some others. Because iodine is a major constituent in contrast agents used in diagnostic radiology, these compounds have had a fair amount of attention.[38-40] It appears that the yield of chromosomal aberrations in peripheral lymphocytes increases when diagnostic x-ray exposure is combined with administration of contrast media. The present theory is that this increase is due to a difference in absorbed dose in the cells caused by the photoelectric effect. A second class of radiosensitizers is those that interact with the DNA metabolism. Such DNA base analogues include 5-fluorouracil, 5-bromouracil, and 5-bromo-2-deoxyuridine. Alkylating agents can form complexes with the DNA bases and influence radiosensitivity; these include radiotherapeutic agents such as 1,3-bis(2-chloroethyl)-1-nitrosurea (BCNU). In addition, methotrexate and cyclophosphamide increase radiosensitivity. Sokol and Maickel published a review of these drugs.[41] Many of these interactions have been described in the individual chapters on direct effects and carcinogenesis of the various organ systems. Additional agents reported by other authors include vincristine,[42] VP16-213 (epipodophylotoxin),[43] and chemotherapy in treatment of Hodgkin's disease.[44]

In general, it is not clear whether most of the chemotherapeutic agents act synergistically or additively because of the differences in time of administration with regard to the radiation and uncertainty about the actual dose delivered to the cells or organ of interest. Some antitumor antibiotics are also known to be active and to have synergistic effects when used in combination with radiation. A prime example is actinomycin D, which has been shown to increase the incidence of radiation pneumonitis and skin erythema.[45–47] Fernando et al. indicated that while some chemotherapeutic agents used with for adjuvant breast cancer therapy can cause an increase in radiation pneumonitis they appear to have little effect on acute skin reactions.[48] Another antitumor antibiotic, bleomycin, appears to inhibit repair of sublethal radiation damage, thus enhancing the action of radiation.[49] Other antitumor antibiotics, including ledermycin and reverine,[50] and interferon-alpha 2B,[51] also appear to enhance radiation effects. When radiation therapy is followed by chemotherapy, subclinical damage from irradiation can be unmasked and clinically manifested as a radiation recall phenomenon. Radiation recall phenomena (usually cutaneous) have been described with anthracyclines (adriamycin), taxanes (paclitaxel), alkylating agents (cyclophosphamide), antimetabolites (methotrexate and 5-fluorouracil), and dacarbazine.[52] One of the newer chemotherapeutic agents, gemcitabine, is unusual in that the radiation recall preferentially involves internal organs.[53,54] Some chemotherapeutic agents known to increase direct radiation effects on various tissues are shown in Table 7-1.

Secondary cancers occur more frequently after treatment of a primary cancer with either radiotherapy, chemotherapy, or a combination than would occur in a control group.[55,56] In general, it appears that certain types of chemotherapeutic agents may cause a large increase in leukemia.[57,58] While radiation tends to

Table 7-1 • Enhanced Deterministic Effects of Radiation on Different Organs by Various Chemotherapeutic Agents

Skin and mucous membranes	Heart
Actinomycin D	Adriamycin (Adria)
Adriamycin (Adria)	Gastrointestinal
Bleomycin sulfate	Actinomycin D
Chlorambucil	Adriamycin (Adria)
5-Fluorouracil	BCNU
Hydroxyurea	Bleomycin sulfate
Methotrexate	5-Fluorouracil
6-Mercaptopurine	Nitrogen mustard
Esophagus	Renal
Actinomycin D	Actinomycin D
Adriamycin (Adria)	Bladder
Bleomycin sulfate	Adriamycin (Adria)
Hydroxyurea	Cyclophosphamide
Procarbazine hydrochloride	Liver
Vinblastine	Actinomycin D
Lung	5-Fluorouracil
Actinomycin D	Eye
Adriamycin (Adria)	5-Fluorouracil
Bleomycin sulfate	Central nervous system
Cyclophosphamide	Methotrexate
Hydroxyurea	
Vincristine	

Adapted from Phillips TL, Fu KK: Quantification of combined radiation therapy effects on critical normal tissues. Cancer 1976;37:1186–1200.

pose a smaller risk, it causes a more general spectrum of neoplasms. The RRs for leukemia after mechlorethamine, vincristine, procarbazine, and prednisone (MOPP) chemotherapy alone can be in the range of 50 to 100. On the basis of the epidemiologic literature and secondary tumor induction, the interaction between most chemotherapeutic agents and radiation does not appear to be synergistic.[59]

In a large series of 82,700 patients treated for breast cancer, 90 secondary leukemia cases were reported. The risk was higher when patients were treated with radiotherapy and alkylating agents (RR 17.4) than with radiotherapy alone (RR 2.4) or with chemotherapy alone (RR 10.0).[60] Later studies, however, have reported a substantial risk reduction associated with chemotherapy, which affects menopausal age, suggesting that ovarian hormones promote tumorigenesis after radiation-induced initiation.[61] In some studies of Hodgkin's disease, there is no increase of chemotherapeutic leukemia risk due to subsequent radiation,[62,63] but at least one other study finds opposite results.[64] Breast cancer risk following Hodgkin's disease treated with radiotherapy may be enhanced due to chemotherapy with alkylating agents.[65] Gilbert et al. studied subsequent lung cancer in treated Hodgkin's patients and reported an additive effect between radiation and chemotherapy.[66] Studies of patients treated for ovarian cancer have reported that combined treatment with radiotherapy and chemotherapy is not associated with a greater risk of leukemia than with chemotherapy alone.[67,68]

Interestingly enough, one report indicates that patients treated with radiation therapy and actinomycin D had a reduced incidence of second neoplasms, that is, that the actinomycin D had a protective effect, although the reason for this effect remains unclear.[69] It is known that the interaction of intrathecal methotrexate with irradiation causes a decrease in IQ of children treated for leukemia with chemotherapy and cranial irradiation. Whereas the mechanism is not clear, Balsom et al. reported that preirradiation intrathecal methotrexate decreases the central nervous system (CNS) radiotoxicity (or has some protective effect), and the IQ was higher than a control group receiving irradiation alone.[70] On the surface this effect would appear biologically implausible, and more research is needed before these results are accepted. Lucanthone hydrochloride (Miracyl D), used in the treatment of parasitic diseases, was shown (1) to reduce the capacity of mammalian cells to accumulate and repair sublethal damage and (2) to act synergistically with radiation, causing developmental abnormalities.[71,72]

Caffeine, when administered after irradiation, reduces the shoulder on the cellular dose-survival curve. This demonstrates that caffeine appears to modify radiation damage in some way. The sensitization of HeLa cells to radiation depends on caffeine concentration: At very high concentrations the slope of the dose-survival curve steepens.[73-75] No interaction of caffeine and radiation has been reported in humans. Many organic chemical compounds are known to be carcinogenic, showing either additive or synergistic effects when combined with radiation. These include benzopyrene, methylcholanthrene, ethylnitrosourea, dimethylbenzanthracene, and 4-nitro-quinoline-1-oxide (4 NQO). Many of these agents have significantly different effects depending on whether the agent is administered before, during, or after irradiation.[76-80] In addition to significant variation of the combined effect produced by the order of administration, some of the compounds (such as ethylnitrosourea) show that administration of the agents together causes a significant shift in the spectrum of tumor types produced from that identified when the radiation is given alone. These types of effects make quantitation and analysis of the compounds exceedingly difficult. A recent study of nuclear workers by Schubauer-Berigan et al. did not find any significant difference for the ERR of chronic myeloid or acute leukemia with various levels of benzene exposure.[81]

In addition to known chemical carcinogens, promoting agents (including phorbol ester and croton oil), when given in combination with radiation, demonstrate results ranging from enhanced effects to absence of enhancement.[82-84] Overall, the number of agents tested

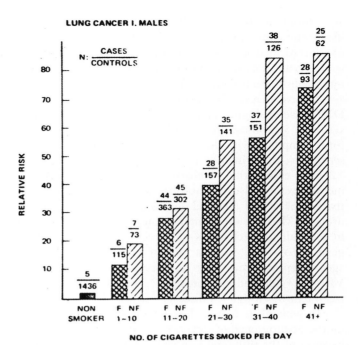

Figure 7-3 • The relative risk of lung cancer in males related to the number of cigarettes smoked daily. F, filtered cigarettes; NF, nonfiltered cigarettes. (From Smoking and health: A report of the Surgeon General. DHEW Publication (PHS) 79-50066, Rockville, Md, U.S. Department of Health, Education, and Welfare, 1979.)

and their response have been extremely variable. Actual results in humans, as compared with tissue culture experiments, are often a matter of conjecture.

Tobacco Smoke

Interaction of tobacco smoke and radiation is a matter of particular interest because of the large number of people who smoke. The incidence of lung cancer and its relationship to the number of cigarettes smoked daily are well known (Fig. 7-3).[85,86] There is also a strong relationship to age at which the individual began smoking (Table 7-2). An increased risk of esophageal, pancreatic, and urinary tract cancers also has been identified in smokers.

Table 7-2 • U.S. Lung Cancer Mortality Ratios for Males by Age They Began Smoking	
Age Began Smoking (yr)	**Mortality Ratio**
Nonsmoker	1.0
25+	4.8 − 5.2
20–24	9.5–10.1
15–19	14.4–19.7
<15	16.8–18.7

From Smoking and health: A report of the Surgeon General. DHEW Publication (PHS) 79-50066, Rockville, Md, U.S. Department of Health, Education, and Welfare, 1979.

The exact interaction between cigarette smoke and radiation is certainly not a simple one, because over 2000 compounds have been identified in cigarette smoke. Among these agents are a number of known carcinogens, cocarcinogens, and promotors.

There is a relatively large animal experience regarding cigarette smoke and radiation.[87–89] Human epidemiologic data come primarily from uranium miners exposed to radon and radon daughters and atomic bomb survivors (discussed in more detail in the section on carcinogenesis and lung cancer in Chapter 5). Exposure to radon is usually measured in WLMs, rather than in a unit of absorbed dose. Lundin et al. indicated that there appears to be a 10-fold synergistic increase in the risk of lung cancer for miners who smoke (a cancer incidence for each year at risk of 1.3×10^{-3} for smokers and 1.7×10^{-4} for nonsmokers).[90] The number of observed cases in the nonsmokers, however, is very low, as is the statistical significance of these results. Larger groups of uranium miners were studied by Archer[91] and others.[92,93] In Archer's group, 207 lung cancers were identified in uranium miners with all but three of the individuals being cigarette smokers (71% of the miners were known to smoke). The various incidences of lung cancer in the groups are shown in Figure 7-4. In a large meta-analysis of 11 underground miner studies, Lubin et al. examined the interaction between radon exposure and smoking.[94] Even though the analysis included over 2750 lung cancer deaths among 68,000 miners, a clear pattern of risk did not emerge. The data were consistent with a risk that was between additive and multiplicative. The most relevant study regarding

residential radon and effects of smoking comes from Pershagen et al.[95] Their conclusion was that the effects appeared more multiplicative than additive; however, this is driven primarily by data at the highest radon levels, and if their highest radon category is omitted, there is almost no evidence against additive effects.

Several mathematical models for interactions have been suggested; they have been examined by UNSCEAR.[96] The additive risk model appears to give results that are closest to the data. Latency time for tumor appearance seems to range between 10 and 15 years. One of the difficulties in analyzing the data is the length of the observation period. For example, if the substances contained in cigarette smoke act predominantly as promoters, and observations are made at a relatively short period, a combination of tobacco smoke and radiation might simply cause the radiation-induced cases to be seen earlier in time: an "apparent synergism." In fact, Lundin et al. do not exclude the possibility that for very long observation times, the yield of lung tumors in nonsmokers might equal that of smokers exposed to radon daughters.[93] With smoking alone, the latent period for lung cancer is about 20 years. In many of the studies, different classification of "high" and "low" smoking exposure categories makes comparison of various studies difficult. The difficulties with radiation dosimetry and estimates of smoking exposure have been discussed previously (in the section on lung cancer in Chapter 5).

Lung cancer has been examined relative to smoking and radiation in the Japanese atomic bomb survivors. The RR function for lung cancer as reported by Kato et al. is compatible with either an additive or multiplicative interaction.[97] Of particular interest in this study, however, is that in persons heavily exposed to both cigarette smoke and radiation, the cancer mortality was significantly lower than the multiplicative RR models would predict for all nonhematologic cancer, stomach cancer, and digestive cancers other than stomach cancer. In fact, the risk for these sites was not only submultiplicative but subadditive. A somewhat later analysis of lung cancer risk by Kopecky et al. indicated that there was no synergism and that the data fit a model in which the excess relative risk (ERR) was the sum of the smoking and the radiation risks.[98] A 2003 report by Pierce et al. evaluated the joint effects of smoking and radiation on lung cancer incidence through 1994 in a subset of 45,000 members of the Life Span Study (LSS) cohort for whom both smoking and radiation dose data were available.[99] The effects were found to be significantly submultiplicative and quite consistent with the additive model, thus they concluded that the effects were almost certainly not multiplicative. An interesting point is that when ERR per Sv (seivert) is examined according to smoking level, the ERR/Sv drops dramatically when the number of cigarettes per day exceeds 16 (Fig. 7-5). This probably

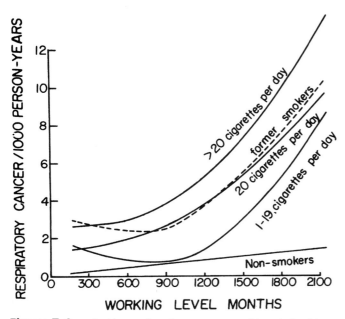

Figure 7-4 • Incidence of respiratory cancer and its relationship to exposure to radon daughter products in WLMs. (From Archer VE, Gillam JD, Wagoner JK: Respiratory disease mortality among uranium miners. NY Acad Sci 1976;271:280–293.)

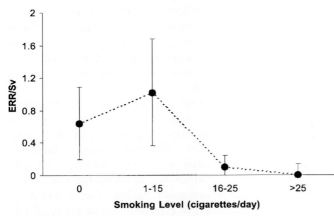

Figure 7-5 • Estimated ERR/Sv relative to background rates for the respective smoking levels represented for ages 60–70. Error bars are ±1 standard error. There is statistically significant evidence that ERR/Sv decreases with smoking level. (From Pierce, DA, et al: Joint effects of radiation and smoking on lung cancer risk among atomic bomb survivors. Radiat Res 2003;159:511–520.)

occurs because tobacco smoke is a much more effective carcinogen than radiation, and in a heavy smoker, any potential risk from radiation exposure is overwhelmed by the smoking risk.

Mabuchi et al.[100] pointed out that the BEIR IV Committee[101] could not reject either an additive or multiplicative interaction model on statistical grounds and, while the early U.S. uranium miner data support a multiplicative interaction, this is not at all clear from the Japanese data or from the combined analysis of the uranium miner studies.[94] Further research is probably needed especially because it seems that the frequency of different tumor cell types may be different with the two agents. The Swedish data on residential radon and lung cancer (see "Lung Cancer," in Chapter 5) suggest that at low levels of radiation, there may be no apparent interaction, and only at very high levels of smoking and radon is there an apparent interaction. It is not clear whether the interaction of radiation and tobacco smoke results directly from a component of the cigarette smoke or whether the effect is indirect. An example of such an indirect effect would be an alteration in the ciliary clearing mechanisms so that the radon absorbed to dust particles is cleared more slowly in smokers than in nonsmokers. There is limited data relative to smoking and medical radiation. Gilbert et al. studied subsequent lung cancer in treated Hodgkin's patients and reported a multiplicative interaction between smoking and radiation.[102]

Overall, epidemiologic data and the multiple chemical agents in tobacco smoke are so complicated that the combined effect of radiation and tobacco smoke remains in doubt. In some studies, it appears to be somewhat more than additive and initially may appear synergistic,

Table 7-3 • Chemical Agents Associated with Cancer	
Organ	**Agent**
Bladder	Aromatic amines (4-aminobiphenyl, benzidine, 2-naphthylamine)
	Auramine
	Chlornaphazine
	Cyclophosphamide
	Cigarette smoke
	Mineral oils
	Soot
	Tar
Gastrointestinal	Asbestos (possible)
Kidney	Aromatic hydrocarbons
Liver	Vinyl chloride, alphatoxin
Larynx	Mustard gas
Lung	Acrylonitrile
	Arsenic
	Asbestos
	Bis-chloromethyl ether
	Cadmium
	Chromium
	Mustard gas
	Cigarette smoke
	Rickel
	Ethylene oxide
	Polycyclic hydrocarbons
Marrow (leukemia and aplastic anemia)	Benzene
	Chlorambucil
	Cyclophosphamide
	Melphalan
Nasal sinuses	Isopropyl oil
	Vinyl chloride
	Nickel
Peritoneum	Asbestos (possible)
Pleura	Asbestos
Prostate	Cadmium
Scrotum	Polycyclic hydrocarbons
Skin	Arsenic
	Polycyclic hydrocarbons
Vagina	Diethylstilbesterol

Adapted from Doll R, Peto R: The causes of cancer: Quantitative estimates of avoidable risks of cancer in the United States today. J Natl Cancer Inst 1981; 66:1192–1308; Schottenfeld D, Haas JF: The workplace as a cause of cancer. Clin Bull 1978;8:54–119.

particularly if the observation period is short. Recent atomic bomb survivor data suggests an additive relationship.

Chemical Occupational Exposures

Many chemical agents known to be carcinogenic are present in various occupational settings. For the most part, the type of interaction, if any, with ionizing radiation is unknown. These agents are listed in Table 7-3 so they will not be overlooked as risk factors when cancer is identified in a given worker.

BIOLOGIC AGENTS

There are few human data regarding the interaction of radiation with biologic agents to indicate whether they act in an additive, synergistic, or antagonistic mode. As pointed out in the section on trauma in combination with radiation, biologic agents may gain entry to the body via trauma and result in substantially higher mortality than either injury alone would indicate. There has been particular interest in studying the interaction of radiation and hormones, particularly because some radiogenic tumors (breast and thyroid) are hormone-dependent. The variable length of the latent period with respect to age at exposure of the individual suggests that hormonal factors may play a prominent role. Most of the experimental animal data concentrate on possible interactions between diethylstilbesterol (DES) and radiation.[103–105] The purpose of these animal experiments has been to ascertain possible effects on women taking contraceptive estrogens. In the animal systems, the total yield of tumors at dose levels of approximately 4 Gy increased in the animals who received combined treatment. Shore et al. examined the effect of childbirth and lactation on the risk of breast cancer in women who received radiotherapy for postpartum mastitis.[106] Even after controlling for age at treatment, women who were irradiated after their second or third pregnancy had a lower risk than those irradiated immediately after their first pregnancy. This confirms data from other studies that early age at first pregnancy lowers the risk of breast cancer. Other animal experimentation has concerned viral and bacterial infections. The viral infections are of interest because viruses are known to act in the induction of various experimental tumors in animals. The animal data in general are very limited; there are essentially no research results at the present time in humans.

ETHNIC FACTORS

There are well-known differences for some cancers by racial and ethnic group. For example, American Indians have very low rates of breast cancer and high rates of cholangiocarcinomas compared with U.S. whites. Japanese have much higher rates of gastric cancers than do Americans. The causes of these differences may be genetic or environmental. Some genetic predispositions to radiation-induced malignancies are discussed in Chapter 3. For the most part, however, racial and ethnic differences appear to have substantially less effect than environmental factors. This assumption is derived from cancer registry data that indicate that cancer rates in immigrants to the United States change to resemble U.S. rates more than the incidence rates in the country of origin. At least with some tumors (e.g., breast cancers in U.S. and Japanese women), the factors responsible for the spontaneous incidence do not appear to interact with radiation except in an additive fashion.[107] The effect of skin pigmentation on the risk of skin cancer is discussed in Chapter 5. In general the risk of radiation-induced skin cancer is much lower in darker-skinned population.

In summary, with the possible exception of chemotherapeutic drugs, there appears to be no clear case of synergistic interaction between radiation and other agents that would be grounds for significant modifications of present risk estimates applied to the population.

REFERENCES

1. United Nations Scientific Committee on the Effects of Atomic Radiation (UNSCEAR), Ionizing radiation: Sources and effects: UNSCEAR report to the General Assembly, in Annex K: Radiation-induced life shortening. 1982, New York: United Nations, p. v.
2. National Council on Radiation Protection and Measurements (NCRP), Comparative carcinogenicity of ionizing radiation and chemicals: Recommendations of the NCRP. NCRP report no. 96. 1989, Bethesda, Md: The Council, p. vii.
3. United Nations Scientific Committee on the Effects of Atomic Radiation (UNSCEAR), Sources and effects of ionizing radiation: UNSCEAR 2000 report to the General Assembly, with scientific annexes. 2000, New York: United Nations.
4. International Agency for Research on Cancer (IARC), Alcohol drinking, in monographs on the evaluation of carcingenic risks to humans. 1988, Lyon, France: IARC.
5. Dewey, W., et al., Cell biology of hyperthermia and radiation. In Radiation Biology and Cancer Research, R. Meyn and H. Withers, eds. 1980, New York: Raven Press.
6. Field, S. and N. Bleehen, Hyperthermia in the treatment of cancer. Cancer Treat Rev, 1979. 6:63–94.
7. Sapareto, S., L. Hopwook, and W. Dewey, Combined effects of x-irradiation and hyperthermia on CHO cells for various temperatures and orders of application. Radiat Res, 1978. 73:211–223.
8. Trujillo, T., J. Spalding, and W. Langham, A study of radiation-induced aging: Response of irradiated and non-irradiated mice to cold stress. Radiat Res, 1962. 16:114–149.
9. Gambino, J., et al., Biological effect of stress following ionizing radiation. Aerospace Med, 1964. 35:220–224.
10. Wordsworth, O.J., Comparative long-term effects of liver damage in the rat after (a) localized x-irradiation and (b) localized x-irradiation in the presence of a strong homogeneous magnetic field. Radiat Res, 1974. 57(3):442–450.
11. Rockwell, S., The influence of a 1400-gauss magnetic field on the radiosensitivity and recovery of EMT 6 cells in-vitro. Int J Radiat Biol, 1977. 31:153–160.
12. Nath, R., R. Schultz, and P. Bongiorni, Response of mammalian cells irradiated with 30 MV x-rays in presence of a uniform 20-kilogauss magnetic field. Int J Radiat Biol, 1980. 38:285–292.
13. Harkanyi, Z., J. Szollar, and Z. Vigvari, A search for an effect of ultrasound alone and in combination with x rays on chromosomes in vivo. Br J Radiol, 1978. 51(601):46–49.
14. Michaelson, S., et al., Influence of microwaves on ionizing radiation exposure. Aerospace Med, 1963. 34:111–117.
15. Stone, R., Polarized debate: EMFs and cancer. Science, 1992. 258(5089):1724–1725.

16. Nair, I., M.V. Morgan, and H. Florig, Biological effects of power frequency electric and magnetic fields: Background paper, Office of Technology Assessment, ed. 1990, Washington, DC: U.S. Congress.

17. Allen, S. and J. Stather, Electric and magnetic fields in the workplace: National Radiological Protection Board. Radiol Protect Bull, 1993. 140:18–22.

18. Sagan, L.A., Epidemiological and laboratory studies of power frequency electric and magnetic fields. JAMA, 1992. 268(5):625–629.

19. Stather, J., Electromagnetic fields and the risk of cancer: Report of an advisory group on non-ionizing radiation. Radiol Protect Bull, 1992. 131:8–14.

20. EMF and cancer. ORAU panel on health effects of low-frequency electric and magnetic fields. Science, 1993. 260(5104):13–16.

21. Leenhouts, H. and K. Chadwick, An analysis of synergistic sensitization. Brit J Cancer, 1978. 37(suppl):S198–S201.

22. Holmberg, M. and J. Jonasson, Synergistic effect of x-ray and UV irradation on the frequency of chromosome breakage in human lymphocytes. Mutat Res, 1974. 23(2):213–221.

23. Holmberg, M., Lack of synergistic effect between x-ray and ultraviolet irradiation on the frequency of chromosome aberration in PHA-stimulated human lymphocytes in the G1 stage. Mutat Res, 1976. 24:141–148.

24. Burnes, F. and R. Albert, Tumor induction by the combination of ultraviolet light and ionizing radiation on rat skin. USDOE Report AT (11–1) 3380. 1980, Washington, DC: U.S. Department of Energy.

25. Shore, R.E., et al., Skin cancer incidence among children irradiated for ringworm of the scalp. Radiat Res, 1984. 100(1):192–204.

26. Modan, B., et al., Factors affecting the development of skin cancer after scalp irradiation. Radiat Res, 1993. 135(1):125–128.

27. Ngo, F., A. Han, and M.M. Elkind, On the repair of sub-lethal damage in V079 Chinese hamster cells resulting from irradiation with fast neutrons or fast neutrons combined with x-rays. Int J Radiat Biol, 1977. 32:507–511.

28. Bird, R., et al., Cell inactivation by a mixture of high and low-LET radiation. In 28th Annual Meeting of Radiation Research Society. 1980, New Orleans: Academic Press.

29. Furncinitti, P. and E.J. Hall, Interaction of high and low-LET sublethal damage: Effect on reproductive capacity of cultured human cells. In 28th Annual Meeting of Radiation Research Society. 1980, New Orleans: Academic Press.

30. Zaider, M. and H.H. Rossi, The synergistic effects of different radiations. Radiat Res, 1980. 83(3):732–739.

31. Panov, D., et al., Radiobiological effects of joint action of alpha radiation and quartz dust in rats' respiratory and renal system. Int Radiat Protect Assoc, 1977. 1:165–168.

32. Sanders, C.L., Jr., Dose distribution and neoplasia in the lung following intratracheal instillation of $^{239}PuO_2$ and asbestos. Health Phys, 1975. 28(4):383–386.

33. Conklin, J., R. Walker, and E. Hirsch, Current concepts in the management of radiation injuries and associated trauma. Surg Gynecol Obstet, 1983. 156:809–829.

34. Ledney, G., et al., Skin wound-enhanced survival and myelocytopoiesis in mice after whole-body irradiation. Acta Radiol Oncol, 1981. 20:29–38.

35. Montague, E.D., Experience with altered fractionation in radiation therapy of breast cancer. Radiology, 1968. 90(5):962–966.

36. Messerschmidt, O., et al., Radiation sickness combined with burn: Report SM-119/34. 1970, Vienna: IAEA.

37. Baker, D. and F. Valeriote, Effects of thermal burns and x-irradiation on early mortality. Proc Soc Exp Biol Med, 1966. 121:1275–1279.

38. Simione, G. and M. Quintiliani, Iodinated radiological contrast media as radiosensitizers. Int J Radiat Biol, 1977. 31:1–10.

39. Norman, A., F.H. Adams, and R.F. Riley, Cytogenetic effects of contrast media and triiodobenzoic acid derivatives in human lymphocytes. Radiology, 1978. 129(1):199–203.

40. Adams, F.H., et al., Effect of radiation and contrast media on chromosomes. Preliminary report. Radiology, 1977. 124(3):823–826.

41. Sokol, G. and R. Maickel, Radiation Drug Interactions in the Treatment of Cancer. 1980, New York: John Wiley and Sons.

42. Hansen, M., et al., Fatal hepatitis following irradiation and vincristine. Acta Med Scand, 1982. 212:171–174.

43. Giever, R.J., et al., Enhanced radiation reaction following combination chemotherapy for small cell carcinoma of the lung, possibly secondary to VP16-213. Int J Radiat Oncol Biol Phys, 1982. 8(5):921–923.

44. Grunwald, H.W. and F. Rosner, Acute myeloid leukemia following treatment of Hodgkin's disease: A review. Cancer, 1982. 50(4):676–683.

45. Wara, W.M., et al., Radiation pneumonitis: A new approach to the derivation of time-dose factors. Cancer, 1973. 32(3):547–552.

46. Phillips, T.L. and K.K. Fu, Quantification of combined radiation therapy and chemotherapy effects on critical normal tissues. Cancer, 1976. 37(suppl 2):1186–1200.

47. D'Angio, G.J., S. Farber, and C. Maddock, Potentiation of x-ray effects of actinomycin D. Radiology, 1959. 73:175–177.

48. Fernando, I.N., et al., An acute toxicity study on the effects of synchronous chemotherapy and radiotherapy in early stage breast cancer after conservative surgery. Clin Oncol (R Coll Radiol), 1996. 8(4):234–238.

49. Henderson, S. and B. Kimler, Response of cultured 9L cells to bleomycin and x-rays. In 28th Annual Meeting of Radiation Research Society. 1980, New Orleans: Academic Press.

50. Michel, C. and H. Fritz-Niggli, Radiation-induced developmental anomalies in mammalian embryos by low doses and interactions with drugs, stress, and genetic factors. In Late Biological Effects of Ionizing Radiation, vol. 2. 1978, Vienna: IAEA.

51. Hazard, L.J., W.T. Sause, and R.D. Noyes, Combined adjuvant radiation and interferon-alpha 2B therapy in high-risk melanoma patients: The potential for increased radiation toxicity. Int J Radiat Oncol Biol Phys, 2002. 52(3):796–800.

52. Kennedy, R.D. and J.J. McAleer, Radiation recall dermatitis in a patient treated with dacarbazine. Clin Oncol (R Coll Radiol), 2001. 13(6):470–472.

53. Jeter, M.D., et al., Gemcitabine-induced radiation recall. Int J Radiat Oncol Biol Phys, 2002. 53(2):394–400.

54. Friedlander, P.A., et al., Gemcitabine-related radiation recall preferentially involves internal tissue and organs. Cancer, 2004. 100(9):1793–1799.

55. de Vathaire, F., et al., Role of radiotherapy and chemotherapy in the risk of second malignant neoplasms after cancer in childhood. Br J Cancer, 1989. 59(5):792–796.

56. Holm, L.E., Cancer occurring after radiotherapy and chemotherapy. Int J Radiat Oncol Biol Phys, 1990. 19(5):1303–1308.

57. Sandoval, C., et al., Secondary acute myeloid leukemia in children previously treated with alkylating agents, intercalating topoisomerase II inhibitors and irradiation. J Clin Oncol, 1993. 11:1039–1045.

58. Boivin, J.F., Second cancers and other late side effects of cancer treatment: A review. Cancer, 1990. 65(suppl 3):770–775.

59. Kaldor, J., Second cancer following chemotherapy and radiotherapy: An epidemiological perspective. Acta Oncol, 1990. 29:647–655.

60. Curtis, R.E., et al., Risk of leukemia after chemotherapy and radiation treatment for breast cancer. N Engl J Med, 1992. 326(26):1745–1751.

61. van Leeuwen, F.E., et al., Roles of radiation dose, chemotherapy, and hormonal factors in breast cancer following Hodgkin's disease. J Natl Cancer Inst, 2003. 95(13):971–980.

62. Kaldor, J.M., et al., Leukemia following Hodgkin's disease. N Engl J Med, 1990. 322(1):7–13.

63. Tucker, M.A., et al., Risk of second cancers after treatment for Hodgkin's disease. N Engl J Med, 1988. 318(2):76–81.

64. Valagussa, P., et al., Second acute leukemia and other malignancies following treatment for Hodgkin's disease. J Clin Oncol, 1986. 4:830–837.

65. Hancock, S.L., M.A. Tucker, and R.T. Hoppe, Breast cancer after treatment of Hodgkin's disease. J Natl Cancer Inst, 1993. 85(1):25–31.

66. Gilbert, E.S., et al., Lung cancer after treatment for Hodgkin's disease: Focus on radiation effects. Radiat Res, 2003. 159(2):161–173.

67. Greene, M.H., et al., Melphalan may be a more potent leukemogen than cyclophosphamide. Ann Intern Med, 1986. 105(3):360–367.

68. Kaldor, J.M., et al., Leukemia following chemotherapy for ovarian cancer. N Engl J Med, 1990. 322(1):1–6.

69. D'Angio, G.J., et al., Decreased risk of radiation-associated second malignant neoplasms in actinomycin-D-treated patients. Cancer, 1976. 37(suppl 2):1177–1185.

70. Balsom, W.R., et al., Intellectual function in long-term survivors of childhood acute lymphoblastic leukemia: Protective effect of pre-irradiation methotrexate? A Children's Cancer Study Group study. Med Pediatr Oncol, 1991. 19(6):486–492.

71. Bases, R., Enhancement of x-ray damage in HeLa cells by exposure to lucanthone (miracyl D) following radiation. Cancer Res, 1970. 30:2007–2011.

72. Michel, C., Combined effects of miracyl D and radiation on mouse embryos. Experientia, 1974. 30:1195–1196.

73. Waldren, C. and I. Rasko, Caffeine enhancement of x-ray killing in cultured cells. Radiat Res, 1978. 73:96–110.

74. Schroy, C., P. Furcinitti, and P. Todd, Caffeine as a potentiator of single hit potentially lethal damage in cultured mammalian cells exposed to ionizing radiations of high and low-LET. In 28th Annual Meeting of Radiation Research Society. 1980, New Orleans: Academic Press.

75. Tolmach, L., P. Busse, and K. Bettham, Concentration dependence of the mode of caffeine-mediated enhancement of HeLa cell killing of x-rays. In 28th Annual Meeting of the Radiation Research Society. 1980, New Orleans: Academic Press.

76. DiPaolo, J., In-vitro transformation: Interactions of chemical carcinogens and radiation. In Biology of Radiation Carcinogenesis, J.M. Yuhas, R. Tennant, and J. Regan, eds. 1976, New York: Raven Press.

77. Furth, J. and M. Boon, Enhancement of leukemogenic action of methylcholanthrene by pre-irradiation with x-rays. Science, 1943. 98:138–139.

78. Cloudman, A., et al., Effects of combined local treatment with radioactive and chemical carcinogens. J Natl Cancer Inst, 1955. 15:1077–1083.

79. Epstein, J., Examination of the carcinogenic and cocarcinogenic effects of Grenz radiation. Cancer Res, 1972. 321:2625–2629.

80. Hoshino, M., H. Tanooka, and F. Fukuoka, Summation of the carcinogenic effect of 4-nitro-quinoline-1-oxide and beta ray. Gan, 1968. 59:43–49.

81. Schubauer-Berigan, M.K., R.D Daniels, D.A. Fleming, et al., Risk of chronic myeloid and acute leukemia mortality after exposure to ionizing radiation among workers at 4 U.S. nuclear weapons facilities and nuclear naval shipyard. Radiat Res, 2007. 167:222–232.

82. Kennedy, A., et al., Enhancement of x-ray transformation by 12-0-tetra-decanoyl-phorbol-13-acetate in a cloned line of C_3H mouse embryo cells. Cancer Res, 1978. 38:439–443.

83. Epstein, J. and H. Roth, Experimental ultraviolet light carcinogenesis: A study of croton oil promoting effects. J Invest Dermatol, 1968. 50:387–389.

84. Brues, A.M., et al., Mechanisms of Carcinogenesis. 1968, Argonne, Ill: Argonne National Laboratory.

85. Doll, R., An epidemiological perspective of the biology of cancer. Cancer Res, 1978. 38(11 Pt 1):3573–3583.

86. Smoking and health: A report of the Surgeon General. DHEW Publication (PHS) 79-50066. 1979, Rockville, Md: U.S. Department of Health, Education, and Welfare.

87. Chameaud, J., et al., Combined effects of inhalation of radon daughter products in tobacco smoke. In Pulmonary Toxicology of Respirable Particles: Proceedings of 19th Hanford Life Sciences Symposium. 1979, Richland, Wash: U.S. Department of Energy, pp. 551–557.

88. Cross, F.T., et al., Study of the combined effects of smoking and inhalation of uranium or dust, radon daughters, and diesel oil exhause in hamsters and dogs. 1978, Richland, Wash: Pacific Northwest Laboratories.

89. Lafuma, J., Pulmonary cancer induced by inhalation of different alpha emitters. In Late Biological Effects of Ionizing Radiation. 1978, Vienna: IAEA.

90. Lundin, F.E., Jr., et al., Mortality of uranium miners in relation to radiation exposure, hard-rock mining and cigarette smoking—1950 through September 1967. Health Phys, 1969. 16(5): 571–578.

91. Archer, V.E., J.K. Wagoner, and F.E. Lundin, Jr., Uranium mining and cigarette smoking effects on man. J Occup Med, 1973. 15(3):204–211.

92. Gillam, J. and J.K. Wagoner, Respiratory disease mortality among uranium miners. Ann NY Acad Sci, 1976. 271:280–293.

93. Lundin, F.E., V.E. Archer, and J.K. Wagoner, An exposure-time response model for lung cancer mortality in uranium miners: Effects of radiation exposure, age, and cigarette smoking. In Energy and Health, N. Breslow and A. Wittemore, eds. 1979, Philadelphia: SIAM Publications.

94. Lubin, J., J.D. Boice, and C. Edling, Radon and lung cancer risk: A joint analysis of 11 underground miner studies. 1994, Washington, DC: U.S. Department of Health and Human Services.

95. Pershagen, G., et al., Residential radon exposure and lung cancer in Sweden. N Engl J Med, 1994. 330(3):159–164.

96. United Nations Scientific Committee of the Effects of Atomic Radiation (UNSCEAR), Sources and effects of ionizing radiation: 2006 Report to the General Assembly with annexes. 2006, New York: United Nations.

97. Kato, H., et al., Studies of the mortality of A-bomb survivors. Report 7. Mortality, 1950–1978: Part II. Mortality from causes other than cancer and mortality in early entrants. Radiat Res, 1982. 91(2):243–264.

98. Kopecky, K., et al., Lung cancer, radiation and smoking among A-bomb survivors, Hiroshima and Nagasaki. 1986, Hiroshima, Japan: Radiation Effects Research Foundation.

99. Pierce, D.A., G.B. Sharp, and K. Mabuchi, Joint effects of radiation and smoking on lung cancer risk among atomic bomb survivors. Radiat Res, 2003. 159(4):511–520.

100. Mabuchi, K., C. Land, and S. Akiba, Radiation, smoking and lung cancer. 1992, Hiroshima, Japan: Radiation Effects Research Foundation.

101. National Research Council (NRC), Committee on the Biological Effects of Ionizing Radiations (BEIR), Health risks of radon and other internally deposited alpha-emitters. BEIR IV. 1988, Washington, DC: NRC Press.

102. Gilbert, E.S., C.E. Land, and S.L. Simon, Health effects from fallout. Health Phys, 2002. 82(5):726–735.

103. Segaloff, A. and W. Maxfield, The synergism between radiation and estrogen in the production of mammary cancer in the rat. Cancer Res, 1971. 31:166–168.

104. Shellabarger, C.J., J.P. Stone, and S. Holtzman, Synergism between neutron radiation and diethylstilbesterol in the production of mammary adenocarcinoma in the rat. Cancer Res, 1976. 36:1019–1022.

105. Bekkum, D., et al. Radiation-induced mammary cancer in the rat. In Proceedings of the 6th International Congress on Radiation Research, Tokyo, Japan. 1979.

106. Shore, R.E., et al., Breast cancer among women given x-ray therapy for acute postpartum mastitis. J Natl Cancer Inst, 1986. 77(3):689–696.

107. Land, C.E., et al., Breast cancer risk from low-dose exposures to ionizing radiation: Results of parallel analysis of three exposed populations of women. J Natl Cancer Inst, 1980. 65(2):353–376.

8 | Radiation Exposure In Utero

In utero radiation exposure of the embryo or fetus generally causes intense anxiety among parents and the public in general. Too often careless statements are made with little or no regard for the actual facts. The in utero effects of radiation on humans have been extensively studied; some of the research findings will be reviewed here. For additional information, the reader may consult the many articles by Brent,[1,2] as well as other existing summary articles in the literature.[3] The 1993 United Nations Scientific Committee on Effects of Atomic Radiation (UNSCEAR) report contains an excellent review of the radiation effects on the central nervous system after in utero radiation exposure.[4] There are also several recent International Commission on Radiological Protection (ICRP) reports on the topic.[5,6]

The great anxiety associated with possible in utero radiation effects has many unfortunate outcomes. Patients often have abortions when there is little or no risk from radiation or they refuse radiographic or nuclear medicine procedures that are medically indicated. If an x-ray is medically indicated, the medical risk to the mother of not having the examination almost always exceeds the radiogenic risk to the fetus. Most diagnostic radiographic examinations can be tailored so that once the diagnosis is obtained, no additional radiation exposure is necessary. In circumstances in which exposure of a female occurs before pregnancy is identified, it is important to counsel both parents, presenting the risks from the radiation in comparison to "normal risks" of pregnancy. This can be done only if the absorbed dose to the embryo or fetus can be estimated and if the appropriate risk factors are available. Such counseling usually relieves the family. When counseling is not performed, not only is there a lot of needless worry, but many such situations ultimately find their way to a legal arena. The public and most physicians are unaware of the in utero effects of radiation and are often quick to blame "spontaneous" malformations and most congenital abnormalities on radiation exposure. As discussed in Chapter 3, the normal incidence of abnormalities in nonexposed pregnancies is between 3% and 10%. Determination of the absorbed dose to the embryo or fetus is difficult but usually can be estimated within a 50% error. For diagnostic radiographic examinations, one can use the mean skin exposure/film (for a given examination) and then estimate the absorbed dose at a certain depth if the technical factors concerning the beam energy are known. If the technical factors are not well known, the mean dose to the ovaries often gives an approximation of fetal dose. When an occupational or accidental exposure occurs and the individual had a film badge, one can assume that the fetal dose is approximately one quarter to one half of the surface dose. In these ways, a reasonable estimate of fetal dose may be obtained. Of course, many individual factors, including machine calibration, direction of the beam, and size of patient may affect this estimate somewhat. The childbearing age in females is historically represented by the age group between 15 and 44 years of age. Data from the late 1960s indicated that approximately 25% of pregnant women received x-rays, and 21% of those received it during the first trimester.[7] The types of examinations were unevenly distributed during pregnancy, with most of the pelvic and abdominal examinations occurring during the third trimester and chest x-rays being evenly distributed throughout pregnancy. In 1970, there were 3.5 million live births in the United States. Approximately 800,000 pregnant women were x-rayed during that year, including about 300,000 fetuses in the direct beam. Of them 22,000 were irradiated during the first trimester; 15,000 during the second trimester; and 263,000 during the third trimester. Thirty-six percent of all x-ray examinations performed on females in 1980 occurred in the 15- to 44-year age group. The distribution of x-rays between men and women is approximately equal. In 1980, approximately 200 to 225 million radiographic examinations were performed; thus, approximately 40 million x-ray examinations are performed annually in the United States on women in the childbearing age group. What percentage of these patients is pregnant at the time of examination is unknown. With the advent of gray scale ultrasound and the increased awareness of possible radiation effects, the percentage of pregnant patients receiving x-rays has undoubtedly markedly decreased. Bonebrake surveyed 1200 cases of prenatal chest x-rays and identified no cases of unsuspected disease.[8] In another smaller study, Mattox found a single benign lesion of the rib cage in

1200 patients surveyed.[8] Pelvic x-rays have been examined in terms of their use and efficacy.[9–11] These early reports indicated that approximately 40% of patients undergoing a cesarean section had received pelvimetry; of those, approximately 30% nevertheless went on to a cesarean section. The correlations between the course of labor and the pelvic measurements are very poor when a statistical analysis is performed. On the basis of the available data, the American College of Radiology, the American College of Obstetricians and Gynecologists, and the U.S. Bureau of Radiological Health have indicated that pelvimetry is not usually necessary or helpful in deciding whether to perform a cesarean section and that in the few instances in which the clinician thinks that pelvimetry may contribute to a treatment decision, the reasons should be clearly delineated. X-ray pelvimetry provides only limited additional information to physicians involved in management of labor and delivery. It appears that although during the 1960s and early 1970s pelvimetry was performed in approximately 5% of deliveries, the current rate may be substantially lower. The mean fetal whole-body dose from pelvimetry is estimated to be approximately 6.2 mGy; in the past, this represented the major single source of ionizing radiation to the fetus.

A number of documents have reviewed prenatal radiation exposure and have produced recommendations or regulations for both medical and occupational exposure. Procedures to minimize diagnostic x-ray exposure of pregnant and potentially pregnant women have been published by the National Council on Radiation Protection and Measurements (NCRP).[12] Maternal occupational exposure leading to fetal exposure has been discussed in an NCRP report.[13] The NCRP recommended that exposure of the fetus be limited to 0.5 mSv per month. The rationale for this limit is that the embryo or fetus should be treated as a member of the general public, since it is involuntarily subjected to the occupational radiation exposure of the mother. In 1975, the Nuclear Regulatory Commission (NRC) issued instructions that all individuals working in or frequenting a portion of a restricted radiation area be instructed in the potential health protection problems associated with radiation exposure (including prenatal radiation exposure).

DETERMINISTIC (NONSTOCHASTIC) EFFECTS

General

Nonstochastic effects of ionizing radiation during pregnancy cover a wide range of identifiable abnormalities, including lethality, cataracts, growth retardation, malformations, and even behavioral disorders. Since the neural system is typically most sensitive, other abnormalities are not seen in humans without neuropathology. Radiation-induced malformations are nonspecific and, of course, can be produced by other noxious agents. Protracted radiation exposures may affect many tissues throughout pregnancy, but in general, such exposures probably have less overall teratogenic effect than a brief radiation exposure of high intensity. It is important to realize that each radiation effect has a temporal relationship to the stage of pregnancy (Table 8-1 and Fig. 8-1). For example, lethality is primarily identified during the preimplantation stage of gestation, and cataracts are predominantly seen when radiation exposure occurs during organogenesis. Developmental postconception stages are shown in Table 8-2, which indicates the tissues that may be susceptible at various times. The following text will discuss direct effects with correlative stages of pregnancy. In some instances, correlating effects with stages of pregnancy is difficult because the epidemiologic studies do not always cover specific stages of pregnancy. Some specific in utero radiation-associated abnormalities are shown in Table 8-3. In general, the radiogenic response of a fetus is related to sensitivity of different structures because the fetus or embryo is usually uniformly irradiated.

Preconception

Several epidemiologic studies have examined the effects of radiation administered prior to conception. Most have

Table 8-1 • Temporal Relationship of Possible Direct Effects of Radiation During Pregnancy*

	Preimplantation	Implantation	Organogenesis Early/Late	Fetal
Days since onset of menses	14–23	24–28	29–64	65–294
Days since conception (gestation)	0–9	9–14	15–50	50–280
Lethality	+++	+	+	—
Gross malformations	—	—	+++	—
Growth retardation (at term)	—	+	+++/++	+
Growth retardation (as adult)	—	+	++/+++	++
Sterility	—	±	—	++
Cataracts	—	—	+	+
Neuropathology	—	—	+++/++	+++/++

*Effects listed in this table have been identified in animals at dose levels of about 1 Gy (100 rad) and are listed with the comparable human gestation period. +++, occurs in high incidence; ++, readily apparent effect; +, demonstrated effect; ±, questionable effect; —, no observed incidence. Timing of some effects (such as neuropathy) in humans does not occur at stages comparable to animals. See text for details.
Adapted from Brent RL: Effects of embryonic and fetal exposure to x-ray, microwaves, and ultrasound. Clinical Obstet Gynecol 1983;26:484–510.

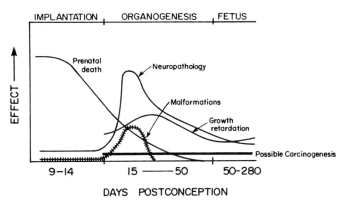

IMPLANTATION   ORGANOGENESIS   FETUS

DAYS POSTCONCEPTION

Figure 8-1 • Schematic presentation of the various adverse effects associated with radiation and their relative incidence at different stages of gestation.

<table>
<tr><td colspan="2">**Table 8-2** • **Postconceptional Stages in Humans**</td></tr>
<tr><td>**Days Postconception**</td><td>**Developmental Activity**</td></tr>
<tr><td>1</td><td>Fertilization</td></tr>
<tr><td>2</td><td>Cleavage: 1–4 cell stage</td></tr>
<tr><td>3</td><td>Cleavage: 5–8 cell stage</td></tr>
<tr><td>7–9</td><td>Early implantation</td></tr>
<tr><td>10–12</td><td>Continued implantation</td></tr>
<tr><td>13–16</td><td>Earliest neurogenesis</td></tr>
<tr><td>17–20</td><td>Neurogenesis: head, eye, thyroid, and heart
Primordia: allantois and first four somite pairs</td></tr>
<tr><td>21–24</td><td>Anterior neuropore: Primitive germ cells hemopoiesis in yolk sac; heart, vitelline vessels, aortic arches; oral membrane and jaw; otic invagination; gut, liver</td></tr>
<tr><td>25–29</td><td>Active organogenesis throughout; brain, myocardial pulsations, all sense organs, optic lens, lung primordia, posterior limb buds, mesonephric tubules</td></tr>
<tr><td>30–34</td><td>Preskeletal chondrification, pharyngeal pouches and pancreas, spinal and sympathetic nerves, semicircular canals, bronchi, corpus callosum</td></tr>
<tr><td>35–39</td><td>Differentiation of appendages and sense organs, all brain parts distinct, cortical differentiation, reflex pathways forming</td></tr>
<tr><td>40–43</td><td>Early fetus, basic organs complete</td></tr>
<tr><td>44–50</td><td>Chondrification of ribs, muscles of esophagus, epithelial cord of testis</td></tr>
<tr><td>51–65</td><td>Cartilage in humerus: 25% gonad differentiation</td></tr>
<tr><td>66–105</td><td>Nucleated red blood cells formed; corpus callosum forms, gastric glands</td></tr>
</table>

Adapted from U.S. Department of Health and Human Services: Effects of ionizing radiation on the developing embryo and fetus: A review. HHS Publication FDA 81–8170, Washington, DC, U.S. Department of Health and Human Services, 1981.

limited themselves to analysis of carcinogenesis rather than direct effects. Effects from preconception irradiation may also be considered genetic effects and are extensively discussed in Chapter 3. Between 1920 and 1940, radiation was used in an attempt to increase fertility. The doses normally used were between 1.5 and 2.25 Gy (gray) over 3 weeks. Subsequent study of these patients yielded no evidence of an increase in malformations in the subsequently conceived children.[14,15] The possibility of conceiving malformed children and the reproductive potential of females treated for Hodgkin's disease have been investigated by Horning et al.[16] Patients usually received both chemotherapy and radiotherapy, and no birth defects were identified. Higher doses of radiation have historically been used to cause sterility, and at least one patient, who received 6.4 Gy, became pregnant two years later and delivered a normal child.[17] Irradiation of the male prior to fertilization has been studied in accidental exposure cases. In one instance, five individuals who received absorbed doses between 2.3 and 3.7 Gy became either aspermic or hypospermic. At least one of these individuals demonstrated "sterility" for several years and then fathered a normal child.[18]

Schull et al. examined the effect of parental exposure on subsequent pregnancies in the survivors of Hiroshima and Nagasaki.[19] Results were divided into the following categories: (1) untoward outcomes (the frequency of pregnancies that terminated in an infant who was grossly abnormal, was stillborn, or died within the first month of life); (2) survival of liveborn children; (3) sex ratio; and (4) cumulative experience of the children of parents who were exposed near the bomb detonation site. For untoward outcomes, 70,082 pregnancies were included in the study. For those not in the city, the frequency of untoward outcomes was 4.71%, and for all those exposed, the frequency was 4.75%. There was a slight increase in untoward outcomes with increasing dose, but it was not statistically significant. With respect to mortality of the liveborn children, no statistically significant evidence

supported an increased mortality within increasing parental dose. No compelling evidence verified that the sex ratio of children subsequently born was altered. Finally, Schull et al. attempted to examine the cumulative effect of the previous three items.[19] Unadjusted data revealed a nonsignificant increase with either maternal or paternal exposure; however, if both parents were exposed, no cumulative effect was seen. Thus, in the survivors of Hiroshima and Nagasaki, no statistically significant radiation effects following preconception irradiation are evident.

Preimplantation

There are few human epidemiologic data available for the preimplantation and implantation periods of gestation. During the preimplantation period, irradiation of animals appears to lead to "all or none" effects. X-ray doses of 2 Gy in mice result in a high incidence of embryonic death; however, those that survive appear to be normal.

Table 8-3 • Anomalies Reported* After High-Dose Human Embryonic and Fetal X-Irradiation†

1. Microcephaly (most frequent)
2. Hydrocephalus
3. Porencephaly (cysts or cavities in the brain cortex)
4. Mental deficiency
5. Mongolism (Down syndrome)
6. Idiocy
7. Head ossification defects
8. Skull malformations
9. Micromelia (small or short limbs)
10. Microphthalmos (small eyes)
11. Microcornea
12. Coloboma (absence or defect of some ocular tissues)
13. Strabismus (deviation of the eye)
14. Cataract
15. Chorioretinitis
16. Nystagmus (involuntary rapid movement of the eyeball)
17. Stillbirth
18. Live birth weight (decrease)
19. Neonatal and infant death (increase)
20. Ear abnormalities
21. Spina bifida
22. Cleft palate
23. Deformed arms
24. Clubfeet
25. Hypophalangism
26. Syndactyly
27. Hypermetropia (farsightedness)
28. Amelogenesis (defective enamel of teeth)
29. Odontogenesis imperfecta (abnormal teeth)
30. Genital deformities

*All anomalies reported caused by human fetal x-irradiation have been experimentally produced in the mouse or rat when they could be recognized and analyzed (obvious exception: 4–6).
†A number of these reports have not been confirmed in subsequent scientific literature as being due to radiation (e.g., Down syndrome).
Adapted from Rugh R: Radiology and the human embryo and fetus. In Dalrymple GV, Gaulden ME, et al (eds): Medical Radiation Biology. Philadelphia, WB Saunders, 1973.

It is possible that spontaneous abortions increase slightly during this early time period; however, this increase has been too small to quantify accurately. Brent suggests that the "normal" incidence of spontaneous abortions in humans may be as high as 30% to 50%.[2] Growth retardation has not been observed as a result of irradiation during the preimplantation period.

Implantation Stage

During implantation (10 to 14 days after conception), the embryo is substantially more resistant to lethal effects than during the preimplantation stage. Transient intra-uterine growth retardation might result from irradiation during this period, but incidence of malformation is orders of magnitude lower at this time than during organogenesis. Since malformations are deterministic in character, they are likely to have a threshold dose. Both human and animal studies indicate that the threshold doses of low-LET ionizing radiation for developmental effects to occur, such as malformations and growth retardation, are about 0.1 to 0.2 Gy.[5,6]

Organogenesis

The period of organogenesis is usually divided into early and late portions. The *early organogenesis* period is 15 to 28 days after conception, whereas *late organogenesis* refers to the time 29 to 50 days after conception. During early organogenesis, the embryo is sensitive to lethal, teratogenic, and growth-retarding effects because of the criticality of cellular activities and the high proportion of radiosensitive cells. Lethal effects in humans have been studied to a very limited extent. Harris examined 138 women irradiated with approximately 5 Gy of 200 kVp x-ray at 6 to 18 weeks of pregnancy.[20] This dose was sufficient to stop fetal growth in 2 weeks and to cause interruption of pregnancy in 129 of the 138 cases within 4 weeks. In a similar study, Mayer et al. indicated that a single exposure of 3.6 Gy caused abortion in a large majority of irradiated women.[21] Some in utero lethal effects were demonstrated at Hiroshima and Nagasaki.[22,23] Of 30 women who were pregnant and demonstrated signs of acute radiation syndromes, 7 (23%) had fetal deaths, and 6 (20%) had neonatal or infant deaths. In 68 women who were exposed at the same distance from the hypocenter but who demonstrated no signs of the acute radiation syndrome, fetal mortality was 10%. This was only slightly greater than the fetal mortality of the control group, which was 6%. In considering teratogenesis, gross congenital malformations, growth retardation, and central nervous system (CNS) and ocular effects should be taken into account. The human data differ from animal data in several respects. In humans, growth retardation, microcephaly, and mental retardation are the predominant effects identified when acute exposures of low-LET radiation exceed absorbed dose levels of 0.5 Gy. There is no report of external radiation inducing a morphologic malformation in humans unless the individual also exhibited either growth retardation or a CNS abnormality.[2] In fact, 80% of malformed children with a history of in utero irradiation in excess of 1 Gy are microcephalic. This is a very important distinguishing factor in analysis of pregnancies in which radiation exposure of the embryo or fetus at term has been followed by the identification of a malformation. One possible reason is that the CNS in humans has a long developmental period extending from day 16 throughout gestation, and neuroblasts in the transitional stage may be destroyed by a dose as low as 0.25 Gy. Dekaban examined more than 200 published cases of therapeutic pelvic irradiation during pregnancy.[24] The indications for the radiation therapy included dysmenorrhea, metrorrhagia, myomata, arthritis, tuberculosis, and malignant tumor. In most instances, the radiation therapy was initiated before the pregnancy was identified, and the absorbed doses usually were in excess of 2.5 Gy. The most

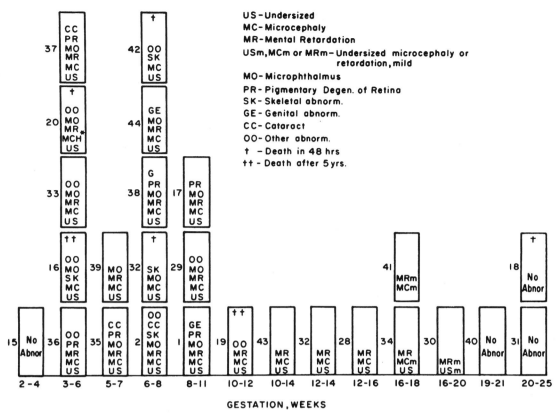

US – Undersized
MC – Microcephaly
MR – Mental Retardation
USm, MCm or MRm – Undersized microcephaly or
                           retardation, mild
MO – Microphthalmus
PR – Pigmentary Degen. of Retina
SK – Skeletal abnorm.
GE – Genital abnorm.
CC – Cataract
OO – Other abnorm.
† – Death in 48 hrs
†† – Death after 5 yrs.

GESTATION, WEEKS

Figure 8-2 • Graphic summary of findings in 26 children who received radiation during different stages of gestation. The number on the left of each rectangle is a reference number of the individual case report. Almost all children received more than 3 Gy. Abnormalities were most marked for the 3rd to 11th week of gestation; mental retardation and growth retardation were seen when exposures occurred as late as 16 to 20 wks of gestation. (From Dekaban AS: Abnormalities in children exposed to x-radiation during various stages of gestation: Tentative timetable of radiation injury to the human fetus. J Nucl Med 1968;9:471–477.)

frequently observed abnormalities were small size at birth, stunted growth, microcephaly (often with mental retardation), cataracts, genital and skeletal malformations, and microphthalmia (Fig. 8-2). The brain was the most consistently affected organ when the radiation was received at 4 to 11 weeks of gestation, although mental retardation and microcephaly were present in a milder form in the 16- to 19-week period (Fig. 8-3).

In another study involving therapeutic radiation, Goldstein and Murphy indicated that 19 of 75 irradiated embryos became either microcephalic or hydrocephalic when the dose received was greater than 1 Gy.[25,26] Most of the children were mentally retarded; other malformations identified included hypoplastic genitalia, cleft palate, hypospadius, and abnormality of the large toe and ear. None of these effects was identified at absorbed dose levels of less than 1 Gy. As was the case with the findings of Dekaban, Goldstein and Murphy identified microphthalmia, cataracts, strabismus, retinal degeneration, and optic atrophy, as well as a case of dwarfism. In that case, high-dose radiation was administered; however, Brent believes the cause was genetic rather than radiogenic.[2]

Several studies have been done to assess the effect of Chernobyl on background incidence of genetic diseases and anomalies. Czeizel et al. reported that in Hungary no increase in anomalies was detected.[27] The International Chernobyl Project reviewed pre- and

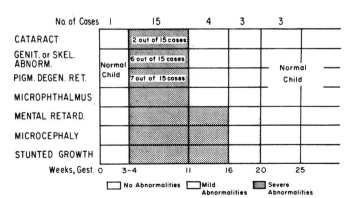

Figure 8-3 • Tentative timetable of abnormalities in humans induced by fetal irradiation at various stages of gestation. (From Dekaban AS: Abnormalities in children exposed to x-radiation during various stages of gestation: Tentative timetable of radiation injury to the human fetus. J Nucl Med 1968;9:471–477.)

post-Chernobyl data from affected republics and concluded that there was no statistically significant increase in malformations that could be attributed to the accident as of 1990.[28] The same conclusions were reached by the Chernobyl Forum in 2005 (discussed in Chapter 3).[29] There was no evidence of an increase in trisomy-21 in Finland as a result of the Chernobyl accident.[30] In addition, there was no evidence of an increase in registered congenital malformations, preterm births, or stillbirths of malformed children.[31] In Norway, Lie et al. reported a positive association with hydrocephaly but not for Down syndrome or other conditions previously reported for radiation such as small head circumference.[32,33]

In another study of environmental radiation, Shields et al. evaluated 13,329 births for 320 kinds of adverse pregnancy outcome in an area of uranium mining.[34] The authors reported that any associations were weak and may be biased. Several researchers have studied in utero exposure at Hiroshima and Nagasaki. Both mental retardation and microcephaly are identified, with the greatest effect from exposure at 8 to 15 weeks of gestation.[35] It should be mentioned that determining the exact fetal age at irradiation in these studies is difficult; age is often calculated in a retrospective manner from the delivery date. This, of course, has inherent inaccuracies. The early studies following in utero exposure at Hiroshima and Nagasaki were limited, and, thus, an exhaustive clinical study known as the PE-86 sample was taken. Subsequently, there has been revision of the PE-86 sample to reduce workload. Both the PE-86 sample and the revised PE-86 include virtually all individuals who received absorbed doses of 0.5 Gy or more. Generally, data on severe mental retardation refer to the smaller revised sample, while data on school performance and intelligence tests usually refer to the unrevised population sample. With the DS86 dosimetry, doses have been calculated to the uterus rather than to the fetus itself. Uncertainties in the risk estimates for radiation effects on the human brain, which have been derived from Hiroshima and Nagasaki data, include a number of factors.[36–38] The estimates are derived from high-dose acute exposure. Other extraneous factors include genetic variation, nutritional deprivation, infection, and hypoxemia. Mole has suggested that the question of the fetal bone marrow and blood-forming capability may have played an important role in the development of mental retardation by reducing oxygen transport to the brain.[39] Whether this is a mechanism that contributed to mental retardation in Japanese children remains unknown. Both linear and linear-quadratic models provide satisfactory approximation to the data, and even threshold models can be fit to the data without difficulty.

Brain Development

Developmental activity of the fetus is an important factor in determining the result of any insult. For purposes of radiation effects on the brain, typically, four age periods have been used: 0 to 7 weeks, 8 to 15 weeks, 16 to 25 weeks, and 26 or more weeks after ovulation. These times are important, because at 0 to 7 weeks the precursors of the neurons and neuroglia become apparent and are dividing. From 8 to 15 weeks, there is a rapid increase in the number of neurons. They migrate to their ultimate sites and lose their capacity to divide. Neuronal migration takes place in two stages. The first stage begins at the 7th week after fertilization and extends to the 10th week. From the 10th week to the 15th week, a second group of cells moves past the first neurons. At 15 to 25 weeks there is more differentiation, formation of connections, and more architectural definition. Brain function ultimately depends on the ability of the neurons to connect properly with each other. Cells that are unable to connect probably die.

Mental Retardation

While mental retardation has been reported in some of the in utero atomic bomb survivors, it is an extremely low frequency effect at low doses and therefore does not represent a major public health problem. The atomic bombs killed almost 100,000 persons but also there were about 100,000 survivors. There was in utero, radiation-induced, severe mental retardation in only 30 individuals among 1544 in utero exposed persons in the revised clinical sample. Three of these with estimated doses of 0, 0.29, and 0.56 Gy are known to have had Down syndrome. A fourth child with an estimated uterine dose of 0.03 Gy had Japanese B encephalitis in infancy, and a fifth individual who received an estimated dose of 0 Gy, had a retarded sibling. Almost certainly, in these five cases, the mental retardation was not radiation-related. When the remaining 25 individuals are examined by developmental age at exposure, the following conclusions emerge:

1. The highest risk of severe mental retardation occurs during major neuronal migration (about 8 to 15 weeks). At this time, the incidence of severe mental retardation increases with dose and 75% (9 out of 12) of fetuses exposed to 1 Gy or more were mentally retarded.
2. At 16 to 25 weeks, the fetus appears less vulnerable with no increase in mental retardation at doses of less than 0.5 Gy.
3. There does not appear to be an increased risk of mental retardation prior to week 8 or after week 25 following ovulation.

Many discussions center on whether there is a threshold for the phenomenon of severe mental retardation (Fig. 8-4). Even though linear and linear-quadratic dose-response relationships are consistent with the data on severe mental retardation in 8- to 15-week fetuses, there could be a threshold. If the two cases of Down syndrome in the 8- to 15-week period are excluded, no definite increase in mental retardation is evident at doses of 0.2 Gy.

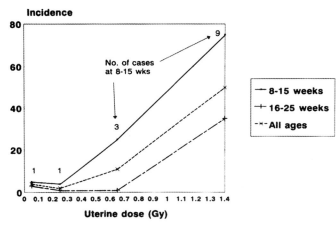

Severe mental retardation (A-bomb)

Figure 8-4 ● Incidence of severe mental retardation in individuals exposed in utero to the atomic bombings in Japan. The data is based on 27 cases. No cases of Down syndrome are included. (From United Nations Scientific Committee on the Effects of Atomic Radiation [UNSCEAR], Sources and effects of ionizing radiation: UNSCEAR 1993 report to the General Assembly, with scientific annexes. New York, United Nations, 1993.)

In the 16- to 25-week group, no cases of severe mental retardation occurred at exposures below 0.5 Gy, and a threshold may exist in the range from 0.2 to 0.7 Gy.[38] The most biologically plausible explanation at this time is that radiation during the sensitive time periods may cause a shift to the left of the normal distribution of intelligence scores. In other words, a dose of radiation in the range of a few tens of mGy will not cause an individual who was destined to have an intelligence quotient (IQ) of 110 to drop to below 70 but potentially could cause a drop from 71 to 69.

IQ

Intelligence test scores in Japanese experience commonly refer to the Koga test. The mean is usually 108, with a standard deviation of 16. A number of authors have described the results of intelligence tests following in utero radiation exposure. Their studies indicate that in the period of 0 to 7 weeks or after the 26th week following ovulation, there is no evidence of a radiation-related decrease in intelligence. At 8 to 15 weeks, and to a lesser extent at 16 to 25 weeks, there is a significant decrease in mean test scores with increasing dose (Fig. 8-5). The risk factor associated with diminution of IQ following radiation exposure in an 8- to 15-week fetus is 21 to 33 points at 1 Gy. This is based on use of a linear model. The regression coefficient appears to be almost the same whether a linear or linear-quadratic model is used and fit to the IQ test scores. School performance also has been evaluated, and the data correspond remarkably well with the IQ data. These findings can be interpreted to signify that there is a dose-related decrease in IQ and that if the dose is high enough, there will be an increase

in cases that are clinically classified as mental retardation.[40,41]

Microcephaly

The In-Utero Mortality Study of the atomic bomb survivors is based on 1600 subjects exposed in utero and on controls.[42–48] Miller analyzed 183 of the subjects exposed in utero at Hiroshima; 78 fetuses were less than 16 weeks of age at the time of irradiation.[45] Of these, 25 were microcephalic, and 11 were mentally deficient. Of 105 fetuses who were 16 weeks or older at the time of irradiation, 7 were microcephalic and 4 were mentally retarded. For those exposed in utero at Hiroshima, there is an extremely strong relationship between radiation dose and microcephaly; although, as mentioned earlier, this also depends on gestational age at irradiation. A significant excess of microcephaly was identified even among those who received only 100 to 190 mGy kerma of mixed neutron and gamma radiation (Table 8-4).[49]

Miller and Mulvihill expressed the relationship among head circumference, dose, and gestational age in a three-dimensional drawing (Fig. 8-6).[50] Table 8-4 demonstrates that the probability of microcephaly from radiation in early pregnancy is approximately 40% at absorbed doses of 1 Gy.

It is not clear whether severe mental retardation and small head size are independent or interdependent of each other. Certainly, the size of the head is dependent on growth of the brain. While a small head may be the result of fewer neurons, this has not been proven, and some individuals with small heads may have reduced size but a normal number of neurons and glial cells. Otake and Schull reexamined the data on small head size using the DS86 doses.[51] For purposes of these studies, an individual with small head size was defined as having a head circumference less than two standard deviations below the mean for the age at measurement. When all ages are considered, 4.2% (62 out of 1473) had small head size. Of 26 mentally retarded individuals, 15 had small head size, and 11 had normal head size. When examined relative to age at exposure, the proportion of individuals with small head size increases with increasing dose, predominantly in the 8- to 15-week period. Seventeen individuals with a small head in the 0- to 7-week period had no evidence of mental retardation. Twelve of 15 individuals (80%) with an atypically small head and severe mental retardation were irradiated in the 8- to 15-week period, and in the 16- to 25-week period, only 1 of the 3 individuals with a small head was mentally retarded. The latter individual had been exposed to a dose of more than 1 Gy. The mean IQ and standard deviation among the 47 individuals having small head size but who did not have severe mental retardation approximated those values seen in the clinical sample. And it is probable that the majority of these individuals are normal persons at the low end of the measurement scale. Ultimately, it appears that there

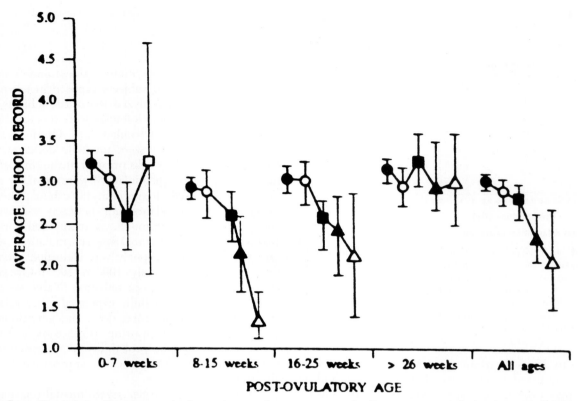

Figure 8-5 • Change in intelligence scores by dose and postovulatory age as a result of in utero exposure during the atomic bombings in Japan. (From United Nations Scientific Committee on the Effects of Atomic Radiation [UNSCEAR], Sources and effects of ionizing radiation: UNSCEAR 1993 report to the General Assembly, with scientific annexes. New York, United Nations, 1993.)

is a correlation between individuals having severe mental retardation and small head size, but the reverse situation is much less clear.

Seizures

Seizures can occur due to a number of causes, one of which is unusual brain development. Seizures are normally classified as febrile, acute symptomatic (as a result of things such as previous head trauma), and unprovoked head seizures. Dunn et al. studied seizures in relationship to the atomic bomb survivors and in utero radiation.[52] No

seizures were identified in the individuals exposed 0 to 7 weeks after ovulation. At 8 to 15 weeks, the incidence of seizures was higher in the group receiving more than 0.1 Gy and increased with the level of fetal exposure. This was true for all types of seizures as well as for unprovoked seizures. Most of the excess seizures were in patients with severe mental retardation. No increase in seizures was identified after radiation at late stages of development. The risk of seizures following exposure during the period of 8 to 15 weeks postovulation was 4.4% (90% confidence interval [CI] 4.1 to 91.6) after doses of 0.5 Gy or more. Two case reports are identified in which patients were exposed during the course of medical treatment and subsequently gave birth to a child with epilepsy.[53] Both of these cases involved women being treated for uterine fibroids, with the actual radiation doses being unknown, but almost certainly in excess of 1 Gy. Both children subsequently born developed epilepsy between the ages of 2 and 4 years.

Structural Neuropathology

There is only a very limited amount of autopsy data with respect to the in utero mortality sample.[54] Four children at Hiroshima who were exposed in utero at less than 2000 m from the hypocenter died but did not have autopsies; all four had mental retardation and were exposed during

Table 8-4 • Relationship of Radiation Dose to Small Head Size in Children Exposed Before the Eighteenth Week of Gestation at Hiroshima	
Radiation Dose (Gy)	**Small Head Size (%)**
0	4
0.01–0.09	7
0.10–0.19	11
0.20–0.29	23
0.30–0.49	36
0.5–1.49	45
>1.5	35

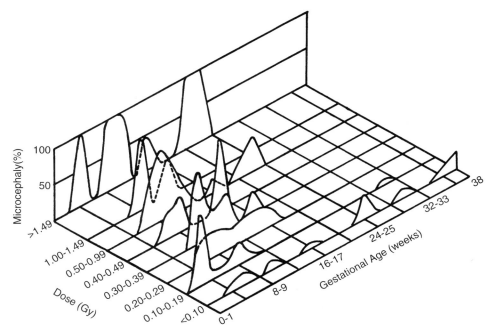

Figure 8-6 ● Incidence of microcephaly at various dose levels and gestational ages at exposure. Incidence approaches 100% when dose level to fetus exceeds 1 Gy or at gestational ages of 6 to 12 weeks. (From Miller RW, Mulvihill JJ: Small head size after atomic irradiation. Teratology 1976;14:355–357.)

the first trimester. In the proximally exposed group at Nagasaki, three deaths were reported, with only one autopsy, performed on a 16-year-old adolescent who had been exposed between the fourth and fifth weeks of gestation. He had a small head circumference, was subnormal in both height and weight, was mentally retarded, and had other abnormalities, including congenital cataracts, strabismus, and microphthalmos. The brain weighed only 860 g, compared with a normal mean of 1275 g. The cerebral hemispheres were symmetrically small, although the brain stem and cerebellum were well developed. The temporal lobes had a polygyric appearance, and the corpora mammalaria could not be identified. There were large islands of heterotopic gray matter about the lateral ventricles, caudate nucleus, and hippocampus. Microscopically, the nerve cell population in the cerebral cortex was reduced, and the laminar arrangement in the cortex was disturbed.[55]

Magnetic resonance imaging (MRI) has been performed on five mentally retarded individuals who were all exposed between 8 and 15 weeks postovulation.[56] In two individuals, both males, who were exposed at 8 to 9 weeks postovulation, the ventricles were slightly larger than normal, and heterotopic gray matter areas were again seen in a periventricular distribution (Fig. 8-7). Two other individuals, who were female and exposed at 12 to 13 weeks after ovulation, did not show heterotopic gray matter but did show faulty brain structure, with sulci that were shallower than normal and a mega cisterna magna. These individuals may not have shown the heterotopic gray matter because exposure occurred late in the

second wave of neuronal migration. Brent questioned why the human CNS appears to be more radiosensitive than that in experimental animals: in experimental animals, many organ systems are more uniformly malformed by irradiation.[2] One possibility that Brent proposes is that the CNS in humans maintains some sensitivity throughout gestation, although the other organ systems have much narrower radiosensitive time periods. Additionally, the time period for multiple system malformations induced by radiation in humans is proportionally quite short: the second to fourth week of gestation, representing only 5% of pregnancy. In the rat, on the other

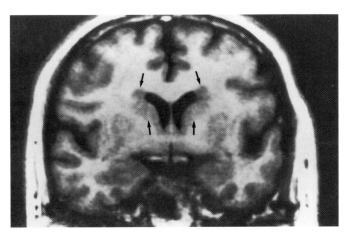

Figure 8-7 ● A coronal MR image of the brain in an atomic bomb survivor prenatally exposed at the eighth to ninth week postovulation. There is ectopic gray matter (*arrows*) at the lateral margins of the ventricles. (Case courtesy of W. Schull.)

hand, the period for multiple malformations is from the ninth to the eleventh day, or 20% of pregnancy.

Fetal Period

Gross abnormalities of the major organ systems do not occur as a result of radiation during this period. However, as indicated by data presented previously, CNS abnormalities may occur, particularly after high doses of radiation received between days 50 and 100 of gestation.

Entire Gestation

In addition to studies of mental retardation and microcephaly, anthropometric data have been collected in the search for radiogenic effects of in utero exposure. The studies of the atomic bomb survivors suggest a general retardation in growth.[57–59] This is true not only for individuals exposed prenatally but also for those exposed in early childhood. The data are difficult to intrepret because the exposed children also suffered substantial physical trauma and nutritional deprivation. The finding of growth retardation appears to have been more pronounced in boys than in girls; the reason for this higher incidence is unknown. Wood et al. studied 1613 Hiroshima and Nagasaki children exposed in utero to identify abnormalities in growth and development.[60] The children were examined at 17 years of age and were divided into groups of 0 m to less than 2000 m from the hypocenter, 3000 m to less than 5000 m from the hypocenter, and not in the city (NIC). Height and weight were lower for the males at Hiroshima and Nagasaki and for the females at Hiroshima who were exposed within 2000 m of the hypocenter. A time of maximal risk for growth retardation has not been observed, and growth retardation may result from substantial fetal dose (greater than 0.2 Gy) at any time during pregnancy. Shohoji and Pasternack also reported on growth retardation.[61] Because the retardation in height and weight appears to be present as a risk from high-dose irradiation throughout pregnancy, whereas mental deficiency occurs only early in pregnancy, the two effects probably have different mechanisms. The major findings of growth retardation in humans include reduced height and reduced head and chest circumferences.[62,63] Burrow et al. examined age at menarchy, degree of epiphyseal closure in the wrist, head circumference, chest circumference, standing and sitting height, and weight.[43] Head size was the single indicator that was most significantly affected. Russell et al. examined the age at epiphyseal closure of the wrist bones in the atomic bomb survivors.[64] Although a delay in epiphyseal closure was identified in both males and females, no correlation between the absorbed dose to the mother and the time of closure of the epiphyses was detected. In a recent publication Otake et al. reported on a longitudinal study of growth, development, and stature among prenatally exposed atomic bomb survivors.[65] Based on repeated

measurements of the stature of 10- and 18-year-old survivors, the analysis indicated a significant retardation of growth in those exposed during the first or second trimester, whether a linear or linear-quadratic dose-response relationship was assumed. However, in those exposed during the third trimester, there was no significant effect using either the linear or linear-quadratic model. Nakashima analyzed the standing height, body weight, sitting height, chest circumference, and intercristal diameter of 1259 subjects at age 18 who were exposed in utero during the atomic bombings.[66] There was a dose response in reduction for most measurements but the interaction between dose and gestational period was not significant.

In 1959, Hammer-Jacobson reported on 11 women who received diagnostic abdominal x-ray examinations during the first trimester.[67] Estimated exposure to the fetus ranged between 3 and 37 mGy. Eight of the women had therapeutic abortions, and three carried the pregnancy to term. No gross malformations appeared in any of the aborted fetuses or term infants. There are some other case reports and studies regarding the role of ionizing radiation in causing brain abnormalities.[68,69] One interesting study of 998 children born to women who had pelvimetry during the course of their pregnancy was performed at Chicago Lying-In Hospital. The estimated dose to the fetus was 0.005 Gy.[70,71] About 90% of the fetuses were exposed in the second half of pregnancy. However, about 120 were exposed prior to the 140th day of the last menstrual cycle. The authors found no statistically significant difference between exposed and comparison groups with regard to CNS abnormalities. Ganrota examined the association between diagnostic x-ray examinations in Finland and defects of the CNS that had suggested abnormalities of the brain.[72] No estimate of fetal absorbed dose was given, and the author indicates that the majority of these infants were exposed because of the clinical suspicion of maternal pelvic or fetal anomaly and that the exposures were unlikely to have been given at a time when the abnormalities that were found should have been induced.[73] Neumeister described 19 children who were prenatally exposed to doses of 0.015 to 0.1 Gy.[74] No instances of severe mental retardation were recorded, and no comparison group was identified. Meyer et al. did not find any evidence of increased frequency among 1455 women who were prenatally exposed as a result of diagnostic pelvic examinations.[75] Most of the exposures occurred late in pregnancy in this particular study. Nokkenteved reported a study from Denmark in 1962 in which 152 children who were exposed in the first 4 months after fertilization to doses of 0.02 to 0.07 Gy were examined.[76] One child in the exposed group was found to be microcephalic. Hu studied 1026 children born in China after prenatal exposure to diagnostic radiation.[77] Absorbed dose to the fetus was estimated to be 12 to 43 mGy. Thirteen children were exposed at 8 to 15 weeks, 41 at 16 to 25 weeks, and most of the remainder subsequent to the 26th week. No significant difference was identified in either physical development or intelligence when comparison was made with a group of 1191 children matched with respect to age, sex, and hospital of birth. Most all of these studies have either very small sample sizes or low doses. In spite of this, the findings are consistent with the findings at Hiroshima and Nagasaki.

Prenatal diagnostic irradiation has been implicated as a cause of heterochromia in the iris of the eye. This relationship was studied by LeJeune et al.[78] and Cheesman and Walby.[79] The LeJeune study indicated a slightly increased incidence of heterochromia; however, the Cheesman study did not demonstrate a statistically significant increase. Jacobsen and Mellemgaard examined 201 female patients who received pelvic irradiation for diagnostic radiologic urinary studies; 184 were examined for ocular defects, which were identified in some cases.[80] Four of 42 individuals irradiated in utero and 7 of 142 children conceived after irradiation had ocular anomalies. Eleven cases of eye malformation in 184 subjects appear to be an unusually high incidence. One of the major limitations of this study is that the absorbed dose was unknown because the patients were irradiated between 1924 and 1930. Such results have not been observed or confirmed by other investigators.

The ICRP has provided the following summary of in utero radiation effects on the CNS.[6] During the period of 8 to 25 weeks postconception, the CNS is very sensitive to radiation. Fetal doses in excess of 100 mGy may result in a decrease of IQ. During this same time, fetal doses in the range of 1000 mGy (1 Gy) result in a high probability of severe mental retardation. The CNS becomes less sensitive to these effects at 16 to 25 weeks of gestational age and is rather resistant after that. Radiation effects on the developing central nervous system are probably the result of cell killing and of changes in cellular differentiation and neuronal migration. Values of IQ lower than expected were reported in some children exposed in utero at Hiroshima and Nagasaki; there were two principal quantitative findings. The first is reduction of IQ with increasing dose (see Fig. 8-5). This effect is very dependent on fetal age. Regardless of the time of gestation, IQ reduction cannot be clinically identified at fetal doses of less than 100 mGy. In the period from 8 to 15 weeks after conception a fetal dose of 1000 mGy (1 Gy) reduces IQ by about 30 points. A similar, but smaller, shift is detectable following exposure in the period from 16 to 25 weeks.

The second finding is of a dose-related increase in the frequency of children classified as "severely retarded." This is not unexpected. If the fetal radiation dose is high and there is a large reduction in IQ, there will be more children born who are severely mentally retarded. At fetal doses of 1000 mGy during 8 to 15 weeks gestational age, the probability of this effect is about 40%. The effects of all levels of dose are less marked following exposure in

the period from 16 to 25 weeks after conception and have not been observed for other periods. All the clinical observations on significant IQ reduction and severe mental retardation relate to fetal doses of about 500 mGy and above and at high-dose rates. Direct use of the observations for chronic exposure of workers probably overestimates the risks. It should be noted that radiation-induced mental retardation may sometimes be distinguished from other forms of retardation. Heterotopic gray matter and microcephaly suggest radiation or maternal alcoholism as a potential cause whereas a child with cerebral palsy, normal head size, and a documented hypoxic episode during delivery would not have irradiation as a likely etiology.

Laboratory Findings

Hematologic findings of persons irradiated in utero at Hiroshima have been studied by several authors.[44,81] The studies demonstrated no significant effects by the time the babies reached childhood or early adolescence. Although hematologic changes may have been present immediately after the bombing, apparently hematologic recovery was complete by the age of 5 years. Increased proteinuria was detected in those exposed at Hiroshima whose mothers were within 1.5 km of the hypocenter.[82] The differences between some of the exposed and unexposed groups did reach significant levels; however, the etiology and biological significance of the proteinuria are unknown.

Sex Ratio

Sex ratio of babies exposed in utero was examined by Meyer et al.[83] The study was performed on black women in Baltimore who were exposed to diagnostic pelvimetry between 1947 and 1949. Doses were estimated to be 10 to 50 mGy. Reproductive capacity of individuals exposed in utero appeared not to be affected; however, it was possible that the mothers exposed at 0 to 29 weeks of pregnancy had a statistically significant excess of male babies. Jablon and Kato did not identify sex ratio change in the offspring (irrespective of the dose group at the time of gestation at irradiation) in the atomic bomb survivors.[84] A study of the reproductive capacity of females exposed in utero, conducted by Meyer et al., concerned diagnostic doses in the range of 10 to 50 mGy and included carefully matched controls.[75] Initially, a 10% to 15% increase in fertility was found in the exposed women even after adjustment for socioeconomic and other factors. Their fertility appeared to be decreasing with time, and the ultimate reproductive capacity of both groups is presently unknown.

Summary

In summary, high doses of radiation, particularly those exceeding 1 Gy to the fetus and delivered early in pregnancy (3 to 17 weeks), may cause nonstochastic effects, particularly a high incidence of microcephaly and mental retardation. Approximately 30 other abnormalities or malformations have been identified and correlated with high-level radiation exposure. With the exception of growth retardation, few of these malformations occur in the absence of neurologic abnormalities or microcephaly. This is a useful aid in sorting out possible radiogenic malformations from the 3% to 10% of live births that have "spontaneous" malformations or congenital abnormalities. Irradiation of the human fetus at doses below 50 mGy has not been observed to cause congenital malformations or growth retardation.[2] The single exception is the one report of ocular abnormalities at low absorbed doses by Jacobsen and Mellemgaard.[80] This finding is at variance with a massive amount of experimental and other epidemiologic literature. At absorbed doses of 0.1 Gy, the risk of spontaneous abortion very early in pregnancy may be increased by 0.1% to 1%. The large "normal" spontaneous abortion rate of 30% to 50% would make the theoretical radiogenic increase difficult, if not impossible, to prove or disprove.

IRRADIATION FROM RADIONUCLIDES DURING PREGNANCY

Irradiation of the embryo or fetus from maternal internal contamination with radionuclides may be divided into two major categories. The first are those radionuclides that do not cross the placenta to the fetus, remaining on the maternal side of the circulation and structure. These radionuclides may irradiate the fetus if the radiation emitted is relatively penetrating (i.e., energetic beta, gamma, and x-rays). Medical radionuclides are often included in this group because most emit energetic gamma rays. Early in pregnancy, when the embryo or fetus is quite small, its irradiation is quite uniform and may be approximated by the dose to the ovary or uterus. Doses to the ovary from various radionuclides are listed in Appendix 2. A second major category of radionuclides causing radiation exposure of the embryo and fetus are those that cross the placenta into the fetal circulation. Many of them are ionic in chemical form. After they cross the placenta, they may be distributed in the body of the embryo or fetus or may concentrate locally if the fetal target organ is mature enough to have a physiologic function. An example of such a radionuclide is radioiodine. Many of the data concerning placental transfer of radionuclides come from animal experimentation; therefore, some animal data are considered in the following discussion. The ICRP has published recent comprehensive reports on doses to the embryo and fetus from intakes of radionuclides by the mother[85] and on doses to infants from ingestion of radionuclides in mother's milk.[86]

Radiostrontium

Several studies have been performed on placental transfer of strontium during gestation. Finkel indicated that, in the mouse, negligible amounts of strontium are transferred across the placenta during the first 15 days of gestation.[87] In the rat, the amount of radionuclide transferred to the fetus is 0.01% to 0.02% early in pregnancy, but later in gestation, the transferral rate is approximately 20-fold higher. With single injections of strontium 90 to pregnant rats, the lethal dose (LD_{50}) is 35 mGy at 4 days after conception and 100 mGy at 15 to 19 days after conception. These rodent studies contrast with studies in pregnant dogs in which injection of strontium 90 at activity levels of 370 to 575 MBq per kg of body weight produced no obvious malformations.[88] Few available human data indicate the percentage of strontium transferred across the placenta, but there does appear to be discrimination between strontium 90 and calcium, with a ratio of 1 to 10.[89] Despite placental discrimination, strontium can cross the placenta readily. Mays and Lloyd have published models for ingestion and resulting dose estimates to the fetus and infant.[90] The newer ICRP report indicates that during pregnancy, absorption of ingested strontium is modeled to increase from 0.3 to 0.4 during the first trimester, 0.4 to 0.6 during the second trimester, and to remain at 0.6 in the third trimester.[85] The dose to the embryo until the end of the eighth week is the same as to the uterus. From the ninth week until birth, rates of transfer from maternal blood to fetal blood are derived on a discrimination factor of 0.6 for transfer of strontium relative to calcium. Highest fetal doses are to the red marrow.

Radioiodine

Internal contamination with radioiodines has been extensively reviewed by NCRP.[12] Pregnancy is associated with increases in iodine by the maternal thyroid and in increases in thyroid hormones. The rate of renal clearance of iodine also increases by a factor of about 2. Radioiodine rapidly and readily crosses the placenta. Before the thyroid starts functioning the iodine mainly accumulates in the liver and intestine. The human fetal thyroid begins to accumulate iodine at about 11 weeks postconception.[91] Between 14 and 22 weeks of gestation, the percentage of uptake of radioiodine by the thyroid is higher than that seen in adults, ranging between 55% and 75%.[92] Toward the end of pregnancy the concentration of radioiodine in the fetal thyroid can exceed that of the mother by 3- to 10-fold. The only well-documented effect of radioiodine in the human fetus is that of hypothyroidism, possibly resulting in cretinism if the abnormality is not promptly recognized and treated. Hypothyroidism following internal fetal irradiation with radioiodine has been reported by several investigators. The administered dose to the mothers reported in these studies ranged from 450 MBq to 8 GBq of iodine 131.[93–96] In one study, nine patients about to undergo medical abortion received tracer doses of iodine 131 12 to 48 hours before surgery.[92] The fetus was sectioned, studied histologically, and assayed for radioactivity. No collection of radioiodine by the fetus before the 12th week of gestation was detected. Beierwaltes et al. reported iodine 131 concentrations in fetal thyroids from fallout.[97,98] These studies also demonstrated that iodine 131 concentration was higher in human fetal thyroids than in adult thyroid glands. In this series, 27 human fetal thyroid glands from 25 pregnancies were obtained at the time of abortion, cesarean section, stillbirth, or neonatal death. No tracer doses were given. The iodine found in the human fetal thyroids was either from weapons testing or other types of environmental contamination. Estimated doses to the fetal thyroid from iodine 131 in fallout are in the range of 7 to 200 Gy per 37 MBq, that is, for gestational ages of 10 to 22 weeks. The total-body fetal dose ranges from 8 to 80 mGy per 37 MBq over the same gestational ages.[99] Other authors have also examined the role of radioiodine during pregnancy.[100–102]

Radioiron

Iron metabolism has been studied since the 1940s in attempts to evaluate nutritional requirements of pregnant women.[103] The mother's body is the largest contributor to the fetal dose of iron 59, accounting for approximately 70% of the dose early in pregnancy and decreasing to 50% of the dose later in pregnancy. Total-body dose to the fetus from internal deposition ranges between 10% and 20% of the total dose, increasing slightly during pregnancy. The dose from iron 59 in the fetal liver as a contributor to the fetal dose accounts for less than 10% at 10 weeks of gestational age but rises rapidly to approximately 30% at 15 weeks. The critical organ in the fetus is the liver, which receives 3 to 6 Gy per 37 MBq administered intravenously to the mother. The dosimetry of iron is complicated because iron is involved in many complex metabolic roles, such as formation of hemoglobin, and composition of enzymes; it also occurs in the form of free iron.

Inert Gases

There is very little experimental evidence concerning the placental transfer of either xenon or krypton, and placental transfer is assumed to be free in both directions. Thus, the dose to the fetus should be quite similar to the maternal dose. The major exception to this may be krypton 81 m, which is used for some pulmonary function tests and has a half-life of only 13 seconds. In this instance, fetal dose is substantially less than that of the mother.

Gallium

Gallium 67 is used widely in nuclear medicine for detection of tumors and abscesses. The fetal dose from gallium may be higher than expected as a result of its active transport across the placenta. The whole-body dose to the fetus is 0.4 mGy per MBq, with five times this dose to the fetal spleen.

Technetium

Technetium 99m is the most widely used radionuclide in nuclear medicine. As a pertechnetate, it rapidly crosses the placenta and localizes in the stomach, colon, and thyroid. Absorbed doses to the fetal thyroid are about 1 mGy per MBq and about a third of this dose to the stomach and colon. Other technetium 99m–labeled radiopharmaceuticals may or may not cross the placenta, depending on the radiopharmaceutical or cell type that has been labeled.

Cesium

Cesium 137 appears to have a metabolic pathway similar to, but not dependent on, that of potassium or rubidium. There is preferential uptake of cesium by human red cells, with the cesium-potassium ratio equaling 3 at equilibrium. Excretion of potassium (and possibly cesium) to a large extent depends on hormones; this dependence may result in decreased fetal concentration during pregnancy. Deposition of cesium during pregnancy was reviewed by Sternberg.[89] Most experiments have used guinea pigs; however, human placentas from Canadian and Japanese women have also been studied. The Japanese women who were studied were present during the 1945 atomic bomb explosion. The data indicate that extrapolations from guinea pigs and observations in humans appear to give comparable results. For cesium 137, the fetal-to-maternal plasma ratio is 0 to 130. It is also apparent from experimental animal data that the placenta is able to discriminate between cesium and potassium, with cesium being more inhibited in transfer to the fetus.[104,105] Bertelli et al. reported that following the radiological cesium contamination accident in Goiania, Brazil, a woman who was 4 months pregnant became contaminated.[106] Concentrations in the mother were very similar to that of her newborn child. A similar report is available from Greece concerning cesium contamination from Chernobyl.[107] Another report from Goiania concerned a female who became pregnant about 4 years after being contaminated and who had a body content of about 300 MBq of cesium 137. At birth the child had concentrations of cesium 13 times lower than the mother because the cesium in the mother was in tissues with a slow turnover rate.[108]

Cerium and Rare Earths of the Lanthanide Group

Radionuclides in the lanthanide group have little clinical importance to the fetus. The target tissue is the maternal reticuloendothelial system, because rare earths precipitate at the pH of body fluids and are then collected by the reticuloendothelial cells. In addition, rare earths are practically insoluble and do not cross the digestive tract. An exception is yttrium 90, which enters the body as strontium 90, subsequently decays to yttrium 90 after absorption, and then becomes concentrated in the skeleton.

Summary

In summary, maternal contamination with radionuclides may cause irradiation of the fetus, even if the radionuclide is not transferred across the placenta. This phenomenon applies mostly to radionuclides, which yield relatively penetrating radiations. A major radionuclide of interest (which causes nonstochastic or somatic effects) is radio-iodine in view of its preferential accumulation by the fetal thyroid after the 13th week of gestation. Other radionuclides may cross the placenta in varying degrees; however, because the mother acts as a discriminator in most instances, their effects, if any, involve induction of neoplasms in the organs of interest rather than nonstochastic effects. The reader is referred to a recent ICRP report for more detailed information and concerning many additional radionuclides.[85]

CARCINOGENESIS

Risk can be expressed either as relative or absolute risk. RR indicates the risk as a function of the "background cancer risk." An RR of 1.0 indicates that there is no effect of irradiation whereas an RR of 1.5 for a given dose indicates that the radiation will cause a 50% increase in cancer above background rates. Absolute risk estimates simply indicate the excess number of cancer cases expected in a population due to a certain radiation dose.

The risk of childhood leukemia and other neoplasms following in utero radiation has been the major concern at low doses (less than 0.1 Gy). Issues regarding preconception radiation and the potential of subsequent leukemia and cancer are discussed in detail in Chapter 3. The major human studies of carcinogenesis after in utero exposure yield varying results. A major category of epidemiologic studies comprises children who received in utero exposure from diagnostic radiologic procedures performed on the mother. The examinations in these series usually include pelvimetries or placentograms, with most performed during the third trimester. As early as 1958, Stewart et al. reported an increased incidence of leukemia in children who had received diagnostic radiologic examinations.[109] This was followed by several similar reports.[110–112] The 1958 study by Stewart (also known as the Oxford Survey of Childhood Cancer) investigated 1299 children in England and Wales who died of leukemia and other cancers prior to 10 years of age. These were matched with controls, and the mothers of both populations were questioned about diagnostic radiation exposure during gestation. In utero exposure was 1.9 times as frequent in the population of children who had leukemia and other cancers as in the control group. In 1975, the Oxford survey was updated by Bithell and Stewart.[113] In this report, the number of cases was increased to 8000 and included children up to 15 years of age. Sixty percent of the children were exposed during the third trimester, and the risk in the exposed group for childhood malignancies

was between 1.4 and 1.5 times that in the nonexposed group. The Oxford survey included nearly 70% of childhood deaths from malignancies in Wales between the years 1953 and 1967. The increased risk identified for each unit of absorbed dose is much higher than would be expected from similar studies of radiation effects in adults. It should be stressed that the poor quality of the information on fetal dose and the possibility that a proportion of the excess risk might be due to factors unrelated to the x-ray exposure preclude an accurate assessment of risk per unit dose. Any such estimates must be interpreted cautiously. Evidence in support of a causal association include the consistency of findings in many studies conducted over a period of 35 years.[114] Case-control studies based on personal interview were initially criticized because of the possibility of response bias, but subsequent large studies based on only review of obstetric records also confirmed the association. The possibility of unidentified conditions that select mothers for x-ray whose children were destined to develop cancer was addressed in a reanalysis by Mole[115,116] of twin data within the Oxford survey and in two case-control studies of twins within population-based tumor registry regions in Connecticut, the United States,[117] and Sweden.[118] Twins were likely to have been x-rayed for reasons unrelated to the mother's health, such as to diagnose the twin pregnancy or to determine fetal position before delivery, and all three evaluations found an association between prenatal x-rays and childhood cancer. Muirhead has pointed out that controlling for maternal illness and drugs taken during pregnancy in the Oxford survey also failed to change appreciably the estimates of relative risk (RR).[119] Stewart's studies have been carefully reviewed and criticized by many authors.[120–122] The criticisms concern several basic issues, particularly methodology and estimate of risk. Many researchers indicated that the population of cancer cases (chosen because they have cancer) is different from the control population. The higher frequency of x-rays performed in the cancer population may be attributable to factors that caused a greater need for medical care. It may be such other factors that caused a higher incidence of leukemia and cancer. Totter examined the Oxford data and pointed out that the dose-response relationship claimed by Stewart could be duplicated or improved by substituting random numbers for the actual values in the survey.[120] In a later paper, Totter and MacPherson clearly demonstrated that (1) the association of x-rays and cancer decreased over the years, (2) the dose-response curves of Stewart were not valid, and (3) the nonexposed siblings of those who received in utero radiation exposure had an almost two times higher probability of developing cancer than the control group; probability of cancer among the control group was 0.0007 versus 0.0018 in siblings of the exposed children.[118] In other words, the retrospective analysis by Stewart did not demonstrate a causal relationship, but rather merely an association between the frequency of x-rays and childhood malignancies. The second major criticism of Stewart's work concerns the estimate of risk. The increase in cancer mortality identified is approximately seven times greater than the estimate of the BEIR 1980 Committee.[123] Webster[122] indicated that there are good reasons to doubt that the fetus is much more sensitive to carcinogenic effects of radiation than the adult; also, Stewart's risk estimates conflict with the data from the atomic bomb survivors.[109,124] According to the Stewart and Kneale risk estimates, 18.4 extra cancer deaths should have been found in the latter group, and, at a minimum, 5.2.[110] There is an additional report by Ishimaru et al. in which 3636 children were studied.[125] This included a control group and survivors from Hiroshima and Nagasaki who were in utero at the time of the bombings. Some of the survivors received over 0.5 Gy. After 34 years of follow-up, only three cases of leukemia were found in the entire group. For a statistically significant increase of in utero radiogenic leukemia, seven cases would have been needed. In a later report, Yoshimoto et al. indicate that after in utero exposure to the bombings in Japan (mean uterine dose, 0.18 Gy), there was no increase in childhood cancer.[126] During the first 14 years of life of the in utero group, no leukemias occurred, and only two cancers were diagnosed: one case of liver cancer at age 6 and one case of Wilms' tumor at age 14.[124]

Many other studies of childhood leukemia and prenatal irradiation have been published; some were reviewed by MacMahon and Hutchinson.[127] The pooled data suggested an increase in leukemia following prenatal exposure, with the average increase in risk being 42%. Court Brown et al. followed 49,000 women exposed to diagnostic abdominal x-ray during pregnancy in the years 1945–1958; they found 9 cases of leukemia versus 10.5 expected from the national statistics of the United Kingdom.[128] This excludes an increase in leukemia by more than 50%, although the 42% increase mentioned earlier appears unlikely but is not excluded.[127] Tabuchi et al. did not demonstrate an increase in leukemia after diagnostic exposure; however, the number of patients involved in their study was relatively small.[129] Most studies of individuals who have received x-rays prenatally report the RR of leukemia to be increased to 1.4 and the RR of all major groups of solid tumors also to be increased to 1.4. This seems strange because cancer and leukemia are known to have dissimilar origins and very different excess relative risks (ERRs) following postnatal exposure. Both MacMahon[130] and Miller[131] pointed out that such a situation is uncharacteristic of any other human or experimental animal exposure, raising questions about biologic plausibility. For example, whereas Japanese children exposed to the atomic bombings under the age of 10 years were at very high risk of developing childhood leukemia (14 cases occurred), no other childhood cancers developed.[132] Finally, it is notable that ERRs have been

found only in case-control studies. No cohort study has detected a significant increase in childhood cancer following prenatal irradiation.[70,124,128,133–135] Indeed, RRs of about 1.0 or less have been found. The cohort studies can be criticized, however, because of small numbers of childhood cases and associated low statistical power to detect an excess. Furthermore, Doll later concluded that there was a strong possibility that ascertainment was incomplete in his investigation, despite the presumed higher frequency of prenatal x-ray exposure among twins compared with single births. Cohort studies of twins in Sweden, Norway, Finland, California, and Connecticut also failed to find an increase in childhood cancer other than leukemia, compared with the general population, and several reported significant deficits. Actual prenatal exposure in the twin studies, however, was not known, and the proportion irradiated may not have been as high as believed. Further, it is not necessarily correct to expect twins to be at the same risk of childhood cancer as singletons. Nevertheless, on the basis of the above discussion, the possibility of a causal association cannot be dismissed, although quantification of risk remains uncertain. Some investigators have suggested that children prone to allergy are more susceptible to in utero irradiation than nonallergic children. This argument was reviewed by NCRP, with the general conclusion that radiation was a "red herring" in such studies.[12] In fact, other unlikely associations for leukemia were also found: use of aspirin by the mother led to a relative leukemia risk factor of 1.9; cold tablets, 2.4; allergy in the mother, 1.6; and allergy in the child, 2.1. If all cancers were studied, pulmonary disease in children leads to an RR of 1.4, and eating fish and chips weekly leads to an RR of cancer of 1.4.[136]

Preconception radiation has been examined with respect to leukemogenesis. Hoshino et al. studied 17,000 children whose parents were atomic bomb survivors and found no increase in leukemia.[137] This report was in contrast to that of Graham, who reported an increased incidence of leukemia from both preconception irradiation and in utero radiation, with identical risk for both.[138] The possibility of preconception irradiation leading to tumors in the offspring is discussed extensively in Chapter 3, and most authors conclude that this does not occur. Some authors have shown various nonradiogenic associations with leukemia in childhood malignancy, including previous maternal history of stillbirth, abortion, maternal smoking, and infants of high birth weight.[139–142] Some genetic or environmental factors may contribute to leukemia, because Miller indicates that siblings of leukemic children have an incidence of leukemia of 1 in 720 up to the age of 10.[141] Stjernfeldt et al. reported an increase in risk of acute lymphocytic leukemia with diagnostic irradiation during pregnancy (RR 1.8 with 95% CI 1.1 to 3.1), with maternal smoking alone (RR 2.2 with 95% CI 1.1 to 4.4), and a combined effect with both together

(RR of 3.6%, CI 1.8 to 7.0).[142] Results of this study should be taken with caution because there are no other reports of maternal smoking causing acute lymphocytic leukemia or of a similar interaction with radiation and smoking in the causation of leukemia. If an assumption is made that fetal doses from medical prenatal exposures were on the order of 10 mSv, then the estimated ERR per sievert (Sv) derived from the various case-control studies is roughly 40 for leukemia and 40 for other cancers. This is in marked contrast to the prenatal or postnatal risk in children derived from the atomic bomb survivor studies. The ERRs per Sv in survivors of the atomic bombing under age 10 years when exposed are approximately 17 for leukemia and 2 for other cancers. Other studies of childhood irradiation found excessive RRs per Sv for leukemia that are generally smaller than those seen in survivors of the atomic bombings. The UNSCEAR committee, in its 1994 report,[143] pointed out that even though there is considerable uncertainty about the mean fetal dose per obstetric examination, estimates of risk have been made by UNSCEAR and others.[119] As expected these estimates vary widely. Some estimates failed to account for the decrease in fetal dose per obstetric examination that occurred over the years. Others relied on the concept of dose per film rather than the more appropriate dose per examination, because more than one film may be taken per examination. Some considered only fatal and not incident cancers; some were computed for the first 10 years of life and others for the first 15 years. One recent analysis of the Oxford survey, with adjustments for many of the previous inadequacies in former computation, indicated a decrease within a year of birth in the excess absolute risk of cancers in those over ages 0 to 14 years, perhaps corresponding, at least in part, to a decrease in fetal dose. Based on the more recent analyses of the Oxford survey, the excess absolute risk of mortality from all cancers for the first 14 years is on the order of $5 \times 10^{-2} Sv^{-1}$. In the only study that has evaluated adult-onset cancers following prenatal exposure, Yoshimoto et al. reported a significantly increased risk of adult cancer among 1630 prenatally exposed survivors of the atomic bombings followed through 1984.[126] However, no cancers occurred in the most recent follow-up interval during 1985–1989, and, although the point estimate of the ERR per unit dose remains quite high (0.9), the increase is no longer statistically significant (95% CI −0.12 to 3.81).[126] The small number of cancer deaths (24) and the limited follow-up during adult life contribute to the uncertainties in the risk estimate. Studies of in utero exposure have thus given a wide range of risk estimates, from high risk to none at all. UNSCEAR concluded that on a biologic basis there is no reason to assume that the fetus is immune to the carcinogenic effects of ionizing radiation and, in particular, leukemogenesis; therefore, a positive finding of a risk after appreciable doses is to be expected.[143] However, on the basis of the present data,

the exact quantification of effects is subject to much uncertainty.

The ICRP provided the following summary relative to carcinogenic effects following in utero radiation exposure.[6] In it, radiation has been shown to cause leukemia and many types of cancer in both adults and children. Throughout most of pregnancy, the embryo/fetus is assumed to be at about the same risk for potential carcinogenic effects of radiation as are children.

As a result of radiation exposure after conception and until delivery there is felt to be an increased risk of childhood cancer and leukemia. The spontaneous incidence of childhood cancer and leukemia from ages 0 to 18, without radiation exposure, is about 2 to 3 per 1000. The magnitude of risk following radiation exposure and whether the risk changes throughout pregnancy has been the subject of many publications, yet interpretation of the data remains open to debate. One type of epidemiological studies (case-control) demonstrated raised risks associated with obstetric x-ray examinations of pregnant women. Similar results were not found in cohort studies. There is some evidence of possibly raised risks of leukemia in the atomic bomb survivors who were irradiated in utero but there was no increasing leukemia trend with dose and the cases did not occur during childhood.

A recent analysis of many of the epidemiological studies conducted on prenatal x-ray and childhood cancer are consistent with an RR of 1.4 (a 40% increase over the background risk) following a fetal dose of 10 mGy. The best methodological studies, however, suggested that the risk is probably lower than this. Even if the RR were as high as 1.4, the individual probability of childhood cancer after in utero irradiation is very low since the background incidence of childhood cancer is so low.

Recent absolute risk estimates for cancer risk from ages 0 to 15 after in utero irradiation were estimated to be in the range of 600 per 10,000 persons each exposed to 1000 mGy (or 0.6% per 100 mGy). This is essentially equivalent to a risk of 1 in 170 per 100 mGy of exposure. Excess lifetime cancer risk as a result of in utero exposure has not been clearly demonstrated among Japanese atomic bomb survivor studies, even though the population has been followed for about 50 years.

COMPARISON OF RISKS DURING PREGNANCY

Minimization of Radiation Exposure During Pregnancy

There have been many attempts to minimize exposure from diagnostic radiologic examinations received by the fetus in pregnancy. One of the earliest was the "10-day rule." This was a recommendation that elective radiographic procedures be postponed so that they could be done only during the first 10 days after the menstrual period.

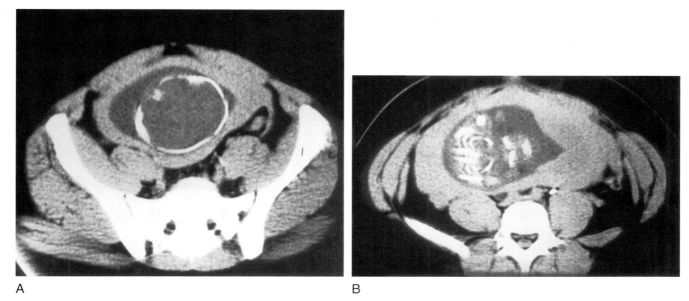

Figure 8-8 • In utero diagnostic medical exposure. Two slices of a computerized tomographic scan done inadvertently on a pregnant patient. The skull (**A**) and the ribs and spine (**B**) of the fetus can easily be seen in the center of the images.

At the present time, most U.S. scientists and physicians do not accept this philosophy for several reasons. Often there is poor patient cooperation and difficulty in scheduling the patients (particularly in those women who have irregular menstrual periods). Additionally, it is possible that a procedure may be postponed in order to wait for the 10-day "window." If the patient is in fact pregnant, the examination may have to be performed when the embryo is more susceptible to potential malformations and CNS effects than it would have been during preimplantation. Current operational philosophy in most radiology departments is to find out which patients believe they may be pregnant before performing a diagnostic radiologic examination. If a non-ionizing technique such as ultrasound cannot provide the information and if the examination is medically indicated, it is usually performed, although careful monitoring of the procedure allows it to be tailored to minimize dose to the fetus while still obtaining necessary diagnostic information.

Termination of Pregnancy After Radiation Exposure

Although an attempt is made to identify pregnant patients and to avoid unnecessary radiation exposure, often a patient has actually received radiation exposure prior to determination of pregnancy (Fig. 8-8). In these circumstances, the patient may be extremely concerned about the outcome of the pregnancy, and a counseling session with the parents may be useful. Counseling can be given after attempting to estimate the dose to the embryo or fetus from the examination and comparing estimated

radiogenic risk with the other risks of pregnancy (Table 8-5). Women exposed to ionizing radiation believe that they have a much higher risk of malformations than a control group, but appropriate counseling can be beneficial.[144] In this context, it usually becomes obvious that the risk from the radiation exposure (particularly for diagnostic examinations) is very low compared to the natural incidence of other abnormalities and diseases. Another useful approach is to indicate to the patient the probability of *not* having a child with either a malformation or cancer (Table 8-6).[145] Brent pointed out that in consideration of most radiation risks, they are generally small compared with the normal incidence of other problems.[146] He also indicated that exposure to microwaves at levels below maximum permissible limits presents no measurable risk to the embryo, and the same is true of diagnostic ultrasound.[147] With regard to ionizing radiation, he reported that the presumed risks of 10 to 50 mGy (1 to 5 rad) are far below the 15% or greater spontaneous abortion rate, the 2.7% to 3.0% major malformation incidence from causes other than radiation, the 4% intrauterine growth retardation rate (mostly due to hypertension), and the 8% to 10% incidence of genetic diseases. Finally, Brent concluded that at fetal doses less than 50 mGy (5 rad), there is no medical justification for terminating a pregnancy because of radiation exposure.

It is quite unusual for any rational combination of diagnostic radiologic procedures to result in a fetal dose in excess of 50 mGy. Brent[2] and the ICRP[6] indicated that irradiation of the human fetus from diagnostic exposure below 50 mGy has not been shown to cause congenital

Table 8-5 • Comparison of Risks During Pregnancy

Risk Factor	Pregnancy Outcome	Risk of Occurrence
Maternal German measles*	Defects of heart, lens of the eye, skeletal muscles, inner ear, teeth	2 in 3
Maternal cigarette smoking[†]	In general, babies weigh 5–9 oz less than average	1 in 5
<1 pack/day	Infant death	1 in 5
>1 pack/day	Infant death	1 in 3
Maternal alcohol consumption[‡]		
2 drinks/day	Babies weigh 2–6 oz less than average	1 in 10
2–4 drinks/day	Signs of fetal alcohol syndrome (growth deficiency, brain dysfunction, characteristic facial signs)	1 in 5
>4 drinks/day		1 in 3
Chronically alcoholic		1 in 2
Maternal age[§]		
20 yr	Down syndrome (mental and physical growth retardation)	1 in 2300
40 yr		1 in 64
High altitude[‖]		
Mean altitude 263 ft	Low birth weight (higher risk); babies weigh less than 5.5 pounds	1 in 15
5000 ft		1 in 10
10,500 ft		1 in 4
Unknown[¶]	Developmental anomaly (natural incidence)	2–4% of live births
Unknown	Intrauterine growth retardation (natural incidence)	2–3%
Genetic[¶]	ABO hemolytic disease	1%
Unknown[¶]	Chromosomal abnormalities (natural incidence)	0.5%
Unknown[¶]	Major malformation rate at delivery	2.75%
Unknown[¶]	Malformations and genetic diseases at 1–2 yr of age	6–10%
Unknown[¶]	Spontaneous abortion during pregnancy	30–50%
Embryo or fetal irradiation		
Childhood cancer		
10 mSv	Childhood leukemia deaths before the age of 12 yr	1 in 3333
10 mSv	Deaths from other childhood cancers before age 10	1 in 3571
A-bomb exposure at 4–13 wk gestation		
>0.5 Gy (Hiroshima)	Small head size, with severe mental retardation at > 0.25 G	1 in 4

*Tondury G: The virus as a danger to human embryos. In Bertelli A, Donati L (eds): Teratology Symposium, Como, Italy, October 1967. Amsterdam, Excerpta Medica Foundation, 1969.
[†]Meyer MB, Tonascia JA: Maternal smoking, pregnancy complications, and perinatal mortality. Am J Obstet Gynecol 1977;128(5):494–502.
[‡]Smith DW: Alcohol effects on the fetus. Prog Clin Biol Res 1980;36:73–82.
[§]Adamson K, Fox HA (eds): Preventability of perinatal injury: Proceedings of a symposium held in New York City, March, 1974. In Progress in Clinical and Biological Research, vol 2. New York, A Liss Publishers, 1975.
[‖]Grahn D, Kratchman J: Variation in neonatal death rate and birth weight in the United States and possible relations to environmental radiation, geology, and altitude. Am J Hum Genet 1963;15:329–351.
[¶]Mossman KL, Hill LT: Radiation risks in pregnancy. Obstet Gynecol 1982;60:237–242.

Table 8-6 • Probability of Birthing Healthy Children

Dose* to Conceptus (mSv)	Child Will Not Develop Cancer (Percentage)
0	99.93
0.5	99.93
1.0	99.92
2.5	99.91
5.0	99.89
10.0	99.84

*Refers to absorbed dose above natural background. This table assumes conservative risk estimates, and it is possible that there is no added risk.
Adapted from Wagner LK, Hayman LA: Pregnancy in women radiologists. Radiology 1982;145:559–562.

malformations or growth retardation. If the lifetime radiogenic risk factor for induction of childhood tumors is 1 in 2000 for each 10 mGy, at 50 mGy to the fetus, the maximal risk factor of having a child with leukemia or childhood cancer would be approximately 1 in 400. In the past, many abortions were recommended when the embryo or fetus had obviously received absorbed doses less than 50 mGy. Such actions are difficult to justify from a philosophical viewpoint. If one is willing to abort a fetus for a maximal estimated risk factor of 1 in 400 of childhood cancer, how does one explain not performing abortions on all pregnant women because the risk of spontaneous congenital malformation approaches 1 in 20? In parents who have a child with leukemia, the risk of having another child with leukemia is in the range of 1 in 400. If one adopts the philosophy that the risk factor associated with a fetal absorbed dose of 50 mGy justifies terminating a pregnancy, then by extension of the same logic, one would be forced to perform abortions on potential siblings of children with leukemia. This has not been common practice, nor is it reasonable. When the dose to the fetus exceeds 50 mGy, the approach to the problem is slightly different. This situation may involve accidental rather than diagnostic exposure, and the estimates of absorbed dose may have a larger factor of uncertainty. If the fetal absorbed dose is high, for example, in excess of 0.5 Gy, and it was incurred during the first trimester, there is a substantial chance of growth retardation and CNS damage. Although it is possible that the fetus may survive doses in this range, the parents should be informed of the risks involved. In the intermediate dose range (50 to 500 mGy), the situation is much less clear-cut, although such circumstances arise relatively infrequently. At this absorbed dose range the risk of mental retardation must be seriously considered if the fetus is between 8 and 15 weeks of gestational age. In such instances, a qualified biomedical or health physicist should calculate the absorbed fetal dose as closely as possible, and the physician should ascertain the individual and personal situation of the parents. For example, if the dose to the fetus were calculated to be in the range of 50 to 100 mGy and the parents had been trying to have a child for several years, then one might suggest that the pregnancy not be terminated.

Summary

Preconception irradiation has not been demonstrated to lead to significant genetic hazards, carcinogenesis, or subsequent fetal malformation in children. In fact, limited studies of patients who have been exposed to high levels of radiation (in some cases causing temporary sterility) have demonstrated normal offspring. Radiation exposure of the embryo at the preimplantation stage probably leads to an all-or-none phenomenon: a spontaneous abortion or a normal pregnancy. The possible radiogenic increase in abortions is very small and has been impossible to quantify accurately in light of the high normal incidence of spontaneous abortions. During the period of organogenesis, absorbed doses exceeding 1 Gy cause a high incidence of CNS abnormalities. Other malformations may occur and are usually accompanied by nervous system abnormalities. During the fetal period, in utero exposure carries a lower risk of nonstochastic or direct effects. Exposures in the range of diagnostic examinations (at absorbed dose levels less than 50 Gy) have not been associated with malformations or congenital abnormalities in humans. The NCRP and ICRP[6] both estimate that a threshold for malformations and growth retardation exists at about 0.1 to 0.2 Gy fetal dose.

There is a vast epidemiologic experience documenting induction of neoplasms after in utero exposure to radiation. The studies show conflicting results and quantitative estimations of risk. A reasonable estimate of the lifetime risk for leukemia and other childhood cancers following in utero radiation would be in the range of 1 excess case in 2000 persons for each 10 mGy. Some researchers postulate a higher risk, but this is effectively excluded by larger statistically significant studies. Overall, the risks associated with diagnostic levels of irradiation, rarely, if ever, justify termination of a pregnancy. In any rational combination of diagnostic procedures, the dose to the fetus should not exceed 50 mGy. Below this level, the radiogenic risk of congenital anomalies and malformations appears to be essentially nonexistent, and the risk of carcinogenesis is much lower than other risks normally associated with pregnancy. When absorbed fetal doses exceed 0.5 Gy, or reach the therapeutic range, termination of pregnancy should be considered seriously. In the range between 50 mGy and 500 mGy, the decision to terminate a pregnancy should be based on careful estimation of the actual absorbed fetal dose, consideration of the other medical factors, and the individual situations of parents. Every effort to reduce radiation exposure to the embryo or fetus should be made whenever reasonably possible; however, it must be remembered that if a radiographic or nuclear medicine procedure is medically indicated, the risk to the mother of not having the procedure is usually substantially greater than the radiation risk to the fetus. Careful evaluation of women undergoing diagnostic or therapeutic procedures will prevent many unnecessary lawsuits. Failure to communicate adequately with the patient may be interpreted in a legal arena as more important than whether the radiation was the etiology of the identified effects.

REFERENCES

1. Brent, R. and R. Gorson, eds. Radiation Exposure in Pregnancy. In 1972, Chicago: Year Book Medical Publishers.
2. Brent, R.L., The effects of embryonic and fetal exposure to x-ray, microwaves, and ultrasound. Clin Obstet Gynecol, 1983. 26(2):484–510.
3. Hoffman, D., R. Felten, and W. Cyr, Effects of ionizing radiation on the developing embryo and fetus: A review. 1981, Washington, DC: U.S. Food and Drug Administration.
4. United Nations Scientific Committee on the Effects of Atomic Radiation (UNSCEAR), Sources and effects of ionizing radiation: UNSCEAR 1993 report to the General Assembly, with scientific annexes. 1993, New York: United Nations.
5. Streffer, C., et al., Biological effects after prenatal irradiation (embryo and fetus): A report of the ICRP. Ann ICRP, 2003. 33(1–2):5–206.
6. International Commission on Radiological Protection (ICRP), Pregnancy and medical radiation. Ann ICRP, 2000. 30(1):iii–viii, 1–43.
7. Brown, M.L., et al., X-ray experience during pregnancy. JAMA, 1967. 199(5):309–314.

8. Bonebrake, C.R., et al., Routine chest roentgenography in pregnancy. JAMA, 1978. 240(25):2747–2748.

9. Mattox, J.H., The value of a routine prenatal chest x-ray. Obstet Gynecol, 1973. 41(2):243–245.

10. Kelly, K.M., et al., The utilization and efficacy of pelvimetry. Am J Roentgenol Radium Ther Nucl Med, 1975. 125(1):66–74.

11. Joyce, D.N., F. Giwa-Osagie, and G.W. Stevenson, Role of pelvimetry in active management of labour. BMJ, 1975. 4(5995):505–507.

12. National Council on Radiation Protection and Measurements (NCRP), Medical radiation exposure of pregnant and potentially pregnant women: Recommendations of the NCRP. 1977, Washington, DC: NCRP, p. iv.

13. National Council on Radiation Protection and Measurements (NCRP), Limitation of exposure to ionizing radiation: Recommendations of the NCRP. NCRP report no. 116. 1993, Bethesda, Md: The Council, p. vi.

14. Kaplan, I., Genetic effects in children and grandchildren of women treated for infertility and sterility by roentgen therapy: A report of the study of 33 years. Radiology, 1959. 72:518–521.

15. Lushbaugh, C. and R. Ricks, Some cytokinetic and histopathological considerations of male and female gonodal tissues. Front Radiat Ther Oncol, 1972. 6:228–248.

16. Horning, S.J., et al., Female reproductive potential after treatment for Hodgkin's disease. N Engl J Med, 1981. 304(23):1377–1382.

17. Jacox, W., Recovery following human ovarian irradiation. Radiology, 1939. 32:528.

18. Andrews, G., et al., Report of 21-year medical follow-up of survivors of the Oak Ridge Y-12 accident. In The Medical Basis of Radiation Accident Preparedness. 1980, New York: Elsevier/North Holland.

19. Schull, W.J., M. Otake, and J.V. Neel, Hiroshima and Nagasaki: A reassessment of the mutagenic effect of exposure to ionizing radiation. In Population and Biological Aspects of Human Mutation. 1981, New York: Academic Press.

20. Harris, S., Therapeutic abortion produced by x-ray. AJR Am J Roentgenol, 1931. 27:415–419.

21. Mayer, M., W. Harris, and S. Wimpfheimer, Therapeutic abortion by means of x-ray. Am J Obstet Gynecol, 1936. 32:945–957.

22. Yamazaki, J., S. Wright, and P. Wright, A study of the outcome of pregnancy in women exposed to the atomic bomb in Nagasaki. J Cell Comp Physiol, 1954. 43:319–328.

23. Yamazaki, J., S. Wright, and P. Wright, Outcome of pregnancy in women exposed to the atomic bomb in Nagasaki. Am J Dis Child, 1954. 87:448–462.

24. Dekaban, A.S., Abnormalities in children exposed to x-radiation during various stages of gestation: Tentative timetable of radiation injury to the human fetus. J Nucl Med, 1968. 9(9):471–477.

25. Goldstein, L. and D. Murphy, Microcephalic idiocy following radium therapy for uterine cancer during pregnancy. Am J Obstet Gynecol, 1929. 18:189.

26. Goldstein, L. and D. Murphy, Etiology of ill health in children born after maternal pelvic irradiation: Defects of children born after post-conceptional maternal irradiation. AJR Am J Roentgenol, 1929. 22:322.

27. Czeizel, A.E., C. Elek, and E. Susanszky, The evaluation of the germinal mutagenic impact of Chernobyl radiological contamination in Hungary. Mutagenesis, 1991. 6(4):285–288.

28. International Atomic Energy Agency (IAEA), The International Chernobyl Project: Report of an international committee. 1991, Vienna: IAEA.

29. Chernobyl Forum, World Health Organization (WHO), Health effects of the Chernobyl accident and special health care programmes. 2005, Geneva: WHO.

30. Harjulehto-Mervaala, T., et al., The accident at Chernobyl and trisomy 21 in Finland. Mutat Res, 1992. 275(2):81–86.

31. Harjulehto, T., et al., Pregnancy outcome in Finland after the Chernobyl accident. Biomed Pharmacother, 1991. 45(6):263–266.

32. Lie, R.T., et al., Birth defects in Norway by levels of external and food-based exposure to radiation from Chernobyl. Am J Epidemiol, 1992. 136(4):377–388.

33. Lie, R.T., I. Heuch, and L.M. Irgens, A temporary increase of Down syndrome among births of young mothers in Norway: An effect of risk unrelated to maternal age? Genet Epidemiol, 1991. 8(4):217–230.

34. Shields, L.M., et al., Navajo birth outcomes in the Shiprock uranium mining area. Health Phys, 1992. 63(5):542–551.

35. Otake, M. and W.J. Schull, In utero exposure to A-bomb radiation and mental retardation: A reassessment. Br J Radiol, 1984. 57(677):409–414.

36. Mole, R.H., Consequences of pre-natal radiation exposure for post-natal development. A review. Int J Radiat Biol Relat Stud Phys Chem Med, 1982. 42(1):1–12.

37. Mole, R.H., The effect of prenatal radiation exposure on the developing human brain. Int J Radiat Biol, 1990. 57(4):647–663.

38. Otake, M., H. Yoshimaru, and W.J. Schull, Severe mental retardation among the prenatally exposed survivors of the atomic bombing in Hiroshima and Nagasaki: A comparison of the T65DR and DA86 dosimetry systems. 1987, Hiroshima, Japan: Radiation Effects Research Foundation.

39. Mole, R.H., Severe mental retardation after large prenatal exposures to bomb radiation. Reduction in oxygen transport to fetal brain: A possible abscopal mechanism. Int J Radiat Biol, 1990. 58(4):705–711.

40. Schull, W.J., M. Otake, and H. Yoshimaru, Effect on intelligence test score of prenatal exposure to ionizing radiation in Hiroshima and Nagasaki: A comparison of the T65DR and DS86 dosimetry systems. 1988, Hiroshima, Japan: Radiation Effects Research Foundation.

41. Otake, M., et al., Effect on school performance of prenatal exposure to ionizing radiation in Hiroshima: A comparison of the T65DR and DS86 dosimetry systems. 1988, Hiroshima, Japan: Radiation Effects Research Foundation.

42. Murphy, D. and L. Goldstein, Micromelia in a child irradiated in utero. Surg Gynecol Obstet, 1930. 50:79.

43. Burrow, G., H.B. Hamilton, and Z. Hrubec, Study of adolescents exposed in utero to the atomic bomb, Nagasaki, Japan. J Am Med Assoc, 1965. 192:357.

44. Burrow, G., et al., Study of adolescents exposed in utero to the atomic bomb, Nagasaki, Japan, general aspects: Clinical laboratory data. Yale J Biol Med, 1964. 36:430.

45. Miller, R., Delayed effects occurring within the first decade of exposure of young individuals to the Hiroshima atomic bomb. Pediatrics, 1956. 18:1.

46. Plummer, G., Anomalies occurring in children exposed in utero to the atomic bomb in Hiroshima. Pediatrics, 1952. 10:687.

47. Tabuchi, A., Fetal disorders due to ionizing radiation, Hiroshima. J Med Sci, 1964. 13:125.

48. Wood, J.W., K.G. Johnson, and Y. Omori, In utero exposure to the Hiroshima atomic bomb. An evaluation of head size and mental retardation: Twenty years later. Pediatrics, 1967. 39(3):385–392.

49. Beebe, G.W., The atomic bomb survivors and the problem of low-dose radiation effects. Am J Epidemiol, 1981. 114(6):761–783.

50. Miller, R.W. and J.J. Mulvihill, Small head size after atomic irradiation. Teratology, 1976. 14(3):355–357.

51. Otake, M. and W.J. Schull, Radiation-related small head sizes among the prenatally exposed survivors in Hiroshima and Nagasaki. 1992, Hiroshima, Japan: Radiation Effects Research Foundation.

52. Dunn, K., et al., Prenatal exposure to ionizing radiation and subsequent development of seizures. Am J Epidemiol, 1990. 131(1):114–123.

53. Guerke, W. and W. Goetze, EEG changes, psychomotor epilepsy and intracranial calcification occurring as late results of radiation therapy. Clin Elec, 1971. 2:146–153.

54. Kato, H., Autopsy rate in F1 mortality sample and PE86 sample. 1968, Hiroshima, Japan: Atomic Bomb Casualty Commission (ABCC).

55. Troup, G.M., II, Growth and development. Hum Pathol, 1971. 2(4):493–499.

56. Schull, W.J., et al., Brain abnormalities among the mentally retarded prenatally exposed survivors of the atomic bombing of Hiroshima and Nagasaki. 1991, Hiroshima, Japan: Radiation Effects Research Foundation.

57. Greulich, W., C. Chrisman, and M. Turner, The physical growth and development of children who survived the atomic bombing of Hiroshima and Nagasaki. J Pediatr, 1953. 43:121.

58. Reynolds, E., Growth and development of Hiroshima children exposed to the atomic bomb, 3-year study (1951–1953). 1959, Hiroshima, Japan: Atomic Bomb Casualty Commission.

59. Nehemias, J.V., Multivariate analysis and the IBM 704 computer applied to ABCC data on growth of surviving Hiroshima children. Health Phys, 1962. 8:165–183.

60. Wood, J.W., et al., Mental retardation in children exposed in utero to the atomic bombs in Hiroshima and Nagasaki. Am J Public Health Nations Health, 1967. 57(8):1381–1389.

61. Shohoji, T. and B. Pasternack, Adolescent growth patterns in survivors exposed prenatally to the A-bombs in Hiroshima and Nagasaki. Health Phys, 1973. 25(1):17–27.

62. Moriyama, I. and H. Kato, Mortality experience of A-bomb survivors, 1970–1972, 1950–1972: 1973, Hiroshima, Japan: Atomic Bomb Casualty Commission (ABCC).

63. Belsky, J.L., K. Tachikawa, and S. Jablon, The health of atomic bomb survivors: A decade of examinations in a fixed population. Yale J Biol Med, 1973. 46(4):284–296.

64. Russell, W.J., et al., Bone maturation in children exposed to the A-bomb in utero. Radiology, 1973. 108(2):367–374.

65. Otake, M., et al., A longitudinal study of growth and development of stature among prenatally exposed atomic bomb survivors. Radiat Res, 1993. 134(1):94–101.

66. Nakashima, E., Relationship of five anthropometric measurements at age 18 to radiation dose among atomic bomb survivors exposed in utero. Radiat Res, 1994. 138(1):121–126.

67. Hammer-Jacobsen, E., Therapeutic abortion on account of x-ray examination during pregnancy. Dan Med Bull, 1959. 6:113–122.

68. Driscoll, S., et al., Acute radiation injury in two human fetuses. Arch Pathol, 1963. 76:125–131.

69. Mole, R.H., Expectation of malformations after irradiation of the developing human in utero: The experimental basis for predictions. Adv Radiat Biol, 1992. 15:217–301.

70. Oppenheim, B.E., M.L. Griem, and P. Meier, Effects of low-dose prenatal irradiation in humans: Analysis of Chicago Lying-In data and comparison with other studies. Radiat Res, 1974. 57(3):508–544.

71. Oppenheim, B.E., M.L. Griem, and P. Meier, The effects of diagnostic x-ray exposure on the human fetus: An examination of the evidence. Radiology, 1975. 114(3):529–534.

72. Granroth, G., Defects of the central nervous system in Finland. IV. Associations with diagnostic x-ray examinations. Am J Obstet Gynecol, 1979. 133(2):191–194.

73. Muller, F. and R. O'Rahilly, Cerebral dysraphia (future anencephaly) in a human twin embryo at stage 13. Teratology, 1984. 30(2):167–177.

74. Neumeister, K., Findings in children after radiation exposure in utero from x-ray examination of mothers, In Late Effects of Ionizing Radiation, 1. 1978, Vienna: IAEA.

75. Meyer, M.B., J.A. Tonascia, and T. Merz, Long-term effects of prenatal x-ray on development and fertility of human females, In Biological and Environmental Effects of Low-Level Radiation, vol. 2. 1976, Vienna: IAEA.

76. Nokkenteved, K., Effects of diagnostic radiation upon the human fetus. 1968, Copenhagen: Munksgaard.

77. Hu, Y. and J. Tao, Effects of prenatal exposure to diagnostic radiation on childhood physical and intellectual development. Chin J Radiol Med Prot, 1992. 12:2–6.

78. LeJeune, J., et al., Results of the first study on the stomatic effects of in-utero irradiation on the embryo and fetus (a particular case of heterochromia of the iris). Rev Franc Etudes Clin Biol, 1960. 6:982–989.

79. Cheesman, E. and A. Walby, Intrauterine irradiation and iris heterochromia. Ann Hum Genet, 1963. 27:23–29.

80. Jacobsen, L. and L. Mellemgaard, A retrospective study of the possible teratogenic effects of diagnostic pelvic x-irradiation. In Progress in Radiology. 1966, Amsterdam: Excepta Medica.

81. Takamura, P. and S. Ueda, Hematologic findings exposed to A-bomb irradiation in utero in Hiroshima. Blood, 1961. 17:728–737.

82. Freedman, L. and R.J. Keehn, Urinary findings of children who were in utero during the bombings of Hiroshima and Nagasaki. Yale J Biol Med, 1966. 39:196–206.

83. Meyer, M.B., T. Merz, and E.L. Diamond, Investigation of the effects of prenatal x-ray exposure of human oogonia and oocytes as measured by later reproductive performance. Am J Epidemiol, 1969. 89(6):619–635.

84. Jablon, S. and H. Kato, Sex ratio in offspring of survivors exposed prenatally to the atomic bombs in Hiroshima and Nagasaki. Am J Epidemiol, 1971. 93(4):253–258.

85. International Commission on Radiological Protection (ICRP), Doses to the embryo and fetus from intakes of radionuclides by the mother: A report of the ICRP. Ann ICRP, 2001. 31(1–3):19–515.

86. International Commission on Radiological Protection (ICRP), A report of doses to infants from ingestion of radionuclides in mothers' milk. Ann ICRP, 2004. 34(3–4):iii, 15–267, 269–280.

87. Finkel, M., The transition of radiostrontium and plutonium from mother to offspring in laboratory animals. Physiol Zool, 1947. 20:405–421.

88. Finkel, M., et al., Strontium 90 toxicity in dogs, In Biomedical Implications of Radiostrontium Exposure, M.B. Goldman and L. Bustad, eds. 1972, Washington, DC: U.S. Atomic Energy Commission, Division of Technical Information.

89. Sternberg, J., Tissular deposition of radionuclide during pregnancy, In Diagnosis and Treatment of Deposited Radionuclides, A. Korngberg and W. Norwood, eds. 1968, Amsterdam: Excerpta Medica.

90. Mays, C.W. and R. Lloyd, ^{90}Sr and Sr dose estimated for the fetus and infant. Health Phys, 1966. 12:1225–1236.

91. Moore, K. and T. Persaud, The Developing Human. 6th ed. 1998, London: W.B. Saunders.

92. Chapman, E., et al., The collection of radioiodine by the human fetal thyroid. J Endocrinol, 1948. 8:717–720.

93. Russell, K., H. Rose, and P. Starr, The effects of maternal and fetal thyroid function during pregnancy. Surg Gynecol Obstet, 1957. 104:560.

94. Hamill, G.C., J.A. Jarman, and M.D. Wynne, Fetal effects of radioactive iodine therapy in a pregnant woman with thyroid cancer. Am J Obstet Gynecol, 1961. 81:1018–1023.

95. Fisher, W.D., M.L. Voorhess, and L.I. Gardner, Congenital hypothyroidism in infant following maternal I-131 therapy with a review of hazards of environmental radioisotope contamination. J Pediatr, 1963. 62:132–146.

96. Green, H.G., et al., Cretinism associated with maternal sodium iodide I 131 therapy during pregnancy. Am J Dis Child, 1971. 122(3):247–249.

97. Beierwaltes, W.H., et al., Radioactive iodine concentration in the fetal human thyroid gland from fall-out. JAMA, 1960. 173:1895–1902.

98. Beierwaltes, W.H., M.T. Hilger, and A. Wegst, Radioiodine concentration in fetal human thyroid from fallout. Health Phys, 1963. 9:1263–1266.

99. Dyer, N.C., et al., Maternal-fetal transport and distribution of 59Fe and 131-I in humans. Am J Obstet Gynecol, 1969. 103(2):290–296.

100. Hodges, R., et al., Accumulation of radioactive iodine by the human fetal thyroid. J Clin Endocrinol, 1955. 15:661–667.

101. Halnan, K.E., The radioiodine uptake of the human thyroid in pregnancy. Clin Sci, 1958. 17:281–290.

102. Evans, T.C., et al., Radioiodine uptake studies of the human fetal thyroid. J Nucl Med, 1967. 8(3):157–165.

103. Hahn, P.F., et al., Iron metabolism in human pregnancy as studied with radioactive isotope, Fe59. Am J Obstet Gynecol, 1951. 61(3):477–486.

104. Sternberg, J., Radioaktive isotope in klinik und Forschung 4, 73. 1960, Munich: Urban and Schwarzenberg.

105. Sternberg, J. and T. Nagai, Radiocontamination of the environment and its effects on the mother and fetus. III. Retention of cesium 137 during pregnancy. J Appl Radiat Isotopes, 1970. 21:351–362.

106. Bertelli, L., et al., A case study of the transfer of cesium 137 to the human fetus and nursing infant. Radiat Prot Dosim, 1992. 41:131–136.

107. Kalef-Ezra, J. and S. Yasumura, Doses and risk estimates to the human conceptus due to internal prenatal exposure to radioactive cesium. Rad Prot Dosim, 1997. 69:205–210.

108. Melo, D.R., J.L. Lipsztein, C.A. Oliveira, et al., Cesium-137 internal contamination involving a Brazilian accident and the efficacy of Prussian blue treatment. Health Phys, 1994. 66(3):245–252.

109. Stewart, A., D. Webb, and B. Hewitt, A survey of childhood malignancies. BMJ, 1958. 1:1495.

110. Stewart, A. and G.W. Kneale, Radiation dose effects in relation to obstetric x-rays and childhood cancers. Lancet, 1970. 1(7658):1185–1188.

111. Stewart, A., Myeloid leukemia and cot deaths. Radiat Med J, 1972. 187:423.

112. Stewart, A., The carcinogenic effects of low level radiation. A re-appraisal of epidemiologists methods and observations. Health Phys, 1973. 24(2):223–240.

113. Bithell, J.F. and A.M. Stewart, Pre-natal irradiation and childhood malignancy: A review of British data from the Oxford Survey. Br J Cancer, 1975. 31(3):271–287.

114. Bithell, J.F., Epidemiological studies of children irradiated in-utero. In Low Dose Radiation: Biological Basis of Risk Assessment, K. Baverstock and J. Strather, eds. 1989, London: Taylor and Francis.

115. Mole, R.H., Antenatal irradiation and childhood cancer: Causation or coincidence? Br J Cancer, 1974. 30(3):199–208.

116. Mole, R.H., Childhood cancer after prenatal exposure to diagnostic x-ray examinations in Britain. Br J Cancer, 1990. 62(1):152–168.

117. Harvey, E.B., et al., Prenatal x-ray exposure and childhood cancer in twins. N Engl J Med, 1985. 312(9):541–545.

118. Rodvall, Y., et al., Prenatal x-ray exposure and childhood cancer in Swedish twins. Int J Cancer, 1990. 46(3):362–365.

119. Muirhead, C. and G.W. Kneale, Prenatal irradiation and childhood cancer. J Radiat Prot, 1989. 9:209–212.

120. Totter, J.R., Some observational bases for estimating the oncogenic effects of ionizing radiation. Nuclear Safety, 1980. 21:83–94.

121. Totter, J.R. and H.G. MacPherson, Do childhood cancers result from prenatal x-rays? Health Phys, 1981. 40(4):511–524.

122. Webster, E.W., Garland Lecture. On the question of cancer induction by small x-ray doses. AJR Am J Roentgenol, 1981. 137(4):647–666.

123. National Research Council (NRC), The effects on populations of exposure to low levels of ionizing radiation. BEIR III. 1980, Washington, DC: National Academy of Sciences, p. xiii.

124. Jablon, S. and H. Kato, Childhood cancer in relation to prenatal exposure to atomic bomb radiation. Lancet, 1970. 2:1000–1003.

125. Ishimaru, T., T. Ishimaru, and M. Mikami, Leukemia incidence among individuals exposed in utero: Children of atomic bomb survivors and their controls (Hiroshima and Nagasaki, 1945–1979). 1981, Hiroshima, Japan: Radiation Effects Research Foundation.

126. Yoshimoto, Y., H. Kato, and W.J. Schull, Risk of cancer among children exposed in utero to A-bomb radiations, 1950-84. Lancet, 1988. 2(8612):665–669.

127. MacMahon, H. and G. Hutchinson, Prenatal x-ray in childhood cancer: A review. Acta Int Contre Cancer, 1964. 20:1172–1174.

128. Court Brown, W.M., R. Doll, and H. Hill, Incidence of leukemia after exposure to diagnostic radiation in utero. BMJ, 1960. 2:1539–1545.

129. Tabuchi, A., et al., Fetal hazards due to x-ray diagnosis during pregnancy. Hiroshima J Med Sci, 1967. 16:49.

130. MacMahon, B., Some recent issues in low-exposure radiation epidemiology. Environ Health Perspect, 1989. 81:131–135.

131. Miller, R.W., Effects of prenatal exposure to ionizing radiation. Health Phys, 1990. 59(1):57–61.

132. Yoshimoto, Y., M. Soda, and W.J. Schull, Studies of children in utero during atomic bomb detonations, In the 203rd National Meeting of the American Chemical Society. 1993, San Francisco: American Chemical Society.

133. Diamond, E.L., H. Schmerier, and A. Lilienfeld, The relationship of intrauterine radiation to subsequent mortality and development of leukemia in children. Am J Epidemiol, 1973. 97:283–313.

134. Inskip, P.D., et al., Incidence of childhood cancer in twins. Cancer Causes Control, 1991. 2(5):315–324.

135. Rodvall, Y., et al., Childhood cancer among Swedish twins. Cancer Causes Control, 1992. 3(6):527–532.

136. National Council on Radiation Protection and Measurements (NCRP), Radiation protection in pediatric radiology: Recommendations of the NCRP report no. 68. 1994, Washington, DC: NCRP, p. vi.

137. Hoshino, T., T. Itoga, and H. Kato, Leukemia in the offspring of parents exposed to the atomic bomb at Hiroshima and Nagasaki. Blood, 1967. 30(6):719–730.

138. Graham, S., M. Levin, A. Lilienfeld, et al., Preconception, intra-uterine and post-natal irradiation as related to leukemia. Natl Cancer Inst Monogr, 1966. 19:347–371.

139. Neutel, C. and C. Buck, Effect of smoking during pregnancy and the risk of cancer in children. J Natl Cancer Inst, 1971. 47:49.

140. Fasal, E., E. Jackson, and M.R. Klauber, Birth characteristics and leukemia in childhood. Natl Cancer Inst Monogr, 1971. 47:501.

141. Miller, R., Epidemiological conclusions from radiation toxicity studies, In Late Effects of Radiation, R. Fry, et al., eds. 1970, London: Taylor and Francis.

142. Stjernfeldt, M., et al., Maternal smoking and irradiation during pregnancy as risk factors for child leukemia. Cancer Detect Prev, 1992. 16(2):129–135.

143. United Nations Scientific Committee on the Effects of Atomic Radiation (UNSCEAR), Sources and effects of ionizing radiation: UNSCEAR 1994 report to the General Assembly, with scientific annexes. 1994, New York: United Nations.

144. Bentur, Y., N. Horlatsch, and G. Koren, Exposure to ionizing radiation during pregnancy: Perception of teratogenic risk and outcome. Teratology, 1991. 43(2):109–112.

145. Wagner, L.K. and L.A. Hayman, Pregnancy and women radiologists. Radiology, 1982. 145(2):559–562.

146. Brent, R.L., The effect of embryonic and fetal exposure to x-ray, microwaves, and ultrasound: Counseling the pregnant and nonpregnant patient about these risks. Semin Oncol, 1989. 16:347–368.

147. Brent, R.L., et al., Reproductive and teratologic effects of electromagnetic fields. Reprod Toxicol, 1993. 7(6):535–580.

9 Uranium, Plutonium, and Radium

Uranium, plutonium, and radium are dealt with here in some detail because they are radionuclides that are commonly a matter of public concern. As will be seen from the following text, uranium and plutonium are quite different in terms of their toxicity, with uranium being predominantly a chemical toxin and plutonium and radium being of concern on a radiologic basis. The effects of plutonium as well as other alpha emitters, including daughter products of uranium and thorium, are covered most extensively in a report of the Biological Effects of Ionizing Radiations (BEIR) IV Committee of the National Academy of Sciences.[1] The reader is referred to this report for more detailed information. There are also proceedings of 1981 and 1988 workshops that contain much detailed information.[2,3]

URANIUM

General

Uranium is a silvery, heavy metal that is ductile and malleable. Uranium is element number 92 and occurs only in radioactive form. Natural uranium is a mixture of three isotopes: uranium 238 (99.28%), uranium 235 (0.715%), and uranium 234 (0.005%). Uranium 238 is a primordial radionuclide and the head of the uranium/radium series. Uranium 234 arises from uranium 238 by radioactive decay. Uranium 235 is of a different origin, and it is the head of the uranium/actinium series. (This is discussed in more detail in Chapter 2.)

The isotopes of uranium have long physical half-lives, as follows: uranium 238, 4.5×10^9 years, uranium 235, 7.1×10^8 years, and uranium 234, 2.5×10^5 years. Natural uranium and its daughters emit alpha, beta, and gamma radiations. By definition of the International Commission on Radiological Protection (ICRP) in 1958, a curie of natural uranium is defined as the sum of 3.7×10^{10} disintegrations per second of uranium 238, 3.7×10^{10} disintegrations per second of uranium 234, and 1.7×10^9 disintegrations per second of uranium 235. This also corresponds to 7.6×10^{10} alpha disintegrations per second. The specific activity of natural uranium is about 1.2×10^{-8} TBq/g. Conversely, 1 g of natural uranium corresponds to 2.5×10^4 alpha disintegrations

per second. The specific activity of uranium 238 is very close to that of natural uranium or 1.2×10^{-8} TBq/g. The specific activity of uranium 235 is 8×10^{-8} TBq/g. Detection of uranium 238 is predominantly done by use of 90 keV emissions from its daughter radionuclides, and detection of uranium 235 can be done by detection of 186 keV emissions. Soluble uranium can be detected through fluorometric analysis of urine. Depleted uranium typically refers to natural uranium that has had most of the uranium 235 removed. It is used for ballast in airplanes and for making armor-piercing projectiles. Depleted uranium is basically a chemical toxin and is covered in more detail later in this section. Uranium oxidizes quickly when exposed to air with formation of a film of uranium oxide (U_3O_8) that is black. Uranium and most of its common salts dissolve readily in most acids, and their solubility in water varies over a wide range, with uranium nitrate and uranyl fluoride (UO_2F_2) being very soluble and uranium tetrafluoride (UF_4) or oxide being relatively insoluble. The most commonly encountered forms of uranium include uranium hexafluoride (UF_6), which is a colorless gas; however, at room temperature and in the presence of water, UF_6 is converted into hydrofluoric acid (HF) and UO_2F_2. Uranium tetraflouride is a green powder insoluble in water that if heated is converted into U_3O_8. Uranium oxide can exist in either the hexavalent or tetravalent state. In nature, this uranium occurs as pitchblende, and it is pitch black and insoluble in water. Tetravalent uranium (UO_2) is a brown-to-black powder insoluble in water.

Uranyl salts form complexes with organic compounds. Under physiologic conditions tetravalent uranium is immediately oxidized to hexavalent uranium, and it is the uranyl ion (UO_2^{2+}) that reacts with biologic entities such as proteins. Protein-bound uranium can be carried by the blood as can uranyl bicarbonate complex. This is often generated as uranium reacts with carbon dioxide in the blood. The ratio of these two complexes in blood remains almost constant, with 40% being protein bound and 60% existing as a carbonate complex, the two being in equilibrium with each other. For natural uranium the quantity of metal absorbed is the dominant issue. After ingestion about 1% to 2% is absorbed, with most being excreted by the kidneys. The kidney is the first organ to show chemical damage, both with nephritis and protein-uria. This happens when concentrations occur on the order of 0.1 mg/kg of body weight. About 70% of soluble uranium is eliminated by the kidneys within 24 hours. Damage to the kidneys appears to be predominantly a result of dissociation of the carbonate complex and uranyl ions causing injury to the proximal convoluted tubules. Between 10% and 30% of uranyl salts are reversibly bound to the surface of bones. The transportability of uranium in the body is a major issue in determining hazard. Highly soluble or transportable forms (class D) include UF_6, UO_2F_2, uranyl nitrate $[UO_2(NO_3)_2]$, uranium sulfates, and uranium carbonates. Moderately transportable forms (class W) include UO_3, UF_4, UCl_4 and uranium nitrates. Compounds of low transportability (class Y) include forms of UO_2, U_3O_8, uranium oxides, uranium hydrides, and uranium carbides. Typically, these refer to transportability patterns after inhalation of uranium compounds. For poorly transportable compounds, the lung, rather than the kidney, is the critical organ. The biologic half-time in the lung is 120 days or more for slightly transportable compounds with particle sizes under 2 μm.[4]

Uranium occurs naturally in body tissues after dietary intake in food and inhalation of dust particles. Some of the values for uranium 238 have been presented in the 1977 United Nations Scientific Committee on Effects of Atomic Radiation (UNSCEAR) report.[5] Dietary intake reported from various different countries generally ranges from 0.3 to 0.5 pCi/day, and urinary excretion typically ranges from 0.003 to 0.13 pCi/day. Activity of uranium 238 in the body is normally in the range of 30 pCi, and skeletal activity is in the range of 20 pCi. It is estimated that a daily dietary intake of 0.4 pCi of uranium 238 leads to concentrations in soft tissues of 0.2 pCi/kg and to a bone concentration of 4 pCi/kg. Values of uranium in both exposed and unexposed human subjects were published by Stannard.[6] In unexposed subjects the concentration of uranium in lung tissue is about 0.01 to 0.09 μg of uranium per gram of wet tissue. Similar values for the kidney are 0.02 to 0.03, for bone 0.01 to 0.03, and for liver 0.01 to 0.08. For activity of uranium 238 and its daughters in various tissues, UNSCEAR uses the following values: lung, 0.2 pCi/kg; testes and ovaries, 0.2; bone, 4.0; red marrow, 0.2; and bone lining cells, 0.2. A large number of papers have dealt with the retention and excretion of various forms of uranium after exposure to relatively low levels of uranium.[7,8] The data suggests that approximate daily urinary excretion after chronic exposure to insoluble uranium at a level of 20 to 50 μg per day corresponds to a burden of 30 mg (0.01 μCi). Thind reported that, in practice, dust particles at fuel fabrication facilities are usually in the range of 5 μm rather than the 1-μm size previously used as a default value by the ICRP.[9]

A number of articles also deal with soluble uranium and its potential effect on the kidneys.[10,11] Renal toxicity due to the chemical effects of uranium is usually manifest as albuminuria during the first days postexposure. Other urinary abnormalities, such as red or white blood cells or casts, should not be considered due to uranium in the absence of frank albuminuria. An extensive review paper by Leggett discusses behavior and chemical toxicity of uranium in the kidney.[12] A concentration of 3 μg of uranium per gram of kidney has been used as a limit relative to chemical toxicity of uranium. This level typically refers to serious tissue damage; however, renal abnormalities are seen in animals from uranium concentrations of about one tenth of this, which can produce biochemical changes and transient elevations in the urinary biochemical indices. Renal effects that are subclinical have been seen at single-dose levels of about 0.1 mg/kg of body weight, but not below such levels. Overall, the chemical hazard to the kidney is the predominant risk when enrichment of uranium is less than 5% to 8%. At higher enrichment levels the ICRP dose limit recommendations for organs become a controlling issue. The annual limit on intake published by the ICRP in 1990 is related to the radiologic hazard and not the chemical hazard; thus, for purposes of management of compounds with low enrichment, the ICRP annual limit is not appropriate for management of an industrial facility.[13]

Experimental Human Data

Uranium-induced renal abnormalities were investigated in six hospital patients in the "Rochester Study," conducted in the late 1940s and reported by Hursh et al.[14] An additional eight terminally ill patients were injected in the "Boston Study," conducted in the mid-1950s and reported by Bernard et al.[15] In these two studies subjects were injected intravenously with either $UO_2(NO_3)_2$ solutions or UO_2 as uranium tetrachloride.. Subjects receiving doses of more than 100 μg of uranium per kilogram of body weight clearly showed renal damage, and the data indicated that an average renal concentration on the order of 2 to 3 μg of uranium per gram of renal tissue was considered to be the threshold for chemical toxicity.

Occupational Exposure

The health effects from occupational exposure to uranium obviously depend on the chemical form of the element, its solubility, and other factors that have already been mentioned. Uranium hexafluoride is a compound that occurs during enrichment of uranium. Fisher reported on the health effects of an accident resulting in exposure to the element in Gore, Oklahoma, in 1986.[16] In this accident a cylinder was ruptured with a release of approximately 13,500 kg of UF_6. The UF_6 and its reaction products, UO_2F_2 and HF, were released into the air, exposing a number of workers. One worker died from massive pulmonary edema due to inhalation of the HF, another was treated for skin irritation and burns from the HF, and an additional 21 were examined and released from the hospital. The estimated inhalation varied over a range of 0.6 to 24 mg of UF_6. The estimated effective dose from these inhalations ranged from 10 to 480 µSv. The highest dose was to the bone surface of one worker and was estimated to be about 530 µSv. In this accident the 40-hour derived intake limit of the Nuclear Regulatory Commission (NRC), which is 9.6 mg of soluble uranium in a work week, was exceeded by 8 of the 31 workers exposed. Estimates of the maximum kidney concentration ranged from 0.048 to 2.5 µg of uranium per gram of kidney tissue, and no toxologic effects were observed, according to clinical laboratory results reported by Fisher.[17]

Boback also reported on workers exposed to UF_6.[18] His reports and subsequent calculations by others indicate that there were probably peak renal uranium concentrations of 4 µg per gram of renal tissue, and an average renal concentration of 1 to 2 µg per gram of renal tissue in the first several days after acute exposure. Urinary excretion was 1.9 to 2.9 mg of uranium per liter. No significant renal abnormalities were identified in the exposed individuals. Eisenbud reported on 130 employees working in a UF_6 plant in 1950, seven of whom had various renal abnormalities and histories of uranium concentrations as high as 3.5 mg/L.[19] However, renal function returned to normal within several months. There is some experience reported relative to an accident in China involving UF_4.[20] In this particular accident, a 23-year-old man was estimated to have inhaled approximately 87 mg of UF_4. The estimated kidney content on day 1 after the accident was 2.6 µg per gram of kidney tissue. Initial examination of the patient was within normal limits; however, by day 6, the patient reported dizziness, nausea, and anorexia, and on day 9 there were additional findings of abdominal pain, diarrhea, tenesmus, and blood in the stool. Oral administration of chloramphenicol produced recovery, and at dismissal from the hospital at 30 days postaccident, all blood and urinary parameters were within normal limits. In a second case reported, a 19-year-old man was severely burned when a thermally hot mixture of $UO_2(NO_3)_2$ and U_3O_8 was spilled onto his body. The total burn area was 71% of body surface. The estimated amount of uranium reaching the transfer compartment was at least 130 mg. The amount estimated to reach the kidney was 50 µg of uranium per gram of kidney. On the second day postaccident the patient had anorexia, nausea, vomiting, and oliguria. By day 7 urinary output was reduced to 10 mL per 24 hours. This was followed by low-grade infection, dizziness, and occasional loss of consciousness as well as hepatomegaly. On the eighth day postaccident, urinary output began to increase, and by 1 month postaccident, various relevant laboratory tests were within normal limits. A few other reports of inhalation of highly soluble uranium compounds appear anecdotally in the literature. Seven persons employed at the National Lead Company of Ohio were estimated to

have inhaled 5 to 12 mg of soluble uranium fluoride compounds. No symptoms of uranium intoxication were identified. In another case reported from the Mallinkrodt Chemical Works in St. Louis, a person who inhaled 70 mg of high-grade uranium concentrate had symptoms of transient damage.[21] Another accident involving the rupture of a cylinder containing UF_6 occurred in the Philadelphia Naval Shipyard on December 2, 1944. There was an estimated release of 182 kg of UF_6, and 20 individuals were exposed in various degrees to the hydrolysis products, which included uranium oxyfluoride (UO_2F_2) and HF.[22] From the chemical cloud there were 2 deaths, 3 seriously injured, 12 hospitalized for observation, and 3 individuals without symptoms. The three seriously injured individuals had urinary findings of abuminuria and casts as well as mental status changes believed to be in excess of what would be caused by fear alone. The seriously injured individuals had first- through third-degree chemical burns on large portions of their bodies, pulmonary edema, and shock. There was also nausea and vomiting, central nervous system overstimulation, and occasional incoherence. Thirty-eight years later in 1982, two of the three seriously injured individuals were still alive and were examined. Clinical laboratory studies relative to renal, bone, and liver function were within normal limits. The best estimate of initial lung deposition was in the range of 40 to 50 mg; however, the confidence limits ranged from approximately 1 to 500 mg.

The incidence of lung cancer in uranium miners is known to be significantly elevated. This has been attributed to both smoking and high levels of radon in the early mines. This matter is discussed extensively in the section "Lung Cancer" in Chapter 5; the reader is referred to that section for more information on lung cancer in uranium workers. There are a number of studies relative to health effects other than neoplasms in uranium miners. Trapp et al. reported on cardiopulmonary function.[23] The authors indicated that respiratory studies on 34 miners showed probable fibrotic changes in the lung, and it was suggested that alpha radiation from daughter products of radon attached to dust may have enhanced the fibrogenic effect of silica in the lung. Several more recent reports have appeared by Samet et al.[24] and Samet and Simpson.[25] It is clear that the air in uranium mines is a complex mixture of agents that can cause lung injury when inhaled. The agents include silica, oxides of nitrogen from diesel engines and blasting, and radon and radon daughters. In addition, epidemiologic studies of uranium miners are complicated by cigarette smoking, which has well-known effects, including epithelial metaplasia, inflammation, and mucous gland hypertrophy, and hyperplasia in the airways as well as emphysema in the alveoli. Summaries of the literature, including those in the BEIR IV report, indicate that nonmalignant respiratory diseases show a relatively broad range of standardized mortality ratios, extending from 1.0 to nearly 5.0 in the study of

Colorado Plateau uranium miners.[1] However, studies of miners in New Mexico reported only a slight excess in mortality. Archer et al. concluded that chronic exposure to airborne radiation as encountered in uranium mines promotes pulmonary emphysema, fibrosis, and chronic bronchitis.[26] As previously cited, Samet et al. and others pointed out the shortcomings of this early study, including inadequate procedures for calibration, not controlling for age, details of test procedure, and other factors. Other studies of uranium miners, which include a 1960 overview of uranium miners and millers, describe the prevalence of silicosis.[27] Of 1589 workers having x-rays, 3.1% had evidence of silicosis. Archer and colleagues noted that only four cases of silicosis occurred in men who had mined only uranium. The remaining 46 had other mining experience in addition to uranium. Little information is available on the silica levels in the uranium mines in the Colorado Plateau; however, some authors have reported that the free-silica content of samples ranges from 40% to 70%, with dust concentrations of 5 to 20 million particles per cubic foot. In the 1984 study by Samet et al., there was investigation of nonmalignant respiratory disease in 192 long-term New Mexico uranium miners.[24] Of the major respiratory symptoms, only the prevalence of dyspnea increased significantly with duration of uranium mining. Chest x-ray findings consisted predominantly of nodular opacities compatible with the diagnosis of silicosis. As a summary of the literature, it appears that silicosis is a well-documented hazard of underground uranium mining in the United States. It is uncertain if simultaneous exposure to radon daughters modifies the relation between silica exposure and the risk of developing silicosis. Whether the uranium miners may develop a pulmonary fibrosis that is distinct from that associated with silicosis still remains unproven. Waxweiler et al. have reported on mortality follow-up in 1977 of white underground uranium miners examined by the U.S. Public Health Service.[28] In this report there was no excess of death due to circulatory system abnormalities, and, in fact, there was a standardized mortality ratio (SMR) of 0.86. An excess risk was identified for only three subcategories of heart disease: rheumatic fever, chronic rheumatic heart disease, and "other" heart disease. The excess risk of nonmalignant respiratory disease appeared to be limited to a twofold excess of bronchitis and a fivefold excess of "other nonmalignant respiratory disease." The latter consisted mainly of silicosis, emphysema, and fibrosis. An excess of mortality due to accidents also was identified. Of interest was an excess of mortality due to chronic nephritis and renal sclerosis, but with only three deaths in this category. One patient died from Goodpasture's disease, which is an immunologically mediated glomerular nephritis. A second person died from glomerular nephritis and a third person from renal tubular degeneration. Wrenn et al. examined both uranium and thorium in lungs of uranium miners.[29] Autopsy data showed concentrations of 0.2 to 3 Bq/kg

for ^{238}U and 0.2 to 3 Bq/kg for ^{234}U. The average radiation dose from ^{234}U, ^{238}U, and ^{230}Th varied from 25 to 142 µGy per year. From these doses there would be little deterministic effect or cancer risk expected on the basis of uranium inhalation alone. The BEIR IV report reviewed the epidemiology of workers exposed to enriched uranium as well as workers at uranium mills.[1] A cohort of 18,869 workers who were employed between 1943 and 1947 at the uranium conversion and enrichment plant in Oak Ridge, Tennessee, was followed for 25 years. Average air concentrations ranged from 25 to 500 µg/m^3. There was no increase in lung cancer identified although the duration of exposure was typically only 1 to 2 years. A later study of those who got lung cancer suggested a risk among white men who were over age 45 at exposure but not in younger men. Studies of uranium mill workers generally show a healthy worker effect, although there is a small excess of deaths due to lymphatic malignancies. No increase in lung cancer death has been identified. Mortality among uranium enrichment workers employed at the Portsmith Uranium Enrichment Plant in Ohio was studied by Brown and Bloom.[30] In this facility there was enrichment of uranium up to 98%. An analysis of the 5773 workers who worked at the plant between 1954 and 1982 indicated that for all causes of death, there was a strong healthy worker effect with an SMR of 0.68. In fact, there were significantly low SMRs in a number of disease categories, for example, circulatory system (SMR 0.72), diseases of the respiratory system (SMR 0.42), diseases of the digestive system (SMR 0.54), and diseases of the genito-urinary system (SMR 0.54).

Since the BEIR IV report there have been four additional occupational studies of populations working in uranium milling and fabrication facilities as well as living nearby. All the studies have yielded negative results.

Ritz studied a population that included 4014 white male workers at the Fernald plant.[31] There was an SMR for all causes of death of 0.84 (95% confidence interval [CI] 0.79 to 0.89) and an SMR for all cancers of 1.09 (95% CI 0.98 to 1.22). None of the SMRs for any site-specific cancer was statistically significantly increased. McGeoghegan and Binks studied the mortality and cancer morbidity experience of workers at the Capenhurst uranium enrichment facility from 1946–1995.[32] This study consisted of a cohort of 12,540 employees and had 334,473 person-years of follow-up. The SMRs for all causes were significantly low at 83 and 91, respectively, for radiation and nonradiation workers. For cancers the SMRs were 88 and 97, respectively. McGeoghegan and Binks also reported on the mortality and cancer morbidity experience of workers at the Springfields uranium production facility from 1946–1995.[33,34] This study included all workers ever employed at the British Nuclear Fuels Springfields site. It included 19,454 current and former employees with 479,146 person-years of follow-up. The SMRs for all causes was 84 and 98, respectively, for radiation and nonradiation workers. For cancers the SMRs were 86 and 96, respectively. There was an association with morbidity, but not mortality, from non-Hodgkin's lymphoma that was not felt to be causal.

Dupree-Ellis et al. reported a study of 2514 male workers employed processing uranium between 1942 and 1966 at the Mallinkrodt Chemical Works.[34] In this study the SMR was statistically significantly below that expected at 0.38 (95% CI 0.12 to 0.89). Pinkerton et al. evaluated the mortality experience of 1484 men employed in seven uranium mills in the Colorado Plateau for at least one year on or after January 1, 1940.[35] Mortality from all causes and all cancers was less than expected based on U.S. mortality rates.

Kathren's recent studies reviewed the mortality and cancer morbidity experience of uranium workers and also included a fresh look at depleted uranium.[36] The overall conclusion reached in the editorial regarding uranium workers is that "The effects of uranium exposure in the study groups are, therefore, likely to be small, if they are present at all."[36] These various studies, which have included more than 100,000 uranium milling or fabrication workers in all, have found no consistent or significant correlations between exposures to uranium and the risks of cancer.[37]

Populations Living Near Nuclear Facilities

Jablon et al. studied cancer in populations living near nuclear facilities in the United States. No excess of cancer was identified.[38] Boice et al. studied cancer mortality over a period of 52 years in a U.S. county with substantial uranium milling and mining activity.[39] There was no difference between the total cancer mortality rates in that county compared to control counties (relative risk [RR] 1.0, 95% CI 0.9 to 1.1). Relative to site-specific cancer data, there were no increases in lung, bone, liver, or kidney cancer compared to control counties in the United States. There was also no temporal change before and after uranium mining occurred. No association was reported between cancer risk and living near uranium facilities in Pennsylvania or Colorado.[40-42] Lopez-Abente et al. reported on mortality in the vicinity of uranium cycle facilities and nuclear power plants of Spain.[43] In contrast to the bulk of literature on the topic they report an increase in lung cancer and kidney cancer around uranium facilities. These results must be interpreted with caution; for example, the risk of kidney cancer was higher the greater the distance from the facilities. A combined analysis of 14 studies, which included over 120,000 uranium workers, was performed by the U.K. Royal Society. Despite large numbers of cancers (7442), there was no elevated RR for any site-specific cancer or all cancers as a group (Table 9-1).[44]

Summary

In spite of the foregoing data, there are some summary toxologic data sheets that include "information" about uranium that is not substantiated in the scientific literature. As an example of this, health and hazard information

Table 9-1 • Site-Specific Cancer Risks from a Pooled Analysis of 120,000 Uranium Workers

Cancer	Relative Risk	95% CI
All cancers	0.91	0.85–0.97
Leukemia	0.90	0.67–1.14
Non-Hodgkin's lymphoma	0.82	0.71–0.92
Brain	0.91	0.65–1.17
Thyroid	0.38	0.00–0.81
Lung	0.94	0.83–1.05
Stomach	0.78	0.62–0.89
Colorectal	0.91	0.78–1.04
Liver	0.84	0.62–1.07
Kidney	0.78	0.59–0.96
Bladder	0.83	0.71–0.96
Bone	0.93	0.53–1.33

Data from The Royal Society: The Health Hazards of Depleted Uranium Munitions, Parts 1 and 2. London, The Royal Society, 2001.

on uranium from the Department of Transportation reports that the chronic effects include the possibility of osteosarcoma. This has been produced only in animals by intravenous or intraskeletal administration of large amounts of uranium. These effects have not been reported in man and remain hypothetical considerations. Other summary sheets indicate that chronic poisoning can develop after exposure to slightly soluble uranium compounds and that the changes include leukopenia, lymphopenia, and symptoms of "vegetative dystonia." These comments come from reports in the early Russian literature and have not been substantiated in any Western scientific literature to date. Soluble uranium at enrichments below 5% is a renal chemical toxin and not a radiological problem. Insoluble uranium that has been inhaled appears to have little direct chemical effect on the lung, and radiation doses to the lung from uranium and its daughter products are unlikely to exceed 0.3 mGy per year, even in uranium miners. The U.S. Agency for Toxic Substances and Disease Registry (ATSDR) of the Centers for Disease Control (CDC) toxicological data profile indicates that large amounts of uranium can react with tissues in the body and damage kidneys but that humans and animals exposed to high levels of uranium do not have higher cancer rates.

DEPLETED URANIUM

Depleted uranium (DU) typically refers to natural uranium from which most of the uranium 235 has been removed. The amount of ^{235}U in DU is typically about one third of that in natural uranium, with the result that the radioactivity of DU is about 60% of the radioactivity of natural uranium. Because of its low specific radioactivity, DU is primarily a chemical toxin; however, as an emitter of alpha, beta, and gamma radiations, it is also a potential radiation hazard if taken into the body. That DU is denser than lead, has a high melting point, and is highly pyrophoric have led to its use in various civilian and military applications.[45] The latter include armor-piercing projectiles, hundreds of tons of which were employed during the 1991 Gulf War and more recently in conflicts in the Balkans, Afghanistan, and Iraq. An estimated 320 tons of DU was used in the First Gulf War, about 15 tons in the Balkans, and probably about 1000 tons in the Second Gulf War. The resulting exposure of military personnel to DU and widespread contamination of the environment in areas where DU munitions were deployed have prompted public concerns about the potential hazards that may be involved.

On external exposure to DU, the potential health effects are limited to those that can be caused by direct contact with a piece of pure DU, which can result in beta-irradiation of the skin at an equivalent dose rate of about 2.5 mSv per hour. Internal exposure to DU, alternatively, may result through the ingestion of contaminated soil, inhalation of contaminated dust, or implantation of embedded fragments by accidental bruising of the skin on contaminated surfaces or by wounding with contaminated shrapnel. Inhalation of dust is considered to be the major pathway of exposure to DU in both combat and noncombat situations. It is noteworthy that a DU penetrating projectile typically ignites on impact (especially with steel), sharpens as it melts, pierces the impacted object (such as heavy armor), and becomes aerosolized, scattering DU fragments and dust into the surrounding environment. The amount of DU that is taken up and deposited in various organs depends on the size and solubility of the DU-containing particles. Chemical toxicity is more likely to be associated with the more soluble forms, and radiotoxicity with the more insoluble forms. As noted above, the kidney is the critical organ for the chemotoxicity of uranium.

On the basis of the available evidence, it is considered unlikely, except under extreme circumstances, that the intakes of DU by soldiers on the battlefield or by those returning to areas where DU munitions were deployed would result in toxic levels of uranium in the kidney or detectable increases in the risks of cancer or other diseases. The extreme circumstances apply to soldiers surviving in tanks struck by DU rounds, those working for extended periods in heavily contaminated vehicles, persons ingesting heavily contaminated water or soil, and children playing in heavily contaminated areas. In each of these cases, although the risks are as yet highly uncertain, it is conceivable that uranium concentrations might lead to short-term kidney dysfunction and/or increased lifetime risks of cancer.[45–48] A small study of Gulf War veterans with retained DU shrapnel fragments did not find adverse effects on renal function even though measurable uranium was found in the urine for up to 12 years.[49] Nonsignificant subtle abnormalities have been suggested in this cohort regarding unspecified neurocognitive and reproductive outcomes, which the authors suggest require more research.[50]

PLUTONIUM

General

The perception that plutonium is the most toxic substance known to humans is inaccurate: only certain forms administered by way of certain routes are toxic. More is known about the toxicology of plutonium than about most other hazardous elements. A review of the subject was published by Bair and Thompson.[51]

Plutonium is a metal of the actinide series, which oxidizes quickly to form plutonium dioxide (PuO_2), the compound most likely to be encountered in accidental situations. Plutonium oxides, hydroxides, and fluorides are moderately inert in the environment, with no known concentration mechanisms that apply to humans. There are 15 isotopes of plutonium, ranging from plutonium 232 to plutonium 246. All are radioactive to some degree and have physical half-lives ranging from less than a second to many years. Plutonium 239 is the radioisotope that has generated most radiobiologic concern. It has a 24,390-year physical half-life and emits energetic alpha particles. These alpha particles have an average energy of 5.15 MeV and a range of 24 μm in bone and 40 μm in tissue. The specific activity of plutonium 239 is 2.3×10^{-3} TBq/g. Plutonium 239 is the radioisotope that is used for fuel in certain types of nuclear power reactors and explosive nuclear devices. While it may be deposited on the skin surface, the alpha radiation does not penetrate through the outer layers of the epithelium. Thus, if exposure is restricted to the skin surface, there is no radiologic hazard. Plutonium 241 emits beta radiation and may represent a skin hazard. Plutonium 238 devices are used as heat sources in cardiac pacemakers and satellites, as well as in many other applications. Plutonium 238 is also an alpha emitter, with a half-life of 86.4 years. The high rate of alpha emissions allows plutonium 238 to be used as a heat source, but it also causes plutonium 238 to be 280 times more hazardous than plutonium 239 when considered on a mass basis. The specific activity of plutonium 238 is 6.3×10^{-1} TBq/g. Early studies with plutonium were conducted in animals. It was quickly found that plutonium injected intravenously was rapidly deposited in the bone and liver; however, the absorption of plutonium administered orally is less than 0.1%. The "toxicity" of plutonium most commonly refers to the induction of lung tumors as a consequence of inhalation deposition of insoluble particulates. The principal experimental animal data presently come from three major studies: (1) evaluation of inhaled PuO_2 in beagle dogs at Battelle's Pacific Northwest Laboratories in Richland, Washington; (2) plutonium aerosol studies in beagles at the Lovelace Foundation in Albuquerque, New Mexico; and (3) administration of plutonium microspheres in the lung capillaries of hamsters at Los Alamos National Laboratory. Recently, Kadhim et al. reported that some animal cells maintained in tissue culture and exposed to alpha particles appear to have transmitted chromosomal instability to their progeny.[52] The authors mentioned that this may have some relationship to leukemia clusters detected around nuclear power plants. Hereditary effects of leukemia clusters are discussed extensively in Chapter 3, and it is clear that not only do leukemia clusters occur at places other than nuclear power plants, but there is often very little plutonium released from most plants. Thus, the reported chromosomal effects of alpha particles, while interesting, remain to be confirmed, and their relevence to human risk assessment remains questionable.[53]

Environmental Aspects

Atmospheric testing of nuclear weapons between 1945 and 1976 released several radionuclides of plutonium into the environment. Careless statements, such as "one pound of plutonium is enough to kill every person in the world" are often made; however, UNSCEAR 1982 estimated that from weapons testing alone, there were approximately 5 tons of plutonium already in the biosphere.[54] Release from atmospheric testing caused plutonium to be deposited on land and in water as insoluble aerosol particles, usually in oxide form. Most of the activity in soil is present in the top 10 cm. In the ocean, about 50% of activity is below the thermocline. Nuclear tests have contributed 0.3 to 0.5 MCi of plutonium 239 and 240, mostly in the northern hemisphere. It is estimated that nuclear tests contributed approximately 9 kCi of plutonium 238 to the fallout, with reentry of a satellite in 1964 adding another 17 kCi. The most important isotopes of plutonium in the environment from weapons testing are plutonium 239, 240, 238, and 241. Although plutonium 241 has a half-life of only 14 years, it is important because it decays to americium 241, an alpha emitter with a half-life of 430 years. Normally, plutonium 239 and 240 are reported together in environmental activity measurements; at the present time, plutonium 239 represents about 60% of the activity measured. These isotopes of plutonium and transplutonium elements are generated in all weapons tests, from activation of uranium 238 and from material that has failed to undergo fission. The transfer coefficient from soil to plants and animals and, subsequently, to humans, was reviewed extensively in UNSCEAR 1977[5] and 1982.[54] It should be pointed out, however, that although plutonium is measurable in most human livers and skeletons, it contributes relatively little radiation exposure.[55] The major radionuclide contributing to the radiation dose commitment from nuclear explosions is carbon 14. Plutonium and the transuranic isotopes contribute less than 1% of the effective dose commitment. The major opportunity for plutonium to enter the environment from nuclear power production is during fuel reprocessing. During reactor operations, plutonium 239 may be formed from neutron activation of uranium 238. Examination of at least two fuel reprocessing facilities demonstrated that a small amount of plutonium may be discharged in the liquid effluent stream into the environment. Plants discriminate against plutonium on the order of 10^{-4} to 10^{-6} and, if the plant is eaten by humans, another factor of 10^{-4} may be applied because of poor intestinal absorption. The extremely poor concentrating ability of plants, combined with the poor absorption from the gut of these radioisotopes, indicates that the ingestion pathway contributes very little to the collective dose commitment.

Human Data

Human data concerning biodistribution of plutonium are from two principal sources: terminally ill patients who were administered small amounts of plutonium[56,57] and a group of workers exposed occupationally during the Manhattan Project.[58]

Various medical considerations will be reviewed here because of the specific attention directed toward this element over the last several years. Experiments involving humans indicate that the method by which plutonium enters the body is the chief determinant of the subsequent effect of the contamination. Vaughan et al. indicated that if various solutions of plutonium are applied to the unbroken skin, absorption ranges between 0.002% and 0.25%.[59] Absorption through the skin generally is a problem only if the skin is damaged. Entry of plutonium into wounds has occurred in various occupational accidents. Once this has happened, the plutonium can be translocated to regional lymph nodes and other tissues, although part of it may remain at the site of the wound, predominantly depending on the chemical nature of the plutonium compound that entered the wound. Descriptions of cases involving plutonium contamination of intact skin, puncture wounds, and inhalation accidents were reviewed by the National Council on Radiation Protection and Measurements (NCRP).[4] To date, no significant adverse effects have been reported from these accidents. In instances in which a wound is contaminated, a fibrous nodule may develop at the site.[60,61] No sarcomas or carcinomas have been reported in such sites. Inhalation is the most common route of internal contamination, with plutonium accounting for 75% of industrial exposures.[62] Deposition patterns and retention of plutonium in the lungs depend on the physical properties and particulate size during the inhalation exposure, as well as the solubility of the specific material inhaled. After inhalation of relatively insoluble particles, a high proportion of plutonium is retained in the tracheobronchial and pulmonary lymph nodes. With such compounds, the retention half-time in the lungs is 150 to 1000 days. Autopsy tissue analysis of occupational workers shows the highest concentration of plutonium to be in the tracheobronchial lymph nodes, followed in decreasing order by lung parenchyma and liver phagocytes.[63-65] Analysis of the PuO_2 aerosol released in an accident at a plutonium facility showed it to have a mean aerodynamic particle size of 4.8 ± 1.5 μm and a dissolution half-time of 900 days, thus providing data that were useful in evaluating the radiation dose to exposed workers.[66]

After entry, some or all of the plutonium may be solubilized; the body distribution of the solubilized plutonium is as follows: skeleton, 45%; liver, 45%; and other tissues, 10%. The half-time in the body is about 200 years, with the retention half-times of plutonium in the liver and skeleton assumed to be 40 and 100 years, respectively. The maximum permissible body burden of plutonium 238 or 239 is 1.4 kBq (0.04 μCi), and the critical organ is the liver.[4] Plutonium uptake and deposition in human tissues at autopsy have been studied by several researchers.[67–69] Bennet estimated that the dose to humans from inhalation of plutonium 239 in fallout through the year 2000 is as follows: cumulative dose to lung, 16 μGy; liver, 17 μGy; bone lining cells, 15 μGy.[70] The distribution of plutonium in workers exposed by chronic inhalation at the Mayak production facility was studied by Suslova,[71] and Khokhryakov et al.,[72] who reported changes in the organ distribution with time and health status.

Preliminary study of a sample of 221 workers employed at the Mayak Production Association facilities for at least one year between 1948 and 1958 found a significant proportion of them to have received annual doses approaching 1 Gy from external and internal sources and to include 14 cases of acute radiation syndrome, 98 cases of "chronic radiation sickness," and 13 cases of "plutonium pneumosclerosis."[73,74] Cytogenetic study of the peripheral lymphocytes of 79 of the plutonium-exposed workers at the facilities showed the frequency of chromosome aberrations in such cells to increase with the plutonium 239 body burden over the range 0 to 4.5 kBq,[75] in keeping with similar findings in plutonium workers at the British Nuclear Fuels plant at Sellafield.[76] Successive cytogenetic examinations over a period of 30 years, however, disclosed no evidence of persistent genomic instability in the bone marrow cells of such workers.[77]

Review of the medical records of five subjects injected experimentally with approximately 11 kBq of plutonium 239, and one injected with 3.5 kBq of plutonium 238 revealed bone lesions in all of them, including osteoporosis, fractures, areas of increased bone density, numerous dystopic calcifications, and one case of widespread pathological calcification on bone surfaces. Nonskeletal findings included labyrinthitis with inflammatory mastoid changes, conduction deafness, and a benign neurofibroma directly adjacent to bone.[78]

There have been a few military accidents involving nuclear weapons in which there has been environmental dispersion of plutonium. Few health effects are reported in workers who cleaned up after these incidents. Juel studied the mortality of 1202 workers employed at the Thule, Greenland, site of a B-52 bomber crash.[79] No differences were found in total mortality or mortality from cancer or heart disease between those employed during the cleanup period and those employed at other times. Occupational exposure experience with plutonium workers is collected by the U.S. Transuranium Registry at Los Alamos National Laboratory and the data were reviewed by Voelz et al.[80] In their review, 224 white male workers with plutonium body burdens of 370 Bq (10 nCi) or more were followed for cause of mortality over 30 years. The average plutonium deposition in those still alive is 21 nCi, with annual dose rates of 10.1 mGy to the lung, 16.9 mGy to the bone surface, and 1.1 mGy to the liver. No excess mortality due to any cause was observed in these male workers. The total cardiovascular and cancer mortality rates were actually lower than expected from age and specific rates for the U.S. white male population. Lung cancer mortality was lower than expected. Goffman proposed an unproven theory that there is an elevated risk of lung cancer in smokers who inhale insoluble plutonium.[81] Voelz et al. applied Goffman's model to the 224 plutonium workers.[82] According to Goffman's theory, 9 to 13 excess lung cancers should have occurred by 1980. No lung cancers occurred in the group of 82 smokers by 1980, and, thus, the available data do not support the hypothetical risk estimates proposed by Goffman. A mortality study of Los Alamos male residents, all of whom worked or lived within a few kilometers of a major plutonium plant or other nuclear facility, showed a possible excess of cancers of the combined lymphatic and hematopoietic tissues, but the incidence data suggest that this excess, if it was real, no longer exists.

The most interesting follow-up of occupationally exposed persons includes 26 Manhattan Project workers heavily exposed to plutonium at the Los Alamos facility between 1942 and 1945. These workers were engaged in the development of methods to process and fabricate plutonium for the atomic bomb. They have been followed since 1953 with routine medical examinations. Plutonium body burden estimates have been obtained from whole-body counting and urine excretion values. The principal mode of exposure was inhalation, although five individuals had contaminated wounds. Their effective doses ranged from 0.1 to 7.2 Sv with a median value of 1.25.

Voelz et al. also reported on a 50-year medical follow-up of these workers.[58] As of 1994, among the 26 workers, 7 persons had died compared to an expected 16 deaths based on mortality rates of U.S. white males. The SMR was 0.43. The causes of death were as follows: one case of lung cancer and one case each of myocardial infarction, automobile/pedestrian accident, pneumonia/congestive heart failure, arteriosclerotic heart disease, prostate cancer, and osteogenic sarcoma. Subject 10 died at the age of 71 of lung cancer, but he had smoked more than one pack per day throughout most of his adult life. Subject 3 died of prostate cancer but also had a large-cell, poorly differentiated carcinoma of the lung and was also a heavy smoker. Subject 25, although dying of severe arteriosclerotic heart disease, had lung cancer as well, but also a 43-year history of cigarette smoking. Three cases of

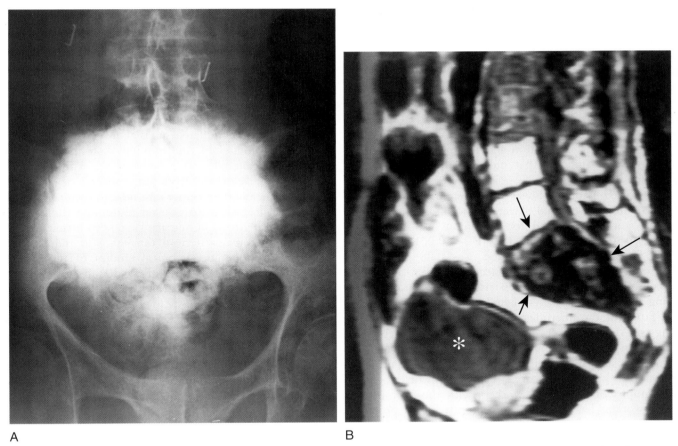

A

B

Figure 9-1 • Osteogenic sarcoma of the sacrum in a plutonium worker. The radiograph of the pelvis (**A**) shows a very dense and large bony tumor near the top of the pelvis. The tumor (*arrows*) is also visualized on a lateral view from an MR scan (**B**). On the scan the bladder is indicated by the *asterisk*.

lung cancer in a group of 26 men over a 44-year period is a higher incidence than expected for the general population but still within the statistical limits of expectation for smokers without plutonium inhalation or exposure. The finding is consistent with the known risks of cigarette smoking, particularly given that all three men had long cigarette-smoking histories. Whether there was additional risk due to plutonium inhalation cannot be determined from these data due to the small numbers involved. Subject 20 died of an osteogenic sarcoma originating in the sacrum (Fig. 9-1). This was the first bone sarcoma apparently reported in a person exposed to plutonium. Bone sarcomas have occurred in persons with internal deposition of radium, as discussed in the section "Bone Tumors" in Chapter 5. Bone tumors have also been observed in beagles exposed to plutonium. Normally, osteogenic sarcomas arise in children or adolescents in the long bones and in adults in areas of Paget's disease. The particular individual mentioned above did not have Paget's disease. The estimated plutonium deposition in this man at the time of death was 560 Bq (15 nCi). The cumulative dose to the bone surface in the man was estimated to be 0.44 Gy through the end of 1986.

A study of workers at the Rocky Flats plant by Wilkinson et al. compared mortality ratios between workers who have plutonium depositions of 74 Bq (2 nCi) or more and unexposed workers with less than 74 Bq.[83] The ratios of lung cancer rates for exposed and unexposed workers were not significantly different. By using 10-year induction times, the ratio was 1.4 (95% CI 0.33 to 4.5), based on only three lung cancer deaths. Similarly, evaluation of the causes of death in a cohort of 260 plutonium workers enrolled in the U.S. Transuranium and Uranium Registries revealed no excess causes of death attributable to radiation.[84] As well, studies of the cancer incidence and mortality in a population residing near two former uranium and plutonium processing facilities in Pennsylvania, analyzed some 40 years after the plants had begun operation, found no significant elevations in the overall cancer rates or the rates of cancers of specific sites.[85,86]

In workers at the Mayak Production Association who were exposed to internally deposited plutonium, as well as external radiation, the rate of mortality from liver cancer has been observed to increase significantly with increasing plutonium body burden, reaching an RR of 17 in those with body burdens estimated to exceed 7.4 kBq.[87]

Similarly, mortality from bone cancer in the same workforce increased with increasing dose.[88]

Mortality from lung cancer in Mayak workers also has been observed to increase with the dose to the lung from plutonium; the excess relative risk (ERR) and excess absolute risk (EAR) both were adequately described by linear functions, the ERR per Gy declining with attained age and the EAR increasing with attained age up to about age 65.[89] Analysis of the interaction between the carcinogenic effects of internal irradiation and those of smoking was interpreted to indicate that most of the lung cancers were due to smoking.[90]

Analyzed under a linear dose-response model, the ERR of lung, liver, and skeletal cancers as a group in Mayak workers, adjusted for plutonium exposure, was estimated to be 0.30 per Gy (P < 0.001) and the ERR for all other solid cancers was 0.08 per Gy.[91] The dose-response for solid cancers, however, appeared to be nonlinear, with the excess risk at doses under 3 Gy being about twice those predicted by the linear model.

Study of the microdistribution of plutonium in the lungs of Mayak workers revealed the long-term retained plutonium to be distributed highly nonuniformly, most being deposited in the parenchyma but a significant portion also in pulmonary scars.[92] Comparison of the chest radiographs of plutonium workers with those of unexposed workers has revealed a significantly higher proportion of abnormal profusion scores among the former (17.5%) than among the latter (7.2%). After controlling for the effects of age, smoking, and asbestos exposure, it was concluded from the findings that lung doses of 10 Sv or more conferred a 5.3-fold risk of an abnormal chest x-ray consistent with pulmonary fibrosis.[93]

Overall rates of cancer mortality in 40,761 employees of three U.K. nuclear facilities, analyzed in relation to doses of internal radiation from plutonium, tritium, or "other radionuclides" (uranium, polonium, actinium, or others), were found to be lower than the national rates. In workers monitored for plutonium, however, the rate increased significantly with the number of years monitored, as did mortality from pleural cancer.[94] Mortality from cancers of the lung and prostate were also increased in workers monitored for "other radionuclides," and cancer of the prostate in workers monitored for tritium. The significance of the findings is limited, however, by the lack of adequate information about the possible influence of exposure to other agents or additional confounding factors.

Study of the mortality of all 14,319 workers employed at the British Nuclear Fuels plant at Sellafield between 1947 and 1975 and followed up to the end of 1992 revealed no statistically significant trend between the risk of death from cancer of any specific site, or from all cancers combined, and the cumulative plutonium and external radiation doses. Trends in cancer incidence, however, showed significant increases in risk with cumulative plutonium plus external doses for all lymphatic and hemopoeitic neoplasms,

analyzed for 0-, 10-, and 20-year lag periods.[95] In 6376 female employees of the facility analyzed separately for the period up to 1998, no statistically significant associations between mortality or cancer morbidity and cumulative assessed organ-specific internal plutonium dose or cumulative external total body dose were found.[96]

In workers employed for 15 to 25 years at the Rocky Flats plant, the risk of lung cancer was found to increase linearly with the cumulative internal dose to the lung from plutonium, americium, and uranium isotopes, and there was a significant association between age at first internal lung dose and mortality from lung cancer.[97]

Estimates of the risk per unit dose to each of the four primary cancer sites for inhaled plutonium (lung, liver, bone, bone marrow) in humans have been formulated by combining estimates derived through four independent approaches: (1) epidemiological studies of plutonium-exposed workers, (2) epidemiological studies of persons exposed to low-LET radiation combined with a factor to adjust for the relative biologic effectiveness of plutonium alpha particles for each site, (3) epidemiological studies of persons exposed to alpha-emitting radionuclides other than plutonium, and (4) extrapolation from controlled studies of animals exposed to plutonium and other alpha emitters. The organ-specific estimates of the risk of cancer mortality per Gy derived by this method were: lung, 0.13 (0.022 to 0.53); liver, 0.0057 (0.011 to 0.47); bone, 0.0013 (0.000060 to 0.025); and bone marrow (leukemia) 0.013 (0.00061 to 0.05).[98]

In a study of a cohort of 26,389 workers employed at the Hanford plutonium production facility during 1944–1978 and followed through 1994, estimates of the ERR for cumulative radiation doses at all ages combined were negative for mortality from all causes and for leukemia, but were positive for mortality from lung cancer and for all cancers combined. The latter risk was attributable primarily to an excess of lung cancer associated with cumulative doses received after age 55, for which the excess risk per Sv was estimated to approximate 9.05 (90% CI 2.96 to 17.92). Plutonium workers at the Hanford site had 15.4 times greater internal deposition than other Hanford workers. As well, plutonium workers had a lower death rate compared to the other workers.[99]

In 801 persons who had lived downwind of the plutonium production facility at Hanford, Washington, a community health survey for the period 1944–1995 revealed greater than expected numbers of cancers of the thyroid gland, central nervous system, uterus, ovary, and breast, suggesting that carcinogenic effects on the population may have resulted from exposure to radioactively contaminated food, water, soil, and/or air; however, the possible influence of confounding factors could not be excluded.[100] The concentrations and ratios of plutonium 239 and plutonium 240 in the tissues of Colorado residents, analyzed in relation to their distance from the Rocky Flats Environmental Technology Site, a potential source of these radionuclides, were interpreted to indicate that the plutonium had come primarily from global radioactive fallout and not from the Rocky Flats site.[101]

The calculation of reasonable risk estimates for workers exposed to plutonium through occupational exposure is based on the following assumptions: Plutonium activity is generally taken to be 50% in the lungs, 40% in the bone, and 10% in the liver, with the plutonium being deposited on the bone's surface only and retained there indefinitely. Twenty-five percent of the alpha energy is assumed to be absorbed in the endosteal cells. A computer program is then used to estimate plutonium deposition on the basis of excretion values in urine.[102]

In summary, the epidemiologic studies of plutonium in humans indicate that the risks are not substantially higher than can be calculated from current UNSCEAR 2006[103] and BEIR VII[37] risk estimates. Extensive epidemiologic studies are continuing to be conducted on the majority of all people in the United States who have worked with transuranic radionuclides, and additional data may be expected to become available in the future. Site-specific cancer for plutonium workers are also presented in Chapter 5.

RADIUM

Radium has the symbol Ra and the atomic number 88. Its appearance is almost white but it rapidly oxidizes to black. It is a decay product of uranium and is therefore found in trace amounts in uranium ores. In the natural environment it is found at very low levels in virtually all rock, soil, water, plants, and animals. Thus, like uranium and plutonium, everyone has some minor exposure to these isotopes.

Radium and its salts are soluble in water and in some areas there are relatively high concentrations in groundwater. Radium is the heaviest of the alkaline earth metals and resembles barium in chemical behavior. Radium is very radioactive (more than one million times the same mass of uranium) and, as a result, radium preparations are usually at a higher temperature than their surroundings. There are 25 different known isotopes found in nature. The most stable and common isotope, radium 226, is a product of uranium 238 decay. It has a physical half-life of 1602 years and decays into radon gas while emitting alpha particles with some gamma radiation. The next longest lived isotope is radium 228 with a physical half-life of 6.7 years. It is predominantly a beta emitter and is a product of thorium 232 decay. Radium 224 has a much shorter half-life of 3.6 days; it has been used to treat tuberculosis and ankylosing spondylitis (see Chapter 5).

Various forms of radium were used during the first half of the 20th century in medical applications (usually to treat cancer). It was also unfortunately added to water, toothpaste, hair creams, and even food for its supposed "healing powers." Spas with radium-rich waters are still in use in some countries around the world. Radium was also mixed with phosphors to make luminous dials for aircraft, watches, and clocks. Many young women were employed as radium dial painters and had a practice of licking their paintbrushes to obtain a fine brush point. This resulted in oral ingestion of large activities of radium. Following ingestion, radium behaves like calcium, about 80% is excreted in feces and much of the residual 20% localizes in bone. Internal ingestion resulted in these young women developing an excess of osteosarcomas, sinus cancers, and osteonecrosis (see Chapters 5 and 6).

Radium is used in some industrial radiography devices, it can be mixed with beryllium to emit neutrons, and it can be used in well-logging devices. Sometimes it is put in the ends of lightning rods to improve their effectiveness by ionizing the air around them. Radium 226 and 228 also have come to recent attention as contaminants in pipe scale. In some communities, elevated levels of radon 222 in the water supplies have been found to result from radium-bearing pipe scale in the water pipes and reservoirs.[104] Such pipe scale, deposited gradually over time on the inner surfaces of underground pipes, typically consists of inorganic solids with traces of naturally occurring radioactive materials. Depending on the geochemical conditions in question, the latter are predominantly radium compounds.[105]

Oil field workers may be exposed to radium 226, which can be present in varying concentrations in the radium-bearing pipe scale that is widely deposited in oil pipes and released from the pipes when they are removed from the oil wells and stored or cleaned. The radium 226 specific activity in such pipe scale has been found to range from 33 to 65 Bq/g. Since the materials are of very low solubility and the scale removed often is of large particle size, the radiation doses are relatively low. The annual committed doses to exposed workers have been estimated to range up to 0.45 mSv for inhalation, 97 μSv for ingestion, and 4.1 mSv for external exposure.[106]

REFERENCES

1. National Research Council (NRC), Committee on the Biological Effects of Ionizing Radiations (BEIR), Health risks of radon and other internally deposited alpha-emitters. BEIR IV. 1988, Washington, DC: National Academies Press. Available from: http://www.netLibrary.com/urlapi.asp?action=summary&v=1&bookid=15940.

2. Rurdo, J., P. Failla, and R. Schlenker, Radiobiology of radium and the actinides in man. In Proceedings of an International Conference, Lake Geneva, Wis., Oct. 11–16, 1981. Health Phys, 1983. 44(suppl 1):1–589.

3. Gerber, G., H. Metivier, and J. Stather, Biological assessment of occupational exposure to actinides. Radiat Prot Dosimetry, 1989. 26:1–4.

4. National Council on Radiation Protection and Measurements (NCRP), Management of persons accidentally contaminated with radionuclides: Recommendations of the NCRP. 1980, Washington, DC: NCRP, p. vi.

5. United Nations Scientific Committee on the Effects of Atomic Radiation (UNSCEAR), Sources and effects of ionizing radiation: Report to the General Assembly, with annexes. 1977, New York: United Nations.

6. Stannard, J., Radioactivity and Health: A History. 1988, Washington, DC: U.S. Department of Energy.

7. West, C.M. and L.M. Scott, Uranium cases showing long chest burden retention—an updating. Health Phys, 1969. 17(6):781–791.

8. Quastel, M.R., et al., Excretion and retention by humans of chronically inhaled uranium dioxide. Health Phys, 1970. 18(3):233–244.

9. Thind, K.S., Determination of particle size for airborne UO_2 dust at a fuel fabrication work station and its implication on the derivation and use of ICRP Publication 30 derived air concentration values. Health Phys, 1986. 51(1):97–105.

10. Cothern, C.R., W.L. Lappenbusch, and J.A. Cotruvo, Health effects guidance for uranium in drinking water. Health Phys, 1983. 44(suppl 1):S377–S384.

11. Kocher, D.C., Relationship between kidney burden and radiation dose from chronic ingestion of U: Implications for radiation standards for the public. Health Phys, 1989. 57(1):9–15.

12. Leggett, R.W., The behavior and chemical toxicity of U in the kidney: A reassessment. Health Phys, 1989. 57(3):365–383.

13. International Commission on Radiological Protection (ICRP), Annual limits on intake of radionuclides by workers based on the 1990 recommendations: A report from Committee 2 of the ICRP. Ann ICRP, 1991. 21(4):1–41.

14. Hursh, J. and N. Spoor, Data on man. In Uranium, Plutonium, Transplutonic Elements: Handbook of Experimental Pharmacology, vol. 36, H. Hodge, J. Stannard, and J. Hursh, eds. 1973, New York: Springer-Verlag.

15. Bernard, S. and E. Struxness, A Study of the Distribution and Excretion of Uranium in Man, 1957, Oak Ridge, Tenn: Oak Ridge National Laboratory.

16. Fisher, D., M.J. Swint, and R.L. Kathren, Evaluation of health effects in Sequoya Fuels Corporation workers from an accidental exposure to uranium hexafluoride. In Nuclear Regulatory Commission Report. 1990, Richland, Wash: Pacific Northwest Laboratory.

17. Fisher, D.R., R.L. Kathren, and M.J. Swint, Modified biokinetic model for uranium from analysis of acute exposure to UF6. Health Phys, 1991. 60(3):335–342.

18. Boback, M., A review of uranium excretion and clinical urinalysis data in accidental exposure cases. Conference on Occupational Health: Experience with Uranium, M. Wrenn, ed. 1975, Arlington, Va: U.S. Energy Research and Development Administration. ERDA-93.

19. Eisenbud, M., Early occupational exposure experience with uranium processing. In Conference on Occupational Health: Experience with Uranium, M. Wrenn, ed. 1975, Arlington, Va: U.S. Energy Research and Development Administration. ERDA-93.

20. Lu, S. and F.Y. Zhao, Nephrotoxic limit and annual limit on intake for natural U. Health Phys, 1990. 58(5):619–623.

21. Uranium (natural) and its compounds; U. Am Ind Hyg Assoc J, 1969. 30(3):313–317.

22. Kathren, R.L. and R.H. Moore, Acute accidental inhalation of U: A 38-year follow-up. Health Phys, 1986. 51(5):609–619.

23. Trapp, E., et al., Cardiopulmonary function in uranium miners. Am Rev Resp Dis, 1970. 101:27–43.

24. Samet, J.M., et al., Prevalence survey of respiratory abnormalities in New Mexico uranium miners. Health Phys, 1984. 46(2):361–370.

25. Samet, J.M. and S. Simpson, Review of silicosis and other pneumoconioses in underground uranium miners. 1992, Washington DC: Centers for Disease Control.

26. Archer, V.E., H.P. Brinton, and J.K. Wagoner, Pulmonary function of uranium miners. Health Phys, 1964. 10:1183–1194.

27. Archer, V.E., et al., Hazards to health in uranium mining and milling. J Occup Med, 1962. 4:55–60.

28. Waxweiler, R.J., R. Roscoe, and V. Archer. Mortality follow-up through 1977 of the white underground uranium miners cohort examined by the United States Public Health Service. In International Conference on Radiation Hazards in Mining: Control, Measurement and Medical Aspects, Golden, Colorado. 1981, Kingsport, Tenn: Kingsport Press.

29. Wrenn, M.E., N.P. Singh, and G. Saccomanno, Uranium and thorium isotopes and their state of equilibria in lungs from uranium miners. Health Phys, 1983. 44(suppl 1):S385–S389.

30. Brown, D. and T. Bloom, Mortality among uranium enrichment workers. In National Institute of Occupational Safety and Health, January, 1987. 1987, Washington, DC: NIOSH.

31. Ritz, B., Radiation exposure and cancer mortality in uranium processing workers. Epidemiology, 1999. 10(5):531–538.

32. McGeoghegan, D. and K. Binks, The mortality and cancer morbidity experience of workers at the Capenhurst uranium enrichment facility 1946–95. J Radiol Prot, 2000. 20(4):381–401.

33. McGeoghegan, D. and K. Binks, The mortality and cancer morbidity experience of workers at the Springfields uranium production facility, 1946–95. J Radiol Prot, 2000. 20(2):111–317.

34. Dupree-Ellis, E., et al., External radiation exposure and mortality in a cohort of uranium processing workers. Am J Epidemiol, 2000. 152(1):91–95.

35. Pinkerton, L.E., et al., Mortality among a cohort of uranium mill workers: An update. Occup Environ Med, 2004. 61(1):57–64.

36. Kathren, R.L., Invited editorial: Recent studies of the mortality and cancer morbidity experience of uranium workers and a fresh look at depleted uranium. J Radiol Prot, 2001. 21(2):105–107.

37. National Research Council (NRC), Committee on the Biological Effects of Ionizing Radiations (BEIR), Health risks from exposure to low levels of ionizing radiation. BEIR VII. 2005, Washington, DC: NRCUSNA Press.

38. Jablon, S., Z. Hrubec, and J.D. Boice, Jr., Cancer in populations living near nuclear facilities: A survey of mortality nationwide and incidence in two states. JAMA, 1991. 265(11):1403–1408.

39. Boice, J.D., Jr., et al., Cancer mortality in a Texas county with prior uranium mining and milling activities, 1950–2001. J Radiol Prot, 2003. 23(3):247–262.

40. Boice, J.P., W.L. Bigbee, M.T. Mumma, et al., Cancer incidence in municipalities near two former nuclear materials processing facilities in Pennsylvania. Health Phys, 2003. 85(6):678–690.

41. Boice, J.P., W.L. Bigbee, M.T. Mumma, et al., Cancer mortality in counties near two former nuclear materials processing facilities in Pennsylvania, 1950–1995. Health Phys, 2003. 85(5):691–700.

42. Boice, J.P., W.L. Mumma, W.J. Blott, et al., Cancer and noncancer mortality in populations living near uranium and vanadium mining and milling operations in Montrose County, Colorado, 1950–2000. Radiat Res, 2007. 167(6):711–726.

43. Lopez-Abente, G., N. Aragones, and M. Pollan, Solid-tumor mortality in the vicinity of uranium cycle facilities and nuclear power plants in Spain. Environ Health Perspect, 2001. 109(7):721–729.

44. The Royal Society, The Health Hazards of Depleted Uranium Munitions. Parts 1 and 2. 2001, London: The Royal Society.

45. Burkart, W., P. Danesi, and J.H. Hendry, Properties, use and health effects of depleted uranium. Int Congress Series, 2005. 1276:133–136.

46. Spratt, B.G., Depleted uranium munitions-where are we now? J Radiol Prot, 2002. 22(2):125–129.

47. The Royal Society: The health effects of depleted uranium munitions: A summary. J Radiol Prot, 2002. 22(2):131–139.

48. McLaughlin, J., Public health and environmental aspects of DU. Intl Congress Series, 2005. 1276:137–140.

49. McDiarmid, M.A., et al., Biological monitoring and surveillance results of Gulf War I veterans exposed to depleted uranium. Int Arch Occup Environ Health, 2006. 79(1):11–21.

50. McClain, D.E., Depleted uranium: A radiochemical toxicant? Mil Med, 2002. 167(suppl 2):S125–S126.

51. Bair, W.J. and R.C. Thompson, Plutonium: Biomedical research. Science, 1974. 183(126):715–722.

52. Kadhim, M.A., et al., Transmission of chromosomal instability after plutonium alpha-particle irradiation. Nature, 1992. 355(6362):738–740.

53. Evans, H.J., Radiation biology. Alpha-particle after effects. Nature, 1992. 355(6362):674–675.

54. United Nations Scientific Committee on the Effects of Atomic Radiation (UNSCEAR), Ionizing radiation: Sources and effects. UNSCEAR report to the General Assembly, in annex K: Radiation-induced life shortening. 1982, New York: United Nations, p. v.

55. Bunzl, K. and W. Kracke, Fallout $^{239/240}$Pu and ^{238}Pu in human tissues from the Federal Republic of Germany. Health Phys, 1983. 44(suppl 1):S441–S449.

56. Langham, W., Determination of internally deposited radioactive isotopes from excretion analyses. Am Ind Hyg Assoc J, 1956. 17:305.

57. Durbin, P., Plutonium: A new look at old data. In Radiobiology of Plutonium, B. Stover and W. Jee, eds. 1972, Salt Lake City: JW Press.

58. Voelz, G.L., J.N. Lawrence, and E.R. Johnson, Fifty years of plutonium exposure to the Manhattan Project plutonium workers: An update. Health Phys, 1997. 73(4):611–619.

59. Vaughan, J., B. Bleaney, and D. Taylor, Distribution, excretion, and effects of plutonium as a bone seeker. In Handbook of Experimental Pharmacology—Uranium, Plutonium, and Transplutonic Elements, H. Hodge, J. Stannard, and J. Hursh, eds. 1973, New York: Springer-Verlag.

60. Lushbaugh, C. and J. Langham, A dermal lesion from implanted plutonium. Arch Dermatol, 1962. 86:461.

61. Lushbaugh, C., R. Cloutier, and G. Humason, Histopathologic studies of intradermal plutonium metal deposits: Their conjectural fate. Ann NY Acad Sci, 1967. 145:791.

62. Ross, D., A statistical summary of United States Atomic Energy Commission contractors' internal exposure experience 1957–1966. In Diagnosis and Treatment of Deposited Radionuclides, H. Kornberg and W. Norwood, eds. 1968, Amsterdam: Excerpta Medica.

63. Campbell, B., et al., Plutonium in autopsy tissue. 1973, Los Alamos, NM: U.S. Energy Research and Development Agency.

64. Lagerquist, C.R., et al., Distribution of plutonium and americium in occupationally exposed humans as found from autopsy samples. Health Phys, 1973. 25(6):581–584.

65. Norwood, W., et al., Preliminary autopsy findings in the U.S. Transuraniuim Registry cases. In Radionuclide Carcinogenesis U.S. Atomic Energy Commission Symposium Series 29. 1973, Springfield, Va: National Technical Information Service.

66. Cheng, Y.S., et al., Characterization of plutonium aerosol collected during an accident. Health Phys, 2004. 87(6):596–605.

67. Nelson, I.C., et al., Plutonium in autopsy tissue samples. Health Phys, 1972. 22(6):925–930.

68. Bair, W.J., C. Richmond, and B. Wachholz, A radiobiological assessment of the spatial distribution of radiation dose from inhaled plutonium. 1974, Washington, DC: U.S. Atomic Energy Commission.

69. Richmond, C. and E. Sullivan, Annual report of the biomedical and environmental research programs of the LASL Health Division. 1974, Los Alamos, NM: Los Alamos Scientific Laboratory.

70. Bennet, B., Fallout of plutonium 239 dose to man. 1974: New York: U.S. Atomic Energy Commission.

71. Suslova, K.G., et al., Extrapulmonary organ distribution of plutonium in healthy workers exposed by chronic inhalation at the Mayak Production Association. Health Phys, 2002. 82(4):432–444.

72. Suslova, K., et al., Modifying effects of health status, physiological, and dosimetric factors on extrapulmonary organ distribution and excretion of inhaled plutonium in workers at the Mayak Production Association. Health Phys, 2006. 90(4):299–311.

73. Claycamp, H.G., et al., Deterministic effects from occupational radiation exposures in a cohort of Mayak PA workers: Data base description. Health Phys, 2000. 79(1):48–54.

74. Okladnikova, N.D., et al., Health status among the staff at the nuclear waste processing plant. Med Tr Prom Ekol, 2000(6):10–14.

75. Okladnikova, N.D., et al., Chromosomal aberrations in lymphocytes of peripheral blood among Mayak facility workers who inhaled insoluble forms of ^{239}PU. Radiat Prot Dosimetry, 2005. 113(1):3–13.

76. Tawn, E.J. and C.A. Whitehouse, Chromosome intra- and inter-changes determined by G-banding in radiation workers with in vivo exposure to plutonium. J Radiol Prot, 2005. 25(1):83–88.

77. Whitehouse, C.A. and E.J. Tawn, No evidence for chromosomal instability in radiation workers with in vivo exposure to plutonium. Radiat Res, 2001. 156(5 Pt 1):467–475.

78. Stebbings, J.H., A case study of selected medical findings among plutonium injectees. Health Phys, 1999. 76(5):477–488.

79. Juel, K., The Thule episode epidemiological follow up after the crash of a B-52 bomber in Greenland: Registry linkage, mortality, hospital admissions. J Epidemiol Community Health, 1992. 46(4):336–339.

80. Voelz, G.L., et al., Studies in persons exposed to plutonium. In Late Biological Effects of Ionizing Radiation. 1978, Vienna: IAEA.

81. Goffman, J., Radiation and Human Health. 1981, San Francisco: Sierra Club.

82. Voelz, G.L., et al. Mortality study of Los Alamos workers with higher exposures to plutonium. In Proceedings of the 16th Mid-Year Topical Meeting: Epidemiology Applied to Health Physics, Albuquerque, NM, January 9–13, 1983. CONF-830101, pp. 318–327.

83. Wilkinson, G.S., et al., Mortality among plutonium and other radiation workers at a plutonium weapons facility. Am J Epidemiol, 1987. 125(2):231–250.

84. Gold, B. and R.L. Kathren, Causes of death in a cohort of 260 plutonium workers. Health Phys, 1998. 75(3):236–240.

85. Boice, J.D., Jr., et al., Cancer mortality in counties near two former nuclear materials processing facilities in Pennsylvania, 1950–1995. Health Phys, 2003. 85(6):691–700.

86. Boice, J.D., Jr., et al., Cancer incidence in municipalities near two former nuclear materials processing facilities in Pennsylvania. Health Phys, 2003. 85(6):678–690.

87. Gilbert, E.S., et al., Liver cancers in Mayak workers. Radiat Res, 2000. 154(3):246–252.

88. Koshurnikova, N.A., et al., Bone cancers in Mayak workers. Radiat Res, 2000. 154(3):237–245.

89. Gilbert, E.S., et al., Lung cancer in Mayak workers. Radiat Res, 2004. 162(5):505–516.

90. Jacob, V., et al., Lung cancer in Mayak workers: Interaction of smoking and plutonium exposure. Radiat Environ Biophys, 2005. 44(2):119–129.

91. Shilnikova, N.S., et al., Cancer mortality risk among workers at the Mayak nuclear complex. Radiat Res, 2003. 159(6):787–798.

92. Hahn, F.F., et al., Plutonium microdistribution in the lungs of Mayak workers. Radiat Res, 2004. 161(5):568–581.

93. Newman, L.S., M.M. Mroz, and A.J. Ruttenber, Lung fibrosis in plutonium workers. Radiat Res, 2005. 164(2):123–131.

94. Carpenter, L.M., et al., Cancer mortality in relation to monitoring for radionuclide exposure in three UK nuclear industry workforces. Br J Cancer, 1998. 78(9):1224–1232.

95. Paquet, F., et al., Efficacy of 3,4,3-LIHOPO for enhancing the excretion of plutonium from rat after simulated wound contamination as a tributyl-n-phosphate complex. Int J Radiat Biol, 1995. 68(6):663–668.

96. McGeoghegan, D., et al., Mortality and cancer morbidity experience of female workers at the British Nuclear Fuels Sellafield plant, 1946–1998. Am J Ind Med, 2003. 44(6):653–663.

97. Brown, S.C., et al., Lung cancer and internal lung doses among plutonium workers at the Rocky Flats plant: A case-control study. Am J Epidemiol, 2004. 160(2):163–172.

98. Grogan, H.A., W.K. Sinclair, and P.G. Voilleque, Risks of fatal cancer from inhalation of ^{239,240}plutonium by humans: A combined four-method approach with uncertainty evaluation. Health Phys, 2001. 80(5):447–461.

99. Wing, S. and D.B. Richardson, Age at exposure to ionising radiation and cancer mortality among Hanford workers: Follow up through 1994. Occup Environ Med, 2005. 62(7):465–472.

100. Grossman, C.M., R.H. Nussbaum, and F.D. Nussbaum, Cancers among residents downwind of the Hanford, Washington, plutonium production site. Arch Environ Health, 2003. 58(5):267–274.

101. Ibrahim, S.A., et al., Plutonium in Colorado residents: Results of autopsy bone samples collected during 1975–1979. Health Phys, 2002. 83(2):165–177.

102. Lawrence, J., A history of PUQFUA, plutonium body burden (Q) from urine assays. 1978, Los Alamos, NM: Los Alamos Scientific Laboratory.

103. United Nations Scientific Committee on the Effects of Atomic Radiation (UNSCEAR), Sources and effects of ionizing radiation; 2006 Report to the General Assembly with annexes. 2006, New York: United Nations.

104. Field, R.W., et al., Radium-bearing pipe scale deposits: Implications for national waterborne radon sampling methods. Am J Public Health, 1995. 85(4):567–570.

105. Hamilton, I.S., et al., Radiological assessment of petroleum pipe scale from pipe-rattling operations. Health Phys, 2004. 87(4):382–397.

10 Attribution of Radiation Effects and Probability of Causation in a Specific Individual

The purpose of this chapter is to discuss the factors that must be considered in assessing the extent to which radiation can be considered to have contributed as a causative agent in the etiology of a given tumor or other lesion in a previously irradiated individual, and to give some examples of how to approach such cases. Ionizing radiation is capable of causing many different effects in humans through a multitude of different mechanisms. The question as to whether a specific observation in an individual or population is due to radiation is a complex one. Generally, the answer is found through an analysis of both general and specific factors related to the nature of the exposure, surrounding circumstances, and the evolution of the subsequent findings. Even though there is a vast scientific literature that can be used to support attribution, each suspected effect must be examined on its own merits and the conclusions may come with varying degrees of certainty.

The term *causation* has a certainty about it, meaning that an effect was indeed partially or wholly due to a certain agent or event. The term *attribution* has less certainty and means the act in which some person or agency has ascribed the effect (correctly or incorrectly) as being due to an agent or event. Factors used to aid in determination of causation/attribution include the "Bradford Hill criteria," medical certainty as judged by a knowledgeable physician, and statistical certainty. General factors in any analysis of radiation causation must include the magnitude, type, penetration, and effectiveness of the incident radiation. The duration of exposure is important with chronic doses having somewhat less effectiveness than acute doses. The time of exposure in relation to when the "effect" is observed is also critical. The volume of tissue or organ exposed needs to be specified and the possibility of interaction between various tissues in the body also must be considered.

There are a number of uncertainties that need to be considered in the analytical process, which include, but are not limited to, the circumstances of the exposure, determination of the actual exposed population, bias factors and confounding issues, and individual variation. The degree of uncertainty is also significantly related to whether the "effect" has happened or is only postulated to occur at some time in the future. Clearly, attribution of future events to radiation exposure is much more uncertain the further in the future the event is expected to occur.

DETERMINISTIC EFFECTS

Attribution of deterministic effects to a radiation exposure requires at least a minimum or threshold dose level. It also often requires observation of a specific set of clinical or laboratory findings in a specific temporal sequence. Acute radiation sickness (ARS) is a good example. Depending on the dose levels, major manifestations of ARS include signs of hematopoietic depression with concurrent infection and hemorrhage (hematopoietic syndrome). The International Atomic Energy Agency has produced useful summary tables on the methods for early diagnosis of radiation injuries, as well as the acute, latent, and critical phases of acute radiation syndrome (also referred to as ARS, see Chapter 6). Even with such classifications, there are essential difficulties in determining the diagnosis and prognosis as well as the outcome, particularly if the situation involves a very uneven distribution of dose or very high doses specifically to the skin, lung, intestine, or hematopoietic tissue.

The possible diagnosis of ARS was initially entertained for 237 persons involved in the Chernobyl accident. After careful retrospective analysis, the diagnosis of ARS was verified in 134 of these patients. In those patients, there is essentially no doubt that 28 deaths occurring during the first months postexposure and clinical findings in the other 106 patients were directly related to radiation exposure during the accident. Over time, whether the cause of death was radiation related has become less clear. Within 14 years after the accident, 14 additional ARS survivors of grades

I to III died from different causes including tuberculosis. Clarification of their deaths is incomplete, because in some cases an autopsy was not performed.

Follow-up of noncancer mortality studies of Russian liquidators who did not suffer from ARS also were performed and the results indicated an overall reduced mortality ratio from all causes but perhaps a slight increase in cardiovascular mortality of the general Russian population. The studies are complicated by many potential factors, which have been difficult to take into account, including ascertainment of both radiation dose and cause of death, and the role of confounding factors such as smoking. In any individual person who was part of a population study, whether their death was partially or not at all related to radiation will be very difficult to ascertain with much certainty. It is typical that as more time passes, the more confounding factors will be present, and without individual analysis, the less certain can be attributability.

STOCHASTIC (PROBABILISTIC) EFFECTS

Cancer is the stochastic effect of most interest related to radiation exposure. Attributability of a cancer to radiation exposure is even more difficult than attribution of nonstochastic effects. One reason is that there is no radiation specific or pathological signature to distinguish radiation-induced tumors from others. Also, in contrast to deterministic effects, no threshold dose is necessary, rather, the probability of neoplasm may rise with absorbed dose up to relatively high dose levels. There are some factors that can provide help in the analytic process, however. These include knowledge of tumor type, time of onset, age of patient at exposure, and radiation dose. Tumor type is important since attributability may be high in patients who develop tumors in those tissues known to be relatively radiation sensitive (e.g., breast, red marrow). Attributability is likely to be low or absent in those patients in whom tumors occur in some other tissues (e.g., prostate, pancreas). In those tissues in which radiation cancers are known to arise, attributability will be higher with increasing radiation dose. Age at exposure plays an important role, particularly when considering tumors of the thyroid, brain, and breast, with attributability being higher when exposure occurs at a young age.

Evaluation of whether radiation caused a cancer or cancers is different depending on whether it involves an individual who has cancer or predicting whether a population will develop cancer. Many groups have tried to wrestle with the concepts of "probability of causation" (PC) or "assigned share" (AS) and to determine, in numeric terms, the probability that a given cancer was due to radiation exposure. For a child who developed thyroid cancer several years after the Chernobyl accident, radiation causation may be ascribed with some confidence, provided the child was known to be in circumstances that may have resulted in significant thyroid absorbed dose.

This confidence (not certainty) is due to the significant increase in childhood thyroid cancer (well above typical background levels) observed in irradiated children, known sensitivity of childrens' thyroids to radiation, and given that the tumor occurred long enough after the accident for the tumor to become clinically evident. The situation would be entirely different if a thyroid cancer occurring in an adult several months after the accident was being considered. In that circumstance, radiation causation would be extremely unlikely. Retrospective determination of whether cases of cancer were produced in a given population by radiation exposure is entirely different from estimating that radiation caused a specific adverse effect such as cancer in a specific individual. In population studies, any radiation effect (especially from low doses) can be obscured by the large number of nonradiation cancers occurring in the population.

Prediction of future cancers in populations is fraught with additional problems regarding uncertainty. These include assumptions regarding future levels of confounding factors (e.g., smoking), continuation of current levels of medical care and efficacy of treatment, some assumptions regarding average life span in future decades, and so forth. In addition to these, there are varying levels of certainty or uncertainty regarding absorbed dose. The Chernobyl Forum and others have estimated the number of cancers and leukemias that might occur in various Chernobyl-exposed populations. Care was taken to make different estimates based on the radiation exposure level. Estimates can be made with more certainty with higher dose. Estimates for those populations receiving doses in excess of those already shown in epidemiological studies to cause a statistically significant increase in cancer (those living close to Chernobyl) are more certain than those at dose levels in which cancer increases are postulated yet have never been detected by current methods (e.g., for those populations living in Western Europe). Despite this, it should be noted that with current dose estimates for both these populations, together with current UNSCEAR radiation risk estimates, it is unlikely that increases in nonthyroid cancer due to radiation will be detectable. Whether there was a radiation-related increase in nonthyroid cancer in the general populations will likely never be known; however, for cancers occurring in these populations, radiation attributability on an individual basis is likely to be extremely low (or possibly even absent).

SECONDARY EFFECTS

Both deterministic and stochastic effects discussed above have a biological basis related to ionizing radiation causing energy deposition in tissue and subsequent phenomena. There are, in addition, profound effects from some radiation exposure situations that are not related to energy deposition. These might be termed *secondary effects* but they are still related to various aspects of the exposures including but not limited to the fear of ionizing radiation. Thus, they in some respects are "attributable" to radiation exposure. In contrast to deterministic and stochastic effects, these effects are often unrelated to the actual magnitude of radiation exposure or absorbed dose. The 2006 Chernobyl Forum, composed of all eight United Nations agencies (including the World Health Organization [WHO]) as well as the governments of Belarus, Russia, and the Ukraine, concluded that stress symptoms, increased levels of depression, anxiety (including post-traumatic stress symptoms), and medically unexplained physical symptoms, have been found in Chernobyl-exposed populations compared to controls. Studies have also found that exposed populations had anxiety symptom levels that were twice as high and that they were three to four times more likely to report multiple, unexplained physical symptoms and subjective poor health. These mental health consequences in the general population mostly were subclinical and did not reach the level of criteria for a psychiatric disorder. Nevertheless, these subclinical symptoms had important consequences for health behavior, specifically medical care use and adherence to safety advisories. It is clear that a significant portion of postaccident behavior was attributable to the Chernobyl accident, if not indirectly to radiation exposure.

CLAIMS OF RADIATION INJURY

Legal claims related to radiation exposure will undoubtedly continue to rise. In the United States from 1995 to 1999 there were approximately 150,000 monitored workers in the nuclear power industry, about 30,000 in the nuclear fuel cycle, more than 30,000 physicians occupationally exposed to radiation, and 100,000 radiologic and 5000 nuclear medicine technologists. There are also many unmonitored persons who have been exposed to radiation, including uranium miners, and military and public persons ("downwinders") exposed to fallout or other radioactive releases.

In these groups there will be approximately 40% who will develop naturally occurring cancers, and if only a small percentage of them file legal claims, there will be an enormous number of litigants. Obviously, there needs to be a way to determine which claims have merit. The initial interaction with radiation-associated problems often occurs when individuals who feel that they may have been injured or affected seek information and guidance from physicians, biomedical physicists, or health physicists. On the basis of the information they receive, they may contact an attorney or the federal government.

Generally, cases can be divided into the following three groups on the basis of the absorbed radiation dose that is assumed:

1. Assumed absorbed doses of less than 0.05 gray (Gy): In these cases, the putative adverse effects that may be identified are more likely to be spontaneous or to have been caused by some other agent rather than the radiation exposure. Claims in this dose range have little or no scientific or medical merit because the dose levels are below those shown in the epidemiological literature to result in a statistically significant increase in cancer.

2. Estimated dose range of 0.05 to 0.5 Gy: The effects may be of legitimate concern and may have a probability of radiogenic causation that is worth considering in relationship to other causal factors. Thus, these cases require careful analysis of the situation and other contributing factors.

3. Estimated doses greater than 0.5 Gy: Again, the situation demands thoughtful analysis. Frequently, however, because of widespread misunderstanding and fear of radiation by the courts and media, a settlement may be in order. At doses in the range of several Gy, the risk may be high enough for some tumors so that radiation may be interpreted "more likely than not" to have caused the tumors.

These are very general categories but may provide a basis for estimation of the likely legal outcome, as indicated later in this chapter. The doses used for assignment to a category should be calculated according to nationally or internationally accepted methodology.

Legal liability is often difficult to evaluate, because court definitions of "proof" and "truth" differ from those normally applied in scientific investigations. Under tort law, four essential components must be included: (1) the injury must be proved, (2) there must be a duty from one party to another, (3) there must be a violation of that duty, and (4) there must be an injury resulting from the violation. The offense may be intentional or unintentional (negligence). The element of fault is very difficult to prove because of the usually low probabilities of causation that are involved in the stochastic effects of radiation and the delayed expression of stochastic and nonstochastic effects. *Proof*, in tort law, "is the persuasion of the mind of the judge or jury by the exhibition of evidence of the reality of an alleged fact."[1] In other words, proof is getting the judge or jury to believe one's version of the facts. In one early case (*Martinez v. University of California*), even fear of radiation has been held to be compensable.[2] Since that time, however, in at least 13 court cases the judges have held that mere exposure to radiation without physical injury is not actionable.[3-15] Recently, there was an allegation that the energy deposited by radiation can be defined as an "injury" even though there are no demonstrable detrimental effects. The position has been rejected (*Ranier v. Union Carbide Corp.*).[16]

Another major issue that has faced courts, not only in radiation cases but in many other technical areas, is how to choose experts and give opinions to the jury that are scientifically correct. Judges often demand that the expert be able to demonstrate to the court that what he or she wants to tell the jury is verifiable in the scientific literature. The courts are also now looking for better-qualified experts, who have published, done research, and are nationally, and preferably internationally, recognized. Many courts have noted the existence of a small but vocal minority of scientists who have opinions that are quite different from those of the majority of scientists but are nevertheless called and used as expert witnesses in various cases. A number of these courts have issued opinions relative to the credibility of some experts in radiation injury cases.

In the 1993 term, the U.S. Supreme Court ruled on the threshold for acceptance of expert witness testimony into evidence under the federal rules of evidence. In the *Daubert et al. v. Merrell Dow Pharmaceuticals* case, the trial judge found that the expert witness provisions of the federal rules of evidence superseded the Frye rule of "general acceptance" in the scientific community promulgated by the D.C. Court of Appeals.[17] As a threshold matter, expert scientific testimony should be scrutinized by the trial judge, including whether it has been subject to peer review and publication as well as the theories known and potential rate of error. The court also stressed that the focus should be on the principles and methodology of the theory and not only its conclusions. Even if the court and the trial judge find expert testimony to be relevant and reliable, the judge can exclude it if it would confuse or mislead the jury.[18] A general overview of this topic has been published by Ayala and Black.[19]

GENETIC INJURIES

The legal liability for genetic injuries from radiation has received relatively little attention, although it has been addressed in several cases. An example of such an "injury" would be a child with Down syndrome (trisomy 21) born to the wife of a patient involved in an accidental radiation exposure. The case of *Troxell v. Bendix Corporation*, one of the few genetic cases reaching trial, involved a 32-year-old woman who alleged permanent genetic damage of her offspring resulting from periodic occupational exposure over a period of 25 months.[20] In such cases, it is important to examine the role of radiation, as well as other mutagens to which the parents of the affected offspring may have been exposed. In addition, the normal incidence of spontaneous mutations, chromosome aberrations, malformations, and other genetic diseases (discussed in Chapter 3) must be considered. The liability for genetic injuries from radiation has been reviewed by Estep and Forgotson.[21] One of the difficulties in the legal management of genetic radiation injuries has been determining whether the affected child, at the time of injury (i.e., prior to its birth), had a legal status that the law will protect. In many circumstances, courts have denied compensation for genetic injury because they reasoned that the unborn child had no existence separate from its mother or that there was difficulty in proving a causal connection between the noxious agent and alleged effect. In the 1991 case of *Coley v. Commonwealth Edison Co.*, a summary judgment was granted against plaintiff children with genetic defects whose fathers received radiation exposure below federal standards.[9]

LIABILITY FOR RADIATION EXPOSURE OF THE EMBRYO AND FETUS

Most claims of legal liability from irradiation of the embryo or fetus arise from diagnostic medical x-ray examinations; less commonly, nuclear medicine, therapeutic irradiation, and accidental exposure also may result in lawsuits. The number of in utero exposure legal cases is substantial and probably is exceeded only by cases involving carcinogenesis. Major reasons for the large number of lawsuits are the high level of spontaneous abnormalities in pregnancy and the high emotional level involved in such instances. Radiation often is the scapegoat for spontaneously occurring abnormalities. In cases in which inadvertent exposure occurs during pregnancy or when purposeful exposure is contemplated, the patient should be counseled about risks and hazards, and such counseling should be documented in writing. An analysis of the physician's role and liability for radiation exposure of the fetus has been written by Perdue.[22] Prior to 1946, under common law, the unborn child was not considered a "person," and an individual who caused harm to the unborn child was not held liable. Of interest in this regard are two cases in which physicians mistakenly diagnosed a pregnancy as a tumor and administered radiation therapy. In both, even though the children were born mentally retarded and severely crippled, the cases were denied (*Smith v. Ruckhardt, Stemmer v. Kline*).[23,24] In 1946, the case of *Bonbrest v. Kotz* was a departure from previous precedent, and recovery for a prenatal injury was allowed.[25]

Under common law, the present interpretation is that the physician has a duty not only to the pregnant patient but also to the unborn child. A child can maintain a tort action for prenatal injuries if negligence can be shown; or, if the child dies, an action can be taken for wrongful death. The *Bonbrest* decision expressed the view that the child should be entitled to recovery for injuries only if the child was indeed viable and capable of sustaining life independent of its mother at the time of injury. The concept of "viability" left open the question of whether an action could be brought for a child before the stage of viability. One of the major difficulties in dealing with such cases at the embryonic and early fetal stages has been the high incidence of spontaneous abortion and chromosomal abnormalities in products of conception. This has compounded the difficulty of demonstrating causation due to radiation. In 1971, the finding in the case of *Delgado v.*

Yandell stated that a cause of action exists for prenatal injury at any stage of pregnancy, but it added that the child must be born alive.[26] This case neatly circumvented the difficult distinction of whether a fetus was viable at the time of injury. To date, most courts have maintained that a stillborn child is not a "person in being"; thus, an action cannot be maintained for wrongful death as the result of an injury (*Hogan v. McDaniel, Drabbels v. Skelly Oil Co., Prates v. Sears, Roebuck & Co.*).[27–29]

With respect to negligent x-ray use, only one case has dealt specifically with injury to the fetus by irradiation. In *Salinetro v. Nystron*, the plaintiff was required to have lumbar spine and abdominal x-rays prior to insurance recovery for an accident.[30] At that time, she was approximately one month pregnant, and the physician did not inquire whether she was pregnant or ask for the date of her last menstrual cycle. On the advice of an obstetrician, a therapeutic abortion was performed because of "possible damage" to the fetus from the x-ray exposure. The fetus was found to be dead at the time of abortion. The legal action failed on the issue of causation because the court concluded that the physician's failure to question the plaintiff about her pregnancy was not the cause for injury: because she did not know she was pregnant, she would have replied in the negative if asked. The *Salinetro* decision appears not to solve all the problems that one is likely to encounter. At present, the burden of determining whether a patient is pregnant before administering irradiation falls on the physician, technologist, or hospital—not the patient. Very few cases involving in utero exposure to radiation have actually reached the appellate level; therefore, one has to rely on the implications of cases of prenatal injury involving other noxious agents. Most of these cases hold that the physician has a duty to live up to the expected standard of medical expertise rather than relying on the oblique reasoning that was used in the *Salinetro* case. It also is obvious from the usual physician negligence liability cases that informed consent is a critical issue and that it is quite likely to be raised in conjunction with any x-ray that may be perceived as resulting in damage.

In a more recent case (*Craft v. Vanderbilt University*), pregnant women were given radioactive iron isotopes as part of an experiment between 1947 and 1956. They were not informed of the risks or when a later follow-up study indicated higher cancer risks in children. The court indicated that the statute of limitations did not apply, that this was not "medical care," and that the physician had an affirmative duty to disclose information.[31]

RADIATION THERAPY AND ACCIDENTS

Most legal controversy concerning entities such as cataracts, radiation myelitis, and tissue necrosis arises from radiation therapy exposures. Often, the litigation focuses on whether there was proper informed consent or whether the dose that was administered was either excessive or delivered in too short a time. The causal relationship of radiation to the abnormalities is usually relatively well defined by the existing literature. Radiation therapy experience has been extensive enough that tolerance doses and the expected incidence of complications are reasonably well known. Prevention of such lawsuits should involve meticulous documentation of machine calibration, informed consent, and the daily records of radiation treatment regimens and dose schedules. Careful clinical examination during the course of treatment often will identify individuals who might otherwise be unusually susceptible to radiation (such as those patients with ataxia telangiectasia). The situation is markedly different in the case of accidental or occupational radiation exposure. In such instances, the exact dose delivered to the organ or site of interest is very difficult to calculate without personnel dosimetry (such as a film badge) or a reconstruction of the events. Even with such reconstructions, dose estimates may be in error by 50% or more, and, thus, one may need to rely on an expert clinical examination of the patient, using the patient response as a biologic dosimeter. Of course, there is some individual variation, but the patient examination often is as useful as, or more useful than, accident reconstruction. The quality of radiation, as well as the dose and time over which it was given, is extremely important. In cases involving internal contamination with radionuclides, bioassay and whole-body counting are very useful for appropriate dose estimates. In cases of accidental external, partial, or whole-body exposure, cytogenetic dosimetry of peripheral lymphocytes can be used, although, as pointed out in Chapter 3, this is only valuable in cases in which the absorbed dose exceeds 0.1 to 0.3 Gy. Cytogenetic analysis may be used as a negative indicator, that is, to demonstrate that the whole-body dose did not exceed a certain level. Once dose estimates are made by both physical measurements and biologic observations, they can be compared with the adverse effect or lesion identified by the patient. Particular attention should be directed toward the possibility of modifying factors, such as individual genetic abnormalities, smoking, alcohol use, and medications (particularly chemotherapy).

RADIATION CARCINOGENESIS

A large number of legal cases have involved the supposition that radiation has induced a particular cancer in a given individual. These cases are quite common, because approximately 40% of the U.S. population will develop cancer, and a large percentage of the population has been exposed to radiation through occupation, accident, or medical treatment. The major difficulty in handling such cases stems from the public perception that a great number of cases of cancer are due to radiation exposure, at the same time overlooking the causes of cancer that are actually much more common. Another problem is that it is impossible to tell whether a cancer was caused by radiation, much less from a particular exposure. Many groups have tried to wrestle with the concepts of PC or AS and to determine, in numeric terms, the probability that a given cancer was due to radiation exposure. The probability of causation is defined as the probability that a specific disease in a person was caused by their exposure to a particular hazardous agent. PC differs from risk in that it is conditional on the occurrence of a disease. The method of estimating PC or AS (PC/AS) is presented later in this chapter.

PC as a term is best used prospectively for cancer risk in a population, and some authors reserve the term *AS* for calculations involving an individual who has developed cancer. In practice, however, both terms are commonly applied to individuals. PC and AS are numerically the same and either can be expressed as a fraction or a percentage, as subsequently noted. As pointed out in Chapter 4, the epidemiologic data concerning radiation carcinogenesis are derived from populations, which in many circumstances are not at all similar to any particular individual who has a specific tumor. One, therefore, must analyze an individual with cancer by determining the following: (1) the relative contributions of the various causes of cancer in the relevant population, (2) the best possible risk estimates for radiation induction of a particular tumor, (3) the probability of the individual's death from or incurring a given tumor under normal circumstances, (4) the actual risk factors incurred by that specific individual, and (5) the temporal events and modifying factors involved. Determining the relative importance of different causes of cancer in a population is difficult. The causes of cancer in the environment have been discussed by Doll and Peto,[32,33] Ames,[34–36] the International Agency for Research on Cancer,[37] and publications by Higginson et al.[38–42] It is thought that 80% to 90% of all cancer deaths in the United States are environmental in origin. These articles point out that the factors to be considered in carcinogenesis in a given individual include as a minimum the following variables: geographic variations of tumor incidence, genetic makeup, individual migration, diet, blood type, age, occupational exposures, chemical exposures including medication, reproductive and sexual behavior, geophysical factors, and infections (particularly viruses). There are, of course, additional unknown causes. Doll and Peto summarize the causes of cancer into three categories: nature, nurture, and luck.[32,33,43] The combination of these factors varies so much worldwide that cancer risks derived from a single population may be of limited value when applied to an individual from a different setting. It is clear that the cancer incidence among people of a given age in different parts of the world often varies by a factor of 10, and possibly as much as 100. The range of geographical variation of tumors is never less than sixfold and is often significantly higher. As an example of

variation in incidence of a common tumor, cancer of the breast affects 6% of U.S. women before the age of 75 and only 1% of non-Jewish Israeli women. Doll and Peto point out that "every type of cancer that is common in one district is rare somewhere else."[33]

"Nature" is essentially the person's genetic makeup, a factor that clearly affects the risk of cancer. A known genetic risk factor is blood type. Those persons having blood type A have a risk of stomach cancer that is 20% greater than that of persons with blood type O. In addition, there are well-known genetic predispositions for some persons to develop cancers such as Wilms' tumor, retinoblastoma, colon cancer, and neuroblastoma. Other factors that can be identified affect the cancer rate, although whether they are related by association or causation is uncertain (e.g., genetic and religious differences). The Mormons of Utah, as well as the Mormons of California, experience very low incidence rates for cancers of the respiratory, gastrointestinal, and genital systems. People of Chinese and Japanese descent have a notable lack of certain lymphoproliferative neoplasms. In spite of such examples, genetic factors in the causation of cancer appear to be largely superseded by environmental factors. The relative importance of environmental over genetic factors can be identified by analysis of cancer incidence rates in populations that have migrated. Black Americans have cancer incidence rates that are much more like those of white Americans than of black populations in West Africa. Similarly, Japanese and white residents of Hawaii have quite similar cancer incidence rates, which are substantially different from the cancer incidence rates in Japan. Other examples also occur (e.g., Indians who went to Fiji or South Africa lost their high risk of developing oral cancer, and Britons who went to Fiji acquired a high risk of skin cancer). Even though environmental factors may be more important than genetic, there are clearly gene-environment interactions. For example, persons with *BRCA*1 or *BRCA*2 genes, or alternations of the p53 tumor suppressor gene, may be affected more by environmental carcinogens.

Another confounding factor in analyzing causative factors is that various anatomic parts of certain organs, such as the colon or skin, may have different risk rates and may, in fact, be affected differently by various noxious agents. As an example, skin cancers have different major causes, depending on whether they occur on the face, abdomen, or other body parts. In addition, biochemical and physiologic considerations also play a substantial role in cancers, particularly skin cancer; for example, blacks have a much lower risk of skin cancer than whites. "Luck" in terms of carcinogenesis is also difficult to deal with. Probabilistic analysis can estimate the overall number of people who might experience a given problem (such as an accident). Unfortunately, there is no way of telling which of those in the population will actually have the accident, and this is matter of luck. The effects under discussion in the present text for legal purposes usually will not include an analysis of this factor because we are dealing with people who already have had the "bad luck" to experience the cancer or other unwanted problem. "Nurture" includes what people do or have had done to themselves from the time of conception to the time of interest; this is the most important category to be analyzed in a person who has developed cancer. Established human carcinogenic agents and circumstances are shown in Tables 10-1 to 10-3. These indicate the best-known occupational, medical, and social agents or circumstances leading to cancer of a given site in humans. Danaei et al. have pointed out that of the 7 million cancer deaths worldwide in 2001 it was estimated that 35% were attributable to nine potentially modifiable factors. In high-income countries, smoking, alcohol use, and being overweight or obese were the most important causes of cancer (Tables 10-4 and 10-5).[44]

With the great variation in cancer incidence among various human populations, it is quite apparent that use of animal data for carcinogenic risk estimates in humans can be performed only by taking a great leap into the realm of uncertainty. Ames points out that carcinogens differ in their potency in rodents by more than a factor of a millionfold and that the levels of particular carcinogens to which humans are exposed can vary in carcinogenicity by more than a billionfold.[35]

Tobacco Smoke

Tobacco smoke is perhaps the best-known carcinogen to which humans expose themselves or are exposed. It is well known that the incidence of lung cancer is more than 10 times greater in regular cigarette smokers than in nonsmokers. In addition, there is accumulating evidence that cigarette smokers have approximately double the

---

Table 10-1 • Established Human Carcinogenic Agents and Circumstances (Occupational)

Agent or Circumstance	Latent Period (yr)	Site of Cancer	Relative Risk
Aromatic amines			
4-Aminodiphenyl	—	Bladder	—
2-naphthylamine		Bladder	
Arsenic	15–35	Skin, lung, bladder	2.3–8.0
Asbestos	15–50	Lung, pleura, peritoneum	1.5–12
Auramine	19	Bladder	4.6
Benzidine	16	Bladder	14
2-Naphthylamine	8.4	Bladder	8
Benzene	6–14	Marrow	2.5
Beryllium	10–15	Lung	1.3–2.0
Bis (chloromethyl) ether	10–15	Lung	100
Cadmium	—	Lung	—
Chromium	10–30	Lung, nasal sinuses	4–20
Dioxin (TCDD)			
Furniture manufacture (hardwood, wood dust)	27–49	Nasal sinuses	500
Ionizing radiations	—	Marrow and many other sites	—
Iron oxides	10+	Respiratory tract	—
Isopropyl alcohol manufacture	—	Nasal sinuses	
Leather goods manufacture	—	Nasal sinuses	
Mustard gas	10–25	Larynx, lung	37
Nickel and compounds	5–40	Nasal sinuses, lung	100–800
Pesticides	—	Blood and lymphatic, brain, skin	5–10
Polycyclic hydrocarbons	—	Skin, scrotum, lung, urinary bladder	—
Tetrachloroethylene (PCE)			
Trichloroethylene (TCE)		Bladder, liver, biliary	—
UV light	5–50	Skin, lip	2.5
Vinyl chloride	12–29	Lung, liver, and brain (angiocarcoma)	1.6

Adapted from Doll R, Peto R: The causes of cancer: Quantitative estimates of avoidable risks of cancer in the United States today. J Natl Cancer Inst 1981; 66:1191–1308; Schottenfeld D, Haas JF: Carcinogens in the workplace. Cancer 1979;29:144–168.

Table 10-2 • Established Human Carcinogenic Agents and Circumstances (Medical Exposure)

Agent or Circumstance	Site of Cancer
Alkylating agents	
Cyclophosphamide	Bladder
Melphalan	Marrow
Arsenic	Skin, lung
Azathioprine	Lymphoma
Busulphan	Marrow
Chlornaphazine	Bladder
Cyclosporin	Lymphoma
Immunosuppressive drugs	Reticuloendothelial system
Ionizing radiations	Marrow and many other sites
Estrogens	
Unopposed	Endometrium
Transplacental (diethylstilbestrol)	Vagina
Phenacetin	Kidney (pelvis)
Polycyclic hydrocarbons	Skin, scrotum, lung
Steroids	
Anabolic (oxymetholone)	Liver
Contraceptives	Liver (hamartoma)

Adapted from Doll R, Peto R: The causes of cancer: Quantitative estimates of avoidable risks of cancer in the United States today. J Natl Cancer Inst 1981;66:1191–1308.

Table 10-3 • Established Human Carcinogenic Agents and Circumstances (Social Circumstances)

Agent or Circumstance	Site of Cancer
Aflatoxin	Liver
Alcoholic drinks	Mouth, pharynx, larynx, esophagus, liver, breast
Chewing (betel, tobacco, lime)	Mouth
Overnutrition (causing obesity)	Endometrium, colon, kidney, esophagus, gallbladder, breast cancer in older women
Reproductive history	
Late age at first pregnancy	Breast
Zero or low parity	Ovary
Parasites	
Schistosoma haematobium	Bladder
Clonorchis sinensis	Liver (cholangioma)
Sexual promiscuity	Cervix (uteri)
Tobacco smoking	Mouth, pharynx, larynx, lung, pancreas, esophagus, bladder
UV light	Skin, lip
Virus (hepatitis B)	Liver (hepatoma)

Adapted from Doll R, Peto R: The causes of cancer: Quantitative estimates of avoidable risks of cancer in the United States today. J Natl Cancer Inst 1981;66:1191–1308.

incidence of bladder and pancreatic cancer, as well as a moderate increase in renal carcinoma.[37,42] This may be the result of the mutagenic chemicals that are absorbed into the bloodstream, circulate throughout the body, and probably are excreted in the urine. Several excellent

Table 10-4 • Proportions of Cancer Deaths Attributed to Various Different Factors

Factor or Class of Factors	PERCENTAGE OF ALL CANCER DEATHS	
	Best Estimate	Range of Acceptable Estimates
Tobacco	30	25–40
Alcohol	3	2–4
Diet	35	10–70
Food additives	<1	−5*–2
Reproductive and sexual behavior	7	1–13
Occupation	4	2–8
Pollution	2	<1–5
Industrial products	<1	<1–2
Medicines and medical procedures	1	0.5–3
Geophysical factors	3	2–4
Infection	10?	1–?
Unknown	?	?

*Allowing for possibly protective effects of antioxidants and other preservatives.
Adapted from Doll R, Peto R: The causes of cancer: Quantitative estimates of avoidable risks of cancer in the United States today. J Natl Cancer Inst 1981;666:1192–1308.

Table 10-5 • Population Attributable Fraction (PAF) for Individual and Joint Risk Factors in High-Income Countries

Cancer	PAF for Individual Factors (%)	PAF Due to Joint Hazards of Risk Factors (%)
Mouth/ Oropharynx	Alcohol (33), smoking (71)	80
Esophagus	Alcohol (41), smoking (71), low fruit and vegetable intake (12)	85
Stomach	Smoking (25), low fruit and vegetable intake (12)	34
Colon/Rectum	Overweight and obesity (14), physical inactivity (14), low fruit and vegetable intake (1)	15
Liver	Smoking (29), alcohol (32), contaminated injections in health care settings (3)	52
Pancreas	Smoking (30)	30
Trachea, bronchus, lung	Smoking (86), low fruit and vegetable intake (8), urban air pollution (3)	87
Breast	Alcohol (9), overweight and obesity (13), physical inactivity (9)	27
Cervix	Smoking (11), unsafe sex (100)	100
Endometrial	Overweight and obesity (43)	43
Bladder	Smoking (41)	41
Leukemia	Smoking (17)	17
Selected other cancers	Alcohol (8)	8
Total		37

Adapted from Danaei G, Vander Hoorn S, Lopez AD, et al: Causes of cancer in the world: Comparative risk assessment of nine behavioral and environmental risk factors. Lancet 2005;366:1784–1793.

reviews of the epidemiology of tobacco smoke in carcinogenesis have been published.[45–49] Doll and Peto have reviewed this literature and concluded in 1980 that in the United States, without tobacco smoking, there would be approximately 12,000 lung cancer deaths annually and that smoking contributed an additional 80,000 to 85,000 lung cancer cases annually.[33] Overall, they indicated that about one third of all U.S. cancer deaths may be attributed to tobacco smoke. Later data from the U.S. Centers for Disease Control indicate that in the period 1995–1999 cigarette smoking annually caused about 125,000 lung cancer deaths, 31,000 other cancer deaths, 17,500 stroke deaths, 82,000 ischemic heart disease deaths, 82,000 deaths from chronic lung disease, and

Table 10-6 • Relative Risks for Esophageal Cancer According to Daily Amounts of Alcohol and Tobacco Consumed

Alcohol Consumption (g/day)	TOBACCO CONSUMPTION (g/day)			
	0–9	10–19	20–29	30
0–40	1.0	3.4	3.2	3.0
41–80	7.3	8.4	8.8	35.0
81–120	11.8	13.6	12.6	83.0
>121	49.6	65.9	137.6	155.6

Adapted from International Agency for Research on Cancer (IARC): IARC monographs on the evaluation of the carcinogenic risk of chemicals to humans: Tobacco smoking, vol 38. Lyon, France, IARC, 1986.

38,000 from secondhand smoke. The attributable risk for cancer of the lung and bronchus from smoking is about 85%. In Western countries 40% to 50% of bladder cancer and about 30% of pancreatic cancer is attributed to smoking. One point of interest is that in the Japanese atomic bomb survivors who smoked, the effect of radiation relative to induction of lung cancer was difficult or impossible to demonstrate, probably because smoking is a much more potent carcinogen.[50]

Alcohol

Alcohol is not known to be a carcinogen, although it does appear to interact with other substances, particularly tobacco. Cancers of the mouth, pharynx, larynx, esophagus, and liver are all known to be increased in men who consume large amounts of alcohol. The relative risks (RRs) of developing cancer of the esophagus with various levels of smoking and drinking are shown in Table 10-6. The relationship in risk is clearly not one of additivity, because alcohol on its own has no carcinogenic effects. Alcohol may be a "carcinogenic sensitizer" for cancers of the mouth, pharynx, larynx, and esophagus. The risk of developing cancer of the esophagus is approximately 150-fold greater in a heavy smoker and drinker than in a nondrinking, nonsmoking individual. There also appears to be a link between alcohol use and breast cancer.

Diet

Diet is a major factor in causation of cancer. Most estimates suggest that dietary habits account for 30% to 40% of all cancers. Several reviews of this area have been published.[34–36,51–53] The carcinogenic effect of dietary components has many factors. Plants themselves contain and are able to synthesize toxic chemicals in large amounts. Ames indicates that the plant materials that humans have available to eat are only those that have not been attacked by bacteria, fungi, insects, and other animals, often because they contain defensive toxins.[40]

To date, the only proven naturally occurring carcinogenic plant that has been shown to affect humans is the bracken fern. Japanese who eat this fern have an increased risk of esophageal carcinoma. Aflatoxin is a product of the fungus *Aspergillus flavus*, which is commonly found in contaminated peanuts and carbohydrate foods. It is one of the most powerful hepatic carcinogens known in animals (and probably humans). Fortunately, in the United States the amount of aflatoxin consumed in the diet is very small. Cooking food may produce a large number of carcinogens not originally present in food. When meat or fish is broiled or smoked, or when any food is fried repeatedly in the same fat, benzo[a]pyrene and other polycyclic hydrocarbons are produced by pyrolysis. Additional mutagens are produced by charcoal broiling. In addition to pyrolysis, the browning action of cooking on food products causes caramelization of sugars, and the brown material on bread crust and toasted bread contains a large variety of DNA-damaging agents and presumptive carcinogens. Coffee contains a considerable amount of burned material, including the mutagens methylglyoxal and caffeic acid. Caffeine is well known to inhibit DNA repair, and it can increase tumor yield and even cause birth defects in some animal species. Some authors suggest that heavy coffee drinking is associated with cancers of the ovary, bladder, pancreas, and colon.[54–58]

The amount of fat in the diet has been associated with breast cancer. Animal studies suggest that a high amount of dietary fat is a promotor and a presumptive carcinogen.[53,59,60] Fat, particularly oxidized fat, accounts for over 40% of the calories in the U.S. diet. Unsaturated fatty acids and cholesterol may be oxidized during cooking, thus exposing the digestive tract to a variety of fat-derived carcinogens. Cholesterol epoxide is an oxidative product of cholesterol present in very high levels in human breast fluid, possibly accounting for the relationship of dietary fat with breast cancer. Quantity of meat consumption is also known to be related to an increase in the incidence of colon cancer.

Another possible mechanism for dietary induction of cancer involves those compounds that become carcinogens once they are ingested. The area that has received the most attention is the formation of *N*-nitroso compounds in the body. Nitrosable compounds occur in many fluids, particularly fish and meat, and may even be formed in the colon from amino acids. Nitrites are often ingested in vegetables as a food preservative, and they may be formed in the body by bacterial action. Increased intake of dietary fiber appears to decrease the risk of colon or rectal cancer. Whether this occurs through decrease in the length of time that the stool remains in contact with the bowel or decrease in the concentration of carcinogens (by increasing bulk) is unknown.

Being overweight is associated with higher than normal incidence of cancer. This has been confirmed by

Table 10-7 • Mortality Ratios from Various Types of Cancer, by Body Weight Index

Type of Cancer	Patient's Sex	BODY WEIGHT INDEX		
		Thin	Average	Large
Endometrium	F	0.89	1.00	5.42
Gallbladder and biliary	F	0.68	1.00	3.58
Cervix	F	0.76	1.00	2.39
Kidney	F	1.12	1.00	2.03
Stomach	M	1.34	1.00	1.88
	F	0.74	1.00	1.03
Colon, rectum	M	0.90	1.00	1.73
	F	0.93	1.00	1.22
Lymphoma	F	0.83	1.00	1.13
Brain	F	0.86	1.00	1.01
Leukemia	F	0.73	1.00	1.24
Breast	F	0.82	1.00	1.53
Prostate	M	1.02	1.00	1.29
Lung	M	1.78	1.00	1.27
	F	1.49	1.00	1.22
Ovary	F	0.86	1.00	1.63
Pancreas	M	1.20	1.00	1.62
	F	1.17	1.00	0.61
All cancers	F	0.96	1.00	1.55
	M	1.33	1.00	1.33

Adapted from Doll R, Peto R: The causes of cancer: Quantitative estimates of avoidable risks of cancer in the United States today. J Natl Cancer Inst 1981;66:1191–1308.

the American Cancer Society study in which 750,000 U.S. men and women were followed for 13 years.[61] Table 10-7 is based on data from this study that indicates a consistent trend toward increasing total risk from cancer with increasing body weight among women. The trend in men is somewhat irregular because thin men and women have the greatest lung cancer risks. One of the clearest relationships between weight and cancer risk is that for endometrial carcinoma. This risk may be related to the level of estrogen in the blood, which may be a major factor in development of endometrial carcinoma, as well as deposition of fat. The strongest links between obesity and cancer are for breast cancer in older women, and cancers of the endometrium, kidney, colon, and esophagus.[62]

As one might suspect, there may also be compounds within the diet that are anticarcinogens, including vitamin E (tocopherol), beta carotene (present in carrots and green vegetables), selenium, glutathione, and ascorbic acid. At what level the optimal effect of the anticarcinogen is achieved is unknown; however, high levels (particularly of selenium) can be extremely toxic and hazardous. Although the contribution of diet to U.S. cancer death rates is uncertain, Doll and Peto indicate that many tumor types can be reduced by dietary means.[33] These issues are important because for a patient with carcinoma of the stomach or colon and a history of radiation exposure,

one would have to examine the dietary history carefully before assigning a probability of causation to the radiation since dietary habits are clearly extremely influential.

Reproductive and Sexual Behavior

The exact reason that patterns of sexual intercourse, childbirth, lactation, and pregnancy cause differences in cancer incidence rates is unknown, although associations have been well defined. The most certain relationship is that between sexual intercourse and cancer of the uterine cervix. Although carcinoma of the cervix is common in women who have had several children, the risk of developing the disease predominantly appears to be related to the number of sexual partners. Cancer of the breast, ovary, and endometrium are less common in women who have had children early in life than those who have had no children. There is good evidence that the risk of breast cancer is less likely as the age at first pregnancy decreases.[63,64]

Current research suggests that for a woman living in North America, the lifetime odds of getting breast cancer are 1 in 8. This is double the risk in 1940. What is responsible for the rise in breast cancer over the last 50 years has remained largely a mystery. It is clear, however, that a number of what are probably hormonal factors as well as genetic factors influence the risk. Known risk factors for breast cancer include old age, upper socioeconomic class, obesity, family history of premenopausal bilateral breast cancer, history of cancer in one breast, fibrocystic disease, primary cancer of the ovary or endometrium, and probably two naturally occurring hormones, estrogen and progesterone.[65,66]

Occupation

It is very difficult to ascertain the proportion of cancer that is attributable to occupational exposure to carcinogens. An early report of occupational carcinogens was that of an increased incidence of scrotal cancer in chimney sweeps. One of the great difficulties in ascertaining the risk of occupational carcinogen hazards is the poor statistical significance of most data. The added risk is usually small compared to other causes, and, in many instances, only a small population group has been exposed. The only occupational hazards that have been easily identified are those that have caused a substantial increase in what is otherwise a rare tumor. Other problems with most occupational studies are that exposure histories are very difficult to obtain and that many chemicals are newly produced and used in occupational situations each year, while others are abandoned. In spite of these difficulties, many authors have attempted to quantify the percentage of cancer cases due to occupational hazards; in general, these suggest figures of less than 5%.[38,42,67] A paper, often referred to as the "OSHA" paper, reached the conclusion that the occurrence of as many as 23% to 28% of cancers may be influenced by occupational causes. Doll and Peto point out, however, that "these estimates of total risk were so grossly in error that no arguments based even loosely on them should be taken seriously" and that the paper appears to have been for political rather than scientific purposes.[33] Of the factors listed in the table is asbestos, which may account for 5% of all present-day lung cancers. Another 5% of lung cancers in males may be due to combustion products of fossil fuels.[39] Doll and Peto estimate that approximately 17,000 of the 400,000 annual cancer deaths (or about 4%) are due to occupational causes. Using a lifetime risk of fatal cancer from radiation of 250 deaths in 1 million people per 10 mSv, Doll and Peto estimated that of the 17,000 occupationally caused cancer deaths, 58 deaths result from exposure to ionizing radiation.[33]

Air Pollution and Environmental Contaminants

Air pollution contains polycyclic hydrocarbons, arsenic, asbestos, radioactive elements, and tobacco smoke. Most of these compounds have been considered carcinogenic in various studies. Overall, the effects of air pollution alone may not be particularly important because the mortality among nonsmokers is extremely low, irrespective of the area in which they live.[68] Doll and Peto estimated that all pollution, including that of air, water, and food, is responsible for approximately 2% of all cancer cases.[32,33] Persons with high exposures to pesticides have higher rates of blood and lymphatic system cancers, cancers of the lip, stomach, lung, brain, and prostate, melanoma, and other skin cancers.[69]

Consumer Products

Included among consumer products are industrial products, as well as medicines and medical procedures. Many industrial products are of recent introduction, and their carcinogenic potential is largely unknown. Certainly, many solvents, metals (arsenic, beryllium, cadmium, chromium), plastics, paints, dyes, and polishes may be carcinogenic. As with other sources, however, the overall impact presently appears to be relatively small compared with that from other causes. Doll and Peto suggest that a nominal value of "less than 1%" of all current cancer deaths are due to industrial products. Many medications have been shown to cause cancer in humans, including azathioprine, cyclophosphamide, cyclosporine, chlorambucil, melphalan, arsenic, busulphan, chlornaphazine, immunosuppressive drugs, estrogens, progesterone, phenacetin, polycyclic hydrocarbons, oxymetholone, and steroid contraceptives. Some of these medications are discussed in Chapter 7, and, of course, many such medications are used to treat cancer.[70] Antineoplastic drugs are a particularly important issue because many legal cases may arise in which the patient has been successfully treated by radiation therapy or chemotherapy for a tumor and subsequently returns with a second malignancy. In such instances, one would need to examine the medication involved, the radiation therapy, and the "natural incidence" of second neoplasms in this population group. Estrogens have been used widely; however, there is good evidence that suggests that they increase the incidence of endometrial carcinoma.[71] Some estimates hold that estrogen may be responsible for one half of the cases of endometrial carcinoma. The role of estrogens in production of breast cancer is uncertain.[65] The effect of steroid oral contraceptives is largely unknown, although large studies are underway to analyze their effects. Ionizing radiation used in medical procedures was estimated by Doll and Peto to cause approximately 0.5% of all cancers and 4500 fatal cancers annually.[33] They do, however, indicate that this may be an overestimate, because much of the medical radiation is received by people with life expectancies lower than the latent period for carcinogenesis. This figure makes no allowance for the abnormal age distribution of the exposed population, and it does not account for potential benefit from diagnosis and treatment. With the markedly increased use of CT scanning in the last two decades, the likely estimate is probably about 10-fold higher.

Geophysical Factors

Geophysical factors usually include natural background radiation and ultraviolet (UV) light. Most of the tumors due to UV (sunlight) are basal cell carcinomas or squamous cell carcinomas of the skin. The survival rate of such patients is very high, approaching 100%. As discussed in Chapter 3, there is a subgroup of individuals with faulty DNA repair mechanisms (such as xeroderma pigmentosum), who have an extremely high incidence of UV-induced skin carcinomas. The number of deaths caused by sunlight and UV light is difficult to ascertain because melanomas, which are rare but almost 100% lethal, are often grouped in the general larger category of skin cancers. It is estimated that approximately 50% of all melanomas may be due to UV light. Additionally, 90% of lip cancers and 80% of other skin cancers, accounting for 1% to 2% of all cancer deaths, may be attributable to sunlight. Natural background radiation is a large contributor of ionizing radiation to the U.S. population (on the order of 200,000 person Sv annually). Using conservative estimates, this would imply production of 5500 cancer deaths annually, or 1.4% of the total. This estimate may be low if exposure to radon and radon daughter products is considered. This latter exposure may account for up to 40% of lung cancers in nonsmokers.

Infection

The role of infection in carcinogenesis appears to be primarily related to viruses. Viruses are known to become integrated into genetic material and to be able to modify the behavior of cells. In high-risk populations 50% to 90% of hepatocellular carcinomas are thought to be the result of hepatitis B virus. The Epstein-Barr virus may cause Burkitt's lymphoma; in epithelial cells of the nasopharynx it causes nasopharyngeal carcinoma. Viruses have also been implicated in cancers of the cervix and penis, acute lymphatic leukemia of childhood, and reticulosarcomas. Infection with parasites or bacteria may affect the rate of converting nitrates into nitrites in the bowel and formation of *N*-nitroso compounds. The sexually transmitted human papilloma virus (HPV) is the primary cause of both cervical and anal cancer. Bacterial infection associated with smoking also may be responsible for decreased pulmonary clearing and longer bronchial epithelial contact with carcinogens. Parasitic infections and their association with neoplasms appear to be of importance only in countries other than the United States. Overall, Doll and Peto give as their best estimate that 10% of all cancer deaths may somehow be attributable to infection.[33] There are possibly other environmental factors that have been overlooked. As an example, prostatic carcinoma accounts for 10% of all cancer deaths in men, although the epidemiologic causes generally remain unknown.

PROBABILITY OF CAUSATION AND ASSIGNED SHARE

Over 95% of cancer is due to causes other than radiation, and these causes cannot be ignored when assigning a probability that a given tumor was induced by radiation.

Many groups have attempted to derive tables assigning the probability of carcinogenesis following a given radiation exposure. Unfortunately, such tables cannot be individualized, owing to the many variables that are involved, and may lead to serious errors in individual cases, particularly if individual age and smoking habits are not considered. Predicting the number of cases of cancer that may be produced in a given population by radiation exposure is entirely different from estimating that radiation caused a specific adverse effect such as cancer in a specific individual.[72]

The probability that a particular cancer may have been caused by a specified irradiation has been dealt with in a statement by the National Council on Radiation Protection and Measurements (NCRP) in 1992.[73] In that statement the NCRP indicates that "... it is impossible to defend, on medical grounds, any statement that a specific cancer was caused by a particular radiation exposure." They indicate that the PC approach should be tailored insofar as possible to a particular individual of a specific age, sex, cancer type, dose, and demographic data. In simplistic terms, the underlying question is whether radiation was responsible for an observed health effect. Either the relative or absolute risk models can be used. Essentially, all the risk before the time of clinical presentation (*Y*) is

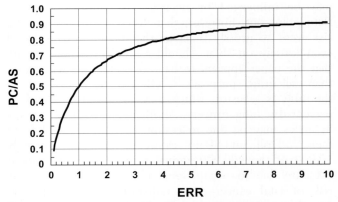

Figure 10-1 • PC/AS as a function of ERR. If the risk from a dose of radiation is 10 times the baseline risk, the PC/AS is 0.91 (i.e., 10/10 + 1). (From National Research Council: Assessment of the scientific information for the radiation exposure screening and education program. Washington, DC, National Academy Press, 2006.)

neglected because the individual has successfully passed those risks. Only the individual excess risk and normal incidence for the year of presentation should be considered. Similarly, the risk in the remaining life span is also neglected. Mathematically, the probability of radiogenic tumor induction (PC or AS) is related to the excess relative risk (ERR) (Fig. 10-1) and may be expressed by the following formula:

$$P_r = \frac{ERR}{I + ERR}$$

In this formula, the probability that radiation caused the effect (P_r) is equal to the excess incidence of effect due to the radiation exposure (*ERR*) divided by the sum of the radiogenic excess (*ERR*) and the natural incidence of the effect in an unexposed population (*I*). To determine the excess risk, one needs to know the radiation dose to the organ of interest (*D*) and an incidence risk coefficient per unit dose (C_r). Thus, the formula now becomes:

$$P_r = \frac{D \times C_r}{I + (D \times C_r)}$$

To apply the formula, one must initially determine the dose to the organ of interest. This has been discussed previously. Often dose determination receives an inordinate amount of attention and can be found with an uncertainty factor of ±50%. Although this initially seems to be a large confidence interval (CI), the majority of this text has been devoted to pointing out the uncertainties that exist in the risk coefficients and in the modeling approaches used. The dose often is one of the smaller uncertainties involved in the ultimate calculation of PC. For multiple radiation doses, one can modify the formula to take into account all exposures from the first to the ith, as follows:

$$P_r = \frac{(D \times C_r)_1 + (D \times C_r)_2 + \cdots (D \times C_r)_i}{I + (D \times C_r)_1 + (D \times C_r)_2 + \ldots (D \times C_r)_i}$$

The incidence risk coefficient per unit dose also has been extensively described in this text. One must decide in the analysis of a given effect which risk factors to use for the radiation exposure. For the nonstochastic or somatic effects, ranges known to cause a given incidence of undesirable side effects are generally available through radiation therapy experience. For evaluations of such abnormalities as mental retardation due to in utero irradiation, there are few attempts to derive risk estimates per unit dose; in fact, many of these effects appear to have a threshold below which the effect is not seen. Thus, for nonstochastic (direct) somatic effects, a risk coefficient per unit dose is not applicable; rather, one should determine the possible threshold and review the existing literature for that particular undesired effect. In terms of carcinogenesis, both absolute and relative risk models (discussed in Chapter 4) are used. Presently, whether to use absolute risk or RR is a matter of debate. Clearly, for leukemia, absolute risk is more appropriate than RR. If one intends to use RR, the risk factors should have been derived from a population base similar to that of the individual concerned. A number of risk estimates compiled from the scientific literature were published by the National Academy of Sciences Biological Effects of Ionizing Radiations (BEIR) VII committee,[74] by the United Nations Scientific Committee on Effects of Atomic Radiation (UNSCEAR) in its 2006 report,[75] and are discussed in Chapter 5. Obviously these summaries present risk estimates from studies in which they can be derived. In quite a few instances no excess is seen, and if such studies are appropriate to the case at hand, they should be considered for use. The "normal" incidence of effects for most abnormalities can be found through a literature search. The baseline incidence rates for specific cancers are usually derived from the Surveillance, Epidemiology, and End Results (SEER) program of the National Cancer Institute. Data in this publication report incidence rates according to sex, race, age, geographic location, anatomic site, and histologic type of cancer. These data represent the baseline cancer incidence rate for various circumstances. Analysis of such PC problems was discussed and published by Voelz.[76]

Modifying factors are very significant for such entities as lung cancer. Unfortunately, most simple PC methods do not allow for the interrelationships of various factors that may have caused the effect. If possible, it would be more appropriate to ask which subset of factors could be responsible for the observed health effect rather than which single factor was responsible. After this has been done, one might ask what share of the responsibility for the observed health effect was due to radiation exposure.

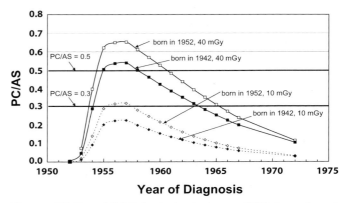

Figure 10-2 ● PC/AS for leukemia (except CLL) for estimated bone marrow doses of 10 and 40 mGy in 1952. (From National Research Council (NRC): Assessment of the scientific information for the radiation exposure screening and education program. Washington, DC, National Academy Press, 2006.)

Such an analysis including modification factors can only be done on an individual basis. In the case of an individual, it is necessary not only to deal with baseline cancer incidence rates, but also to adjust them for the individual differences and modifying factors that may be present. Day proposed a method combining RRs.[77] If a certain factor, X, occurs in $p\%$ of a population and is associated with an RR of r for a particular effect, the cumulative risk for the whole population, R, and the cumulative risk, R^I, for those with factor X is given by:

$$R^1 = \frac{rR}{(1 + rp - p)}$$

As an example, if $R = 10$ and 10% of a population engaged in an activity that caused a risk for lung cancer five times higher than that for the rest of the population, then the % risk for such persons of developing lung cancer is given by:

$$R^1 = \frac{10 \times 5}{1 + 0.5 - 0.1} = 35.7$$

This method allows calculation of the risk for subgroups of a population with a specific factor that increases the risk above normal. Age, dose, as well as the time after exposure all have a significant impact on PC/AS (Fig. 10-2).

When more than one etiologic factor is involved, the situation is complicated by the difficulty of assessing the interactions among the agents. The most common question that arises is how to deal with the potential interactive effect of smoking and lung cancer. As an example of how to do this, let us suppose an individual who has smoked enough to have an RR of 15 compared to the nonsmoking population. In this case if the RR_s is 15, then the ERR from smoking (ERR_s) is $15 - 1$, or 14. Let us also assume a lung dose of 0.2 Sv, which would give an RR from radiation (RR_r) of 1.072 or an ERR from radiation (ERR_r) of

0.072. If the interaction between smoking and radiation were multiplicative it would be appropriate to use RR as follows: $15(RR_s) \times 1.072 (RR_r) = 16.08$ total RR. If the interaction between the two agents is additive the ERR should be used as follows: $14 (ERR_s) + 0.072 (ERR_r) = 14.072$ (total ERR). We must then add 1.0 to include the baseline incidence so that now we have an RR of 15.072. Overall, it is still clear that it is much more likely than not that lung cancer would have been due to smoking regardless of whether the risks from smoking and radiation are additive or multiplicative.

LEGISLATIVE COMPENSATION PROGRAMS

Over the years, a large number of persons with suspected radiogenic cancer and other conditions have been unable to win remediation in the U.S. court system and have turned to political avenues for compensation through legislation. There have been four somewhat confusing pieces of legislation that deal with radiation exposure compensation. All of these have weakened the legal definition of causation as a basis for compensation. These legislative programs are the product of legal, political, and social "justice" advocates rather than being based purely on science. The lists of compensated malignant conditions include many neoplasms that can clearly be related to radiation exposure but also some neoplasms that have had little, if any, evidence of being radiation-induced, especially at low radiation levels (e.g., non-Hodgkin's lymphoma, and pancreatic, small intestine, and adult brain cancers). As of 2005, awarded compensation from these legislative compensation programs has exceeded $2 billion.[78]

The Radiation Exposure Compensation Act (RECA) of 1990 with amendments in 2000 and 2002 covers uranium miners with certain exposure levels, specific aboveground groups dealing with uranium, groups present during aboveground nuclear detonations, and "downwinders" who could demonstrate residence in specific counties. For the RECA program there is no need to demonstrate any level of radiation dose but merely a presence at a location at some time or a specific occupation. There is no distinction made between smokers and nonsmokers. Compensated conditions include nonchronic lymphocytic leukemia (non-CLL); cancer of the brain, bile duct, breast, colon, esophagus, gallbladder, liver, and lung; multiple myeloma; non-Hodgkin's lymphoma; and cancer of the ovary, pancreas, pharynx, kidney, salivary gland, small intestine, stomach, thyroid, and urinary bladder. Compensated conditions vary by class; for example, multiple myeloma is compensable for downwinders but not for uranium miners or millers. RECA also covers a number of nonmalignant conditions for those exposed to uranium including chronic renal disease, cor pulmonale, pneumoconiosis, pulmonary fibrosis, and silicosis. Payments are $100,000 to uranium miners, millers, and ore transporters; $75,000 to onsite nuclear test participants; and $50,000 to downwinders. These payments are described as "partial" and as "compassionate payments." Why there should be different monetary awards for the same condition is unclear. As of November 2004 almost a billion dollars ($835 million) had been approved under this program.

Two radiation compensation programs apply to military veterans, the 1984 Veterans' Dioxin and Radiation Exposure Compensation Act and the Radiation Exposure Veterans' Compensation Act (REVCA). Covered "presumptive" conditions include non-CLL; cancer of the bile ducts, bone, brain, breast, bronchoalveolar, colon, esophagus, gallbladder, small intestine, liver, and lung; lymphoma (except Hodgkin's); multiple myeloma; cancer of the ovary, pancreas, pharynx, thyroid, salivary gland, stomach; and any cancer of the urinary tract. It also includes compensation for those persons with tumors of the head and neck who had received nasopharyngeal radium radiotherapy. For presumptive conditions, no radiation dose level is necessary to obtain compensation. The claimant must only show that they participated in atmospheric nuclear tests or underground tests at Amchitka Island, Alaska, prior to 1974 or served in Hiroshima or Nagasaki from August 1945 to July 1946, were prisoners of war in Japan, or worked at gaseous diffusion plants in Paducah, Kentucky, Portsmouth, Ohio, or at area K25 at Oak Ridge, Tennessee.

The U.S. Department of Veterans Affairs (VA) compensation programs also include a category of "nonpresumptive" diseases or conditions that include all other cancers, cataracts, thyroid nodular disease, parathyroid adenoma, and tumors of the brain and central nervous system. These conditions are compensated if the 99% upper CI of the PC/AS is 0.5 or 50%. This would obviously take the estimated radiation dose into account. The amount of payment under the VA system depends on the assigned degree of disability. The total amount awarded under this program is not available.

An additional program applies to U.S. Department of Energy workers, the Energy Employees Occupational Illness Compensation Program Act of 2000 (EEOICPA). This program provides compensation for specified diseases including non-CLL; cancer of the brain, bile duct, breast, colon, esophagus, gallbladder, liver, and lung; multiple myeloma; non-Hodgkin's lymphoma; cancer of the ovary, pancreas, pharynx, kidney, salivary gland, small intestine, stomach, thyroid, and urinary bladder; chronic renal disease; cor pulmonale; pneumoconiosis; pulmonary fibrosis; silicosis; and chronic beryllium disease. For the neoplasms listed compensation is provided if the dose received results in a 99% upper CI for a PC/AS of 0.5 or 50% based on National Institutes of Health (NIH) radioepidemiological tables. Smoking history is taken into consideration. Awards are generally a $150,000 lump sum payment and the total awarded as of December 31, 2004, was just under a billion dollars ($975,640,617).

Table 10-8 • Approximate Absorbed Dose (mGy) That Cause the PC/AS to Exceed 50%			
Tumor	Geometric Mean of Organ dose (Gy) That Causes the Central Estimate of PC/AS) to Exceed 50%	Geometric mean of Organ Dose (Gy) That Causes the 99th Percentile of PC/AS to Exceed 50%	Ratio of the Two Doses
Oral cavity and pharynx	4.1	0.5	8.2
Esophagus	1.7	0.2	8.5
Lung			
Never smoked	1.5	0.3	5.0
10–19 cigarettes/ day	5.8	0.5	11.6
Former smoker	3.5	0.4	8.8
Female breast	1.4	0.2	7.0
Pancreas	5.6	0.5	11.2
Stomach	2.5	0.2	6.2
Colon	1.3	0.2	12.5
Rectum	7.3	0.6	12.2
Bladder	1.7	0.3	5.7
Thyroid	1.6	0.1	16.0
Leukemia	0.3	0.05	6.0
Lymphoma and multiple myeloma	5.3	0.4	13.3

Scenario postulates a male (except for breast cancer) born in 1940, acutely exposed to x-rays in 1980 at age 40, who developed cancer in 2000 at age 60.
For all cancers and leukemia, estimates obtained using the NIH Interactive Radio-Epidemiological Program (IREP) available from http://www.irep.nci.nih.gov/ (accessed Sept. 12, 2007). Values vary somewhat based upon choice of geometric standard deviation of uncertainty.

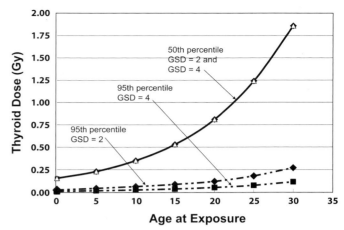

Figure 10-3 • Estimated thyroid dose (Gy) for which the PC/AS = 0.5 for different ages at exposure. Dose is given for the 50th and 95th percentile uncertainty. The geometric standard deviation was assumed to be 2 and 4. Curves for the 50th percentile GSD = 2 and GSD = 4 coincide with each other. (From National Research Council (NRC): Assessment of the scientific information for the radiation exposure screening and education program. Washington, DC, National Academy Press, 2006.)

There are some serious issues that should be raised about these types of legislative compensation programs. As can be noted from the above list, there is not uniformity in the list of covered conditions and there is not uniformity of amount awarded, even for the same condition in a given program. That the programs award compensation for conditions that are not likely to be radiation related has been pointed out in the past. Tumor sites included in one program were not selected based on radiogenic nature of the tumors but rather on the criteria that there were at least 50 incident cases in atomic bomb survivors who received at least 5 mSv. Thus a common tumor that was not radiogenic would be included. The 2006 report by the National Research Council on assessment of scientific information for the radiation exposure and screening program indicated, for example, that multiple myeloma is classified as having very low or no susceptibility to radiation induction yet it is included as a compensable condition in all the programs.[78]

As mentioned earlier, the legislative compensation programs have shifted from the legal definition of causation using "more likely than not" or using the best estimate of a PC/AS of 50%, to now compensate when there is a PC/AS of 50% at the 99% CI. The BEIR VII committee has stated, "with the exception of sampling variability, the uncertainty distributions for the individual sources were based on informed but nevertheless subjective decisions."[74]

Using the "subjective" 99th percentile upper bound for the PC/AS has two significant effects. The first effect is probably intentional and is a marked relaxation in the strength of association with radiation dose needed in order to be compensated (Table 10-8). For example, a white nonsmoking male born in 1940, who was exposed to x-rays in 1980 and developed lung cancer in 2000, would need a lung dose of about 1.5 Gy to be compensated in a court of law but in the legislative programs that invoke the 99% CI, he would be compensated at a lung dose 5-fold lower (0.3 Gy). Interestingly, if this compensation scheme were applied to medical exposures, any individual who had had two computerized tomography (CT) scans and later developed leukemia would be compensated. Even using the 95% CI has a significant effect on reducing the required dose for PC/AS (Fig. 10-3).

The other effect of using the 99% CI for the PC/AS was likely unintended. CIs for a PC/AS are based on the confidence of the dose level as well as the CIs from the epidemiological literature. Use of the confidence limits in awarding compensation then results in inequity based on tumor type. For tissues that have a relatively high radiation sensitivity for cancer induction (such as lung or breast) confidence limits will be relatively small.

With tumors that are very rare or not likely due to radiation, the confidence limits are large due to small numbers of observed tumors. Thus, for a given radiation dose, a person with a truly radiogenic cancer of the lung might not be compensated, while a person with a rare likely nonradiogenic cancer would be compensated at the same dose simply because of wider CIs. The same would occur if the dose was more uncertain for one person than another. A person living close to a fallout monitoring station would have less uncertainty in dose than a person living farther away. If they both actually received the same dose but there was more uncertainty for the person living at a greater distance, the first person might not be compensated and the second could be compensated. Because of these and other objections a number of authors and even the American Medical Association have suggested the PC/AS approach not be used for compensation.[79–82]

There are a number of other possible compensation schemes that have been suggested and used. In the United Kingdom, the Compensation Scheme for Radiation-Linked Diseases (CSRLD) is used. This covers all cancers except non-CLL, malignant melanoma, mesothelioma, and Hodgkin's lymphoma. A sliding scale for compensation and those with estimated values of PC/AS that are 0.5 (50%) or higher receive full awards, and those between 0.2 and 0.5 (20% to 50%) receive partial awards (Fig. 10-4).[83] Other ideas have included compensation based on years of life lost.[84] Ultimately the question of what is the best way to compensate when a disease has a number of causes and for which assignment can only be expressed on a probabilistic basis remain debatable. Upton and Wilson suggested a sum be decided for the disease in question and then compensation be made on the sum multiplied by the PC/AS with a de minimus cutoff at some level.[85]

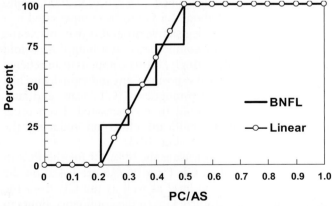

Figure 10-4 • Percentage of full compensation based on PC/AS used in the British Nuclear Fuels compensation scheme in the UK. (From National Research Council: Assessment of the scientific information for the radiation exposure screening and education program. Washington, DC, National Academy Press, 2006.)

PC OR AS CALCULATORS

Both the U.S. NIH and the National Institute of Occupational Safety and Health (NIOSH) have online calculators that can be used to estimate the probability that a cancer was caused by radiation exposure (available at www.irep.nci.nih.gov). Both Institutes use the Interactive Radioepidemiological Program (IREP), which has gone through several versions (version 5.5 as of 2006). The program allows for inputs such as patient age, sex, condition, year of diagnosis, year of exposure, acute versus chronic exposure, type and energy of radiation, and organ dose.[86] A sample of results is shown in Table 10-8. The program as it is currently structured has a number of flaws. The program uses data from the atomic bomb survivors almost exclusively (with the exception of thyroid and lung cancer). It assumes a generally linear relationship of all solid cancers from 0.01 Gy to 500 Gy. There is no scientific basis at this time to believe that a linear relationship is true at low doses for bone cancer. In addition, the probability of cancer actually decreases at doses higher than 3 to 5 Gy due to cell killing. The program does not take into account deterministic effects that would modify cancer risk. As pointed out above, the program also includes cancers (such as pancreas) that most scientific reviews have concluded are not likely to be radiation induced.

EXAMPLE CASES

Case 1: Lung Cancer in a Radiation Worker

Background

S. E. is a 55-year-old black male who had a 3-month history of fatigue, weight loss, and coughing. An x-ray demonstrated a lesion in the right upper lobe of his lung, which was biopsied; it was judged to be undifferentiated carcinoma of the lung, probably adenocarcinoma. He had worked at various jobs; however, he was predominantly a welder. During the course of this occupation, he worked for a period of approximately 10 years at a plant in which radiation was used, terminating his employment at the facility 10 years before the diagnosis of lung cancer was made. His recorded film badge radiation dose was 0.14 mSv. Over the last 10 years, he had worked for various construction companies in which there was exposure to asbestos insulation and also to triethylene, which was used as a cleaning solvent. His past history of smoking was at least one pack of unfiltered cigarettes daily; these cigarettes were high in both tar and nicotine.

Risk Analysis

This case is somewhat difficult to analyze for risk because of several individual factors: the patient was black, smoked cigarettes, was exposed to asbestos, and had the possibility of both internal and external radiation exposure. The first question to be answered is what this individual's chances of having lung cancer at age 55 were without the asbestos, smoking, or radiation histories. The "naturally occurring" incidence of cancer of the lung and bronchus can be found in the SEER data. It is important to use the correct incidence table because substantially different results may be obtained from the wrong table. If one examines the annual risk rate for developing cancer of the lung and bronchus at age 55 for all races and both sexes, one determines that the risk is 130 per 100,000. This, of course, is unrealistic because the lung cancer incidence rates are substantially different in males and females. The risk for age 55 for males of all races is 192 in 100,000. If one now examines the risk for cancer of the lung and bronchus for black males, the figure is 341 in 100,000. This example indicates that failure to individualize the risk factors may cause the estimate of the natural incidence of cancer to be wrong by as much as a factor of 3. Thus, the "normal" risk of this patient getting cancer of the lung or bronchus at age 55 was 341 in 100,000. Obviously, this incidence rate is derived from individuals who are both smokers and nonsmokers. At this point, one must try to determine the incidence rate in black males who smoke. An approximation can be made by using the natural incidence multiplied by some modifying factor. It is known that smoking is responsible for over 80% of lung cancer cases in men. The probability of developing lung cancer depends not only on the number of cigarettes smoked, but also on the age at which smoking began; the patient indicated that he began smoking during his teens. Data from several different studies indicate that the mortality ratio for such individuals may be 12 times that expected for nonsmokers; light smokers (who smoke fewer than 20 cigarettes daily) have a risk 7 times that of nonsmokers of developing lung cancer, whereas heavy smokers (smoking more than 20 cigarettes daily) have a risk of up to 25 times that of nonsmokers.[47] One can determine from the same data that about 50% of all black males smoke. Thus, our patient has a risk of developing lung cancer 10 to 20 times that of a nonsmoker. If we now use the formula given by Day[77] for combination of RR with the cumulative risk:

$$p = 50\%$$
$$r = 10$$
$$R = \frac{341}{100,000}$$

The formula for the cumulative risk of these individuals who smoke is given by:

$$R' = \frac{10 \times \frac{341}{100,000}}{1 + 10(0.5) - 0.5} = \frac{620}{100,000}$$

The risk factor of nonsmokers developing lung cancer would be substantially less (approximately 60 in 100,000).

Before identifying the risk attributable to occupational radiation exposure alone, one could consider other sources of radiation. The first of these is natural background. The background radiation exposure may be calculated, but the effect of such exposure is already included in the "natural" incidence of the SEER tables. Medical diagnostic and therapeutic radiation are other sources of radiation exposure. Records indicated that several chest x-rays were obtained during the course of his employment at various companies and that the dose to the lung from medical sources was approximately 1 mSv. This dose is close to the national average, so its effect again would be included in the natural incidence. If the patient had received substantially more, this would have to be considered as an extra risk. External exposure measurements are usually derived from film badge measurements that record exposure at the surface of the body; however, for conservative purposes, one might assume that this figure would represent the dose to the lung in this instance. Approximately 0.14 Sv whole-body, low-LET radiation from occupational sources was recorded in occupational exposure records. It would be best, however, to correct this for depth dose to the organ of interest; in this case, calculated absorbed dose to the lung was 0.1 Gy. In risk analysis for radiation carcinogenesis of lung tumors, one must initially consider the latent period. In this particular instance, the lung cancer did occur some 10 years or more after most of the occupational exposure, and, therefore, the occupational exposure must be considered. Using BEIR VII committee risk age-specific estimates for lung cancer, one concludes that *risk*, or the lifetime attributable risk of developing lung cancer from the occupational radiation received 10 years earlier, was about 100 in 100,000.[74] The lifetime risk would be spread out over his remaining 20 to 30 years of expected life and therefore would be about 5 in 100,000 per year. The risk could be smaller than that quoted because the radiation exposure was chronic rather than acute, and the risk estimates were based on linear extrapolation to low doses rather than using a linear-quadratic curve. Thus, at this point, one could conclude that the radiation accounted for less than 1% (5 in 620) probability of causation of developing cancer in that specific year. The percentage does not change much even if a multiplicative interaction is assumed between radiation and smoking (see earlier text for methodology).

Case Summary

If we consider the individual's total risk of developing lung cancer, one can conclude that there is a 90% probability that the lung cancer was due to cigarette smoking, more than a 9% chance that it was due to causes other than occupational radiation exposure, and less than a 1% chance that it was due to occupational radiation exposure. An important point is to note the age and smoking effect on the outcome of this example. Had this worker been exposed in his early 20s, was 30 to 34 years old when he developed cancer, and if he had not been a smoker, the chances would have been greater than 50% that the cancer was caused by radiation exposure.

Case 2: Cataracts in an X-Ray Technologist

Background

C. M. is a 55-year-old diabetic white male who had worked as an x-ray technician in a cardiac catheterization laboratory for the past 10 years. He demonstrated bilateral cataract formation, requesting compensation on the basis of alleged radiation induction of the cataracts. The cataracts were examined by an ophthalmologist, who described them as nonspecific. Specific questioning and reexamination by another ophthalmologist indicated that it is not possible to ascertain whether these cataracts began in the anterior or posterior pole of the lens.

Risk Analysis

Estimation of normal incidence must be calculated first. Cataracts are the most common cause of blindness in the world, with an estimated 17 million persons affected. In the United States, the Framingham Study indicated that 15% of persons in the age range of 52 to 85 years are affected by cataracts.[87] Modifying factors of the normal incidence also must be taken into account: diabetes and diastolic hypertension have a long-accepted association with senile cataracts. A list of associations that should be evaluated as modifying factors in cataract formation includes the following:

1. Drugs: allopurinol, ethylene oxide, Dilantin (Parke-Davis), chlorpromazine, corticosteroids, barbiturates, monoamine oxidase inhibitors, and tricyclic antidepressants.
2. Trauma: lasers, UV light, microwaves, and penetrating physical injuries.
3. Systemic abnormalities: diabetes, riboflavin deficiency, and hypocalcemia.
4. Genetic syndromes: congenital cataracts; Down, Marfan's, and Cockayne's syndromes; 13-15 trisomy, and so on.

In this patient, the history of diabetes obviously is a modifying factor raising the nonradiogenic incidence for cataracts in this individual to above 15%. Estimation of the actual absorbed radiation dose received by the lens of the eye during the occupational exposure is difficult. There have been several studies of the subject, and it appears that the exposure reported ranges between 30 and 450 μSv for each cardiac catheterization procedure.[88] The individual in this particular case wore his film badge on the collar, and it is reasonable to estimate that the dose to the lens of the eye might be 75% of that found on the

collar. A confounding factor in this particular instance was that the individual normally wore glasses. The effectiveness of glass lenses in reducing exposure to the eye has been examined by several authors.[89,90] Overall, for normal prescription glasses, a radiation attenuation factor of 50% may also be introduced. There are several alternative methods for calculating the dosimetry in this case. Total film badge readings taken on the collar indicated a total occupational exposure value of 0.2 Sv. Although the value to the lens of the eye may be slightly lower, a conservative measure would be to assume that the collar dose was indeed the dose to the lens of the eye. If film badge readings had not been available, one might have assumed that the individual had not exceeded the allowable whole-body maximum limit of 0.05 Sv annually. Thus, over the 10 years of employment, it would be extremely unlikely that the dose to the eye would have exceeded 0.5 Sv. A third method of calculation would be to review the number of procedures performed weekly (in this case, five catheterization procedures). Allowing for vacations, sick time, and so on, this would be approximately 2300 examinations performed over the 10-year period. Using the average dose per procedure in the literature, this would indicate a dose to the lens of the eye of approximately 0.4 to 0.6 Sv. With the attenuation for the prescription glasses, by all three methods, the dose to the eye is unlikely to have exceeded 0.1 to 0.3 Sv over this time period.

Radiation as a Cause of Cataracts

Radiation as a cause of cataracts has been discussed by many authors and is reviewed in Chapter 6. One cannot use the point of origin of the cataracts in this case; as mentioned earlier, early radiation cataracts are relatively specific lesions that begin in the posterior pole of the lens, whereas senile cataracts begin in the anterior pole. Unfortunately, in this case, the cataracts were too advanced to allow for differentiation and thus were classed as nonspecific. The latent period for manifestation of radiation-induced cataracts varies between several months and 20 years. Thus, one cannot exclude radiation-induced cataracts on the basis of the latent period. There has, however, been extensive study of the threshold dose to cause clinically significant cataracts. For fractionated, protracted radiation exposure, the lowest threshold dose reported by any investigator is about 6 Sv, with the quoted range in the literature 6 to 14 Sv.[91]

Summary

Unless the dose to the lens of the eye approaches 6 Sv, clinically significant radiation-induced cataracts from fractionated or protracted radiation exposures are unlikely. In this particular individual with diabetes, the normal probability of developing cataracts is well in excess of 15%, and the possibility of radiation-induced cataracts cannot be seriously considered.

Case 3: Mental Retardation Following In Utero Radiation Exposure

Background

C. Z., a 26-year-old mother of two children, took her 2-year-old son to the hospital after a head injury. A skull film was ordered, and the mother was asked to hold the child during the procedure, although there is some doubt as to whether she was asked to wear a lead apron. Subsequently, she discovered that she was approximately 9 weeks pregnant at the time. Consultation with her obstetrician resulted in the suggestion that an abortion be performed on the basis of the radiation exposure; however, she elected not to have a therapeutic abortion and carried the pregnancy to term without incident. Following a "normal" delivery of a female infant, the child was subsequently diagnosed to be mentally retarded. No physical stigmata were associated with the retardation. The legal situation concerned whether the mental retardation resulted from the radiation exposure incurred by the pregnant mother while holding her son for the skull film.

Risk Analysis

The normal incidence of mental retardation in the population depends on the definition used. At the present time, most organizations define an IQ below 70 as *mental retardation*. Current prevalence figures range from 2.4% to 2.5%. The incidence figures related to live birth may be slightly higher, if mentally retarded persons do not have a normal life span. Modifying factors that may be considered are many. At the present time, over 250 causes of mental retardation have been identified, including malnutrition, lead poisoning, rubella infections during pregnancy, and alcoholism. No definite predisposing causes or modifying factors other than radiation exposure were identified in this particular patient. Thus, one might assume that the "normal" incidence of mental retardation, which is approximately 3%, is applicable in this case.[92,93]

Radiation as a Cause of Mental Retardation

The items to be considered in this particular case are an analysis of the radiation dose to the fetus, evaluation of the time of the exposure during pregnancy, and identification of other physical abnormalities in the retarded child. Analysis of the exact dose is difficult, although estimates can be made within an order of magnitude. In this particular case, the mother claims that she was not given a lead apron to wear during the procedure. As an extremely conservative estimate, one might suppose that the mother's pelvis was in the direct x-ray beam and received the same absorbed skin dose that the son's head did. Most skull films are taken at 80 kVp; assuming that the uterus was 8 cm deep in the tissue, a maximal depth dose to the fetus is 2 mSv. If the mother's pelvis had not been in the direct beam, a much more reasonable value would be 1% of this, or 10 to 20 µSv. During the course of the pregnancy, the fetus received not only the exposure implicated in this case, but also radiation exposure due to natural background sources, approximately 0.1 Sv. If there is a risk of mental retardation from "natural" radiation exposure, this would be already included in the natural incidence. The next point to be addressed is whether the radiation exposure occurred at a time in pregnancy when mental retardation has been identified as a possible effect (discussed in Chapter 8). On the basis of radiation exposure at 9 weeks of pregnancy, mental retardation induced by radiation cannot be excluded on a temporal basis. Had the exposure occurred at 2 to 3 weeks of pregnancy or, for example, late in the third trimester, radiogenic mental retardation could essentially have been excluded. The data from Hiroshima and Nagasaki, as well as subsequent reports of the International Commission on Radiological Protection (ICRP), suggest that while high doses of radiation may damage enough neurons to cause severe mental retardation, there is essentially a shift to the left of the normal distribution of IQ. While a low dose of radiation may theoretically reduce IQ by a few points, it is extremely unlikely to cause severe mental retardation in a person who was destined to have an average IQ in the absence of radiation exposure.[94]

Associated physical findings are important in analysis of this case because most cases of radiogenic mental retardation are also accompanied by microcephaly and occasionally by intrauterine growth retardation. Neither was present in this particular case, thus additionally lowering the possibility that the mental retardation was due to radiation exposure. In the literature concerning in utero exposure and atomic bomb survivors, the exposures were substantially higher; however, 95% of those mentally retarded also demonstrated microcephaly. No case of mental retardation due to radiation exposure has ever been documented in cases in which the fetal radiation dose was less than 0.1 Gy.

Summary

With the data presented in this case, one would conclude that there is virtually no chance that the radiation, even under "worst case assumptions," would have been responsible for severe mental retardation. Whether the radiation may have caused a drop in IQ by 1 or 2 points is a moot point.

REFERENCES

1. Riley, P., Radiation risk in the context of liability for injury. J Radiol Prot, 2003. 23(3):305–315.
2. *Martinez v. University of California*, 601 P2d 425. 1979, N.M.
3. *Landry v. Florida Power and Light Corp.*, 779F. Supp. 94. 1992, S.D., Fla.
4. *Brown v. Centerior Energy Corp.*, Slip Op. No. 1:91 CV 0332. 1992.
5. *Laswell v. Brown*, 683 F. 2nd 261. 1982, 8th Cir.
6. *Prunett v. Carter*, 621 F. 2nd 578. 1980, 3rd Cir.
7. *Whiting v. Boston Edison Co.*, No. 88-2125. 1991, D. Mass.
8. *Hennessy v. Commonwealth Edison Co.*, 764 F. Supp. 495, 501. 1991, N.D., Ill.
9. *Coley v. Commonwealth Edison Co.*, 768 F. Supp. 625. 1991, N.D., Ill.
10. *Caputo v. Boston Edison Co.*, Slip op. No. 88-2126-Z 1990 WL 98694. 1990, D. Mass.
11. *Jurka v. Commonwealth Edison Co.*, 88 C 7852. 1990, N.D. Ill.
12. *Kesecker v. United States Department of Energy*, 679 F. Supp. 726. 1988, S.D., Ohio.
13. *Timothy v. United States*, 612 F. Supp. 160. 1985, D. Utah.
14. *Crowther v. Seaborg*, 312 F. Supp. 1234. 1970 D. Colo.
15. *Akins v. Sacramento Utility District*, 6 Cal. App. 4th 1605, * Cal. Rptr. 2d 785 1992.
16. Sen, M., Defining the boundaries of "personal injury": *Rainer v. Union Carbide Corp.* Stanford Law Rev, 2006. 58(4):1251–1266.
17. *Daubert et al. v. Merrell Dow Pharmaceuticals, Inc.*, 113 S. Ct. 2786. 1993.
18. Masten, J. and J.J. Strzelczyk, Admissibility of scientific evidence post-Daubert. Health Phys, 2001. 81(6):678–682.
19. Ayala, F. and B. Black, Science and the courts. American Scientist, 1993. 81:230–239.
20. *Troxell v. Bendix Corp.*, 12660 F XXX. 1963, Dist. C. Mo.
21. Estep, S.D. and E.H. Forgotson, Legal liability for genetic injuries from radiation. Louisiana Law Rev, 1963. 24:1–53.
22. Perdue, J., An analysis of the physicians professional liability for irradiation of the fetus. In Bilogical Risks of Medical Irradiation, G. Fullerton, D. Kopp, and R.G. Waggener, eds. Monograph 5. 1980, New York: American Association of Physicists in Medicine.
23. *Smith v. Ruckhardt*, 19 NE2d 446. 1939, App C Ill.
24. *Stemmer v. Kline*, 26 A2d 489. 1942, C Err App N.J.
25. *Bonbrest v. Kotz*, 65 FS 138. 1946, U.S. Dist C, Wash. D.C.
26. *Delgado v. Yandell*, 468 SW2d 475. 1971, C Civ App Tex.
27. *Hogan v. McDaniel*, 319 SW 2d 221. 1958, Tenn.
28. *Drabbels v. Skelly Oil Co.*, 50 NW2d 229. 1951, Neb.
29. *Prates v. Sears Roebuck & Co.*, 118 A2d 633. 1955, Sup C Conn.
30. *Salinetro v. Nystrom*, 341 S2d 1059. 1977, Dist C App Fla.
31. *Craft v. Vanderbilt University*. Fed Suppl, 1998. 18:786–798.
32. Doll, R., The causes of cancer. Rev Epidemiol Sante Publique, 2001. 49(2):193–200.
33. Doll, R. and R. Peto, The causes of cancer: Quantitative estimates of avoidable risks of cancer in the United States today. J Natl Cancer Inst, 1981. 66(6):1191–1308.
34. Ames, B.N., Dietary carcinogens and anti-carcinogens. J Toxicol Clin Toxicol, 1984. 22(3):291–301.
35. Ames, B.N., Dietary carcinogens and anticarcinogens: Oxygen radicals and degenerative diseases. Science, 1983. 221(4617):1256–1264.
36. Ames, B.N. and L.S. Gold, Dietary carcinogens, environmental pollution, and cancer: Some misconceptions. Med Oncol Tumor Pharmacother, 1990. 7(2–3):69–85.
37. International Agency for Research on Cancer (IARC), Cancer: Causes, occurrence and control, L. Tomatis, ed. 1990, Lyon, France: IARC.
38. Higginson, J., From geographical pathology to environmental carcinogenesis: A historical reminiscence. Cancer Lett, 1997. 117(2):133–142.
39. Higginson, J., Environmental carcinogenesis. Cancer, 1993. 72(suppl 3):S971–S977.
40. Higginson, J., Everything is a carcinogen? Regul Toxicol Pharmacol, 1987. 7(1):89–95.
41. Higginson, J., O.M. Jensen, and C.S. Muir, Environmental carcinogenesis—A global problem. Curr Probl Cancer, 1981. 5(7):1–43.
42. Higginson, J., C. Muir, and N. Munoz, Human Cancer: Epidemiology and Environmental Causes. 1992, Cambridge, UK: Cambridge University Press.
43. Armitage, P., et al., Dose-response relationship in radiation leukaemia. Nature, 1959. 184(suppl 21):S1669–S1670.
44. Danaei, G., et al., Causes of cancer in the world: Comparative risk assessment of nine behavioural and environmental risk factors. Lancet, 2005. 366(9499):1784–1793.
45. Cori, G. and B.S. Bock, A safe cigarette? Banbury Report 3. 1980, Cold Spring Harbor, NY: Cold Spring Harbor Laboratory.
46. Report of the Surgeon General on Smoking. 1979: Washington, DC: U.S. Department of Health.
47. Smoking and health: A report of the Surgeon General of the U. S. Public Health Service. 1979: Washington, DC: U.S. Public Health Service.
48. The health consequences of smoking for women: A report of the Surgeon General of the U.S. Public Health Service. 1980: Washington, DC: U.S. Public Health Service.
49. The health consequences of smoking: A changing cigarette. A report of the Surgeon General of the U.S. Public Health Service, 1981, Washington, DC: U.S. Government Printing Office.
50. Pierce, D.A., G.B. Sharp, and K. Mabuchi, Joint effects of radiation and smoking on lung cancer risk among atomic bomb survivors. Radiat Res, 2003. 159(4):511–520.
51. Ames, B.N. and L.S. Gold, The causes and prevention of cancer: The role of environment. Biotherapy, 1998. 11(2–3):205–220.
52. Ames, B.N. and L.S. Gold, The causes and prevention of cancer: Gaining perspective. Environ Health Perspect, 1997. 105(suppl 4):S865–S873.
53. National Research Council (NRC), Diet, nutrition and cancer. 1982, Washington, DC: N.A. Press.
54. Rebelakos, A., et al., Tobacco smoking, coffee drinking, and occupation as risk factors for bladder cancer in Greece. J Natl Cancer Inst, 1985. 75(3):455–461.
55. Trichopoulos, D., M. Papapostolou, and A. Polychronopoulou, Coffee and ovarian cancer. Int J Cancer, 1981. 28(6):691–693.
56. Cuckle, H.S. and L.J. Kinlen, Coffee and cancer of the pancreas. Br J Cancer, 1981. 44(5):760–761.
57. Phillips, R.L. and D.A. Snowdon, Association of meat and coffee use with cancers of the large bowel, breast, and prostate among Seventh-Day Adventists: Preliminary results. Cancer Res, 1983. 43(suppl 5):S2403–S2408.
58. Marrett, L.D., S.D. Walter, and J.W. Meigs, Coffee drinking and bladder cancer in Connecticut. Am J Epidemiol, 1983. 117(2):113–127.
59. Kinlen, L.J., Fat and cancer. BMJ (Clin Res Ed), 1983. 286(6371):1081–1082.
60. Kritchevsky, D. and D.J. Fink, Introduction to the workshop on fat and cancer. Cancer Res, 1981. 41(9 Pt 2):3684.
61. Lew, E.A. and L. Garfinkel, Variations in mortality by weight among 750,000 men and women. J Chronic Dis, 1979. 32(8):563–576.
62. National Cancer Institute, National Institute of Environmental Health Sciences (NIEHS), Cancer and the environment. 2003, Washington DC: National Cancer Institute, NIEHS.
63. MacMahon, B., Epidemiology and the causes of breast cancer. Int J Cancer, 2006. 118(10):2373–2378.

64. MacMahon, B., P. Cole, and J. Brown, Etiology of human breast cancer: A review. J Natl Cancer Inst, 1973. 50(1):21–42.

65. Hoover, R., et al., Menopausal estrogens and breast cancer. N Engl J Med, 1976. 295(8):401–405.

66. Marshall, E., Search for a killer: Focus shifts from fat to hormones. Science, 1993. 259:618–621.

67. Wynder, E.L. and G.B. Gori, Contribution of the environment to cancer incidence: An epidemiologic exercise. J Natl Cancer Inst, 1977. 58(4):825–832.

68. Doll, R., Atmospheric pollution and lung cancer. Environ Health Perspect, 1978. 22:23–31.

69. Heidenreich, W.F., et al., Age and time patterns in thyroid cancer after the Chernobyl accidents in the Ukraine. Radiat Res, 2000. 154(6):731–732; discussion, 734–735.

70. Harris, C.C., A delayed complication of cancer therapy—Cancer. J Natl Cancer Inst, 1979. 63(2):275–277.

71. Jick, H., A.M. Walker, and K.J. Rothman, The epidemic of endometrial cancer: A commentary. Am J Public Health, 1980. 70(3):264–267.

72. National Research Council (NRC), Assigned share for radiation as a cause of cancer: A view of radioepidemiologic tables assigning probabilities of causation. 1984, Washington, DC: N.A. Press.

73. National Council on Radiation Protection and Measurements (NCRP), The probability that a particular malignancy may have been caused by a specified irradiation. NCRP Statement No. 7. 1991, Bethesda, Md: NCRP.

74. National Research Council (NRC). Committee on the Biological Effects of Ionizing Radiations (BEIR), Health risks from exposure to low levels of ionizing radiation. BEIR VII. 2005, Washington, DC: NRCUSNA Press.

75. United Nations Scientific Committee of the Effects of Atomic Radiation (UNSCEAR), Sources and effects of ionizing radiation: 2006 Report to the General Assembly with annexes. 2006, New York: United Nations.

76. Voelz, G. What is the probability that radiation caused a particular cancer? In Epidemiology Applied to Health Physics: Sixteenth Mid-year Topical Meeting. 1983. Albuquerque, NM: Health Physics Society.

77. Day, N., Cumulative rate and cumulative risk: Cancer incidence on 5 continents. 1982, Geneva: International Agency for Research on Cancer (IARC).

78. National Research Council (NRC), Assessment of the scientific information for the radiation exposure screening and education program. 2006, Washington, DC: National Academy Press.

79. Wagner, L.K., et al., Probability of causation for cancers potentially induced by ionizing radiation. Med Phys, 1989. 16(3):406–413.

80. Gray, J.E., Clinical viewpoint on NCRP probability of causation statement. Health Phys, 1993. 64(5):550–551.

81. Parascandola, M., Uncertain science and a failure of trust: The NIH radioepidemiologic tables and compensation for radiation-induced cancer. Isis, 2002. 94(4):559–584.

82. Beljan, J.R., et al., Radioepidemiological tables. Council on Scientific Affairs. JAMA, 1987. 257(6):806–809.

83. Wakeford, R., B. Antell, and W. Leigh, A review of probability of causation and its use in a compensation scheme for nuclear industry workers in the United Kingdom. Health Phys, 1998. 74(1):1–9.

84. Robins, J. and S. Greenland, Estimability and estimation of expected years of life lost due to a hazardous exposure. Stat Med, 1991. 10(1):79–93.

85. Upton, A.C. and R. Wilson, Compensating government workers exposed to radiation. Harvard Center for Risk Analysis. Risk in Perspective, 2000. 8(7):1–4.

86. Kocher, D.C. and A. Apostoaei, Radiation effectiveness factors for use in calculating probability of causation of radiogenic cancers. Health Phys, 2005. 89(1):3–32.

87. Kahn, H.A., et al., The Framingham Eye Study. II. Association of ophthalmic pathology with single variables previously measured in the Framingham Heart Study. Am J Epidemiol, 1977. 106(1):33–41.

88. Wold, G.J., R.V. Scheele, and S.K. Agarwal, Evaluation of physician exposure during cardiac catheterization. Radiology, 1971. 99(1):188–190.

89. Agarwal, S.K., et al., The effectiveness of glass lenses in reducing exposure to the eyes. Radiology, 1978. 129(3):810–811.

90. Young, R.G. and W.H. Carlton, X-ray attenuation by prescription lenses. Radiology, 1978. 129(3):811.

91. Bendel, I., W. Schuttmann, and B. Arndt, Cataract of the lens as a late effect of ionizing radiation in occupationally exposed persons, In Late Biological Effects of Ionizing Radiation. 1978, Vienna: IAEA.

92. Ingalls, R., Mental Retardation: The Changing Outlook. 1978, New York: John Wiley and Sons.

93. United Nations Scientific Committee on the Effects of Atomic Radiation (UNSCEAR), Sources and effects of ionizing radiation: UNSCEAR 1993 report to the General Assembly, with scientific annexes. 1993, New York: United Nations.

94. Streffer, C., et al., Biological effects after prenatal irradiation (embryo and fetus): A report of the International Commission on Radiological Protection. Ann ICRP, 2003. 33(1–2):5–206.

11 Perception of Radiation and Psychological Effects

Radiation is frightening to most people. This chapter attempts to analyze the reasons for this fear, related psychological issues, and the decision-making process involved in acceptance or rejection of radiation-related risks. This chapter is concerned with radiation doses that are below those known to cause deterministic effects. The well-documented neuropsychological effects following high-dose radiation therapy are discussed in Chapter 6 and those associated with in utero exposure are discussed in Chapter 8.

The public is constantly assaulted with news headlines and stories related to the safety of all sorts of items (ranging from cosmetics to toys from China). Lowrance has pointed out that debates over consumer products often seem to result in a large amount of confusion and public anxiety.[1] It often is unclear to the public why one group of eminent "experts" may indicate that medical x-rays are not a problem, whereas another group may suggest that there is a major and obvious problem that has been overlooked. Most issues related to hazards are scientifically complex enough that the public has no personal knowledge of these matters and therefore relies on other people's opinions. Despite all the hazards around us, humankind is undoubtedly much safer today than ever before. In 1900, more than 13% of all American children died before their first birthday with the principal fatal diseases being pneumonia, influenza, and tuberculosis. At the same time, there were 150,000 horses decorating the streets of New York with horse manure, and the air was filled with coal dust and cinders.[1] It was probably not until the 1900s that medicine cured more people than it injured. With the rapid advancement of technology, we have replaced some of the previous hazards, which were quite well known, with a myriad of newer, less well-known potential problems.

The terms *risk* and *safety* are often used without a clear understanding of their meanings, and they therefore need to be defined relative to their use in this text. In general, something is said to be "safe" if its risks are judged to be acceptable. Because nothing is free from risk, the concept of safety is a matter of judging acceptability of a risk (either on a personal or social basis).

Determination of safety is a judgment process and therefore cannot be directly measured. The term *risk* is often used to connote the potential of an undesirable event. More properly it is used to mean the probability of a specific undesired event occurring within a given period of time or under a certain set of circumstances. Sometimes there is an attempt to add more dimensions to risk by multiplying the probability by the severity of the events in hopes of determining how to plan for efficient use of resources. This approach may or may not be useful, especially if one is considering a low-probability catastrophic event such as a major earthquake. The ICRP in its 1990 recommendations has used length of life lost in addition to cancer probability to express detriment.[2] One can envision other parameters as well, including cost of treatment, loss of income, pain, and so forth. The reader is also referred to a broader summary of the issues published by the National Council on Radiation Protection and Measurements (NCRP).[3]

Measurement of risk is a scientific activity that can be done in many ways. Once a risk has been scientifically measured, it can then be presented to the individual or society. As a risk measurement is presented to society it may be amplified, attenuated, colored, or influenced by outside factors such as the media. Finally, the risk is judged by the individual or by society to be acceptable or unacceptable (safe or unsafe). As mentioned in other chapters, medical effects of radiation may be classified either as genetic or somatic. *Genetic effects* affect the individual's offspring, as well as future generations. Genetic effects are *stochastic*, meaning that the occurrence of genetic effects is a function of probability, and that probability increases with increasing dose. The severity of a genetic effect, however, is unrelated to the magnitude of the radiation dose that caused the effect. *Somatic effects* occur in the body of the individual who has been exposed to ionizing radiation. Somatic effects may be either stochastic or nonstochastic (deterministic). The typical stochastic effect is cancer induction. *Nonstochastic* somatic effects are those that are associated with cellular and functional abnormalities in specific tissues, for example, radiation-induced skin ulcer. In contrast with stochastic effects,

459

the severity of nonstochastic effects is directly related to the absorbed dose. In development of radiation standards, as well as in the public perception of radiation, both somatic and genetic effects and risks are usually (and perhaps inappropriately) merged.

MEASUREMENT OF RISK

Lines of evidence that are sometimes used to evaluate risk come from a variety of sources, including folk knowledge, common sense, analogy to similar situations, and experiments on either the risk-causing agent or its effects on organisms. Clearly, the most desirable and most difficult information to obtain concerns the effect of a particular agent on humans. This information may be drawn from direct experiments on humans, accidents, epidemiologic studies, or even reviews of occupational exposures. Statistical principles have been applied to both epidemiologic and occupational exposures to extract as much information as possible without resorting to human experimentation. The process usually involved in determining specific risk estimates includes the following steps: (1) definition of the conditions of exposure, (2) identification of adverse effects, (3) evaluation of the statistical probability that the exposure indeed caused the identified effects, (4) assessment to determine whether there is a dose-response relationship, and (5) estimation of overall risk.[1] This book has emphasized identifying and quantifying the medical effects of radiation exposure and pointed out that drastically different risk estimates for a given effect may be obtained for exposures to different types of radiation. Even the same type of radiation when delivered in different time–dose schedules may have markedly different effects. Thus, potential ill effects or risk should be measured and expressed under specific and defined circumstances.

Adverse effects are probably better documented for radiation than for almost any other type of noxious agent. Although some questions as to the exact quantification of radiation risk at very low doses remain, the order of magnitude of adverse effects is reasonably well known. There is little question of the effect when radiation dose levels exceed 1 Gy, and there are some reasonably accurate data for the dose range of 0.1 to 1 Gy. Relating adverse effects to radiation doses below 0.1 Gy has proven difficult; estimates of risk are usually based on mathematical extrapolation models. In general, any such statistical methods that are used at low-dose levels do not establish scientific proof of a causal relationship between radiation and a given effect. To evaluate whether radiation actually caused an effect, one must rely on other factors, including consistency, statistical strength, temporal relationship, and comparison with other known associations. In any case, the statistical methods employed are probabilistic; therefore, there will always remain room for some debate within confidence limits about low-level radiation effects.

Although radiation effects at low doses are not precisely known, it is possible to quantify radiation risk estimates within limits. This problem was discussed and presented in an eloquent lecture by Pochin, who points out that quantification of risk estimates is the initial step necessary in proposing limits of radiation exposure.[4] It is unlikely that quantitative information will ever be adequate to prove the exact effects of low levels of radiation conclusively; however, great accuracy is not needed. It is unlikely that even if one could distinguish differences in risk of some adverse effect, for example, between one and two chances in a million, that such accuracy would have a significant impact on acceptance of risk. Risk estimates of the genetic effects of radiation are discussed extensively in Chapter 3; as was pointed out, the majority of the genetic data come from animals. The applicability of these data to humans has been uncertain, although some significant human data concerning genetic effects in the children of atomic bomb survivors and radiation therapy patients (see Chapter 3) have been published. It is clear that at this point genetic risks from radiation are substantially less than those from radiation-induced cancer.

Somatic risks are somewhat more difficult to quantify because they include nonstochastic abnormalities (due to cell killing) and stochastic effects such as carcinogenesis. When very high dose levels are reached, for example, tens of gray (Gy), the nonstochastic direct effects of cell killing and tissue death predominate. At low-dose levels, the only concern is usually that of the stochastic or probabilistic effect of carcinogenesis. In the intermediate dose ranges, both the risk of carcinogenesis and cell-killing effects must be considered as risks. Thus, overall measurement of radiation risk should include a genetic component, a carcinogenic component, and, at high dose levels, risk due to cell killing. The question of which risk "measurement" to use in relating various radiation effects has been the subject of intense study. The problems involved in developing an "index of harm" have been set forth by reports of the International Commission on Radiological Protection (ICRP), which indicate that measurement of such diffuse end points as anxiety and fear is practically impossible.[5,6] Measurement of illness is somewhat easier but still has great inherent difficulties. For example, how can one equate a short, painful illness with a chronic illness that is less painful? Most radiation risk estimates in the literature have therefore used one or more of three parameters: (1) time lost from a full and normal working life, (2) fatality rate, or (3) cancer incidence/mortality. Risks for various occupations expressed in these ways are shown in Tables 11-1 and 11-2.

Time of life lost, or fatality rate, is often used for comparing risks associated with various conditions or activities. In this way, the risks from diverse activities can be compared (Tables 11-3 and 11-4).[7] Pochin has used the same type of calculation to consider the average risk from radiation exposure involved in nuclear power production.[4]

Table 11-1 • Average Reduction in Life Span (Days) in Various Occupations

	For 1 Year of Working Life	For 35 Years of Working Life
Deep sea fishing	32	923
Coal mining	3.6	103
Oil refinery	2.6	74
Railways	22	63
Construction	2.1	62
Industry (average value)	0.5	13.5
Occupational exposure to radiation at the annual dose limit of 50 mSv	1.3	32
Occupational exposure to radiation at 5 mSv	0.1	3

From the International Atomic Energy Agency (IAEA): Bulletin vol. 22, nos. 5–6. Vienna, IAEA, 1980, p. 117.

Estimates of total dose range from 0.02 to 0.06 man Sv per megawatt year for the entire nuclear fuel cycle. In a population deriving 1 kilowatt per person from nuclear sources, there is an estimated mean dose equivalent of 40 μSv per year, or an average individual risk equal to smoking one cigarette every 2 years.

RISK PERCEPTION AND ACCEPTABILITY

After risks have been measured, one is in a position to judge the acceptability of risk, either to oneself or to society. Judging the acceptability of the risk is essentially assessing the safety of an activity. Obviously, the acceptability of any risk depends on the surrounding circumstances: what is "safe" for one person may not be for another. The perception of acceptability of risks by individuals is a very complex and often inaccurate procedure.

Table 11-2 • Mean U.S. Fatal Occupational Accident Rates

Industry	Death/Million Persons/Year
Mining and quarrying	994
Construction	717
Agriculture	613
Transport and public utilities	373
Service in government	131
Manufacturing	103
Trade	83
Industry (average)	200

From Pochin E: Why be quantitative about radiation risk estimates? NCRP Annual Meeting. Crystal City, MD: NCRP, 1978.

Table 11-3 • Average Life Span Shortening Associated with Various Conditions or Etiologies

Condition or Etiology	Days
Unmarried (male)	3500
Cigarette smoking	
Male	2400
Female	1420
Heart disease	2100
30% overweight	1560
Cancer	980
Stroke	700
Unemployment	500
Motor vehicle accidents	207
Large cars	145
Small cars	290
Alcohol (U.S. average)	125
Accidents in home	74
Accidents at workplace	60
AIDS	55
Jogging (for 30 yr)	50
Radon in homes	29
Drowning	24
Illicit drugs (U.S. average)	18
Natural radiation (other than radon)	9
Medical x-rays	6
Reactor accidents	0.02–2
Smoke alarm in home	−9
Seat belts in cars	−69

Adapted from Cohen EL, Lee IS: A catalog of risks. Health Phys 1979; 36:707–722; Cohen B: Catalog of risks extended and updated. Health Phys 1991;61:317–335.

If the activity involved is something that the person is familiar with (such as crossing the street), the individual usually has a substantial amount of personal experience and knowledge with which to judge the situation. Unfortunately, most safety decisions that reach public attention, such as radiation effects, health effects of air pollutants, and adverse effects of pharmaceuticals or pesticides, require a very detailed knowledge that the individual usually does not possess. Recent experience plays a significant role in judging the acceptability, or safety, of a risk. For example, somebody who has been injured in a recent automobile accident may well decide that it is unacceptable to travel in a car without a seatbelt, whereas previously that individual might have regarded driving without a seatbelt as quite safe. Other factors entering into assessment and perception of risk are the type and nature of the injury or adverse effect expected, for example, whether the injury is expected to be fatal, crippling, or merely a temporary inconvenience. Whether the adverse effect occurs immediately or is delayed also has a substantial impact on individual perception and acceptance of risk. A classic example of this is cigarette smoking: although almost everybody is aware of the well-documented hazards, many people persist in smoking, knowing that the effect is not likely to happen

Table 11–4 • Activities Estimated to Increase Risk of Death by One Chance in a Million

Activity	Cause of Death
Smoking 1 cigarette	Cancer, heart disease
Drinking half liter of wine	Cirrhosis of the liver
Spending 1 hr in a coal mine	Black lung disease
Spending 3 hr in a coal mine	Accident
Living 2 days in New York or Boston	Air pollution
Rock climbing for 1.5 min	Accident
Traveling 6 min by canoe	Accident
Traveling 10 miles by bicycle	Accident
Traveling 30–60 miles by car	Accident
Flying 1000 miles by jet	Accident
Flying 6000 miles by jet	Cancer caused by cosmic radiation
Living 2 mo in Denver	Cancer caused by cosmic radiation
Living 2 mo in an average city	Cancer caused by natural radioactivity
Being a man age 60 for 20 min	Illness
One chest x-ray taken in a good hospital	Cancer caused by radiation
Living 2 mo with a cigarette smoker	Cancer, heart disease
Eating 40 tsp of peanut butter	Liver cancer caused by aflatoxin B
Drinking Miami drinking water for 1 yr	Cancer caused by chloroform
Drinking 30 cans (12 oz) of diet soda	Cancer caused by saccharin
Living 5 yr at site boundary of a typical nuclear power plant in the open	Cancer caused by radiation
Drinking 1000 soft drinks from recently banned (24 oz) plastic bottles	Cancer from acrylonitrile monomer
Living 20 yr near PVC plant	Cancer caused from vinyl chloride (1976 standard)
Living 150 yr within 20 miles of a nuclear power plant	Cancer caused by radiation
Eating 100 charcoal-broiled steaks	Cancer from benzopyrene
Risk of accident by living within 5 miles of a nuclear reactor for 50 yr	Cancer caused by radiation

From Pochin E: Why be quantitative about radiation risk estimates? NCRP Annual Meeting. Crystal City, MD: NCRP, 1978; Cohen EL, Lee IS: A catalog of risks. Health Phys 1979;36:707–722; Wilson R: Analyzing the daily risks of life. Technol Rev 1979;81(4):40.

immediately. Covello and others have pointed out that there are some more specific factors that influence how people perceive risk.[8] In general, hazards are regarded as having higher risk if they are unfamiliar, poorly understood, involuntary, irreversible, affect children, may be associated with potentially unethical activities (such as war), and those that have a potential for inequitable distribution of benefits and risks. Other factors leading to high-risk perception occur if the risk is uncontrollable by the person, involves the person or their family directly, has identifiable victims, has immediate effects, has catastrophic potential, may affect future generations, has poorly defined benefits, is associated with institutions that are not trusted, or receives a lot of media attention. Slovic asked North Americans to rate 90 hazards on a set of 18 dimensions.[9] From the resulting data he was able to plot a cognitive map (Fig. 11-1), which to a large extent corroborates Covello's observations.

The presence of alternatives also plays a significant role in acceptability. If there are no practical alternatives in sight, many adverse conditions are easily accepted. Along the same line, whether the exposure to the noxious agent is essential or a luxury (voluntary or involuntary) is usually factored into acceptability. On one hand, food additives and cosmetics are usually regarded as luxuries, and dangers associated with them are easily regarded as being unsafe. On the other hand, the carcinogenic potential of many pharmaceuticals is often deemed acceptable if the pharmaceutical is essential to the person at a given time. Whether the expected consequences are reversible also has some bearing on acceptability; people may easily accept a risk if, when the adverse effect occurred, it could be reversed. On a larger societal scale, other factors are considered, and they may be more important than those normally factored in by the individual.[10] These have been well described by Lowrance.[1] One guide to acceptability on this larger scale is "reasonableness." This criterion is often included in various safety statements, although it is rarely, if ever, defined. Customs of usage and prevailing professional practice also are guides to acceptability; even though adverse effects may be manifested at some later time, the prevailing professional opinion is usually deemed to be acceptable. In the same manner, exposure to an agent in relation to natural background is sometimes proffered as a guide to acceptability; for example, if a particular radiation exposure adds a negligible amount of radiation dose to the population in comparison with natural background, this relationship is often an argument for acceptability. Finally, whether something will be used as intended or is likely to be misused is also often taken into account. One of the major public fears of nuclear power plants centers around the question of sabotage by terrorist groups. Thus, misuse or diversion from an original purpose may lead some people to decide that a certain activity is not acceptable. There are two major areas in which perception of measured risks becomes very distorted. These deal with what may be referred to as "dread" hazards and to crisis situations. Radiation certainly is regarded by some as a mysterious and dreaded hazard; this aura may be because radiation is difficult to perceive with the senses. Interestingly enough, the same type of radiation from different sources may be regarded very differently. For example, natural background radiation is rarely regarded as a dreaded hazard, whereas a much smaller amount of the same type of radiation from

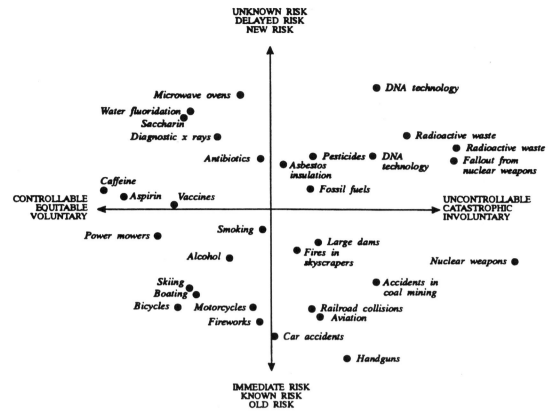

Figure 11-1 • Cognitive map of hazards derived from interviews conducted in North America. (From Slovic, P: Perception of risk. Science 1987;236(4799):280–285.)

nuclear weapons or from a nuclear power plant can cause a much higher level of anxiety. An atmosphere of crisis often surrounds acceptance of risk and safety problems. The crisis may either be media-generated or real.

The management of nuclear waste is an issue sometimes clouded by the media, politics, and perceived, rather than measured, risks. The issues, of course, relate to disposal of any potentially toxic substance and a predominant public attitude that is often referred to as "NIMBY" or "not in my backyard." In a large survey by Flynn et al., the closest median distance that most people were willing to live to a nuclear waste repository was 200 miles.[11] This was twice the distance that they wanted to be from a chemical waste landfill, and this is three to eight times the distance that they were willing to locate relative to an oil refinery, nuclear power plant, or pesticide manufacturing plant. Slovic et al. pointed out that in addition to standard concerns, nuclear waste conjures up fear and dread due to radioactivity, links with the use of nuclear weapons, and distrust due to reports of mishandling of radioactive wastes at the nation's military weapons facilities and laboratories.[12] It is also clear that people's attitude toward a potentially hazardous installation depends on whether the facility already exists. People living near an existing hazardous plant tend to consider the risks to be less probable and less serious than those living farther away.

The opposite is true when a hazardous facility is being planned. For these, opposition is greatest for the persons living closest to the designated site. Few people (1%) associate radiation with the natural environment.[13] After recognition of potentially high radon levels in some homes, there was an attempt by many government agencies to conduct awareness campaigns and to set action levels for mitigation. These efforts allowed a number of studies to be performed relative to perception and action of the public relative to this "radiation risk." A number of these studies were reviewed by Fisher, and the results show that people are generally apathetic.[14] Even though the risk may involve themselves and their families, few people test for radon, and even fewer take any remedial action. A number of factors involved in the apathy appear to be personal cost to take action, delayed rather than immediate effect, apparently equitable exposure, and the natural origin of the radiation. Finally, radon is part of one's home, which is often recognized as a safe place. The longer a person has lived in a home, the less likely he or she is to be concerned about radon.[15] Burger et al. pointed out that even though there are persons who hunt and fish near nuclear sites, only about half feel the game or fish are actually not safe to eat.[16]

The individual's perception of radiation undoubtedly deals with most of the factors mentioned in a complex way.

Once this aspect is considered, actual perception can be measured and compared to the perceived risk from other activities (Table 11-5). In this table, estimated numbers of annual deaths for different activities are shown in parentheses, and activities are ranked in decreasing order of hazard. Although the number of deaths attributed to some activities is difficult to estimate and the range of uncertainty is quite large, the table is quite useful in providing a ranking in terms of risk. Ranking of the risks associated with the various activities by three groups of educated persons revealed large discrepancies between reality and perception. Nuclear power, pesticides, and spray cans have been highlighted in the news at various times. The survey showed that all of the population groups substantially overestimated the actual risk for these items.[17,18] Both the League of Women Voters and college students ranked nuclear power as a risk greater than smoking, alcoholic beverages, and motor vehicles. The timing of such questionnaires with respect to current areas highlighted in the news media and the way in which questions are posed in the survey may substantially affect the result obtained. Thus, some skepticism is warranted in interpreting such survey results.

Slovic et al. performed a large survey in Canada about the perception of risks to health.[19] The interview sample included 1500 persons who were matched to the 1992 Canadian population in terms of household size, community size, age, and gender (Fig. 11-2). It is clear that females generally perceive risks to be higher than do males. There was much less difference relative to age group although older individuals tended to rate a health risk as high (such as asbestos). Another interesting finding was that risks were perceived to be higher by persons with only a high-school education than by those with a college degree (Fig. 11-3). The survey also has useful information about the sources of information Canadians use to learn about health risks and their confidence in those sources. As might be expected, about 90% indicate that they get much or a fair amount of information from the media, and about 70% thought it was reasonably reliable. About 65% got information from medical doctors, who were regarded as reliable by 90% of persons. About 20% to 40% got information from various government agencies and 25% to 75% thought it was reliable (depending on the agency). Private industry fared the worst. Only 20% of persons used this as an information source, and only 25% thought it was reliable. Political association was also an interesting issue. In general, people voting for conservative parties tended to minimize risks, while persons voting for left-wing parties tended to magnify risks. Mihai et al. found similar results in a recent Romanian study.[20]

Another approach to the perception of risk was outlined by Watson and Walsh.[21] The specific questions posed to members of health physics organizations throughout the United States and Canada was, "If you had to choose between loss of a limb(s) or part of a limb

Table 11-5 • Risk: How People See It (Ranking of Hazards by Three Different Groups)

Activity and Deaths per Year (Estimate)	League of Women Voters	College Students	Business and Professional Club Members
1. Smoking (150,000)	4	3	4
2. Alcoholic beverages (100,000)	6	7	5
3. Motor vehicles (50,000)	2	5	3
4. Handguns (17,000)	3	2	1
5. Electric power (14,000)	18	19	19
6. Motorcycles (3000)	5	6	2
7. Swimming (3000)	19	30	17
8. Surgery (2800)	10	11	9
9. X-rays (2300)	22	17	24
10. Railroads (1950)	24	23	20
11. General (private) aviation (1300)	7	15	11
12. Large construction (1000)	12	14	13
13. Bicycles (1000)	16	24	14
14. Hunting (800)	13	18	10
15. Home appliances (200)	29	27	27
16. Firefighting (195)	11	10	6
17. Police work (160)	8	8	7
18. Contraceptives (150)	20	9	22
19. Commercial aviation (130)	17	16	18
20. Nuclear power (100)	1	1	8
21. Mountain climbing (30)	15	22	12
22. Power mowers (24)	27	28	25
23. High school and college football (23)	23	26	21
24. Skiing (18)	21	25	16
25. Vaccinations (10)	30	29	29
26. Food coloring*	26	20	30
27. Food preservatives*	25	12	28
28. Pesticides*	9	4	15
29. Prescription antibiotics*	28	21	26
30. Spray cans*	14	13	23

*Data on mortality from these sources are too uncertain to estimate.
When the 3 groups were asked to rank 30 products or activities from most to least risky, they gave the order listed.
Adapted from Slovic P, Flynn J, Mertz C, et al: Health risk perception in Canada: Report for the Department of Health and Welfare, Ottawa, Department of National Health and Welfare, 1992; Sinclair WK: Effects of low-level radiation and comparative risk. Radiology 1981;138:1–8; Howard N, Antilla S: What price safety? The zero risk debate. Duns Review 1979;114: 48–57.

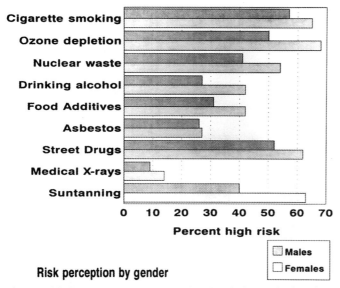

Risk perception by gender

Figure 11-2 • Perception of some health risks by gender based on interviews conducted in Canada. (From Slovic P, et al: Health risk perception in Canada. Ottawa, Department of Health and Welfare, 1992.)

(e.g., by amputation) and a delivered acute dose of whole-body radiation (uniform energy deposition), what is the highest dose you would accept in lieu of the specified injury?" The replies are shown in Figure 11-4. The data indicated a reasonable trend with an expected increase of acceptable equivalent exposure as the severity of the bodily injury increased. The distribution in extremes of the replies is shown in Table 11-6. The results here are

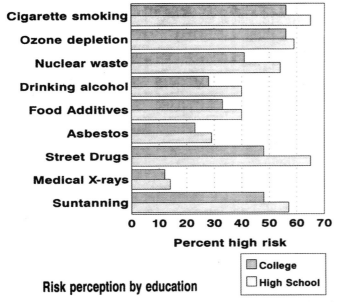

Risk perception by education

Figure 11-3 • Perception of some health risks by education based on interviews conducted in Canada. (From Slovic P, et al: Health risk perception in Canada. Ottawa, Department of Health and Welfare, 1992.)

rather surprising and disquieting, considering that the population questioned was supposedly knowledgeable concerning radiation effects. If one examines the first line, it is clear that some people (0.67%) would rather lose a small finger than incur a clinically insignificant whole-body dose of 0.05 Gy. The only suggested somatic effect at this dose level is a lifetime risk of radiogenic cancer of about 1 chance in 2000, compared with a "normal" chance of dying from cancer of about 1 in 5. The upper end of the distribution is equally disturbing; a significant number of respondents (greater than 6%) indicated that they would rather be exposed to 3 Gy than lose a finger. It certainly seems strange that some supposedly knowledgeable health physicists would prefer a radiation dose that carries a 1 in 5 chance of losing one's life over loss of a finger by amputation.

In a similar manner many people refuse a medically indicated x-ray examination because of the fear of carcinogenesis. Webster has given conservative estimates of this risk for several examinations.[22] The risk of leukemia or carcinogenesis is extremely low compared with the risk of "spontaneous" cancer. Broadbent and Hubbard published a short review of perception of radiation risk in relation to radiology and radiologic practice.[23] Patients and the population at large cannot easily be blamed for not understanding risks associated with medical uses of radiation. The public expects that physicians and health professionals will know and be able to communicate potential risks of the radiation procedures they are ordering or performing.[24] Among U.S. physicians and even radiologists the actual risk is very poorly understood.[25,26] Even among U.S. military medical personnel the fear of radiation and poor knowledge base has been a cause for concern.[27,28]

Potential risks following in utero radiation are discussed in detail in Chapter 8. Bentur et al. reported on a Motherisk program for counseling about diagnostic radiation exposure during pregnancy.[29] Fifty exposed women were compared with 48 women exposed to nonteratogenic drugs and chemicals. Prior to counseling, the women exposed to radiation assigned a teratogenic risk to themselves of about 25%. Counseling was effective in preventing unnecessary terminations of pregnancy. Perceptions about the risks of in utero radiation exposure after the Chernobyl accident in 1986 were thought to result in a large number of unnecessary abortions in Western European countries. This aspect was examined in the former Soviet Union by the International Chernobyl Project.[30] No increase in abortion rate was identified in the official statistics; however, the abortion rate was very high to begin with (70 to 100 abortions per year per 1000 fertile-age females) because abortion was the major form of birth control. It appeared that the average woman had about 6 to 8 abortions during her fertile life as a means of birth control even before the accident. It was clear, however, that the birth rates in highly contaminated

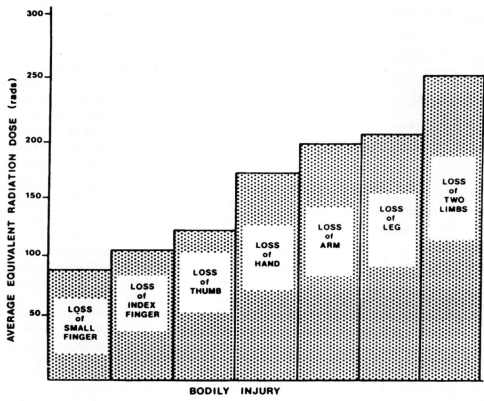

Figure 11-4 • Average equivalent acceptable exposure in lieu of various bodily injuries. (From Watson DA, Walsh ML: The perception of harm from radiation exposure. Health Phy 1980;38:845–846.)

settlements decreased in the first years after the accident, but they returned to preaccident levels by 1989 or 1990, even though the contamination was still present and relatively unchanged.

PSYCHOLOGICAL EFFECTS

The accident at the Three Mile Island (TMI) Nuclear Generating Station is an example of inappropriate responses fueled by the media; for example, in one incident, medical personnel refused to attend to patients in a nursing home, who subsequently were evacuated because of lack of medical attention. The maximum radiation dose at the plant boundary for the course of the entire "accident" was less than 1 mGy, substantially lower than the dose from an abdominal x-ray. In contrast, during actual crisis situations, very large risks are often accepted. In the SL-1 reactor accident in Idaho Falls and at Chernobyl, workers were willing to accept doses well in excess of 250 mGy to retrieve their comrades. The psychologic response to nuclear reactor accidents has been studied at Three Mile Island and Chernobyl. Baum et al. pointed

Table 11-6 • Distribution of Acceptable Doses versus Bodily Injuries

Bodily Injury	PERCENTAGE OF REPLIES TO WHOLE-BODY DOSE (Sv)							
	0.005	0.05	0.25	0.5	1.0	1.5	2.0	2.5
Loss of small finger	0.67	8.8	25.2	19.7	22.5	12.2	4.8	6.1
Loss of index finger		4.0	22.2	14.1	27.5	15.4	8.1	8.7
Loss of thumb		2.0	18.0	15.3	22.0	13.3	18.0	11.3
Loss of hand		2.0	3.3	17.3	12.7	20.0	17.3	27.3
Loss of arm			2.8	7.6	17.9	13.8	22.1	35.9
Loss of leg			2.8	4.2	15.4	13.3	25.2	39.2
Loss of two limbs			2.8	2.8	4.9	7.8	19.7	62.0

Adapted from Watson DA and Walsh ML: The perception of harm from radiation exposure. Health Phys 1980;38(5):845–846, Slovic P: Perception of risk. Science 1987;236:280–285.

out that the suddenness, personal uncontrollability, lack of reliable information, and an accident, in what was thought to be a relatively safe technology, all contributed to problems.[31] However, while there was stress in the local community during and immediately after the TMI accident, this dissipated rapidly, with only a few manifestations present a year later. This is in contrast to the reactions at Chernobyl.[30] Five years after the accident, the majority of people attributed almost all health problems to the accident. Persons living in contaminated villages reported the following symptoms: fatigue, 89%; headache, 81%; and depression, 42%. Of interest was that in clean villages the percentages were also high and were reported as 81%, 77%, and 42%, respectively. In the contaminated villages, 45% of persons thought they had an illness due to radiation, and another 46% were not sure. In the clean settlements, 30% of persons thought they had an illness due to radiation, and another 44% were not sure. The fatigue issue is discussed in Chapter 6.

Fatigue was a common complaint in the atomic bomb survivors but appears to have a large psychologic component, because the frequency of complaints was not found to be dose-related, and it was present in a large number of persons in the Adult Health Study Sample who received 0 dose.[32] An additional follow-up study concluded that the atomic bomb radiation had no apparent effect on cognitive function[33] although psychological effects were more prevalent among those who suffered from acute radiation effects and who were in the city at the time of the bombing.[34]

Existing data show that the psychological effects can extend well beyond any measurable radiation or contamination. The psychological responses to accidents at TMI and Chernobyl, as well as a number of other radiation accidents, were published in a book edited by Ricks et al.[35] Unfortunately, the papers were proffered and not peer-reviewed. Some of the included papers regarding TMI either do not have control groups[36] or do not give the sample size of the group studied.[37] In addition, some of the conclusions are conflicting. Data from the Chernobyl survivors of the acute radiation syndrome express fear and anxiety particularly relative to the potential long-term consequences.[38] Having examined a number of the patients ourselves, it appears that some have adapted very well and are leading productive lives, while others are satisfied with being classified as invalids. Much of this may relate to their personality type prior to the accident. The response to the Chernobyl accident has pointed out a few items that deserve more discussion.

The concept of social and media amplification has been studied in relation to other issues.[39] One theory that has been proposed for amplification is the "availability heuristic," which suggests that a direct or recent experience of a single accident results in an exaggerated assessment of the likelihood of similar accidents in the future. The media coverage of an accident stimulates "availability." Media attention and unsubstantiated claims about health effects were widely disseminated after Chernobyl and may have made the population more stressed and caused more complaints to be registered and led to more trips to the doctor. This increase could then be reported in the media and lead to a cycle of amplifying concern. How much an effect this had is unknown; however, we cannot blame the media for everything. This phenomenon of amplification of risk perception did not occur when the residential radon issue was picked up by the media. Psychologists who examined the population around Chernobyl did not feel that the people suffered from an unreasonable fear of radiation or "radiophobia" but rather, that in addition to the accident, the population was involved in nationalism, perestroika, food shortages, media distortion, distrust of the government, economic hardships, as well as disruption of traditions and lifestyle.[40,41] While there was clearly psychologic stress associated with the accident, it was not thought that the population was suffering from post-traumatic stress disorder as defined by the American Psychiatric Association. Clear and concise communication of the risk and potential effects would have helped to alleviate some of the problems. This has been pointed out as a necessary ingredient in management of all risk communication.[42-44]

The 2006 Chernobyl Forum composed of all eight United Nations agencies (including the World Health Organization [WHO]), as well as the governments of Belarus, Russia, and the Ukraine, reached the conclusions set forth in the next six paragraphs.[45] Findings of stress symptoms, increased levels of depression, anxiety (including post-traumatic stress symptoms), and medically unexplained physical symptoms, were found in Chernobyl-exposed populations compared to controls.[46,47] Studies also found that exposed populations had anxiety symptom levels that were twice as high and they were three to four times more likely to report multiple, unexplained physical symptoms and subjective poor health.[48,49]

Mostly these mental health consequences in the general population were subclinical and did not reach the level of criteria for a psychiatric disorder.[48] Nevertheless, these subclinical symptoms had important consequences for health behavior, specifically, medical care use and adherence to safety advisories.[46] To some extent, these symptoms were driven by the belief that the people's health was adversely affected by the disaster and that they were diagnosed by a physician with a "Chernobyl-related health problem."[40,49,50]

In general, the findings on the psychological consequences of Chernobyl have been consistent with other exposure studies, such as research on the atomic bombings of Hiroshima and Nagasaki, the TMI accident, other neurotoxic exposures in work environments, and other toxic environmental contaminations.[33] Nevertheless, the context in which the Chernobyl accident occurred makes the findings difficult to interpret because of the complicated series of events unleashed by the accident, the multiple extreme stresses that occurred before and after the event, and the culture-specific ways of expressing distress. In addition, the affected population was officially given the label "Chernobyl victim," and frequently took on the role of "invalid" or disabled. It is well known that if a situation is perceived as real, it is likely to be real in its consequences. Thus, rather than perceiving themselves as "survivors," the affected population perceived themselves as "victims" and not strong or having control over their future.

The mental health impact of Chernobyl is the largest public health problem caused by the accident to date. The magnitude and scope of the disaster, the size of the affected population, and the long-term consequences make it, by far, the worst industrial disaster on record. Chernobyl unleashed a complex web of events and long-term difficulties, such as massive relocation, loss of economic stability, and long-term threats to health in current and, possibly, future generations, that resulted in an increased sense of anomie and diminished sense of physical and emotional balance. It may never be possible to disentangle the multiple Chernobyl stressors from those following in its wake, including the dissolution of the Soviet Union. However, the high levels of anxiety and medically unexplained physical symptoms continue to this day. The studies also reveal the importance of understanding the role of perceived threat to health in epidemiological studies of health effects. There is one recent report of increased suicide among Estonians who worked as recovery workers at Chernobyl.[51] The standardized mortality rate (SMR) was 1.32 (5% confidence interal [CI] 1.03 to 1.67) and continued for the study period of 17 years. There are no other reports of increased suicide in other Chernobyl-exposed populations nor have there been reports of increased suicide among atomic bomb survivors.

The Chernobyl accident had a serious impact on mental health and well-being in the general population. Importantly, however, it appears that this impact is demonstrable mainly at a subclinical level. Although the empirical studies do not support the view that the public anxiety bears a resemblance to clinical psychiatric disorders such as phobia or psychosis, the disaster did have a psychological effect that is not limited to mental health outcomes. It also has ramifications for other areas of subjective health and health-related behavior, especially reproductive health and medical service use, and the level of trust in authorities. Further, it may influence people's willingness to adopt safety guidelines issued by the authorities.

What the Chernobyl disaster clearly demonstrated is the central role of information and how it is communicated in the aftermath of radiation or toxicological incidents.[43] Nuclear activities in Western countries have also tended to be shrouded in secrecy. The Chernobyl experience has raised the awareness among disaster planners and health authorities that the dissemination of timely and accurate information by trusted leaders is of the greatest importance.

Psychological effects are clearly important with reference to terrorist events. These events are purposely designed to evoke fear and uncertainty. Addition of radiation or radioactivity to such an event can only be expected to heighten the psychological consequences. To date, no large-scale radiation terrorist events have occurred, but many groups and authors have stressed the lesson from Chernobyl and other events in terms of planning emergency response.[52–54]

Psychological effects also are important to consider when proposals are made to conduct medical monitoring or screening of populations that were exposed to ionizing radiation.[45,55] Some authors suggest that instituting a screening program may reduce psychological stress, however, there is little or no evidence to support such claims. In fact, such programs may increase stress and psychological effects. There are not only stigmatization issues related to having been identified as "exposed" but also worries about being a person identified as "at risk." Any medical monitoring or screening program also must consider as a cost the well-documented issues related to false positive results when multiple tests are being performed. False positive results usually occur between 5% to 15% of the time depending on the test. In addition to false positive results, there are incidental findings found (e.g., on 10% to 50% of CT scans), which may require additional workup and most of which are of no clinical importance. Of interest is a 2006 report of the National Research Council (NRC), which recommended screening for depression in persons exposed to ionizing radiation due to nuclear testing or who are/were uranium miners or millers.[56] This recommendation was not based on any scientific evidence related to radiation effects, but rather as a social justice issue and as an easy and effective test to do on a condition that is common in many populations.

The importance and consideration of psychological effects has also been stressed during the medical uses of ionizing radiation. Usually there is little concern about radiation effects when patients receive diagnostic medical x-ray examinations, however, patients and their families become much more concerned when patients receive larger radiation doses associated with radiotherapy.[57] This issue becomes even more acute when patients are either injected with, or ingest, large amounts of unsealed radionuclides (such as iodine 131) for therapeutic purposes. Patients are usually told that the treatments are "safe" but then they are often put in strict isolation in a hospital for a period of days. They do express their confusion at the seemingly conflicting actions but no definite long-lasting adverse psychological effects have been demonstrated.

SOCIAL DECISIONS

After risk has been measured, and individuals have perceived the risk and appraised it according to ambient and personal factors, they must decide whether to accept or reject the risk. Who decides what level of risk is acceptable, both for the individual and for society? Expressed another way, what standard should be established, and how much harm can be tolerated? There are national and international groups that deal with radiological protection, including the NCRP and the ICRP. Most of these organizations develop and recommend radiation protection standards. Generally, the standards are chosen to keep the risk as low as is reasonably achievable under the circumstances that necessitate the practice. The ICRP indicates that all the practices involving radiation exposure should be justified by the benefits that they convey. Occupational limits recommended by these organizations are not decided solely on radiobiological issues but also include factors to ensure that the total fatality rate in radiation-associated industries is comparable with that of existing "safe" industries. This usually corresponds to a fatality rate of less than 100 deaths in 1 million persons annually. Once exposure limits have been recommended, they are usually reviewed and adopted by governmental regulatory agencies. The "recommended" limits then become regulations. Throughout the governmental acceptance process, cost versus benefit may be discussed; however, the benefits are often so difficult to measure that they are usually excluded from consideration. In the United States, the governmental philosophy for radiation protection practices has been to keep the doses "as low as reasonably achievable" (ALARA); this has been defined as meaning that the doses should be kept "as low as reasonably achievable, taking into account the state of technology and economics of improvement in relation to benefit to the public health and safety as well as inclusion of other societal and socioeconomic considerations." This rather complex and elusive philosophy is also difficult to define, but in theory it has been used. Current radiation dose limits in the United States are listed in Chapter 2. At the point when "regulatory" limits are being considered, there is usually an opportunity for public input. Although individuals may express their views, the majority of input is provided by position or organizational advocates. Sometimes, these advocates are less than honest in presenting the measured risk. They do, however, perform an important function of providing input that indicates the perception of risk by various groups. Public hearings are often made complex and difficult to understand when participants begin to debate the validity of various radiation protection models and concepts such as hormesis[58] or synergistic effects.[59] If public perception is substantially

different from measured risk, the regulatory limit-setting process may include reaction from public interest groups and lobbyists. Finally, after the regulations have been issued, the judicial systems and courts are the forum available to the public for appealing what is considered to be an unacceptable regulation or risk. Comparison of risks due to chemical exposures and ionizing radiation was examined by the NCRP.[60] In broad terms, the principles of assessment can be applied to both. It is interesting to compare the regulatory decisions of limits related to chemical carcinogens with those for ionizing radiation. As with radiation, it does appear that the model used by the public to judge chemical exposure risk is substantially different from that used by toxicologists.[61]

Travis et al. reviewed 132 decisions of the federal government related to carcinogenic factors.[62] Usually three measures of risk are considered: individual risk, size of population exposed, and population risk. Individual risk is an upper-limit estimate of the probability that the highest exposed person will develop cancer as a result of lifetime exposure. The exposed population size is needed to determine population risk, which is an upper-limit measure of the number of additional cases of cancer in the exposed population. Two additional terms are used by regulators: de manifestis and de minimus risk. The former refers to a level of risk or danger that is easily recognized by a person of ordinary intelligence; the latter term refers to a level of risk that is below regulatory concern. In between these levels, judgment is needed to establish exposure limits. Travis et al. also pointed out that if one examines preregulatory risk levels, virtually every chemical with an individual cancer risk above 4×10^{-3} (1 in 250) with chronic exposure was regulated, whereas if the risk was below 1×10^{-6} (1 in a million), no regulatory action was taken.[62] This de minimus risk corresponds to about the same cancer risk that might be projected from a dose of 20 μSv. This is close to the range of what the NCRP has referred to as a negligible risk level (NRL) of 10 μSv annual effective dose per source.[63]

Population size and aggregate harm have modified regulatory decisions somewhat. The U.S. Environmental Protection Agency has declined to regulate natural radionuclide emissions from elemental phosphorus plants. The individual risk of 1×10^{-3} for workers only resulted in a predicted 0.06 cancer deaths per year due to the small size of the exposed population, and, thus, the cost of regulation was not justified. Since 1983, the de minimus level used by the government for exposure of small populations is an individual lifetime risk of 1×10^{-4}. For most chemical exposure limits, the federal agencies usually assume a maximum exposure and a linear-no-threshold dose-response function. This is considered to usually overestimate risk and is the same approach used by many radiation protection advisory groups. There are many areas, however, where chemicals and ionizing radiation are regulated differently.

Chemical carcinogens are regulated individually. Radiation is regulated as a cumulative dose or risk from a number of sources. Chemicals are also regulated on the basis of quantities released into the environment, whereas radiation is regulated by absorbed dose to a person. Travis et al. also examined the relative stringency of chemical and radiation regulations.[64] Often, a much wider margin of risk is accepted between public and occupational risk for chemicals than for radiation. As an example, the postregulatory public lifetime risk limit for benzene is about 80 fatal cancers per 100,000 and for occupational exposure it is 15,200 per 100,000. This difference is a factor of about 200, while the range allowed for the difference between the dose of ionizing radiation for the public and the dose for the occupationally exposed worker is in the range of a factor of 10 to 20. Results of comparison with chemical regulations show that estimated maximum public lifetime cancer risk for any given exposure to ionizing radiation is about 2 to 21 times higher than the median upper-bound lifetime public cancer risk to chemical carcinogens. Thus, if individuals are exposed to only one or two carcinogens then the nuclear industry is less controlled than the chemical industry; however if individuals are exposed to many chemical carcinogens then the nuclear industry is more tightly controlled.

SUMMARY

Perception and acceptance of risks are very complex problems. Risks are difficult to compare with one another because they differ in kind and circumstance. Because they can be easily measured, the usual measure of risk that most researchers use is time lost from work, cancer incidence, or fatality rate. These have some inherent problems, but they are probably the best parameters available. Even though risks can be measured, individual and public perceptions of risks and safety are likely to be markedly different from those measured by experts. Such judgments are colored by the person's general viewpoint of the world, society, surrounding circumstances, attention in the media, and other related perceptions about the activity itself. Stigma, perceived risk, and potential adverse economic issues are very relevant issues to be considered.[11] The decision to expose an individual or society to a given level of risk usually results from recommendations by recognized scientific committees and commissions. Such "recommended limits" are turned into "regulatory limits" by governmental agencies. The public has a chance to affect these decisions, either personally or through advocates and lobbyists. Once the regulations are in place, the judicial system becomes the final arbiter of acceptable risk.

Psychological effects have been observed following radiation exposure and even to perceived radiation exposure when none actually occurred. These effects typically are of a subclinical nature and usually result in more self-reported illnesses and hospital admissions even though no actual change in disease incidence is epidemiologically evident. Persons with a prior history of mental illness or depression appear to be at greater risk of psychological consequences as are females who were pregnant during exposure, mothers of young children, or first responders.

REFERENCES

1. Lowrance, W., Of acceptable risk. In Science and the Determination of Safety. 1976, Los Altos, Calif: W. Kaufman.
2. International Commission on Radiological Protection (ICRP), 1990 Recommendations of the ICRP. Ann ICRP, 1991. 21(1–3): 1–201.
3. National Council on Radiation Protection and Measurements (NCRP). Radiation science and the public: Can the gap be bridged? In 29th Annual Meeting. 1994. Crystal City, Md: NCRP.
4. Pochin, E. Why be quantitative about radiation risk estimates? Annual Meeting. 1978. Crystal City, Md: National Council on Radiation Protection and Measurements.
5. International Commission on Radiological Protection (ICRP), Problems involved in developing an index of harm. 1977, Oxford: Pergamon Press.
6. International Commission on Radiological Protection (ICRP), Quantitative bases for developing a unified index of harm. Ann ICRP, 1985. 15(3):1–64.
7. Cohen, B.L., Catalog of risks extended and updated. Health Phys, 1991. 61(3):317–335.
8. Covello, V., Social and behavioral research on risk: Uses in risk management decision making. NATO ASI series G, vol. 4. *Environmental impact risk assessment: Technology and risk analysis*, V. Covello, ed. 1985, Berlin: Springer-Verlag.
9. Slovic, P., Perception of risk. Science, 1987. 236(4799):280–285.
10. Southwood, R., Risks from radiation: Perception and reality: The 1993 Crookshank Lecture. Clin Oncol, 1993. 5:302–308.
11. Flynn, J., et al., Evaluations of Yucca mountain: Survey findings. 1990, Carson City, Nev: Nevada Nuclear Waste Project.
12. Slovic, P., J. Flynn, and M. Layman, Perceived risk, trust and the politics of nuclear waste. Science, 1991. 254:1603–1607.
13. Brown, J. and H. White, The public's understanding of radiation and nuclear waste. J Soc Radiol Prot, 1987. 7:61–70.
14. Fisher, A. and F. Johnson, Radon risk communication research: Practical lessons. J Air Waste Management Assoc, 1990. 40:738–739.
15. Johnson, F. and R. Luken, Radon risk information and voluntary protection: Evidence from a natural experiment. Risk Anal, 1987. 7:97–107.
16. Burger, J., J. Sanchez, et al., Risk perception, federal spending, and the Savannah River Site: Attitudes of hunters and fisherman. Risk Anal, 1997. 17(3):313–320.
17. Sinclair, W.K., Effects of low-level radiation and comparative risk. Radiology, 1981. 138(1):1–9.
18. Howard, N. and S. Antilla, What price safety? The zero risk debate. Duns Review, 1979. 114:48–57.
19. Slovic, P., et al., Health risk perception in Canada. 1992, Ottawa: Department of Health and Welfare.
20. Mihai, L.T., et al., Ionizing radiation—Understanding and acceptance. Health Phys, 2005. 89(4):375–382.

21. Watson, D.A. and M.L. Walsh, The perception of harm from radiation exposure. Health Phys, 1980. 38(5):845–846.
22. Webster, E., Risks of diagnostic radiology: A physicist's viewpoint. Radiology, 1959. 72:493–507.
23. Broadbent, M. and L. Hubbard, Science and perception of radiation risk. Radiographics, 1992. 12:381–392.
24. Ludwig, R. and L. Turner, Effective patient education in medical imaging: Public perceptions of radiation exposure risk. J Allied Health, 2002. 31(3):159–164.
25. Correia, M.J., et al., Lack of radiological awareness among physicians working in a tertiary-care cardiological centre. Int J Cardiol, 2005. 103(3):307–311.
26. Lee, C.I., et al., Diagnostic CT scans: Assessment of patient, physician, and radiologist awareness of radiation dose and possible risks. Radiology, 2004. 231(2):393–398.
27. Pastel, R. and J. Mulvaney, Fear of radiation in U.S. military medical personnel. Mil Med, 2001. 166(suppl 2):S80–S82.
28. Landauer, M., E. Young, and A.L. Hawley, Physiological and psychological impact of low-level radiation: An overview. Mil Med, 2002. 167(suppl 1):S141–S142.
29. Bentur, Y., N. Horlatsch, and G. Koren, Exposure to ionizing radiation during pregnancy: Perception of teratogenic risk and outcome. Teratology, 1991. 43(2):109–112.
30. International Atomic Energy Agency (IAEA), The International Chernobyl Project: Report of an international committee. 1991, Vienna: IAEA.
31. Baum, A., R. Gatchel, and M. Schaeffer, Emotional, behavioral and psychological effects of chronic stress at Three Mile Island. J Consult Clin Psychol, 1983. 51(4):565–572.
32. Yamada, M., K. Kodama, and F. Wong, The long term psychological sequelae of atomic bomb survivors in Hiroshima and Nagasaki. In The Medical Basis of Radiation Accident Preparedness. III. Proceedings of a Conference, December 5–7, 1990, Oak Ridge, Tennessee, R. Ricks, M. Berger, and F. M. O'Hara, Jr., eds. 1991, New York: Elsevier.
33. Yamada, M., et al., Study of cognitive function among the Adult Health Study (AHS) population in Hiroshima and Nagasaki. Radiat Res, 2002. 158(2):236–240.
34. Yamada, M. and S. Izumi, Psychiatric sequelae in atomic bomb survivors in Hiroshima and Nagasaki two decades after the explosions. Soc Psychiatry Psychiatr Epidemiol, 2002. 37(9):409–415.
35. Ricks, R.C., S.A. Fry, and U.S. Radiation Emergency Assistance Center/Training Site (REAC/TS), The medical basis for radiation accident preparedness. II. Clinical experience and follow-up since 1979. Proceedings of the Second International REAC/TS Conference on the medical basis for radiation accident preparedness, held October 20–22, 1988. 1990, New York: Elsevier, p. xli.
36. Bromet, E., Psychological effects of the radiation accident at TMI: The medical basis for radiation accident preparedness. III. The psychological perspective. Proceedings of a conference, December 5–7, 1990, Oak Ridge, Tennessee. R. Ricks, M. Berger, and F.J. O'Hara, eds. 1991, New York: Elsevier.
37. Collins, D., Stress at Three Mile Island: Altered perceptions, behaviors, and neuroendocrine measures: The medical basis for radiation accident preparedness. III. The psychological perspective. Proceedings of a conference, December 5–7, 1990, Oak Ridge Tennessee. R. Ricks, M. Berger, and F.J. O'Hara, eds. 1991, New York: Elsevier.
38. Chinkina, O., Psychological characteristics of patients exposed to accidental irradiation at the Chernobyl atomic power station: The medical basis for radiation accident preparedness. III. The psychological perspective. Proceedings of a conference, December 5–7, 1990, Oak Ridge Tennessee. R. Ricks, M. Berger, and F.J. O'Hara, eds. 1991, New York: Elsevier.
39. Kasperson, R., The social amplification of risk: A conceptual framework. Risk Anal, 1988. 8:177–187.
40. Havenaar, J., et al., Perception of risk and subjective health among victims of the Chernobyl disaster. Soc Sci Med, 2003. 56(3):569–572.
41. Pastel, R., Radiophobia: Long-term psychological consequences of Chernobyl. Mil Med, 2002. 167(suppl 1):S134–S136.
42. National Research Council (NRC), Improving risk communication. 1989: Washington, DC: N.A. Press.
43. Becker, S., Emergency communication and information issues in terrorist events involving radioactive materials. Biosecurity Bioterrorism: Biodefense Strategy, Prac Sci, 2004. 2:195–207.
44. Becker, S., Responding to the psychological effects of toxic disaster: Policy initiatives, constraints and challenges. In Toxic Turmoil: Psychological and Societal Consequences of Ecological Disasters, J. Havenaar, J. Cwikel, and E. Bromet, eds. 2002, New York: Plenum, pp. 199–216.
45. Chernobyl Forum and World Health Organization (WHO), Health effects of the Chernobyl accident and special health care programmes. 2005, Geneva: WHO.
46. Havenaar, J., et al., Health effects of the Chernobyl disaster: Illness or illness behavior? A comparative general health survey in two former Soviet regions. Environ Health Perspect, 1997. 105(suppl 6):S1533–S1537.
47. Bromet, E., et al., Children's well-being 11 years after the Chernobyl catastrophe. Arch Gen Psychiatry, 2000. 57:563–571.
48. Havenaar, J., et al., Long-term mental health effects of the Chernobyl disaster: An epidemiologic survey in two former Soviet regions. Am J Psychiatry, 1997. 154:1605–1607.
49. Bromet, E., et al., Somatic symptoms in women 11 years after the Chernobyl acident: Prevalence and risk factors. Environ Health Perspect, 2002. 110(suppl 4):S625–S629.
50. Havenaar, J., et al., Perception of risk and subjective health among victims of the Chernobyl disaster. Soc Sci Med, 2003. 56:569–572.
51. Rahu, K., et al., Suicide risk among Chernobyl cleanup workers in Estonia still increased: An updated cohort study. Ann Epidemiol, 2006. 16(12):917–919.
52. Becker, S., Meeting the threat of weapons of mass destruction terrorism: Toward a broader conception of consequence management. Mil Med, 2001. 166(suppl 12):S13–S16.
53. Valentin, J., Protecting people against radiation exposure in the event of a radiological attack. A report of the International Commission on Radiological Protection. Ann ICRP, 2005. 35(1):1–110.
54. National Council on Radiation Protection and Measurements (NCRP), Management of terrorist events involving radioactive material: Recommendations of the NCRP. NCRP report no. 138. 2001, Bethesda, Md: NCRP, p. xiii.
55. Mettler, F.A., et al., Potential radiation exposure in military operations: Protecting the soldier before, during, and after. 1999, Washington, DC: National Academy Press.
56. National Research Council (NRC), Assessment of the scientific information for the radiation exposure screening and education program. 2006, Washington DC: National Academy Press.
57. International Commission on Radiological Protection (ICRP), Release of patients after therapy with unsealed radionuclides. Ann ICRP, 2004. 34(2):1–79.
58. Flynn, J. and D. MacGregor, Commentary on hormesis and public risk communicaton; Is there a basis of public discussions? Hum Exp Toxicol, 2003. 22(1):31–34.
59. Hampson, S., et al., Lay understanding of synergistic risk: The case of radon and cigarrette smoking. Risk Anal, 1998. 18(3):343–350.
60. National Council on Radiation Protection and Measurements (NCRP), Comparative carcinogenicity of ionizing radiation and chemicals: Recommendations of the NCRP. NCRP report no. 96. 1989, Bethesda, Md: The Council, p. vii.

61. MacGregor, D.G., P. Slovic, and T. Malmfors, "How exposed is exposed enough?" Lay inferences about chemical exposure. Risk Anal, 1999. 19(4):649–659.

62. Travis, C.C., et al., Cancer risk management: A review of 132 federal regulatory decisions. Environ Sci Technol, 1987. 21:415–420.

63. National Council on Radiation Protection and Measurements (NCRP), *Limitation of exposure to ionizing radiation: Recommendations of the NRCP. NCRP report no. 116.* 1993, Bethesda, Md: The Council, p. vi.

64. Travis, C.C., S.R. Pack, and H.A. Hattemer-Frey, Is ionizing radiation regulated more stringently than chemical carcinogens? Health Phys, 1989. 56(4):527–531.

12 Hormesis

The term *hormesis* is used in a number of ways, but for purposes of radiation effects it generally refers to a process whereby low doses of radiation may result in beneficial or stimulatory effects. Another use of the term is a physiologic, or stimulatory, effect that cannot be anticipated by linear downward extrapolation from toxic levels of exposure.[1-4] Chapter 12 is placed intentionally at the end of the book because it deals with a concept that is controversial at best. It appears to have little use in radiation protection even though some authors suggest that as a result of hormesis, radiation protection standards should be relaxed.[5,6] At least the concept should be considered on an intellectual basis.[7,8]

Hormesis should be distinguished from the broader term of "adaptive responses," which have been found in some experimental systems. The term *adaptive response* refers to a reduced response to a second dose of radiation when the cells have been "primed" with an initial radiation dose. The reduced response may be in the form of DNA repair, transformation frequency, or cell lethality. This phenomenon is not found in all cells either in vivo or in vitro and there is considerable variability among individuals of the same species. The response requires initial priming doses above several tens of milligrays (mGy) and challenge doses on the order of 1 to 2 Gy. To date, no consistent reduction in tumor yield or immune effect has been identified in humans or animals attributable to an adaptive response.[9]

The most vocal proponent of the hormesis concept is Luckey, who wrote articles as well as a book on the topic.[10-14] He claims that minute doses of radiation benefit animal growth, development, fecundity, health, and longevity. He also states that there are specific improvements in neurologic function, survival of the young, wound healing, immune competence, resistance to infection, and protection from radiation morbidity and tumor induction. His book contains a large number of points selected from the scientific literature that are presented together to support his hypothesis of radiation hormesis. Obviously, in the statistical uncertainty, population variation, bias factors, and the data scatter present in many studies, there are points that by chance will occur below the expected effects. Selective presentation of these data points can cause the appearance of a beneficial effect.

In the book there are also misquotes and figures (that we do not recognize) ascribed to us in the first edition of this textbook. For a more balanced viewpoint, the reader is referred to an overview of an international conference on the topic published in *Health Physics*[8] and reports by United Nations Scientific Committee on Effects of Atomic Radiation (UNSCEAR)[15] and Biological Effects of Ionizing Radiations (BEIR) Committee VII.[9] The concept of hormesis has been applied over a wide variety of effects ranging from radiation stimulation of plant seed, increased fertility in animals, augmentation of the immune system, and others.[2,16-20]

In this chapter, effects on humans will be discussed. The pharmacologic and physiologic background of hormesis has been discussed by Furst and Totter.[21,22] In simplistic terms, the concept is not as foreign as it first may seem. There are chemicals that are used by us every day that have beneficial, and even necessary, effects at low doses but are toxic at high doses. Examples of such compounds are aspirin, vitamins, and trace metals. With ionizing radiation the situation is more complex because of the wide variety of tissues that can be affected by radiation, the different spatial distributions of energy with various radiations, and a myriad of other factors. For radiation it is probable that stimulatory or adaptive effects may occur in a number of different ways, and a unifying hypothesis or mechanism is not necessarily needed. In a few areas, such as with the immune system, augmentation can occur in specific circumstances where the biologic basis is plausible.

ENVIRONMENTAL EXPOSURES

The effect of natural background radiation and its relation to cancer incidence has been studied by a number of authors. Early studies in the United States seemed to suggest a hormetic effect, or at least there were areas of higher radiation background that had lower cancer incidence.[23,24] In a more recent article, Nambi et al. reported that in areas of India where radiation levels are elevated, cancer risk is reduced.[25] A number of other studies have emerged that have not found an inverse correlation and have pointed out the potential bias factors in such studies, including chemical pollution, dietary variations, different social habits, genetic differences, and others.[9,26–30]

Luckey uses other nondisease data relative to natural background to support hormesis.[12,13] He points out that Kerala, India (which has one of the highest natural background radiation levels in the world), has a higher fertility rate and a lower neonatal death rate than any other state in India. He also indicated that in high-background areas of China, women have had more children than control groups. Of course, there are large natural variations in these rates based on other factors such as incidence of infection, water supply, nutrition, and tradition. What these observations may represent is unclear; however, it is unlikely that the difference is related to radiation. There have been a large number of articles and television programs related to the reactor accident at Chernobyl. They suggest that there has been an increase in fetal malformations. Luckey points out that no evidence of an increase above control areas was reported and uses this as an argument for hormesis. The International Chernobyl Project,[31] UNSCEAR 2000,[32] the 2005 Chernobyl Forum,[33] and the BEIR VII[9] committees examined this issue and reported that no increase was identified but did not conclude that it was an argument in favor of hormesis. The Chernobyl accident also has been used as a platform for rather amazing statements relative to potential radiation carcinogensis. Luckey stated, "Radiation hormesis insures decreased cancer incidence and mortality in northern and eastern Europe compared with what those areas would have experienced without Chernobyl. If the exposures had been greater the biopositive effects would be more evident."[12] In other words, he believes that Chernobyl was good for the population of Europe.

ATOMIC BOMB SURVIVORS

In 1984 Stewart and Kneale reported a U-shaped dose-response curve for noncancer mortality in atomic bomb survivors.[34] Mine et al. also reported that Nagasaki atomic bomb survivors (not in the Radiation Effects Research Foundation [RERF] cohort) with doses in the intermediate dose range of 0.5 to 1.49 Gy had less noncancer disease than age-matched unexposed controls.[35] This was seen in males but not females. Whether these results are statistical aberrations, results of some selection bias, or due to other causes is unknown. Analysis of the RERF cohort by Shimizu et al. in 1991 showed a slight decrease in noncancer mortality for those over the age of 40 at the time of the bombing who were exposed to doses between 1 and 2 Gy.[36] When specific disease categories are examined, the decrease is related only to digestive and "other disease" categories. It is not seen for stroke, heart disease, respiratory disease, or cancer. Thus, as an argument for hormesis these data are at best inconsistent. In addition, more recent data suggest a possible increase in noncancer mortality over all age groups.[37,38] Whereas the vast majority of scientific literature shows dose-dependent increases in the cancer rate of the atomic bomb survivors, Luckey indicates that at doses in the range of 0.03 Gy there is less than expected cancer mortality.[12] Most scientists agree that the data below 0.10 Gy is statistically too weak to permit inferences. Kato et al. specifically examined the atomic bomb survivors in the less than 0.5 Gy group using the end points of cancer mortality, cancer incidence, frequency of chromosomal aberrations, and phytohemagglutinin response of peripheral lymphocytes, as well as frequency of mental retardation after in utero exposure.[39] In general, the dose-response relations for these indices of radiation damage were varied but failed to suggest the existence of radiation hormesis.[9] Changes in the immune system of atomic bomb survivors are discussed in Chapter 6. In general, no dose-related difference is seen in T-cell activity, but some data show a reduction in the number of T-cells in those who were over 30 years old at exposure and who received more than 1 Gy.[40] Studies of atomic bomb survivors who now reside in the United States show that several parameters of cellular immune function were enhanced in the exposed group compared with the nonexposed group.[41] The reason for this is obscure, and studies performed on A-bomb survivors residing in Hiroshima do not confirm this difference.[42]

OCCUPATIONAL EXPOSURE

As pointed out in the sections related to occupational exposure, workers typically show less mortality than would be expected in comparison with the general population. This is a well-recognized phenomenon in epidemiologic studies and is referred to as the "healthy worker effect." Luckey uses this as an argument for hormesis, but clearly sick persons are unlikely to work, with the result that workers tend to appear healthier than the population as a whole. As an example, Tietjen reported that the lung cancer mortality in the National Plutonium Workers Study is surprisingly low when compared with national averages.[43] He points out the difficulties that occur with selection bias, definition of exposure, and smoking. All of these confound the situation, and while the reason for the lower incidence of lung cancer remains a matter of speculation, this is not proof of the existence of a beneficial effect of plutonium. Matanoski et al. analyzed the mortality patterns of radiologists.[44] It is clear that early radiologists received high radiation doses and suffered from a higher incidence of leukemia and other tumors than nonradiologist physicians. Radiologists entering practice later have experienced lower mortality than other physicians (but only until they were 50 years old). A multitude of bias factors may account for this difference rather than hormesis.[9] The major issues are selection bias for entering radiology and the sedentary nature and lifestyle differences of the profession, all of which cannot be easily accounted for. Tuschl et al. reported that after ultraviolet irradiation, there is an increase in unscheduled DNA synthesis induced in cultured lymphocytes obtained from occupationally exposed persons.[45] They also reported a reduced rate of mitomycin C–induced sister chromatid exchanges in such cells.[46] More recently they investigated the profile of lymphocytic T-cells in the blood of occupationally exposed persons, in which no influence of very low radiation exposure was established.[47]

FUTURE RESEARCH

Evaluation of the concept of hormesis appears to center on the immune system and particularly on the role of lymphocytes.[48–55] Most of the data and reports are concerned with in vitro experiments and have not been shown to have significant clinical implications. Some of the most interesting areas of research are the experiments of Shadley et al., who showed that cultured human lymphocytes pretreated with 0.01 Gy of x-rays become somewhat refractory to the induction of chromatid deletions by subsequent doses of 1.5 Gy.[56–59] This adaptive response is also achieved by pretreatment with tritiated thymidine.[60] The magnitude of the effect is not only dependent on dose but dose rate as well. The overall importance of this adaptive response has been put into question by some work of Bosi et al.[61] They examined the adaptive response using lymphocytes from different individuals and found that in some persons, there was no adaptive response, in others an increased synergistic response, and in some an adaptive response. In another different type of cell culture experiment, dealing with potential hormetic effects, Watanabe et al. reported that human embryo fibroblast-like cells had a prolonged in vitro life span after low-dose gamma irradiation.[62]

SUMMARY

With the vast scientific literature on the effects of ionizing radiation, clearly there are instances in which the potential effects of low-dose radiation are not identified. In addition to variability in populations, statistical uncertainties, potential bias factors, and chance, on one hand there will be instances in which there was less effect than predicted. This is all understandable without invoking a unifying hypothesis of hormesis. On the other hand, there are biologically plausible instances in which there may be regulatory processes in the body with the suppressor and augmentation portion being of different radiosensitivities. With the immune system, there are specific circumstances in which immune augmentation may occur transiently. At the present time, none of the observed effects have been proven to be of sufficient magnitude to alter radiation protection limits or to be of much use in the clinical arena. The BEIR VII report indicates that on the basis of current information, the assumption is unwarranted that any stimulatory effects of low doses of ionizing radiation substantially reduce long-term deleterious radiation effects in humans.[9]

REFERENCES

1. Koppenol, W. and P. Bounds, Hormesis. Science, 1989. 245:311.
2. Calabrese, E.J. and L.A. Baldwin, Radiation hormesis: The demise of a legitimate hypothesis. Hum Exp Toxicol, 2000. 19(1):76–84.
3. Calabrese, E.J. and L.A. Baldwin, Radiation hormesis: Its historical foundations as a biological hypothesis. Hum Exp Toxicol, 2000. 19(1):41–75.
4. Calabrese, E.J. and L.A. Baldwin, Tales of two similar hypotheses: The rise and fall of chemical and radiation hormesis. Hum Exp Toxicol, 2000. 19(1):85–97.
5. Loken, M.K. and L.E. Feinendegen, Radiation hormesis: Its emerging significance in medical practice. Invest Radiol, 1993. 28(5):446–450.
6. Cohen, B.L., Cancer risk from low-level radiation. AJR Am J Roentgenol, 2002. 179(5):1137–1143.
7. Sagan, L.A., What is hormesis and why haven't we heard about it before? Health Phys, 1987. 52(5):521–525.
8. Sagan, L.A., Radiation hormesis, overview of an international conference held in Oakland, CA, August 14–16, 1985. Health Physics, 1987. 52:517–680.
9. National Research Council (NRC), Committee on the Biological Effects of Ionizing Radiations (BEIR), Health risks from exposure to low levels of ionizing radiation. BEIR VII. 2006: Washington, DC: NRCUSNA Press.
10. Luckey, T.D., Beneficial physiologic effects of ionizing radiation. Strahlenschutz Forsch Prax, 1985. 25:184–196.
11. Luckey, T.D., Physiological benefits from low levels of ionizing radiation. Health Phys, 1982. 43(6):771–789.
12. Luckey, T.D., Radiation hormesis. 1991, Boca Raton, Fla: CRC Press.
13. Luckey, T.D., The evidence for radiation hormesis. 21st Century Sci Technol, 1996. 9:12–20.
14. Luckey, T.D., Nurture with ionizing radiation: A provocative hypothesis. Nutr Cancer, 1999. 34(1):1–11.
15. United Nations Scientific Committee on the Effects of Atomic Radiation (UNSCEAR), Sources and effects of ionizing radiation: UNSCEAR 1994 report to the General Assembly, with scientific annexes. 1994, New York: United Nations.
16. Calabrese, E., Risk communication and the challenge of hormesis. Hum Exp Toxicol, 2003. 22(1):1.
17. Calabrese, E.J., Should hormesis be the default model in risk assessment? Hum Exp Toxicol, 2005. 24(5):243.
18. Calabrese, E.J. and R.R. Cook, Hormesis: How it could affect the risk assessment process. Hum Exp Toxicol, 2005. 24(5):265–270.
19. Callahan, B.G., Can hormesis be a default for dose-response? Hum Exp Toxicol, 2005. 24(5):271–273.
20. Pickrell, J.A. and F.W. Oehme, Invited response to definition of hormesis (E.J. Calabrese and L.A. Baldwin). Hum Exp Toxicol, 2002. 21(2):107–109; discussion, 113–114.
21. Furst, A., Hormetic effects in pharmacology: Pharmacological inversions as prototypes for hormesis. Health Phys, 1987. 52(5):527–530.

22. Totter, J.R., Physiology of the hormetic effect. Health Phys, 1987. 52(5):549–551.

23. Frigerio, N. and R. Stowe, Carcinogenic and genetic hazard from background radiation. In Proceedings on Biological Effects of Low-Level Irradiation Pertinent to Protection of Man and his Environment, vol. 2. 1976, Vienna: IAEA.

24. Hickey, R.J., et al., Low level ionizing radiation and human mortality: Multi-regional epidemiological studies. A preliminary report. Health Phys, 1981. 40(5):625–641.

25. Nambi, K.S. and S.D. Soman, Environmental radiation and cancer in India. Health Phys, 1987. 52(5):653–657.

26. Hatch, M. and M. Susser, Background gamma radiation and childhood cancers within ten miles of a US nuclear plant. Int J Epidemiol, 1990. 19(3):546–552.

27. Jacobson, A., P. Plato, and N. Frigerio, The role of natural radiations in human leukemogenesis. Am J Public Health, 1976. 66:31–37.

28. Shimizu, M., et al., Correlation between natural radiation exposure and cancer mortality. J Nihon Univ Sch Dent, 1987. 29:314–320.

29. Tirmarche, M., et al., Epidemiologic study of regional cancer mortality in France and natural radiation. Radiat Prot Dosim, 1988. 24:479–482.

30. Walter, S.D., J.W. Meigs, and J.F. Heston, The relationship of cancer incidence to terrestrial radiation and population density in Connecticut, 1935–1974. Am J Epidemiol, 1986. 123(1):1–14.

31. International Atomic Energy Agency (IAEA), The International Chernobyl Project: Report of an international committee. 1991, Vienna: IAEA.

32. United Nations Scientific Committee on the Effects of Atomic Radiation (UNSCEAR), Sources and effects of ionizing radiation. II. Effects: UNSCEAR 2000 report to the General Assembly, with scientific annexes. 2000, New York: United Nations.

33. Chernobyl Forum and World Health Organization (WHO), Health effects of the Chernobyl accident and special health care programmes. 2005, Geneva: WHO.

34. Stewart, A.M. and G.W. Kneale, Non-cancer effects of exposure to A-bomb radiation. J Epidemiol Community Health, 1984. 38(2):108–112.

35. Mine, M., et al., Apparently beneficial effect of low to intermediate doses of A-bomb radiation on human lifespan. Int J Radiat Biol, 1990. 58(6):1035–1043.

36. Shimizu, Y., H. Kato, and W.J. Schull, Non-cancer mortality in the Life Span Study, 1950–1985. RERF Update, Summer. 1991, Hiroshima, Japan: Radiation Effects Research Foundation.

37. Preston, D.L., D.A. Pierce, and Y. Shimizu, Age-time patterns for cancer and noncancer excess risks in the atomic bomb survivors. Radiat Res, 2000. 154(6):733–734; discussion, 734–735.

38. Preston, D.L., et al., Studies of mortality of atomic bomb survivors. Report 13: Solid cancer and noncancer disease mortality: 1950–1997. Radiat Res, 2003. 160(4):381–407.

39. Kato, H., et al., Dose-response analyses among atomic bomb survivors exposed to low-level radiation. Health Phys, 1987. 52(5):645–652.

40. Kusunoki, Y., et al., Age-related alteration in the composition of immunocompetent blood cells in atomic bomb survivors. Int J Radiat Biol Relat Stud Phys Chem Med, 1988. 53(1):189–198.

41. Bloom, E.T., et al., Delayed effects of low-dose radiation on cellular immunity in atomic bomb survivors residing in the United States. Health Phys, 1987. 52(5):585–591.

42. Bloom, E.T., et al., Immunological responses of aging Japanese A-bomb survivors. Radiat Res, 1988. 116(2):343–355.

43. Tietjen, G.L., Plutonium and lung cancer. Health Phys, 1987. 52(5):625–628.

44. Matanoski, G.M., A. Sternberg, and E.A. Elliott, Does radiation exposure produce a protective effect among radiologists? Health Phys, 1987. 52(5):637–643.

45. Tuschl, H., et al., Effects of low-dose radiation on repair processes in human lymphocytes. Radiat Res, 1980. 81(1):1–9.

46. Tuschl, H., R. Kovac, and H. Altmann, UDS and SCE in lymphocytes of persons occupationally exposed to low levels of ionizing radiation. Health Phys, 1983. 45(1):1–7.

47. Tuschl, H., R. Kovac, and A. Wottawa, T-lymphocyte subsets in occupationally exposed persons. Int J Radiat Biol, 1990. 58(4):651–659.

48. Anderson, R.E. and I. Lefkovits, In vitro evaluation of radiation-induced augmentation of the immune response. Am J Pathol, 1979. 97(3):456–472.

49. Liu, S.Z., W.H. Liu, and J.B. Sun, Radiation hormesis: Its expression in the immune system. Health Phys, 1987. 52(5):579–583.

50. Akiyama, M., et al., Age and dose related alteration of in vitro mixed lymphocyte culture response of blood lymphocytes from A-bomb survivors. Radiat Res, 1989. 117(1):26–34.

51. Kelsey, K.T., et al., Human lymphocytes exposed to low doses of x-rays are less susceptible to radiation-induced mutagenesis. Mutat Res, 1991. 263(4):197–201.

52. Makinodan, T. and S.J. James, T cell potentiation by low dose ionizing radiation: Possible mechanisms. Health Phys, 1990. 59(1):29–34.

53. Planel, H., et al., Investigations of the biological effects of very low doses of ionizing radiations. In Low Dose Irradiation and Biological Defense Mechanisms, T. Sugahara, L.A. Sagan, and T. Aoyama, eds. 1992, Amsterdam: Elsevier Science.

54. Pereira, L., J. Povoa, and V. Povoa, Individual variability of adaptive response of human lymphocytes primed with low dose gamma rays. In Low Dose Irradiation and Biological Defense Mechanisms, T. Sugahara, L.A. Sagan, and T. Aoyama, eds. 1992, Amsterdam: Elsevier Science.

55. Youngblom, J.H., J.K. Wiencke, and S. Wolff, Inhibition of the adaptive response of human lymphocytes to very low doses of ionizing radiation by the protein synthesis inhibitor cycloheximide. Mutat Res, 1989. 227(4):257–261.

56. Shadley, J.D., Chromosomal adaptive response in human lymphocytes. Radiat Res, 1994. 138(suppl 1):S9–S12.

57. Shadley, J.D., V. Afzal, and S. Wolff, Characterization of the adaptive response to ionizing radiation induced by low doses of x rays to human lymphocytes. Radiat Res, 1987. 111(3):511–517.

58. Shadley, J.D. and J.K. Wiencke, Induction of the adaptive response by x-rays is dependent on radiation intensity. Int J Radiat Biol, 1989. 56(1):107–118.

59. Shadley, J.D. and S. Wolff, Very low doses of x-rays can cause human lymphocytes to become less susceptible to ionizing radiation. Mutagenesis, 1987. 2(2):95–96.

60. Sanderson, B.J. and A.A. Morley, Exposure of human lymphocytes to ionizing radiation reduces mutagenesis by subsequent ionizing radiation. Mutat Res, 1986. 164(6):347–351.

61. Bosi, A. and G. Olivieri, Variability of the adaptive response to ionizing radiations in humans. Mutat Res, 1989. 211(1):13–17.

62. Watanabe, M., et al., Effect of multiple irradiation with low doses of gamma rays on morphological transformation and growth ability of human embryo cells in vitro. Int J Radiat Biol, 1992. 62:711–718.

Appendix 1 Glossary

ABCC. *See* RERF.

Absolute risk. *See* Risk, absolute.

Absorbed dose. When ionizing radiation passes through matter, some of its energy is imparted to the matter. The amount absorbed per unit mass of irradiated material is called the absorbed dose, and it is measured in gray or rad. *See* Threshold dose.

Absorbed dose equivalent. *See* Dose equivalent.

Accelerator. Device imparting high kinetic energy to a charged particle, causing it to undergo nuclear or particle reaction.

Acrocentric. Having the centromere near one end of the replicating chromosome so that one arm is much longer than the other.

Actinide series. The series of elements beginning with number 89 and continuing through number 105, which together occupy one position in the periodic table. The series includes uranium, element 92, and all the synthetic transuranic elements. The group is also referred to as the *actinides. Compare* Lanthanide series.

Activation. The process of making a material radioactive by bombardment with neutrons, protons, or other nuclear particles.

Activity. *See* Radioactivity; Specific activity.

Activity mean aerodynamic diameter (AMAD). The diameter in an aerodynamic particle size distribution for which the total activities on particles above and below this size are equal. A lognormal distribution of particle sizes is usually assumed.

Acute exposure. An exposure that took place over a short period of time (minutes or hours).

Acute radiation injury. Refers to deterministic effects that occur as a result of direct cell killing. For whole-body exposure this usually refers to clinical manifestation of the acute radiation syndrome. For local exposure it refers to erythema, skin blistering, and other findings. Most acute effects are expressed within the first 6 months after exposure.

Acute radiation sickness (ARS). Clinical findings after whole-body exposure to radiation doses in excess of 0.75 Gy. Usually classified in grades from mild to severe based on the spectrum of symptoms and clinical findings.

Acute radiation syndrome (ARS). Often confused with acute radiation sickness but really relates to syndromes related to specific organ systems (e.g., hematopoietic, gastrointestinal, cardiovascular, neurological, and cutaneous).

Adaptive response. An effect observed when a conditioning radiation dose lowers the biological effect of a subsequent (usually higher) radiation exposure.

Aerosol. Extremely small liquid or solid particles suspended in air.

ALARA. NRC operating philosophy for maintaining occupational radiation exposures "as low as is reasonably achievable," taking into account social and economic factors.

Allele (allelomorph). Alternative forms of a gene derived by mutation or duplication. In a single normal individual, each locus is represented only twice. No more than two different alleles can be found.

Alpha particle. Nucleus of a helium atom emitted by certain radioisotopes on disintegration. Contains two protons and two neutrons.

AMU. *See* Atomic mass unit.

Aneuploid. A chromosome number that deviates from the normal for a species. It may be more or less than the diploid number but is not an exact multiple of the basic haploid number found in germ cells.

Annihilation. Reaction between a pair of particles resulting in their disintegration and the production of an equivalent amount of energy in the form of photons.

Annual dose limits. Any of the annual dose limits for individual members of the public or workers; recommended by the ICRP or NCRP as part of its system of radiation protection.

Annual limit on intake (ALI). The activity of a radionuclide that, when taken alone, would irradiate a person to the limit set for each year of occupational exposure.

ARS. *See* Acute radiation sickness, Acute radiation syndrome.

Assigned share (AS). The individual's share of total risk of a disease that is due to a specific agent. Numerically the same as probability of causation.

Atmospheric testing. Detonation of nuclear weapons or devices in the atmosphere or close to the top of the earth's surface as part of the nuclear weapons testing program.

Atom. Smallest unit of an element that can exist and still maintain the properties of the element.

Atomic bomb. A nuclear weapon that relies on fission only, in contrast with a thermonuclear "hydrogen" bomb that uses fission and fusion.

Atomic mass. Mass of a neutral atom, usually expressed in atomic mass units.

Atomic mass unit (AMU). Exactly one twelfth the mass of carbon 12; 1.661×10^{-24} g.

Atomic number (Z). Number of protons in an atom.

Atomic weight. Average weight of the neutral atoms of an element.

Attributable risk percent. The percentage of disease that could be eliminated if a particular exposure was stopped.

Auger electron. An orbital electron ejected by a characteristic x-ray that is usually emitted after electron capture or internal conversion.

Autoimmune disease. A disease caused by one's immune system attacking the cells of one's own body rather than attacking foreign cells, such as bacteria.

Autoimmune hypothyroidism. An autoimmune disease that prevents the thyroid from producing enough thyroid hormone.

Autoimmune thyroiditis. Damage to the thyroid caused when the body's immune system attacks and destroys cells in the thyroid gland. It can be radiation induced (at least at high dose levels). Has not been reliably associated with radiation at low dose levels. If damage is substantial enough, a person may develop signs and symptoms of hypothyroidism.

Autosome. Chromosomes other than the sex (X or Y) chromosomes. Humans carry 22 pairs of autosomes.

Average life. The mean time during which an atom exists in a particular form. The average life is 1.44 times the physical half-life.

Avogadro's number. Number of atoms is the gram atomic weight of a given element or the number of molecules in the gram molecular weight of a given substance: 6.02×10^{23} per g mole.

Background. Detected disintegration events not emanating from the sample.

Background radiation. Natural background is that ionizing radiation that is a natural part of a person's environment, primarily terrestrial radioactivity and cosmic rays.

Basal cells. A cell in the epidermis that gives rise to more specialized cells.

Basal cell carcinoma. A malignant growth originating from basal cells that is most common in fair-skinned persons and sun-exposed areas of skin. The most common form of skin cancer.

Becquerel (Bq). The SI unit of radioactivity equaling one disintegration per second; approximately 2.7×10^{-11} curies (Ci), or 27 picocuries (pCi).

BEIR. Biological Effects of Ionizing Radiation: A series of reports by a committee of the National Academy of Sciences.

Benign tumor. A general category of tumors that do not invade the surrounding tissue. Characterized by slow growth through expansion. They are not malignant or cancerous.

Beta particle. An electron of positive or negative charge.

Bias. The systematic tendency of a measurement of prediction of a quantity to overestimate or underestimate the actual value on the average.

Bioassay. An assessment of radioactive materials that may be present inside a person's body. Assessment may be based on analysis of the person's urine, blood, feces, sweat, or through use of an external whole-body counter.

Body burden. The amount of radioactive material present in a human or animal.

Bremsstrahlung x-rays. Photonic emissions caused by the slowing down of beta particles in matter.

By-product material. Radioactive material arising from controlled fission.

Bystander effect. Various deleterious (and occasionally beneficial) effects that an irradiated cell has on nearby nonirradiated cells. This may involve induction of mutations, micronuclei formation, cell killing, changes in signal transduction, genomic instability, or malignant transformation.

Cancer. A malignant tumor of potentially unlimited growth that expands locally by invasion and systemically by metastasis.

Cancer risk. A theoretical risk of getting cancer if exposed to a substance every day for 70 years (a lifetime exposure). The true risk might be lower.

Carcinogen. An agent or substance capable of causing induction of a cancer. A complete carcinogen may contain both initiating and promoting capabilities.

Carcinogenesis. The process of induction of cancer in a cell.

Carcinoma. A malignant tumor that occurs in epithelial tissues that cover the body or body parts and enclose and protect those parts, produce secretions and excretions, and function in absorption.

Carrier. (1) An individual who possesses and can transmit the gene for a given trait but does not exhibit the trait, or (2) quantity of stable isotopes of an element mixed with radioactive isotopes of that element.

Carrier-free. Adjective describing a radionuclide that is free of its stable isotopes.

Case-control study. An epidemiologic investigation in which patient cases are selected on the basis of having a disease or condition, and they are compared in terms of a particular exposure to controls who are selected because they do not have the condition. These studies are efficient for rare diseases with long latency periods, but they are particularly susceptible to selection bias.

Case study. A medical or epidemiological evaluation of one person or a small group of persons to gather information about specific health conditions and exposures.

Cataract. A clouding of the lens or its capsule that obstructs the passage of light to some extent.

Cell cycle. The cycle undergone by the nuclear DNA from one cell division to the next. It consists of *GI*, a period of growth; *S*, a period of chromosomal DNA replication; *G2*, a period of further growth; and mitosis *(M)*. G indicates "gap" in DNA replication activity; *S* stands for "synthesis."

Central estimate. A "best" estimate of the dose received or other value as distinct from the upper bound that accounts for uncertainty in that estimate.

Centromere. The small constricted region on a chromosome at which identical chromatids are joined and by which the chromosome is attached to a spindle fiber. The position of the centromere determines the length of the arms of the chromosome and, for any particular chromosome, is constant in location.

Chance. A situation in which something happens unpredictably without discernable human intention or observable cause.

Chromatids. The individual strands of a chromosome that result from its lengthwise duplication. When the centromere that joins the two chromatids separates, each chromatid becomes a separate chromosome.

Chromosome aberration. Alteration from normal structure or number.

Chromosomes. Various-sized structural elements in the cell nucleus, composed of deoxyribonucleic acid (DNA) and proteins, which carry the genes that convey the genetic information. Chromosomes have a species-specific morphology and number.

CI. *See* Confidence interval.

Cocarcinogen. An agent that can cause cancer by itself but that, when combined with another carcinogen, produces an effect greater than the sum of either individually (i.e., it is synergistic).

Cohort. A group of individuals that has a common association or factor.

Cohort study. An epidemiologic investigation or follow-up of a group of individuals who are known to

have had an exposure and are followed to see if they develop a disease or condition. Usually are expensive and time-consuming because they typically follow a large number of individuals for many years.

Collective dose. The estimated dose for an area, region, or group of people multiplied by the number of exposed population.

Collective dose equivalent. The collective dose equivalent to a population in units of man-sievert (man Sv) or man-rem that is the sum of the products of the individual (or per capita dose equivalent) and the number of individuals in each exposed group in a population.

Confidence interval (CI). A range of numbers giving a probability that the true answer lies within the range. For example, an epidemiologic data point of 4.3 is subject to a number of uncertainties based on sample size and other factors. The value should not be assumed to represent the "truth" but rather an approximation of it. If 95% CI of 2.3 to 7.8 are given with the data presented, this means that one can be 95% sure that the true value lies in this range.

Confidence limits. The highest and lowest boundaries in a confidence interval.

Confounding factors. Any characteristic that makes it difficult to compare two or more distinct groups in an epidemiological study. Confounding factors can mask a health effect so that the relationship of the effect and the exposure is not recognized. They can also make it appear as though there is an effect when there is none.

Congenital. Present at birth. Does not imply either genetic or nongenetic causation.

Contamination (radioactive). A radioactive substance in a material or place where it is undesirable.

Correlation. Most generally, the degree to which one phenomenon or variable is associated with or can be predicted from another. In statistics, usually refers to the degree to which a predictive relationship exists between variables.

Cosmic rays. Radiation of many sorts, but mostly atomic nuclei (protons) with very high energies originating outside the earth's atmosphere. Cosmic radiation is part of the natural background radiation. Some cosmic rays are more energetic than any synthetic forms of radiation.

Criticality. The state of a nuclear reactor when it is sustaining a chain reaction.

Critical mass. The smallest mass of fissionable material that will support a self-sustaining chain reaction under a stated condition.

Critical organ. Organ (1) of interest or (2) most radiobiologically affected by a technique. Usually the organ with the highest absorbed dose.

Cross section (symbol Σ [sigma]). A measure of the probability that a nuclear reaction will occur. Usually measured in barns. It is the apparent or effective area presented by a target nucleus, or particle, to an oncoming particle or other nuclear radiation, such as a neutron.

Cumulative dose. The total dose resulting from repeated or continuous exposure of the same portion of the body or of the whole body to ionizing radiation.

Curie. Standard measure of rate of radioactive decay, based on the disintegration of 1 g of radium or 3.7×10^{10} disintegrations per second; expressed in SI units as 3.7×10^{10} Bq.

Cutaneous radiation syndrome (CRS). The complex syndrome resulting from radiation exposure of more than 2 Gy to the skin. The immediate effects can be reddening, blisters, ulceration, hair loss, and pain.

Cyclotron. A device consisting of two hollow D-shaped chambers for accelerating charged particles to energies up to 15 MeV or more by periodic accelerations through a potential difference.

Daughter radionuclide. Decay product of a radionuclide. The element from which the daughter was produced is called the parent.

DDREF. Dose and dose-rate effectiveness factor. A factor used to adjust for the different biologic effect with different doses and dose rates of low-LET radiation from those at which original data were obtained. Typically, the factor refers to the possible reduction in carcinogenesis at low doses (<200 mGy) or with low dose rates (<0.1 mGy per minute averaged over 1 hour). Biologically the value may range from 1 to 10, but for most risk estimates a value between 1.5 and 2 is used. For high-LET radiation, a DDREF of 1 is used.

Decay. Radioactive disintegration of a nucleus of an unstable nuclide.

Decay constant (λ). The probability per unit of time that a given radionuclide atom will undergo a radioactive transformation.

Decay, radioactive. *See* Radioactive decay.

Decay schemes. Diagram showing the decay mode or modes of a radionuclide.

Decontamination. The removal of radioactive contaminants from surface or equipment, for instance, by cleaning and washing with chemicals.

Decorporation. Removal of radioactive isotopes from the body using specific drugs.

Delayed neutrons. Neutrons emitted by radioactive fission products in a nuclear reactor over a period of seconds or minutes after a fission takes place. Fewer than 1% of the neutrons are delayed; more than 99% are prompt neutrons. Delayed neutrons are important considerations in reactor design and control.

Deletion. Loss of a portion of a chromosome as a result of chromosome breakage.

de minimus. An expression derived from the Latin *deminimus non jurat lex* ("the law is not concerned with trivialities"). A de minimus level is one that is so low as to be trivial. The NCRP has indicated that an annual absorbed dose of less than 10 µSv from a source should not be of concern.

Deoxyribonucleic acid (DNA). The nucleic acid primarily contained within the cell nucleus that carries the genetic information.

Depleted uranium. Uranium containing less than 0.7% uranium 235.

Deuterium (^{2}H or D). An isotope of hydrogen whose nucleus contains one neutron and one proton and, therefore, is about twice as heavy as the nucleus of normal hydrogen, which is only a single proton. Deuterium is often referred to as *heavy hydrogen*; it occurs in nature as 1 atom to every 6500 atoms of normal hydrogen. It is nonradioactive. *Compare* Tritium.

Deuteron. The nucleus of deuterium containing one proton and one neutron.

Diploid. Possessing a paired set of chromosomes, one set from the father and one set from the mother (2n). Characteristic of all somatic cells.

Disintegration. General process of radioactive decay, usually measured for each unit of time, for example, disintegrations per second.

DNA. *See* Deoxyribonucleic acid.

Dominant. A trait that is expressed in individuals who are heterozygous for a particular gene.

Dose. A term denoting the amount of energy absorbed. *Absorbed dose* is the energy imparted to matter by ionizing radiation for each unit of mass of irradiation material at the point of interest. Usually expressed in rad (conventional unit) or gray (SI unit). *Cumulative dose* is the total dose resulting from repeated exposures to radiation.

Dose coefficient. The factor used to convert radionuclide intake to dose. Usually expressed as dose per unit intake (e.g., sieverts per Becquerel).

Dose equivalent (H). A unit of biologically effective dose, defined by the ICRP in 1977 as the absorbed dose in rads multiplied by the quality factor (Q). For all x-rays, the gamma rays, beta particles, and positrons likely to be used in nuclear medicine, the quality factor is 1. The dose equivalent *(H)* is given by the equation $H \times DQN$, where D is absorbed dose, Q is the quality factor, and N is the product of modifying factors (N is usually 1). *See also* Equivalent dose.

Dose equivalent commitment. For any specified decision, practice, or operation, the infinite time integral of the per capita dose equivalent rate for a specified population. In other words, the dose committed over a certain time period resulting from an action.

Dose ranges. Arbitrary designations of dose. Low dose range is roughly 0 to 0.2 Gy in a single dose or 10 mGy per year of uniform whole-body radiation.

Intermediate dose is roughly 0.2 to 2.5 Gy; high dose is above 2.5 Gy.

Dose rate. The radiation dose delivered for each unit of time and measured, for instance, in rad per hour. *See* Absorbed dose.

Dose-response analysis. A statistical analysis to estimate values of parameters that describe the relationship between the dose of a hazardous agent (such as ionizing radiation) and an increase in a specified biologic response (such as cancer) above the normal background incidence.

Dosimeter. A device that measures radiation dose, such as a film badge or thermoluminescent dosimeter (TLD).

Doubling dose (genetic). That radiation dose estimated to double the spontaneous or natural incidence of any given effect.

DREF. *See* DDREF.

DS86. A 1986 system of dosimetry used to describe the exposure of atomic bomb survivors.

Duplication. A chromosome abnormality in which a segment of the chromosome is represented more than once as a result of breakage and refusion.

EAR. *See* Excess absolute risk.

Effective dose. A quantity that takes into account the difference in sensitivity of various body tissues and effectiveness of different radiations to obtain a uniform expression of risk for stochastic effects. It has been defined by the ICRP in 1990 as the sum of equivalent doses that have been multiplied by a tissue-weighting factor (W_T). The unit of effective dose is the sievert or rem.

Effective dose equivalent. An older version of effective dose using slightly different weighting factors.

Effective half-life. *See* Half-life, effective.

Electromagnetic radiation. Radiation consisting of associated and interacting electric and magnetic waves that travel at the speed of light, such as light, radio waves, gamma rays, and x-rays. All electromagnetic radiation can be transmitted through a vacuum. *Compare* Ionizing radiation.

Electron capture. Method of radioactive decay in which the nucleus captures an orbital electron, which then interacts with a proton, effectively negating the proton and transmuting the nucleus to that of another element.

Electron volt (eV). A unit of energy equal to the kinetic energy required by an electron when accelerated through a potential difference of 1 volt ($1eV = 1.60 \times 10^{-19}$ joule).

Element. Pure substance, consisting of atoms of the same atomic number that cannot be decomposed by ordinary chemical means.

Embryo. The organism in the first stages of development. In humans, this is generally considered to be the period from the end of the second week through the eighth week of gestation.

Enriched uranium. Uranium in which the proportion of uranium 235 has been increased above 0.7% by removing uranium 238 mechanically.

Epidemiologic studies. Studies designed to examine associations or commonly hypothesized causal relations. These are usually concerned with identifying or measuring the effects of risk factors or exposures.

Epidemiology. The study of incidence, distribution, and causes of health conditions and events in populations.

Epigenetic effect. Genomic or cellular effects without the requirement for directly induced DNA damage. Such effects are termed epigenetic and are often divided into two classes: (1) genomic instability and (2) bystander effects.

Equivalent dose. A newer version of dose equivalent. Defined by the ICRP in 1990, it uses radiation-weighting factors (W_R) instead of the older quality factor (*Q*).

ERR. *See* Excess relative risk.

Erythema. Reddening of the skin. May come in waves over a few weeks after doses in excess of several gray.

Etiology. The study of the origins and causes of disease.

Euploid. A chromosome number that is the exact multiple of the haploid number.

Euploidy. Presence in a cell of an exact whole-number multiple of the gametic (haploid) chromosome number.

Excess absolute risk (EAR). The increase in risk of disease posed by exposure to a specified dose, or the arithmetic difference in risk of disease between exposed and unexposed subjects.

Excess relative risk (ERR). Relative risk minus 1.0.

Exposure. A term relating to the amount of ionizing radiation that is incident on living or inanimate material.

Exposure rate. Increment of exposure expressed for each unit of time.

Fast neutrons. Neutrons with energy greater than approximately 100,000 electron volts. *Compare* Delayed neutrons.

Fertile material. A material, not itself fissionable by thermal neutrons, that can be converted into a fissile material by irradiation in a nuclear reactor. There are two basic fertile materials, the uranium isotope ^{238}U and the thorium isotope ^{232}Th. When these fertile materials capture neutrons, they are partially converted into the fissile plutonium isotope ^{239}Pu and the fissile uranium isotope ^{233}U, respectively.

Fetus. Unborn offspring; in humans, the period from 8 weeks after fertilization until birth.

Film badge. Photographic film shielded from light; worn by an individual to measure radiation exposure.

Fissile material. Although used as a synonym for *fissionable material*, this term has acquired a more restricted meaning, that is, any material fissionable by neutrons of all energies, especially thermal, or slow, neutrons as well as fast neutrons. The uranium isotope ^{235}U and the plutonium isotope ^{239}Pu are examples of fissile material.

Fission. The splitting of a heavy nucleus into two approximately equal parts (which are nuclei of lighter elements), accompanied by the release of a relatively large amount of energy and generally one or more neutrons. Fission can occur spontaneously, but usually it is caused by nuclear absorption of gamma rays, neutrons, or other particles.

Fission products. The nuclei (fission fragments) formed by the fission of heavy elements plus the nuclides formed by the fission fragments' radioactive decay. *See* Radioactive decay.

Fissionable material. *See* Fissile material.

Fuel cycle. The series of steps involved in supplying fuel for nuclear power reactors. It includes mining, refining, fabricating the fuel elements, using them in a nuclear reactor, chemical processing to recover the fissionable materials remaining in the spent fuel, re-enriching the fuel material, and refabricating it into new fuel elements.

Fuel element. A rod, tube, plate, or other mechanical shape or form into which nuclear fuel is fabricated.

Fusion, nuclear. The formation of a heavier nucleus from two lighter ones, such as hydrogen isotopes, with the attendant release of energy. It takes energy input to get fusion fuel to fuse, but once fused, it releases much more energy than that put in. *Compare* Fission.

Fusion fuel. Commonly used fusion fuels for laboratory experiments are isotopes of hydrogen, that is, deuterium and tritium. Hydrogen itself is the fusion fuel of the sun. Other "futuristic" fusion fuels include helium and lithium.

Gamete. A mature male or female germ cell (sperm or egg) containing a haploid number of chromosomes.

Gamma emission. Nuclear process in which an excited nuclide de-excites by emission of a nuclear photon.

Gamma ray. Radiation emitted from the nucleus having a wavelength range of 10^{-9} to 10^{-12} cm.

Geiger-Müller counter (tube). A high-voltage (>1000 V) gas tube to detect ionizing particles. It is based on the avalanche effect observed when ions are accelerated by an electric field under appropriate conditions.

Gene. The basic unit of heredity. A finite segment of DNA that controls the production of a specific polypeptide.

Genetic code. The triplet sequence of nucleotide bases in the DNA chain, as reflected in messenger RNA (mRNA), that determines the sequence of amino acids during protein synthesis.

Genetic effects of radiation. Radiation effects that can be transferred from parent to offspring. Any radiation-caused changes in the genetic material of germ cells. *Compare* Somatic effects of radiation.

Genetically significant dose (GSD). The gonad dose from a given radiation source that if received by every member of the population would be expected to produce the same total genetic effect on the population as the sum of the individual doses actually received.

Genomic instability. An initial chromosomal aberration that results in an increase in chromosomal aberrations, gene mutations, or apoptosis (cell death) occurring many generations later. (In contrast, conventional DNA damage from radiation is usually expressed within 1 to 2 cell cycle divisions.)

Genotype. The genetic constitution of an individual that determines the physical and chemical characteristics of that individual.

Giga- (G). A prefix that multiples a basic unit by one billion (10^9).

Gigaelectron volt (GeV). One billion electron volts; also written as BeV. *See* Electron volt.

G-M tube. *See* Geiger-Müller counter (tube).

Gray (Gy). The international (SI) unit of radiation absorbed dose. One gray is equal to an energy deposition of 1 J/kg (100 rad).

Ground state. The state of lowest energy of a system.

H. *See* Dose equivalent.

Half-life, biologic. The time required for the amount of a particular substance in a biologic system to be reduced to half of its initial value by biologic processes when the rate of removal is approximately exponential.

Half-life, effective. The time required for the amount of a particular specimen of a radionuclide in a system to be reduced to half its initial value as a consequence of both radioactive decay and other processes such as biologic elimination.

Half-life, radioactive. For a single radioactive decay process, the time required for the activity of a given sample to decrease to half its initial value by that process.

Half-value layer (HVL). Thickness of absorbing material necessary to reduce the intensity of radiation by one half.

Haploid. Having a single set of unpaired chromosomes (*N*); there are 23 in humans.

Health physics. The science concerned with the recognition, evaluation, and control of health hazards from ionizing radiation.

Heteroploidy. Any alteration of chromosome number from the orthoploid state.

Heterozygous. Having dissimilar alleles at the same locus on homologous chromosomes.

HEU. *See* Highly enriched uranium.

High dose. More than 2 Gy (200 rad).

Highly enriched uranium (HEU). Uranium that is enriched to above 20% uranium 235. Weapons grade HEU is enriched to more than 90% of uranium 235.

Homozygous. Having the same genes at a given locus on homologous chromosomes.

Hormesis. The term *hormesis* is used in a number of ways, but for purposes of radiation effects it generally refers to a process whereby low doses of radiation may result in beneficial or stimulatory effects.

HVL. *See* Half-value layer.

ICRP. International Commission on Radiological Protection.

ICRU. International Commission on Radiation Units.

Incidence. The number of persons who have developed a disease in a given period of time divided by the total population at risk.

Initiator. A substance or agent that primes a cell to the development of a tumor. Usually it will not cause a tumor by itself.

Intermediate dose. Intermediate dose is 0.2 to 2.0 Gy.

Intermediate neutrons. Neutrons having energy greater than thermal neutrons but lower than fast neutrons. The range is between 0.5 and 100,000 electron volts. Also called *epithermal neutrons*.

Internal conversion. The transition between two energy states of a nucleus in which the energy difference is not emitted as a photon but is given to an orbital electron, which is thereby ejected from the atom.

Internal dose. The dose to tissue or organs due to sources of ionizing radiation in the body.

In utero. In the uterus or womb.

Inverse-square law. The radiation intensity of any source decreases inversely as the square of the distance between the source and the detector (e.g., doubling the distance from a source decreases the intensity by one-fourth).

Inversion. A chromosomal abnormality in which a segment of the chromosome recombines in an inverted relationship after breakage.

Ionization. The process whereby a charged portion (usually an electron) of an atom or molecule is given enough kinetic energy to dissociate.

Ionization chamber. A closed vessel used for the detection of radiation energy and containing a gas and two electrodes maintained at a potential difference. Any radiation incident on this container forms ions that move to the appropriate electrode, producing a current that can be measured.

Ionizing radiation. Radiation that produces ion pairs along its path through a substance.

Ion pair. A closely associated position ion and negative ion (usually an electron) having charges of the same magnitude and formed from a neutral atom or molecule by radiation.

Irradiation. Exposure to radiation.

Isobar. Nuclides that have the same total number of neutrons and protons but are different elements.

Isomer. One of two or more nuclides having the same number of neutrons and protons in their nuclei but having different energies. A nuclide in the excited state and a similar nuclide in the ground state are isomers.

Isomeric states. States of a nucleus having different energies and observable half-lives.

Isomeric transition (IT). A transition between two isomeric states of a nucleus. No elementary change of species is involved.

Isotones. Nuclides having the same number of neutrons but a different number of protons.

Isotopes. Nuclides having the same number of protons but a different number of neutrons.

IT. *See* Isomeric transition.

Karyotype. A systemized array of chromosomes from a single cell, prepared by photography, that demonstrates the number and morphology of the chromosome complement.

Kerma. Kinetic energy released in material. A unit of quantity that represents the kinetic energy transferred to charged particles by the uncharged particles for each unit of mass of a medium. Expressed in rad or gray.

keV. One thousand electron volts (10^3 eV).

Lanthanide series. The series of elements beginning with lanthanum, element number 57, and continuing through lutetium, element number 71, that together occupy one position in the periodic table of the elements. These are the *rare earths*, all having chemical properties similar to lanthanum. Also called the *lanthanides*.

Latent period. Usually refers to the time elapsed between radiation exposure and the clinical appearance of an effect (such as appearance of a cancer).

LET. *See* Linear energy transfer.

Lethal dose. A dose of ionizing radiation sufficient to cause death. Median lethal dose (*ML*, or LD_{50}) is the dose required to kill, within a specified period of time (usually 30 days), half the individuals in a large group of organisms similarly exposed. The $LD_{50/30}$ for humans without medical treatment is about 2.5 to 4.5 Gy.

Life Span Study (LSS). Continuing follow-up of the population exposed to atomic bomb detonations in Hiroshima and Nagasaki and their progeny. Conducted by the Radiation Effects Research Foundation (RERF).

Linear energy transfer (LET). Amount of energy lost by ionizing radiation by way of interaction with matter for each unit of path length through the absorbing material.

Linear model. The assumption that the effect of exposure to ionizing radiation is directly and simply proportional to dose.

Linear nonthreshold model (LNT). An empirical equation used to assign risk of cancer induction by ionizing radiation. The equation has the form, risk = A + kD where k is a risk coefficient, D is a measure of dose, and A represents the baseline risk, absent radiation. With this empirical model, any dose in excess of 0 is presumed to be associated with an increased risk of cancer. Further, use of this model implies that doubling the dose will double the calculated excess risk.

Linear-quadratic model. The assumption that the effect of exposure is related not only to the dose received but also to the square of the dose.

Locus. The site occupied by a specific gene, or allele, on a particular chromosome.

Low dose. Less than 0.2 Gy.

Low-dose rate. Less than 0.1 mGy per minute averaged over about 1 hour. Sometimes also refers to less than 10 mGy per year.

LSS. *See* Life Span Study.

Lugol's solution. An iodine solution.

Malignant. Tending to infiltrate, metastasize, and terminate fatally.

Man rem. A unit of collective population dose calculated by multiplying the number of persons exposed times their average individual whole-body dose in rems.

Maximum permissible concentration (MPC). An obsolescent term for the amount of radioactive material in the air, water, or food that might cause a maximum permissible dose at a standard rate of intake.

Maximum permissible dose (MPD). The maximum amount of radiation that may be received by an individual within a specified time period with expectation of no significantly harmful result. MPD is a regulatory concept. A dose above this level does not mean that harm has been done.

Mean. The arithmetic average of a set of values, given by the sum of the values divided by the number of values. The mean of a distribution of values is the weighted average of possible values, each value weighted by its probability of occurrence in the distribution.

Median dose. The central estimate in a dose range estimate. Half the possible doses are above the median and half are below it.

Medical monitoring. A program to screen a group of people who are at risk for specific diseases or conditions and to refer individuals for additional evaluation and treatment if needed. Monitoring does not include medical care.

Megaton (Mt). The energy of an explosion that is equivalent to an explosion of 1 million tons of TNT. One megaton is equivalent to 10^{18} calories.

Meiosis. The special type of cell division of gametogenesis by which a mother cell with a diploid set of chromosomes divides to produce gametes with a haploid, or single, set of chromosomes; reductional division.

Meson. One of a class of medium-mass, short-lived elementary particles with a mass between that of the electron and the proton.

Messenger RNA (mRNA). RNA that serves as a template for protein synthesis.

Metaphase. The stage of mitosis or meiosis in which the centromeres of the contracted chromosomes are arranged on the equitorial plate.

Metastable state. An excited nuclear state of a particular isotope that has a finite half-life and decays by gamma emission. Examples: ^{99m}Tc, ^{99}Tc (6 hours); ^{38m}Cl, ^{38}Cl (0.74 seconds).

MeV. One million (10^6) electron volts.

Micro- (μ). A prefix that divides a basic unit by one million (10^{-6}).

Microcurie (μCi). That quantity of radioactive material having 3.7×10^4 disintegrations per second. One-millionth part of a curie (37 kBq).

Micrometer (μm). One millionth of a meter; formerly micron.

Milli- (m). A prefix that divides a basic unit by 1000 (10^{-3}).

Millicurie (mCi). That quantity of radioactive material having 3.7×10^7 disintegrations per second. One-thousandth part of a curie (37 MBq).

Mill tailing. Naturally radioactive residue from the processing of uranium ore into yellowcake in a mill. The residue contains uranium, thorium, radium, polonium, and radon.

Minisatellite. Repeated segments of the same sequence of multiple triplet codons, each segment varying between 14 and 100 base pairs, useful as linkage markers because of their highly polymorphic nature and that they are usually situated near genes. Minisatellites are inherently unstable and susceptible to mutation at a higher rate than other sequences of DNA.

Mitosis. Somatic cell division by which the mother cell produces two daughter cells, each with the identical chromosome complement to the original cell.

Monosomy. Loss of one member of a chromosome pair so that there is one less than the diploid number of chromosomes (2n−1).

Monozygotic. Refers to twins derived from a single fertilized ovum; identical twins.

Morbidity. A measure of a diseased condition or state; refers to illness not death.

Morbidity rate. The rate at which people get a disease, usually expressed as the number of cases per 100,000 people per year.

Mortality. A measure of the number of people who die from a specific disease or condition.

Mortality rate. The rate at which people die from a disease (such as a specific type of cancer), usually expressed as the number of cases per 100,000 people per year.

Mosaicism. The presence in the same individual of two or more genotypically different cell lines.

MPC. *See* Maximum permissible concentration.

MPD. *See* Maximum permissible dose.

Mutation. A hereditary change in genetic material. A mutation can be a change in a single gene (*point mutation*) or a change in chromosome characteristics.

Mutation rate. The rate at which mutations occur at a given locus; expressed as mutations/gamete for each locus in a generation.

N. *See* Neutron number. Also used as the abbreviation for the haploid number of chromosomes in the human.

Nano- (n). A prefix that divides a basic unit by one billion (10^{-9}).

National Academy of Sciences (NAS). A private nonprofit group of scholars engaged in scientific research. Congressionally chartered with a mandate to advise the federal government.

NCRP. National Council on Radiation Protection and Measurements. A nongovernmental congressionally chartered agency focusing on issues related to radiation protection and measurement.

Neutron number (N). Number of neutrons in a nucleus.

Noble gas. Any group of rare gases (helium, neon, argon, krypton, xenon, and radon) that exhibit great stability and low chemical reaction rates.

Nondisjunction. Failure of two chromatids or two homologous chromosomes to separate or disjoin so that both pass to the same daughter cell.

Nonstochastic effect. Also called a *deterministic effect*. Describes an effect whose severity is a function of dose. Some may have an apparent clinical threshold. Examples of nonstochastic effects include skin erythema, cataracts, and bone marrow depression.

Nuclear Regulatory Commission (NRC). United States government agency regulating by-product material. (NRC also stands for National Research Council, a part of the National Academy of Sciences.)

Nuclear weapon. A weapon that derives its explosive force from nuclear fission or fusion.

Nucleons. Any particle commonly contained in the nucleus of an atom.

Nucleus. The small, positively charged core of an atom. It is only about one ten-thousandth the diameter of the atom but contains nearly all the atom's mass. All nuclei contain both protons and neutrons, except the nucleus of ordinary hydrogen, which consists of a single proton.

Nuclides. A general term applicable to all atomic forms of the element. The term is often used incorrectly as a synonym for isotope, which properly has a more limited definition. Whereas isotopes are the various forms of a single element (hence, are a family of nuclides) and all have the same atomic number and number of protons, nuclides comprise all the isotopic forms of all the elements. Nuclides are distinguished by their atomic number, atomic mass, and energy state.

Nullisomy. Absence from a cell of both members of a pair of chromosomes.

Odds. A measure of the likelihood that an event will occur. For example, the odds of developing a particular disease.

Odds ratio (OR). Used as an estimation of relative risk (RR). Primarily used for case-control studies and is calculated from the odds of exposure among the cases to that among controls.

Oncogene. A cancer-causing gene arising from a cellular gene (proto-oncogene) concerned with normal growth and development.

Operator gene. A gene that is responsible for regulating the function of a group of genes closely linked to it.

Operon. A group of linked genes that are under control of a single operator gene.

Organ dose. The energy absorbed in a specific organ divided by its mass. This quantity is expressed in gray (Gy) or its submultiples.

Orthoploid. Normal number of chromosomes.

Parent radionuclide. Radionuclide that decays to a specific daughter nuclide either directly or as a member of a radioactive series.

Personnel monitor. *See* Thermoluminescent dosimeter; Film badge.

Photon. A quantum of electromagnetic radiation, having no mass or electrical charge, that exhibits both particle and wave behavior, especially a gamma ray or an x-ray.

Photopeak. The peak (maximum intensity) in a gamma spectrum as measured by a scintillation detector.

Pico- (p). A prefix that divides a basic unit of one trillion (10^{-12}). Same as micromicro.

Pipescale. Relatively insoluble deposit on the inside of pipes (usually oil wells) that often contains naturally occurring radioactive material (predominately radium).

Pitchblende. A brown to black mineral that has a distinctive luster. It consists mainly of urananite (UO_2) but also contains radium.

Positron. A particle equal in mass to the electron but having a positive electronic charge.

Power. The probability that a study can distinguish between a true exposure-to-disease relationship and a coincidence. The power of a study depends on the size of its population, the amount of radiation exposure, and the number of cases of disease under investigation.

Prevalence. The proportion of individuals in a population who have a disease at a specific time. For example, the number of people in the United States who have lung cancer. It is not the number of new cases in that year. Prevalence is the incidence multiplied by the average duration of disease.

Probability. The likelihood (chance) that a specified event will occur. Probability can range from 0, indicating that the event is certain not to occur, to 1, indicating that the event is certain to occur.

Probability of causation (PC). The probability that a specific disease in a person was caused by their exposure to a particular hazardous agent (such as ionizing radiation). PC is estimated as the quotient of two risks: PC = R divided by ($R + B$), where R is the estimated risk of the disease in a person due to the exposure and B is the estimated baseline (background) risk of the disease in that person from all other causes (that is, the risk in the absence of exposure to that agent). PC differs from risk in that it is conditional on the occurrence of the disease.

Progeny. The decay products resulting after a series of radioactive decay. Progeny can also be radioactive, and decay continues until a stable nuclide is formed.

Promotor. A substance or agent that will not cause a tumor by itself but will once an initiator has acted on the cell of interest.

Prospective study. A study in which two groups of people, one exposed and one unexposed, are followed forward in time to determine the possible linkage between exposure and health effects.

Protective clothing. Special clothing worn to prevent radioactive contamination.

Proton. An elementary particle with a mass 1873 times that of an electron and a positive charge equal to the basic electronic charge.

Quadratic model. The assumption that the effect of exposure to ionizing radiation is related to the square of the dose received.

Quality factor (QF). Dependent factor by which absorbed doses are to be multiplied to account for the varying effectiveness of different radiations. QF for 250-kVp x-rays is equal to 1. *See also* Weighting factor (radiation).

Rad. Radiation absorbed dose. The unit of absorbed dose of ionizing radiation. One rad is equal to 100 erg/g. *See* Gray.

Radiation. Energy propagated through space or matter as waves (gamma rays, ultraviolet light) or as particles (alpha or beta rays). External radiation is from a source outside the body, whereas internal radiation is from a source inside the body (such as radionuclides deposited in tissues).

Radiation area. Any accessible area in which the level of radiation is such that a major portion of an individual's body could receive in any one hour a dose in excess of 5 mrem or in any five consecutive days a dose in excess of 150 mrem.

Radiation Effects Research Foundation (RERF). The nonprofit Japanese-American research foundation which supervises the studies of atomic bomb survivors. The successor in 1975 to the Atomic Bomb Casualty Commission (ABCC).

Radiation therapy. Treatment of disease with any type of radiation. Often called *radiotherapy*.

Radioactive contamination. Deposition of radioactive material in any place where it may harm persons, spoil experiments, or make products or equipment unsuitable or unsafe for some specific use; the presence of unwanted radioactive matter. Also, radioactive material that is found on the walls of vessels in spent-fuel processing plants or has leaked into a reactor coolant. Often called *contamination*.

Radioactive decay. The spontaneous transformation of one nuclide into a different nuclide or into a different energy state of the same nuclide. The process results in a depletion, with time, of the radioactive atoms in a sample. Radioactive decay involves (1) the emission from the nucleus of alpha particles, beta particles (electrons), or gamma rays; (2) the nuclear capture or ejection of orbital electrons; or (3) fission. Also called *radioactive disintegration*. *See* Half-life.

Radioactivity. The property of certain nuclides of emitting radiation by the spontaneous transformation of their nuclei.

Radioepidemiological tables. A tabulation of the estimated probabilities of causation of specific cancers in a person who receives various doses of ionizing radiation.

Radiogenic disease. A type of disease assumed on the basis of scientific studies to have an association with radiation exposure. A statement that a cancer is radiogenic does not imply that radiation is the only cause of the cancer but rather that radiation has been shown to be one of its causes.

Radionuclide. Unstable nucleus that transmutes by way of nuclear decay.

Radionuclide purity. Amount of total radioactive species in a sample that is the desired radionuclide.

Radiopharmaceutical. Radioactive drug used for therapy or diagnosis.

Radiophobia. Abnormal fear of radiation.

Radioprotector. Compound that inhibits the radiation response of biologic systems.

Radioresistance. A relative resistance of cells, tissues, organs, or organisms to the harmful action of radiation.

Radiosensitivity. A relative susceptibility of cells, tissues, organs, or organisms to the harmful action of radiation.

Radiosensitizer. Substance that enhances the radiation response of biologic systems.

Radiotherapy. *See* Radiation therapy.

Radium (Ra). A radioactive metallic element with atomic number 88. As found in nature, the most common isotope has an atomic weight of 226. It occurs in minute quantities associated with uranium in pitchblende, carnotite, and other minerals. Uranium decays to radium in a series of alpha and beta emissions. By virtue of being an alpha and gamma emitter, radium is a source of luminescence and a radiation source in medicine and radiography.

Radon (Rn). A radioactive element and the heaviest gas known. Its atomic number is 86, and its atomic weight varies from 200 to 226. It is a daughter of radium in the uranium radioactive series.

Radon progeny. The radioactive products formed in the radioactive decay of radon; radionuclides which when inhaled can expose cells to alpha particles.

Rare earths. A group of 15 chemically similar metallic elements, numbers 57 through 71 in the periodic table; also known as the *lanthanide series.*

Rate meter. Device used in conjunction with a detector that measures the rate of activity of a radioisotope, usually in units of counts per minute or counts per second.

RBE. *See* Relative biologic effectiveness.

Recessive. Refers to a gene that produces its effect (is expressed) only when it is present in the homozygous state.

Reference man. An "ideal or standard man" used for radiation protection purposes. Has defined anatomic and physiologic specifications. Originally defined in ICRP, Reference man: Anatomical, physiological and metabolic characteristics. Report No. 23, Oxford, Pergamon Press, 1975.

Relative biologic effectiveness (RBE). Ratio of the biologic response derived from a particular radiation as compared to another radiation exposure.

Rem. *See* Roentgen equivalent man.

RERF. *See* Radiation Effects Research Foundation.

Risk, absolute. The excess risk attributed to irradiation and usually expressed as the numeric difference between irradiated and nonirradiated populations (e.g., 1 excess case of cancer in 1 million people irradiated annually for each rad). Absolute risk may be given on an annual basis or lifetime (70-year) basis.

Risk, relative (RR). The ratio between the number of cancer cases in the irradiated population to the number of cases expected in the unexposed population. An RR of 1.1 indicates a 10% increase in cancer due to radiation, compared with the "normal" incidence. Relative risk is more appropriate to use when considering selected population groups.

RNA (ribonucleic acid). A nucleic acid formed on a DNA template and taking part in the synthesis of polypeptides. Instead of thymine, RNA contains uracil. Three forms are recognized: (1) messenger RNA (mRNA), which is the template on which polypeptides are synthesized; (2) transfer RNA (sRNA, soluble RNA), which, in cooperation with the ribosomes, brings activated amino acids into position along the mRNA template; (3) ribosomal RNA (rRNA), a component of the ribosomes, which function as nonspecific sites of polypeptide synthesis.

Robertsonian translocation. A translocation between two acrocentric chromosomes by fusion at the centromeres and loss of the respective short arms.

Roentgen (R). Quantity of x- or gamma ray radiation per cubic cm of air that produces one electrostatic unit of charge.

Roentgen equivalent man (rem). The unit of dose equivalent. The absorbed dose in rad multiplied by the quality factor of the type of radiation. *See* Sievert.

RR. *See* Risk, relative.

Satellite. A small chromatin knob attached to the short arm of some chromosomes.

Scattered radiation. Radiation that during its passage through a substance has been deviated in direction, possibly with an energy loss.

Screening. The application of a test to detect potential disease or condition in a person who has no known signs or symptoms of a condition or disease.

Sealed source. A radioactive source, sealed in an impervious container that has sufficient mechanical strength to prevent contact with and dispersion of the radioactive material under conditions of use and wear for which it was designed. Generally used for industrial radiography or radiation therapy.

Sex chromosomes. Chromosomes that determine the sex of the individual; in humans, the X chromosome in the female, the X and Y chromosomes in the male.

Sex-linked. A gene located on a sex chromosome. Often used to describe genes on the X chromosome, although *X-linked* is the more accurate term.

Shield (shielding). A body of material used to reduce the intensity of radiation.

Shielding. Any material used to absorb beta, x-, and gamma ray radiation.

Sievert (Sv). The SI unit of dose equivalent. The absorbed dose in gray multiplied by the quality factor or radiation-weighting factor of the type of radiation. l sievert equals 100 rem.

SIR. *See* Standardized incidence ratio.

SI units. International system of units. SI refers to *Systeme International d'Unites.* Radiation units include joule/kg, gray, sievert, and becquerel.

SMR. *See* Standardized mortality ratio.

Somatic effects of radiation. Effects of radiation limited to the exposed individual, as distinguished from genetic effects, which also affect subsequent unexposed generations. Large radiation doses can cause somatic effects that are fatal. Lower doses may make the individual noticeably ill, produce temporary changes in blood-cell levels detectable only in the laboratory, or have no detectable effects.

Somatic mutation. A mutation occurring in a somatic cell (i.e., one that is not passed on to future generations).

Specific activity. Unit pertaining to the disintegrations per g of a radioisotope.

Spectrum. A range or distribution of wavelengths of radiation with a lower and upper limit of energy. Particulate radiation may also be included in the designation.

Spent fuel. Nuclear reactor fuel that has been irradiated (used) to the extent that it can no longer effectively sustain a chain reaction.

Standardized incidence ratio (SIR). Number of observed cases divided by the number of expected cases. The word *standardized* means that there has been adjustment for one or more potential bias factors such as age and sex.

Standardized mortality ratio (SMR). Number of observed deaths divided by the number of expected deaths. The word *standardized* means that there has been adjustment for one or more potential bias factors such as age and sex.

Standard man. *See* Reference man.

Statistical significance. The likelihood that an association between exposure and disease risk that a study finds did not occur by chance.

Stochastic effect. An effect whose probability of occurrence in an irradiated population or individual is a function of dose. Commonly regarded as having no threshold dose. An example is radiation carcinogenesis.

Survey meter. Meter that measures rate of radioactive exposure, usually in units of milliroentgens per hour.

Survival curve. Obtained by plotting the number or the percentage of organisms surviving at a given time against the dose of radiation or the number surviving at different intervals after a particular dose of radiation.

Teratogenic effect. Birth defects that are not passed on to future generations. Caused by exposure to a toxin as a fetus.

Thermal neutrons. Neutrons in thermal equilibrium with their surrounding medium. Thermal neutrons are those that have been slowed down by a moderator to an average speed of about 220 m per second at room temperature from the much higher initial speeds they had when expelled by fission. *Compare* Fast neutrons; Intermediate neutrons.

Thermoluminescent dosimeter (TLD). Type of crystal used to monitor radiation exposure by emitting light; often used in a body, wrist, or ring badge. Must be processed to be "read."

Thorium (Th). A naturally radioactive element with atomic number 90 and, as found in nature, an atomic weight of approximately 232. The fertile thorium isotope ^{232}Th is abundant and can be transmuted to the fissionable uranium isotope ^{233}U by neutron irradiation. *See* Fertile material.

Threshold dose. The minimum dose of radiation that will produce a detectable biologic effect.

Tissue-weighting factor. *See* Weighting factor.

Transient equilibrium. Equilibrium reached by a parent-daughter radioisotope pair in which the half-life of the parent is longer than that of the daughter.

Translocation. The transfer of genetic material from one chromosome to another, nonhomologous chromosome. An exchange of genetic material between two chromosomes is referred to as a *reciprocal translocation*. When a small fragment, which is usually lost, is formed (*centric fusion*), this is referred to as a *Robertsonian translocation*.

Transuranic nuclide. A nuclide having an atomic number greater than that of uranium (92). Includes neptunium, plutonium, americium, and curium.

Triplet. In molecular genetics, a unit of three successive bases in DNA or RNA, coding for a specific amino acid.

Triploid. A cell with three times the haploid number of chromosomes (i.e., 3n).

Trisomy. A state in which there are three members of a given chromosome instead of the normal pair.

Tritium (^{3}H or T). A radioactive isotope of hydrogen with two neutrons and one proton in the nucleus. It is made synthetically and is heavier than deuterium (heavy hydrogen). Tritium is used as a label in chemical and biologic experiments. Its nucleus is a triton.

Tumor-suppressor gene. A gene that normally acts to inhibit cell proliferation.

UF conversion. The process of converting the solid uranium oxide (commonly called *yellowcake*) that comes from uranium mining and milling into a uranium fluoride gas.

UNSCEAR. United Nations Scientific Committee on the Effects of Atomic Radiation. A committee of the U.N. General Assembly charged with evaluating the sources and effects of ionizing radiation on behalf of the member nations.

Uranium (U). A radioactive element with atomic number 92 and, as found in natural ores, an average atomic weight of approximately 238. The two principal natural isotopes are ^{235}U (0.7% of natural uranium), which is fissionable, and ^{238}U (99.3% of natural uranium), which is fertile. Natural uranium also includes a minute amount of ^{234}U. Uranium is the basic raw material of nuclear energy.

Weighting factor. A number of values that is used to adjust for the various sensitivities of tissues and effectiveness of radiations to express risk. The values listed here were derived by the ICRP (2007) and refer to stochastic effects only.

Tissue (W_T)
  0.01 bone
  0.01 brain
  0.01 salivary gland
  0.01 skin

0.04 bladder
0.04 esophagus
0.04 liver
0.04 thyroid
0.08 gonads
0.12 bone marrow
0.12 breast
0.12 colon
0.12 lung
0.12 remainder organs
0.12 stomach
Radiation (W_R)
1.0 photons
1.0 electrons, and muons
5–20 neutrons, value depends on energy
5.0 protons
20.0 alpha particles

Whole-body counter. A device used to identify and measure radionuclides in the body (*body burden*) of humans and animals. It uses heavy shielding (to keep out background radiation), ultrasensitive scintillation detectors, and electronic equipment.

Working level (WL). Any combination of radon and radon daughters in 1 L of air that will result in the emission of 1.3×10^{-5} megaelectron volts of alpha particle energy.

Working level month (WLM). One working level incurred over 170 working hours. A WLM is approximately equal to an absorbed dose of 5 mGy and an effective dose of 12 mSv.

X chromosome. A sex chromosome found in duplicate in the normal female and singly in the male.

X-linkage. A gene carried on the X chromosome.

Y chromosome. One of the sex chromosomes found in the normal male. The Y chromosome is essential for the development of male gonads.

Yellowcake. The semirefined product from uranium mining and milling operations that is sent to conversion plants.

Z number. *See* Atomic number.

Zygote. The diploid cell found by the fusion of the haploid male and female gametes; the fertilized ovum.

Appendix 2 Radiation Source Term Table

Radionuclides Listed Alphabetically

Radionuclide	Physical Half-Life	Effective Half-Life	Radiation
Americium 241	458 yr	139 yr	α, e^-, γ
Americium 243	7950 yr	194 yr	α, γ
Antimony 122	67 hr	—	β^-, β^+, γ
Antimony 124	60 days	—	β^-, γ
Antimony 125	2.7 yr	—	β^-, e^-, γ
Argon 37	35 days	—	γ
Arsenic 74	18 days	17 days	β^-, β^+, γ
Arsenic 76	26.5 hr	—	β^-, γ
Arsenic 77	39 hr	24 hr	β^-, γ
Barium 131	12 days	—	γ, e^-
Barium 133	7.2 yr	—	γ, e^+
Barium 137m	2.55 min	—	γ, e^-
Barium 140	13 days	11 days	β^-, e^-, γ
Beryllium 7	53 days	—	γ
Bismuth 207	30 yr	—	e^-, γ
Bismuth 210	5.01 days	—	α, β^-, γ
Bromine 82	35.34 hr	—	β^-, γ
Cadmium 109	453 days	140 days	e^-, γ
Cadmium 115	53.5 hr	—	β^-, γ
Cadmium 115	43 days	—	β^-, γ
Calcium 45	165 days	162 days	β^-
Calcium 47	4.5 days	4.5 days	β^-, γ
Californium 242	2.6 yr	2.2 yr	γ, α, N
Carbon 11	20.3 min	—	β^+, γ
Carbon 14	5730 yr	12 days	β^-
Cerium 141	33 days	30 days	β^-, e^-, γ
Cerium 144	284 days	280 days	β^-, e^-, γ
Cesium 131	9.70 days	—	γ
Cesium 134	2.05 yr	—	β^-, γ
Cesium 137	30.0 yr	70 days	β^-, e^-, γ
Chlorine 36	3.1×10^5 yr	—	β^-, γ
Chromium 51	27.8 days	27 days	e^-, γ
Cobalt 57	270 days	9 days	e^-, γ
Cobalt 58	71.3 days	8 days	β^+, γ
Cobalt 60	5.26 yr	10 days	β^-, γ
Copper 64	12.8 hr	—	$\beta^-, e^-, \beta^+, \gamma$
Curium 242	163 days	155 days	α, N, γ
Curium 243	32 yr	27.5 days	α, γ
Curium 244	17.6 yr	16.7 yr	α, N, γ
Dysprosium 159	144 days	—	e^-, γ

Continued

Radionuclides Listed Alphabetically—cont'd

Radionuclide	Physical Half-Life	Effective Half-Life	Radiation
Erbium 169	9.4 days	—	β^-, e^-, γ
Europium 152	13 yr	3 yr	β^-, β^+, e^-, γ
Europium 154	16 yr	3 yr	β^-, e^-, γ
Europium 155	2 yr	1.3 yr	β^-, e^-, γ
Fluorine 18	2 hr	2 hr	β, γ
Gadolinium 153	242 days	—	e^-, γ
Gallium 67	78.1 hr	—	γ
Gallium 68	68.3 min	—	β^+, γ
Gallium 72	14.1 hr	12 hr	β, γ
Germanium 71	11.4 days	—	γ
Gold 195	183 days	—	e^-, γ
Gold 198	2.7 days	2.6 days	β^-, e^-, γ
Gold 199	75.6 hr	—	β^-, e^-, γ
Hafnium 181	42.5 days	—	β^-, e^-, γ
Holmium 166	26.9 hr	—	β^-, e^-, γ
Hydrogen 3	12 yr	12 days	β^-
Indium 111	2.8 days	—	γ
Indium 113m	100 min	—	e^-, γ
Indium 114	72 sec	—	β^-, β^+, γ
Indium 114m	49 days	27 days	e^-, γ (DR)
Iodine 123	13 hr	—	γ
Iodine 125	60 days	42 days	e^-, γ
Iodine 129	1.7×10^7 yr	—	β^-, e^-, γ
Iodine 130	12.4 hr	—	β^-, γ
Iodine 131	8.05 days	8 days	β^-, e^-, γ
Iridium 192	74 days	—	β^-, e^-, γ
Iridium 194	17.4 hr	—	β, γ
Iron 52	8.3 hr	—	β^-, χ, γ
Iron 55	2.6 yr	1 yr	γ
Iron 59	45 days	42 days	β^-, γ
Krypton 81m	13.0 sec	—	γ
Krypton 85	10.76 yr	—	β^-, γ
Lanthanum 140	40.22 hr	—	β^-, γ
Lead 210	22.3 yr	1.3 yr	α, β^-, e^-, γ
Lutetium 177	6.7 days	—	β^-, e^-, γ
Magnesium 28	21 hr	—	β^-, e^-, γ
Manganese 54	303 days	—	e^-, γ
Mercury 197	2.7 days	2.3 days	e^-, γ
Mercury 197m	24 hr	—	e^-, γ
Mercury 203	46 days	11 days	β^-, e^-, γ
Molybdenum 99	67 hrs	1.5 days	β^-, γ
Neodymium 147	11.1 days	—	β^-, e^-, γ
Neptunium 237	2×10^6 yr	200 yr	α, γ (DR)
Neptunium 239	2.3 days	2.3 days	β, γ
Nickel 63	92 yr	—	β^-
Niobium 95	35 days	—	β^-, γ
Nitrogen 13	10 min	—	β^+, γ
Osmium 191	15 days	—	β^-, e^-, γ
Oxygen 15	124 sec	—	β^+, γ
Palladium 103	17 days	—	γ
Palladium 109	13.47 hr	—	β^-, e^-, γ
Phosphorus 32	25.6 days	14 days	β^-
Plutonium 238	88 yr	63 yr	γ, α
Plutonium 239	2.4×10^4 yr	197 yr	γ, α
Polonium 210	138 days	46 days	α, γ
Potassium 42	12 hr	12 hr	β^-, γ
Praseodymium 142	19.2 hr	—	β^-, γ
Praseodymium 143	13.6 days	—	β^-
Praseodymium 144	17.3 min	—	β^-, γ
Promethium 147	2.6 yr	1.6 yr	β^-

Radionuclides Listed Alphabetically—cont'd

Radionuclide	Physical Half-Life	Effective Half-Life	Radiation
Promethium 149	2.2 days	2.2 days	β^-, γ
Protactinium 233	27.0 days	—	β^-, e^-, γ
Protactinium 234	6.75 hr	—	β^-, e^-, γ
Radium 224	3.6 days	3.6 days	γ, α (DR)
Radium 226	160 yr	44 yr	α, e^-, γ (DR)
Rhenium 186	90 hr	—	β^-, e^-, γ
Rhodium 106	30 sec	—	β^-, γ
Rubidium 82	1.3 min	—	β^+, γ
Rubidium 86	19.0 days	13.2 days	β^-, γ
Ruthenium 97	2.9 days	—	e^-, γ
Ruthenium 103	39.6 days	—	β^-, γ
Ruthenium 106	367 days	2.5 days	β^- (DR)
Samarium 151	87 yr	—	β^-, e^-, γ
Samarium 153	47 hr	—	β^-, e^-, γ
Scandium 46	84 days	40 days	β^-, γ
Selenium 75	120.4 days	—	e^-, γ
Selenium 77m	17.5 sec	—	γ
Silver 110	24.4 sec	—	β^-, γ
Silver 110m	253 days	5 days	β^-, e^-, γ
Silver 111	7.5 days	—	β^-, γ
Sodium 22	2.60 yr	11 days	β^+, γ
Sodium 24	15 hr	14 hr	β^-, γ
Strontium 85	64 days	64 days	e^-, γ
Strontium 87m	2.83 hr	—	e^-, γ
Strontium 89	52 days	—	β^-, γ
Strontium 90	28 yr	15 yr	β^- (DR)
Sulfur 35	88 days	44 days	β^-
Tantalum 182	115 days	—	β^-, e^-, γ
Technetium 99	2.12×10^5 yr	20 days	β^-
Technetium 99m	6.0 hr	—	e^-, γ
Tellurium 132	78 hr	—	β^-, e^-, γ
Terbium 160	72.1 days	—	β^-, e^-, γ
Thallium 201	73 hr	—	γ (DR)
Thallium 204	3.8 yr	—	β^-, γ
Thorium 230	8×10^4 yr	200 yr	α, γ
Thorium 232	1.4×10^{10} yr	200 yr	α, γ (DR)
Thulium 170	130 days	—	β^-, e^-, γ
Tin 113	115 days	—	γ
Tin 119m	250 days	—	e^-, γ
Titanium 44	48 hr	—	e^-, γ (DR)
Tungsten 185	75 days	—	β^-
Tungsten 187	23.9 hr	—	β^-, e^-, γ
Uranium 235	7.1×10^8 yr	15 days	α, γ (DR)
Uranium 238	4.51×10^9 yr	—	α, e^-, γ (DR)
Xenon 127	36.4 days	—	e^-, γ
Xenon 133	5.27 days	—	β^-, e^-, γ
Ytterbium 169	32 days	—	e^-, γ
Yttrium 90	64 hr	64 hr	β^-
Yttrium 91	58.8 days	—	β^-, γ
Zinc 65	245 days	194 days	β^+, e^-, γ
Zinc 69	57 min	—	β^-
Zirconium 95	66 days	56 days	β^-, γ (DR)

DR, daughter radiation; N, neutron.
From Mettler FA, Moseley RD (eds): Medical Effects of Ionizing Radiation, New York, Grune and Stratton, 1985.

Appendix 3 Conversion Tables

Table A3-1 • Conventional and International (SI) Unit Conversions

Factor	Prefix	Symbol	Factor	Prefix	Symbol
10^{18}	exa	E	10^{-1}	deci	d
10^{15}	peta	P	10^{-2}	centi	c
10^{12}	tera	T	10^{-3}	milli	m
10^{9}	giga	G	10^{-6}	micro	u
10^{6}	mega	M	10^{-9}	nano	n
10^{3}	kilo	k	10^{-12}	pico	p
10^{2}	hecto	h	10^{-15}	femto	f
10^{1}	deka	da	10^{-18}	atto	a

Table A3-2 • Conversion of Exposure Units

Coulomb/kg		Roentgen (R)
10 C/kg	=	38,000 R
1 C/kg	=	3,880 R
10^{-1} C/kg	=	388 R
10^{-2} C/kg	=	38.8 R
10^{-3} C/kg	=	3.88 R
10^{-4} C/kg	=	0.388 R (388 mR)
10^{-5} C/kg	=	3.88×10^{-3} R (38.8 mR)
10^{-6} C/kg	=	3.88×10^{-3} R (3.88 mR)
10^{-7} C/kg	=	3.88×10^{-4} R (388 μR)
10^{-8} C/kg	=	3.88×10^{-5} R (38.8 μR)
10^{-9} C/kg	=	3.88×10^{-6} R (3.8 μR)
10^{-10} C/kg	=	3.88×10^{-7} R (388 nR)
10^{-11} C/kg	=	3.88×10^{-8} R (38.8 nR)

Table A3-3 • Conversion of Absorbed Dose Units

SI Units		Conventional
100 Gy (10^{2} Gy)	=	10,000 rads (10^{4} rads)
10 Gy (10^{1} Gy)	=	1,000 rads (10^{3} rads)
1 Gy (10^{0} Gy)	=	100 rads (10^{2} rads)
100 mGy (10^{-1} Gy)	=	10 rads (10^{1} rads)
10 mGy (10^{-2} Gy)	=	1 rad (10^{0} rads)
1 mGy (10^{-3} Gy)	=	100 mrad (10^{-1} rads)
100 uGy (10^{-4} Gy)	=	10 mrad (10^{-2} rads)
10 uGy (10^{-5} Gy)	=	1 mrad (10^{-3} rads)
1 uGy (10^{-6} Gy)	=	100 μrad (10^{-4} rads)
100 nGy (10^{-7} Gy)	=	10 μrad (10^{-5} rads)
10 nGy (10^{-8} Gy)	=	1 μrad (10^{-6} rads)
1 nGy (10^{-9} Gy)	=	100 nrad (10^{-7} rads)

Table A3-4 • Conversion of Dose Equivalent Units

SI Units		Conventional
100 Sv (10^{2} Sv)	=	10,000 rem (10^{4} rem)
10 Sv (10^{1} Sv)	=	1,000 rem (10^{3} rem)
1 Sv (10^{0} Sv)	=	100 rem (10^{2} rem)
100 mSv (10^{-1} Sv)	=	10 rem (10^{1} rem)
10 mSv (10^{-2} Sv)	=	1 rem (10^{0} rem)
1 mSv (10^{-3} Sv)	=	100 mrem (10^{-1} rem)
100 μSv (10^{-4} Sv)	=	10 mrem (10^{-2} rem)
10 μSv (10^{-5} Sv)	=	1 mrem (10^{-3} rem)
1 μSv (10^{-6} Sv)	=	100 μrem (10^{-4} rem)
100 nSv (10^{-7} Sv)	=	10 μrem (10^{-5} rem)
10 nSv (10^{-8} Sv)	=	1 μrem (10^{-6} rem)
1 nSv (10^{-9} Sv)	=	100 nrem (10^{-7} rem)

Table A3-5 • Conversion of Radioactivity Units

SI Units		Conventional
100 Tbq (10^{14} Bq)	=	2.7 kCi (2.7×10^3 Ci)
10 TBq (10^{13} Bq)	=	270 Ci (2.7×10^2 Ci)
1 TBq (10^{12} Bq)	=	27 Ci (2.7×10^1 Ci)
100 GBq (10^{11} Bq)	=	2.7 Ci (2.7×10^0 Ci)
10 GBq (10^{10} Bq)	=	270 mCi (2.7×10^{-1} Ci)
1 GBq (10^9 Bq)	=	27 mCi (2.7×10^{-2} Ci)
100 MBq (10^8 Bq)	=	2.7 mCi (2.7×10^{-3} Ci)
10 MBq (10^7 Bq)	=	270 μCi (2.7×10^{-4} Ci)
1 MBq (10^6 Bq)	=	27 μCi (2.7×10^{-5} Ci)
100 kBq (10^5 Bq)	=	2.7 μCi (2.7×10^{-6} Ci)
10 kBq (10^4 Bq)	=	270 nCi (2.7×10^{-7} Ci)
1 kBq (10^3 Bq)	=	27 nCi (2.7×10^{-8} Ci)
100 Bq (10^2 Bq)	=	2.7 nCi (2.7×10^{-9} Ci)
10 Bq (10^1 Bq)	=	270 pCi (2.7×10^{-10} Ci)
1 Bq (10^0 Bq)	=	27 pCi (2.7×10^{-11} Ci)
100 mBq (10^{-1} Bq)	=	2.7 pCi (2.7×10^{-12} Ci)
10 mBq (10^{-2} Bq)	=	270 fCi (2.7×10^{-13} Ci)
1 mBq (10^{-3} Bq)	=	27 fCi (2.7×10^{-14} Ci)

Table A3-6 • Radon Conversion Chart*

Working Level	pCi/L	Bq/m^3
0.01	1	37
0.028	2.75	100
0.04	4	148
0.055	5.5	200
0.1	10	370
0.11	11	400
1	100	3700

*Values are approximate. Actual values depend upon assumptions related to equilibrium, attached fraction, and other factors.
WL = any combination of short-lived daughters in one L of air that will release 1.3×10^5 of potential alpha energy.
1 WLM = exposure to 1 WL for 170 hr.
1 WLM = 3.51 mJ/h/m^{-3}.
1 mJ/h/m^{-3} = 0.285 WLM.
Epidemiological studies indicate that 1 WLM of radon gives about the same risk as an effective dose of about 5 mSv.
In homes 400 MBq^{-3} corresponds to an annual effective dose of about 10 mSv while at work 1000 MBq^{-3} corresponds to an annual effective dose of about 6 mSv. The difference is based upon occupancy times of 7000 hr at home and 2000 hr annually at work.

Appendix 4 Absorbed Dose Estimates from Radionuclides

These charts can be used to estimate absorbed dose from a variety of accidental situations involving radionuclides.

Table A4-1 is derived from data from the International Commission on Radiological Protection (ICRP): Dose coefficients for intakes of radionuclides by workers, ICRP report no. 68. Oxford, Pergamon Press, 1995. For age-dependent doses to members of the public from intake of radionuclides, the reader is referred to ICRP report nos. 67, 69, 71, and 72.

Tables A4-2 to A4-4 contain corrected data from the National Council on Radiation Protection and Measurements (NCRP): Developing Radiation Emergency Plans for Academic, Medical or Industrial Facilities, NCRP report no. 111. Bethesda, MD, NCRP, 1991. (These latter tables do not use the new ICRP models.)

Table A4-1 • Dose Coefficients for Intakes of Radionuclides by Workers (Sv/Bq)

Nuclide	Physical $t_{1/2}$	Type*	Inhalation[†] 1 μm AMAD	Inhalation[†] 5 μm AMAD	Ingestion[†]
Americium 241	4.32E+02 yr	M	3.9E-05	2.7E-05	2.0E-07
Americium 243	7.38E+03 yr	M	3.9E-05	2.7E-05	2.0E-07
Arsenic 74	17.8 days	M	2.1E-09	1.8E-09	1.3E-09
Arsenic 77	1.62 days	M	3.8E-10	4.2E-10	4.0E-10
Barium 140	12.7 days	F	1.0E-09	1.6E-09	2.5E-09
Cadmium 109	1.27 yr	F	8.1E-09	9.6E-09	2.0E-09
Cadmium 109	—	M	6.2E-09	5.1E-09	—
Cadmium 109	—	S	5.8E-09	4.4E-09	—
Calcium 45	163 days	M	2.7E-09	2.3E-09	7.6E-10
Calcium 47	4.53 days	M	1.8E-09	2.1E-09	1.6E-09
Californium 252	2.63 yr	M	1.8E-05	1.3E-05	9.0E-08
Carbon 14	5.7E+03 yr	—	—	—	5.8E-10
Cerium 141	32.5 days	M	3.1E-09	2.7E-09	7.1E-10
Cerium 141	—	S	3.6E-09	3.1E-09	—
Cerium 144	284 days	M	3.4E-08	2.3E-08	5.2E-09
Cerium 144	—	S	4.9E-08	2.9E-08	—
Cesium 134	2.06 yr	F	6.8E-09	9.6E-09	1.9E-08
Cesium 137	30.0 yr	F	4.8E-09	6.7E-09	1.3E-08
Chromium 51	27.7 days	F	2.1E-11	3.0E-11	3.8E-11
Chromium 51	—	M	3.1E-11	3.4E-11	3.7E-11
Chromium 51	—	S	3.6E-11	3.6E-11	—
Cobalt 57	271 days	M	5.2E-10	3.9E-10	2.1E-10
Cobalt 57	—	S	9.4E-10	6.0E-10	1.9E-10
Cobalt 58	70.8 days	M	1.5E-09	1.4E-09	7.4E-10
Cobalt 58	—	S	2.0E-09	1.7E-09	7.0E-10
Cobalt 60	5.27 yr	M	9.6E-09	7.1E-09	3.4E-09
Cobalt 60	—	S	2.9E-08	1.7E-08	2.5E-09
Curium 242	163 days	M	4.8E-06	3.7E-06	1.2E-08

Continued

Table A4-1 • Dose Coefficients for Intakes of Radionuclides by Workers (Sv/Bq)—cont'd

Nuclide	Physical $t_{1/2}$	Type*	Inhalation[†] 1 μm AMAD	Inhalation[†] 5 μm AMAD	Ingestion[†]
Curium 243	28.5 yr	M	2.9E-05	2.0E-05	1.5E-07
Curium 244	18.1 yr	M	2.5E-05	1.7E-05	1.2E-07
Europium 152	13.3 yr	M	3.9E-08	2.7E-08	1.4E-09
Europium 154	8.8 yr	M	5.0E-08	3.5E-08	2.0E-09
Europium 155	4.96 yr	M	6.5E-09	4.7E-09	3.2E-10
Flourine 18	1.83 hr	F	3.0E-11	5.4E-11	4.9E-11
Flourine 18	—	M	5.7E-11	8.9E-11	—
Flourine 18	—	S	6.0E-11	9.3E-11	1.9E-10
Gallium 67	3.26 days	F	6.8E-11	1.1E-10	—
Gallium 67	—	M	2.3E-10	2.8E-10	—
Gallium 72	14.1 hr	F	3.1E-10	5.6E-10	1.1E-09
Gallium 72	—	M	5.5E-10	8.4E-10	—
Gold 198	2.69 days	F	2.3E-10	3.9E-10	1.0E-09
Gold 198	—	M	7.6E-10	9.8E-10	—
Gold 198	—	S	8.4E-10	1.1E-09	—
Hydrogen 3	12.3 yr	—	—	—	1.8E-11
Indium 114m	49.5 days	F	9.3E-09	1.1E-08	4.1E-09
Indium 114m	—	M	5.9E-09	5.9E-09	—
Iridium 192	74.0 days	F	1.8E-09	2.2E-09	1.4E-09
Iridium 192	—	M	4.9E-09	4.1E-09	—
Iridium 192	—	S	6.2E-09	4.9E-09	—
Iodine 123	13.2 hr	F	7.6E-11	1.1E-10	2.1E-10
Iodine 125	60.1 days	F	5.3E-09	7.3E-09	1.5E-08
Iodine 131	8.04 days	F	7.6E-09	1.1E-08	2.2E-08
Iron 52	8.3 hr	F	4.1E-10	6.9E-10	1.4E-09
Iron 52	—	M	6.3E-10	9.5E-10	—
Iron-55	2.7 yr	F	7.7E-10	9.2E-10	3.3E-10
Iron-55	—	M	3.7E-10	3.3E-10	—
Iron 59	44.5 days	F	2.2E-09	3.0E-09	1.8E-09
Iron 59	—	M	3.5E-09	3.2E-09	—
Lead 210	22.3 yr	F	8.9E-07	1.1E-06	6.8E-07
Mercury 197 (inorganic)	2.67 days	F	6.0E-11	1.0E-10	2.3E-10
Mercury 197 (inorganic)	—	M	2.9E-10	2.8E-10	—
Mercury 203 (inorganic)	46.6 days	F	4.7E-10	5.9E-10	5.4E-10
Mercury 203 (inorganic)	—	M	2.3E-09	1.9E-10	—
Molybdenum 99	2.75 days	F	2.3E-10	3.6E-10	7.4E-10
Molybdenum 99	—	S	9.7E-10	1.1E-09	1.2E-09
Neptunium 237	2.14E+06 yr	M	2.1E-05	1.5E-05	1.1E-07
Neptunium 239	22.36 days	M	9.0E-10	1.1E-09	8.0E-10
Phosphorus 32	14.3 days	F	8.0E-10	1.1E-09	2.4E-09
Phosphorus 32	—	M	3.2E-09	2.9E-09	—
Plutonium 238	87.7 yr	M	4.3E-05	3.0E-05	2.3E-07
Plutonium 238	—	S	1.5E-05	1.1E-05	8.8E-09
Plutonium 239	2.41E+04y	M	4.7E-05	3.2E-05	2.5E-07
Plutonium 239	—	S	1.5E-05	8.3E-06	9.0E-09
Polonium 210	138 days	F	6.0E-07	7.1E-07	2.4E-07
Polonium- 210	—	M	3.0E-06	2.2E-06	—
Potassium 42	12.4 hr	F	1.3E-10	2.0E-10	4.3E-10
Promethium 147	2.62 yr	M	4.7E-09	3.5E-09	2.6E-10
Promethium 147	—	S	4.6E-09	3.2E-09	—
Promethium 149	2.21 days	M	6.6E-10	7.6E-10	9.9E-10
Promethium 149	—	S	7.2E-10	8.2E-10	—
Radium 224	3.66 days	M	2.9E-06	2.6E-06	6.5E-08
Radium 226	1.60E+03 yr	M	1.6E-05	1.2E-05	2.8E-07
Rubidium 86	18.6 days	F	9.6E-10	1.3E-09	2.8E-09
Ruthenium 106	1.01 yr	F	8.0E-09	9.8E-09	7.0E-09
Ruthenium 106	—	M	2.6E-08	1.7E-08	—
Ruthenium 106	—	S	6.2E-08	3.5E-08	—
Scandium 46	83.8 days	S	6.4E-09	4.8E-09	1.5E-09
Silver 110m	250 days	F	5.5E-09	6.7E-09	2.8E-09

Table A4-1 • Dose Coefficients for Intakes of Radionuclides by Workers (Sv/Bq)—cont'd

Nuclide	Physical $t_{1/2}$	Type*	Inhalation[†] 1 μm AMAD	Inhalation[†] 5 μm AMAD	Ingestion[†]
Silver 110m	—	M	7.2E-09	5.9E-09	—
Silver 110m	—	S	1.2E-08	7.3E-09	—
Sodium 22	2.6 yr	F	1.3E-09	2.0E-09	3.2E-09
Sodium 24	15.0 hr	F	2.9E-10	5.3E-10	4.3E-10
Strontium 85	64.8 days	F	3.9E-10	5.6E-10	5.6E-10
Strontium 85	—	S	7.7E-10	6.4E-10	3.3E-10
Strontium 90	29.1 yr	F	2.4E-08	3.0E-08	2.8E-08
Strontium 90	—	S	1.5E-07	7.7E-08	2.7E-09
Sulfur 35 (inorganic)	87.4 days	F	5.3E-11	8.0E-11	1.4E-10
Sulfur 35 (inorganic)	—	M	1.1E-09	1.1E-09	1.9E-10
Technetium 99m	6.02 hr	F	1.2E-11	2.0E-11	2.2E-11
Technetium 99m	—	M	1.9E-11	2.9E-11	—
Technetium 99	2.13E+05 yr	F	2.9E-10	4.0E-10	7.8E-10
Technetium 99	—	M	3.9E-09	3.2E-09	—
Thallium 201	3.04 days	F	4.7E-11	7.6E-11	9.5E-11
Thorium 230	7.7E+04 yr	M	4.0E-05	2.8E-05	2.1E-07
Thorium 230	—	S	1.3E-05	7.2E-06	8.7E-08
Thorium 232	1.4E+10 yr	M	4.2E-05	2.9E-05	2.2E-07
Thorium 232	—	S	2.3E-05	1.2E-05	9.2E-08
Uranium 235	7.04E+08 yr	F	5.1E-07	6.0E-07	4.6E-08
Uranium 235	—	M	2.8E-06	1.8E-06	8.3E-09
Uranium 235	—	S	7.7E-06	6.1E-06	—
Uranium 238	4.47E+09 yr	F	4.9E-09	5.8E-07	4.4E-08
Uranium 238	—	M	2.6E-06	1.6E-06	7.6E-09
Uranium 238	—	S	7.3E-06	5.7E-06	—
Yttrium 90	2.67 days	M	1.4E-09	1.6E-09	2.7E-09
Yttrium 90	—	S	1.5E-09	1.7E-09	—
Zinc 65	244 days	S	2.9E-09	2.8E-09	3.9E-09
Zirconium 95	64.0 days	F	2.5E-09	3.0E-09	8.8E-10
Zirconium 95	—	M	4.5E-09	3.6E-09	—
Zirconium 95	—	S	5.5E-09	4.2E-09	—

*Type F (fast lung clearance), type M (moderate), type S (slow).
[†]Expressed as 50-year committed effective dose.
AMAD, activity median aerodynamic diameter.

Table A4-2 • Skin Contamination Dose Equivalent Rate Factors at a Depth of 7 mg/cm²

Radionuclide	Infinite Area Source*,† (mSv/cm/MBq/hr)	Point Source‡ (mSv/MBq/hr)
^{14}C	305	2.45×10^6
^{22}Na	1870	3.3×10^6
^{24}Na	2357	2.3×10^6
^{32}P	2397	2.2×10^6
^{35}S	332	2.4×10^6
^{36}Cl	2178	2.8×10^6
^{45}Ca	884	3.6×10^6
^{57}Co	78	NV
^{59}Fe	1283	3.6×10^6
^{60}Co	1146	3.7×10^6
^{67}Ga	322	NV
^{90}Sr–^{90}Y (equilibrium)	4272	5.4×10^6
^{99m}Tc	243	NV
^{111}In	367	NV
^{123}I	360	NV
^{125}I	417	NV
^{131}I	1694	3.3×10^6
^{137}Cs–^{137}Ba (equilibrium)	1941	3.5×10^6
^{147}Pm	612	3.0×10^6
^{192}Ir	1592	3.2×10^6
^{201}Tl	343	NV
^{204}Tl	1803	3.0×10^6

*Appropriate for sources with average radii larger than the range of the radiation in water.
†Multiply by 3.7 to obtain the dose equivalent rate in rad/cm²/mCi/hr.
‡Multiply by 3.7 to obtain the dose equivalent rate in rad/mCi/hr.
NV, no value provided.

Table A4-3 • Maximum External Photon and Electron Dose Equivalent Factors for Any Organ for Selected Radionuclides for Point and Infinite Area Sources

Radionuclide	Point Sources (mSv/cm²/Bq/hr)	Area Source* at 1m†-photons (mSv/cm²/Bq/hr)	Area Source* at 1m†-electrons (mSv/cm²/Bq/hr)
^{22}Na	3.1×10^{-6}	8.5×10^{-5}	$5.1 \times 10^{-6‡}$
^{24}Na	4.8×10^{-6}	1.4×10^{-4}	2.1×10^{-4}
^{32}P	NV	NV	2.7×10^{-4}
^{51}Cr	4.2×10^{-8}	1.7×10^{-6}	0
^{57}Co	2.3×10^{-7}	8.7×10^{-6}	0
^{59}Fe	1.7×10^{-6}	4.5×10^{-5}	5.3×10^{-7}
^{60}Co	3.4×10^{-6}	9.3×10^{-5}	7.5×10^{-8}
^{67}Ga	2.9×10^{-7}	NV	NV
^{90}Sr–^{90}Y (equilibrium)	NV	2.4×10^{-10}	3.8×10^{-4}
^{99m}Tc	1.5×10^{-7}	8.7×10^{-6}	0
^{111}In	5.1×10^{-7}	NV	NV
^{123}I	1.9×10^{-7}	NV	NV
^{131}I	5.8×10^{-7}	1.9×10^{-5}	6.2×10^{-6}
^{137}Cs–^{137}Ba (equilibrium)	8.6×10^{-7}	2.5×10^{-5}	3.9×10^{-5}
^{192}Ir	1.3×10^{-6}	NV	NV
^{201}Tl	2.1×10^{-8}	NV	NV

*Specific gamma factors were multiplied by the factors for converting from roentgens to rads in water given and assuming a Q of 1. To obtain mSv/hr, multiply by activity in Bq and divide by the square of the distance in cm. From National Council on Radiation Protection and Measurements (NCRP): Dosimetry of x-ray and gamma ray beams for radiation therapy in the energy range 10 keV to 50 MeV. NCRP report no. 69. Washington, DC: NCRP, 1981.
†Value is maximum at 1 meter above contaminated surface. To obtain mSv/hr, multiply by the surface contamination in Bq/cm².
‡Value is at 70 μm. Dose calculated to basal layer. Assume bare source dispersed on ground.
NV, no value has been provided.

Table A4-4 • Maximum Photon Dose Equivalent Rate Conversion Factors for Any Organ and Electron Dose Equivalent Rate Conversion Factors for Skin for Submersion in Contaminated Air

Radionuclide	Photon Dose Equivalent Rate $(mSv/cm^3/Bq/hr)$*	Electron Dose Equivalent Rate[†]
^{14}C	0	7.8×10^{-4}
^{22}Na	4.5×10^{-1}	4.0×10^{-2}
^{24}Na	9.2×10^{-1}	1.2×10^{-1}
^{32}P	0	1.6×10^{-1}
^{35}S	0	9.5×10^{-4}
^{57}Co	3.9×10^{-2}	9.8×10^{-3}
^{59}Fe	2.4×10^{-1}	2.0×10^{-2}
^{60}Co	0.5×10^{-2}	1.5×10^{-6}
^{85}Kr	4.8×10^{-4}	4.4×10^{-2}
$^{90}Sr-^{90}Y$ (equilibrium)	1.4×10^{-8}	2.5×10^{-1}
^{99m}Tc	3.9×10^{-2}	3.2×10^{-4}
^{131}I	9.0×10^{-2}	3.0×10^{-2}
^{133}Xe	1.2×10^{-2}	9.6×10^{-3}
$^{137}CS-^{137}Ba$ (equilibrium)	1.2×10^{-1}	4.3×10^{-2}
^{147}Pm	1.1×10^{-6}	6.0×10^{-3}

*Value is the maximum over all organs, excluding skin, semi-infinite cloud.
[†]Value is for infinite medium dose to basal layer, 70 μm depth, and does not include the photon skin dose. Photon skin dose is approximately equal to the value in the photon dose column.

Appendix 5 Specific Gamma Ray Constants

Nuclide	Γ	Nuclide	Γ	Nuclide	Γ
Actinium 227	∼2.2	Gold 198	2.3	Potassium 43	5.6
Antimony 122	2.4	Gold 199	∼0.9	Radium 226	8.25
Antimony 124	9.8	Hafnium 175	∼2.1	Radium 228	∼5.1
Antimony 125	∼2.7	Hafnium 181	∼3.1	Rhenium 186	∼0.2
Arsenic 72	10.1	Indium 114m	∼0.2	Rubidium 86	0.5
Arsenic 74	4.4	Iodine 124	7.2	Ruthenium 106	1.7
Arsenic 76	2.4	Iodine 125	∼0.7	Scandium 46	10.9
Barium 131	∼3.0	Iodine 126	2.5	Scandium 47	0.56
Barium 133	∼2.4	Iodine 130	12.2	Selenium 75	2.0
Barium 140	12.4	Iodine 131	2.2	Silver 110m	14.3
Beryllium 7	∼0.3	Iodine 132	11.8	Silver 111	∼0.2
Bromine 82	14.6	Iridium 192	4.8	Sodium 22	12.0
Cadmium 115m	∼0.2	Iridium 194	1.5	Sodium 24	18.4
Calcium 47	5.7	Iron 59	6.4	Strontium 85	3.0
Carbon 11	5.9	Krypton 85	∼0.04	Tantalum 182	6.8
Cerium 141	0.35	Lanthanum 140	11.3	Technetium 99m	0.60
Cerium 144	∼0.4	Lutecium 177	0.09	Tellurium 121	3.3
Cesium 134	8.7	Magnesium 28	15.7	Tellurium 132	2.2
Cesium 137	3.3	Manganese 52	18.6	Thulium 170	0.025
Chlorine 38	8.8	Manganese 54	4.7	Tin 113	∼1.7
Chromium 51	0.16	Manganese 56	8.3	Tungsten 185	∼0.5
Cobalt 56	17.6	Mercury 197	∼0.4	Tungsten 187	3.0
Cobalt 57	0.9	Mercury 203	1.3	Uranium 234	∼0.1
Cobalt 58	5.5	Molybdenum 99	.9	Vanadium 48	15.6
Cobalt 60	13.2	Neodymium 147	0.8	Xenon 133	0.1
Copper 64	1.2	Nickel 65	∼3.1	Ytterbium 175	0.4
Europium 152	5.8	Niobium 95	4.2	Yttrium 88	14.1
Europium 154	∼6.2	Osmium 191	∼0.6	Yttrium 91	0.01
Europium 155	∼0.3	Palladium 109	0.03	Zinc 65	2.7
Gallium 67	∼1.1	Platinum 197	∼0.5	Zirconium 95	4.1
Gallium 72	11.6	Potassium 42	1.4		

Adapted from Bureau of Radiological Health: Radiological Health Handbook. PHS pub. no. 2016. Washington, DC, U.S. Department of Health, Education and Welfare, 1970.

Γ, gamma ray constant. Γ/10 = R/hr at 1 m/Ci. The following gives examples of the use of specific gamma ray constants. The conventional constant gives the exposure in R/mCi/hr at 1 cm; the constant divided by 10 gives exposure in R/hr at 1 m from 1 Ci. The specific gamma ray constant can be used to find the exposure rate (R/hr) for a source of activity A (mCi) at any distance d (cm) by using the following formula:

$$\text{Exposure rate} = \frac{\Gamma A}{d^2}$$

As an example, to calculate the exposure rate at 92 cm (3 feet) from a 1 Ci (1000 mCi) source of cobalt 60, the calculation would be as follows:

$$\text{Exposure rate} = \frac{13.2 \times 1000}{(92)^2} = \frac{13,200}{8464} = 1.56 \text{ R/hr}$$

The gamma constant can be multiplied by 3×10^{-5} to give dose in mSv/hr/MBq.

Appendix 6 SOMA Normal Tissue Radiotoxicity Tables

Note: These tables were derived for high doses associated with radiotherapy; they are not appropriate for use at doses below several Gy. If these symptoms or findings occur in persons exposed to lower doses, radiation is almost certainly not the cause. All tables are adapted from LENT SOMA tables. Radiother Oncol 1995; 35(1):17–60.

Brain

	Grade 1	Grade 2	Grade 3	Grade 4
Subjective				
Headache	Occasional and minimal	Intermittent and tolerable	Persistent and intense	Refractory and excruciating
Somnolence	Occasional, able to work or perform normal activity	Intermittent, interferes with work or normal activity	Persistent, needs some assistance for self-care	Refractory, prevents daily activity, coma
Intellectual deficit	Minor loss of ability to reason and judge	Moderate loss of ability to reason and judge	Major loss of ability to reason and judge	Complete loss of reasoning and judgment
Functional competence	Perform complex tasks with minor inconvenience	Cannot perform complex tasks	Cannot perform simple tasks	Incapable of self-care/ supervision, coma
Memory	Decreased short term, difficult with learning	Decreased long term, loss of short term	Loss of short and long term	Complete disorientation
Objective				
Neurological deficit	Barely detectable neurological signs, able to perform normal activities	Easily detectable neurological abnormalities, interferes with normal activities	Focal motor signs, disturbances in speech, vision, etc., interfering with daily activities	Hemiplegia, hemisensory deficit, aphasia, blindness, etc., requires continuous care, coma
Cognitive functions	Minor loss of memory, reason and/or judgment	Moderate loss of memory, reason and judgment	Major intellectual impairment	Complete memory loss and/or incapable of rational thought
Mood and personality changes	Occasional and minor	Intermittent and minor	Persistent and minor	Total disintegration
Seizures	Focal, without impairment of consciousness	Focal, with impairment of consciousness	Generalized, tonic-clonic or absence attack	Uncontrolled with loss of consciousness >10 min
Management				
Headache, somnolence	Occasional non-narcotic medication	Persistent non-narcotic medication, intermittent low-dose steroids	Intermittent high dose steroids	Parenteral high-dose steroids, mannitol and/or surgery
Seizures	Behavioral modification	Behavioral modification and occasional oral medication	Permanent oral medication	Intravenous anticonvulsive medication
Cognition, memory	Minor adaption	Psychosocial and educational intervention	Occupational and physiotherapy	Custodial care

Continued

Brain—cont'd

	Grade 1	Grade 2	Grade 3	Grade 4
Analytic				
Neuropsychologic	Minor deficits in memory, IQ, and/or attention	10–19 point decrease in IQ level	20–29 point decrease in IQ level	≥30-point decrease in IQ level, but can learn simple tasks
MRI	Focal white matter changes; dystrophic cerebral calcification	White matter changes affecting ≤ 1 cerebral lobe; limited perilesional necrosis	Focal necrosis with mass effect	Pronounced white matter changes; mass effect requiring surgical intervention
CT	Assessment of swelling, edema, atrophy*			
MRS	Assessment of chemical spectra*			
PET	Assessment of metabolic activity*			
Magnetic mapping	Assessment of cognitive function*			
Serum	Assessment of myelin basic protein levels*			
CSF	Assessment of total protein and myelin basic protein*			

*Applies to all grades.

Spinal Cord

	Grade 1	Grade 2	Grade 3	Grade 4
Subjective				
Paresthesia (tingling sensation, shooting pain, Lhermitte's syndrome)	Occasional and minimal	Intermittent and tolerable	Persistent and intense	Refractory and excruciating
Sensory (numbness)	Minimal change	Mild unilateral sensory loss; works with some difficulties	Partial unilateral sensory loss; needs assistance for self-care	Total loss of sensation, danger of self-injury
Motor (weakness)	Minor loss of strength	Weakness interfering with normal activities	Persistent weakness preventing basic activities	Paralysis
Sphincter control	Occasional loss	Intermittent loss	Incomplete control	Complete incontinence
Objective				
Neurological evaluation	Barely detectable decrease in sensation or motor weakness on one side, no effect on function	Easily detectable decrease in sensation or motor weakness on one side, disturbs but does not prevent function	Full Brown-Sequard syndrome, loss of sphincter function, prevents function	Complete transection, disabling, requiring continuous care
Management				
Pain	Occasional non-narcotic medication	Persistent non-narcotic medication, intermittent low dose steroids	Intermittent high dose steroids	Persistent high dose steroids
Neurological function	Needs minor adaption to continue working	Regular physiotherapy	Intensive physiotherapy plus regular supervision	Intensive nursing and/or life support
Incontinence	Occasional use of incontinence pads	Intermittent use of incontinence pads	Regular use of incontinence pads or self-catheterization	Permanent use of pads or catheterization
Analytic				
MRI	Edema	Localized demyelination	Extensive demyelination	Necrosis
CT	Assessment of swelling, edema, atrophy*			
MRS	Assessment of chemical spectra*			
PET	Assessment of metabolic activity*			
Serum	Assessment of myelin basic protein levels*			
CSF	Assessment of total protein and myelin basic protein*			

*Applies to all grades.

Peripheral Nerves

	Grade 1	Grade 2	Grade 3	Grade 4
Subjective				
Pain	Occasional and minimal	Intermittent and tolerable	Persistent and intense	Refractory and excruciating
Strength		Detectable weakness	Persistent weakness	Paralysis, transverse myelitis
Sensory	Occasional paresthesia, hyperthesia	Intermittent paresthesia	Persistent paresthesia	Paralysis
Motor paresis	Occasional	<50% decrease from baseline capabilities	≥50% decrease from baseline capabilities	Paralysis
Objective				
Motor dysfunction	<20% loss	20–30% loss	>30–50% loss	>50% loss
Sensory dysfunction	Paresthesia	Vibration decrease	Decrease to pin prick	Complete anesthesia
Reflex	Decreased deep tendon reflex	Absent deep tendon reflex	—	—
Management				
Pain	Occasional non-narcotic	Regular non-narcotic	Regular narcotic	Surgical intervention
Motor dysfunction	—	—	Physical or medical intervention	Surgical intervention
Sensory dysfunction	—	—	Physical or medical intervention	Surgical intervention
Sensory	—	—	—	Neurosurgical intervention
Analytic				
MRI	Assessment of associated muscle atrophy, changes in nerve intensity*			
Nerve conduction studies	Assessment of speed, absence of conduction of electrical impulse*			

*Applies to all grades.

Male Hypothalamic-Pituitary-Gonadal Axis

	Grade 1	Grade 2	Grade 3	Grade 4
Subjective				
Libido	Occasionally suppressed	Intermittently suppressed	Persistently suppressed	Refractory and excruciating
Objective				
Fertility	—	—	—	Impotent
Libido	Occasional loss	Intermittent loss	Persistent loss	—
Management				
Libido	—	Hormone replacement	—	—
Analytic				
FSH/LH	Normal limits or borderline decreased	Decreased	—	—
Testosterone	Normal limits or borderline decreased	Decreased	—	—
Stimulated FSH/LH	Assessment of testes responsiveness and hypothalamic-pituitary-testes axis integrity*			

*Applies to all grades.

Female Hypothalamic-Pituitary-Gonadal Axis

	Grade 1	Grade 2	Grade 3	Grade 4
Subjective				
Hot flashes	Occasional	Intermittent	Persistent	—
Dysmenorrhea	Occasional	Intermittent	Persistent	—
Menstruation		Oligomenorrhea	Amenorrhea	—
Libido	Occasionally suppressed	Intermittently suppressed	Persistently suppressed	—
Objective				
Ovulation	—	—	Anovulation in premenopausal women	—
Involuntary infertility	—	—	—	Infertile
Osteoporosis	—	—	Radiographic evidence	Fracture
Management				
Dysmenorrhea, hot flashes	—	Persistent hormone replacement	—	—
Menstruation	—	Hormone replacement	—	—
Osteoporosis	—	Hormone replacement, calcium supplements	—	—
Analytic				
FSH/LH/Estradiol	Assessment of hypothalamic-pituitary-gonadal axis integrity*			
Bone densitometry	Quantify bone density*			
Stimulated FSH/LH	Assessment of pituitary responsiveness*			

*Applies to all grades.

Hypothalamic-Pituitary-Adrenal Axis

	Grade 1	Grade 2	Grade 3	Grade 4
Subjective				
Activity level	Occasional fatigue	Intermittent fatigue and drowsiness	Drowsiness and weakness	Paralysis/coma
Appetite	Occasional anorexia	Anorexia/nausea	Persistent vomiting	Refractory vomiting
Skin color	Darkened scars	Darkened mucosa, palmar creases	Darkened skin	—
Objective				
Strength	—	—	Muscle weakness	Paralysis
Cardiovascular	—	BP 20% below baseline	BP 20–50% below baseline	BP > 50% below baseline
Metabolic	Occasional salt craving and muscle cramping	Intermittent salt craving and muscle cramping, light headedness	Persistent salt craving and muscle cramping, dizziness, syncope	Refractory muscle cramping, coma
Skin color	Darkened scars	Darkened mucosa, palmar creases	Darkened skin	—
Management				
Hypoadrenalism	Hydrocortisone replacement	—	—	—
Analytic				
Corticotrophin–stimulation test	Assessment of adrenal responsiveness and hypothalamic-pituitary-adrenal axis integrity*			
Corticotrophin–releasing hormone stimulation test	Assessment of adrenal responsiveness and hypothalamic-pituitary-adrenal axis integrity*			

*Applies to all grades.

Skin and Subcutaneous Tissue

	Grade 1	Grade 2	Grade 3	Grade 4
Subjective				
Scaliness/roughness	Present/asymptomatic	Symptomatic	Require constant attention	—
Sensation	Hypersensitivity, pruritus	Intermittent pain	Persistent pain	Debilitating dysfunction
Objective				
Edema	Present/asymptomatic	Symptomatic	Secondary dysfunction	Total dysfunction
Alopecia (scalp)	Thinning	Patchy, permanent	Complete, permanent	—
Pigmentation change	Transitory, slight	Permanent, marked	—	—
Ulcer/necrosis	Epidermal only	Dermal	Subcutaneous	Bone exposed
Telangiectasia	Minor	Moderate, <50%	Gross, ≥50%	—
Fibrosis/scar	Present/asymptomatic	Symptomatic	Secondary dysfunction	Total dysfunction
Atrophy/contraction (depression)	Present/asymptomatic	Symptomatic, <10%	Secondary dysfunction/ 10–30%	Total dysfunction, >30%
Management				
Dryness	—	—	Medical intervention	—
Sensation	—	Intermittent medical intervention	Continuous medical intervention	—
Ulcer	—	—	Medical intervention	Surgical intervention/ amputation
Edema	—	—	Medical intervention	Surgical intervention/ amputation
Fibrosis/scar	—	—	Medical intervention	Surgical intervention/ amputation
Analytic				
Color photographs	Assessment of changes in appearance*			

*Applies to all grades.

Eye

	Grade 1	Grade 2	Grade 3	Grade 4
Subjective				
Vision	Indistinct color vision	Blurred vision, loss of color vision	Severe loss of vision, symptomatic visual field defect with decrease in central vision, some ability to perform daily living activities	Blind, inability to perform daily living activities
Light sensitivity	Photophobia, no change in vision	Increased photophobia, decreased vision	Photophobia, major loss of vision	—
Pain/dryness	Occasional and minimal	Intermittent and tolerable	Persistent and intense	Refractory and excruciating
Tearing	Occasional	Intermittent	Persistent	—
Objective				
Best corrected vision	>20/40	20/50 – 20/200	<20/200 Count fingers at 1 m	Cannot count fingers at 1 m
Cornea	Increased tearing on examination	Noninfectious keratitis	Infectious keratitis, corneal ulcer	Panophthalmitis, corneal scar, ulceration leading to perforation/loss of globe
Iris	Rubeosis only	Rubeosis, increased intraocular pressure	Neovascular glaucoma with ability to count fingers at 1 m	Neovascular glaucoma without ability to count fingers at 1 m, complete blindness

Continued

Eye—cont'd

	Grade 1	Grade 2	Grade 3	Grade 4
Objective—cont'd				
Sclera	Loss of episcleral vessels	≤50% scleral thinning	>50% scleral thinning	Scleral or periosteal graft required due to perforation
Optic nerve	Afferent pupillary defect with normal appearing nerve	≤¼ pallor with asymptomatic visual field defect	>¼ pallor or central scotoma	Profound optic atrophy, complete blindness
Lens	Asymmetric lenticular opacities, no visual loss	Moderate lenticular changes with mild-moderate visual loss	Moderate lenticular changes with severe visual loss	Severe lenticular changes
Retina	Microaneurysms, nonfoveal exudates, minor vessel attenuation, extrafoveal pigment changes	Cotton wool spots	Massive macular exudation, focal retinal detachment	Opaque vitreous hemorrhage, complete retinal detachment, blindness
Facial bones	Cosmetically undetectable fascial asymmetry	Minimal cosmetic asymmetry	Moderate orbital contracture	Severe hypoplasia of orbital bones
Management				
Tearing, cornea, lacrimation	Lubrication as needed	Lubrication with or without pressure patch, antibiotics	Topical antibiotics with or without cycloplegia	Corneal graft, enucleation
Pain	Occasional non-narcotic	Regular non-narcotic	Regular narcotic	Parenteral narcotics
Neovascularization	Pan-retinal photocoagulation for neovascular changes	Medical management of glaucoma, pan-retinal photocoagulation	Surgical management of glaucoma, cytodestructive procedure	Enucleation
Lens	—	—	Cataract extraction depending on visual potential	—
Retina	—	Medical management of glaucoma, focal photocoagulation	Surgical management of glaucoma, with or without pan-retinal photocoagulation	Cytodestructive procedure, repair of retinal detachment
Facial bones	—	—	Cosmetic repair ± orbital augmentation for anophthalmic socket	Enucleation, orbital augmentation for anophthalmic socket

Analytic	
Slit lamp examination	Assessment of intraocular pressure, pupils, ocular motility, dilated funduscopic exam and gonioscopy*
Cultures and stains	Assessment of corneal infiltrates*
Ultrasound	Examination of posterior pole if opaque media.(i.e. cornea, lens, vitreous)*
Fluorescein angiogram	Evaluation of retinal neovascularization, macular edema/exudates*
Color vision	Assessment if afferent pupillary defect, or optic nerve asymmetry*
Automated visual field	Bilateral—assessment of optic nerve, pupillary, or color vision abnormality*
MRI	Assessment of sudden visual loss and abnormal optic disc or normal appearing optic disc and no other visible reason for visual loss*

*Applies to all grades.

Ear

	Grade 1	Grade 2	Grade 3	Grade 4
Subjective				
Pain	Occasional and minimal	Intermittent and tolerable	Persistent and intense	Refractory and excruciating
Tinnitus	Occasional	Intermittent	Persistent	Refractory
Hearing	Minor loss, no impairment in daily activities	Frequent difficulties with faint speech	Frequent difficulties with loud speech	Complete deafness
Objective				
Skin	Dry desquamation	Otitis externa	Superficial ulceration	Deep ulceration, necrosis, osteochondritis
Hearing	<10 decibel loss in one or more frequencies	10–15 decibel loss in one or more frequencies	>15–20 decibel loss in one or more frequencies	>20 decibel loss in one or more frequencies
Management				
Pain	Occasional non-narcotic	Regular non-narcotic	Regular narcotic	Parenteral narcotics
Skin	Occasional lubrication/ ointments	Regular eardrops or antibiotics	Eardrums	Surgical intervention
Hearing loss	—	—	Hearing aid	—
Analytic				
Pure tone audiometry	Assessment of characteristics of sensorineural perception*			
Speech audiometry	Assessment of characteristics of speech perception*			

*Applies to all grades.

Mucosa—Oral and Pharyngeal

	Grade 1	Grade 2	Grade 3	Grade 4
Subjective				
Pain	Occasional and minimal	Intermittent and tolerable	Persistent and intense	Refractory and excruciating
Dysphagia	Difficulty eating solid food	Difficulty eating soft food	Can take liquids only	Totally unable to swallow
Taste alteration	Occasional, slight	Intermittent	Persistent	
Objective				
Mucosal integrity	Patchy atrophy or telangiectasia	Diffuse atrophy or telangiectasia, superficial ulcer	Deep ulcer, no bone or cartilage exposure	Deep ulcer with bone or cartilage exposure
Weight	≤5% loss	>5–10% loss	>10–15%	>15% loss
Management				
Pain	Occasional non-narcotic	Regular non-narcotic	Regular narcotic	Surgical intervention
Ulcer	—	Cleanse	Antibiotics or oxidants	Debridement and other surgical intervention
Dysphagia	Lubricants, diet modification	Non-narcotic	Narcotic	PEG tube and/or surgical intervention
Taste alteration	Minor diet changes (non acidic)	Minor diet changes (semi-soft)	Major diet changes (soft)	Major diet changes (liquid)
Analytic				
Color photo	Assessment of changes in appearance*			
Cytology, biopsy, imaging	Rule out persistent tumor*			
Smear, culture, antifungal trial	Rule out candidiasis*			

*Applies to all grades.

Salivary Gland

	Grade 1	Grade 2	Grade 3	Grade 4
Subjective				
Xerostomia	Occasional dryness	Partial but persistent dryness	Complete dryness, nondebilitating	Complete dryness, debilitating
Objective				
Saliva	Normal moisture	Scant saliva	Absence of moisture, sticky, viscous saliva	Absence of moisture, coated mucosa
Management				
Xerostomia	—	Occasional saliva substitute; sugarless candy or gum, sialogogues	Frequent saliva substitute or water; sugarless candy or gum, sialogogues	Needs saliva substitute or water to eat sugarless candy or gum, sialogogues
Analytic				
Salivary flow quantity/ stimulation	76–95% of pretreatment	51–75% of pretreatment	26–50% of pretreatment	0–25% of pretreatment

Mandible

	Grade 1	Grade 2	Grade 3	Grade 4
Subjective				
Pain	Occasional and minimal	Intermittent and intolerable	Persistent and intense	Refractory and excruciating
Mastication	—	Difficulty with solids	Difficulty with soft foods	—
Denture use	—	Loose dentures	Inability to use dentures	—
Trismus	Noted but unmeasurable	Preventing normal eating	Difficulty eating	Inadequate oral intake
Objective				
Exposed bone	—	≤2 cm	>2 cm or limited sequestration	Fracture
Trismus	—	1–2 cm opening	0.5–1 cm opening	<0.5 cm opening
Management				
Pain	Occasional non-narcotic	Regular non-narcotic	Regular narcotic	Surgical intervention or resection
Exposed bone	—	Antibiotics	Debridement HBO_2	Resection
Trismus and mastication	—	Soft diet	Liquid diet, antibiotics, muscle relaxant medications	NG tube, gastrostomy
Analytic				
Mandibular radiograph	Questionable changes or none	Osteoporosis (radiolucent), osteosclerosis (radiodense)	Sequestra	Fracture
Panograph x-rays/CT	Assessment of necrosis progression*			

*Applies to all grades.

Teeth

	Grade 1	Grade 2	Grade 3	Grade 4
Subjective				
Pain	Occasional and minimal	Intermittent and tolerable	Persistent and intense	Refractory and excruciating
Objective				
Caries	DMF <25%	DMF 25–50%	DMF >50%	Fracture
Management				
Pain	Occasional non-narcotic	Regular non-narcotic	Regular narcotic	Extraction
Caries	Prescribed fluorides	Restoration	Selected extraction	Total extraction
Analytic				
Dental x-rays	Assessment of necrosis progression with periapical, bite wing, panograph x-rays*			
Probe for softness	Assessment of teeth for decalcification and caries*			
Pulp test	Assessment of pulp integrity with heat, cold, electric current*			
Percussion	Assessment for tenderness and pain*			
Mobility	Assessment of alveolar bone for loss and infection*			

DMF, number of decayed, missing, filled teeth compared to pre-RT.
*Applies to all grades.

Larynx

	Grade 1	Grade 2	Grade 3	Grade 4
Subjective				
Pain	Occasional and minimal	Intermittent and tolerable	Persistent and intense	Refractory and excruciating
Voice/hoarseness	Occasional hoarseness on prolonged use	Intermittent hoarseness, voice unreliable, varies in day-to-day communication	Persistent hoarseness, incapable of normal communication	Complete loss of voice
Breathing	Occasional difficulty	Intermittent difficulty	Labored breathing	Stridor
Objective				
Edema	Arytenoids only	Arytenoids and aryepiglottic folds	Diffuse edema of supraglottis, airway adequate	Diffuse with significant narrowing of airway, <½ normal
Mucosal integrity	Patchy atrophy, telangiectasia	Complete atrophy, extensive telangiectasia	Ulcer, cartilage not exposed	Necrosis, cartilage exposed
Respiration		Dyspnea on exertion	Labored at rest	Stridor at rest
Management				
Pain	Occasional non-narcotic	Regular non-narcotic	Regular narcotic	Surgical intervention
Hoarseness		Rest voice, or whisper only	No talking or whispering	Laryngectomy
Respiration		Humidifier, steroids	Temporary tracheostomy	Permanent tracheostomy
Analytic				
Indirect laryngoscopy	Assessment of edema, mucosal integrity, vocal cord motion, ulcer, and necrosis*			
Direct laryngoscopy	Assessment of edema, mucosal integrity, vocal cord motion, ulcer, and necrosis*			
CT	Assessment of edema, necrosis, asymmetry*			
MRI	Assessment of edema, necrosis, asymmetry*			

*Applies to all grades.

Thyroid and Hypothalamic-Pituitary-Thyroid Axis

	Grade 1	Grade 2	Grade 3	Grade 4
Subjective				
Metabolic	Occasional chilliness[†]	Intermittent chilliness	Needs supplemental heat	—
Gastrointestinal	Occasional constipation[†]	Intermittent constipation	Persistent constipation	—
Weight	≥5% gain[†]	<10% gain	≥10% gain	—
Skin texture	—	Intermittent sensation of dryness	Persistent sensation of dryness	—
Energy level	Occasional fatigue[†]	Intermittent fatigue	Persistent fatigue	—
Objective	—			
Facies	—	Barely noticeable puffiness and thickened lips	Obvious puffiness and thickened lips	—
Speech quality	—	Barely noticeable hoarseness and slowed speech	Obvious hoarseness and slowed speech	—
Skin temperature	—	Cool	Cold	—
Hair texture	—	Difficult to comb	Brittle, splitting, hair loss	—
Nodules	—	—	—	Palpable
Heart rate	—	—	Slowed	—
Management				
All SOM Symptoms	—	Thyroid replacement therapy	—	—
Nodules	—	—	Surgery/radionuclide therapy	—
Analytic				
Basal T4	Normal limits	0–50% decrease	>50% decrease	—
Basal TSH*	Increased	—	—	—
Basal TSH[†]	Decreased	—	—	—
Stimulated TSH*	Assessment of thyroid responsiveness[‡]			
Stimulated TSH[†]	Assessment of pituitary responsiveness and hypothalamic/pituitary-thyroid axis integrity[‡]			

*Primary thyroid.
[†]Hypothalamic-pituitary-thyroid axis.
[‡]Applies to all grades.

Breast

	Grade 1	Grade 2	Grade 3	Grade 4
Subjective				
Pain	Occasional and minimal hypersensation, Pruritus	Intermittent and tolerable	Persistent and intense	Refractory and excruciating
Objective				
Edema	Asymptomatic	Symptomatic	Secondary dysfunction	—
Fibrosis*/fat necrosis	Barely palpable increased density	Definite increased density and firmness	Very marked density, retraction and fixation	—
Telangiectasia	<1 cm^2	$1–4$ cm^2	>4 cm^2	—
Lymphedema, arm (circumference)	$2–4$ cm increase	$>4–6$ cm increase	>6 cm increase	Useless arm, angiosarcoma
Retraction/Atrophy†	$10–25\%$	$>25–40\%$	$>40–75\%$	Whole breast
Ulcer	Epidermal only, ≤ 1 cm^2	Dermal, >1 cm^2	Subcutaneous	Bone exposed, necrosis
Management				
Pain	Occasional non-narcotic	Regular non-narcotic	Regular narcotic	Surgical intervention
Edema	—	—	Medical intervention	Surgical intervention/ mastectomy
Lymphedema, arm	—	Elevate arm, elastic stocking	Compression wrapping, intensive physiotherapy	Surgical intervention/ amputation
Atrophy	—	—	—	Surgical intervention/ mastectomy
Ulcer	—	Medical intervention	Surgical intervention, wound debridement	Surgical intervention/ mastectomy
Analytic				
Photographs	Assessment of skin changes as atrophy, retraction or fibrosis, ulcer‡			
Tape measure	Assessment of breast size and forearm diameter‡			
Mammogram	Assessment of skin thickness and breast density‡			
CT/MRI	Assessment of breast size, fat atrophy, and fibrosis density‡			

*Compare exposed area to contralateral non-irradiated skin according to defined parameters
†Volume loss due to surgery and/or RT (compared to opposite breast).
‡Applies to all grades.

Heart

	Grade 1	Grade 2	Grade 3	Grade 4
Subjective				
Angina pectoris	Occasional, only with intense exertion	With moderate exertion	With mild exertion	At rest
Pericardial pain	Occasional and minimal	Intermittent and tolerable	Persistent and intense	Refractory and excruciating
Palpitation	Occasional	Intermittent	Persistent	Refractory
Dyspnea	SOB on intense exertion	SOB on mild exertion	SOB at rest, limits all activity	Prevents any physical activity
Pedal edema	—	Asymptomatic	Symptomatic	Prevents daily activities
Objective				
Pedal edema	1+	2+	3+	4+
Cardiomegaly	Minimal enlargement of cardiosilhouette (ECS)	ECS without pulmonary congestion	ECS with minimal pulmonary congestion	ECS with frank pulmonary edema
Cardiac dysrhythmia	Occasional, asymptomatic	Intermittent ECG changes	Persistent ECG changes	Refractory
Myocardial CHF	Asymptomatic decline of resting ejection fraction by ≤20% of baseline	Decline of resting ejection fraction by >20% of baseline	Reversible CHF	Irreversible CHF
Myocardial ischemia	Abnormal stress test NL resting EKG	Asymptomatic, ST, and T-wave changes without stress test	Angina without evidence for infarction	Acute myocardial Infarction
Pericardial disease	Asymptomatic effusion	Rub, chest pain, ECG changes	Tamponade	Constriction
Management				
Pain (pericarditis)	Occasional non-narcotic	Regular non-narcotic	Regular narcotic	Coronary artery bypass
Angina	Present but no therapy	Nitroglycerin PRN	Long acting agents	Coronary artery bypass
Pericardial disease	—	Present but no therapy	Pericardiocenthesis	Pericardiectomy
Cardiac dysrhythmia	—	—	Medical intervention	Requires monitoring or cardioversion
Myocardial infarction	—	—	Medical intervention	Coronary bypass
Myocardial CHF	—	—	Medical intervention	Cardiac transplant
Analytic				
Equilibrium radionuclide angiography (ERNA)	Abnormal, <20% decrease in left ventricle ejection fraction	20–40% decrease in left ventricle ejection fraction	<40% decrease in left ventricle ejection fraction	—
Exercise tolerance test (ETT)	Assessment of pulse rate, blood pressure, and EKG polarization changes*			
Cardiac catheterization	Assessment of coronary artery blood flow*			
Thallium scintigraphy	Assessment of myocardial perfusion*			
Coronary angiography	Assessment of number of vessels involved and extent of stenosis*			

*Applies to all grades.

Vessels

	Grade 1	Grade 2	Grade 3	Grade 4
Subjective				
Arterial	No clinical symptom	Clinical symptoms of ischemia during exertion	Clinical symptoms of ischemia at rest	Necrosis
Venous	Asymptomatic	Thrombosis requiring no systemic anticoagulant therapy	Thrombosis requiring systemic anticoagulant therapy	Pulmonary embolism and/or thrombosis requiring surgical intervention
Objective				
Arterial	Minor ischemia	Intermittent ischemia	Intense ischemia	Necrosis
Venous	Minor edema	Intermittent edema	Ulcus or active thrombosis	Pulmonary embolism
Management				
Arterial	Behavioral changes	Permanent medicam treatment	Conservative surgery	Amputation
Venous	Elastic bandage	Elastic bandage and regular antibiotics/anticoagulant treatments	Regular parenteral Anticoagulant treatment	Surgery
Analytic				
Doppler ultrasound	Assessment of blood flow and detection of abnormalities*			
Angiography	Assessment of lumen size and collateralization*			

*Applies to all grades.

Lung

	Grade 1	Grade 2	Grade 3	Grade 4
Subjective				
Cough	Occasional	Intermittent	Persistent	Refractory
Dyspnea	Breathless on intense exertion	Breathless on mild exertion	Breathless at rest, limits all activities	Prevents any physical activity
Chest pain/discomfort	Occasional and minimal	Intermittent and tolerable	Persistent and intense	Refractory and excruciating
Objective				
Pulmonary fibrosis	Radiological abnormality	Patchy dense abnormalities on radiograph	Dense confluent radiographic changes limited to radiation field	Dense fibrosis, severe scarring and major retraction of normal lung
Lung function	10–25% reduction respiration volume and/or diffusion capacity	>25–50% reduction of respiration volume and/or diffusion capacity	>50–75% reduction of respiration volume and/or diffusion capacity	>75% reduction of respiration volume and/or diffusion capacity
Management				
Pain	Occasional non-narcotic	Regular non-narcotic	Regular narcotic	Surgical intervention
Cough	—	Non-narcotic	Narcotic, intermittent corticosteroids	Respirator, continuous corticosteroids
Dyspnea	—	Occasional O_2	Continuous O_2	—
Analytic				
PFT	Decrease to >75–90% of preTx value	Decrease to >50–75% of preTx value	Decrease to >25–50% of preTx value	Decrease to ≤25% of preTx value
DLCO	Decrease to >75–90% of preTx value	Decrease to >50–75% of preTx value	Decrease to >25–50% of preTx value	Decrease to ≤25% of preTx value
% O_2/CO_2 saturation	>70% O_2, ≤50% CO_2	>60% O_2, ≤60% CO_2	>50% O_2, ≤70% CO_2	≤50% O_2, >70% CO_2
CT/MRI	Assessment of lung volume and zones of fibrosis*			
Perfusion scan	Assessment of pulmonary blood flow and alveolar filling*			
Lung lavage	Assessment of cells and cytokines*			

*Applies to all grades.

Esophagus

	Grade 1	Grade 2	Grade 3	Grade 4
Subjective				
Dysphagia	Difficulty eating solid foods	Difficulty eating soft foods	Can take liquids only	Totally unable to swallow
Pain	Occasional and minimal	Intermittent and tolerable	Persistent and intense	Refractory and excruciating
Objective				
Weight loss from time of treatment	$\geq$5–10%	>10–20%	>20–30%	>30%
Stricture	>$\frac{2}{3}$ normal diameter with dilatation	>$\frac{1}{3}$–$\frac{2}{3}$ normal diameter with dilatation	$\leq\frac{1}{3}$ normal diameter	Complete obstruction
Ulceration	Superficial, $\leq$1 cm^2	Superficial, >1 cm^2	Deep ulcer	Perforation, fistulae
Bleeding (melena or hematemesis)	Occult	Occasional, normal hemoglobin	Intermittent, 10–20% decrease in hemoglobin	Persistent, >20% decrease in hemoglobin
Anemia	—	Fatigue	Exhaustion	—
Management				
Dysphagia/stricture	Diet modification or antacids	Diet modification and occasional dilatation	Temporary NG tube or regular dilatation	Parenteral feeding, prosthesis, gastrostomy or permanent NG tube
Weight loss	Diet modification	Nutritional supplements	Tube feeding	Surgical bypass, PEG
Pain/ulceration	Occasional non-narcotic	Regular non-narcotic	Regular narcotic	Surgical intervention
Bleeding	Iron therapy	Occasional transfusion	Frequent transfusions	Surgical intervention
Analytic				
Barium esophagram	Assessment of esophageal lumen, stricture, dilatation*			
Endoscopy	Assessment of esophageal lumen, mucosal integrity, ulceration*			
CT	Assessment of esophageal wall thickness, stricture, dilatation*			
MRI	Assessment of esophageal wall thickness, lumen, stricture, dilatation*			
Ultrasonography	Assessment of esophageal wall thickness, lumen, stricture, dilatation*			
Mobility esophagram	Assessment of motility of bolus and peristalsis*			
Electromyogram	Assessment of motility of bolus and peristalsis*			

*Applies to all grades.

Stomach

	Grade 1	Grade 2	Grade 3	Grade 4
Subjective				
Epigastric distress	Occasional and minimal	Intermittent and tolerable	Persistent and intense	Refractory and excruciating
Emesis	Occasional	Intermittent	Persistent	Refractory
Pain	Occasional and minimal	Intermittent and tolerable	Persistent and intense	Refractory and excruciating
Objective				
Hematemesis	Occasional	Intermittent	Persistent	Refractory
Weight loss from time of treatment	$\geq$5–10%	>10–20%	>20–30%	>30%
Melena	Occult/occasional, normal hemoglobin	Intermittent, <10% decrease in hemoglobin	Persistent, 10–20% decrease in hemoglobin	Refractory or frank blood, >20% decrease in hemoglobin
Ulceration	Superficial, $\leq$1 cm^2	Superficial, >1 cm^2	Deep ulcer	Perforation, fistulae
Stricture (antropyloric region)	> ⅔ normal diameter	⅓–⅔ normal diameter	<⅓ normal diameter	Complete obstruction
Management				
Epigastric distress/ emesis	Diet modification, antacids	Intermittent prescription medication	Persistent medial management	Surgical intervention
Pain	Occasional non-narcotic	Regular non-narcotic	Regular narcotic	Surgical intervention
Bleeding	Iron therapy	Occasional transfusion	Frequent transfusions	Embolization, coagulation, or surgical intervention
Ulceration	—	—	Medical intervention	Surgical intervention
Stricture	—	—	Medical intervention	Surgical intervention
Analytic				
Barium radiography	Assessment of lumen and peristalsis*			
Endoscopy	Assessment of lumen and mucosal surface*			
CT	Assessment of wall thickness, sinus and fistula formation*			
MRI	Assessment of wall thickness, sinus and fistula formation*			

*Applies to all grades.

Small Intestine and Colon

	Grade 1	Grade 2	Grade 3	Grade 4
Subjective				
Stool frequency	2–4 day	5–8 day	>8 per day	Refractory diarrhea
Stool consistency	Bulky	Loose	Mucous, dark, watery	
Pain	Occasional and minimal	Intermittent and tolerable	Persistent and intense	Refractory/rebound
Constipation	3–4 per wk	Only 2 per wk	Only 1 per wk	No stool in 10 days
Objective				
Melena	Occult/occasional	Intermittent and tolerable, normal hemoglobin	Persistent, 10–20% decrease in hemoglobin	Refractory or frank blood, >20% decrease in hemoglobin
Weight loss from time of treatment	≥5–10%	>10–20%	>20–30%	>30%
Stricture	> ⅔ normal diameter with dilatation	⅓–⅔ normal diameter with dilatation	<⅓ normal diameter	Complete obstruction
Ulceration	Superficial, ≤1 cm^2	Superficial, >1 cm^2	Deep ulcer	Perforation, fistulae
Management				
Pain	Occasional non-narcotic	Regular non-narcotic	Regular narcotic	Surgical intervention
Stool consistency/ frequency	Diet modification	Regular use of non-narcotic antidiarrheal	Continuous use of narcotic antidiarrheal	—
Bleeding	Iron therapy	Occasional transfusion	Frequent transfusions	Surgical intervention
Stricture	Occasional diet adaption	Diet adaptation required	Medical intervention, NG suction	Surgical intervention
Ulceration	—	—	Medication intervention	Surgical intervention
Analytic				
CT	Assessment of wall thickness, sinus and fistula formation*			
MRI	Assessment of wall thickness, sinus and fistula formation*			
Absorption studies	Assessment of protein and fat absorption and metabolic balance*			
Barium radiograph	Assessment of lumen and peristalsis*			

*Applies to all grades.

Rectum

	Grade 1	Grade 2	Grade 3	Grade 4
Subjective				
Tenesmus	Occasional urgency	Intermittent urgency	Persistent urgency	Refractory
Mucosal loss,	Occasional	Intermittent	Persistent	Refractory
Sphincter control	Occasional	Intermittent	Persistent	Refractory
Stool frequency	2–4 per day	4–8 per day	>8 per day	Uncontrolled diarrhea
Pain	Occasional and minimal	Intermittent and tolerable	Persistent and intense	Refractory and excruciating
Objective				
Bleeding	Occult	Occasionally >2 per wk	Persistent/daily	Gross hemorrhage
Ulceration	Superficial, ≤ 1 cm^2	Superficial, >1 cm^2	Deep ulcer	Perforation, fistulae
Stricture	>⅔ normal diameter with dilatation	⅓–⅔ normal diameter with dilatation	<⅓ normal diameter	Complete obstruction
Management				
Tenesmus and stool frequency	Occasional, ≤2 antidiarrheals per wk	Regular, >2 antidiarrheals per wk	Multiple, >2 antidiarrheals perday	Surgical intervention/ permanent colostomy
Pain	Occasional non-narcotic	Regular non-narcotic	Regular narcotic	Surgical intervention
Bleeding	Stool softener, iron therapy	Occasional transfusion	Frequent transfusions	Surgical intervention/ permanent colostomy
Ulceration	Diet modification, stool softener	Occasional steroids	Steroids per enema, hyperbaric oxygen	Surgical intervention/ permanent colostomy
Stricture	Diet modification	Occasional dilatation	Regular dilatation	Surgical intervention/ permanent colostomy
Sphincter control	Occasional use of incontinence pads	Intermittent use of incontinence pads	Persistent use of incontinence pads	Surgical intervention/ permanent colostomy
Analytic				
Barium enema	Assessment of lumen and peristalsis*			
Proctoscopy	Assessment of lumen and mucosal surface*			
CT	Assessment of wall thickness, sinus and fistula formation*			
MRI	Assessment of wall thickness, sinus and fistula formation*			
Anal manometry	Assessment rectal compliance*			
Ultrasound	Assessment of wall thickness, sinus and fistula formation*			

*Applies to all grades.

Liver

	Grade 1	Grade 2	Grade 3	Grade 4
Subjective				
Pain RUQ	Occasional and minimal	Intermittent and tolerable	Persistent and intense	Refractory and excruciating
Objective				
Abdominal findings	Hepatomegaly	Soft ascites	Tense ascites	—
Edema	Occasional leg edema	Intermittent leg edema	Anasarca responsive to diuretics	Anasarca unresponsive to diuretics
Weight gain	—	≤5%	>5–10%	>10%
Alertness	—	Change in attentiveness and sleep pattern	Confusion	Coma
Bleeding	—	—	Correctable	Unresponsive
Management				
Pain	Occasional non-narcotic	Regular non-narcotic	Regular narcotic	Continuous narcotic
Abdominal findings	—	Intermittent diuretics	Permanent diuretics	—
Bleeding	—	Iron therapy	Occasional transfusion of fresh frozen plasma	Frequent transfusions
Analytic				
AST/ALT/Alk phos	<2.5 × normal	2.5 × 5.0 normal	>5–20 × normal	>20.0 × normal
Bilirubic	<1.5 × normal	1.5–5.0 × normal	>5.–10 × normal	>10.0 × normal
PT/PTT	<1.25 × normal	1.25–1.5 × normal	>1.50–2 × normal	>2 × normal
Serum alb (gm/dL)^3	>3	>2.5–3	>2–2.5	≤2
Platelets (1000)	>75	>50–75	>25–50	≤25

*Applies to all grades.

Kidney

	Grade 1	Grade 2	Grade 3	Grade 4
Subjective				
Symptoms	—	—	Fatigue, headache	Obtundation, oliguria, edema
Objective				
Blood pressure	—	Systolic ≤20 over normal, diastolic ≤10 over normal	Systolic >20 over normal, diastolic >10 over normal	Malignant hypertension
Hematuria	Microscopic	Intermittent macroscopic	Persistent macroscopic	Refractory
Edema	None or transient	Pedal; 2+ – 3+	Pedal 4+, edema of lower legs(s)	Uremic coma, anasarca
Specific gravity	—	Urine SpG decreased	—	
Management				
Blood pressure/renal failure	Diet	Antihypertension medication	Dialysis, unilateral nephrectomy	Permanent dialysis or renal transplant
Hematuria	Iron therapy	Occasional transfusion or single cauterization	Persistent transfusion or coagulation	Surgical intervention
Analytic				
Proteinuria	<3 g/L	3–10 g/L	>10 g/L	Nephrotic syndrome
Creatinine clearance	5–10% decrease	>10–30 decrease	>30–60% decrease	>60% decrease
Creatinine	1.25 × normal to 2.5 x normal	>2.5 × normal to 5 × normal	>5 × normal to 10 × normal	>10 × normal
B2 Microglob	—	—	>2 × normal to 4 × normal	>4 × normal
Glomerular filtration rate	Quantification of filtration rate*			
Renal scanning	Assessment of renal size and radioisotope clearance*			

*Applies to all grades.

Ureter

	Grade 1	Grade 2	Grade 3	Grade 4
Subjective				
Pain	Occasional and minimal	Intermittent and tolerable	Persistent and intense	Refractory and excruciating
Objective				
Obstruction	Ureteral narrowing without hydronephrosis	Ureteral narrowing with hydronephrosis	Unilateral obstruction	Bilateral obstruction
Renal function	1+ proteinuria	2+ proteinuria	4+ proteinuria	—
Management				
Pain	Occasional non-narcotic	Regular non-narcotic	Regular narcotic	Surgical intervention
Obstruction	—	—	Unilateral stent or nephrostomy	Bilateral nephrostomy or diversion
Analytic				
Intravenous pyelography	Assessment of ureter integrity*			

*Applies to all grades.

Bladder and Urethra

	Grade 1	Grade 2	Grade 3	Grade 4
Subjective				
Dysuria	Occasional and minimal	Intermittent and tolerable	Persistent and intense	Refractory and excruciating
Frequency	3–4 hour intervals	2–3 hour intervals	1–2 hour intervals	Hourly
Hematuria	Occasional	Intermittent	Persistent with clot	Refractory
Incontinence	< weekly episodes	< daily episodes	≤2 pads/undergarments per day	Refractory
Decreased	Occasionally weak	Intermittent	Persistent but incomplete obstruction	Complete obstruction
Objective				
Hematuria	Microscopic, normal hemoglobin	Intermittent macroscopic, <10% decrease in hemoglobin	Persistent macroscopic, 10–20% decrease in hemoglobin	Refractory, >20% decrease in hemoglobin
Endoscopy	Patchy atrophy or telangiectasia without bleeding	Confluent atrophy or Telangiectasia with gross bleeding	Ulcerations into muscle	Perforation, fistula
Maximum volume	>300–400 mL	>200–300 mL	>100–200 mL	≤100 mL
Residual volume	25 mL	>25–100 mL	>100 mL	—
Management				
Dysuria	Occasional non-narcotic	Regular non-narcotic	Regular narcotic	Surgical intervention
Frequency	Alkalization	Occasional antispasmodic	Regular narcotic	Cystectomy
Hematuria/ telangiectasia	Iron therapy	Occasional transfusion or single cauterization	Frequent transfusion or coagulation	Surgical intervention
Incontinence	Occasional use of incontinence pads	Intermittent use of incontinence pads	Regular use of pad or self-catheterization	Permanent catheter
Decreased stream	—	< Once-a-day self-catheterization	Dilatation, > once-a-day self-catheterization	Permanent catheter, surgical intervention
Analytic				
Cystography	Assessment of mucosal surface*			
Volumetric analysis	Assessment of bladder capacity in millimeters*			
Contrast radiography	Assessment for ulcers, capacity, and contractility*			
Ultrasound	Assessment of wall thickness, sinus and fistula formation*			
Electromyography	Assessment of sphincter activity using intraluminal pressure transducer, contraction pressure, and volume curves*			

*Applies to all grades.

Testes

	Grade 1	Grade 2	Grade 3	Grade 4
Subjective				
Libido	Occasionally suppressed	Intermittently suppressed	Persistently suppressed	—
Objective				
Fertility	—	—	Oligospermia	Azoospermia
Appearance	—	—	—	Atrophy
Management				
Fertility	—	—	In vitro fertilization	Sperm retrieval if previously banked
Libido	—	Testosterone	—	—
Analytic				
FSH/LH	Increased FSH/nl LH	Increased FSH/ increased LH	—	—
Testosterone	—	—	—	Decreased
Spermatoanalysis	Assessment of sperm number, motility, and morphology*			
Flow cytometric analysis	Assessment of sperm integrity*			
DNA chromatin analysis	Assessment of sperm chromatin integrity*			

*Applies to all grades.

Vulva

	Grade 1	Grade 2	Grade 3	Grade 4
Subjective				
Dryness	Occasional	Intermittent	Persistent	—
Pruritus	Occasional and minimal	Intermittent and tolerable	Persistent and intense	Refractory and excruciating
Pain	Occasional and minimal	Intermittent and tolerable	Persistent and intense	Refractory and excruciating
Objective				
Pigmentation Change	Patchy	Confluent	—	—
Alopecia	Partial	Complete	—	—
Atrophy	Patchy	Confluent	—	—
Appearance	Telangiectasia without bleeding	Telangiectasia with gross bleeding	—	—
Ulceration/necrosis	Superficial, ≤ 1 cm^2	Superficial, >1 cm^2	Deep	Fistulae
Fibrosis	—	—	Partial	Complete
Edema	—	—	Partial	Complete
Introital stenosis	—	—	Partial	Complete
Serous transudate	Occasional	Intermittent	Persistent	Refractory
Management				
Pruritus/atrophy	Occasional hormone cream	Intermittent hormone cream	Regular hormone cream	—
Pain	Occasional non-narcotic	Regular non-narcotic	Regular narcotic	Surgical intervention
Ulceration	Conservative	Wound care	Debridement	Graft
Introital stenosis	Occasional dilation	Intermittent dilation	Persistent dilation	Surgical repair
Analytic				
Color photograph	Assessment of changes in skin, mucous, and telangiectasia*			

*Applies to all grades.

Vagina

	Grade 1	Grade 2	Grade 3	Grade 4
Subjective				
Dyspareunia	Occasional and minimal	Intermittent and tolerable	Persistent and intense	Refractory and excruciating
Dryness	Occasional	Intermittent	Persistent	Refractory
Bleeding	Occasional	Intermittent	Persistent	Refractory
Pain	Occasional and minimal	Intermittent and tolerable	Persistent and intense	Refractory and excruciating
Objective				
Stenosis/length	> ⅔ normal length	⅓–⅔ normal length	< ⅓ normal length	Obliteration
Dryness	Asymptomatic	Symptomatic	Secondary dysfunction	—
Ulceration/necrosis	Superficial, ≤1 cm^2	Superficial, >1 cm^2	Deep ulcer	Fistulae
Atrophy	Patchy	Confluent	Nonconfluent	Diffuse
Appearance	Telangiectasia without bleeding	Telangiectasia with gross bleeding	—	—
Synechiae	—	Partial	Complete	—
Bleeding	—	On contact	Intermittent	Persistent
Management				
Dyspareunia/pain	Occasional non-narcotic	Regular non-narcotic	Regular narcotic	Surgical intervention
Atrophy	Occasional hormone cream	Intermittent hormone cream	Regular hormone cream	—
Bleeding	Iron therapy	Occasional transfusion	Frequent transfusions	Surgical intervention
Stenosis	Occasional dilation	Intermittent dilation	Persistent dilation	Surgical reconstruction
Dryness	Hormone replacement	Artificial lubrication	—	—
Ulceration	Conservative	Debridement	HBO$_2$	Graft, surgical repair
Analytic				
MRI	Assessment of wall thickness, sinus and fistula formation*			
Ultrasound	Assessment of wall thickness, sinus and fistula formation*			
EUA Cytology/biopsy	Assessment of wall diameter and length and mucosal surface*			

*Applies to all grades.

Uterus and Cervix

	Grade 1	Grade 2	Grade 3	Grade 4
Subjective				
Amenorrhea	Asymptomatic	Symptomatic	—	Infertility
Dysmenorrhea	Asymptomatic	Symptomatic	—	—
Pain	Occasional and minimal	Intermittent and tolerable	Persistent and intense	Refractory and excruciating
Bleeding	Occasional, normal hemoglobin	Intermittent, <10% decrease in hemoglobin	Persistent, 10–20% decrease in hemoglobin	Refractory, >20% decrease in hemoglobin
Objective				
Pyometra	Asymptomatic	Symptomatic	—	—
Hematometra	Asymptomatic	Symptomatic	—	—
Necrosis	Asymptomatic	Symptomatic	—	—
Ulceration	Superficial, ≤ 1 cm^2	Superficial, >1 cm^2	Deep ulcer	Fistulae
Incompetent	—	—	—	Infertility
Cervical os stenosis	Asymptomatic	Symptomatic	—	—
			—	—
Management				
Pain	Occasional non-narcotic	Regular non-narcotic	Regular narcotic	Surgical intervention
Amenorrhea, dysmenorrhea, hematometra	Occasional hormone replacement	Intermittent hormone replacement	Persistent hormone replacement	—
Pyometra	—	D and C, antibiotics	—	—
Necrosis	—	Debridement	D and C	Hysterectomy
Bleeding	Iron therapy	Occasional transfusion	Frequent transfusions	Surgical intervention
Cervical os stenosis	—	—	D and C	Surgical intervention
Ulceration	Conservative	Antibiotics	Debridement, surgical management	Hysterectomy
Incompetent	—	—	—	Obstetrical management
Analytic				
MRI	Assessment of wall thickness, perametrial infiltrates, sinus and fistula formations*			
Ultrasound	Assessment of wall thickness, perametrial infiltrates, sinus and fistula formation*			
EUA cytology/biopsy	Assessment of mucosal surfaces and ulcers*			

*Applies to all grades.

Ovary and Reproductive Organs

	Grade 1	Grade 2	Grade 3	Grade 4
Subjective				
Hot flashes	Occasional	Intermittent	Persistent	—
Dysmenorrhea	Occasional	Intermittent	Persistent	—
Menstruation	—	Oligomenorrhea	Amenorrhea	—
Objective				
Ovulation	—	—	Anovulation in premenopausal women	—
Involuntary infertility	—	—	Infertility	—
Osteoporosis	—	—	Radiographic evidence	Fracture
Management				
Dysmenorrhea, hot flashes	—	Hormone replacement	—	—
Menstruation	—	Hormone replacement	—	—
Osteoporosis	—	Hormone replacement, calcium supplements	—	—
Analytic				
FHS/LH/estradiol	Assessment of hormonal production*			
Bone densitometry	Quantify bone density*			

*Applies to all grades.

Sexual Dysfunction—Female

	Grade 1	Grade 2	Grade 3	Grade 4
Subjective				
Dyspareunia	Occasional	Intermittent	Persistent	Refractory
Dryness	Occasional	Intermittent	Persistent	Refractory
Desire	Occasional	Intermittent	Seldom	Never
Satisfaction	Occasional	Intermittent	Seldom	Never
Objective				
Vaginal stenosis/length	> ⅔ normal length	⅓–⅔ normal length	< ⅓ normal length	Obliteration
Synechiae	—	—	Partial	Complete
Frequency	—	Decreased from normal	Rare	Never
Orgasm	Occasional	Intermittent	Seldom	Never
Management				
Dryness	Hormone replacement	Artificial lubricant	—	—
Stenosis/synechiae	Occasional dilation	Intermittent dilation	Persistent dilation	Surgical reconstruction
Dyspareunia	Occasional hormone cream	Intermittent hormone cream	Persistent hormone cream	—
Analytic				
Psychosocial	Evaluate quality of life/sexual satisfaction*			
Vaginal measurement	Evaluate degree of vaginal stenosis*			

*Applies to all grades.

Muscle and Soft Tissue

	Grade 1	Grade 2	Grade 3	Grade 4
Subjective				
Pain	Occasional and minimal	Intermittent and tolerable	Persistent and intense	Refractory and excruciating
Function	Interferes with athletic recreation	Interferes with work	Interferes with daily activity	Complete lack
Objective				
Edema	Present/asymptomatic	Symptomatic	Secondary dysfunction	Total dysfunction
Mobility and extremity function	Present/asymptomatic	Symptomatic	Secondary dysfunction	No mobility, frozen
Fibrosis	Detectable	≤20% of muscle	>20–50% of muscle	>50% of muscle
Atrophy	≤10%	>10–20%	>20–50%	>50%
Contracture	—	≤10 linear field	>10–30% linear field	>30% linear field
Management				
Pain	Occasional non-narcotic	Regular non-narcotic	Regular narcotic	Surgical intervention
Edema	—	Compression	Medical intervention	Surgical intervention
Mobility and extremity function	Occasional physiotherapy	Intermittent physiotherapy	Persistent physiotherapy or medical intervention	Surgical intervention
Fibrosis	Occasional physiotherapy	Intermittent physiotherapy	—	Surgical intervention
Atrophy	—	Intermittent physiotherapy	—	Surgical intervention
Analytic				
MRI	Development of investigational testing suggested*			

*Applies to all grades.

Growing Bone

	Grade 1	Grade 2	Grade 3	Grade 4
Subjective				
Pain	Occasional and minimal	Intermittent and tolerable	Persistent and intense	Refractory and excruciating
Abnormal gait	Slight	Noticeable limp	Severe limp	Unable to walk
Disfigurement	Slight, not cosmetically significant	Mild cosmetic deformity	Moderate cosmetic deformity	Severe disfigurement
Objective				
Extremities	Mild curvature or length discrepancy <2 cm	Moderate curvatureor length discrepancy 2–5 cm	Severe curvature or length discrepancy >5 cm	Epiphysiodesis, severe functional deformity
Spine				
Sit/standing height	Mild disproportion	Moderate	Severe	—
Scoliosis	<5 degrees	5–10 degrees	>10–20 degrees	>20 degrees, interfering with cardiopulmonary function
Kyphosis/lordosis	Mild radiographic changes	Moderate accentuation	Severe accentuation	Severe slipped capital femoral epiphysis >60 degrees; avascular necrosis
Femoral heads	Mild valgus/varus deformity	Moderate valgus/varus deformity	Mild slipped capital femoral epiphysis/ epiphyseal widening	—
Flat/facial bones	Slight changes, not cosmetically significant	Mild cosmetic deformity	Moderate cosmetic deformity	Profound hypoplasia or functional problem
Management				
Extremities	—	Minimal shoe lift	Moderate shoe lift	Surgical intervention
Scoliosis	—	—	Brace	Surgical intervention
Femoral heads	—	—	Pinning	Hip replacement
Flat/facial bones	—	—	—	Surgical intervention
Analytic				
Measurement growth	No growth retardation	Growth retardation ≤1 percentile	Growth retardation >1 percentile	Growth arrest
Radiograph/CT	Assessment of bone integrity*			

*Applies to all grades.

Mature Bone (Excluding Mandible)

	Grade 1	Grade 2	Grade 3	Grade 4
Subjective				
Pain	Occasional and minimal	Intermittent and tolerable	Persistent and intense	Refractory and excruciating
Function	Interferes with athletic recreation	Interferes with work	Interferes with daily activity	Complete lack of function
Joint movement	Stiffness interfering with athletic recreation	Stiffness interfering with work	Stiffness interfering with daily activity	Complete fixation, necrosis
Objective				
Fracture	—	—	Partial thickness	Full thickness
Mucosa soft tissue	—	—	Sequestration	—
Skin over bone	Erythema	Ulcer	Sinus	Fistula
Joint movement	<10% decrease	> 10–30% decrease	>30–80% decrease	>80% decrease
Management				
Pain	Occasional non-narcotic	Regular non-narcotic	Regular narcotic	Surgical intervention
Function	Occasional physiotherapy	Intermittent physiotherapy	Persistent physiotherapy or medical intervention	Surgical intervention
Joint movement	Occasional physiotherapy	Intensive physiotherapy	Corrective surgery	—
Analytic				
Density imaging	Assessment for osteosclerosis and osteoporosis*			
X-ray	Assessment of bone and joint integrity including linear fracture and displaced fracture*			
Arthropathy	Assessment of joint integrity*			
Arthroscopy	Evaluation for joint abnormalities*			

*Applies to all grades.

Bone Marrow

	Grade 1	Grade 2	Grade 3	Grade 4
Subjective				
Anemia symptoms	—	Fatigue	Exhaustion	—
Leukopenia symptoms	—	—	Fever	—
Thrombocytopenia symptoms	—	—	Easy bruisability	Spontaneous bleeding
Objective				
Anemia	—	Abnormal Hgb/Hct <10/<30	Pallor	Tachypnea
Leukopenia	—	Abnormal WBC <2000	Infection	Sepsis
Thrombocytopenia	Abnormal aspirate/ biopsy	Platelets > 20–100K	Platelets >5–20K, petechia	Platelets <5K, hemorrhage
Management				
Anemia	—	—	Occasional use of red blood products	Frequent use of red blood products
Leukopenia	—	—	Antibiotics/cytokines	—
Thrombocytopenia	—	—	Platelets/RBCs	Bone marrow transplant
Analytic				
Assays	Assessment of bone marrow reserves with:* Hematopoietic progenitor cell assays in common use (CFU-GM, BFU-R, CFU-GEMM, CFU-blast, etc.) Stromal cell assays (CRU-F, support of long-term bone marrow cultures) Growth factor production Primitive stem cell assays (HPP-CRL, CFU-Dexter, LTC-IC, somatic mutation analysis/DWA analysis)			
Chimerism, clonality	In setting of bone marrow transplant (studies of mixed [donor/host] chimerism, studies of clonality [donor vs host])* Future consideration: challenge with growth factors to assay stem cell reserve*			

*Applies to all grades.

Index

Note: Page numbers followed by the letter f refer to figures; those followed by the letter t refer to tables.

A

Abdomen, postradiotherapy
  bloating of, 323
  CT scan of changes in, 325f
  obstruction of, 323
  pain in, 323
Abortion, spontaneous
  legal liability for, 440–441
  after in utero exposure, 411–412
Absolute risk, definition of, 81
Absorbed dose coefficients, for radionuclide
      intakes by workers, 497t–499t
Absorbed doses, 20, 389–390. *See also* Dose
      and dose rate effectiveness factor
      (DDREF)
  average outdoor from terrestrial sources, 35
  definition of, 20
  equivalent dose and, 20
  from nuclear power plants, 42
  of radon, 37–38
    ventilation affecting, 38
  of terrestrial radiation, worldwide annual
      rates of, 31–32
  total, in rads, 17
  units of, 7–8
    conversion table for, 495t
Absorption of radiation. *See* Radiation,
      absorption of
Accidental exposure situations, dose limits in,
      23–24
Acneiform changes, after radiotherapy, 289
ACTH. *See* Adrenocorticotropin (ACTH)
Actinium series, 30
  radiation energies and intensities of, 33t
Actinomycin D
  enhancing skin radiosensitivity, 290
  in hepatic radiosensitivity, 327
  in predisposition to radiation pneumonitis,
      313
  in radiation pneumonitis and skin erythema,
      393
  in radiation toxicity of intestine, 323
  in radiation-induced esophagitis, 321
  radiosensitizing effect of, 9
  reducing second neoplasm risk, 394
Actinoranium, radiation energies and
      intensities of, 33t
Activated charcoal canisters, in measuring
      radon, 34–35
Activation products, 6
Acute lymphocytic leukemia (ALL). *See*
      Leukemia, acute lymphocytic (ALL)
Acute myeloid leukemia (AML). *See*
      Leukemia, acute myeloid (AML)
Acute radiation sickness (ARS)
  assessment of, 357
  cataracts in, 308
  in Chernobyl patients, 359
    degree of and percentage skin burns and
        dose in, 360t
    doses, number, and outcome of, 360t
  severity of, 359–360

Acute radiation sickness (ARS) *(Continued)*
  criteria for, 356
  critical phase of, 357t
  diagnosis of, 437–438
  latent phase of, 357t
  lymphocyte count changes in, 359t
  manifestations of, 356, 437
  phases in, 356
  prodromal phase of, 356t
  registries for, 356
  after whole-body irradiation, 355–360
Acute radiation syndrome
  after Chernobyl accident, 359
    in children exposed to, 352
  combined injuries with, prognosis of, 392
  degrees of various types of, 358t
  diagnosis of, 437
  hematopoietic form of, 340
  after organogenesis period radiation
      exposure, 404–405
  subgroups of, 357–358
  after whole-body irradiation, 355–360
Adaptive responses, 11, 473
  lymphocytes in, 475
Additive effects, 390f
  of chemotherapy and radiotherapy, 393
  of electromagnetic fields and radiation, 391
  of smoking and radiation exposure, 395
Additive risk projection models, 82
  ICRP, 82
  versus multiplicative risk projection
      models, 83
  problems with, 82
Additivity, definition of, 389
Adenine (A), 47
Adenocarcinoma
  esophageal, 215
  of lung, 173
    in uranium miners, 184
  of stomach, Thorotrast injection and, 224
Adrenal glands, deterministic radiation effects
      in, 299
Adrenocorticotropin (ACTH)
  deficiency of
    after high-dose pituitary irradiation, 293
    after pituitary irradiation, 294
  radiotherapy effects on, 299
Adriamycin (doxorubicin hydrochloride)
  cardiotoxicity of, 317
  enhancing skin radiosensitivity, 290
  in hepatic radiosensitivity, 327
  in predisposition to radiation pneumonitis,
      313
  in radiation recall phenomena, 393
  in radiation toxicity of intestine, 323
  in radiation-induced esophagitis, 321
Adult respiratory distress syndrome, radiation
      induced, 312
Adverse effects
  documenting, 460
  identifying, 460
  risk perception and, 461–462

AET. *See* S-(2-aminoethyl) isothiuronium
      (AET)
Aflatoxin
  carcinogenic effect of, 445
  in hepatobiliary system cancers, 236
  in stomach cancer incidence, 223–224
Africa, terrestrial radiation in, 31–32
Age
  affecting skin reaction to radiation, 290
  at exposure, radiation-induced breast cancer
      and, 165
  in leukemia risk, 118
  in nonmelanoma skin cancer after
      radiotherapy, 262
Aging, premature. *See* Life shortening,
      radiation-induced
Aggregate harm, 469–470
Air pollution, in cancer risk, 447
Air travel, cosmic ray doses from, 38, 38t
Airline crews/pilots
  bladder cancer in, 195
  bone tumors in, 250
  colon cancer in, 227
  increased natural cosmic irradiation in, 119
  lung cancer incidence in, 175
  occupational exposures of, 42–43
  pancreatic cancer in, 243
  rectal cancer in, 233
  stomach cancer in, 220
Airplane travel, cancer risk from, 99
Airport scanners, cosmic radiation from, 40
ALARA (as low as reasonably achievable)
      doses, 22, 469
Albinism, squamous cell skin cancer and,
      259–260
Albuminuria, radiation-induced, 329
Alcohol consumption
  carcinogenic sensitizing effect of, 445
  in esophageal cancer, 215
  in hepatobiliary system cancers, 236
  in oral and pharyngeal cancers, 147
  in relative risk of esophageal cancer,
      358
  with tobacco smoking, 389–390
Alkaline phosphatase, secretion of, 310
Alkylating agents
  in bone tumors, 248–249
  cancer risk from, 443
  for childhood cancer, 55–56
  in germ cell depletion with radiotherapy,
      334
  in leukemia, 393–394
  in radiation brain injury, 302
  in radiation recall phenomena, 393
  radiosensitizing effect of, 392–393
  radiosensitizing effects of
    on reproductive organs, 331
  in xeroderma pigmentosum, 75–76
ALL. *See* Leukemia, acute lymphocytic (ALL)
Alleles, 47–48
  homologous, 47–48
Allelic expansion, 47–48

Alpha radiation, 1–2
  bone tumors related to, 249–250, 253, 256
  combined with nitro-oxides, 392
  in cosmic rays, 27
  dicentric chromosomes induced by, 54t
  lung cancer risk with, 188
    in plutonium workers, 187
  particulate radiation of, 4–5, 4t
  range of, 5t
  RBE of, 3t
Alpha/beta ratios, 17–18
Alpha-emitting radionuclides, 5–6
  cardiac complications from, 320
  cesium 137, 290
  from radium, 30–31
  to tracheobronchial region, 32–34
  from uranium isotopes, 30
Altitude
  cosmic radiation and, 27–28
  incremental increases in cosmic dose rates
    and, 29t
Americium 241, in smoke detectors, 39
Americium radionuclides, dose coefficients for
    worker intakes of, 497t–499t
Amifostine (WR-2721), radioprotective effect
    of, 9
Amino acids, coding for, 47
AML. See Leukemia, acute myeloid (AML)
Anemia
  aplastic. See also Fanconi anemia
    in atomic bomb survivors, 341
    cataracts after treatment for, 308–309
    as myelodysplasia syndrome, 137
    after radiation exposure, 344
    from radiation exposure, 137
  pernicious, as myelodysplasia syndrome, 137
Anemia, fatigue and, 364
Angelman syndrome, 48
Angioplasty, inhibiting coronary artery
    restenosis after, 318
Angiosarcoma
  after radiotherapy, 256, 258–259
  vinyl chloride-induced, 74
Ankylosing spondylitis radiotherapy, 101
  bone sarcomas after, 252
  bone tumors after, 249–250, 253–254
  breast cancer related to, 169
  CNS tumors related to, 140
  colon cancer after, 229
  esophageal cancer after, 217–218
  hepatobiliary system cancer after, 240, 241
  kidney cancer after, 193
  leukemia risk from, 121–123
  liver injury after, 327–328
  lung cancer after, 178, 188
  nonmelanoma skin cancer after, 262–263
  oropharyngeal cancer after, 149–150
  pancreatic cancer after, 246
  prostate cancer after, 211–212
  radiation-induced life shortening after,
    361–362
  rectal cancer after, 236
  stomach cancer after, 223, 224
  thyroid cancer after, 158
Anoxia, 9
Anoxic tumors, oxygen enhancement ratio
    and, 9, 9f
Antagonism, 389, 390f
  of electromagnetic fields and radiation, 391
Anthracyclines
  cardiomyopathy and, 317
  for childhood cancer, coronary
    complications after, 318–319
  in radiation recall phenomena, 393

Antibiotics
  broad-spectrum, to reduce radiation
    pneumonitis severity, 312
  cardiotoxicity of, 317
Antibody production, in immune response,
    349
Antigen
  B-cells and, 349
  produced by immune competent cells, 347
Antihypertensive drugs, cardiotoxicity of, 317
Antimetabolites, in radiation recall
    phenomena, 393
Antineoplastic drugs
  carcinogenic effects of, 447
  in hepatic radiosensitivity, 327
Antistatic devices, radioactive substances in,
    39
Antithyroid peroxidase (ATPO; thyroid
    antimicrosomal antibodies)
  in atomic bomb survivors, 295
  in children exposed to Chernobyl fallout,
    297
  in populations exposed to Chernobyl
    fallout, 297
Anxiety, after nuclear accidents, 467
Aortic atherosclerosis, with fallout exposure,
    361
APC gene, in tumor initiation, 72
Apoptosis (programmed cell death), 11–12
  in deterministic effects of radiation, 285
  radiation induced genomic instability and, 7
Ara C, in radiation myelopathy, 304
ARS. See Acute radiation sickness
Arsenic radionuclides
  cancer risk from, 443, 447
  dose coefficients for worker intakes of,
    497t–499t
  medical exposure to, carcinogenic effects of,
    447
Arterioles
  radiation injury of, 286f
  skin ulceration with radiation of, 288
Arteriosclerotic heart disease
  in plutonium workers, 430–431
  in radiation brain injury, 302
Artery
  radiation injury of, 286f
  radiation-induced stenosis of, 319
Arthritis radionuclide treatment, bone effects
    with, 338
AS calculator, 452
As low as reasonably achievable (ALARA)
    standard, 22, 469
Asbestos exposure
  cancer risk from, 447
  lung cancer after, 452–454
  mesothelioma after, 74
Ascorbic acid, anticarcinogenic effect of, 446
Assigned share (AS), 438
  estimating, 441–442, 448–450
  probability of, 448–450
Astatine, radiation energies and intensities of,
    33t
Astronauts, cataract formation in, 308
Ataxia-telangiectasia (A-T)
  clinical features of, 76t
  genetic predisposition to, 73
  nonmelanoma skin cancer and, 259
  radiation susceptibility in, 441
  radiation-induced, 76–77
Atherosclerosis, radiation-induced, 319
ATM genes
  in ataxia-telangiectasia, 76, 77
  mutations of, 76

Atmosphere
  carbon 14 concentrations in, 29–30
  coal-fired power plant emissions into, 35–36
  cosmic ray reaction with, 27
  shielding effect of, 27
Atomic bomb survivors
  adverse pregnancy outcomes in, 406
  bladder cancer in, 195
  bone tumors in, 250–251, 256
  brain and CNS tumors in, 138
  breast cancer in
    incidence of, 166–167
    susceptibility to, 73–74
  cancer risk in, 56, 85–86
    estimates for, 85
    after in utero exposure, 416
  cataracts in, 307
  chromosomal studies in, 57–58
  CNS cancer incidence in, 138f
  colon cancer in, 228, 231
  congenital malformations in, 403, 410
  deaths by cancer site and sex in, 84t
  dementia in, 303
  depressed immunocompetence in, 90–92
  dose-translocation frequency in, 62f
  epidemiologic studies of, 88–92
    weaknesses of, 88
  esophageal cancer in, 215–216, 218–220
    excess relative risk for, 216f
  estimated cancer risk for, 89t
  expected and radiation excess cancer
    mortality in, 88f
  fatigue in, 467
  genetic disorders in, 50–51
  genetic studies of, 53–55
  granulosa cell proliferation in, 332
  hematopoietic symptoms in, 341
  hepatobiliary system cancers in, 236–238
  hormetic effects on, 474
  hprt gene mutation frequency in, 58f
  hyperparathyroidism in, 146
  hypertension in, 319–320
  hypothyroidism in, 295–296
  immune function in, 350–351
  in utero radiation exposure in
    carcinogenic effects and, 416
    CNS abnormalities after, 411
    CNS tumors after, 142
    congenital abnormalities after, 410
    leukemia with, 414–415
    structural neuropathology and, 408–409
  kidney cancer in, 189
  lens radiosensitivity in, 307
  leukemia in, 117–118
    with benzene exposure, 394
    in children of, 99–100
    incidence of, 117, 118
    RR estimates of, 91f
  Life Span Study of, 88
  lung cancer in, 173–175
    mortality rates of, 81f
    smoking and, 174
  lymphatic system changes in, 345–346
  lymphocyte chromosome aberrations in, 64
  male genital tumors in, 212
  melanoma in, 263
  mental retardation in children of, 407f, 455
  microcephaly in children of, 407
  multiple myeloma in, 133
  natural background radiation levels in, 92
  non-Hodgkin's lymphoma risk in, 130–131
  nonmelanoma skin cancers in, 260, 260f
  obstetrical prenatal irradiation effects
    compared to, 100

Atomic bomb survivors *(Continued)*
  oral cavity cancer incidence in, 147, 148f
  ovarian cancer in, 200, 203–204
    at different dose levels, 202f
  pancreatic cancer in, 243
  prostate cancer in, 209
  radiation-induced cancer deaths in, 88
  radiation-induced life shortening in, 361
  rectal cancer in, 233
  renal and ureteral stones in, 330
  salivary gland tumors in, 144–145
  sex ratio of babies born to after in utero
    exposure, 411
  smoking and radiation effects on, 395–396
  solid tumors in
    death rates for, 175
    ERR estimates of, 91f
  status of in 2001, 88f
  stomach cancer in, 220–221, 224–225
  T-cell receptor (TCR) gene mutations in,
    58
  threshold analysis of, 80–81
  thyroid cancer in, 153
    ERR of, 153f
    incidence of, 81f
  thyroid nodules or adenomas in, 161
  tumor doubling time in, 78–79
  tumors in
    ERR for incidence by tumor type, 89f
    ERR for mortality by tumor type, 90f
  uterine cancer in, 205
Atomic energy facilities. *See* Nuclear energy
    facilities
Atomic mass number, 5
Atomic mass unit (AMU), 1
Atomic structure, 1
Atoms, splitting of, 6
ATPO. *See* Antithyroid peroxidase (ATPO;
    thyroid antimicrosomal antibodies)
Atrioventricular block, after breast carcinoma
    radiotherapy, 318–319
Attributability, of cancer to radiation
    exposure, 438
Attribution, definition of, 437
Aurora borealis, 27
Australian aboriginal newborns, incidence of
    congenital anomalies in, 52
Authorized limits, 23–24
Autoimmune disease, with accidental radiation
    exposure, 352
Autoimmune thyroiditis
  in Chernobyl fallout populations, 297
  in populations near Hanford plant, 297
Autosomal aneuploidy, in atomic bomb
    survivors, 57
Autosomes, 47
Availability heuristic, 467
Axillary skin, radiosensitivity of, 290
Azathioprine, cancer risk from, 443, 447
Azoospermia, after Hodgkin's disease
    radiotherapy, 334

B

Background radiation
  acceptability of, 462–463
  in bladder cancer, 195
  in bone tumors, 250
  brain and CNS tumors from, 138
  in breast cancer incidence, 167
  carcinogenic effect of, 447
  in colon cancer, 227
  epidemiologic studies in high levels of, 92

Background radiation *(Continued)*
  in esophageal cancer, 215
  in hepatobiliary system cancers, 236
  hormetic effects of, 473–474
  in hypothyroidism, 295
  in kidney cancer, 189
  leukemia incidence from, 119
  lung cancer from, 175
  in melanoma, 263
  multiple sclerosis and, 303
  in non-Hodgkin's lymphoma, 130
  in nonmelanoma skin cancers, 260
  in oral cavity cancers, 147
  in ovarian cancer, 200
  in pancreatic cancer, 243
  in prostate cancer, 208–209
  in radiation-induced cancer, 78–79
  in rectal cancer, 233
  in stomach cancer, 220
  terrestrial, average annual doses and
    effective dose equivalents of by
    state, 36t
  in thyroid cancer risk, 153
  thyroid nodules or adenomas from,
    160–161
  in uterine cancer, 205
Bacterial infections, carcinogenic effect of,
    447–448
Banding analysis
  of *ATM* genes, 76
  for dicentric lymphocyte chromosome
    aberrations, 61–62
  for incidence of chromosomal anomalies in
    live-born children, 52
  for incidence of naturally occurring
    chromosome abnormalities, 51
Barium imaging, of radiation-induced colon
    injury, 324
Barrett's esophagus
  adenocarcinomas and, 215
  interactive mechanisms in, 389–390
Basal cell carcinoma
  caretaker genes in, 72–73
  genetic factors in, 72
  incidence of, 259
    at low radiation dose levels, 259–260
  modifying factors in, 259
  mortality rate from, 259
  risk factors in, 263
  UV light in, 447
Basal cell layer
  blister formation beneath, 288
  injury below, 288–289
Basement membrane, 287
B-cells
  in atomic bomb survivors, 350–351
    differentiation of, 351
  circulating, 59
  count of after accidental radiation
    exposure, 352
  differentiation of, 347
  functions and subtypes of, 347–353
  in humoral immunity, 349
  radiosensitivity of, 348
BCNU
  in pulmonary fibrosis incidence, 315–316
  radiosensitizing effect of, 392–393
Becquerel, Henri, 287–288
Becquerels (Bq, Curie), 34
  definition of, 7, 8
Behavioral disorders
  radiation-induced, 302
  radiotherapy-induced, 302
Belarus, congenital anomalies registry in, 55f

Belarus-Russia-International Agency for
    Research on Cancer, Chernobyl fallout
    studies of, 159–160
Benign disease radiotherapy
  carcinogenic effects of, 101–102
  gynecologic, 102
  in postpartum mastitis, 101
  prostate and seminal vesicle effects of,
    359–360
Benzene exposure, in leukemia risk in atomic
    bomb survivors, 394
Benzopyrene, carcinogenic effect of, 394
Bergonié-Tribondeau law, 14, 333–334
Beryllium
  in air and rainwater, 29
  contributing to background radiation, 28–29
Beta burns, 291
  after Chernobyl accident, 359–360
  in Chernobyl fireman, 293f
Beta carotene, anticarcinogenic effect of, 446
Beta negative decay, 6
Beta particles, 1–2
  maximum range of, 291
  particulate radiation of, 4
Beta radiation
  in cataract formation, 308
  cataract formation after, 309
  inhibiting coronary artery restenosis, 318
  maximum penetration of, 4t
  penetrating skin, 287
  RBE of, 3t
  skin reaction to, 290–291
Beta-aminoisobutyric acid (BAIBA), urinary
    output of after radiation exposure,
    363–364
Beta-emitting radionuclide irradiation
  gastrointestinal effects of, 325–326
  skin changes from, 291–293
Beta-gamma emitting particles, skin changes
    from, 291–293
Betatrons, 4–5
Bile, in intestine, 359
Bile duct cancer, incidence of, 236
Biliary system
  cancer of in nuclear industry workers, 239
  high-LET radiation effects on, 327
  low-LET radiation effects on, 326–327
  radionuclide irradiation effects on, 327–328
Bioacids, tumor promoting, 71–72
Biochemical indicators, 363–364
Biologic agents, in radiation effects, 396–397
Biologic half-life, 7
Biological Effects of Ionizing Radiations
    (BEIR) committees
  fallout estimates of, 93–94
  leukemia mortality statistics of, 117
  lifetime attributable risk for solid cancer
    incidence and mortality estimates
    of, 90t
  lifetime attributable risk for solid cancers
    and leukemia, 104, 104t
Biological Effects of Ionizing Radiations
    (BEIR) reports, 11
  on chromosomal abnormalities, 51–52
  on hereditary radiation-induced cancer
    risk, 56
  on kidney cancer risk, 193
  on leukemia risk from radiotherapy, 123
  on lung cancer rates in miners, 185
  in radiation risk assessment, 54
  on radon risk for lung cancer, 181
  risk estimates of, 82
Biologically effective dose (BED), 17–18
Birth defects, radiotherapy and, 332

Bladder (urinary)
  cancer of
    etiology and epidemiology of, 193, 195
    external radiation-induced, 195–198
    incidence of, 193
    internal radiation-induced, 198–200
    radioiodine injection in, 100–101
    risk estimates for, 200, 201t
    risk factors in, 193, 200
    smoking as risk factor in, 443–445
    spontaneous, estimated lifetime risk
        of, 83t
  chemotherapeutic agents enhancing
      radiation effects on, 392t
  deterministic radiation effects on, 330–331
  high-LET radiation effects on, 331
  radiation tolerance of, 330
  radionuclide radiation effects on, 331
  radiosensitivity of, 200, 330
  SOMA normal tissue radiotoxicity for, 523t
  ulceration and telangiectasia of, 331
Bleomycin
  enhancing skin radiosensitivity, 290
  inhibiting repair of radiation damage, 393
  in predisposition to radiation pneumonitis,
      313
  in pulmonary fibrosis incidence, 315–316
  in radiation-induced esophagitis, 321
Blindness, cataracts in, 454
Blistering, with high radiation doses, 288
  beneath basal cell layer, 288
Blobs, 10
Blood bactericidal activity, in atomic bomb
    survivors, 341
Blood cells, after acute whole-body radiation,
    342f
Blood vessels
  high-LET and radionuclide radiation of,
      320
  internal irradiation of, 320
  large, radiation damage to, 319
  low-LET radiation of, 316–320
  radiation-induced damage to, 319
  SOMA normal tissue radiotoxicity for, 517t
Bloom's syndrome
  clinical features of, 76t
  radiosensitivity in, 77
Bodily injuries
  appreciable, 22
  average equivalent acceptable exposure in
      lieu of, 466f
  distribution of acceptable doses versus, 466t
Body weight
  in cancer risk, 445–446
  mortality ratios from various cancer by,
      445t
Bonbrest v. Kotz, 140, 440–441
Bone
  cancer of
    multiplicative versus additive risk
        projections for, 83
    plutonium occupational exposure in,
        431–432
    from radiotherapy for skin hemangiomas
        in childhood, 102
  decreased infection resistance of, 336
  density of, after radiotherapy in children,
      336
  hypoplasia of after radiotherapy in children,
      336
  low-LET radiation effects on, 335–338
  necrosis of
    with neutron therapy, 338
    radiation-induced, 336

Bone (Continued)
  in radium dial painters, 338
  neutron or high-LET radiation effects
      on, 338
  radiation-induced demineralization of, 337
  radionuclide accumulation in, 338
  radionuclide radiation effects on, 338–339
  sarcomas of
    dose-response relation for, 256f
    latent period for, 250
    versus sinus carcinomas, 144
    threshold for radium burden in, 254–256
  SOMA normal tissue radiotoxicity for
    in growing bone, 528t
    in mature bone, 529t
  tumors of (See also Chondrosarcomas;
        Ewing's sarcoma; Fibrosarcomas;
        Osteosarcomas)
    epidemiology of, 256
    external radiation-induced, 250–253
    incidence and mortality from, 257t
    incidence of, 248
    internal radiation-induced, 253–256
    latent period for, 250
    modifying factors in, 249–250
    plutonium exposure and, 430–431
    in radium dial painters, 338
    risk estimates for, 256
    risk factors in, 248–249
    secondary after radiation therapy, 258
    threshold dose-response data for, 80–81
    types of, 248
  uranium and thorium radionuclide
      concentrations in, 34t
Bone marrow
  fatty change in 342, 342f
  after fractionated radiotherapy, 342
  hematopoietic syndrome after radiation
      of, 343
  in immune response, 346–347
  measurement of radiation dose in, 8
  postradiotherapy changes in, 342
  radiation doses in ablation of, 343
  recovery of after whole-body
      irradiation, 343
  reduced lymphocyte count in, 342–343
  shielding active portions of, 354
  SOMA normal tissue radiotoxicity for,
      529t
Bone marrow (bursa) cells. See B-cells
  radiosensitivity of, 14–15
Bone marrow depression, 285
  after cesium 137 ingestion, 345
  after Chernobyl accident, 360
  from Chernobyl accident
      contamination, 291
  treatment of, 343–344
Bone marrow transplantation
  in children, thyroid cancers in, 156
  gonadal failure after, 334
  growth retardation after whole-body
      radiation before, 294
  liver dysfunction with radiotherapy
      before, 326
  lung cancer after, 179
  myeloablation before, 345
  in population exposed to Chernobyl
      accident fallout, 343–344
  secondary infections after, 360
  unnecessary, deaths from, 360
  veno-occlusive disease after, 327
  whole-body irradiation with, 343
Brachial plexus damage, low-LET radiation
    induced, 305

Brachytherapy
  bladder cancer after, 199–200
  dysuria after, 331
  intracoronary, inhibiting restenosis
      after, 318
  penis, urethra, and scrotum effects of, 335
  radiation exposure from, 45
  testicular effects of, 335
Bragg peak, 2, 5
Brain
  in atomic bomb survivor prenatally
      exposed, 409f
  background radiation in cancer of, 138
  calcification of and neuropsychological
      impairment, 302–303
  delayed hemorrhage of after radiotherapy,
      300–301
  genetic anomalies of, 50–51
  hemorrhage of after Chernobyl
      accident, 360
  mineralizing microangiopathy in, 301–302
  parenchyma of, 299–300
  postradiation necrosis in, 300
  radiation effects on development of,
      406–410
  radiation necrosis of
    imaging of, 300–301
    MRI and CT images of, 301f
  radiation-induced changes in, 299, 300
    deterministic, modifying factors in, 302
    early delayed, 300
    high-LET, 303
    from internal radiation exposure, 303
    low-LET, 300–303
    parenchymal, 302
    vascular, 302
  radioiodine implant effects in, 303
  SOMA normal tissue radiotoxicity for,
      505t–506t
  tolerance dose of, 300
  tumors in
    with high-LET radiation, 303
    radiation induced, 137–144
BRAVO thermonuclear tests
  fallout on Marshall Islands population
      from, 94
  thyroid nodules or adenomas in population
      near, 162
Brazil, terrestrial radiation in, 31–32
Brazil nut trees, radium concentration in,
    30–31
BRCA1/BRCA2 genes, 72–73
  in breast cancer susceptibility, 73
  chromosome 18q region on, 73
  environmental carcinogens and, 442
Breast
  benign disease treatment of
    lung cancer after, 178
    rectal cancer after, 234–235
    secondary cancers after, 156
    small intestinal cancer after, 225
    stomach cancer after, 223
  deterministic radiation effects on, 311–312
  hypoplasia of after childhood
      irradiation, 311f
  radiation-induced ulceration of, 312
  SOMA normal tissue radiotoxicity
      for, 515t
Breast cancer
  annual radiogenic risk of, 84
  associated with ovarian cancer, 200
  atomic bomb survivor susceptibility
      to, 73–74
  correlated to fission products in diet, 92

Breast cancer (*Continued*)
with family history of ataxia-telangiectasia, 77
genetic predisposition to, 397
incidence of
geographic and racial variations in, 164
pregnancy and, 164
within-country variances in, 164
lactation and radiotherapy in risk of, 397
latent period for
age at radiation exposure and, 77–78
with various radiation-induced tumors, 76t–78t
lifetime risk of in North American women, 446
modifying factors in, 165–166
postnatal irradiation and, 100
radiation-induced
dose-incidence data on, 171
from external exposure, 166–170
in females and males, 171
fractionation effects in, 171
from internal exposure, 170–171
risk estimates for incidence and mortality from, 172t
radioiodine injection in, 100–101
after radiotherapy
for benign postpartum mastitis, 101
for cervical carcinoma, 103
for skin hemangiomas in childhood, 102
radiotherapy for
angiosarcomas of breast after, 258–259
bladder cancer after, 197
bone tumors after, 258
breast cancer recurrence after, 170
cardiac and coronary complications after, 318
ECG changes after, 318–319
leukemia after, 123, 393–394
lung cancer after, 179
second cancer after, 102–103
T-cell depression after, 350
reproductive and sexual behavior in risk of, 446
risk factors for, 165, 446
spontaneous, estimated lifetime risk of, 83t
x-ray examinations and risk of, 100
Breast ducts, radiation effects on, 311–312
Breast-conserving radiation therapy, lung cancer after, 179
Bremsstrahlung, 8
British National Radiological Protection Board, weapons fallout studies of, 93, 120
5-Bromo-2-deoxyuridine, radiosensitizing effect of, 392–393
5-Bromouracil, radiosensitizing effect of, 392–393
Bronchial tree, radiosensitivity of, 173
Bronchiolitis obliterans, radiation induced, 312
Brown-Séquard syndrome, 304
Buccal cancer
in atomic bomb survivors, 147
in medical diagnostic workers, 149
from medical radiation exposure, 149–150
from radar exposure, 149
in uranium workers, 149
Building materials, radon concentrations in and lung doses, 37t
Buildings
in cosmic ray attenuation, 28
as modified natural radiation source, 37–38
phosphate usage in, 37
Bullae
high radiation doses and, 288

Bullae (*Continued*)
infected, 288
Bureau of Radiological Health, video display terminal working conditions recommendations of, 39
Burns
radiation combined with, 392
from uranium exposure, 424–425
Busulfan
carcinogenic effects of, 443, 447
in hepatic radiosensitivity, 327
in predisposition to radiation pneumonitis, 313
in pulmonary fibrosis incidence, 315–316
Bystander effect (postirradiation bystander signaling), 10–11

C

Cadmium radionuclides, dose coefficients for worker intakes of, 497–499t
Caffeine
carcinogenic effects of, 445
after irradiation, 394
Calcitonin levels, with radioiodine therapy, 298–299
Californium, 4–5, 252,
dose coefficients for worker intakes of, 497t–499t
Cancer. *See also* Childhood cancer; Metastatic cancer; *specific types and sites of*
attributability of to radiation exposure, 438
background radiation in, 473–474
calculating probability of causation/assigned share for, 448–450
carcinogenic risk animal data on, 443
carcinogens and circumstances in risk of
from medical exposure, 443
from occupational exposure, 442t
chemical agents associated with, 395t
clusters of near nuclear facilities, 95
congenital anomalies and etiology of, 52
determining cause of
biochemical and physiologic considerations in, 442–443
individual nature in, 442
electromagnetic fields and, 391
with family history of ataxia-telangiectasia, 76, 77
fatal, probability of, 104t
fatigue after treatment of, 364–365
genetic abnormalities in, 72
high temperatures in treatment of, 390–391
incidence of
in atomic bomb survivors, 474
in medical diagnostic workers, 133
in offspring of parents with germ-cell mutations, 56
induction of, 71
epidemiological aspects of, 83–86
in populations living near nuclear facilities, 94–96
induction thresholds for, 71
legislative compensation programs for, 450–452
lifetime mortality from, 82t
by type, 104f
molecular and cellular aspects of, 71–73
mortality rates for
in nuclear facility workers, 98, 432
in atomic bomb survivors, 89t
in populations near nuclear facilities, 95
multicausal, multistage development of, 71

Cancer (*Continued*)
nature-nurture concerns in, 442–443
nominal probability coefficients for, 82t
in Portsmouth Naval Shipyard workers, 97
prediction of future cases of in populations, 438
probability of causation and assigned share for, 442
radiation-induced
as cause of death in Hiroshima and Nagasaki, 88
evaluation of, 438
legal liability for, 441–448
from occupational exposure, 96–99
retrospective determination of, 438
risk estimates for, 87–88
radiogenic versus spontaneous, 79–80, 80f
after radiotherapy
for benign gynecologic diseases, 102
for cervical carcinoma, 103
for childhood cancer, 170
with combined chemotherapy, 393
for peptic ulcer, 101–102
for polycythemia vera, 102
for primary malignancies, 122–123
for skin hemangiomas in childhood, 102
for tinea capitis in children, 101
rates of
in atomic energy facility workers, 96–97
in radiologists, 121
relative importance of causes of, 442
with retinoblastoma, 77
risk of
with Bloom's syndrome, 77
from cervical carcinoma radiotherapy, 103
collective dose equivalents in, 22
dietary factors in, 74
etiologic factors in, 449–450
with Fanconi anemia, 77
in high-natural background radiation areas, 92
incidence risk coefficient in, 449
from iodine 131 treatment for hyperthyroidism, 102
from jet travel, 99
from medical exposure, 135
modifying factors in, 449
in offspring of patients receiving Thorotrast injections, 56
radiogenic versus spontaneous, 85
radioiodine injection in, 100–101
after radioiodine treatment for thyroid cancer, 103
with radiotherapy for ankylosing spondylitis, 101
systemic and population aspects of, 77–79
spontaneous
due to high natural background radiation, 92
estimated lifetime risks of, 83t
spontaneous mutations and, 74
steps in growth and spread of, 73f
for subgroups of population, 449
systemic factors in, 73–74
from thyrotoxicosis therapy, 102
transfer of from population to population, 87
underreporting of, 86–87
in uranium workers, 427
viral infection in, 71–72
Cancer endpoints, DDREF for, 16–17
Cancer genes, low penetrance, 75

Cancer-prone genetic disorders,
  spontaneous, 73–75
Capenhurst uranium enrichment facility
  bladder cancer in workers at, 198
  bone tumors in workers at, 254
  breast cancer in workers at, 168
  cancer mortality in workers at, 135
  CNS cancer incidence among workers
    at, 140
  colon cancer in workers at, 230
  esophageal cancer in workers at, 217
  hepatobiliary system cancer in workers
    at, 239
  Hodgkin's disease risk for workers at, 130
  kidney cancer in workers at, 192
  leukemia from occupational exposure
    at, 127
  melanoma in workers at, 265
  non-Hodgkin's lymphoma risk to
    workers at, 132
  oropharyngeal cancer in workers at, 149
  ovarian cancer in workers at, 202
  pancreatic cancer in workers at, 247–248
  prostate cancer in workers at, 211
  salivary gland tumors in workers at, 145
  small intestinal cancer in workers at, 225
  stomach cancer in workers at, 222
  uterine cancer in workers at, 206
Capillary
  dilatation of in radiation therapy, 288
  radiation injury of, 286f
  radiation-induced degeneration of, 319–320
Carbon
  average body burden of, 32
  contributing to background radiation, 28–29
Carbon 14
  atmospheric, 29–30
    from nuclear power plants, 41–42
  dose coefficients for worker intakes of,
    497t–499t
  in fallout irradiation, 40–41
  in weapons testing fallout, 41
Carcinogenesis
  changes in, 72
  in utero exposure and, 414–416
  of radiation, 441–448
  risk for versus time after irradiation, 81–83
  of specific sites (See specific cancer types and
    sites)
Carcinogenic sensitizers, 445
Carcinogens
  in cancer risk
    from medical exposure, 443
    from occupational exposure, 442t
  chemical, combined with radiation,
    389–390, 392
Carcinoma
  after childhood cancer radiotherapy, 170
  of lungs, 173
  risk of with Fanconi anemia, 77
Cardiac complications
  after breast cancer radiotherapy, 318
  after Hodgkin's disease radiotherapy, 318
Cardiomyopathy, radiation-induced, 317
Cardiovascular disease
  incidence of in nonexposed populations, 363
  ionizing radiation and, 363
  radiotherapy in risk of, 362
Cardiovascular system
  high-LET and radionuclide radiation of,
    320
  internal irradiation of, 320
  late radiotherapy effects of, 316
  low-LET radiation of, 316–320

Caretaker genes, in carcinogenesis, 72–73
Cargo container scanners, cosmic radiation
  from, 40
Carmustine, in pulmonary fibrosis incidence,
  315–316
Carotid stenosis, radiation-induced, 319
Cartilage
  low-LET radiation effects on, 335–338
  neutron or high-LET radiation effects
    on, 338
  radionuclide radiation effects on, 338–339
  radionuclide-induced necrosis of, 339
  radioresistance of, 337–338
Cascade, 27
Case-control studies, 84
  for age-related radiation-induced cancer
    risk, 86
  of populations affected by Chernobyl
    fallout, 94
  of prenatal irradiation effects, 99
    versus atomic bomb survivor studies,
      100
    versus cohort study results, 100
Cataracts
  with acute radiation sickness, 308
  in astronauts, 308
  in atomic bomb survivors
    exposed in utero, 408–409
    types of, 307
  causes of, 307
  from Chernobyl accident fallout, 308
  in children treated for leukemia, 308–309
  lens sensitivity and, 307
  modifying factors in, 454
  with neutron exposure, 309
  probability of, 307f
  radiation induced, 306–308
  radiation threshold dose in, 308
  after radionuclide irradiation, 309
  senile, 306–307
  after in utero radiation, 309
  in x-ray technologists, 454–455
    case summary of, 454–455
    radiation as cause of, 454
    risk analysis of, 454
Cathode ray tubes, cosmic radiation from, 39
Causation
  in compensation programs, 451
  definition of, 437
  probability of (PC), 448–450
Cavernous hemangioma treatment, breast
  tissue effects of, 311–312
CD cell counts, after accidental radiation
  exposure, 352
CD4 cells, radiosensitivity of, 348
CD4+/CD8+ ratio
  after chest radiotherapy, 350
  after lymphoma radiotherapy, 350
  after occupational radiation exposure, 349
Cell cycle, 11–12
  inverse dose rate effect in, 17
  radiosensitivity and stage of, 12f
Cell cycle checkpoint genes, 11–12
Cell survival curves, 12–13
  decreasing dose rate and, 13f
  fractionation and, 13f
Cells
  generation cycle in, 11
  programmed death of (apoptosis),
    7, 11–12, 285
  radiation dose lethality to, 473
  radiation effects on, 14–16
    morphologic, 14
  radiosensitivity of, 14–15

Cells (Continued)
  in different phases, 11
  reduced cloning efficiency of, 7
Cellular death, 13–14
  double-stranded DNA breaks in, 10
Cellular homeostasis, promoting agents
  disturbing, 71–72
Cellular immunity, lymphocytes in, 347
Central nervous system (CNS)
  abnormalities of
    with radiation exposure during fetal
      period, 410
    from radiation exposure during
      pregnancy, 416–417
    after radiation exposure throughout
      gestation, 410–411
    after in utero radiation exposure,
      417–419
  cancer of in atomic bomb survivors, 138f
  radiation-induced changes in, 299
    chemotherapeutic agents enhancing, 392t
    after organogenesis period radiation
      exposure, 404–405
  radiosensitivity of, 409–410
    in thoracic segments, 304
  tumors of, radiation induced, 137–144
    from external exposure, 138–141
    from internal exposure, 141–142
    from prenatal exposure, 142
    radioiodine injection in, 100–101
Central nervous system syndrome, 299
Cerebrospinal fluid pressure, elevated, 300
Cerium 144, in weapons testing fallout, 41
Cerium radionuclides
  dose coefficients for worker intakes
    of, 497t–499t
  exposure to during pregnancy, 413
Cervical cancer (carcinoma)
  epidemiology of, 207–208
  incidence and risk factors for, 204–205
  nonmelanoma skin cancer after, 263
  radiation-induced
    from external exposure, 205–207
    from internal exposure, 207
Cervical cancer (carcinoma) radiotherapy
  bladder cancer after, 197–198
    by time after treatment, 197f
  bone tumors after, 252
  breast cancer related to, 170
  case-control study of, 103
  CNS tumors related to, 141
  colon cancer after, 230
    relative risk of, 230f
  esophageal cancer after, 217–218
  hepatobiliary system cancer after, 240
  kidney cancer after, 191–192, 191f
  leukemia risk from, 122f
  lung cancer after, 178–179
  melanoma after, 265
  non-Hodgkin's lymphoma risk from,
    132–133
  obstructive uropathy after, 331
  oropharyngeal cancer related to, 150
  ovarian cancer after, 202–203
    relative risk of, 203f
  pancreatic cancer after, 246–247
    relative risk for, 247f
  radium exposure in, 333
  rectal cancer after, 235
    relative risk of, 230f–235f
  second cancers after, 102–103, 206–207
    relative risk for, 207f
Cervix, SOMA normal tissue radiotoxicity
  for, 526t

Cesium 137 exposure
  bone marrow depression after, 345
  colon cancer after, 230
  skin reaction to, 290
Cesium 157 exposure, in weapons testing, 41
Cesium radionuclide exposure, during
    pregnancy, 413
c-fins gene mutation, Thorotrast and, 74–75
Chapelcross plant of British Nuclear Fuel
    workers
  bladder cancer in, 196
  bone tumors in, 251
  cancer mortality and morbidity in, 133–135
  CNS cancers rate in, 139
  colon cancer in, 228
  esophageal cancer in, 216
  hepatobiliary system cancers in, 238
  Hodgkin's disease risk to, 129
  kidney melanoma in, 190
  lung cancer in, 176
  male genital cancer in, 212
  melanoma in, 264
  non-Hodgkin's lymphoma risk to, 131–132
  occupational exposure of, 123
  oropharyngeal cancer in, 148
  pancreatic cancer in, 244
  prostate cancer in, 209
  rectal cancer in, 233
  salivary gland tumors in, 145
  small intestinal cancer in, 225
  stomach cancer in, 221
Characteristic radiation, 3
c-Ha-RAS gene mutations, codon 61, 74–75
Charge, 2
Chelyabinsk nuclear reactor
  lung cancer in workers at, 178
  occupational exposure at, 124–125
Chemical agents
  carcinogenic, 75
    regulation of, 469–470
    in xeroderma pigmentosum, 75–76
  occupational exposures to, 396
  in radiation effects, 392–396
Chemical exposure limits, federal regulation
    of, 469–470
Chemotherapeutic agents
  carcinogenic effects of, 447
  in esophagitis, 321
  leukemia risk from, 123, 393–394
  in radiation toxicity of intestine, 323
  radiosensitizing effect of, 393
    on different organs, 392t
    hepatic, 327
    in reproductive organs, 331
Chemotherapy
  in atomic bomb survivors, dose-response
      relationship of, 58–59, 58f, 59f
  chronic radiation nephritis and, 330
  in cognitive function, 302
  fatigue after, 364–365
  radiosensitizing effect of, 389–390, 392–393
    in kidney, 329
    with radioiodine therapy, 345
    in skin, 290
  with radiotherapy, 389
    in germ cell depletion, 334
    ototoxic, 310
    in ovarian radiosensitivity, 332
    in radiation brain injury, 302
    in radiation myelopathy, 304
    in radiation pneumonitis, 313
  second cancers after, 393
  in soft-tissue sarcoma risk, 256–258
Chernobyl Forum (2006), 55

Chernobyl nuclear accident, 42
  acute health effects of total-body exposure
      from, 359–360
  acute radiation sickness after, percentage
      skin burns and dose and, 360t
  amplification of risk perception of, 467
  burn and radiation injury in firemen at, 392
  cesium contamination from, 413
  cleanup workers at
    beta burns in, 293f
    bone tumors in, 251
    CNS cancer incidence in, 139–140
    colon cancer in, 228
    esophageal cancer in, 216
    Hodgkin's disease risk to, 129–130
    immune function in, 352
    kidney cancer in, 192
    male genital cancer in, 212
    melanoma in, 264
    non-Hodgkin's lymphoma risk to, 132
    nonmelanoma skin cancer in, 260
    oropharyngeal cancer in, 148
    prostate cancer in, 210
    small intestinal cancer in, 225
    solid cancer mortality ratio in, 94f
    stomach cancer in, 221
  combined radiation and chemical
      carcinogen exposure after, 392
  congenital malformation incidence in
      survivors of, 55f
  Down syndrome risk in survivors of, 57
  effective dose from, 20–21
  fallout patterns following, 92–93
  genetic diseases and anomalies after,
      405–406
  genetic studies on survivors of, 55
  GPA assays of survivors of, 58–59
  immune status of children around, 352
  immunological effects of, 352
  LD50 doses from, 354
  in lymphocyte chromosome aberrations, 64
  mental health effects of, 467
  perceptions of in utero exposure risks from,
      465–466
  population near, 94–95
    bladder cancer in, 199
    bone marrow transplantation in, 343–344
    cataracts in, 308
    Down syndrome incidence in, before and
        after, 56f
    fallout effects on, 94
    fatigue in, 365
    hematologic effects in, 341–342
    hypothyroidism in, 296–297
    immune function in, 351–353
    leukemia in, 120
    thyroid nodules or adenomas in, 162
  psychological effects of, 466–468
  radiation hormesis and, 474
  secondary effects of fallout from, 438–439
  skin and bone doses from, 359–360
  skin contamination from, 291
  T-cell receptor (TCR) gene mutations in
      survivors of, 58
  thyroid cancer after, 438
    cell type of in children, 151
    genetic signature of, 151
    in population near, 159–160
    in recovery workers at, 160
Chernobyl nuclear plant, occupational
    exposure at, 125
Chest radiotherapy, breast tissue effects of,
    311–312
Chest x-rays, prenatal, fetal effects of, 401–402

Childbirth
  in breast cancer risk, 397
  healthy, probability of, 418t
  patterns of in cancer incidence rates, 446
Childhood cancer
  colon cancer after, 230
  genetic studies on survivors' offspring,
      55–56
  low-dose obstetric x-rays and, 99
  Oxford Survey of, 414–416
  preconception irradiation and, 415–416
  prenatal irradiation and, 415, 416
  radiotherapy for
    bone tumors after, 252, 253
    breast cancer after, 170
    coronary complications after, 318–319
    hepatobiliary system cancer after, 240
    lung cancer after, 179
    second cancer after, 103
    thyroid cancers related to, 156–157
    tumors after, 123
  after in utero radiation exposure, 416–419
  case-control and cohort studies of, 100
Childhood irradiation
  bones effects of, 336
  brain neoplasms from, 140
  late intestinal complications of, 323–324
  radiation-induced excess relative risk from,
      86
Childhood radiotherapy
  bone effects of, 336
  colon cancer after, 230
  pulmonary reactions after, 315
  salivary gland tumors after, 145
  soft-tissue tumors after, 258
  T-cells effects of, 349
  thyroid cancer after, 156
  thyroid nodules or adenomas after, 161
Children
  affected by Chernobyl fallout, 94
    immune status of, 352
    thyroid dose in, 297
  cataracts after leukemia therapy in, 308–309
  fallout studies of in Utah, 93
  hepatobiliary system cancer in after Wilms'
      tumor treatment, 240
  lens opacities after skin hemangioma
      treatment in, 309
  living near nuclear facilities, leukemia rates
      among, 95–96
  nervous system radiosensitivity in, 302
  radiation nephropathy in, 329
  thyroid cancer risk in, 162
Chimney sweeps, scrotal cancers in, 212
Chlorambucil
  carcinogenic effects of, 447
  in hepatic radiosensitivity, 327
Chlornaphazine
  cancer risk from, 443
  carcinogenic effects of, 447
Cholangiocarcinoma, after Thorotrast
    injection, 241
Cholesterol epoxide, carcinogenic effect of,
    445
Chondroblast proliferation, reduced, 336–337
Chondrosarcoma
  age as factor in, 248–249
  after Hodgkin's disease treatment, 252
  leukemia risk from radiotherapy for,
      126–127
  sulfur 35 treatment of, 345
Chordoma treatment, leukemia risk from,
    126–127
Chromatid type aberrations, 59

Chromium radionuclides, dose coefficients for worker intakes of, 497t–499t
Chromosomal aberrations, 49
  in atomic bomb survivors, 57–58, 64
    frequency of, 474
    rate of, 55
  clinical peripheral studies of, 62–64
  contrast media in, 392–393
  identifying, 49–50
  in infants dying in perinatal period, 51–52
  in live-born children, 52
  normal incidence of, 51
  in peripheral lymphocytes, 59–62
  radiation exposure and, 56–57
  radiation-induced genomic instability and, 7
  varieties of, 50f
Chromosome breaks
  in genetic disorders, 49–50
  single and double, 50, 50f
Chromosome painting technique, for lymphocyte chromosome aberrations, 61–62
Chromosomes, 47
  euploid structural arrangement of, 51–52
  instability of in carcinogenesis, 73
  metaphase
    karyotype of, 49f
    morphology of, 48f
Chronic fatigue syndrome, after radiation exposure, 364
Chronic lymphocytic leukemia. See Leukemia, chronic lymphocytic (CLL)
Chronic myeloid leukemia (CML). See Leukemia, chronic myeloid (CML)
Chronic obstructive pulmonary disease (COPD), radiotherapy in, 313–314
Circulatory disease, in atomic bomb survivors, 319–320
Cirrhosis
  increased incidence of with fallout exposure, 361
  after Thorotrast injection, 327–328
Cisplatinum
  ototoxicity of, 310
  in radiation myelopathy, 304
  in radiation-induced esophagitis, 321
Clinical peripheral chromosome studies, of radiation-induced aberrations, 62–64
Clodronate, for radiation osteonecrosis, 336–337
Clonal growths, cancers as, 71
Clusters of differentiation, 347
c-mos gene mutations, 74–75
CNS. See Central nervous system (CNS)
Coal, as modified natural radiation source, 35–36
Coal mining, occupational exposures from, 42
Cobalt 60, 290
  central nervous system effects of, 299
  immune function effects of, 351
  penis, urethra, and scrotum effects of, 335
Cobalt radionuclides, dose coefficients for worker intakes of, 497t–499t
Cockayne's syndrome
  clinical features of, 76t
  radiosensitivity in, 77
Codons, strings of, 47
Coffee, carcinogens in, 445
Cognitive function
  impaired after cutaneous hemangioma treatment, 303
  radiation and chemotherapy effects on, 302

Cohort studies
  of combined nuclear facilities workers, 97
  of populations affected by Chernobyl fallout, 94
Colitis
  acute radiation, 324
  long-standing ulcerative, 324–325
Collagen bundles, 287
Collagen formation, in deterministic effects of radiation, 286
Collective dose equivalent, limitations of, 21–22
Collective effective doses, from nuclear accidents, 42
Collective equivalent dose, 21–22
Collective equivalent or effective dose, 22
Collective equivalent or effective dose commitment concept, 22
Colon
  epithelium of, 324
  hyperemic mucosa of, 324
  low-LET radiation effects on, 324–325
  mucosal cells of, 324
  neutron radiation effects on, 325
  radionuclide radiation effects on, 325–326
  radiosensitivity of, 324
    rectosigmoid portion of, 324–325
  shortening and fibrosis of, 324–325
  SOMA normal tissue radiotoxicity for, 520t
  ulceration of, 324
    with high-dose radiation, 325
Colon cancer
  incidence and etiology of, 227
  radiation-induced
    dose-response relationship in, 231
    from external exposure, 227–230
    from internal exposure, 230–231
  risk estimates for, 231, 232t
  spontaneous, estimated lifetime risk of, 83t
  steps in induction of, 73f
Colorectal cancer
  genetic factors in, 72, 73
  incidence and types of, 227
Combine effects, classes of, 389
Combined actions, problems examining, 389–390
Comedones, localized, after radiotherapy, 289
Committed equivalent or effective dose, 22
Compensation programs, 450–452
  PC/AS-based, 452, 452f
Compensation Scheme for Radiation-Linked Diseases (CSRLD), UK, 452
Compton effect, 3
Computed tomography (CT)
  radiation exposure from, 43, 44
  of radiation necrosis of brain, 300–301
  temporary epilation after, 290
Computer image analysis, of circulating lymphocytes, 59–60
Concrete dwellings, gamma radiation from, 119
Conditions of exposure, defining, 460
Confidence interval (CI), 84
Congenital abnormalities
  in atomic bomb survivors, 57
  after Chernobyl accident, 405–406
  after high embryonic and fetal x-ray doses, 404t
  incidence of in live-born children, 52
  normal incidence of, 51–52
  transmissibility of, 51
  after in utero exposure, 401–402, 411–412
    during fetal period, 410
    in organogenesis period, 404–405

Congenital abnormalities (Continued)
  tentative timetable of, 405f
  at various gestational stages, 405f
Conjunctival carcinoma, radiation-induced, 305–306
Connective tissue
  cancer of
    in atomic bomb survivors, 250–251
    uranium contamination in, 250
  multipotential cells of, radiosensitivity of, 14–15
  stromal degeneration of, 289
  tumors of, 257t
Consumer products
  in cancer risk, 447
  as modified natural radiation source, 38–39
  radiation exposure from in United States, 40t
Contrast media, radiosensitizing effects of, 392–393
Conversion tables
  of absorbed dose units, 495t
  of dose equivalent units, 495t
  of exposure units, 495t
  of radioactivity units, 496t
  of radon, 496t
  SI unit, 495t
Cooking, carcinogenic effects of, 445
Cooperative Thyrotoxicosis Follow-up Study Group, 157–158
Cooperative Thyrotoxicosis Therapy Follow-up Study, 102
Cor pulmonale, compensation for, 450
Cornea
  radiation effects on, 305
  radiation-induced ulceration of, 305–306
Corneocytes, 287f
Coronary artery
  disease in after breast carcinoma radiotherapy, 318–319
  inhibition of stenosis of, 318
  narrowing of
    after Hodgkin's disease radiotherapy, 317–318
    after radiotherapy, 319
Coronary heart disease
  after breast cancer radiotherapy, 318–319
  after radiotherapy, 362
Corticosteroids
  long-term use of in cataract formation, 308
  to reduce radiation pneumonitis severity, 312
Cosmic protons, sea-level effective dose rate of, 27
Cosmic radiation, 27–28. See also Background radiation exposure
  absorbed dose rate at sea level of, 27–28
  annual effective dose from
    contribution of sources to, 28f
    worldwide collective, 28
  annual effective doses from, 27–28
    average, 37t
    by location, 29t
    per caput in United States, 28f
    in U.S. population, 28t
  attenuation of, 27, 28
  average annual doses and effective dose equivalents of by state, 36t
  bone tumors related to, 250
  colon cancer related to, 227
  dose rates of
    incremental increase in with altitude, 29t
    variation in with latitude at sea level, 29t
  in esophageal cancer, 215

Cosmic radiation (*Continued*)
  factors affecting, 27
  galactic, 27
  as modified natural radiation source, 38
  as natural radiation source, 35
  radionuclides produced by, 29t
  reacting with atmosphere, 27
  rectal cancer related to, 233
  at sea level versus high altitude, 27–28
  solar, 27
Craft v. Vanderbilt University, 441
Cranial irradiation
  gonadotrophin deficiency and premature puberty after, 331
  mineralizing microangiopathy after, 301–302
  neuropsychological impairment after, 302–303
Cranial sinus
  carcinomas of, 144
  radiation-induced tumors of, 144
    in radium dial painters, 338
Cranial tumor radiotherapy
  growth hormone deficiency in children after, 293–294
C-reactive protein (CRP), in atomic bomb survivors, 351
Creatine excretion, after radiation exposure, 364
Creatinine clearance, after radiotherapy, 329
Croton oil, enhanced radiation effect with, 394
Crypts of Lieherkühn, mucosal epithelial cell proliferation in, 322–323
Crysotile asbestos fiber inhalation, 391–392
Curie, Marie, 287–288
Curies (Ci, becquerel), 8, 34
Curium radionuclides, dose coefficients for worker intakes of, 497t–499t
Cutaneous hemangioma treatment, cognitive impairment after, 303
Cutaneous radiation syndrome, 287–288
Cutaneous syndrome, 357–359
  degrees of, 358t
Cyclophosphamide
  carcinogenic effects of, 447
  leukemia risk from, 123
  in pulmonary fibrosis incidence, 315–316
  in radiation myelopathy, 304
  in radiation recall phenomena, 393
  radiosensitizing effect of, 392–393
Cyclosporine, carcinogenic effects of, 443, 447
Cyclotron workers, cataracts in, 309
Cyclotrons, 4–5
Cysteamine, radioprotective effect of, 9
Cysteic acid excretion, after radiation exposure, 363–364
Cysteine, radioprotective effect of, 9
Cystic hygroma treatment, breast hypoplasia after, 311f
Cystitis, acute, radiation-induced, 330
Cytarabine, in hepatic radiosensitivity, 327
Cytogenetic analysis
  of circulating lymphocytes, 59–60
  of incidence of chromosome abnormalities, 51
  in legal documentation, 441
Cytokines
  in bone marrow transplantation, 343–344
  in cell development, 340
Cytomegalovirus, after Chernobyl accident, 360
Cytoplasmic inheritance, 47–48
Cytosine (C), 47

Cytotoxic chemotherapy, plasma taurine levels after, 364

D

Dacarbazine, in radiation recall phenomena, 393
Dactinomycin
  in predisposition to radiation pneumonitis, 313
  in soft-tissue sarcoma risk, 256–258
Daily tolerance dose, 22
Daubert et al. v. Merrell Dow Pharmaceuticals, 440
Daunomycin, cardiomyopathy and, 317
Delgado v. Yandell, 440–441
Dementia, radiation exposure and, 303
Demyelinating disorder, radiation-induced, 299
Demyelination
  radiotherapy induced, 301
  of white matter, 299–300
DEN repair deficiencies, 73
Dental abnormalities, radiation-induced, 337
Dental x-rays
  CNS cancer incidence from exposure to, 140
  salivary gland tumors related to, 145
Denver, absorbed dose rates of terrestrial radiation in, 31–32
Deoxycytidine excretion, after radiation exposure, 363–364
Department of Energy workers, compensation programs of, 450
Depigmentation, after radiotherapy, 289
Depression
  after nuclear accidents, 467
  screening programs for, 468
Derived limits, 23–24
Dermal plexus, 287f
Dermatitis
  chronic radiation, 290
  exudative, with low-LET radiation, 288
Dermatosis, benign, treatment of, nonmelanoma skin cancer after, 262
Dermis, 286–287
  injury to, 288–289
DeSanctis-Cacchione syndrome, 75–76
Desquamation
  of eyes, 305–306
  from uranium exposure, 291–293
Deterministic effects of radiation, 437–438
  acute, 286
  apoptosis in, 285
  biochemical indicators of, 363–364
  of bone, cartilage, and muscle
    with low-LET radiation, 335–338
    with neutron or high-LET radiation, 338
    with radionuclide irradiation, 338–339
  of breast tissue, 311–312
  classification of, 286
    modifying factors in, 286
  delayed, 286
  of ear, 309–310
    low-LET radiation in, 310
  of endocrine glands, 293–299
    adrenal, 299
    parathyroid, 298–299
    pituitary, 293–294
    thyroid, 294–298
  of eye, 305–309
    high-LET radiation in, 309
    low-LET radiation in, 305–309

Deterministic effects of radiation (*Continued*)
    radionuclide irradiation in, 309
  fatigue in, 364–365
  of gastrointestinal tract, 320–326
    in colon, sigmoid, and rectum, 324–326
    esophageal, 321–322
    oral cavity and pharynx, 320–321
    small intestinal, 322–324
    stomach, 322
  general aspects of, 286
  of heart and vessels
    with high-LET radiation, 320
    with internal irradiation, 320
    with low-LET radiation, 316–320
    with radionuclide irradiation, 320
  of hematopoietic system, 340–345
    with high-LET radiation, 344
    with internal irradiation, 344–345
    with low-LET radiation, 341–344
  historic background of, 285–286
  of immune system, 346–353
    cell types and function in, 347–353
  of larynx, 312
  life-shortening, 360–363
    in atomic bomb survivors and persons exposed to fallout, 361
    with occupational exposure, 362–363
    in radiotherapy patients, 361–362
  of liver and biliary system
    with high-LET radiation, 327
    with LET radiation, 326–327
    with radionuclide irradiation, 327–328
  of lung, 312–316
    with high-LET radiation, 316
    with low-LET radiation, 312–316
    with radionuclide irradiation, 316
  of lymphatic system, 345–346
    of high-LET and radionuclide irradiation, 346
    with low-LET radiation, 345–346
  of nervous system, 299–305
    brain, 300–303
    peripheral, 305
  of pancreas, with low-LET radiation, 328
  of reproductive organs, 331–335
    ovarian, 331–332
    in penis, urethra, and scrotum, 335
    in prostate and seminal vesicles, 335
    testicular, 333–335
    uterine, 332–333
    vaginal, 333
  reviews and observation of, 285
  of salivary glands, 310–311
    high-LET radiation in, 311
    low-LET radiation in, 310–311
    radionuclide irradiation in, 311
  of skin and mucosa, 286–293
    with low-LET radiation, 288–290
    neutron irradiation and, 290
    radionuclide radiation in, 290–293
  threshold dose in, 285
  tissue radiosensitivity and, 285
  of total-body irradiation, 353–360
    acute syndromes and sickness in, 355–360
  toxicity scoring systems for, 285
  of urinary system
    in kidney, 328–330
    in ureter and bladder, 330–331
Deuterons, particulate radiation of, 4–5, 4t
Developmental stages, postconception, 403t
Diabetes, cataracts in, 454

Diagnostic medical radiation, 99–101. *See also* Medical radiation exposure; Medical radiation workers
absorbed doses from, 43
bladder cancer related to, 197
bone tumors related to
with external exposure, 252
with internal exposure, 253
epidemiologic risk studies of, 88
fetal exposure to, 401–402
kidney cancer related to, 191
leukemia incidence from, 121
lung cancer related to, 178
nonmelanoma skin cancer after, 261
postnatal, 100–101
pregnancy termination after, 417–419
prenatal, 99–100
thyroid cancer related to external exposure in, 154
uterine cancer after, 206
Diagnostic x-radiation
abdominal, during gestation, 410–411
breast cancer related to, 168
in cataract formation, 308
effective doses from, 44t
prenatal, 402
Diarrhea
radiation-induced, bile in, 359
after radiotherapy, 323
treatment of, 324
after whole-abdominal radiation in children, 323–324
Diet
anticarcinogens in, 446
carcinogenic effects of, 74, 445–446
fission products in, correlated to breast cancer rats, 92
high-protein, high-caloric, for liver disease, 326–327
low-residue, 324
tumor promoting, 71–72
Diethylstilbestrol (DES), radiation interaction with, 397
Differentiating intermitotic cells, radiosensitivity of, 14–15
Digestive system disease, in uranium miners and mill workers, 425–426
Dimethylbenzathracene, carcinogenic effect of, 394
Dimethylbusulfan, in hepatic radiosensitivity, 327
Diploid number, 49–50
Disease frequency measures, in epidemiological studies, 84
Disomy, uniparental, 47–48
Diuretics, for liver disease, 326–327
DNA
breakdown of after radiation exposure, 363–364
genetic sequences of, 47
integrity of, 47
mitochondrial mutations of, 47–48
as radiation target, 9
replication of, cell cycle phases based on, 11f
synthesis of, 11
high temperature inhibiting, 390–391
DNA analogs, radiosensitizing effect of, 9, 392–393
DNA breaks
double-strand (DSBs), 9–10
in cellular death, 10, 13–14
in locally multiply damaged sites, 10
ionizing radiation-induced, 9–10

DNA breaks (*Continued*)
single-strand (SSBs), 9–10
in cellular death, 13–14
in locally multiply damaged sites, 10
DNA code, 47
DNA cross-linking agents
in Fanconi anemia, 77
in xeroderma pigmentosum, 75–76
DNA cross-linking repair, defective, 77
DNA deletions, 49
spontaneous, 74
DNA methylation, 73
DNA radical formation, 8–9
DNA repair, 11
caffeine inhibiting, 445
defect in with Bloom's syndrome, 77
modifiers affecting, 9
with radiation dose, 473
subcellular, 13
sublethal, 13
DNA viruses, oncogenic, 74
DNA-DNA covalent cross-links, 9–10
DNA-protein crosslinks, 9–10
Dominant lethal gene, 49
Dominant traits, 47–48
Dose and dose-rate effectiveness factor (DDREF), 16–17
in uncertainty of cancer risk estimates, 87
Dose equivalent, 20
conversion table for units of, 495t
maximum external photon and electron for organs, 500t
Dose equivalent rate factors, for skin radionuclide contamination, 500t
Dose limits, 22–24
application of, 23–24
Dose range estimates, 460–461
Dose rate, in cell survival curve, 13f
Dose-effect relationship, 79–81
common mathematical models for, 79f
epidemiological data for, 79
linear model for, 79–80
linear-quadratic model for, 80
quadratic model for, 80
threshold model for, 80–81
Dose-rate effectiveness factor (DREF), in uncertainty of cancer risk estimates, 87
Dose-response curve, for leukemia, 117
Dose-response relationship, 79–81
assessment of, 460
epidemiologic data on, 83–84
sample size for statistical precision in, 82t
sensitive population response and, 77
Dosimetry
chromosome aberrations in peripheral lymphocytes in, 59–62
genetic markers used for, 58–62
at Hiroshima and Nagasaki, 89–90
in uncertainty of risk estimates, 87
Dot deletion, 49–50
Doubling dose
with chronic radiation exposure, 55
in estimating radiation-induced genetic disease risk, 53–54
for infant deaths in atomic bomb survivors, 57
for protein phenotype mutations in atomic bomb survivors, 57–58
Doubling time, for radiation-induced tumors, 78–79
Dounreay nuclear installation, leukemia clusters around, 56, 95

Down syndrome, 49–50
in high natural background areas, 63
incidence of, 52
incidence of in Belarus before and after Chernobyl accident, 56f
incidence of in populations near Chernobyl nuclear accident, 55, 57
maternal age and, 57
radiation-induced hereditary risk of, 56–57
after in utero radiation exposure, 406
in utero radiation threshold for, 406
Downwinders, 439
compensation for, 450
Doxorubicin
cardiomyopathy and, 317
radiosensitizing effect of, 9
second tumors after, 123
Doxorubicin hydrochloride. *See* Adriamycin (doxorubicin hydrochloride)
Drabbels v. Skelly Oil Co., 440–441
Drosophila
radiation risk data from, 53
x-ray induced mutations in, 47
DS86 dose
contribution to total radiation dose, 87
at Hiroshima and Nagasaki, 89–90
DS02 dosimetry, in leukemia risk, 117
Duodenum, radiation injury in, 322–323
Dwarfism, after radiotherapy during pregnancy, 405
Dyspepsia, radiation-induced, 322
Dysphasia, with low-LET radiation, 321
Dysuria, after brachytherapy, 331

E
Ear
deterministic effects of radiation in, 309–310
from low-LET radiation, 310
external, radiation sensitivity of, 309–310
inner, radiation sensitivity of, 309–310
middle, radium-induced damage to, 309–310
SOMA normal tissue radiotoxicity for, 511t
Ectoderm, embryonic, 286–287
Edema, of larynx, 312
Effective dose, 20–22
Effective dose equivalent, 20–21
Effective half-life, 7
Elastic scattering, 4–5
Electroencephalography, 299–300
Electromagnetic radiation, 1–5
particulate, 4–5
in radiation effects, 391
Electromagnetic spectrum, 1
wavelength, frequency, and energy of, 2f
Electron affinic agents, radiosensitizing effect of, 392–393
Electron capture, 6
Electron packets, 10
Electronic equipment, cosmic radiation from, 39
Electrons, 1
fast, gamma or x-rays combined with, 391
particulate radiation of, 4t
Emanation actinon, radiation energies and intensities of, 33t
Emanation thoron, radiation energies and intensities of, 32t
Embryo
absorbed dose in, 401–402
anomalies after high-dose x-irradiation of, 404t

Embryo (*Continued*)
liability for radiation exposure of, 440–441
nervous system radioresistance of, 299–300
radionuclide irradiation of, 412–414
Embryonic yolk sac, immune stem cell production in, 346–347
Emergent situations, dose limits in, 23–24
Emphysema, in uranium miners, 425–426
Encephalitis, Japanese B, after in utero radiation exposure, 406
Endocardium, late fibrosis changes in, 318
Endocrine system
deterministic radiation effects on, 293–299 (*See also specific glands*)
neoplasms of
multiple, DNA sequence loss for, 73
in pancreatic cancer risk, 243
radioresistance of, 293
Endometrial cancer
incidence of, 204–205
risk factors for, 446
Endoscopy, for radiation proctitis, 324
Energetic beta-particle emitters, skin reaction to, 290–291
Energy deposition, 10
in secondary effects, 438–439
into tissue, 2
Energy Employees Occupational Illness Compensation Program Act of 2000 (EEOICPA), 450
Entrance skin dose, 8
Environment
contaminants of in cancer risk, 447
individual genetics and carcinogens in, 442
radiation exposure from
hormetic effects of, 473–474
plutonium in, 429
Epicardial fibrosis, mechanisms of, 319
Epidemiological studies
criteria in, 84–85
disease frequency measures in, 84
in high natural background radiation areas, 92
of populations living near nuclear facilities, 94–96
of radiation-induced cancer risk, 88–103
reporting no radiation link, 85
sample size required for, 82t, 83–84
Epidemiology
of radiogenic cancers, 83–86
in uncertainty of risk estimates, 86–87
Epidermis, 286–287
injury to, 288–289
sloughing of, 288
Epigenetic responses, 10–11
Epilation (hair loss)
after accidental whole-body exposure, 289f
with radiation-induced skin erythema, 288
temporary, 288–289
post-CT scan, 290
Epiphyseal closure, delayed, after gestational radiation exposure, 410
Epipodophyllotoxin (VP16-213)
enhancing skin radiosensitivity, 290
in secondary leukemia, 123
Epstein-Barr virus
carcinogenic effect of, 447–448
reactivation of in atomic bomb survivors, 350–351
Equivalent dose, 20
Erbium 169 citrate, in cartilage necrosis, 339
Erectile dysfunction, after brachytherapy, 331

Erythema
with beta-particle emitter exposure, 290–291
initial and secondary, 288–289
with low-LET radiation
early phase, 288
late phase, 288
with neutron irradiation, 290
from uranium exposure, 291–293
Erythroblasts, radiosensitivity of, 340
Erythrocytes, depletion of, 340–341
Erythropoiesis, radiosensitivity of, 340
Esophageal cancer (carcinoma)
alcohol and tobacco use in relative risk for, 358
in atomic bomb survivors, 85–86
cell types in, 215
dietary carcinogens in, 445
epidemiology of, 218–220
incidence of, 214–215
interactive mechanisms in combined agents in, 389–390
radiation-induced
from external exposure, 215–218
from internal exposure, 218
risk estimates for incidence and mortality from, 219t
risk factors for, 215
Esophagitis
chemotherapeutic agents and, 321
with low-LET radiation, 321
Esophagus
chemotherapeutic agents enhancing radiation effects on, 392t
epithelial regeneration of after radiotherapy, 321–322
impaired motility of, radiotherapy-related, 321
low-LET radiation effects on, 321–322
radiation stricture of, 322f
radiation-induced ulceration of, 321, 322
SOMA normal tissue radiotoxicity for, 518t
squamous epithelium of, 321
strictures of, radiation-induced, 321
Estrogens
in breast tissue radiosensitivity, 311–312
cancer risk from, 443
carcinogenic effects of, 447
radiation cataracts and, 308–309
radiation interaction with, 397
radiation interference with, 332
Etched track detector, in measuring radon, 34–35
Ethnicity
in hepatobiliary system cancers, 236
in radiation effects, 397
Ethnicity/race, in nonmelanoma skin cancer, 259
Ethylnitrosourea, carcinogenic effect of, 394
Europe, Chernobyl fallout in, 64
Europium radionuclides, dose coefficients for worker intakes of, 497t–499t
Evidence, sources of in risk measurement, 460
Ewing's sarcoma, 248–249
Ewing's tumor, after radiotherapy for Wilms' tumor, 252
Excess cancer. *See* Radiation-induced tumors
Excess lifetime risk, 82–83
Excess relative risk (ERR), 84
in atomic bomb survivors, 85
in calculating PC/AS, 448f
considerations in calculating, 85–86
with irradiation in childhood, 86
in radiation-induced and spontaneous cancer risk, 85

Exon, 47–48
Exophthalmos, after radioiodine therapy, 309
Expert witness testimony
selecting experts for, 439–440
threshold for acceptance of, 440
Exposure
definition of, 389–390
length of, 389–390
Exposure units, conversion table for, 495t
External beam radiotherapy
radiation exposure from, 45
for skin hemangiomas in childhood, 102
thyroid cancer after, 158
Extrapolated dose response (ERD) model, 18
Extremity swelling, late radiation, 288
Exudative epidermatitis, 288–289
Eye
chemotherapeutic agents enhancing radiation effects on, 392t
deterministic effects of radiation in, 305–309
from high-LET radiation, 309
from low-LET radiation, 305–309
from radionuclide irradiation, 309
malformations of after radiation exposure throughout gestation, 411
radiosensitivity of, 305
SOMA normal tissue radiotoxicity for, 509t–510t
Eyebrows, radiation effects on, 305–306

F
Facial bone, SOMA normal tissue radiotoxicity for, 509t–510t
Fallout exposure, 40–41
average effective doses from, 41
from various radionuclides, 41t
bone tumors related to, 250
in breast cancer incidence, 167
cataract formation from, 308
from Chernobyl accident, 64
colon cancer related to, 227
epidemiologic risk studies of, 88
esophageal cancer in populations near, 215
kidney cancer in workers exposed to, 189
larynx cancer related to, 146–147
leukemia incidence from, 119–120
lung cancer related to, 175–176, 179–180
melanoma related to, 263
multiple myeloma in populations exposed to, 133
in nonmelanoma skin cancers, 260
pancreatic cancer related to, 247
patterns of, 92–93
plutonium exposure from, 429
radiation-induced life shortening from, 361
skin changes with, 291
stomach cancer in workers exposed to, 221
studies of populations exposed to, 92–94
thyroid cancer related to, 158–160
thyroid nodules or adenomas related to, 162
Familial cancer
radiation induced, 75
specific syndromes of, 75–77
Fanconi anemia
clinical features of, 76t
radiosensitivity in, 77
Fat
dietary, carcinogenic effect of, 74, 445
subcutaneous, 287f

Fatality rate, measuring, 460–461
Fatigue
    after accidental radiation exposure, 365
    in atomic bomb survivors, 467
    in cancer patients, 364–365
    definition of, 364
    radiation-induced, 364–365
Fatty diet, in colon cancer, 227
Favre-Racouchot syndrome, after
    radiotherapy, 289
Femoral epiphysis slippage, after radiotherapy
    in children, 336
Fernald uranium processing plant
    renal damage in populations near, 331
    workers at
        bladder cancer in, 198
        bone tumors in, 254
        CNS cancer incidence in, 140
        colon cancer in, 230
        esophageal cancer in, 217
        hepatobiliary system cancer in, 239
        kidney cancer in, 192
        leukemia in, 125
        lung cancer in, 186
        male genital cancer in, 214
        nonmelanoma skin cancer in, 261
        oropharyngeal cancer in, 149
        prostate cancer in, 211
        rectal cancer in, 234
        stomach cancer in, 222
        uranium-induced illness in, 426–427
Fertilizers, phosphate, as modified natural
    radiation source, 37
Fetal period, radiation exposure during, 410
Fetus
    absorbed dose in, 401–402
    brain development in, 406–410
    radiation exposure of, 401–402
        liability for, 440–441
        radionuclide, 412–414
    x-irradiation of
        diagnostic, 402
        high-dose, anomalies after, 404t
Fibrin deposition, in deterministic effects of
    radiation, 286
Fibrinous exudate, in deterministic effects of
    radiation, 286
Fibroadenomatosis treatment, breast cancer
    related to, 169
Fibroblasts, radiosensitivity of, 340
Fibrosarcomas
    age as factor in, 248–249
    after pelvic tumor radiation, 258–259
    after radiotherapy, 256
Fibrosis
    after breast irradiation, 312
    edema and, 286
    late subcutaneous radiation, 290
    skin, from Chernobyl accident
        contamination, 291
Fibrous histiocytomas
    after breast or pelvic cancer
        radiotherapy, 258
    after radiotherapy, 256
Film badges
    for atmospheric weapons test personnel,
        93–94
    in estimating radiation doses, 63–64
    for legal documentation, 441
FISH analysis. See Fluorescence in situ
    hybridization technique (FISH)
Fission, 6
Fission product fallout, skin changes and,
    291

Fixed postmitotic cells
    death of, 16f
    radiosensitivity of, 14–15
Fluorescence in situ hybridization technique
    (FISH)
    in chromosome aberration analysis in
        Chernobyl accident survivors, 64
    for dicentric lymphocyte chromosome
        aberrations, 61–62
Fluorine radionuclides. dose coefficients for
    worker intakes of, 497t–499t
Fluoroscopy
    bone tumors after, 252
    breast cancer after, 168–169
    colon cancer after, 229
    kidney cancer after, 191
    lung cancer after, 173, 178
    nonmelanoma skin cancer after, 261
    pancreatic cancer after, 246
    postnatal effects of, 100
    rectal cancer after, 234–235
    stomach cancer after, 223
    thyroid nodules or adenomas after, 161
5-Fluorouracil
    cataractogenic effect of, 309
    for hepatic metastases, 327–328
    in hepatic radiosensitivity, 327
    in radiation brain injury, 302
    in radiation recall phenomena, 393
    in radiation-induced esophagitis, 321
    radiosensitizing effect of, 9, 392–393
Flurospar miners, lung cancer in, 185
Fly ash, as modified natural radiation source,
    35–36
Foamy cells, 319–320
    intimal, 330
Follicle-stimulating hormone (FSH)
    deficiency, after pituitary irradiation, 294
Food preservatives, carcinogenic effect of,
    445
Fossil fuel, as modified natural radiation
    source, 35–36
Fractionated radiation, 16–18
    bone marrow changes after, 342
    cardiac complications of, 319
    chronic radiation nephritis after, 330
    gastric ulceration with, 322
    gastrointestinal effects of, 320
    liver tolerance of, 326
    myocarditis in, 317
    nausea and vomiting after, 322
    penis, urethra, and scrotum effects of, 335
    radiation pneumonitis and, 313
    skin erythema threshold and, 288
    skin ulceration with, 288
Fractionation
    in bone tumors, 249–250
    in cell survival curve, 13f
Fragile sites, in carcinogenesis, 73
Fragile-X syndrome, 47–48
Free electron, 3
Free radicals
    formation of, 8–9
    induction of, 9, 392–393
Frontal sinus carcinoma, in radium dial
    painter, 144f

G
G2 molecular checkpoint gene mutations,
    17
G1 phase, 11
G2 phase, 11

Gallbladder cancer
    in atomic bomb survivors, 236–237, 238f
    incidence of, 236
    from internal radiation exposure, 240–241
    from medical radiation exposure, 240
    from occupational radiation exposure, 238–240
Gallium 67 citrate scans, salivary gland effects
    of, 310–311
Gallium radionuclide exposure
    dose coefficients of in workers, 497t–499t
    during pregnancy, 413
Gallstones, in gallbladder cancer, 236
Gamete production, reduction or obliteration
    of, 331
Gamma brachytherapy, inhibiting coronary
    artery restenosis, 318
Gamma knife radiosurgery, neuropsychologic
    impairment after, 302
Gamma photons, maximum range of, 291
Gamma radiation, 1–2
    absorption of, 3
    background, 30
    in cataract formation, 308
    dicentric chromosomes induced by, 54t
    electromagnetic wavelengths of, 3
    half-value layer of, 3–4
    with heavy ions, 391
    in lung cancer risk in plutonium
        workers, 187
    lung cancer risk with, 188
    lymphocyte chromosome aberration
        induction by, 60–61, 60f
    photon emissions of, 6
    from radon decay, 433
    RBE of, 3t
    sensitivity to in ataxia-telangiectasia, 76–77
    terrestrial, annual effective dose from,
        31–32, 34t, 37t
    total body, lymphocyte chromosome
        aberrations with, 60–61, 60f
Gamma ray constants, for radionuclides, 503t
Gamma-emitting radionuclides, 30–31
    skin reaction to, 290
Gastric acidity, reduction of, 322
Gastric motility, radiation-induced impairment
    of, 322
Gastric reflux, in esophageal cancers, 215
Gastric ulceration, radiation-induced, 322
Gastritis, chronic atrophic, radiation-induced,
    322
Gastrointestinal syndrome, 320, 357–358
    absorbed skin doses in, 358–359
    after Chernobyl accident, 359–360
    degrees of, 358t
    human data on, 359
    manifestations of, 358–359
    with radiation of small intestine, 323
Gastrointestinal system
    chemotherapeutic agents enhancing
        radiation effects on, 392t
    deterministic radiation effects on, 320–326
    hypermotility of, radiation-induced, 323
    long-term radiotherapy complications of,
        325–326
    radiosensitivity of, 15, 320
    SOMA normal tissue radiotoxicity for, 520t
Gastrointestinal tract cells, radiosensitivity of,
    14–15
Gatekeeper genes, in tumor initiation, 72
G-banding method, for chromosome
    aberration estimates in atomic bomb
    survivors, 64
Gemcitabine, in radiation recall phenomena of
    internal organs, 393

Gene amplification, 47–48
Gene-environment interactions, 442
Genes
    definition of, 47
    dominant and recessive, 47–48
    "hot spots" on, 50
    radiation-induced genomic instability and
        mutation of, 7
Genetic abnormalities, 440
    normal incidence of, 51–52
    in radiation carcinogenesis, 72
    from radiation exposure, 53–54
Genetic code, 47
    in human genome, 47–48
Genetic disorders
    alleles in, 47–48
    Chernobyl fallout effect on, 405–406
    environmental factors in, 50–51
    estimated risks of from chronic low-LET
        radiation, 52t
    mutation component of, 53–54
    with serious health consequences, natural
        incidence of, 52t
Genetic effects
    definition of, 459–460
    risk estimates for, 460
Genetic expansion, 47–48
Genetic mutations
    alleles in, 47–48
    direct and indirect methods of
        estimating, 53
    heterozygous, 49
    lethal, 49
    potential recoverability conversion factor
        for, 53–54
    radiation-induced, 64–65
        background of, 47–49
        clinical peripheral chromosome studies
            of, 62–64
        discovery of, 47
        genetic markers for, 58–62
        long generation time for, 47
        types of, 49–58
    rate of radiation-induced, 53
    spontaneous versus induced rates of, 53–54
    sublethal, 49
    tumor-specific, 74–75
    UNSCEAR data on, 65
Genetic predispositions
    to natural versus radiogenic cancers, 83
    in radiation-induced breast cancer, 165
    in radiation-induced malignancies, 397
Genetic studies, on radiation-exposed
    populations, 54–58
Genetics
    in cancer, 442
    in nonmelanoma skin cancer, 259
    in ovarian cancer, 200
    in thyroid cancers in Chernobyl accident
        survivors, 151
Genomic imprinting, 47–48
Genomic instability
    bystander effect and, 10–11
    radiation induced, 10
Geophysical factors, in cancer risk, 447
Germ-cell depletion, with radiation and
    chemotherapy, 334
Germ-cell mutations, causing cancer in
    offspring, 56
Germinal cell necrosis, postradiation, 334
Gestation, radiation exposure throughout,
    410–411
Gestational stages, radiation adverse effects at,
    403f

Glasses, thorium in manufacture of, 39
Glial cells, 299
    radiation damage to, 300
Glomerular filtration
    postradiotherapy, 329
    radiation effects on, 329
Glomerulus cells, 328–329
Glutathione, anticarcinogenic effect of, 446
Glycophorin A (GPA) assay
    for atomic bomb survivors, 58
    for Chernobyl accident survivors,
        58–59
Goiania cesium contamination accident,
    413
    chromosome aberrations in survivors of,
        64
Goiter
    immune function after treatment of, 350
Goiters, 160
    nodular, after thyroid irradiation, 295
Gold 198 colloid treatment
    in cartilage necrosis, 339
    for serosal metastatic carcinoma, 345
Gold 198 therapy, of pituitary lesions, 294
Gold jewelry, radioactive, 290
Gold radionuclides, dose coefficients for
    worker intakes of, 497t–499t
Gonadal function, radiotherapy effects on,
    331–335
Gonadotropin
    abnormal levels of after radiotherapy, 332
    deficiency of
        after cranial irradiation, 331
        after high-dose radiation of pituitary,
            293
        indicating hypopituitarism, 293
GPA variant erythrocytes
    in atomic bomb survivors, 64
    with occupational exposure, 63–64
Granisetron
    to prevent nausea and vomiting with whole-
        body irradiation, 354–355
Granulocyte macrophage-colony stimulating
    factor (GM-CSF)
    in bone marrow transplantation, 343–344
    healing radiation-induced esophageal
        ulceration, 321
Granulocytes
    depression of after bone marrow ablation,
        343
    reserves of in atomic bomb survivors, 341
Granulocytopenia, postradiation, 340–341
Granulosa cells, 331–332
    radiation effects on, 332
Graphite reactor accident, 42
Graves' disease
    iodine 131 treatment of, 298
    misclassification of cancer in, 187
    radiotherapy for
        cataract formation after, 309
        immune function after, 350
        thyroid cancer after, 157–158
    thyroid antibodies in, 295
Gray (rad), 7–8. *See also* Kerma
Groin area skin, radiosensitivity of, 290
Growth factors
    in cell development, 340
    tumor promoting effects of, 71–72
Growth hormone-releasing factor, damage to
    cells producing, 293
Growth hormones
    deficiencies of
        with high-dose radiation of pituitary,
            293

Growth hormones (*Continued*)
    in hypopituitarism, 293
    after leukemia radiotherapy in children,
        293–294
    threshold for radiation damage to, 293
Growth retardation
    after organogenesis period radiation
        exposure, 404–405
    after radiation exposure throughout
        gestation in, 410
    radionuclide-induced, 339
    radiotherapy-induced, 335, 336
    after in utero radiation exposure,
        417–419, 455
    after whole-body radiation, 294
Guanine (G), 47
Gulf War, First, depleted uranium munitions
    in, 427–428
Gynecologic disorder radiotherapy
    bladder cancer after, 197
    urinary RNase output after, 363–364
Gypsum, from phosphate rock, 37

H
Hair follicles, 287f
    epilation sensitivity of, 288–289
Hair loss, temporary, 288–289
Half-life
    definition of, 7
    with radionuclide decay, 7
Half-value layer (HVL), 3–4, 4t
    of neutrons in water, 4–5
Hanford National Laboratory
    populations near
        bladder cancer in, 195
        carcinogenic effects on, 432–433
        colon cancer in, 227
        esophageal cancer in, 215
        hypothyroidism and autoimmune
            thyroiditis in, 297
        lung cancer in, 175–176
        non-Hodgkin's lymphoma risk in, 130
        pancreatic cancer in, 243
        stomach cancer in, 220
        thyroid nodules or adenomas in, 162
        uterine cancer in, 205
    workers at
        bladder cancer in, 196
        bone tumors in, 251
        cancer mortality in, 97
        colon cancer in, 228
        combined cohort study of, 97
        esophageal cancer in, 216
        hepatobiliary system cancers in, 239
        Hodgkin's disease risk in, 127–129
        kidney cancer in, 190
        lung cancer in, 177
        lung cancer risk in, 186, 432
        male genital cancer in, 212–214
        nonmelanoma skin cancer in, 261
        occupational exposure of, 55, 124
        pancreatic cancer in, 245
        rectal cancer in, 233–234
        stomach cancer in, 222
        thyroid cancer in, 159
        uterine cancer in, 206
Haploid number, 49–50
Hashimoto's thyroiditis, after thyroid
    irradiation, 294–295
Hazards
    acceptable risk of, 461–462
    alternatives to, 462–463

Hazards *(Continued)*
  cognitive map of, 463f
  ranked by different groups, 464t
Head
  circumference of
    after radiation exposure throughout gestation in, 410
    related to radiation dose and gestational age, 407
  meningioma incidence after injuries to, 140
Head and neck radiation, nonmelanoma skin cancer after, 262–263
Health risk perception, 464
  by education level, 465f
  by gender, 465f
  by physicians and radiologists, 465
Health warnings, psychological effects of, 459
"Health-worker" effect, 96
Hearing loss, radiation-induced, 310
Heart
  blood vessel and connective tissue radioresistance of, 318–319
  chemotherapy-enhanced radiation effects on, 392t
  high-LET and radionuclide radiation of, 320
  internal irradiation of, 320
  low-LET radiation of, 316–320
  SOMA normal tissue radiotoxicity for, 516t
Heart disease. *See also* Ischemic heart disease
  genetic, natural incidence of, 52
  radiation-induced, 317
  in uranium miners, 425–426
Heat-radiation synergism, 390–391
Heavy ions
  gamma or x-rays combined with, 391
  particulate radiation of, 5
Hemangioendotheliomas, after Thorotrast injection, 241
Hemangioma treatment, in infancy, pancreatic cancer after, 246
Hemangiosarcomas, after pelvic tumor radiation, 258–259
Hematopoietic syndrome, 343, 357–358
  degrees of, 358t
Hematopoietic system
  deterministic radiation effects of, 340–345
    from high-LET radiation, 344
    from internal radiation, 344–345
    from low-LET radiation, 341–344
  kinetics of, 340
    postradiation, 340–341
Hematuria, postradiation, 329, 330
Hemizygosity, 47–48
Hemorrhage, in gastrointestinal syndrome, 359
Heparin, radiation cataracts and, 308–309
Hepatic cells
  loss of, 327
  radiation-induced changes in, 326
  radioresistance of, 326
Hepatic necrosis, radiation-induced, 326
  after massive doses, 327
Hepatic veno-occlusive lesions, postradiotherapy, 327
Hepatitis
  chronic, in hepatobiliary cancers, 236, 241–243
  radiation-induced, 326
    temporary, 327–328
    vincristine and, 327
Hepatitis B virus, carcinogenic effect of, 447–448

Hepatobiliary system cancers
  epidemiology of, 241
  incidence of, 236
  radiation-induced
    from external exposure, 236–240
    from internal exposure, 240–241
  risk estimates for, 241–243
  types of, 236
Hepatomas, after Thorotrast injection, 241
Herbal tea, in esophageal cancer, 214–215
Heredity, nontraditional types of, 47–48
Heterozygosity, 47–48
Hiroshima
  dosimetry at, 89–90
  genetic population studies at, 54–55
  lung cancer in, 174
  major causes of death at, 88
  salivary gland tumor incidence in, 144–145
  skin cancer incidence in, 260
Histohematic barrier (HHB)
  edema and inflammation in, 16f
  fibrosis of
    edema and inflammation following, 15f
    parenchymal atrophy from, 15f
Hodgkin's disease
  additive effects of radiotherapy and chemotherapy for, 393–394
  definition of, 127
  in populations near nuclear facilities, 95
  radiotherapy for
    bone tumors after, 252
    breast cancer after, 170
    cardiac function after, 318
    cardiovascular disease after, 362
    hyperthyroidism after, 296
    immune function after, 350
    leukemia risk from, 123
    lymphocyte depletion after, 345
    ovarian effects of, 332
    pericardial effusions after, 317
    pericardial thickening after, 318
    pericarditis after, 317–318
    pneumonitis after, 315
    preconception, congenital malformations after, 402–403
    radiation stricture of esophagus after, 322f
    radiation-induced heart disease after, 317
    small intestinal late complications of, 323–324
    testicular effects of, 334
    thyroid nodules or adenomas after, 161
  risk of from external and internal radiation exposures, 127–130
Hogan v. McDaniel, 440–441
Homozygosity, 47–48
Hormesis
  adaptive response and, 473
  in atomic bomb survivors, 474
  criticisms of, 473
  definition of, 473
  from environmental exposure, 473–474
  future research on, 475
  from occupational exposure, 474–475
  theory of, 348–349
hprt gene mutations
  DS86 dose and frequency of in atomic bomb survivors, 58f
  induction of, 58
  from nuclear accident fallout, 64
Human genome, 47–48
Human papilloma virus (HPV), carcinogenic effect of, 447–448

Human tissues, uranium and thorium radionuclide concentrations in, 34t
Humoral immunity
  B-cells in, 349
  lymphocytes in, 347
Hydrocephaly
  after Chernobyl accident, 405–406
  after radiotherapy during pregnancy, 405
Hydrofluoric acid (HF), 423
Hydrogen, average body burden of, 32
Hydrogen 3, dose coefficients for worker intakes of, 497t–499t
5-Hydroxyindoleacetic acid (5-HIAA) excretion, after radiation therapy, 364
Hydroxyl (OH.) radical
  clusters of, 10
  in free-radical formation, 8–9
5-Hydroxytryptamine, to prevent nausea and vomiting, 354–355
Hyperbaric oxygen therapy
  neuropsychological impairment after, 302
  for radiation osteonecrosis, 336–337
Hyperemia, postradiotherapy, 330
Hyperparathyroidism
  in atomic bomb survivors, 146
  after radiotherapy, 146
Hyperpigmentation, after radiotherapy, 289
Hyperprolactinemia, after pituitary irradiation, 294
Hypertension
  in atomic bomb survivors, 319–320
  incidence of after fallout exposure, 361
  after radiotherapy, 329, 330
    benign and malignant, 330
Hyperthermia
  radiosensitizing effect of, 9
  total-body, 390–391
Hyperthyroidism
  affecting skin reaction to radiation, 290
  after Graves' disease treatment, 298
  after medical external exposure, 296
  modifying thyroid response to radiation, 298
  radioiodine therapy-induced, 146
  radioiodine treatment for, 102, 298
    bladder cancer after, 199
    bone tumors after, 253
    breast cancer after, 170–171
    colon cancer after, 231
    hepatobiliary system cancer after, 241
    immune function after, 350
    kidney cancer after, 193
    lung cancer after, 187
    mediastinal hemorrhage after, 320
    oropharyngeal cancer after, 150
    ovarian cancer after, 203
    pancreatic cancer after, 248
    prostate cancer after, 211
    rectal cancer after, 236
    salivary gland effects of, 311
    stomach cancer after, 224
    uterine cancer after, 207
Hypopituitarism
  with high-dose radiation of pituitary, 293
  indicators of, 293
Hypoproteinemia, postradiotherapy, 323
Hypothalamic-pituitary-adrenal axis, SOMA normal tissue radiotoxicity for, 508t
  female, 508t
  male, 507t
Hypothalamic-pituitary-thyroid axis, SOMA normal tissue radiotoxicity for, 514t
Hypothyroidism
  in atomic bomb survivors, 295–296
  after Chernobyl accident, 296–297

Hypothyroidism (*Continued*)
    in Chernobyl fallout populations, 297
    after Graves' disease treatment, 298
    after nuclear weapons fallout exposure,
        296
    after pituitary irradiation, 294
    in populations near Hanford plant, 297
    after radioiodine treatment, 170–171, 298
    radioiodine treatment of during pregnancy,
        412–413
    after radiotherapy, 296
    after thyroid irradiation, 294
        clinical and subclinical, 295

I

Idaho Falls reactor accident, psychological
    effects of, 466–467
Ileum, terminal, radiation injury in, 322–323
Ilium, hypoplasia of, with radiotherapy in
    children, 336
Immune competent cells, antigen production
    of, 347
Immune response
    after accidental radiation exposure,
        351–353
    in atomic bomb survivors, 350–351
    augmentation of, 348–349
    cell types and function in, 347–353
    depression and regeneration of, 348
    deterministic radiation effects on, 346–353
    functional, 348–349
    after occupational exposure, 349
    after radiotherapy, 349–350
    of skin, 286–287
    T-cell-related, in atomic bomb
        survivors, 351
    after total and partial-body irradiation,
        349–353
Immune stem cells, 346–347
Immune system
    depression of after Chernobyl accident
        contamination, 291
    hormetic effects on, 475
Immunocompetence, depressed, in resistance
    to disease in atomic bomb survivors,
        90–92
Immunoglobulins
    in atomic bomb survivors, 351
    in immune response, 346–347
    lymphocyte secretion of after radioiodine
        therapy, 350
    serum level of after radiotherapy, 350
Immunologic memory, 346
Immunomodulation, 348–349
Immunosuppressive agents, 348–349
    cancer risk from, 443
    carcinogenic effects of, 447
Implantation stage, radiation exposure
    during, 404
Incontinence (urinary), after prostatic
    carcinoma radiotherapy, 331
Index of harm, 460
Indium radionuclides, dose coefficients for
    worker intakes of, 497t–499t
Individual risk, 469
Industrial products, in cancer risk, 447
Inert gas exposures, during pregnancy,
    413
Infants
    chest radiation of, 101
    chromosome abnormalities and mortality
        of, 51–52

Infections
    in cancer risk, 447–448
    with combined radiation and trauma, 392
    in gastrointestinal syndrome, 359
Informed consent issues, 441
Intelligence quotient (IQ)
    after leukemia therapy, 302
    microcephaly and, 407–408
    by radiation dose and postovulatory age at
        exposure, 408f
    after radiation exposure throughout
        gestation, 411
    radiation-induced decline in, 302,
        407
Interactive agents, 389–390
    additive and antagonistic, 390f
    in sensitization, 390f
Interactive Radioepidemiological Program
    (IREP), 452
Interferon-alpha 2B, enhancing radiation
    effects, 393
Interferon-gamma, for late subcutaneous
    radiation fibrosis, 290
Interleukin-2, in radiation brain injury, 302
Interleukin-3, in bone marrow transplantation,
    343–344
Interleukin-6, in atomic bomb survivors, 351
Internal conversion, 6
Internal radiation
    carcinogenic effects of, 99
    from fallout, 40–41
International Chernobyl Project data, 55, 64
    on thyroid function, 296–297
    on thyroid nodules, 162
International Commission on Radiation
    Protection (ICRP)
    additive and multiplicative risk
        recommendations of, 82
    on cancer-predisposing mutations, 75
    DDREF for cancer endpoints of, 16–17
    on hereditary radiation-induced cancer risk,
        56
    loss of life expectancy estimate of, 82–83
    radiation limits of, 22
    recommendations of for radiation exposure,
        127
    recommended dose limits (2006) of, 23t
    reports of, 460
    tissue weighting factors of, 20–21, 21t
International Commission on Radiologic
    Units (ICRU), exposure units proposed
    by, 7
Interphase, 11
Interphase death, 13–14
Interstitial deletion, 49–50
Intestinal bleeding
    postradiotherapy, 323
    after whole-abdominal radiation in children,
        323–324
Intestinal malabsorption, postradiotherapy,
    323
Intestinal obstruction, after whole-abdominal
    radiation in children, 323–324
Intron, 47–48
In utero radiation exposure
    anxiety associated with, 401–402
    carcinogenesis of, 414–416
    cataract formation after, 309
    CT scan showing fetus in, 417f
    deterministic (nonstochastic) effects of,
        402–412
        during entire gestation, 410–411
        in fetal period, 410
        at implantation stage, 404

In utero radiation exposure (*Continued*)
    at organogenesis, 404–406
        preconception, 402–403
        preimplantation, 403–404
    laboratory findings for, 411
    mental retardation after, 455
    minimizing during pregnancy, 416–417
    potential risks of, 465–466
    radionuclides in, 412–414
    sex ratio of, 411
    terminating pregnancy after, 417–419
Iodine
    deficiency of
        in fallout exposed population, 160
        genetic mutations and, 74–75
        in radiation-induced thyroid cancer,
            74–75, 152,160
    radiosensitizing effect of, 392–393
Iodine 125
    penis, urethra, and scrotum effects of, 335
    thyroid cancer related to, 159
Iodine 131 therapy
    bladder cancer after, 199
    cataract formation after, 309
    CNS tumors related to, 141
    esophageal cancer after, 218
    follow-up study of, 102
    GPA mutation frequency and, 59
    for hyperthyroidism, 102
    hypothyroidism and autoimmune thyroiditis
        after, 297–298
    immune function after, 350
    in internal irradiation from fallout, 40–41
    leukemia risk and, 125–126
    lung cancer after, 187
    multiple myeloma risk from, 136
    non-Hodgkin's lymphoma risk from, 133
    parathyroid changes after, 298–299
    parotid gland lymphoma related to, 145
    during pregnancy, 412–413
    rectal cancer after, 236
    thyroid cancer after, 157–159
    thyroid nodules or adenomas after,
        161–162
Iodine radionuclides
    atmospheric release of from nuclear power
        plants, 41–42
    brain effects of, 303
    after Chernobyl accident, 159–160
    dose coefficients for worker intakes of,
        497t–499t
Ionization process, 1–3
Ionizing radiation
    adaptive responses to, 11
    atomic structure of, 1
    biologic effect of, 8–9
    biologic effectiveness of, 2–3
    biologic factors in, 9–16
    cancer risk from, 443
    chemical factors of, 8–9
    combinations of, 391
    energy deposition from, 10
    epigenetic responses to, 10–11
    indirectly and directly, 1–2
    modifiers of, 9
    physical factors of, 1–7
    target of, 9–11
    ultraviolet light and, 391
Iridium 192, 290
    inhibiting coronary artery restenosis in
        brachytherapy, 318
    penis, urethra, and scrotum effects of, 335
Iridium radionuclides, dose coefficients for
    worker intakes of, 497t–499t

Iris, radiation effects on, 305–306
Iron miners
 bladder cancer in, 199
 hepatobiliary system cancer in, 240–241
 kidney cancer in, 192–193
 melanoma in, 264
 stomach cancer in, 224
Iron radionuclides
 dose coefficients for worker intakes of, 497t–499t
 exposure to during pregnancy, 413
 with myeloablation before bone marrow transplantation, 345
Ischemia, in skin ulceration, 288
Ischemic heart disease
 incidence of with fallout exposure, 361
 smoking as risk factor in, 443–445
Isomeric transition, 6
Isotopes
 carrier-free, 6
 stable and unstable, 5
 uranium, 30–31

J
Jaundice, radiation-induced, 326
Jejunum, radiation injury in, 322–323

K
Kaons, produced by spallation, 27
Kaposi's sarcoma, viral infection in, 71–72
Karyotype, 49
 in identifying chromosomal aberrations or mutations, 49–50
 of metaphase chromosome, 49f
Keratin, 287f
Keratitis, radiation induced, 305–306
Kerma, 8
Kidney
 calcium deposition in, 329
 cell groups of, 328–329
 increased capillary permeability of, 329
 radiation effects on
  chemotherapy-enhanced, 392t
  deterministic, 328–330
 recurrent tumor or metastases to, 329
 SOMA normal tissue radiotoxicity for, 522t
 tolerance dose for, 329
 uranium and thorium radionuclide concentrations in, 34t
 uranium concentrations in tissues of, 424–425
 uranium effects on, 424
 vascular supply system of, 328–329
Kidney cancer
 genetic factors in, 72
 incidence of, 188–189
 radiation-induced
  from external exposure, 189–192
  from internal exposure, 192–193
  risk factors in, 193
 radioiodine injection in, 100–101
 risk estimates for incidence and mortality from, 194t
 risk factors for, 189
Kidney stones, with uranium exposure, 331
KL-6 antigen, after radiation therapy, 364
Korean War Navy veterans, oropharyngeal cancer in, 149
K-RAS mutations, 74–75

Krypton
 atmospheric release of from nuclear power plants, 41–42
 average effective doses of from fallout, 41t
 placental transfer of, 413

L
Lacrimal glands, 305
 dysfunction of after radioiodine therapy, 311
Lactate dehydrogenase (LDH), secretion of, 310
Lactation
 in breast cancer risk, 397
 in cancer incidence rates, 446
Lactose malabsorption, radiation-induced, 323
Langerhans cells, in immune function, 286–287
Lanthanide
 pulmonary fibrosis with inhalation of, 316
 radionuclide exposure to during pregnancy, 413
Lapps (Swedish)
 bladder cancer in, 198
 colon cancer rates in, 230
 fallout studies of, 93
 hepatobiliary system cancer rates in, 240–241
 leukemia in, 120
 male genital cancers in, 214
 nonmelanoma skin cancer incidence in, 263
 pancreatic cancer rates in, 247
 prostate cancer in, 211
 rectal cancer rate in, 235
 stomach cancer rates in, 223–224
Large intestine. See also Colon; Rectum
 low-LET radiation effects on, 324–325
 mucosal cells of, 324
 neutron radiation effects on, 325
 radionuclide irradiation effects on, 325–326
Larynx
 atypic of squamous epithelium of, 312
 cancer of
  causes and incidence of, 146–147
  risk factors in, 147
 deterministic radiation effects on, 312
 SOMA normal tissue radiotoxicity for, 513t
Late Effects Study Group (LSEG), for childhood cancer survivors, 156
Lawrence Livermore Laboratory, melanoma in workers at, 264
Lead 210, dose coefficients for worker intakes of, 497t–499t
Learning disabilities, after cranial radiotherapy, 302–303
Leber optic atrophy, 47–48
Ledermycin, enhancing radiation effects, 393
Legal cases
 classification of, 439
 of radiation-induced cancer, 441–448
Legal liability
 for documentation and informed consent in, 441
 evaluation of, 439
 for genetic injuries, 440
 for radiation exposure of embryo and fetus, 440–441
 for radiation injury, 439–440
Legislative compensation programs, 450–452
Lens
 opacities of
  incidence of, 309

Lens (Continued)
 radiation induced, 307
 radiosensitivity of in children, 307
 SOMA normal tissue radiotoxicity for, 509t–510t
LENT (Late Effects Normal Tissue) system, 285
Lentigo, from Chernobyl accident contamination, 291
Leukemia
 acute lymphocytic (ALL), 117
  expression of radiation effects in, 118
  maternal smoking and, 415–416
  preleukemic translocation and, 75
  relative risk of, 119t
  in weapons test personnel, 93–94
 acute myelocytic (AML), in weapons test personnel, 93–94
 acute myeloid (AML), 117
  expression of radiation effects in, 118
  myelodysplasia and, 137
  relative risk of, 119t
 age as risk factor in, 78
 in airline crews, 119
 in atomic bomb survivors
  benzene exposure and, 394
  calculating ERR and RR in, 85–86
  excess absolute risk in, 118
  incidence of, 88–89
  mortality rates from, 89t
  RR estimates for, 91f
 after breast cancer treatment, 393–394
 case-control versus cohort studies of in utero exposure effects on, 100
 after cervical cancer radiotherapy, 103, 246–247
 after chemotherapy, 393
 childhood
  after cancer radiotherapy, 170
  cancer risk in offspring of survivors of, 56
  in populations near nuclear facilities, 95–96
  prenatal irradiation and, 415
  after in utero radiation exposure, 416
 chronic granulocytic (CGL), in atomic bomb survivors, 118
 chronic lymphocytic (CLL), 117
  expression of radiation effects in, 118
  factors in, 74
  in nuclear power workers, 98
  radiation effects on, 71
  in radiation workers, 97
  radiogenic, mortality data for, 79
 chronic myeloid (CML), 117
  expression of radiation effects in, 118
  relative risk of, 119t
 clusters of
  near nuclear facilities, 94–95
  plutonium exposure in, 428–429
 congenital anomalies in offspring of survivors of, 55–56
 definition of, 117
 epidemiological risk data for, 84
 with family history of ataxia-telangiectasia, 77
 gatekeeper genes in pathogenesis of, 72
 genetics of, 117
 hairy-cell
  in weapons test personnel, 93–94
 in high-natural background radiation areas, 92
 incidence of, 117
 induction period and risk of as function of age, 78f

Leukemia (Continued)
  latent period for, 77
  lifetime attributable risk for, 104, 104t
  lifetime attributable risk of, 91t
  lymphocytosis and, 347–348
  from medical exposure, 135
  modifying factors in, 117–118
  multiplicative versus additive risk
      projections for, 83
  in nuclear workers, 96–97
      international collaborative retrospective
          study of, 98
      mortality from, 89t, 98
  from occupational exposure, 96
  PC/AS for, 449f
  in population near Sellafield Nuclear Plant,
      56
  in Portsmouth Naval Shipyard workers, 97
  preconception irradiation and, 415–416
  prenatal irradiation effects and, 99–100
  radiation effects by type of, 118
  in radiation workers, 97
      combined cohort study of, 97
      death rate from, 362
  radiation-induced
      age-time patterns in risk of, 87f
      from external exposure, 118–125
      from internal exposure, 125–127
      from neutron exposure, 127
      risk estimates for, 128t–129t
  radioiodine injection in, 100–101
  after radioiodine treatment for thyroid
      cancer, 103
  after radiotherapy, 217–218, 361–362
  after radium exposure, 362–363
  radon and, 125
  relative risk of after radiotherapy, 122f
  risk factors for, 117
  risk of after in utero radiation exposure,
      414–415
  spontaneous
      due to high natural background radiation,
          92
      estimated lifetime risk of, 83t
      incidence of, 82
  T-cell, viral infection in, 71–72
  from Techa River contamination, 94
  treatment for
      brain delayed injury after, 300
      cataracts after, 308–309
      cognitive impairment after, 303
      growth hormone deficiency after,
          293–294
      mineralizing microangiopathy after,
          301–302
      nervous system radiosensitivity after,
          302
      neuropsychological impairment after, 302
  types of, 117
  in weapons test personnel, 93–94
  whole-body irradiation with bone marrow
      transplantation for, 343
  x-ray examinations and, 100
Leukocytes, 347
Leukoencephalopathy, radiotherapy induced,
      301
Lhermitte's sign, 304
Life lost, measuring, 460–461
Life shortening, radiation-induced, 360–363
  animal data on, 361
  in atomic bomb survivors and persons
      exposed to fallout, 361
  descriptions of, 360
  human epidemiologic data on, 361

Life shortening, radiation-induced (Continued)
  from occupational exposure, 362–363
  in radiotherapy patients, 361–362
Life Span Study (LSS), of atomic bomb
      survivors, 88
Lifespan reduction
  associated with various conditions or
      etiologies, 461t
  average in various occupations, 461t
Linear accelerators, 4–5
  heavy ions in, 5
Linear dose-response models, 79–80
Linear energy transfer (LET) radiation, 2
  in cell survival curve, 12–13, 12f
  in cellular death, 13–14
  oxygen enhancement ratio and, 9, 9f
  passing through chromatin, 2f
  relative biologic effectiveness and, 3f
  for various radiation types, 2t
Linear-no-threshold (LNT) risk model, 79–80
Linear-quadratic dose-response models, 80
Liquid crystal watch displays, cosmic radiation
      from, 38–39
Liquidators
  cataract formation in, 308
  noncancer mortality studies of, 438
Liver
  atrophy of, 327
  cancer of
      alcohol in, 236
      in atomic bomb survivors, 236–238, 238f
      epidemiology of, 241
      from internal radiation exposure, 240–241
      from medical radiation exposure, 240
      occupational radiation exposure in, 238–240
      risk estimates for incidence and mortality
          from, 242t
  chemotherapeutic agents enhancing
      radiation effects on, 392t
  disease of
      radiation-induced, 326
      after Thorotrast injection, 327–328
  high-LET radiation effects on, 327
  low-LET radiation effects on, 326–327
  pathologic changes in, 326–327
  radionuclide irradiation effects on, 327–328,
      327f
  radiosensitivity of, 326
  SOMA normal tissue radiotoxicity for, 522t
  uranium and thorium radionuclide
      concentrations in, 34t
Locally multiply damaged sites (LMDS), 10
Los Alamos National Laboratory plutonium
      workers
  bladder cancer in, 196
  bone tumors in, 251
  colon cancer in, 228–231
  esophageal cancer in, 216–217
  hepatobiliary system cancers in, 239
  kidney cancer in, 190, 192
  lung cancer in, 186
  pancreatic cancer in, 245, 248
  prostate cancer in, 270
  pulmonary fibrosis in, 316
  rectal cancer in, 233–235
  stomach cancer in, 222
Loss of life expectancy estimate, 82–83
Low-linear energy transfer (LET) radiation
      risk, 79–80
Lucanthone hydrochloride (Miracyl D),
      synergism of with radiation, 394
Lung
  chemotherapy-enhanced radiation effects
      on, 392t

Lung (Continued)
  chronic disease of and smoking, 443–445
  deterministic radiation effects on, 312–316
      from high-LET radiation, 316
      from low-LET radiation, 312–316
      from radionuclide irradiation, 316
  fibrosis of, with polonium 210 and quartz
      dust inhalation, 391
  nodules of, radiation-induced, 315–316
  radiosensitivity of, 312
  radon doses in, 37t
  SOMA normal tissue radiotoxicity for, 517t
  uranium and thorium radionuclide
      concentrations in, 34t
  uranium deposition in, 425
  uranium half-life in, 423–424
Lung cancer
  additive effects of radiotherapy and
      chemotherapy for, 393–394
  age started smoking and mortality rate
      from, 393t
  in atomic bomb survivors, 81f
  calculating cumulative risk for, 452–453
  case example in radiation worker, 452–454
  cigarette smoking in, 180
      in atomic bomb survivors, 395–396
      and relative risk of, 395f
      as risk factor, 443–445
  epidemiology of, 173
  excess relative risk and smoking levels in,
      396f
  incidence of, 173
      and number of cigarettes smoked,
          394–395
  latent period of, 173
  linear dose-response relationship in, 180
  modifying factors for, 173–174
  mortality risk estimates for in underground
      miners, 188t
  in National Plutonium Workers Study,
      474–475
  in plutonium workers, 431, 432
  pooled case-control study data on, 188t
  radiation combined with nitro-oxides in,
      392
  radiation myelitis after radiotherapy for, 304
  in radiation worker, 452
      case summary of, 453–454
      risk analysis of, 452–453
  radiation-induced, 173
      acute versus fractionated exposure in, 173
      cell type of, 173
      from external exposure, 174–180
      from internal exposure, 181–188
      radiation type in, 173–174
      risk estimates for incidence and mortality
          for, 180t–181t
      risk versus exposure rate in, 174
  after radiotherapy for testicular cancer, 103
  risk estimates for, 180
  risk-dose relationship in, 173
  in Rocky Flats plant workers, 432
  small and large cell, 173
  spontaneous, estimated lifetime risk of, 83
  in uranium miners, 425–426
Luteinizing hormone (LH) deficiency, after
      pituitary irradiation, 294
Luteinizing hormone-releasing hormone
      (LRH) deficiency, after pituitary
      irradiation, 294
Lymph nodes, 345
  cells of, 347
Lymphangiography, after radiotherapy,
      345–346

Lymphatic system, 345–346
  high-LET radiation and radionuclide
    radiation effects on, 346
  low-LET radiation effects on, 345–346
  malignancies of in uranium miners and mill
    workers, 425–426
Lymphatic tissue
  atrophy of after Hodgkin's disease
    radiotherapy, 345
  regeneration of, 348
Lymphatic vessels
  late radiation occlusion of, 288
  radiation dose tolerance of, 345–346
Lymphocyte chromosome aberrations
  in atomic bomb survivors, 64, 64f
  background frequency of, 60
  clinical studies of, 62–64
  dicentric, 61–62, 60f
    induced by gamma rays and alpha
      particles, 54t
  dosimetric estimates of, 60
  high natural background incidence of, 63
  induction of, 60–61
  nuclear accidents in, 64
  occupational exposure in, 63–64
  stable and unstable, 60
Lymphocyte counts
  after accidental radiation exposure, 352
  in acute radiation sickness, 359t
  after whole-body irradiation, 343, 355f
Lymphocytes. *See also* B-cells; T-cells
  antigen-activated, 347–348
  in atomic bomb survivors, 350–351
  circulating, 59–60
  depletion of, 340–341
    after Hodgkin's disease radiotherapy, 345
  in hormetic effect, 475
  in immune response, 346–347
  irradiated, dose-response relationships for, 54t
  LD50 changes in, 347–348
  low radiation exposure of, 474–475
  motility and morphology changes in, 347
  peripheral, chromosome aberrations in, 59–62
  radiation effects on, 347–348
  reactive, 348
  refractive, 348
  subtypes of, 346–353
Lymphocytosis, 348
  as precursor of leukemia, 347–348
Lymphoid follicles, 347
Lymphoid hyperplasia treatment, thyroid
  nodules or adenomas after, 161
Lymphoid organs
  in immune response, 346
  T-cell changes after radiation of, 349–350
Lymphoma. *See also* Hodgkin's disease
  in atomic bomb survivors, 88–89
  childhood survivors of, cancer risk in
    offspring of, 56
  clusters of near nuclear facilities, 95
  differential diagnosis of, 127
  with family history of ataxia-telangiectasia,
    77
  gatekeeper genes in pathogenesis of, 72
  non-Hodgkin's
    external radiation exposure in, 130–133
    incidence and mortality risk from with
      radiation exposure, 134t
    internal exposure in, 133
  in nuclear energy facility workers, 96–97
  of parotid gland, after thyroid radiotherapy,
    145
  in population near Sellafield Nuclear
    Plant, 56

Lymphoma *(Continued)*
  radiotherapy for
    hyperthyroidism after, 296
    immune function after, 350
    small intestinal late complications of,
      323–324
    viral infection in, 71–72
    in weapons test personnel, 93–94
Lymphopoiesis, pathway to, 340

M

Macrophages, radiosensitivity of, 340
Magnetic fields
  affecting cosmic radiation, 27
  in radiation effects, 391
Magnetic resonance imaging (MRI)
  of brain injury after radiotherapy, 301
  in radiation myelitis diagnosis, 304–305
Malacia, of white matter, 299–300
Male genital tumors. *See also* Penis, cancer of;
  Scrotal cancer; Testicular cancer
  radiation-induced, 212
Male gonads, radiation damage to, 16
Malformation registries, increasing number of,
  52
Malformations
  congenital
    after Chernobyl accident, 405–406
    in Chernobyl accident survivors, 55, 55f
    in pregnancies of atomic bomb survivors,
      403
    with in utero radiation exposure,
      401–402
  genetic, normal incidence of, 51–52
  handicapping, normal incidence of, 51
  after high embryonic and fetal x-ray doses,
    404t
  with implantation-stage radiation exposure,
    404
  lethal, normal incidence of, 51
  after organogenesis period radiation
    exposure, 404–405
  after radiation exposure during pregnancy,
    417–419
  from radiation exposure during pregnancy,
    416–417
  radiation-induced
    after Hodgkin's disease treatment,
      402–403
    from in utero exposure, 402
  after in utero exposure, 411–412, 417
Malignancy
  radiation-induced
    genetic predisposition to, 397
    predisposition to, 73–75
    radiotherapy for, 103–104
      hepatobiliary system cancer after, 240
      leukemia incidence with, 122–123
      melanoma after, 265
      nonmelanoma skin cancer after, 263
      stomach cancer after, 223
      treatment options for, 361–362
Malignant conversion, genetic factors in, 73
Malignant fibrous histiocytoma, after
  Hodgkin's disease treatment, 252
Malignant progression, 71, 72
Malignant transformation, bystander effect
  and, 10–11
Mallinkrodt Chemical Works workers
  bladder cancer in, 198
  bone tumors in, 254
  CNS cancer incidence among, 140

Mallinkrodt Chemical Works
  workers *(Continued)*
  esophageal cancer in, 217
  hepatobiliary system cancer in, 239
  kidney cancer in, 192
  leukemia and occupational exposure of,
    125
  lung cancer in, 186
  male genital cancer in, 214
  non-Hodgkin's lymphoma risk to, 132
  nonmelanoma skin cancer in, 261
  pancreatic cancer in, 247–248
  prostate cancer in, 211
  rectal cancer in, 234
  stomach cancer in, 222
  thyroid cancer in, 157
  uranium-induced illness in, 427
Mammalian cell
  radiation survival curves for, 12–13
  survival dose-response curve for, 12f
Mandible
  osteoradionecrosis of, 337
  radiation-induced necrosis of, 337f
  SOMA normal tissue radiotoxicity for,
    512t
Manganese 54, in internal irradiation from
  fallout, 40–41
Manhattan Project plutonium workers
  bone tumors in, 254
  colon cancer in, 230–231
  esophageal cancer in, 218
  hepatobiliary system cancer in, 240–241
  pancreatic cancer in, 248
  plutonium body burden in, 430
  plutonium exposure of, 429
  prostate cancer in, 270
  pulmonary fibrosis in, 316
Mantle field treatment, after Hodgkin's
  disease therapy, 296
Marriage, consanguinous, 47–48
Marshall Islanders
  fallout studies in, 92–94
  fallout-induced leukemia in, 119
  radiation-induced life shortening on, 361
  skin changes in, 291
  thyroid cancer in, 158
    multiparous women, 152
  thyroid nodules or adenomas in, 162
  thyroid radiation doses in, 296
Martinez v. University of California, 439
Masothorium, radiation energies and
  intensities of, 32t
Mass, 2
Massachusetts tuberculosis fluoroscopy study,
  121
Mastectomy irradiation
  lung cancer after, 179
  spontaneous rib fractures after, 336–337
Mastitis radiotherapy
  breast cancer related to, 169
  nonmelanoma skin cancer after, 262–263
Maxillary sinuses, osteonecrosis of, 336
Maximum permissible body burden
  (MPBB), 24
Maximum permissible doses, 22–24
Mayak Production Association facility
  fallout-related thyroid cancer in residents
    around, 94
  workers at
    lung cancer in, 178, 187
    lung cancer mortality in, 432
    plutonium body burden in, 431–432
    plutonium contamination in, 430
    plutonium microdistribution in, 432

Mayak Production Association facility (*Continued*)
  pulmonary fibrosis in, 316
  radiation risk to, 98
  solid cancers in, 432
Mean bone marrow dose, 8
Meat, carcinogenic effect of, 445
Mechlorethamine, leukemia risk after, 393
Media amplification, of radiation risk, 467
Mediastinal hemorrhage, after radioiodine therapy, 320
Medical monitoring, for psychological effects of radiation risk, 468
Medical radiation exposure, 43
  brain and CNS tumors from, 140–141
  categories of, 43
  effective doses from, 44t
  epidemiologic risk studies of, 88
  external
    bone tumors from, 252
    colon cancer from, 229–230
    esophageal cancer from, 217–218
    hepatobiliary system cancers from, 240
    hyperthyroidism from, 296
    ovarian cancer from, 202–203
    prostate cancer from, 211
    rectal cancer from, 234–235
    stomach cancer from, 223
    thyroid nodules or adenomas from, 161
    uterine cancer from, 206–207
  frequency and absorbed doses from, 43
  frequency of x-ray examinations and, 43
  global, 43–44
  internal
    lung cancer from, 187–188
    thyroid cancer from, 157–158
    thyroid nodules or adenomas from, 161–162
  leukemia incidence from, 125–127
  multiple myeloma risk from, 135
  in nuclear medicine, 44–45
  pancreatic cancer from, 246–247
  psychological effects of, 468–469
  from radiation therapy, 45
  salivary gland tumors from, 145
Medical radiation workers. *See also* Diagnostic medical radiation; Radiologists/radiology technicians; x-ray technicians
  bladder cancer in, 197
  bone tumors in, 251–252
  breast cancer in, 167–168
  cancer incidence in, 133
  CNS cancer incidence in, 139–140
  colon cancer in, 229
  esophageal cancer in, 217
  hepatobiliary system cancer in, 239–240
  kidney cancer in, 190–191
  leukemia incidence in, 121
  lung cancer in, 177
  non-Hodgkin's lymphoma risk in, 131
  occupational exposure of, 99
  occupational exposures of, 42–43
  oropharyngeal cancer in, 149
  ovarian cancer in, 202
  pancreatic cancer in, 245–246
  prostate cancer in, 210
  rectal cancer in, 234
  stomach cancer in, 222–223
  uterine cancer in, 206
Medications, carcinogenic, 447
Megalokaryoblasts, radiosensitivity of, 340
Megavoltage radiation therapy, soft-tissue tumors after, 258
Meibomian glands, 305

Melanocytes, increased enzymatic activity of, 289
Melanoma, 263
  in atomic bomb survivors and populations exposed to fallout, 263
  caretaker genes in, 72–73
  genetic factors in, 72
  incidence of in Swedish Lapps, 263
  malignant, after testicular cancer radiotherapy, 103
  occupational radiation exposure in, 264–265
  radiation from background exposure and nuclear facilities in, 263
  risk estimates for incidence and mortality from, 265t
  risk factors in, 265–266
  in weapons test personnel, 93–94
Melatonin, radiation cataracts and, 308–309
Melphalan
  carcinogenic effects of, 447
  leukemia risk from, 123
Mendelian hereditary patterns, 50–51
Meniere's disease, radiation-induced, 310
Meningioma, after severe head injury, 140
Menopause
  postradiotherapy, 331
  radiation-induced, 332–333
Mental function
  after cranial radiotherapy, 303
  radiation brain injury, 301
Mental health, nuclear accident effects on, 467
Mental retardation
  euploid structure in, 51–52
  incidence of, 52
  in utero radiation threshold for, 406
  modifying factors in, 455
  in offspring of atomic bomb survivors, 406
  after postovulation exposure, 409–410
  radiation and, 302, 406–407
  radiation dose threshold for, 406
  severe
    microcephaly and, 407–408
    after radiation exposure throughout gestation, 411
    after in utero exposure to atomic bombing, 407f
  after in utero radiation exposure, 455
    in atomic bomb survivors, 408–409
    case summary of, 455
    during organogenesis period, 404–405
    radiation as cause in, 455
    from radiotherapy, 405
    risk analysis of, 455
    seizures and, 408
    throughout gestation, 410
Mercury radionuclides, dose coefficients for worker intakes of, 497t–499t
Mesenchyme, embryonic, 286–287
Mesons, sea level, 27
Mesothelioma
  asbestos-induced, 74
  after chest wall radiotherapy, 179
Metastatic cancer
  after breast cancer treatment, 103
  from radiotherapy for peptic ulcer, 102
Methotrexate
  with cranial radiation, mineralizing microangiopathy after, 301–302
  enhancing skin radiosensitivity, 290
  gliomas linked to, 141
  interaction of with radiation, 394
  in predisposition to radiation pneumonitis, 313
  in radiation brain injury, 301, 302

Methotrexate (*Continued*)
  in radiation myelopathy, 304
  in radiation recall phenomena, 393
  in radiation-induced esophagitis, 321
  radiosensitizing effect of, 9, 392–393
Methylcholanthrene, carcinogenic effect of, 394
Metronidazole, radiosensitizing effect of, 9
Metropathia hemorrhagica treatment, leukemia incidence and, 122
Microcephaly
  incidence of by dose level and gestational age, 409f
  in offspring of atomic bomb survivors, 406
    radiation dose and expsure before 18th gestational week in, 408t
  after organogenesis period radiation exposure, 404–405
  radiation effects on, 407–408
  after radiation exposure throughout gestation, 410
  after radiotherapy during pregnancy, 405
  severe mental retardation and, 407–408
Micronucleus frequencies, in lymphocyte chromosome aberrations, 62
Microphthalmos, in atomic bomb survivors exposed in utero, 408–409
Microwave exposure, in utero, 417
Midline tissue dose (MTD), 8
Military veterans, radiation compensation programs for, 450
Mineral oils, in scrotal cancer, 212
Mineralizing microangiopathy, after cranial radiation and methotrexate, 301–302
Miners. *See also* Iron miners; Uranium miners
  lung cancer in, 183–186
    mortality from, 188t
    risk for, 185
  occupational exposure of, 99
Mining. *See also* Miners; *specific materials*
  lung cancer in workers in, 183–186
  occupational exposures in, 42
  radon dosimetry in, 183–184
  radon effective doses in, 38
  radon exposure from, 92
  radon levels in, 184
Miracyl D (lucanthone hydrochloride), synergism of with radiation, 394
Misonidazole
  in radiation brain injury, 302
  radiosensitizing effect of, 9
Mitochondrial genes, in genetic inheritance, 47–48
Mitomycin C, in predisposition to radiation pneumonitis, 313
Mitosis phase, 11
Mitotic activity, cellular radiosensitivity and, 14
MLH1 gene, 72–73
MM mutant frequency, in atomic bomb survivors, 58–59, 59f
Modifiers, 9
Moist desquamation, in low-LET radiation, 288
Moll's glands, 305
Molybdenum 99, dose coefficients for worker intakes of, 497t–499t
Monazite sands, terrestrial radiation from, 31–32
Mongolism (Down syndrome), 49–50
Monocytes, radiosensitivity of, 340
Monosomy, 49–50
Morphologic cell changes, radiation-induced, 14

Mosaicism, 47–48
Mound Nuclear Facility
    occupational study at, 97
    prostate cancer in, 210
    stomach cancer in, 222
    workers at
        bladder cancer in, 196
        bone tumors in, 251
        colon cancer in, 228
        esophageal cancer in, 216–217
        kidney cancer in, 190
        lung cancer in, 177
        nonmelanoma skin cancer in, 261
        occupational exposure of, 124
        pancreatic cancer in, 245
MSH2 gene, 72–73
Mucosa
    deterministic effects of radiation on,
        286–293
        with low-LET radiation, 288–290
        with neutron irradiation, 290
        with radionuclide irradiation, 290–293
    oral and pharyngeal, SOMA normal tissue
        radiotoxicity for, 511t
Mucosa-associated lymphoid tissue (MALT),
    in immune response, 346
Mucositis, of esophagus, 321
Muller, H. J., discovery of x-ray induced
    mutations by, 47
Multibit multitarget model, 9
Multibit single-target model, 9
Multiglandular endocrine neoplasia (MEN),
    Types I and II, differential diagnosis of,
    145
Multiorgan failure, after bone marrow
    transplantation, 343–344
Multiple sclerosis
    cranial radiation and, 303
    radiation-accelerated, 299
Multiplicative effect, 389–390
    of smoking and radiation exposure in lung
        cancer, 395–396
Multiplicative risk projection models, 81
    versus additive risk projection model,
        82, 83
    problems with, 82
    transfer of risks in, 87
Muons, 27
Muscle
    acute radionecrosis of, 338
    low-LET radiation effects on, 335–338
    neutron or high-LET radiation effects on,
        338
    radiation-induced atrophy of, 340f
    radionuclide effects on, 338–339
    SOMA normal tissue radiotoxicity for,
        527t
    uranium and thorium radionuclide
        concentrations in, 34t
Mutation component (MC), 53–54
    occlusion of
        parenchymal atrophy from, 15f
        in radiation injury, 16f
    in radiation risk assessment, 54
Myelin sheath, 299
Myelitis
    acute transient, 304
    radiation-induced, 303–304
        diagnosis of, 304–305
        after lung cancer radiotherapy, 304
    thoracic, 304
Myelodepression, after whole-body irradiation,
    343–344
Myelodysplasia, radiation-induced, 137

Myelodysplasia syndrome (MDS), 137
    in acute myeloblastic leukemia development,
        137
    etiological factors for, 137
Myeloma, multiple
    in atomic energy facility workers, 96–97
    from occupational exposure, 97
    risk estimates for from radiation exposure,
        136t
    treatment of, 343
        from external radiation exposure, 133–135
        from internal exposure, 135–136
        leukemia risk from, 123
        non-Hodgkin's lymphoma risk from, 133
Myelopathy
    assessing risk of, 304
    modifying factors in, 304
Myelopoiesis, radiosensitivity of, 340
Myelosuppression, after phosphorus 32
    exposure, 345
Myocarditis
    with fractionated radiotherapy, 317
    radiation and, 317
Myocardium
    fibrosis of after radiotherapy, 319
    radiation effects on, 317
    structure of, 316–317
Myoclonic epilepsy, 47–48
Myotonic muscular dystrophy, 47–48

N

Nagasaki, atomic bomb survivors of
    dosimetry in, 89–90
    genetic studies of, 54–55
    lung cancer in, 174
    major causes of death in, 88
    salivary gland tumor incidence in, 144–145
    skin cancer incidence in, 260
    thyroid nodules or adenomas in, 161
Nasopharyngeal carcinoma, viral infection in,
    71–72
Nasopharyngeal tumor radiotherapy,
    hypopituitarism after, 293
National Council on Radiation Protection and
    Measurements (NCRP), 459
    radiation limits of, 22
    radiation protection limits of, 22
    Recommended Dose Limits (1990) of, 23t
    reports of, 389
National Dose Registry of Canada data
    on bladder cancer, 196
    on bone tumors, 251
    on breast cancer, 167
    on cancer risk from occupational
        exposure, 135
    on CNS cancers rate, 139
    on colon cancer, 228
    on esophageal cancer, 216–217
    on hepatobiliary system cancers, 239
    on Hodgkin's disease risk from occupational
        exposure, 129
    on kidney cancer, 190
    on lung cancer, 176
    on male genital cancer, 212
    on melanoma, 264
    on non-Hodgkin's lymphoma risk, 132
    on nonmelanoma skin cancer, 261
    on oropharyngeal cancer, 149
    on ovarian cancer, 202
    on pancreatic cancer, 244–245
    on prostate cancer, 209–210
    on radiation exposure, 123–124

National Dose Registry of Canada
    data *(Continued)*
    on rectal cancer, 233
    on salivary gland tumor, 145
    on stomach cancer, 221–222
    on thyroid cancer, 154
    on uterine cancer, 206
National Institutes of Health (NIH)
    projection models, 82
National Research Council 2006 radiation
    exposure and screening program
    report, 451
Natural background radiation. *See* Background
    radiation exposure
Natural killer (NK) cells, 347
    in atomic bomb survivors, 350–351
Nausea and vomiting
    with abdominal radiation, 323
    drugs to prevent, 354–355
    with fractionated abdominal ratiation, 322
    postradiotherapy, 323
    after whole-body irradiation, 354–355
Navy veterans
    esophageal cancer in, 216–217
    male genital cancer in, 212–214
Necrosis, of white matter, 299–300
Negligible risk level (NRL), 469
Neoplasms
    genetic susceptibility to, 74
    induction rate of, 348
    malignant
        colon cancer after treatment of, 229
        radiation therapy for, 45
    predisposition to in xeroderma
        pigmentosum, 75–76
    progressive cell dedifferentiation in, 72
    radiotherapy for
        bone tumors after, 252–253
        central nervous system effects of, 299
        leukemia risk from, 123
    second, actinomycin D reducing risk of, 394
    spinal, radiotherapy induced, 303–304
    after in utero radiation exposure, 419
Neoplastic conversion, 71
Nephritis
    acute radiation, 329
        treatment of, 330
    chronic radiation, 330
    CT scan for, 329
    severe radiation, 329
Nephrons, hypertrophy of, 328–329
Nephropathy, radiation, 329
Nephrosclerosis, radiation-induced, 329
Neptunium radionuclides, dose coefficients for
    worker intakes of, 497t–499t
Nervous system. *See also* Brain; Central
    nervous system
    cells of, 299
    deterministic radiation effects on, 299–305
        in brain, 300–303
        in peripheral nerves, 305
        in spinal cord, 303–305
    functional disturbances of, 391
    increased radiosensitivity of in children, 302
Neural sheath tumors, after radiotherapy, 256
Neural tube defects, 50–51
Neuroblastoma, treatment of, 343
Neurofibromatosis, genetic factors in, 72
Neurofibrosarcoma
    after pelvic tumor radiation, 258–259
    after radiotherapy, 258
Neuroglia, 299
Neurologic abnormalities, after in utero
    exposure, 411–412

Neurons, 299
migration of, 406
Neuropathology, structural, in utero radiation effects on, 408–410
Neuropsychological abnormalities
after cranial radiotherapy, 302–303
after high-dose radiation therapy, 459
after leukemia therapy, 302
radiotherapy-induced, 302
Neurovascular syndrome, 299, 357–358
degrees of, 358t
Neutrino, formation of, 6
Neutron irradiation
bone, cartilage, and muscle effects of, 338
brain tumors and, 303
in cataract formation, 309
large intestinal effects of, 325
oral cavity and pharyngeal effects of, 321
particulate, 4–5, 4t
pneumonitis after, 316
skin reaction to, 290
of testes, 335
thyroid response to, 298
Neutron-deficient nuclide, 6
Neutron-proton ratios, 6–7
Neutrons, 1
fast, gamma or x-rays combined with, 391
fission, 4–5
formation of, 6
produced by spallation, 27
RBE of, 3t
Neutrophils
count of after whole-body irradiation, 344f
phagocytosis of in atomic bomb survivors, 341
Nevada nuclear weapons test fallout
doses from, 93
effects on personnel at, 93–94
studies of children exposed to, 93
thyroid cancer from in population near, 158
Nevoid basal cell carcinoma syndrome (NBCS), nonmelanoma skin cancer and, 259
Nijmegen breakage syndrome, radiosensitivity in, 75
NIMBY (not in my backyard), 463
Niobium workers, nonmelanoma skin cancer in, 261
Nitrites, carcinogenic effect of, 445
Nitrogen mustard, in radiation brain injury, 302
Nitroimidazoles, radiosensitizing effect of, 9
Nitro-oxides, combined with alpha irradiation, 392
4-Nitroquinoline-1-oxide (4 NQO) carcinogenic effect of, 394
Nitrosamines
in esophageal cancer, 214–215
in stomach cancer, 220
N-nitroso compounds, infections and, 447–448
Nitrosourea, in predisposition to radiation pneumonitis, 313
Nitrostable compounds, carcinogenic effect of, 445
Nodule, definition of, 160
Nominal standard dose (NSD), 17
Nonlethal genetic mutations, 49
Nonstochastic effects. See Deterministic effects of radiation
Noxious agents, inhalation of, 391
Nuclear accidents, 41–42
collective effective doses from, 42
in lymphocyte chromosome aberrations, 64

Nuclear accidents (Continued)
media amplification of risk from, 467
psychological effects of, 466–467
Nuclear facilities
bladder cancer in populations near, 195
bone tumors in populations near, 250
brain and CNS tumors in populations near, 138
breast cancer in populations near, 167
colon cancer in populations near, 227
combined cohort study of, 97
epidemiologic risk studies of populations near, 88
esophageal cancer in populations near, 215
hepatobiliary system cancers in populations near, 236
kidney cancer in populations near, 189
leukemia in populations around, 120–121
lung cancer in populations near, 175–176
melanoma in populations near, 263
multiple myeloma in populations near, 133
nonmelanoma skin cancers in populations near, 260
occupational studies at, 96–97
oral cavity cancers in population near, 147
ovarian cancer in populations near, 200
pancreatic cancer in populations near, 243
prostate cancer in populations near, 208–209
rectal cancer in populations near, 233
stomach cancer in populations near, 220
thyroid cancer in populations near, 153–154
uterine cancer in populations near, 205
Nuclear facility workers
bladder cancer in, 195–196
bone tumors in, 251
cancer mortality in, 135, 432
colon cancer in, 228, 229
esophageal cancer in, 216–217
estimated cancer risk for, 89t
hepatobiliary system cancers in, 238–239
immune function in, 349
international collaborative retrospective study of, 98
kidney cancer in, 189, 190
larynx cancer in, 146–147
leukemia incidence in, 123–125
lung cancer in, 176, 179–180
lung cancer risk in, 432
male genital cancer in, 212, 214
melanoma in, 264–265
multiple myeloma risk in, 133–135
non-Hodgkin's lymphoma risk in, 131–132
nonmelanoma skin cancer in, 260–261
oral cavity cancers in, 148
ovarian cancer in, 202
pancreatic cancer in, 244–245, 247–248
prostate cancer in, 209–210
rectal cancer in, 233–234
small intestinal cancer in, 225
stomach cancer in, 221, 222
uranium-induced illness in, 426–427
uterine cancer in, 205–206
Nuclear fuel cycle, occupational exposures from, 42
Nuclear instability, 5
Nuclear medicine examinations
absorbed doses from, 43
collective doses from, 44–45
effective doses from, 44t
estimated number of in United States, 45t
medical exposure from, 44–45

Nuclear power
fear of misuse of, 462–463
production of, 41–42
Nuclear power plants
bladder cancer in workers at, 196
during World War II, 196
cancer risk in populations near, 56
colon cancer in workers in, 228–229
immune function in population near, 351–352
occupational exposure and chromosome aberration rates at, 63–64
occupational exposures at, 42–43
occupational risk at, 98
occupational studies at, 96–97
oropharyngeal cancer in workers at, 148–149
perceived risk of, 463
plutonium exposure from, 429
skin changes in populations near, 291–293
studies of populations living near, 94–96
Nuclear reactions, of cosmic rays with atmospheric nuclei, 27
Nuclear Regulatory Commission (NRC), occupational radiation dose limits of, 22, 23t
Nuclear waste, management of, 463
Nuclear weapons
fallout from, 40–41
hypothyroidism and, 296
thyroid cancer related to, 158–159
fallout studies on, 93
military accidents involving, 430
skin changes from, 291
trauma and radiation exposure from, 391–392
Nuclear weapons facility workers
bone tumors in, 251
CNS cancers in, 138–139
liver cancer risk in, 241
lung cancer in, 176–177
oral cavity cancer in, 148
pancreatic cancer in, 244, 245
rectal cancer in, 233
small intestinal cancer in, 225
stomach cancer in, 221
thyroid cancer in, 154
Nuclear weapons tests
atmospheric, fallout effects on personnel participating in, 93–94
bladder cancer in populations near, 198
bone tumors in populations near, 250
compensation for participants in, 450
fallout effects on personnel participating in, 93–94
fallout from, 40–41
kidney cancer related to, 192
leukemia incidence from, 119–120
melanoma in participants in, 264
melanoma in populations near, 263
nonmelanoma skin cancer in participants in, 260
plutonium exposure from, 429
risk hepatobiliary system cancers in populations near, 236
stomach cancer in populations near, 220
thyroid nodules or adenomas related to, 162
workers involved in
bladder cancer in, 195–196
esophageal cancer in, 216
kidney cancer in, 189
pancreatic cancer in, 244
Nucleic acid metabolites, after radiation exposure, 363–364

Nucleotides, coding for amino acids, 47
Nulliparity, ovarian cancer and, 200
Nullisomy, 49–50
Nutritional deprivation. with radiation
    exposure throughout gestation, 410

O

Oak Ridge National Laboratory
    BAIBA levels of after accidental radiation
        exposure in, 363–364
    breast cancer in populations near, 167
    occupational study at, 97
    temporary aspermia after accidents at, 334
    workers at
        bladder cancer in, 196
        CNS cancers in, 138–139
        colon cancer in, 228–229
        esophageal cancer in, 216–218
        hepatobiliary system cancers in, 239
        Hodgkin's disease risk in, 129
        kidney cancer in, 190
        leukemia mortality for, 124
        lung cancer in, 177
        male genital cancer in, 212–214
        non-Hodgkin's lymphoma risk to, 132
        occupational exposure of, 124
        oropharyngeal cancer in, 148–149
        pancreatic cancer in workers at, 245, 248
        prostate cancer in, 210
        rectal cancer in, 233–235
        stomach cancer in, 222
        uranium contamination of, 425–426
        uterine cancer in, 206
Obesity
    in cancer risk, 445–446
    in uterine cancer, 204–205
Obstetric x-radiation, low-dose, childhood
    cancers and, 99
Occupation, in cancer risk, 446–447
Occupational accident rates, fatal, mean U.S.,
    461t
Occupational exposure, 42–43
    bladder cancer related to, 195–197
    brain and CNS tumors from, 138–140
    breast cancer related to, 167
    cancers related to, 96–99
    carcinogenic agents and cancer risk from,
        442t
    chemical agents and radiation effects from,
        396
    epidemiologic risk studies of, 88
    external
        bone tumors related to, 251–252
        colon cancer related to, 228–229
        esophageal cancer related to, 216–217
        hepatobiliary system cancers related to,
            238–240
        ovarian cancer related to, 200–202
        prostate cancer from, 209–210
        rectal cancer related to, 233–234
        stomach cancer related to, 221–223
        thyroid cancer related to, 154
        uterine cancer related to, 205–206
    hormetic effects of, 474–475
    immune function after, 349
    internal
        bone tumors related to, 254–256
        thyroid cancer related to, 157
    kidney cancer related to, 189–191
    leukemia incidence from, 125, 127
    leukemia risk from, 123–125
    lung cancer related to, 176–178

Occupational exposure (Continued)
    in lymphocyte chromosome aberrations,
        63–64
    in melanoma, 264–265
    in multiple myeloma risk, 133–135
    non-Hodgkin's lymphoma risk from, 131–132
    nonmelanoma skin cancer after, 260–261
    from nuclear power production, 41–42
    oral cavity cancers from, 148–149
    pancreatic cancer from, 244–246
    to plutonium, 430
    in radiation-induced cancer, 78–79
    radiation-induced life shortening from,
        362–363
    salivary gland tumors from, 145
    to uranium, 424–427
Occupational radiation dose limits, NRC, 22,
    23t
Odds ratio (OR), 84
Oil field workers
    radium 226 exposure in, 433
    radium exposure of, 433
Oligodendrocytes, radiation changes of, 300
Oligodendrogliocytes, abnormal myelin
    synthesis of, 304
Oligospermia
    after Hodgkin's disease radiotherapy, 334
    postradiation, 334
Oncogene tumor genes, 72
Oncogenes, signals activating, 73
Ondansetron, to prevent nausea and vomiting
    with whole-body irradiation, 354–355
Oocytes, 331–332
Operation Hardtack, fallout effects on
    personnel participating in, 93–94
Optic nerve, SOMA normal tissue
    radiotoxicity for, 509t–510t
Optic neuropathy, radiation, 306
Oral cavity
    cancer of
        in atomic bomb survivors, 148f
        incidence of, 147
        radiation-induced from external exposure,
            147–150
        radiation-induced from internal exposure,
            150
        risk factors in, 147
    low-LET radiation effects on, 320–321
    mucosa of, SOMA normal tissue
        radiotoxicity for, 511t
    neutron radiation effects on, 321
    radiation-induced ulceration of, 322
Organ radiation damage
    clinicopathologic course of, 16f
    mechanism of, 16f
Organ radiosensitivity, 15–16
Organ system abnormalities, with fetal
    radiation exposure, 410
Organic compounds
    carcinogenic, 394
    radiosensitizing, 392–393
Organogenesis period, radiation exposure
    during, 404–406
Ossicles, necrosis of, radiation-induced, 310
Osteochondromas
    benign, in CT scan, 253f
    after childhood cancer radiotherapy, 253
Osteonecrosis
    contributing factors in, 336
    treatment of, 336–337
Osteosarcoma
    age as factor in, 248–249
    after breast or pelvic cancer radiotherapy,
        258

Osteosarcoma (Continued)
    after childhood cancer treatment, 103
    extraosseous
        after radiotherapy, 256
        after Thorotrast injection, 258–259
    after Hodgkin's disease treatment, 252
    latent period for, 250
    modifying factors in, 249–250
    in plutonium workers, 431f
    radionuclides in, 253
    after radiotherapy, 256–258
        for neoplasms, 252–253
        for Wilms' tumor, 252
    in radium dial painters, 338
    after radium exposure, 362–363
Otitis media
    radiation-induced, 310
    thyroid cancer after radiotherapy for, 156
Otosclerosis, radiation-induced, 310
Ovarian cancer
    additive effects of radiotherapy and
        chemotherapy for, 393–394
    in atomic bomb survivors at different dose
        levels, 202f
    incidence of, 200
    radiation-induced
        from external exposure, 200–203
        from internal exposure, 203
        risk estimate for, 203–204
    risk estimates for incidence and mortality
        from, 204t
    risk factors for, 200, 446
Ovarian follicles, 331–332
Ovary
    cells of, 331–332
    chemotherapeutic and alkylating agent
        toxicity in, 331
    deterministic radiation effects on, 331–332
    radiation-induced failure of, 332
    radiosensitivity of, 332
    SOMA normal tissue radiotoxicity for,
        526t
Overweight, in cancer risk, 445–446
Ovum (ova), 331–332
Oxygen, radiosensitizing effect of, 392
Oxygen effect, 9
Oxygen enhancement ratio (OER), 9
    LET and, 9, 9f

P

p73 immunoglobulins, in atomic bomb
    survivors, 351
p53 tumor suppressor gene, environmental
    carcinogens and, 442
P value, in epidemiological studies, 84
Pacemaker failure, after radiotherapy, 318–319
Paclitaxel
    in predisposition to radiation pneumonitis,
        313
    in radiation recall phenomena, 393
Paget's disease
    bone tumors and, 248–249
    predisposing to osteogenic sarcomas, 254
Pair production, 3
Palladium 103 seed implants, 335
Pancarditis, radiation and, 317
Pancreas
    low-LET radiation effects on, 328
    necrosis of, 328
    radiation-induced fibrosis of, 328
    radioresistance of, 328
    structures and composition of, 328

Pancreatic cancer
   in atomic bomb survivors, excess relative
      risk for, 244f
   in atomic energy facility workers, 96–97
   epidemiology of, 248
   incidence of, 243
   from occupational exposure, 97
   radiation-induced
      from external exposure, 243–247
      from internal exposure, 247–248
   risk estimates for, 243, 249t
   smoking in, 443–445
   survival rates in, 243
Pancreatic islet cell tumors, risk factors in, 243
Pancreatitis, chronic radiation-induced, 328
Panhypopituitarism, after pituitary irradiation,
   294
Panophthalmitis, radiation-induced, 305–306
Pantex nuclear weapons facility
   bladder cancer in workers at, 196
   pancreatic cancer in workers at, 245
Papillary adenocarcinoma, well-differentiated,
   151
Papillary carcinoma, occult, 151
Parasitic infections, carcinogenic effect of,
   447–448
Parathyroid glands
   deterministic radiation effects in, 298–299
   radioiodine therapy-induced cancer of, 146
   radiotherapy-induced adenomas of, 146
   tumors of, radiation-related, 145
      from external exposure, 145–146
      from internal exposure, 146
Parenchyma
   periods of damage to, 15–16
   vascularity and secondary degeneration of,
      16
Parenchymal cells
   deterministic effects of radiation on, 285
   periods of radiation damage to, 15–16
   radiosensitivity of, 15
Parotid glands, 310
Particulate radiation, 4–5, 4t
PC calculator, 452
PC/AS, subjective 99th percentile upper
   bound of, 451–452
Pelvic cancer radiotherapy
   genital effects of, 331
   prostate and seminal vesicle effects of,
      359–360
   second tumors after, 258–259
      of bone, 258
Pelvic inflammatory disease, in ureteral
   stenosis, 330
Pelvic irradiation
   angiosarcomas of breast after, 258–259
   blood vessel damage from, 319
   bone changes after, 342–343
   chronic pancreatitis after, 328
   radiation necrosis after, 339f
   rectal complications with, 325
   thyroid cancer related to, 156
Pelvimetry, x-ray, fetal radiation exposure
   from, 401–402
Penile angiosarcoma, after radiotherapy, 214
Penis
   cancer of
      epidemiology of, 214
      incidence of, 212
      radiation-induced, 212–214
   deterministic radiation effects on, 335
Pentoxyphilline
   for late subcutaneous radiation fibrosis, 290
   for radiation osteonecrosis, 336–337

Peptic ulcers
   pancreatic cancer after, 246
   radiotherapy for, 101–102
      bladder cancer after, 197
      breast cancer after, 169
      coronary heart disease after, 318
      coronary heart disease risk after, 362
      esophageal cancer after, 217–218
      gastric acidity after, 322
      hepatobiliary system cancer after, 240
      leukemia after, 122
      prostate cancer after, 211
      thyroid cancer after, 156
   after whole-abdominal radiation in children,
      323–324
Pericardial effusions, after Hodgkin's disease
   radiotherapy, 317
Pericardial fibrosis, 317, 319
   late changes in, 318
Pericarditis
   fibrinous, after radiotherapy, 319
   after Hodgkin's disease radiotherapy,
      317–318
Peripheral ganglia, 299
Peripheral lymphoid tissue, in immune
   response, 346
Peripheral nerves
   deterministic radiation effects on
      high-LET, 305
      low-LET, 305
      with radionuclide exposure, 305
   sheath around, 299
   SOMA normal tissue radiotoxicity for,
      507t
Peripheral neuropathy, low-LET radiation
   induced, 305
Personnel dosimetry, in legal liability, 441
Peterostor therapy, bone tumors after,
   253–254
Pharynx
   cancers of
      incidence of, 147
      after occupational exposure, 148–149
      risk factors in, 147
   low-LET radiation effects on, 320–321
   neutron radiation effects on, 321
   radiotherapy for malignancies of, 310
   SOMA normal tissue radiotoxicity for
      mucosa of, 511t
   tumors of after cervical cancer treatment,
      150
Phenacetin, cancer risk from, 443
Phenobarbital, tumor promoting effects of,
   71–72
Pheochromocytoma, genetic factors in, 72
Philadelphia chromosome, 50
Phlebotomy, leukemia risk from, 126–127
Phorbol esters
   enhanced radiation effect with, 394
   tumor promoting effects of, 71–72
Phosphate
   lung cancer and, 182
   natural radiation from, 37
Phosphate mills, lung cancer and, 182
Phosphorus 32 chromic phosphate, in
   cartilage necrosis, 339
Phosphorus 32 exposure
   dose coefficients for worker intakes of,
      497t–499t
   hematopoietic change with, 345
   immune function after, 350
Phosphorus 32 phosphate colloid, hepatic
   injury after, 327–328
Photoelectric absorption, 3

Photons
   half-value layer for, 4t
   produced by spallation, 27
Photosynthesis, carbon 14 concentrations and,
   29–30
Physical agents, in radiation effects, 390–392
Physical half-life, 7
Phytohemagglutinin (PHA) response, in
   atomic bomb survivors, 350–351
Pigmentation sequence, after radiotherapy,
   289
Pi-mesons
   brain tumors and, 303
   pneumonitis and, 316
Pions, produced by spallation, 27
Pituitary glands
   deterministic radiation effects on, 293–294
      with high-LET radiation, 294
      with radionuclide irradiation, 294
   fibrosis of after high-LET irradiation, 294
   radioresistance of, 293
Placental transfer
   of strontium, 412
   of xenon and krypton, 413
Plant alkaloids, in radiation brain injury, 302
Plants
   carbon 14 concentrations in, 29–30
   carcinogenic toxins of, 445
Plasma cells
   in immune response, 349
   radioresistance of, 347–348
   radiosensitivity of, 340
Platelets
   counts of
      after bone marrow ablation, 343
      after whole-body irradiation, 343, 344f
Platelets
   depression of with radioiodine therapy,
      345
   radiosensitivity of, 340
Pleural effusions, in radiation pneumonitis,
   312–313
Plummer-Vinson syndrome, 215
Pluripotent stem cells, radiosensitivity of, 340
Plutonium
   accumulated in bone, 338
   average effective doses of from fallout, 41t
   beneficial effect of, 474–475
   body burdens of from occupational
      exposure, 63–64, 431–432
   in bone tumors, 430–431
   cardiac complications with inhalation of,
      320
   characteristics of, 428–429
   crysotile asbestos inhalation and, 391
   dose coefficients for worker intakes of,
      497t–499t
   entry of into wounds, 429–430
   environmental exposure to, 429
   human data on biodistribution of, 429–433
   inhalation of, 186, 429–430
   isotopes of, 428–429
   maximum permissible body burden of, 430
   microdistribution of in plutonium workers,
      432
   in nonmelanoma skin cancer, 263
   in nuclear weapons, 40–41
   risk per unit dose of, 432
   toxicology of, 428
   in tracheobronchial lymph nodes, 429–430
Plutonium 238/239 radionuclides, 428–429
   experimental injection of, 430
   inhalation of in lung cancer risk, 186–187
Plutonium hydroxides, 428–429

Plutonium oxides, 428–429
Plutonium pneumosclerosis, 430
Plutonium production facilities
  accident at, 42
  prostate cancer in workers at, 270
Plutonium workers
  bladder cancer in, 198–199
  bone tumors in, 254
  breast cancer in, 171
  chronic radiation sickness in, 430
  colon cancer in, 230–231
  esophageal cancer in, 218
  hepatobiliary system cancer rates in,
    240–241
  hepatobiliary system cancers in, 239
  Hodgkin's disease risk in, 129
  kidney cancer in, 192
  leukemia from occupational exposure of,
    127
  lung cancer in, 176–177, 186–187
    incidence of, 474–475
    mortality from, 432
    risk for, 432
  male genital cancers in, 214
  melanoma in, 265
  mortality rates in, 430–431
  occupational exposure of, 430
  oropharyngeal cancer in, 150
  osteogenic sarcoma in, 431f
  pancreatic cancer in, 248
  plutonium microdistribution in, 432
  pulmonary fibrosis in, 316
  rectal cancer in, 235
  risk estimate for, 433
  small intestinal cancer in, 225–227
  solid cancers in, 432
  stomach cancer in, 223–224
  thyroid cancer in, 154, 157
  uterine cancer in, 207
PMS gene, 72–73
Pneumoconiosis, compensation for, 450
Pneumonia, radiation, KL-6 levels with, 364
Pneumonitis
  after high-LET radiation, 316
  radiation, 312
    with actinomycin D and radiotherapy,
      393
    characteristics of, 312–313
    after Chernobyl accident, 359–360
    in chest radiograph CT scans, 314f
    chronic or late effects of, 315
    dose-volumetric parameters for
      fractionated radiotherapy and, 313
    dose-volumetric parameters for
      predicting, 313
    latent period for, 313
    permanent changes in, 313–314
    predisposing factors in, 312
    radiographic changes in, 313
    reducing severity of, 312
    with Thorotrast administration, 316
    time course in, 314f
  after radiotherapy in children, 315
  "recall," 313
Point mutations
  classification of, 49
  definition of, 47
  spontaneous, 49, 74
Pollution, in cancer risk, 447
Polonium 210
  combined with quartz dust inhalation,
    391–392
  dose coefficients for worker intakes of,
    497t–499t

Polycyclic hydrocarbons
  in cancer risk, 447
  cancer risk from, 443
  in scrotal cancer, 212
Polycythemia
  after phosphorus 32 exposure, 345
  from radiation exposure, 137
Polycythemia vera
  in atomic bomb survivors, 341
  after radiation exposure, 344
  radiotherapy for, 102
    immune function after, 350
    leukemia risk from, 126–127
Polygenic disorders, 50–51
Polyploidy, 49–50
Pooled analysis, time and age patterns in risk
    of radiation-induced cancers, 87–88
Population
  mobility of affecting studies of
    populations living near nuclear
    facilities, 94–95
  risk to, 469
  size of, 469
    aggregate harm and, 469–470
Porcelain, thorium in manufacture of, 39
Portsmith Uranium Enrichment Plant,
    uranium-induced illness in workers of,
    426
Portsmouth Naval Shipyard
  cancer rates in populations near, 95–96
  occupational exposure study at, 97
Positron
  emission of, 6
  particulate radiation of, 4t
Positron emission tomography (PET)
  radiation exposure from, 44
  of radiation necrosis of brain, 300–301
Postirradiation bystander signaling
    (bystander effect), 10–11
Postnatal irradiation exposure, 100–101
Potassium radionuclides
  average body burden of, 32
  dose coefficients for worker intakes of,
    497t–499t
  as internal radiation source, 35
Potential recoverability conversion factor
    (PRCF), 53–54
  in radiation risk assessment, 54
Power plants, coal-fired, as radiation source,
    35–36
Prader-Willi syndrome, 47–48
Prates v. Sears, Roebuck & Co., 440–441
Precambrian granite, high radon levels in, 182
Preconception irradiation, 419
  in childhood leukemia and malignancies,
    415–416
Prednisone (MOPP), leukemia risk after, 393
Pregnancy
  in breast tissue radiosensitivity, 311–312
  in cancer incidence rates, 446
  carcinogenesis during, 414–416
  comparison of risks during, 418t
  outcomes of in atomic bomb survivors, 57
  ovarian cancer and, 200
  after ovarian radiation, 332
  radiation exposure during
    carcinogenic effects of, 416
    minimizing, 416–417
    temporal relationship of effects of, 402t
    termination of, 417–419
  radionuclide irradiation during, 412–414
Preimplantation period, radiation exposure
    during, 403–404
Preleukemic changes, 137

Premature chromosome condensation (PCC),
    59–60
Premature puberty, after cranial irradiation,
    331
Prenatal irradiation, 100–99
  CNS tumors related to, 142
Prenatal x-radiation, in childhood cancer, 416
Probabilistic analysis, 442–443
Probabilistic effects, 438
Probability
  of causation (PC), 438
    estimating, 442, 448–450
    versus risk, 441–442
  evaluating, 460
Procarbazine
  leukemia risk after, 393
  in radiation brain injury, 302
  in soft-tissue sarcoma risk, 256–258
Proctitis, radiation, 324
Proctosigmoiditis, radiation, 324
Prodromal period, 354
Progesterone, carcinogenic effects of, 447
Programmed cell death. See Apoptosis
    (programmed cell death)
Progressive external ophthalmoplegia, 47–48
Progressive fibrosis, 286
Projection models, in uncertainty of risk
    estimates, 87
Promethium radionuclides, dose coefficients
    for worker intakes of, 497t–499t
Proof, court definition of, 439
Prostate, low-LET radiation effects on, 335
Prostate cancer
  epidemiology of, 212
  incidence and causes of, 208
  radiation-induced
    from external exposure, 208–211
    from internal exposure, 211–212
  radiotherapy for
    colon cancer after, 230
    incontinence after, 331
    rectal cancer after, 235
    renal injury after, 331
    soft-tissue sarcomas after, 258–259
    testicular effects of, 335
  risk estimates for incidence and mortality
    from, 213t
  spontaneous, estimated lifetime risk of, 83t
Protection, definition of, 389
Protein phenotype mutations, in atomic bomb
    survivors, 57–58
Protoactinium, radiation energies and
    intensities of, 33t
Protons, 1
  in cosmic rays, 27
  particulate radiation of, 4t
Psoriasis, radiation exacerbating, 290
Psychiatric disorders, nuclear accidents and,
    468
Psychological effects, 466–469
Psychotherapy, for postradiotherapy fatigue,
    364–365
PTCH (Patched) gene, in tumor initiation, 72
Puberty, early, after pituitary irradiation, 294
Public health and safety
  health hazards and, 459
  nuclear accident impact on, 468
Pulmonary artery occlusion, radiation-
    induced, 319
Pulmonary edema, from uranium exposure,
    424–425
Pulmonary fibrosis
  compensation for, 450
  drugs increasing incidence of, 315–316

Pulmonary fibrosis (Continued)
  permanent changes in, 313–314
  radiation induced, 312
  after radionuclide irradiation, 316
  after whole-lung radiotherapy, 315
Pulmonary hypertension, with mediastinal
    irradiation, 315–316
Pulmonary metastasis
  lung after irradiation for, 315f
  pneumonitis after treatment for, 316
Pyloric stenosis, incidence of, 52
Pyrimidine
  excretion of after radiation exposure,
    363–364
  halogenated, radiosensitizing effect of, 9

Q

Quadratic dose-response models, 80
Quartz dust inhalation, polonium 210 and,
    391

R

Rad (gray), 7–8. See also Kerma
Radar exposure
  breast cancer related to, 167
  oropharyngeal cancer related to, 149
  skin changes after, 291
Radiation. See also Ionizing radiation;
    Radiotherapy
  absorption of, 31–32
  and biologic agents, 396–397
  in cataracts, 454
  and chemical agents, 392–396
  chronic low-LET, genetic disease risk from,
    52t
  combined with burns, 392
  compensation for disease induced by, 130
  DDREF of, 16–17
  dose-response relationship for in
    lymphocytes, 54t
  effects of
    adverse, at different gestational stages,
      403f
    carcinogenic, 71
    deterministic, 437–438 (See also
      Deterministic effects of radiation)
    heritable, 47, 53–54
    hormetic (See also Hormesis)
    immunomodulatory, 353
    measuring risk of, 460–461
    nomenclature for, 389–390
    perception and acceptability of, 461–466
    psychological, 459, 466–469
    secondary, 438–439
    social decisions about, 469–470
    stochastic (probabilistic), 438
    subcellular and cellular mechanisms in,
      12
  of embryo and fetus, liability for, 440–441
  and ethnic factors, 397
  fractionation of, 16
  genetic studies on populations exposed to,
    54–58
  genomic instability induced by, 10
  in Hodgkin's disease, 127–130
  in immune response, 346
  inverse dose rate effect of, 17
  legislative compensation programs for
    exposure to, 450–452
  in leukemia, 117

Radiation (Continued)
    risk estimates for incidence and mortality
      from, 128t–129t
  lymphocyte chromosome aberration
      frequency with, 60
  in mental retardation, 455
  multiple myeloma incidence and mortality
      from, 136t
  natural (background), 27
  non-Hodgkin's lymphoma risk estimates
      from, 134t
  nonionizing, from video display terminals,
      39
  with other agents, 389
  perception and acceptability of levels of,
      464–465
  with physical agents, 390–392
  preconception, 402–403
  during pregnancy
    minimizing, 416–417
    pregnancy termination after, 417–419
  protection from, concepts and quantities in,
      20–24
  protection limits of, collective dose
      equivalents and, 22
  risk estimates for, 53–54
    based on spontaneous and induced
      mutation rates, 53–54
    data used in, 53
    direct and indirect methods of, 53
  specific quantities of, 8
  subcellular repair of damage from, 13
  sublethal damage from, capacity to repair,
      13
  technologically induced, 27
  tolerance doses for, 19t
  toxicity scoring system for, 285
  units and quantities of, 7–8
Radiation accidents, 441
  deterministic effects in, 285–286
Radiation carcinogenesis, 441–448
  genetic abnormalities in, 72
Radiation compensation acts, U.S., 130
Radiation compensation programs, absorbed
    doses used in, 450t
Radiation dermatitis, 287–288
  with nonmelanoma skin cancer after
    radiotherapy, 262
Radiation doses
  in legal claims, 439
  levels of in nonmelanoma skin cancers,
    259–260
  limits of, in special situations, 23–24
  maximum permissible and limits for, 22–24
  in radiation-induced breast cancer,
    165–166
  regulation of limits for, 469
  units and quantities of, 14t–21t
Radiation Exposure Compensation Act
    (RECA), 450
Radiation Exposure Veterans' Compensation
    Act (REVCA), 450
Radiation injury
  biochemical indicators of, 363–364
  claims of, 439–440
  early diagnosis methods for, 437
  functional response of body to, 363
  involving capillary, arteriole, and small
    artery, 286f
  periods of clinical manifestation of, 15–16
Radiation myelopathy, 304
Radiation protection philosophy
  in accidental and emergent situations, 23–24
  cancer induction thresholds in, 71

Radiation protection philosophy (Continued)
  genetic damage data and, 53
Radiation recall phenomena, 393
Radiation sickness
  acute (ARS) (See Acute radiation sickness)
  chronic, in plutonium workers, 430
  after whole-body irradiation, 355–360
Radiation sources
  medical, 43–45
  natural
    cosmic, 27–28
    cosmogenic, 28–30
    modification of, 35–40
    terrestrial, 30–35
  technological, 40–43
  technologically modified, 35–40
    natural, 35–40
Radiation therapy. See Radiotherapy
Radiation weighting factors, 20, 20t
Radiation workers
  bladder cancer in, 197
  bone tumors in, 254
  cancer mortality in, 97
  cancer rates among, 96
  colon cancer in, 228
  hepatobiliary system cancers in, 238
  kidney cancer in, 189–190
  lung cancer in, 452–454
  melanoma in, 264
  occupational studies of in U.S., 97
  pancreatic cancer in, 244
  salivary gland tumors in, 145
  small intestinal cancer in, 225
  stomach cancer in, 221–222
  U.K. registry of, 96–97
  uterine cancer in, 205–206
Radioactinium, radiation energies and
    intensities of, 33t
Radioactive decay, 7
  mechanisms of, 5–6
    alpha emission in, 5–6
    beta negative, 6
    electron capture in, 6
    isomeric transition in, 6
    positron emission in, 6
  of primordial radionuclides, 30
Radioactivity, 5
  physical factors of, 5–6
Radioactivity units, conversion table for, 496t
Radiobiology, four R's of, 17
Radiocesium exposure, from Chernobyl
    accident, 199
Radiography source, skin lesions from, 292f
Radioiodine exposure
  breast cancer after, 170–171
  carcinogenic effects of, 100–101
  from Chernobyl fallout, 159, 199
    thyroid dose from, 296–297
  CNS tumors related to, 141
  colon cancer after, 231
  hepatobiliary system cancer after, 241
  inhalation of in thyroid neoplasms, 152
  lung cancer after, 187
  ovarian cancer after, 203
  during pregnancy, 412–413
  thyroid cancer from, 158, 159
Radioiodine therapy
  autoimmune thyroiditis after, 295
  bladder cancer after, 199
  bone tumors after, 253
  brain effects of, 303
  brain necrosis after, 303
  cataract formation after, 309
  esophageal cancer after, 218

Radioiodine therapy *(Continued)*
  hematopoietic system changes after, 345
  hyperthyroidism after, 146
  hypothyroidism and autoimmune thyroiditis after, 297–298
  immune function after, 350
  kidney cancer after, 193
  male genital cancers after, 214
  mediastinal hemorrhage after, 320
  nonmelanoma skin cancer after, 263
  oropharyngeal cancer after, 150
  pancreatic cancer after, 248
  parathyroid changes after, 298–299
  parotid gland lymphoma related to, 145
  prostate cancer after, 211
  pulmonary fibrosis after, 316
  rectal cancer after, 236
    high-dose, 236
  salivary gland effects of, 311
  second cancer after, 103
  stomach cancer after, 224
  testicular effects of, 335
  thyroid cancer after, 157, 158
  uterine cancer after, 207
Radioiron irradiation, during pregnancy, 413
Radioisotope contamination, in bone tumors, 249–250, 254
Radiologists/radiologic technologists. *See also* Diagnostic medical workers; Medical radiation workers; x-ray technologists
  bladder cancer in, 197
  bone tumors in, 251–252
  breast cancer in, 168
  cancer incidence in, 133
  CNS cancer incidence among, 140
  colon cancer in, 229
  esophageal cancer in, 217
  hepatobiliary system cancer in, 239–240
  Hodgkin's disease risk in, 130
  hormetic effects in, 474–475
  incidence of leukemia and AML in, 137
  kidney cancer in, 190–191
  larynx cancer in, 146–147
  leukemia incidence in, 121
  lung cancer in, 177–178
  male, cancer mortality in, 98
  male genital cancer in, 212–214
  myelodysplasia risk in, 137
  non-Hodgkin's lymphoma risk in, 131
  nonmelanoma skin cancer in, 260, 261
  oropharyngeal cancer in, 149
  ovarian cancer in, 202
  pancreatic cancer in, 245, 246
  prostate cancer in, 210
  radiation-induced life shortening in, 362
  rectal cancer in workers at, 234
  small intestinal cancer in, 225
  stomach cancer in, 222–223
  uterine cancer in, 206
Radioluminous timepieces, cosmic radiation from, 38–39
Radionuclide irradiation
  bladder and ureteral effects of, 331
  bone, cartilage, and muscle effects of, 338–339
  in bone tumors, 249–250
  bone tumors after, 256
  cancer mortality from, 432
  cardiac complications after, 320
  cataracts after, 309
  after Chernobyl accident, 159
  colon cancer after, 230–231
  cosmogenic, 28–30
    in cosmic rays, 27

Radionuclide irradiation *(Continued)*
  interacting with atmosphere, 29t
    as natural radiation source, 35
  deterministic effects of on pituitary glands, 294
  esophageal cancer after, 218
  of heart and vessels, 320
  large intestinal effects of, 325–326
  leukemia risk from, 125
  of lymphatic system, 346
  male genital cancers after, 214
  melanoma after, 265
  nephritis after, 329
  nonmelanoma skin cancer after, 263
  pancreatic cancer after, 248
  parathyroid changes after, 298–299
  peripheral nerve effects of, 305
  during pregnancy, 412–414
  prostate cancer after, 211, 270
  pulmonary fibrosis after, 316
  rectal cancer after, 235
  salivary gland effects of, 311
  skin reaction to, 290–293
  small intestinal cancer after, 225–227
  stomach cancer after, 223–224
  of testes, 335
  from worldwide fallout, 40–41
Radionuclides. *See also* Alpha-emitting radionuclides; Radionuclide irradiation
  annual collective dose of in U.S. population, 45t
  average body burden of, 32
  beta-emitting, skin reaction to, 290–291
  from burning coal, 35–36
  in CNS tumors, 141–142
  decay schemes of from unstable to stable states, 5f
  dose coefficients for worker intakes of, 497t–499t
  in fallout, 40–41
  half-lives of, 7
    and type of radiation, 491t–493t
  hepatobiliary system cancer related to, 240–241
  in lung cancer in plutonium workers, 186
  maximum external photon and electron dose equivalent factors for organs, 500t
  maximum photon dose equivalent and electron dose equivalent rate conversion factors for, 501t
  in measuring circulation reduction, 288
  in osteosarcoma, 253
  physical factors of, 5
  primordial, 30–35
    actinium series of, 30
    as natural radiation source, 35
    physical half-lives of, 30t
    thorium series of, 30
    uranium series of, 30, 31t
  production of, 6–7
  radioactivity of, 5
  released in nuclear power production, 41–42
  skin contamination dose equivalent rate factors for, 500t
  soil content of in United States, 33t
  specific gamma ray constants for, 503t
  stomach cancer after, 224
  thyroid cancer in population exposed to, 157
Radiopharmaceuticals
  during pregnancy, 413
  radiation exposure from, 44, 45
Radioprotective agents, 9

Radiosensitivity
  in ataxia-telangiectasia, 76
  cell oxygenation and, 13f
  cellular, 14–15
  as function of cell cycle stage, 12f
  as function of cell type, 14f
  genetic disorders associated with, 76t
  interactive agents in, 390f
  of normal cells, 14t
  of organ tissue, 15–16
  peak period of, 16
Radiosensitizers, 9, 389
Radiostrontium irradiation, during pregnancy, 412
Radiotellurium exposure, after Chernobyl accident, 159
Radiotherapy, 441
  abdominal, pancreatic cancer after, 243
  absorbed doses from, 43
  adrenal effects of, 299
  in atherosclerosis and arterial stenosis, 319
  basal cell carcinoma after, 259
  for benign diseases, 101–102
    breast cancer after, 169–170
  bladder cancer after, 197–198
  bone, cartilage, and muscle effects of, 335–338
  bone marrow changes after, 342
  bone tumors after, 252–254
  breast cancer after, 170
  breast tissue effects of, 311–312
  carcinogenic effects of, 447
  cardiac and coronary complications after, 318
  cataracts after, 308
  with chemotherapy, 389
  for childhood cancer, 55–56
  CNS tumors related to, 140–141
  in cognitive function, 302
  colon cancer after, 229–230
    in children, 230
  congenital anomalies after, 405
  curative regimes in, 45
  early and late effects of, 18
  epidemiologic risk studies of patients exposed to, 88
  esophageal cancer after, 217–218, 321–322
  fatigue after, 364–365
  fractionation in, 17–18
  hepatobiliary system cancer after, 240
  high-dose
    neuropsychological effects after, 459
    rectal cancer after, 235
  hyperparathyroidism related to, 146
  immune function after, 349–350
  kidney cancer after, 191–192
  large intestinal effects of, 324–325
  leukemia incidence from, 121–123
  liver and biliary complications after, 326–327
  low-dose, rectal cancer after, 234–235
  lung cancer after, 178–179
  lymphatic system effects of, 345–346
  for malignant disease, 103–104
  medical exposure from, 45
  megavoltage, soft-tissue tumors after, 258
  melanoma after, 265
  multiple sclerosis and, 303
  nonmelanoma skin cancer after, 262–263
  oropharyngeal cancer after, 149–150
  ovarian cancer after, 202–203
  pancreatic cancer after, 246–248
  pancreatic effects of, 328
  penile angiosarcoma after, 214

Radiotherapy (Continued)
  penis, urethra, and scrotal effects of, 335
  pericardial effusions after, 317
  pericardial thickening after, 318
  pericarditis after, 317–318
  prostate cancer after, 211
  pulmonary reactions after in children, 315
  radiation-induced life shortening from, 361–362
  renal injury after, 329–330
  salivary gland effects of, 310–311
  salivary gland tumors in children receiving, 145
  second tumors after, 258
  skin changes with, 288
  small intestinal cancer after, 225
  soft-tissue tumors after, 256–259
  spinal cord injury after, 303–304
  stomach cancer after, 223, 225
  stomach effects of, 322
  with surgery, 391–392
  testicular effects of, 333–334
  thyroid cancer related to, 154–157
  in utero, cataract formation after, 309
Radiothorium, radiation energies and intensities of, 32t
Radiothyroid therapy, thyroid cancer after, 157–158
Radium, 433
  average body burden of, 32
  in Brazil nuts, 30–31
  carcinogenic effects of, 99
  in CNS tumors, 141
  in cranial sinus tumors, 144
  energies and intensities of, 31t
  in industrial radiography devices, 433
  isotopes of, 30–31
  in medical applications, 433
  metabolism of, 144
  in natural environment, 433
  oil field workers exposure to, 433
  pancreatic cancer in workers exposed to, 248
  in tumor deaths, 362–363
  in water, lung cancer risk and, 182
Radium 224
  bone changes from, 339
  in bone tumors, 249–250, 253–256
  in breast cancer, 171
  decay of, 32–34
  in hepatobiliary system cancer, 241
  leukemia risk with intravenous administration of, 126
  in liver injury, 327–328
  in lung cancer, 188
  in pancreatic cancer, 248
  in renal insufficiency, 331
  in stomach cancer, 224
  in thyroid cancer, 158
Radium 226
  in bone tumors, 253, 254
  in cranial sinus carcinoma, 144
  in hematopoietic system changes, 344–345
  in nonmelanoma skin cancer, 262–263
  occupational exposure to, 433
Radium applicators, thyroid cancer related to, 156
Radium burn, 287–288
Radium dial painters
  bone changes in, 338
  bone tumors in, 254–256
    dose-response relation in, 256f
  breast cancer in, 171
  frontal sinus carcinoma in, 144f

Radium dial painters (Continued)
  hematopoietic system changes in, 344–345
  leukemia risk in, 126
  osteogenic sarcoma in
    with pelvic ischium destruction, 255f
    with tarsal bone destruction, 255f
  photo of, 255f
  radiation-induced life shortening in, 362–363
  rectal cancer in, 235
Radium Hill miners, lung cancer mortality in, 185
Radium osteitis, of vertebral body and proximal tibia, 341f
Radium radionuclides, 433
  in colon cancer, 231
  dose coefficients for worker intakes of, 497t–499t
  hematopoietic system changes in, 344–345
Radium salts, 433
Radium therapy
  for ankylosing spondylitis, 101
  bladder cancer after, 197, 199
  breast cancer after, 169
  cataract formation after, 309
  intrauterine, colon cancer after, 229–230
  kidney cancer after, 191, 193
  lung cancer after, 178
  middle ear damage after, 309–310
  nasopharyngeal, pituitary effects of, 294
  uterine effects of, 333
  for uterine hemorrhage, leukemia risk with, 126
Radon
  average annual doses and effective dose equivalents of by state, 36t
  average annual effective doses from, 37t
  biodistribution of, 133
  in building materials, 37–38
  in CNS tumors, 141–142
  conversion chart for, 496t
  cumulative doses of and lung cancer rates, 185
  decay of, 433
  in fluorspar mines, 185
  in hepatobiliary system cancer, 240–241
  indoor concentration of, 35
  indoor sources of exposure to, 37–38
  inverse dose-rate effect in lung cancer rates and, 185–186
  leukemia incidence from, 125
  long-term measurement of, 34–35
  in lung cancer, 181, 188
    from geological exposure, 182
    from residential exposure, 182–183
  measurement of activity of, 34
  in multiple sclerosis, 303
  natural background exposure to, 45
  occupational exposures to, 42
  outdoor concentrations of, 32–35
  in pancreatic cancer in uranium miners, 247
  perception and acceptability of risk of, 463
  residential and mining exposure studies of, 92
  in respiratory cancer, 395f
  smoking and effects of, 395
  in stomach cancer from occupational exposure, 224
  in uranium 238 decay chain, 34
  in uranium mines, 184–185
  variation in building concentrations and lung doses of, 37t
  in water, lung cancer risk and, 182

Radon 222, internal body burden of, 32–34
Radon daughters
  lung cancer mortality risk with, 188t
  measurement of, 34
Radon miners, 183–184
  exposure of, 185
  leukemia risk in, 125
  melanoma in, 264
Radon seed brachytherapy, of pituitary lesions, 294
Radon thermal spring, Badgastein, Austria, chromosome aberrations at, 63
Ranier v. Union Carbide Corp., 439
Rapid renewal system, postradiation events of, 15f
Rare earth radionuclide exposure, during pregnancy, 413
RAS gene mutations, 74–75
RB tumor suppressor gene defect, 74–75
RBl gene, in tumor initiation, 72
Reading Prong, radon levels and lung cancer rates in, 182
Reasonableness, in risk acceptability, 462–463
Reassortment, 17
Recessive traits, 47–48
Rectal cancer
  epidemiology of, 236
  incidence of, 231–232
    increased, 227
    risk estimates for mortality and, 237t
  in medical diagnostic workers, 229
  in radiation and nuclear workers, 228
  radiation-induced
    from external exposure, 233–235
    from internal exposure, 235–236
    medical, 234–235
Rectosigmoid, postradiation narrowing of, 325f
Rectum
  low-LET radiation effects on, 324–325
  neutron radiation effects on, 325
  painless, postradiation bleeding in, 324
  radionuclide radiation effects on, 325–326
  radiosensitivity of, 324–325
  SOMA normal tissue radiotoxicity for, 521t
  telangiectasia of, 324f
  ulceration and stricture of, 324f
Relative biologic effectiveness (RBE), 2–3
  linear energy transfer and, 3f
  oxygen enhancement ratio and, 9
  for various radiation types, 2t
Relative risk (RR), 84
  in cohort studies of radiation-induced and spontaneous cancer risk, 85
  concept of, 81, 82
  considerations in calculating, 85–86
  problems with, 82
Rem (sievert), 8
Renal abnormalities, uranium-induced, 424
Renal adenocarcinoma, risk factors for, 189
Renal calculi, in atomic bomb survivors, 330
Renal carcinoma, smoking as risk factor in, 443–445
Renal failure, after radiotherapy, 330
Renal function, long-term radiation effects of, 329
Renal insufficiency
  after Chernobyl accident, 360
  after radionuclide irradiation, 331
Renal pelvic tumors, risk factors for, 189
Renal plasma levels, radiation effects on, 329
Renal stones, in atomic bomb survivors, 330
Renal transplant radiotherapy, immune function after, 349–350

Renal tubules
cells of, 328–329
degeneration of in uranium miners, 425–426
Renal-cell carcinoma, incidence of, 188–189
Reoxygenation, 17
Repair, of sublethal damage, 17
Repopulation, 17
Reproductive behavior, in cancer risk, 446
Reproductive death, 11
with low-LET radiation, 13–14
Reproductive system
deterministic radiation effects on, 331–335
female, SOMA normal tissue radiotoxicity for, 526t
Respiratory disease, in uranium miners, 425–426
Respiratory tract
deterministic radiation effects on, 312–316
radiosensitivity of, 173
radon-related cancer of, 395f
RET gene, in tumor initiation, 72
Reticular cells, radiosensitivity of, 340
Reticular dermis, 287
Retina
hemorrhage of, 306
SOMA normal tissue radiotoxicity for, 509t–510t
Retinoblastoma
DNA sequence loss for, 73
gene mutations in, 77
genetic factors in, 72
paternally transmitted, 47–48
radiotherapy for
nonmelanoma skin cancer after, 263
soft-tissue sarcomas after, 256–258
RB tumor suppressor gene defect in, 74–75
Retinoids, antipromoter effect of, 71–72
Retinopathy, radiation, 306
Reverine, enhancing radiation effects, 393
Reverting postmitotic cells (RPM)
radiation effect on, 15f
radiosensitivity of, 14–15
Rhabdium (Rb), as internal radiation source, 35
Rhenium 186 sulfide, in cartilage necrosis, 339
Rheumatoid arthritis radiotherapy, T-cell changes after, 349–350
Rib fractures, postmastectomy irradiation, 336–337
Ribonuclease (RNase), increased urinary output of after radiation exposure, 363–364
Risk
acceptability of, 461–466
presence of alternatives and, 462–463
activities estimated to increase, 462t
definition of, 459
of exposure-induced death, 82–83
measurement of, 459–461
measures of, 469
perception of, 461–466
amplification of, 467
ranking of, 463–464
by different groups, 464t
uncertainties in estimating, 86–88
Risk projection models
for lifetime risk, 82–83
problems with, 81, 82
Rocky Flats Nuclear Weapons Facility workers
bladder cancer in, 196
bone tumors in, 251
colon cancer in, 228–231

Rocky Flats Nuclear Weapons Facility workers *(Continued)*
esophageal cancer in, 216–218
hepatobiliary system cancer in, 239, 240–241
kidney cancer in, 190, 192
lung cancer in, 176–177
lung cancer risk in, 186, 432
mortality ratios in, 431
occupational exposure at, 124
occupational study of, 97
pancreatic cancer in, 245, 248
prostate cancer in, 210, 270
pulmonary fibrosis in, 316
rectal cancer in, 233–234
stomach cancer in, 222
Roentgen, 7
Roentgen ulcers, chronic, 287–288
Rubidium 86, dose coefficients for worker intakes of, 497t–499t
Rubrum, average body burden of, 32
Ruthenium 106
dose coefficients for worker intakes of, 497t–499t
in weapons testing fallout, 41

S
Safety
determination of, 459
risk perception and, 461–462
Salinetro v. Nystron, 441
Salivary gland ducts
diminished filling of, 310–311
necrotic cell debris in, 310
Salivary glands
amylase levels in after radiation exposure, 364
deterministic radiation effects of, 310
from high-LET radiation, 311
from low-LET radiation, 310–311
from radionuclide irradiation, 311
ducts of, 310
SOMA normal tissue radiotoxicity for, 310, 512t
tumors of, 144
from external radiation exposure, 144–145
from internal exposure, 145
radiation risk factors for, 145, 146t
risk factors for, 145
Salty diets, in stomach cancer incidence, 223–224
S-(2-aminoethyl) isothiuronium (AET), radioprotective effect of, 9
Sarcomas
bone. *See* Bone, sarcomas of; Osteosarcoma
maternally transmitted, 47–48
Savannah River plant workers
bladder cancer in, 196
bone tumors in, 251
colon cancer in, 228
esophageal cancer in, 216–217
hepatobiliary system cancers in, 239
kidney cancer in, 190
nonmelanoma skin cancer in, 261
oropharyngeal cancer in, 149
pancreatic cancer in, 245
rectal cancer in, 233–234
Scandium 46, dose coefficients for worker intakes of, 497t–499t
Schizophrenia, radiation exposure and, 303
Schneeberger Lung Disease, in miners, 183

Schwann cells, 299
Science technicians
breast cancer in, 168
CNS cancer incidence among, 140
Sclera
radiation effects on, 305
SOMA normal tissue radiotoxicity for, 509t–510t
Scleroderma, localized radiation-induced, 290
Sclerosis, permanent changes in, 313–314
Scoliosis
breast cancer related to diagnostic x-rays for, 168
rate of with chronic radiation exposure, 55
with Wilms' tumor radiotherapy in children, 336
Screening programs, for psychological effects of radiation risk, 468
Scrotal cancer
epidemiology of, 214
incidence of, 212
radiation-induced, 214
from external exposure, 212–214
from internal exposure, 214
Scrotum, deterministic radiation effects on, 335
Seascale cluster study, 95
Sebaceous glands, radiosensitivity of, 289
Secondary effects, 438–439
Security screening devices
cosmic radiation from, 40
as modified natural radiation source, 40
Seizures
after cranial radiotherapy, 302–303
in utero radiation effects on, 408
Selenium
anticarcinogenic effect of, 446
radioprotective effect of, 392
Sellafield Plant of British Nuclear Fuels
leukemia and lymphoma in population surrounding, 56
non-Hodgkin's lymphoma risk to workers at, 131–132
workers at
bladder cancer in, 196
bone tumors in, 251, 254
breast cancer in, 171
cancer mortality in, 432
colon cancer in, 228, 230–231
esophageal cancer in, 216, 218
hepatobiliary system cancer in, 238, 240–241
immune function in, 349
kidney cancer in, 192
leukemia in, 127
lung cancer in, 176
lung cancer risk in, 186
male genital cancer in, 212, 214
occupational exposure and chromosome aberration rate in, 63–64
occupational exposure of, 123
oropharyngeal cancer in, 150
ovarian cancer in, 203
pancreatic cancer in, 244, 248
plutonium contamination in, 430
prostate cancer in, 209, 270
rectal cancer in, 235
small intestinal cancer in, 225–227
stomach cancer in, 223–224
thyroid cancer in, 153–154, 157
uterine cancer in, 205–207
Seminal vesicles, low-LET radiation effects on, 335

Seminoma
  radiation-induced, 319
  radiotherapy for
    pericardial thickening after, 318
    small intestinal late complications of,
      323–324
Semipalatinsk nuclear test site
  chromosome aberrations in workers at, 63
  esophageal cancer in populations near, 215,
    218
  fallout-induced leukemia in populations
    near, 120
  lung cancer in populations near, 175–176
  stomach cancer in populations near, 220
Sensitization, 390f
  definition of, 389
Sensorineural hearing loss, radiation-induced,
  310
Serosal metastatic carcinoma, treatment of,
  345
Serum amylase
  elevated levels of, 311
  increases in after radiation exposure, 364
Serum glutamic-oxaloacetic transaminase
  (SGOT), secretion of, 310
Serum glutamic-pyruvic transaminase (SGPT),
  secretion of, 310
Sex chromosomes, 47
  aneuploids of, doubling dose for in atomic
    bomb survivors, 57
  in genetic inheritance, 47–48
Sexual behavior, in cancer risk, 446
Sexual dysfunction, female, SOMA normal
  tissue radiotoxicity in, 527t
Sexual intercourse patterns, in cancer
  incidence rates, 446
Sexual maturation, in boys after Hodgkin's
  disease radiotherapy, 334
Shale oils, in scrotal cancer, 212
Short tracks, 10
SI unit conversions, 495t
Sicca syndrome, 311
Sievert (rem), 8
Sigmoid
  low-LET radiation effects on, 324–325
  neutron radiation effects on, 325
  radionuclide radiation effects on, 325–326
Silicosis
  compensation for, 450
  in uranium miners, 391, 425–426
Silver 110m, dose coefficients for worker
  intakes of, 497t–499t
Single photon emission computed tomography
  (SPECT), of radiation necrosis of brain,
  300–301
Single-bit multitarget model, 9
Single-target model, 9
Skeletal cancer. See Bone tumors; specific
  tumors
Skeleton, radiosensitivities in different
  portions of, 252
Skin
  atrophy of, 290
    from Chernobyl accident contamination,
      291
  basal cell layer of, 286–287
  characteristics of, 286–287
  clinical injury of, Types I, II, and III,
    288–289
  deterministic effects of radiation on,
    286–293
    with low-LET radiation, 288–290
    with neutron irradiation, 290
    with radionuclide irradiation, 290–293

Skin (Continued)
  dose limits for in special situations, 23–24
  erythema of, with actinomycin D and
    radiotherapy, 393
  functions of, 286–287
  immune and barrier functions of, 346, 359
  irradiation of, dose equivalent rate factors
    for, 500t
  lesions of, post-radiation, 292f
  moist desquamation of, 288
  necrosis of, 288–289
    of chest wall, 291f
  radiation exposure at surface of, 8
  radiation penetrating, 287–288
  radiation reaction of
    atypical, 290
    chemotherapy-enhanced, 392t
    factors affecting, 290
  regenerative capacity of, 288
  second- and third-degree thermal burns of,
    288
  SOMA normal tissue radiotoxicity for, 509t
  structures of, 286–287, 287f
  ulceration of, 288–289
    from Chernobyl accident contamination,
      291
    late radiation, 288
    with low-LET radiation, 288
    from radiography source, 292f
Skin cancer
  nonmelanoma
    cell types of, 259
    fatality rate for, 259
    geographic variation in, 259
    incidence and mortality risk estimates
      from, 264t
    incidence of, 259
    modifying factors in, 259–260
    radiation risk estimates for, 263
    radiation-induced from external exposure,
      260–263
    radiation-induced from internal exposure,
      263
    risk factors for, 259, 263
  ultraviolet exposure in, 391, 447
Skin erythema dose, 7
Skin folds, radiosensitivity of, 290
Skin graft, radiosensitivity of, 290
Skin hemangioma
  in childhood
    CNS tumors related to radiotherapy for,
      141
    radiotherapy for, 102
  therapy for
    colon cancer after, 229
    lens opacities after, 309
    leukemia incidence after, 122
    lung cancer after, 178
Slipped capital epiphyses, after radiotherapy in
  children, 336
Slow renewal system
  postradiation events of, 15f
  radiation damage in, 16f
Small intestine
  cancer of
    from external radiation exposure, 225
    incidence and etiology of, 225
    from internal radiation exposure, 225–227
    risk estimates for, 227
  late radiation injury of, 323
    in children, 323–324
  low-LET radiation effects of, 322–324
  mucosal reaction to radiotherapy in,
    322–323

Small intestine (Continued)
  mucosal regeneration of after radiation
    exposure, 322–323
  mucosal sloughing of, 322–323
  nodular filling defects of, 323
  radiosensitivity of, 322–323
  SOMA normal tissue radiotoxicity for, 520t
Smith v. Ruckhardt, Stemmer v. Kline, 440
Smoke, secondhand, 443–445
Smoke detectors, radioactive emissions from,
  39
"Smokey" bomb test, fallout effects on
  personnel participating in, 93–94
Smokey study, 97
Smoking
  in cancer risk, 443–445
  delayed adverse effects of, 461–462
  in esophageal cancer, 215, 218–220
  in esophageal cancer relative risk, 358
  in genetic disorders, 50–51
  in heart disease and cancer incidence, 52
  in lung cancer, 173, 174, 180
    among metal miners, 185
    among miners, 185
    among plutonium workers, 186
    among uranium miners, 425–426
    in atomic bomb survivors, 174
    mortality ratios for by age started, 393t
    number of cigarettes smoked and,
      395f
    radiation exposure and, 174
    in radiation workers, 452
    risk of, 452–454
  maternal, acute lymphocytic leukemia and,
    415–416
  in oral and pharyngeal cancers, 147
  in osteonecrosis, 336
  in pancreatic cancer, 243
  plutonium exposures and, 430–431
  and radiation effects, 389–390, 394–396
  and radiation risk in miners, 185
  radon exposure and
    in lung cancer incidence, 182
    in lung cancer risk, 183
  in uterine cancer, 204–205
Social decisions, 469–470
Sodium
  annual absorbed dose of, 30
  contributing to background radiation, 28–29
Sodium iodide 131, therapeutic use of, 45
Sodium radionuclides, dose coefficients for
  worker intakes of, 497t–499t
Soft tissue
  heterotropic calcification of, 338
  SOMA normal tissue radiotoxicity for, 527t
Soft-tissue sarcomas, right temporal, after
  radiotherapy, 258f
Soft-tissue tumors
  of breast, 258–259
  at low-level radiation, 256
  radiation-induced
    megavoltage, 258
    risk factors in, 256–258
    types of, 256
  after radiotherapy, 258–259
    for childhood skin hemangiomas, 102
Soil
  radionuclide content of in United States,
    33t
  radium in as source of indoor radon
    exposure, 30–31
Solid cancers
  in atomic bomb survivors, 174–175
    radiation dose and, 89–90

Solid cancers *(Continued)*
 in Chernobyl emergency workers, 94f
 in plutonium workers, 432
 in residents of contaminated versus
  uncontaminated Russian counties, 94f
Solid tumors
 in atomic bomb survivor life span study, 83t
 in atomic bomb survivors
  estimates for based on DS02 dosimetry,
   91f
  BEIR VII committee incidence and
   mortality estimates for, 90t
 cancer-predisposing mutations in, 75
 case-control versus cohort studies of in
  utero exposure effects on, 100
 excess relative risk of, 80f
 incidence and deaths from by sex and colon
  dose, 90t
 lifetime attributable risk for, 104t
  site-specific incidence and mortality from,
   90t
  site-specific incidence of, 89t
  site-specific mortality from, 105t
 in populations near nuclear facilities, 138
 prenatal irradiation effects and, 99–100
 radiogenic
  age-time patterns in risk of, 86f
  mortality data for, 79
 threshold dose-response data for, 80–81
Solvents, in cancer risk, 447
SOMA (subjective, objective, management,
 and analytic) normal tissue radiotoxicity,
 285, 287–288
 for bladder and urethra, 523t
 for blood vessels, 517t
 for bone marrow, 529t
 for brain, 505t–506t
 for breast, 515t
 for cardiovascular system, 316
 for ears, 511t
 for esophagus, 518t
 for eyes, 509t–510t
 in female sexual dysfunction, 527t
 for growing bone, 528t
 for heart, 516t
 for hypothalamic-pituitary-adrenal axis, 508t
 for kidney, 522t
 for larynx, 513t
 for liver, 522t
 for lung, 517t
 for male hypothalamic-pituitary-gonadal
  axis, 507t
 for mandible, 512t
 for mature bone, 529t
 for muscle and soft tissue, 527t
 for oral and pharyngeal mucosa, 511t
 for ovary and reproductive system, 526t
 for peripheral nerves, 507t
 for rectum, 521t
 for salivary glands, 512t
 for skin and subcutaneous tissue, 509t
 for small intestine and colon, 520t
 for spinal cord, 506t
 for stomach, 519t
 for teeth, 513t
 for testes, 524t
 for thyroid, 294
 for thyroid and hypothalamic-pituitary-
  thyroid axis, 514t
 for ureter, 523t
 for uterus and cervix, 526t
 for vagina, 525t
 for vulva, 524t

Somatic cells, 47
Somatic effects
 acceptability of risk of, 464–465
 definition of, 459–460
 nonstochastic, 459–460
Somatic mutations, in biologic dosimetry,
 58–62
Somatic risks, measuring, 460
Space radiation, in cataract formation, 308
Space travel
 cancer risk from, 99
 cosmic ray doses in, 38
Spallation, 27
Spanish Nuclear Energy Board workers
 bone tumors in, 251
 CNS cancers rate in, 139
 colon cancer in, 228
 hepatobiliary system cancers in,
  238–239
 Hodgkin's disease risk in, 129–130
 lung cancer in, 176
 mortality of, 135
 oropharyngeal cancer in, 148
 prostate cancer in, 210
 stomach cancer in, 221
Spatullation particles, high-energy, 27
Specific activity, 7
Sperm production, 333–334
Spermatogenesis, impaired by radionuclide
 exposure, 335
Spermatogonia
 postradiation regeneration of, 334
 types A and B, 333–334
Spermidine, reduction of after radiation
 exposure, 364
Spermine, reduction of after radiation
 exposure, 364
Spinal bulbar atrophy, x-linked, 47–48
Spinal cord
 genetic anomalies of, 50–51
 low-LET radiation effects on, 303–305
 parenchyma of, 299–300
 RBE of neutrons for, 305
 SOMA normal tissue radiotoxicity for,
  506t
 tolerance dose of, 304
Spine
 decreased activity of, 338f
 deformity of after Wilms' tumor
  radiotherapy in children, 336
 lumbar
  decreased activity of, 338f
  myelopathy radiation-induced myelopathy
   of, 304
 thoracic, decreased activity of, 338f
Spironolactone, for liver disease, 326–327
Spleen, 345
 atrophy and fibrosis of, 346
 fractionated radiotherapy of, 345–346
 in immune response, 346
 thorium retained in, 346f
Springfields uranium production facility
 workers
 bladder cancer in, 198
 bone tumors in, 254
 CNS cancer incidence among, 140
 colon cancer in, 230
 esophageal cancer in, 217
 kidney cancer in, 192
 male genital cancer in, 214
 pancreatic cancer in, 247–248
 prostate cancer in, 211
 rectal cancer in, 234

Springfields uranium production facility
 workers *(Continued)*
 small intestinal cancer in, 225
 stomach cancer in, 222
 uranium-induced illness in, 426–427
Spurs, 10
Squamous cell carcinoma
 bladder cancer after radiotherapy for,
  199–200
 caretaker genes in, 72–73
 esophageal, 215
 incidence of, 259
 of lungs, 173
 mortality rate from, 259
 risk factors in, 263
 UV light in, 447
Squamous cell skin cancer, modifying factors
 in, 259–260
SR 2509, radiosensitizing effect of, 9
Standardized incidence ratios (SIRs), in
 radiation workers, 96
Standardized mortality ratio (SMR), with
 irradiation in childhood, 86
Statistical significance
 definition of, 84
 limitation of, 84–85
Stent placement, inhibiting coronary artery
 restenosis after, 318
Sterility
 male, postradiation, 334
 radiation doses causing, 332–333
 temporary radiation, 332
Steroids
 for acute radiation nephritis, 330
 cancer risk from, 443
 cataract formation with long-term use of, 308
 contraceptive, carcinogenic effects of, 447
 for liver disease, 326–327
 radiation cataracts and, 308–309
 for radiation proctosigmoiditis, 324
Stillbirths, in atomic bomb survivors, 57
Stochastic (probabilistic) effects, 438, 459–460
Stomach
 cancer of
  in atomic bomb survivors, excess relative
   risk for, 221f
  from external radiation exposure, 220–223
  incidence and mortality estimates
   for, 226t
  incidence of, 220
  from internal radiation exposure,
   223–224
  risk estimates for, 224–225
  risk factors for, 220, 225
  spontaneous, estimated lifetime risk of, 83t
  types of, 220
 low-LET radiation effects on, 322
 nonspecific wall thickening of, 322
 perforation of, radiation-induced, 322
 SOMA normal tissue radiotoxicity for, 519t
Strabismus, in atomic bomb survivors exposed
 in utero, 408–409
Stratosphere, radionuclide particles in,
 40–41
Stratum corneum, 286–287
Stratum germinativum, 286–287
Stratum granulosum, 286–287
Stratum spinosum, 286–287
Stress
 from nuclear accidents, 467
 tumor-promoting effects of, 71–72
Stress-rest myocardial perfusion examination,
 radiation exposure from, 44

Strontium 90
for pituitary lesions, 294
in weapons testing fallout, 41
Strontium radionuclides
dose coefficients for worker intakes of, 497t–499t
placental transfer of during pregnancy, 412
Subatomic particles, acceleration of, 4–5
Subclinical symptoms, 438–439
Subcutaneous tissue, SOMA normal tissue radiotoxicity for, 509t
Sublingual gland, 310
Submaxillary gland, 310
Sucralfate
for radiation proctosigmoiditis, 324
radioprotective effects of, 323
Sulfonamides, cardiotoxicity of, 317
Sulfur 35
for chondrosarcomas, 345
dose coefficients for worker intakes of, 497t–499t
leukemia risk from, 126–127
Sunlight
carcinogenic effect of, 447
in nonmelanoma skin cancer, 259
Superficial papillary dermis, 287
Suppressor genes, in tumor initiation, 72
Surface seekers, 338
Surface water, tritium in, 29
Surgery, combined with radiation therapy, 391–392
Sweat glands, radiosensitivity of, 289
Swedish cancer registry
colon cancer data of, 231
in radioiodine carcinogenic effect study, 100–101
rectal cancer data of, 236
Synergism, 390f
of chemotherapy and radiotherapy, 393
definition of, 389
of radiation and heat, 390–391
of radiation and trauma, 392
of smoking and radiation exposure, 395
Synovial sarcomas, after radiotherapy, 256

T

T bands, hot spots on, 50
Tamoxifen, in predisposition to radiation pneumonitis, 313
Target, of ionizing radiation, 9–11
Taurine plasma levels, after radiation exposure or chemotherapy, 364
Taxanes, in radiation recall phenomena, 393
T-cell receptor (TCR) gene mutations, 58
T-cells
in atomic bomb survivors, 350–351
circulating, 59–60
count of after accidental radiation exposure, 352
depression of after radiotherapy, 350
functions and subtypes of, 347–353
helper and suppressor, 347
radiosensitivity of, 348, 349
response of to total lymphoid radiotherapy, 349–350
subtypes of in immune response, 346–347
suppressor, 348–349
Techa River contamination studies, 94

Technetium 99/99m exposure
dose coefficients for worker intakes of, 497t–499t
during pregnancy, 413
Technetium 99m-labeled radiopharmaceuticals, 44
Teeth
radiosensitivity of, 337
SOMA normal tissue radiotoxicity for, 513t
Telangiectasia
of bladder, 331
conjunctival, 306
diffuse, with low-LET radiation, 290
of rectum, 324f
of retinal vessels, 306
of skin, from Chernobyl accident contamination, 291
small-vessel, 312
Television sets, cosmic radiation from, 39
Temperature, in radiation effects, 389–391
Teratogenic radiation effects, in organogenesis period, 404–405
Teratoma radiotherapy, small intestinal late complications of, 323–324
Terminal deletion, 49–50
Terrorist events, psychological effects of, 468
Testes
high-LET radiation effects on, 335
low-LET radiation effects on, 333–334
radionuclide radiation effects on, 335
radiosensitivity of, 333–334
SOMA normal tissue radiotoxicity for, 524t
tumor radiotherapy for
gastric ulceration after, 322
nonmelanoma skin cancer after, 263
Testicular cancer
in atomic energy facility workers, 96–97
epidemiology of, 214
incidence of, 212
radiation-induced
from external exposure, 212–214
from internal exposure, 214
after radiotherapy, 217–218
radiotherapy for
lung cancer after, 179
second tumors after, 103
soft-tissue sarcomas after, 258–259
stomach cancer after, 223
ureteral obstruction after, 331
Tetraploidy, 49–50
Thallium 201, accumulation of in brain necrosis, 300–301
Thallium radionuclides, dose coefficients for worker intakes of, 497t–499t
T-helper cell antibody response, to diphtheria or tetanus toxin, 349–350
Theophylline, cardiotoxicity of, 317
Thermoregulation, skin in, 287
Thioguanine, in hepatic radiosensitivity, 327
Thorium dioxide
leukemia risk and, 126
splenic dose of, 346
Thorium plant workers, lung cancer in, 187
Thorium series radionuclides, 30
accumulated in bone, 338
average body burden of, 32
in consumer products, 39
in cranial sinus tumors, 144
dose coefficients for worker intakes of, 497t–499t
occupational exposure to, 99
radiation energies and intensities of, 32t
reference values for in human tissues, 34t

Thoron
in building materials, 37–38
from radium 224 decay, 32–34
Thorotrast injection
bladder cancer after, 199
bone tumors after, 253
dose-response relation in, 256f
breast cancer after, 100, 171
CNS tumors related to, 141
colon cancer after, 231
in cranial sinus carcinoma, 144
esophageal cancer after, 218
genetic mutations and, 74–75
hepatic injury after, 327–328
hepatobiliary system cancer after, 241
in heritable cancer risk, 56
kidney cancer after, 193
larynx cancer after, 146–147
leukemia risk and, 126
lung cancer after, 187–188
lymphatic system changes after, 346
melanoma after, 265
myelodysplasia after, 137
nonmelanoma skin cancer after, 263
ovarian cancer after, 203
pancreatic cancer after, 248
postnatal, 100
prostate cancer after, 211–212
pulmonary fibrosis after, 316
rectal cancer after, 236
small intestinal cancer after, 225–227
in soft tissues of neck, 147f
soft-tissue sarcomas after, 258–259
stomach cancer after, 224
TCR gene mutations in patients receiving, 58
uterine cancer after, 207
Three Mile Island accident, 42
leukemia in population around, 120–121
psychological effects of, 466–467
Threshold dose-response models, 80–81
Thrombocytic purpura, after radiation exposure, 344
Thrombocytopenia
postradiotherapy, 326
rapid development of, 340–341
Thymine (T), 47
Thymus, 345
cells of, 347
hypertrophy of, chest radiation of infants for, 101
in immune response, 346–347
irradiation of, 349
breast cancer after, 169–170
Thymus-derived cells. See T-cells
Thyroglobulin agglutination, with thyroid irradiation, 295
Thyroid antibodies
in populations exposed to Chernobyl fallout, 297
with thyroid irradiation, 295
Thyroid antimicrosomal antibodies. See Antithyroid peroxidase (ATPO; thyroid antimicrosomal antibodies)
Thyroid autoantibodies, in children exposed to Chernobyl fallout, 297
Thyroid cancer
anaplastic, 151
in atomic bomb survivors, 81f
in atomic energy facility workers, 96–97
characteristics of, 151
chemotherapy for and GPA mutation frequency, 59

Thyroid cancer *(Continued)*
  after Chernobyl accident, 94, 151, 438
    in children, 94
  after childhood cancer treatment, 103
  genetic/mutational signature of, 151
  incidence of, 150
  latent period for, 77
  in Marshall Islanders, 94
  modifying factors in, 151–152
  mortality from, 150–151
  occult, 151
  radiation-induced
    estimating probability of, 152
    ethnic background in, 152
    ethnicity in, 155
    exposure sources and rates of, 151–152
    from external exposure, 153–157
    gender differences in, 152
    from internal exposure, 157–160
    iodine deficiency and, 152
    latent period in, 151
    risk estimates for incidence and mortality
      of, 163t–164t
    thyroid-stimulating hormone in, 152
    types and duration of exposure in, 151
  after radioiodine therapy, 100–101
    follow-up studies in, 103
    pathological specimen of, 159f
  risk factors for, 151
  spontaneous, estimated lifetime risk of,
    83t
  therapy for
    bladder cancer after, 199
    breast cancer after, 171
    kidney cancer after, 193
    male genital cancers after, 214
    pulmonary fibrosis after, 316
    stomach cancer after, 224
    uterine cancer after, 207
  5-year survival rate for, 150
Thyroid dose, estimated, 451f
Thyroid gland
  adenomas and nodules of, 160
    in children, 162
    diagnosis of, 160
    gender differences in, 164
    incidence of, 160
    radiation-induced, 160–164
  benign radiation-induced neoplasms of, 160
  carcinomas of
    genetic factors in, 72
    well-differentiated, 151
  dental x-ray sensitivity of, 145
  fallout-related disease of, 361
  radiosensitivity of in children versus adults, 152
  SOMA normal tissue radiotoxicity for, 514t
Thyroid irradiation, 294–298
  high-dose, nodules after, 156
  high-LET, 298
  internal
    from Chernobyl accident, 296–297
    from Hanford nuclear facility, 297
    from nuclear weapons fallout, 296
    from radioiodine thyroid therapy, 297–298
  low-LET
    in atomic bomb survivors, 295–296
    in high background radiation areas, 295
    from medical external exposure, 296
  parotid gland lymphoma with, 145
  testicular effects of, 335
Thyroid scanning
  lung cancer after, 187
  male genital cancers after, 214
  nonmelanoma skin cancer after, 263

Thyroid scanning *(Continued)*
  oropharyngeal cancer after, 150
  ovarian cancer after, 203
Thyroid storm, after Graves' disease
    treatment, 298
Thyroiditis
  in atomic bomb survivors, 295, 296
  autoimmune
    from nuclear weapons fallout, 296
    with thyroid irradiation, 294–295
  with thyroid irradiation, 294
Thyroid-stimulating hormone (TSH)
  deficiency of, 293
    after pituitary irradiation, 294
  in thyroid radiation carcinogenesis, 152
Thyrotoxicosis therapy
  follow-up study for, 102
  leukemia risk and, 125–126
Thyrotropin-releasing hormone deficiency,
    294
Tibia, radium osteitis of, 341f
Time, dose, and fractionation (TDF) factors,
    18
Tinea capitis treatment
  in bone tumors, 249–250
  bone tumors after, 252
  effects of, 101
  leukemia incidence and, 122
  nonmelanoma skin cancer after, 262
  thyroid nodules or adenomas after, 161
Tinnitus, radiation-induced, 310
Tissue breakdown, generalized skin reaction
    to, 288
Tissue polypeptide antigen (TPA), 364
Tissue wounding, tumor promoting effects of,
    71–72
T-lymphocytes. *See* T-cells
Tobacco products. *See also* Smoking
  in oral and pharyngeal cancers, 147
  radiation doses from, 39
Tocopherol
  for late subcutaneous radiation
    fibrosis, 290
  for radiation osteonecrosis, 336–337
Tolerance dose (TD), 18, 285–286
  for various organs, 19t
Tonsils, 345
Total-body irradiation. *See* Whole-body
    irradiation
TP53 gene, 72–73
Tracheobronchial lymph nodes, plutonium
    accumulation in, 186
Transformation frequency, 473
Translocation, 50
Trauma, in radiation effects, 391–392
Triethylene exposure, in lung cancer, 452
Triplet frames, 47
Triploidy, 49–50
Trisomy, incidence of, 52
Trisomy 21, 49–50
  after Chernobyl accident, 405–406
  radiation-induced hereditary risk of, 56–57
Tritium radionuclides
  contributing to background radiation, 28–29
  in fallout, 40–41
  in hepatobiliary system cancer, 240–241
  in melanoma, 265
  in nonmelanoma skin cancer, 263
  nuclear facility release of, 41–42
    leukemia in population around, 121
  in pancreatic cancer, 248
  in rectal cancer, 235
  in small intestinal cancer, 225–227
  source of, 29

Tritium radionuclides *(Continued)*
  in stomach cancer, 223–224
  in weapons testing fallout, 41
Tropisetron, with whole-body irradiation,
    354–355
Troxell v. Bendix Corporation, 440
Truth, court definition of, 439
Tryptophan metabolism abnormalities, 364
Tuberculosis treatment
  bladder cancer after, 197
  bone tumors after, 252, 254
  breast cancer related to, 169
  colon cancer after, 229
  hepatobiliary system cancer after, 240
  kidney cancer after, 191
  liver injury after, 327–328
  lung cancer after, 178
  non-Hodgkin's lymphoma risk from, 132
  pancreatic cancer after, 246
  prostate cancer after, 211–212
  stomach cancer after, 224
  thyroid cancer after, 158
Tumor cell modifiers, 9
Tumor genes, in radiation carcinogenesis, 72
Tumor promoting agents, 71–72
Tumor registries, population-based, 414–415
Tumors, radiation-induced
  age as risk factor in, 77–78
  carcinogenic risk for versus time after
    exposure, 81–83
  common mathematical models for induction
    of, 79f
  epidemiological aspects of, 83–86
  initiation phase of, 71–72
    genetic determinants in, 72
  latent period of, 77
    age as factor in, 77–78
    doubling time in, 78–79
    by tumor type, 76t–78t
  malignant, in high versus low natural
    background radiation areas, 92
  mortality data for, 79
  promotion phase of, 71–72
  secondary after testicular cancer
    radiotherapy, 103
Tumor-suppressor genes
  caretaker type, 72
  gatekeeper type, in carcinogenesis, 72
  loss of negative signals from, 73

U
Ulceration, of larynx, 312
Ulcerative colitis, in colon cancer risk, 227
Ultrasound
  in utero exposure to, 417
  radiation effects and, 391
  video display terminal emission of, 39
Ultraviolet (UV) irradiation
  carcinogenic effects of, 447
  in melanoma, 265–266
  in nonmelanoma skin cancer, 259, 263
  in radiation effects, 391
  in skin cancer induction, 391
  in xeroderma pigmentosum, 75–76
Uncertainty of risk estimates
  dosimetry issues in, 87
  epidemiological issues in, 86–87
  extrapolating from high to low-dose rates
    in, 87
  in low-dose associated cancer, 86–88
  projection model in, 87
  risk transfer in, 87

Uniparental disomy, 47–48
United Kingdom Atomic Energy Authority, pancreatic cancer in workers at, 244
United Kingdom Compensation Scheme for Radiation-linked Diseases, 130
United Kingdom National Registry of Radiation Workers
  colon cancer data of, 228
United Kingdom National Registry of Radiation Workers data, 123
  on bladder cancer, 196
  on bone tumors, 251
  on breast cancer, 167
  on CNS cancers rate, 139
  on esophageal cancer, 216
  on hepatobiliary system cancers, 238
  on Hodgkin's disease risk, 129
  on kidney cancer, 189–190
  on lung cancer, 176
  on male genital cancer, 212
  on melanoma, 264
  on multiple myeloma risk, 133
  on non-Hodgkin's lymphoma risk, 131–132
  on nonmelanoma skin cancer, 260–261
  on oral cavity cancer, 148
  on ovarian cancer, 200–202
  on pancreatic cancer, 244
  on prostate cancer, 209
  on rectal cancer, 233
  on stomach cancer, 221
  on thyroid cancer, 154
  on uterine cancer, 205–206
United Nations Scientific Committee on the Effects of Atomic Radiation (UNSCEAR)
  1982 report of, 389
  2006 report of, 27
  chromosome abnormalities reports of, 51–52
  DDREF for cancer endpoints 2000 report of, 16–17
  genetic mutation data of, 65
  loss of life expectancy estimate of, 82–83
  radiation protection limits of, 22
  radiation-induced death estimates of, 82–83
United States workforce, occupational exposures of, 42–43, 43t
Uranium, 30
  activity of, 423
  biodistribution of, 133
  in body tissues, 424
  bone tumors in populations near processing of, 250
  cardiac complications with inhalation of, 320
  characteristics of, 423
  depleted (DU), 427–428
    external exposure to, 427–428
    inhalation of, 428
    internal exposure to, 428
    soldiers' exposure to, 427–428
  fission of, 6
  half-life of in lung, 423–424
  inhalation of, 424–425
  isotopes of, 423
    half-lives of, 423
  larynx cancer related to, 146–147
  occupational exposure to, 424–427
    leukemia after, 125
  oxidation of, 423
  protein-bound, 423–424

Uranium (*Continued*)
  radiation energies and intensities of, 33t
  radionuclides of, 32–34
    dose coefficients for worker intakes of, 497t–499t
    energies and intensities of, 31t
    reference values for in human tissues, 34t
    reprocessing workers risk from, 98
  renal abnormalities induced by, 424
  renal damage related to, 331
  renal toxicity of, 424
  skin changes related to, 291–293
  soluble, 424
  tetravalent (UO2), 423–424
  thyroid nodules or adenomas from waste disposal of, 160–161
  transportability of, 423–424
  uterine cancer in populations near processing facilities for, 205
Uranium 238
  decay chain of, 34
  decay products of, 35
  detection of, 423
  half-life of, 433
  from phosphate usage, 37
Uranium enrichment/processing workers
  breast cancer in, 168
  cancer incidence in, 427
  cancer morbidity and mortality in, 427
  cancer mortality in, 135
  CNS cancer incidence in, 140
  colon cancer in, 228–230
  compensation for, 450
  esophageal cancer in, 217
  hepatobiliary system cancer in, 239
  Hodgkin's disease risk in, 130
  leukemia in, 127
  lung cancer in, 186
  male genital cancers in, 214
  melanoma in, 265
  non-Hodgkin's lymphoma risk to, 132
  nonmelanoma skin cancer in, 261
  oropharyngeal cancer in, 149
  ovarian cancer in, 202
  rectal cancer in, 234
  salivary gland tumors in, 145
  small intestinal cancer in, 225
  stomach cancer in, 222
  thyroid cancer in, 157
  uranium-induced illness in, 427
  uterine cancer in, 206
Uranium hexafluoride, 424–425
Uranium miners
  bone tumors in, 254
  CNS tumors in, 141–142
  colon cancer in, 230–231
  esophageal cancer in, 218
  heart disease in, 425–426
  hepatobiliary system cancer in, 240–241
  kidney cancer in, 192
  lung cancer in, 173, 184
  lung cancer incidence in, 425–426
  nonmelanoma skin cancer in, 260, 261
  occupational exposure of, 99
  oropharyngeal cancer in, 149
  pancreatic cancer in, 247–248
  prostate cancer in, 211
  pulmonary fibrosis in, 316
  rectal cancer in, 235
  renal degeneration in, 425–426
  respiratory cancer incidence in, 395f

Uranium miners (*Continued*)
  smoking and lung cancer risk in, 395
  smoking effects on, 395
  stomach cancer in, 223–224
  uranium inhalation by, 391
Uranium mining/milling facilities
  agents causing lung injury in, 425–426
  occupational exposures at, 42
  populations near
    bladder cancer in, 195, 198
    bone tumors in, 250
    colon cancer in, 227
    esophageal cancer in, 215
    hepatobiliary system cancers in, 236
    Hodgkin's disease in, 127–129
    leukemia in, 121
    melanoma in, 263
    non-Hodgkin's lymphoma risk in, 130
    nonmelanoma skin cancers in, 260
    pancreatic cancer in, 243, 247
    prostate cancer in, 208–209
    stomach cancer in, 220
  radon levels in, 184–185
  workers at
    pancreatic cancer in, 247–248
    smoking and lung cancer risk in, 185
    thyroid cancer in, 153–154
Uranium nitrate, 423
Uranium tetrafluoride, 423
Uranium-containing alum shale, gamma radiation from, 119
Uranyl bicarbonate complex, 423–424
Uranyl fluoride, 423
Uranyl salts, 423–424
Ureter
  deterministic radiation effects on, 330–331
  high-LET radiation effects on, 331
  obstruction of after testicular carcinoma radiotherapy, 331
  radionuclide radiation effects on, 331
  radiosensitivity of, 330
  SOMA normal tissue radiotoxicity for, 523t
  stenosis of, 330
  stones of in atomic bomb survivors, 330
  stricture of
    and hydronephrosis of, 330
    after pelvic carcinoma radiotherapy, 359–360
Urethra
  deterministic radiation effects on, 335
  radiation-induced stenosis of, 335
  SOMA normal tissue radiotoxicity for, 523t
  strictures in after brachytherapy, 331
Urinary bladder. *See also* Bladder (urinary)
Urinary tract
  carcinomas of in atomic bomb survivors, 85–86
  deterministic radiation effects on, 328–331
Urogenital abnormalities, 52
Uropathy, obstructive, after cervical cancer radiotherapy, 331
U.S. Environmental Protection Agency, measuring population size exposed to risk, 469–470
Utah fallout studies, 93
Uterine bleeding treatment
  breast cancer after, 169
  colon cancer after, 229–230
  hepatobiliary system cancer after, 240
  pancreatic cancer after, 246
  stomach cancer after, 223
Uterine cancer. *See also* Cervical cancer (carcinoma)
  epidemiology of, 207–208

Uterine cancer (*Continued*)
incidence and risk factors in, 204–205
radiation-induced
from external exposure, 205–207
from internal exposure, 207
risk estimates for incidence and mortality
from, 208t
Uterus
atrophy of, 333
deterministic radiation effects on, 332–333
encapsulated radium treatment for
hemorrhage of, 126
endometrial burns of, 333
impaired growth of, 332–333
myoma of
after fallout exposure, 361
pancreatic cancer and, 246–247
postradiotherapy atrophy of, 333
radioresistance of, 332–333
seizures in infants exposed to in utero
radiotherapy of, 408
SOMA normal tissue radiotoxicity for, 526t
spontaneous cancer of, estimated lifetime
risk for, 83t
ulceration of, 333

V

Vagina
low-LET radiation effects of, 333
mucosa of, 333
necrosis of, 333
SOMA normal tissue radiotoxicity for,
525t
Vascular changes, with radiation damage,
15–16
Vascular endotheliitis, 288–289
Vasculature, renal, 328–329
Vasculopathy, radiation-induced, 319–320
Vegetative intermitotic cells, radiosensitivity
of, 14–15
Veno-occlusive disease, after liver radiation,
327
Venous vessel occlusion, late radiation, 288
Ventilation
and absorption rate of radon, 38
building material radiation and, 37, 38
Vertebral body, radium osteitis of, 341f
Veterans Affairs, U.S. Department of,
compensation programs of, 450
Veteran's Dioxin and Radiation Exposure
Compensation Act, 450
VHL gene, in tumor initiation, 72
Video display terminals
cosmic radiation from, 39
nonionizing radiation from, 39
Vinblastine, in radiation myelopathy, 304
Vincristine
in hepatic radiosensitivity, 327
leukemia risk from, 393
in radiation brain injury, 302
radiosensitizing effect of, 392–393
Vinyl chloride, in angiosarcoma, 74
Viral infections
carcinogenic effect of, 447–448
neoplastic effects of, 71–72
radiation interaction with, 397
Vitamin C, protective effect of against
gliomas, 140
Vitamin E (tocopherol), anticarcinogenic
effect of, 446

Vitreous hemorrhage, 306
Volume seekers, 338
Vomiting. *See* Nausea and vomiting
VP16-213 (epipodophyllotoxin)
enhancing skin radiosensitivity, 290
radiosensitizing effect of, 392–393
Vulva, SOMA normal tissue radiotoxicity for,
524t

W

Watches, cosmic radiation from, 38–39
Weapons. *See* Nuclear weapons; Nuclear
weapons tests
White matter
asymptomatic periventricular changes of,
300
radiation effects on, 299–300
radiotherapy-induced injury of, 301
Whole-body irradiation
acute radiation syndromes and sickness
after, 355–360
with bone marrow transplantation, 343
deterministic effects of, 353–360
growth retardation after, 294
in utero, central nervous system effects of,
299
LD50 doses of, 353–355
lethal doses of, 354
lung radiosensitivity and, 312
lymphocyte count after, 355f
midline tissue dose (MTD) in, 354, 355
myelodepression after, 343–344
neutrophil and platelet count after,
344f
prodromal symptoms of, 354–355
sources of, 353
spectrum of sources and effects of, 353f
survival chances after, 343, 343t
symptoms after, 355t
Whole-lung radiotherapy, pneumonitis after,
315
Wilms' tumor
after childhood cancer treatment, 103
DNA sequence loss for, 73
genetic factors in, 72
incidence of, 188–189
in utero radiation exposure and, 414–415
radiotherapy for
bladder cancer after, 198
bone effects of, 336
bone tumors after, 252
hepatic fibrosis after, 326
hepatobiliary system cancer after,
240
kidney cancer after, 192
muscle atrophy after, 340f
pneumonitis after, 315
small intestinal late complications of,
323–324
WT gene in, 74–75
Windscale graphite reactor accident, 42
Working level months (WLM), chromosome
aberration rates and, 63–64
Wound healing
prolonged with combined radiation and
trauma, 392
in radiation therapy, 392
WR-2721. *See* Amifostine (WR-2721)
WT gene mutations, in Wilms' tumors,
74–75

X

X chromosome, in genetic inheritance, 47–48
Xenon, placental transfer of, 413
Xeroderma pigmentosum (XP)
clinical features of, 76t
genetic predisposition to, 73, 75–76
Xerostomia, after salivary gland irradiation,
310–311
XPA-G gene, 72–73
X-ray examinations
absorbed doses from, 43
breast cancer risk and, 100
estimated number of in United States, 44t
frequency of, 43, 44t
X-ray technologists
bone tumors in, 251–252
cancer mortality in, 98
cataracts in, 454–455
lung cancer in, 177
occupational exposures of, 42–43
ovarian cancer in, 203–204
radiation-induced life shortening in, 362
thyroid cancer in, 152
X-ray therapy
of head and neck
brain tumor incidence with, 140–141
hyperthyroidism after, 296
oropharyngeal cancer after, 149–150
X-rays, 1–2
absorption of, 3
combined with contrast media, 392–393
combined with heavy ions and fast neutrons
and electrons, 391
discovery of, 285–286
electromagnetic wavelengths of, 3
embryonic and fetal exposure to, 401–402
anomalies from, 404t
non-Hodgkin's lymphoma risk from, 132
genetic mutations caused by, 47
half-value layer of, 3–4
high-energy, 7
multiple myeloma risk from, 135
negligent, 441
during preimplantation period, 403–404
RBE of, 3t
from televisions, 39

Y

Y chromosome, in genetic inheritance,
47–48
Yttrium 90
dose coefficients for worker intakes of,
497t–499t
of pituitary lesions, 294
resin microspheres of
for hepatic metastases, 327–328
liver scans after, 328
Yttrium 90 silicate citrate, in cartilage
necrosis, 339

Z

Zinc 65, dose coefficients for worker intakes
of, 497t–499t
Zirconium 95
dose coefficients for worker intakes of,
497t–499t
in weapons testing fallout, 41
Zygote, homozygous for malformations, 51